es the b
er ti

Oxford Textbook of
Primary Medical Care

Project Administrator	Janet Whitehouse
Project Manager	Kate Martin
Project Editor	Newgen Imaging Systems (P) Ltd
Indexer	Newgen Imaging Systems (P) Ltd
Design Manager	Andrew Meaden
Illustrations	Newgen Imaging Systems (P) Ltd
Publisher	Alison Langton

volume **2** **Clinical Management**

Oxford Textbook of
Primary Medical Care

Edited by

Roger Jones
Nicky Britten
Larry Culpepper
David A. Gass
Richard Grol
David Mant
and Chris Silagy

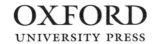

OXFORD

UNIVERSITY PRESS

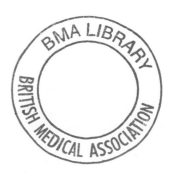

OXFORD
UNIVERSITY PRESS

Great Clarendon Street, Oxford OX2 6DP

Oxford University Press is a department of the University of Oxford.
It furthers the University's objective of excellence in research, scholarship,
and education by publishing worldwide in

Oxford New York

Auckland Bangkok Buenos Aires Cape Town Chennai
Dar es Salaam Delhi Hong Kong Istanbul Karachi Kolkata
Kuala Lumpur Madrid Melbourne Mexico City Mumbai Nairobi
São Paulo Shanghai Taipei Tokyo Toronto

Oxford is a registered trade mark of Oxford University Press
in the UK and in certain other countries

Published in the United States
by Oxford University Press Inc., New York

British Library Cataloguing in Publication Data

Data available

ISBN 0 19 852963 5 (vol 1)
       0 19 852964 3 (vol 2)
       0 19 263219 1 (set)
       (Available as a set only)

10 9 8 7 6 5 4 3 2 1

Typeset by Newgen Imaging Systems (P) Ltd, Chennai, India
Printed in Italy
on acid-free paper by Legoprint.

Section editors

Volume 1: Sections 1–16

Richard Baker
Professor, Clinical Governance Research and Development Unit, University of Leicester, Leicester General Hospital, Leicester, UK
Section 13: Quality improvement

Jozien Bensing
Director and Professor, NIVEL (Netherlands Institute for Health Services Research), Utrecht, The Netherlands
Section 5: The consultation

Nicky Britten
Professor of Applied Health Care Research, Institute of Clinical Education, Peninsula Medical School, Universities of Exeter and Plymouth, St Luke's Campus, Exeter, UK
Section 3: Reasons for consultation
Section 5: The consultation
Section 14: Research

Thomas L. Campbell
Professor, Family Medicine and Dentistry, University of Rochester School of Medicine and Dentistry, Rochester, New York, USA
Section 9: Family medicine

Larry Culpepper
Professor and Chairman of Family Medicine, Boston University, Boston, USA
Section 1: Primary medical care
Section 8: Integrated management
Section 9: Family medicine

Geert-Jan Dinant
Professor, University of Maastricht, Maastricht, The Netherlands
Section 6: Diagnosis and decision-making

Len Doyal
Professor of Medical Ethics, St Bartholomew's and The Royal London School of Medicine and Dentistry, Queen Mary College, University of London, UK
Section 16: Ethics and law

David A. Gass
Professor, Department of Family Medicine, Dalhousie University, Halifax, Canada
Section 15: Education and professional development
Section 16: Ethics and law

Richard Grol
Professor and Director, Centre for Quality of Care Research (WOK), Nijmegen University Medical Centre, Maastricht University, The Netherlands
Section 2: Primary care around the world
Section 8: Integrated management
Section 12: Practice management
Section 13: Quality improvement

Roger Jones
Wolfson Professor of General Practice and Primary Care, Guy's, King's and St Thomas' School of Medicine, London, UK
Section 1: Primary medical care
Section 2: Primary care around the world
Section 6: Diagnosis and decision-making

J.A. Knottnerus
Professor of General Practice, Netherlands School of Primary Care Research, Maastricht and President of the Health Council of the Netherlands, The Hague, The Netherlands
Section 4: Descriptive epidemiology

Michael M. Kochen
Professor of General Practice, University of Göttingen, Germany
Section 7: Management of individuals

David Mant
Professor of General Practice, University of Oxford, UK
Section 4: Descriptive epidemiology
Section 10: Managing the practice population
Section 11: Prevention and health promotion

Chris Silagy*
Professor and Director, Institute of Public Health and Health Services Research, Monash University, Monash Medical Centre, Clayton, Australia
Section 7: Management of individuals
Section 10: Managing the practice population
Section 11: Prevention and health promotion
Section 14: Research

Eloy H. van de Lisdonk
General Practitioner and Senior Lecturer, University of Nijmegen, Nijmegen, The Netherlands
Section 3: Reasons for consultation

Valerie Wass
Professor of Community Based Education, University of Manchester, School of Primary Care, Rusholme Health Centre, Manchester, UK
Section 15: Education and professional development

* It is with regret that we must report the death of Chris Silagy during the preparation of this Textbook.

Volume 2: Sections 1–17

Willem J.J. Assendelft
Head, Department of Guideline Development and Research Policy, Dutch College of General Practitioners, Utrecht, The Netherlands
Section 13: Musculoskeletal problems

Larry Culpepper
Professor and Chairman of Family Medicine, Boston University, Boston, USA
Section 3: Ear, nose, and throat problems
Section 5: Metabolic problems
Section 10: Child health

Niek J. de Wit
Senior Lecturer, General Practitioner, Julius Center for Health Sciences and Primary Care, University Medical Center, Utrecht, The Netherlands
Section 4: Digestive problems

Isser Dubinsky
Director of Emergency Services, The Toronto Hospital, Ontario, Canada
Section 14: Common emergencies and trauma

Peggy Frith
Consultant Medical Ophthalmologist, Oxford Eye Hospital, Radcliffe Infirmary, Oxford, UK
Section 12: Eye problems

David A. Gass
Professor, Department of Family Medicine, Dalhousie University, Halifax, Canada
Section 9: Mental health problems
Section 16: Old age
Section 17: Palliative care

Irene J. Higginson
Professor and Head, Department of Palliative Care and Policy, King's College London, Weston Education Centre, London, UK
Section 17: Palliative care

Richard Hobbs
Professor and Head of Primary Care and General Practice, Primary Care Clinical Sciences Building, University of Birmingham, Edgbaston, Birmingham, UK
Section 1: Cardiovascular problems

Roger Jones
Wolfson Professor of General Practice and Primary Care, Guy's, King's and St Thomas' School of Medicine, London, UK
Section 1: Cardiovascular problems
Section 4: Digestive problems
Section 7: Women's health
Section 8: Conception, pregnancy, and childbirth
Section 14: Common emergencies and trauma

Tony Kendrick
Professor of Primary Medical Care, Director of Community Clinical Sciences Division, University of Southampton Medical School, Aldermoor Health Centre, Southampton, UK
Section 9: Mental health problems

Michael C. Klein
Professor of Family Practice and Paediatrics and Head, Division of Maternity and Newborn Care, University of British Columbia, Vancouver, Canada
Section 8: Conception, pregnancy, and childbirth

David Mant
Professor of General Practice, University of Oxford, Oxford, UK
Section 12: Eye problems
Section 13: Musculoskeletal problems
Section 15: Skin and soft tissue problems

Kenneth Marshall
Professor of Family Medicine (retired), University of Western Ontario, Ontario, Canada
Section 3: Ear, nose, and throat problems
Section 6: Genito-urinary problems

Thomas Nicholas
Department of Family Medicine, University of Missouri Kansas City, Missouri, USA
Section 15: Skin and soft tissue problems

Mary Pierce
Senior Lecturer in General Practice, University of Warwick, UK
Section 5: Metabolic problems

Leone Ridsdale
Senior Lecturer in Neurology and Reader in General Practice, Guy's, King's, and St Thomas' School of Medicine, King's College School of Medicine, London, UK
Section 11: Neurological problems

Walter W. Rosser
Chair, Department of Family Medicine, Queens University, Kingston, Ontario, Canada
Section 10: Child health

Chris Silagy*
Professor and Director, Institute of Public Health and Health Services Research, Monash University, Monash Medical Centre, Clayton, Australia
Section 2: Respiratory problems
Section 6: Genito-urinary problems
Section 11: Neurological problems

Paul Wallace
Professor of Primary Health Care, University College London, London, UK
Section 16: Old age

Chris van Weel
Professor and Chairman, University Medical Center, Nijmegen, The Netherlands
Section 2: Respiratory problems

Ruth Wilson
Professor, Department of Family Medicine, Queen's University, Kingston, Ontario, Canada
Section 7: Women's health

*It is with regret that we must report the death of Chris Silagy during the preparation of this Textbook.

Summary of contents

Volume 1: Principles and Concepts

Section 1 Primary medical care
Edited by Larry Culpepper and Roger Jones

Section 2 Primary care around the world
Edited by Roger Jones and Richard Grol

Section 3 Reasons for consultation
Edited by Nicky Britten and Eloy H. van de Lisdonk

Section 4 Descriptive epidemiology
Edited by David Mant and J.A. Knottnerus

Section 5 The consultation
Edited by Nicky Britten and Jozien Bensing

Section 6 Diagnosis and decision-making
Edited by Roger Jones and Geert-Jan Dinant

Section 7 Management of individuals
Edited by Chris Silagy and Michael M. Kochen

Section 8 Integrated management
Edited by Richard Grol and Larry Culpepper

Section 9 Family medicine
Edited by Thomas L. Campbell and Larry Culpepper

Section 10 Managing the practice population
Edited by David Mant and Chris Silagy

Section 11 Prevention and health promotion
Edited by David Mant and Chris Silagy

Section 12 Practice management
Edited by Richard Grol

Section 13 Quality improvement
Edited by Richard Grol and Richard Baker

Section 14 Research
Edited by Chris Silagy and Nicky Britten

Section 15 Education and professional development
Edited by David A. Gass and Valerie Wass

Section 16 Ethics and law
Edited by Len Doyal and David A. Gass

Volume 2: Clinical Management

Contents

Volume 2: Clinical Management

Preface

The concept of a definitive textbook for primary care physicians, general practitioners, and family physicians, published by Oxford University Press, has been under discussion for many years. The present work is the result of these detailed deliberations and the hard work of an almost unprecedented number of editors and authors, representing primary care medical expertise from around the globe. The final decision to produce the Textbook was based on a broad consensus that a fixed reference point in the maelstrom of information about primary medical care and primary care services was essential. Whilst many have argued that the volume and constantly changing content of information may render traditional paper-based textbooks redundant, in many ways it is the very extent of this information, and the difficulties of finding a way through it, that persuaded us to embark on this ambitious project.

Over the three or four years that it has taken to produce the Textbook, the need for it has become even more apparent. Paradoxically, in health care systems with well-developed primary care sectors, there has been a recent tendency to 'de-construct' primary care and general practice through the provision of multiple points of entry into the primary and secondary care systems, changing roles for primary care professionals, fragmentation of both personal and organizational continuity of care, and a policy focus on activity and volume rather than on quality and patient-centred outcomes. At the same time, the value of a strong primary care sector is increasingly appreciated in developing health care systems, where the generalist function in medicine is recognized as crucial to the delivery of effective and efficient care for populations.

Design issues

Even before drawing up the terms of reference that would inform the content of the Textbook, the editors spent many hours agonizing about the title, which would predicate these. 'General practice' is well-understood to be pretty well synonymous with primary medical care in northern European countries, and in parts of Australasia and the Pacific rim, but has a different connotation in North America. 'Family medicine' has a specific North American connotation, which is not widely shared and which, in other settings, has a specific, restrictive meaning. 'Primary care' was judged to be over-inclusive, with implications for public health, community development, and political structures and initiatives. We believe that 'primary medical care' sits reasonably comfortably at the interstices between these terms, and provides a conceptual framework that is both broad enough to ensure that primary care physicians and their teams practising medicine in a range of health care and geographical settings will find the book valuable, whilst being sufficiently focused to ensure adequate coverage of key topics within manageable constraints of space and cost.

We were particularly concerned to assemble a core Editorial Board, which, through selection of appropriate topics and authors, would ensure full coverage of the field from multiple disciplinary and cultural perspectives. This has resulted in the engagement of 400 authors from some 20 different countries.

The decision to produce this Textbook in two distinct volumes, of approximately equal length, stems from the need to adequately describe both the principles underlying the establishment and delivery of high-quality primary care and the clinical information and skills required for patient management in that setting. The first volume describes the fundamentals of primary care and the second focuses on clinical management in primary care, taking an approach based on the management of presenting symptoms, embedded in a systems-based framework.

Principles and concepts

The first volume, 'Principles and Concepts', provides a systematic overview of the nature, structure and functions of primary medical care, with a strong focus on the consultation and the doctor–patient interactions that are at the core of primary care medicine. We have described both individual and population approaches to the delivery of primary medical care and emphasized the wide range of disciplines involved. As well as clinical sciences, the basic sciences of primary medical care include medical sociology, health psychology, epidemiology, and the principles of organizational management. We have highlighted the importance of ensuring and enhancing the quality of care and provide concise, detailed sections on research, education, and ethics and law.

In many ways, the essays that make up the first volume of the Textbook represent the 'eternal verities' of primary medical care. Although health care systems and political priorities will shift and change, new diseases will emerge, patients will become increasingly well-informed and empowered, and the traditional role of primary health care professionals will be transformed, many of the fundamental principles of doctor–patient interaction within the consultation, and the means of studying and teaching them, will doubtless endure.

Clinical management

In the second volume of the Textbook, we have taken an approach based on presenting problems within a comprehensive systems framework. In our guidance to authors we emphasized the importance of taking a broad perspective on each topic, attempting to assure its relevance for physicians and health care systems at different levels of development, emphasizing core clinical principles of diagnosis and management and considering the broader public health and health economic implications of each problem. We identified, through section co-editors, individuals in a number of countries who were able to provide an expert primary care perspective on each problem, often by writing in conjunction with specialist colleagues. We recognize that this contemporary account of good practice in primary care medicine will, inevitably, change as new diagnostic technologies and therapeutic interventions are developed, and the introductory essay on genomic medicine reflects the pace of change in medical science and looks ahead at the extraordinary potential that it possesses for improving health and health care in the future.

Using the Textbook

The *Oxford Textbook of Primary Medical Care* has been written as a definitive account of primary care medical practice, and to act as a reference
point for all those involved in teaching, learning, researching, and delivering primary medical care. We hope that practising physicians around the
world will find the clinical sections a valuable source of contemporary
advice and guidance, and that undergraduate medical students—
tomorrow's doctors—will find not only the clinical problems directly relevant to their studies, but will also benefit from reading many of the sections
in the 'Principles and Concepts' volume, providing them with a broadly
based understanding of primary care medicine.

We would like to think that the Textbook will find its way into all those
practices where undergraduate and postgraduate teaching and training are
carried out. Vocational trainees, in particular, should find the level of detail
in both volumes appropriate for their studies, and undergraduate teachers
and postgraduate trainers will, we hope, find much here to inform and
inspire the development and delivery of their curricula. There is much here
too, we believe, for university departments of general practice and family
practice; many of the essays in 'Principles and Concepts' are state-of-the-
art, in-depth and fully referenced sources on key topics. The sections on
research and education provide a substantial basis for engaging with the
academic facets of primary care medical practice. Planners and policy
makers will find valuable guidance in the Textbook about the essential components of high-quality primary care and its role within health services.

Acknowledgements

Any new literary venture, T.S. Eliot pointed out, is no more or less than an
attempt to re-discover 'what has been lost and found and lost again and
again' by those 'whom one cannot hope to emulate'. Whilst the authorship
of this Textbook includes many of the most influential figures in primary
medical care—and we are particularly proud that Professor Ian
McWhinney has written its Foreword—we pay tribute to other giants of
primary medical care who have not been able to contribute. We were privileged to have numbered Professor Chris Silagy amongst our core editorial
team, and his death during the preparation of the Textbook represented a
massive blow to primary care across the world.

I would like to take this opportunity to acknowledge the tremendous
support and commitment that I have received from my co-editors,
Professors Nicky Britten, Larry Culpepper, David Gass, Richard Grol,
David Mant, and Chris Silagy and from all the section editors who joined
us in putting together the second volume of the Textbook. I would also like
to express profound thanks to all the authors involved in producing this
Textbook, and to acknowledge their contributions of wisdom, expertise,
experience, and passion.

It has been a pleasure working with Oxford University Press. Special
thanks are due to Janet Whitehouse, the project administrator for the
Textbook, who has displayed remarkable patience and tenacity coupled
with highly developed author management skills, and Alison Langton,
Editorial Director for Medicine at Oxford University Press, who was a constant source of wisdom, encouragement, and firm guidance. None of us
could have contemplated undertaking this work without administrative
and secretarial support from our own institutions but I would like to say a
very special thank you, on behalf of all of us, to Pat Taylor, my personal
assistant at King's College, London, without whom this enterprise would
have been impossible.

Roger Jones
London, 2003

Foreword

Ian R. McWhinney

Emeritus Professor of Family Medicine, the University of Western Ontario

Recognition of a scientific discipline or body of knowledge by the academic community requires that it should not be entirely derived from other disciplines, that it should have its own scholarly and scientific literature, and that research should be generated within the discipline. The publication of scientific textbooks marks the articulation of a newly defined body of knowledge. The same could be said of the creation of new academic units and of listings in indices compiled by academic libraries. Kuhn[1] described the publication of textbooks as marking the emergence of a dominant paradigm, his term for the tacit assumptions and theoretical principles that form the basis of research and the organization of knowledge. According to Kuhn, textbooks usually treat the new paradigm as given, systematically disguising the scientific revolution which gave rise to it. Textbooks thus begin by 'truncating the scientist's sense of [the] discipline's history and then proceed to supply a substitute for what they have eliminated'. Osler's *Textbook of Medicine*, published in 1892, marked the culmination of almost a century of descriptive research, clinical and pathological, based on the revolution in medical thought that took place around the turn of the nineteenth century. Today, we might call it 'the medical model'. Osler saw no need to inform his readers about the origins of this paradigm, or to explain its concepts and vocabulary. Chapter 1 of Osler's textbook launches immediately into a description of infectious diseases and all the other chapters have diseases as their subject matter. For all his interest in the history of medicine, Osler in his textbook presented a medicine that was both unhistorical and a theoretical. This book promises to be different.

In his seminal lectures on diagnosis in 1926, Crookshank[2] remarked that every discipline sooner or later must define its fundamental concepts, and that for medicine the need was imperative. The medicine of Crookshank's time, and after, might well have been considered derivative from the laboratory sciences and therefore not a truly independent discipline. However, experience showed that no knowledge of basic science could predict all the phenomena of human illness: the application of this knowledge depended on a great body of taxonomic clinical knowledge accumulated over the years. Medicine derives from the laboratory sciences, but is also a descriptive science in its own right.

For many years, general practice was considered entirely derivative. It was assumed that the methods learned in one context—the teaching hospital—could be applied unmodified in the very different context of general practice. Even in these days, there were some who challenged these assumptions. In *The Future of Medicine*, Mackenzie[3] described the experience of the general practitioner as unique and maintained that general practice should be represented in the medical school. Mackenzie's research on the natural history of heart disease depended on such features of general practice as experience of the earliest stages of illness, observation over long periods, and personal knowledge of patients. His books became foundation texts for the emerging discipline of cardiology and his *Symptoms and their Interpretation*[4] could be regarded as a precursor text of general practice, even though it dealt only with one particular aspect.

From general practice to primary medical care

The first British textbooks of general practice appeared in the 1950s, a time when increasing specialization, and the need to teach the new trainee assistants, was forcing general practitioners to define their body of knowledge. When I entered general practice in 1954, two textbooks had recently become available. Both of these broke new ground and were remarkable achievements.[5,6] They were written by general practitioners using their own experience, backed up by data collected in their own practices. Both were insistent on the unique perspective of general practice, but there was little conceptual analysis, or indication that general practice might have distinctive methods and modes of thought. Both texts were organized according to conventional disease categories and nomenclature.

In the years since publication of these early texts, many more books have appeared, some of them research-based monographs on specific aspects of general practice, others covering the field as a whole. It is now customary to refer to the field as primary medical care, rather than general or family practice. The Institute of Medicine in the United States has described the four cornerstones of primary care as accessibility, comprehensiveness, continuity, and coordination. In some jurisdictions, general paediatrics and internal medicine share these features with general practice. Emergency medicine shares accessibility but not continuity. Bringing them together under one roof has administrative and pedagogic utility, but it would be a mistake to allow these disciplines to be submerged and disappear into a loose confederation. As well as sharing a great deal, each has a distinct culture, which is worth preserving. General practice, for example, has a long tradition and a unique outlook on medicine. It is not simply an amalgam of all the specialties, nor is it simply clinical medicine, plus epidemiology plus sociology. Its essence is an unconditional commitment to patients whatever may befall them. The commitment is to a person, not to a person with a certain disease. Since they cannot foresee all their patients' future needs, family doctors have to be generalists. Being generalists does not preclude a special interest in a single aspect of practice. Indeed, we need generalists who can speak with authority at consensus conferences, and who can write clinical chapters in textbooks. But generalists who make their patients their body of knowledge should be valued no less.

Primary care paediatricians and internists restrict their practices by age, but continue to be generalists capable of providing comprehensive care. If, however, primary care were to split into disease-specific specialties and become a mirror image of hospital medicine, two of the cornerstones (comprehensiveness and coordination) would collapse and the logic of a primary care sector would no longer apply.

Undifferentiated illness

Any textbook of general practice or primary care medicine faces a difficult problem. Family doctors are usually the first physicians to assess their patients' illnesses. These present as undifferentiated symptoms and, as Mackenzie understood, their assessment is a different process from the diagnosis of disease in its typical and fully developed form. In many patients the symptoms are self-limiting illnesses or short-lived responses to life's traumas, in some they are the earliest harbingers of a chronic illness, in others they are danger signals of an acute and life-threatening disease. The primary care physician must be adept at differentiating these conditions. A diagnosis of a spurious disease at this stage may set the stage for life-long invalidism. Misdiagnosis of an acute curable condition may result in disability or death. The importance of the primary assessment of symptoms, in the context of their meaning for the patient, cannot be over-emphasized. Primary care physicians have to work at all levels of abstraction and all levels of certainty, though paucity of data in the early stages of illness often obliges them to make clinical judgements in conditions of high uncertainty. High uncertainty requires fail-safe strategies, such as robust rule-out tests and watchful waiting.

Necessary as they are in a textbook, the conventional divisions into the abstractions of disease and system categories do not fully represent the experience of the family doctor. Moreover, it is not sufficient for the textbook to include only the commoner diseases. If a patient with pheochromocytoma or cranial arteritis is misdiagnosed, it is no excuse to say that the disease is rare.

If a textbook of primary care has to be so inclusive, how can it avoid looking like a watered down textbook of internal medicine? Only by taking the perspective of the primary care clinician. Much progress has been made in our understanding of such aspects as clinical method, critical appraisal, preventive practice, doctor–patient relationships, working relationships with other professions, home care, and practice management.

Clinical epidemiology has given us tools for evaluating the relevance of evidence. We cannot assume that assessment or management protocols developed in other fields are appropriate in primary care. The predictive value of symptoms and tests varies with the prevalence of the target disorder. The harm done to disease-free patients who test positive may outweigh, in the primary care population, the benefits to patients with the target disorder. The sensitivity of a test varies with the stage of the illness. A test that is a good 'rule-out' test in a fully developed illness may not be sensitive enough in the early stages seen by the family doctor. Textbooks of internal medicine tend to deal with the later stages of illness.

Primary care clinicians have to be critical in their application of guidelines derived from randomized controlled trials. Clinical trials are done in highly selected populations. The elderly, the uneducated, the non-compliant, and patients with co-morbidity or borderline conditions are under-represented: yet these are common in primary care. Clinical trials are rarely long enough or large enough to reveal the long-term effects of drugs. To be useful in primary care, evidence-based guidelines should pass the scrutiny of well-informed primary care clinicians. We should expect this in a textbook such as this one. Even when evidence is universally accepted, it is often interpreted differently in different countries. An international text has the difficult task of dealing with such issues as the critical levels for prescription of cholesterol-lowering and antihypertension drugs, the management of otitis media, and the indications for a PSA test. A set of guidelines that makes sense in terms of one specialty may look very different when added to those of all the other specialties and viewed from the perspective of the primary care physician who has to apply them.

The importance of relationships

In most fields of primary medical practice, relationships are of prime importance. These may be relationships with patients, with families, with colleagues in other professions, and with communities. These values are embodied in the concept of continuity of care, by a physician or small practice team who know the patient. They are based on the well-founded belief that a personal relationship, when combined with professional competence, provides the best context for long-term care. Every new illness or episode is then interpreted in the context of knowledge of the patient. Continuity of care is now under siege from many quarters: from fragmentation of care, from consumer and commercial values, from the difficulty of reconciling accessibility with continuity.

To be healers for their patients, family doctors have to be involved, person to person. But there are right ways and wrong ways of being involved. The wrong way is to be involved at the level of the doctor's unexamined negative emotions: fear, helplessness, self-interest, likes and dislikes, self-centred attachments. The right way is to reconcile the seeming opposites of involvement and detachment.

Primary care physicians usually work closely with members of other professions, often in small close-knit teams, at other times by referral and collaboration. The nurse–physician relationship is important in the medical centre, the home, and the community, as are relationships with social workers, counsellors, psychologists, and others, especially for practices in areas of deprivation. Although primary care medicine includes only physicians, a textbook must address these roles and relationships, and convey the skills and attitudes required of team members.

Of all fields of medicine, general practice has traditionally been closest to where people live, and therefore vividly aware of the impact of poverty on health and on access to medical care. Although physicians cannot directly determine social policy, they can address difficulties of access, support their patients in obtaining their entitlements, and help them to adopt preventative practices.

A different world view

A primary care text should provide an alternative to the paradigm that still dominates biology and medicine. General practice, for example, has never fitted well into the low context, mechanistic, and reductionist approach to medicine. The person is not a machine, even though the body has some machine-like features. We can for practical purposes reduce a patient's problem to a simple linear causal chain, as when we prescribe an antibiotic or diagnose appendicitis. Medicine has achieved great success by treating the body as a machine, but everything we do for patients depends on their qualities as organisms. Mechanistic and organismic thinking are complementary not mutually exclusive—two perspectives on the same reality. Organisms have qualities possessed by no machine: growth, regeneration, learning, healing, intentionality, and self-transcendence. At its most successful, medicine works by supporting these natural processes. Our therapy often consists of removing the obstacles to healing whether they are psychological or physical. The traditional regimens of balanced nutrition, rest, sound sleep, exercise, relief of pain, personal support, and peace of mind are all measures that support the organism's natural healing powers. Immunization, the most effective of all scientific advances, strengthens the body's own powers of resistance. There is now convincing evidence that personal support works in the same way, justifying our belief in the power of the doctor–patient relationship.

An organism reacts to the traumas of life as a whole. 'The manner in which an organism copes with a defect is always characteristic of its individual nature.'[7] All significant illness affects the organism at every level, from the molecular to the cognitive and affective. The essence of the clinical method in general practice is that the body, the emotions, and the patient's experience of illness are attended to in every case, the degree of attention obviously depending on the individual circumstances. General practice is at the same time a clinical and existential medicine. The patient-centred clinical method requires us to make a clinical diagnosis and to attend to the patient's experience. A large part of general practice is helping patients to cope with and adapt to chronic illness and disability. No two patients are the same in their response. If we are to be healers, we have to understand the meaning of the illness in the life of each patient, and often in the life of the family. General practice has led the way in including the human experience of illness as a necessary part of medical knowledge. There is now a rich literature on the experience of illness and a textbook of primary care should find a place for it. It can teach us what it is like to become blind, to have multiple sclerosis, or to care for a spouse with

Alzheimer's disease or a child with diabetes. A textbook can mine this literature for the meanings that are common to all or most patients with a specific disability or disease; it can describe the tools and devices available to the disabled; and, by including case reports, it can stimulate the imagination of readers and help them to empathize with their patients. It is more difficult for a textbook addressed to a global readership to deal adequately with the power of a patient's and family's culture of origin to shape the meaning illness has for them. At least it should sensitize readers to the importance of culture.

The transition from mechanistic to organismic thinking requires a radical change in our notion of disease causation. Medicine has been dominated by a doctrine of specific aetiology: a cause for each disease. We have learned to think of a causal agent as a force acting in linear fashion on a passive object. In self-organizing systems such as organisms, causation is nonlinear. The multiple feedback loops between patient and environment, and between all levels of the patient as organism, require us to think in causal networks, not straight lines. Moreover, the patient as organism is not a passive object. The 'specific cause' of an illness may only be the trigger, which releases a process that is already a potential of the organism. The causes that maintain an illness and inhibit healing may be different from the causes that initiated it, and these may include the patient's own maladaptive behaviours, or even the doctor's actions.

Organismic thinking is thinking in terms of complementarity rather than duality: both/and rather than either/or. As organismic thinkers, either/or questions, such as 'is migraine organic or psychogenic?' become meaningless to us.[8] In this context, it is disappointing to see tiredness and fatigue, sleeping disorders and somatization—all of them complex and multifactorial illnesses—categorized as mental health problems. What message will this convey to our trainees? Primary care physicians have to know where they are on the scale of the complementarities between organismic and mechanistic, uncertainty and precision, involvement and detachment, concrete and abstract, and the particular and the general. The dominance of the mechanistic, reductionist world view has not been unchallenged. An undercurrent of organismic thought has continued and is now finding new acceptance in the sciences of complexity.[7,9,10] Publication of the *Oxford Textbook of Primary Medical Care* will, I hope, be a milestone in the development of primary care medicine.

Acknowledgements

I thank the Canadian Library of Family Medicine for bibliographic support and Joanna L. Asuncion for preparing the manuscript.

References

1. Kuhn, T.S. *The Structure of Scientific Revolutions*. Chicago: University of Chicago Press, 1967.
2. Crookshank, F.G. (1926). The theory of diagnosis. *Lancet* **2**, 939.
3. Mackenzie, J. *The Future of Medicine*. London: Henry Frowde, Hodder and Stoughton, 1919.
4. Mackenzie, J. *Symptoms and their Interpretation*. London: Shaw, 1920.
5. Fry, J., ed. *Clinical Medicine in General Practice*. London: J&A Churchill, 1954.
6. Craddock, D. *A Short Textbook of General Practice*. London: HK Lewis, 1953.
7. Goldstein, K. *The Organism*. New York: Zone Books, 1995.
8. McWhinney, I.R. (1996). The importance of being different. *British Journal of General Practice* **46**, 433–6.
9. Dubos, R. *Man Adapting*. London: Yale University Press, 1965.
10. Boyd, C.A.R. and Noble, D., ed. *The Logic of Life: The Challenge of Integrative Physiology*. Oxford: Oxford University Press, 1993.

Contributors

Samuel B. Adkins Residency Director, East Carolina University, Greenville, South Carolina, USA
Volume 2: 13.6 Hip problems

Bert Aertgeerts Associate Professor, University of Leuven, Leuven, Belgium
Volume 2: 6.2 Haematuria and proteinuria

Mohammed Ali Lecturer, Centre for International Health, Curtin University of Technology, Perth, Western Australia
Volume 1: 1.8 First contact care in developing health care systems

Keith P. Allison Specialist Registrar in Plastic Surgery and Burns, University Hospital Birmingham, NHS Trust, Birmingham, UK
Volume 2: 14.6 Burns

Jeremy Anderson Professor of Epidemiology and Biostatistics, School of Population Health, University of Melbourne, Melbourne, Australia
Volume 1: 10.5 Community interventions—mental health

Richard Anstett Professor of Dermatology, University of Wisconsin-Madison, Wisconsin, USA
Volume 2: 15.6 Chronic skin rashes

Willem J.J. Assendelft Head, Department of Guideline Development and Research Policy, Dutch College of General Practitioners, Utrecht, The Netherlands
Volume 2: 13.8 Tennis elbow

Jo Baggen University of Maastricht, Maastricht, The Netherlands
Volume 1: 8.4 Clinical specialization

Macaran A. Baird Department Head, Family Practice and Community Health, University of Minnesota, USA
Volume 1: 9.3 Family interviewing and assessment
Volume 1: 10.7 Allocating and managing resources

Richard Baker Professor, Clinical Governance Research and Development Unit, University of Leicester, Leicester General Hospital, Leicester, UK
Volume 1: 13.1 Principles and models for quality improvement

Sally Baldwin Research Professor, The University of York, Heslington, York, UK
Volume 1: 10.6 Social care and its place in primary care

Kevin Barraclough General Practitioner, Painswick, Gloucestershire, UK
Volume 2: 1.3 Palpitations and silent arrhythmias

Marie-Dominique Beaulieu Professeur titulaire Chaire Dr Sadok Besrour en Medecine Familiale, Département de Médecine Familiale et Centre de Recherche du CHUM, Université de Montréal, Montréal, Quebec, Canada
Volume 2: 7.12 Screening for cancer in women

Justin Beilby Professor of General Practice, University of Adelaide, Adelaide, Australia
Volume 2: 2.3 Acute non-infective respiratory disorders

Kathleen A. Bell-Irving Clinical Instructor, University of British Columbia, Vancouver, Canada
Volume 2: 16.7 Functional assessment of the elderly

Eugene Bereza Director, Medical Ethics Program, Faculty of Medicine, McGill University, Montréal, Canada
Volume 1: 16.3 Truth-telling in family medicine

Howard Bergman The Dr Joseph Kaufmann Professor of Geriatric Medicine, McGill University, Jewish General Hospital, Montréal, Canada
Volume 2: 16.4 Non-specific presentations of illness
Volume 2: 16.5 Dementia

Thomas M. Best Associate Professor of Orthopedics and Rehabilitation and Family Medicine, University of Wisconsin Medical School, Madison, Wisconsin, USA
Volume 2: 13.3 Acute joint pain

Jo Betterton Team Leader, Consultancy Liaison Service, Hurley Clinic, London, UK
Volume 2: 9.5 Alcohol misuse and primary care

Alison Blenkinsopp Professor of the Practice of Pharmacy, Keele University, Staffs, UK
Volume 1: 3.5 Self-care and self-medication

Wienke G.W. Boerma Senior Researcher, NIVEL (The Netherlands Institute for Health Services Research), Utrecht, The Netherlands
Volume 1: 2.1 Health care systems: understanding the stages of development
Volume 1: 12.7 General practitioners' use of time and time management

Christine Bond Professor of Primary Care, Head of Teaching, University of Aberdeen, Foresterhill Health Centre, Aberdeen, UK
Volume 1: 3.5 Self-care and self-medication

Jeffrey M. Borkan Sackler Faculty of Medicine, Tel Aviv University, Tel Aviv, Israel
Volume 1: 1.4 Community primary care
Volume 1: 9.5 Working with families with chronic medical disorders

Peter Bower Senior Research Fellow, National Primary Care Research and Development Centre, University of Manchester, UK
Volume 1: 1.3 The health care team

Colin Bradley Professor of General Practice, University College Cork, Cork, Ireland
Volume 1: 16.6 Ethics of resource allocation

Suzanne F. Bradley Associate Professor of Internal Medicine, University of Michigan and Veterans Affairs, Ann Arbor Healthcare System, Ann Arbor, Michigan, USA
Volume 2: 16.3 Infections

Nicky Britten Professor of Applied Health Care Research, Institute of Clinical Education, Peninsula Medical School, Universities of Exeter and Plymouth, St Luke's Campus, Exeter, UK
Volume 1: 7.5 Concordance and compliance

Howard Brody Professor, Family Practice and Center for Ethics and Humanities in the Life Sciences, Michigan State University, Michigan, USA
Volume 1: 16.7 End-of-life decisions

Carlos Brotons Unitat d'Epidemiologia, Hospital General Vall d'Hebron, Barcelona, Spain
Volume 1: 11.7 Anticipatory care of established illness: vascular disease

Judith Belle Brown Professor, Center for Studies in Family Medicine, UWO Research Park, Ontario, Canada
Volume 1: 5.6 Time and the consultation

Frank Buntinx Professor, Catholic University of Leuven, Belgium, University of Maastricht, The Netherlands
Volume 2: 6.2 Haematuria and proteinuria

Frederick I. Burge Faculty of Medicine, Dalhousie University, Halifax, Canada
Volume 2: 17.5 Hospice and home care

Sandra K. Burge Professor, University of Texas Health Science Center, San Antonio, Texas, USA
Volume 1: 9.6 Family violence

Peter Burke General Practitioner, St Bartholomew's Medical Centre, Oxford, UK
Volume 1: 11.3 Screening

John L. Campbell Professor of General Practice and Primary Care, Peninsula Medical School, Postgraduate Medical Centre, Exeter, UK
Volume 1: 2.6 Primary care and general practice in Europe: West and South
Volume 1: 12.5 Organization of services

Thomas L. Campbell Professor, Family Medicine and Dentistry, University of Rochester School of Medicine and Dentistry, Rochester, New York, USA
Volume 1: 9.1 Working with families in primary care

Yvonne H. Carter Professor of General Practice & Primary Care, Director, Institute of Community Health Sciences, Barts and the London, Queen Mary's School of Medicine and Dentistry, London, UK
Volume 1: 14.1 History and structure

Francoise P. Chagnon Director of Professional Services, McGill University Health Centre, Montréal, Canada
Volume 2: 3.1 Epistaxis
Volume 2: 3.5 Hoarseness and voice change

Carlos A. Charles Wound Healing Fellow, University of Miami School of Medicine, Florida, USA
Volume 2: 15.4 Pigmented skin lesions

Ian Charlton Associate Professor of Medicine, Newcastle University; Chairman, Asthma Watch, NSW Central Coast, New South Wales, Australia
Volume 2: 2.4 Asthma

Rodger Charlton Director of General Practice, Undergraduate Medical Education, Warwick Medical School, University of Warwick, Coventry, UK
Volume 2: 17.2 Pain concepts and pain control in palliative care

Howard Chertkow Director, Bloomfield Centre for Research in Aging, Lady Davis Institute for Medical Research, S.M.B.D. Jewish General Hospital, Montréal, Canada
Volume 2: 16.5 Dementia

G. Kheng Chew Subspecialty Fellow, Aberdeen Royal Infirmary, Aberdeen, UK
Volume 2: 7.10 Abnormal cervical smear

Joseph L. Chin Professor and Chair, Division of Urology, University of Western Ontario, London Health Sciences Centre, Ontario, Canada
Volume 2: 6.3 Acute urinary retention in adults
Volume 2: 6.4 Testicular and scrotal problems

Katia Cikurel Consultant Neurologist, King's College Hospital, London, UK
Volume 2: 11.7 Coma

A. Mark Clarfield Chief of Geriatrics, Soroka Hospital; Professor and Sidonie Hecht Chair of Gerontology, Faculty of Health Sciences, Ben Gurion University of the Negev, Beersheva, Israel
Volume 2: 16.4 Non-specific presentations of illness
Volume 2: 16.5 Dementia

Lyn Clearihan Senior Lecturer, Monash University, Melbourne, Australia
Volume 2: 15.5 Acute skin rashes
Volume 2: 15.7 Acne

Matthew K. Cline AnMed Family Practice Center, Anderson, South Carolina, USA
Volume 2: 8.8 Caring for women in labour

Kathleen Cole-Kelly Professor, Family Medicine, Case Western Reserve University School of Medicine, Cleveland, Ohio, USA
Volume 1: 9.5 Working with families with chronic medical disorders

Colin Coles Professor, Institute of Health and Community Studies, Bournemouth University, Hampshire, UK
Volume 1: 15.4 Personal growth and professional development

Matthew W. Cooke Reader in Emergency Care, Warwick Medical School, University of Warwick, Warwick, UK
Volume 2: 14.4 Head and neck injuries

Massimo Costantini Senior Epidemiologist, Hospice Medical Director, Servizio di Epidemiologia Clinica, Istituto Nazionale per la Ricerca sul Cancro, Genova, Italy
Volume 1: 7.8 Terminal and palliative care
Volume 2: 17.1 The dying patient and their family

Angela Coulter Chief Executive, Picker Institute Europe, Oxford, UK
Volume 1: 3.4 Medicine and the media

Sarah Cox Consultant in Palliative Medicine, Chelsea and Westminster Hospital, London, UK
Volume 1: 7.8 Terminal and palliative care
Volume 2: 17.6 Symptoms and palliation

Benjamin F. Crabtree Professor and Research Director, University of Medicine and Dentistry of New Jersey, Robert Wood Johnson Medical School, New Brunswick, USA
Volume 1: 14.2 Methods: qualitative

Marilyn A. Craven Associate Clinical Professor, McMaster University, Hamilton, Ontario, Canada
Volume 2: 9.2 Anxiety

Margaret E. Cruickshank Senior Lecturer in Gynaecology and Oncology, Aberdeen Maternity Hospital, Aberdeen, UK
Volume 2: 7.10 Abnormal cervical smear

Alicia Curtin Clinical Assistant Professor, Brown University School of Medicine, Memorial Hospital of Rhode Island, Pawtucket, Rhode Island, USA
Volume 2: 16.1 Falls in the elderly

Jeremy Dale Professor of Primary Care, Warwick Medical School (LWMS), University of Warwick, Coventry, UK
Volume 1: 1.5 Primary care in the emergency department

Maaike Dautzenberg Senior Researcher, Centre for Quality of Care Research (WOK), Universiteit Maastricht/Universitair Medisch Centrum, Nijmegen, The Netherlands
Volume 1: 8.7 Collaboration between professional and lay care

David Davis Associate Dean, University of Toronto, Ontario, Canada
Volume 1: 15.3 The professional development of the family physician: managing knowledge

Jan de Maeseneer Professor and Head of Department, Department of General Practice and Primary Health Care, Ghent University, Gent, Belgium
Volume 1: 4.5 Socio-economic differences in health

Ruut A. de Melker Former Head of the Department of Family Medicine, Emeritus Professor of General Practice, University of Utrecht, Utrecht, The Netherlands
Volume 1: 4.1 The iceberg of illness

Marc De Meyere Vakgroep Huisartsgeneeskunde, Gent, Belgium
Volume 2: 2.5 Chronic lower respiratory disorders

Peter A.G.M. de Smet Clinical Pharmacologist and Professor in Pharmaceutical Care, Scientific Institute Dutch Pharmacists, The Hague, The Netherlands
Volume 1: 1.6 Traditional healers as health care providers: Africa as an example

An de Sutter Department of General Practice and Primary Health Care, Ghent University, Ghent, Belgium
Volume 2: 2.5 Chronic lower respiratory disorders

Niek J. de Wit Senior Lecturer, General Practitioner, Julius Center for Health Sciences and Primary Care, University Medical Center, Utrecht, The Netherlands
Volume 2: 4.3 Acute abdominal pain
Volume 2: 4.11 Constipation

Chris Del Mar Professor and Director, Centre for General Practice, Medical School, University of Queensland, Queensland, Australia
Volume 2: 3.2 Ear pain in adults

F.W. Dijkers General Practitioner, Teacher in Practice Organization, Leiden University Medical Center, Leiden, The Netherlands
Volume 1: 12.3 Equipment and premises in general practice

Geert-Jan Dinant Professor, University of Maastricht, Maastricht, The Netherlands
Volume 1: 6.1 Undifferentiated illness and uncertainty in diagnosis and management
Volume 1: 6.2 Clinical diagnosis: hypothetico-deductive reasoning and other theoretical frameworks

Sean Dinneen Community Diabetologist, Addenbrooke's Hospital, Cambridge, UK
Volume 2: 5.2 Diabetes—Type 1 and Type 2

Anna Donald Chief Executive, Bazian Ltd, London, UK
Volume 1: 13.3 Evidence-based medicine as a tool in quality improvement

Len Doyal Professor of Medical Ethics, St Bartholomew's and The Royal London School of Medicine and Dentistry, Queen Mary College, University of London, UK
Volume 1: 16.1 Ethics in primary care

Gordon W. Duff Florey Professor of Molecular Medicine, Director, Division of Genomic Medicine, School of Medicine and Biomedical Science, University of Sheffield, UK
Volume 2: Introduction—genomic medicine

Tzvi Dwolatzky Director, Geriatric Department, Mental Health Hospital, Beersheva, Israel
Volume 2: 16.4 Non specific presentations of illness

Kathi Earles Assistant Director of Pediatric Residency Program, Morehouse School of Medicine, SW Atlanta, Georgia, USA
Volume 2: 10.2 Childhood respiratory infections

Martin Eccles Professor of Clinical Effectiveness and The William Leech Professor of Primary Care Research, Centre for Health Services Research, University of Newcastle, Newcastle upon Tyne, UK
Volume 1: 13.4 Using and developing clinical guidelines

Polly Edmonds Consultant/Honorary Senior Lecturer, Palliative Care Team, King's College Hospital, London, UK
Volume 1: 7.8 Terminal and palliative care
Volume 2: 17.1 The dying patient and their family
Volume 2: 17.6 Symptoms and palliation

Adrian Edwards Reader, Primary Care Group, Swansea Clinical School, University of Wales Swansea, Swansea, UK
Volume 1: 5.5 Shared decision-making in clinical practice
Volume 1: 7.3 Communication about risks and benefits of treatment and care options

Helena Elkington Research Fellow and General Practitioner, Guy's, King's and St Thomas' School of Medicine, King's College, London, UK
Volume 2: 2.6 Chronic cough

Glyn Elwyn Senior Lecturer in General Practice, University of Wales College of Medicine, Llanedeyrn Health Centre, Cardiff, UK
Volume 1: 5.5 Shared decision-making in clinical practice
Volume 1: 7.3 Communication about risks and benefits of treatment and care options
Volume 1: 14.1 History and structure

Jon Emery Cancer Research UK, Clinician Scientist General Practice & Primary Care Research Unit, University of Cambridge, Institute of Public Health, Cambridge, UK
Volume 1: 6.6 Computerized decision support
Volume 1: 9.4 Assessment and management of genetic risk

Michael Francis Evans Principal Investigator, Knowledge Translation Program, Assistant Professor and Research Scholar, Family & Community Medicine, University of Toronto, Toronto, Canada
Volume 1: 15.3 The professional development of the family physician: managing knowledge

Wes E. Fabb Honorary Clinical Associate Professor, Department of General Practice, Monash University, Melbourne, Australia
Volume 1: 2.13 International organizations

Tom Fahey Professor of Primary Care Medicine, Tayside Centre for General Practice, University of Dundee, Dundee, UK
Volume 2: 1.10 High blood pressure
Volume 2: 2.7 Haemoptysis

Steven R. Feldman Professor of Dermatology, Pathology, and Public Health Sciences, Wake Forest University School of Medicine, Medical Center Boulevard, North Carolina, USA
Volume 2: 15.8 Psoriasis

Ian S. Fentiman Professor of Surgical Oncology, Guy's Hospital, London, UK
Volume 2: 7.11 Abnormal mammogram

Richard A. Figler Assistant Clinical Instructor, Assistant Clinical Professor, Co-coordinator of Procedural Skills, East Carolina University School of Medicine, Brody School of Medicine, East Carolina University, North Carolina, USA
Volume 2: 13.7 Foot problems

Gerda Fijten General Practitioner and Medical Teacher, Skillslab, University of Maastricht, Maastricht, The Netherlands
Volume 2: 4.8 Rectal bleeding

Denise Findlay Caulfield Community Care Centre, Victoria, Australia
Volume 2: 1.8 Varicose veins
Volume 2: 1.9 Leg ulcers

David A. Fitzmaurice Professor of General Practice, The University of Birmingham Medical School, Birmingham, UK
Volume 1: 6.5 Diagnostic tests and use of technology
Volume 2: 1.6 Thrombosis and thromboembolism

Douglas M. Fleming Director, Birmingham Research Unit, Royal College of General Practitioners, Birmingham, UK
Volume 1: 10.3 Health surveillance

Sander Flikweert Senior Scientific Staff Member of Dutch College of General Practitioners (Nederlands Huisartsen Genootschap (NHG)), Utrecht, The Netherlands
Volume 2: 8.6 Vaginal bleeding in early pregnancy

Signe Flottorp Researcher, Directorate for Health and Social Affairs, Oslo, Norway
Volume 1: 13.5 Tools for quality improvement and change in practice

Colleen Fogarty Assistant Professor and Director of Psychosocial Medicine, Department of Family Medicine, Boston University Medical Center, Boston, Massachusetts, USA
Volume 1: 9.6 Family violence

Walter A. Forred Director, Family Practice Residency Program, Kansas City, USA
Volume 2: 15.3 Pruritus

Robbie Foy Clinical Senior Lecturer in Primary Care, Centre for Health Services Research, University of Newcastle upon Tyne, Newcastle, UK
Volume 1: 14.3 Methods: quantitative

Gerri Frager Medical Director, Pediatric Palliative Care, IWK Health Centre, Halifax, Nova Scotia, Canada
Volume 2: 17.4 Death of a child

Deborah A. Frank Professor of Pediatrics, Boston University School of Medicine, Boston, Masssachusetts, USA
Volume 2: 10.5 Failure to thrive

Caroline Free Research Fellow, Guy's, King's, and St Thomas's School of Medicine, Department of General Practice and Primary Care, London, UK
Volume 2: 8.5 Teenage pregnancy

George K. Freeman Professor of General Practice, Centre for Primary Care and Social Medicine, Imperial College London, London, UK
Volume 1: 8.1 Coordination and continuity of care

Peggy Frith Consultant Medical Ophthalmologist, Oxford Eye Hospital, Radcliffe Infirmary, Oxford, UK
Volume 2: 12.4 Ptosis and unequal pupils

Yvonne Fry Chief, Maternal and Child Health Team, Instructor of Clinical Pediatrics, National Center for Primary Care, Morehouse School of Medicine, Atlanta, Georgia, USA
Volume 2: 10.2 Childhood respiratory infections

George E. Fryer Analyst, The Robert Graham Center for Policy Studies in Family Practice and Primary Care, Washington DC, USA
Volume 1: 1.1 The nature of primary medical care

John M. Galloway General Practitioner, St James' House Surgery, Norfolk, UK
Volume 2: 4.2 Dysphagia

Goh Lee Gan Associate Professor, Department of Community, Occupational, and Family Medicine, National University of Singapore, Singapore
Volume 1: 2.3 Primary care and general practice in East and Southeast Asia

B.C. Gee Specialist Registrar in Dermatology, Queen's Medical Centre, Nottingham, UK
Volume 2: 15.1 Hair-related problems

Clare Gerada Director, Royal College of General Practitioners Drugs Training Programme; General Practitioner, London, UK
Volume 2: 9.4 Drug misuse and dependence
Volume 2: 9.5 Alcohol misuse and primary care

Dwenda Kay Gjerdingen University of Minnesota, St Paul, Minneapolis, USA
Volume 2: 8.11 Postpartum care

Hein G. Gooszen Professor of Surgery, University Medical Centre, Utrecht, The Netherlands
Volume 2: 4.5 Abdominal mass

Amy A. Gorin Assistant Professor of Psychiatry and Human Behavior, Brown Medical School, Weight Control and Diabetes Research Center, The Miriam Hospital, Providence, Rhode Island, USA
Volume 2: 5.1 Obesity

Kees J. Gorter General Practitioner, Lecturer and Senior Researcher, Julius Center for Health Sciences and Primary Care, University Medical Center (UMC), Utrecht, The Netherlands
Volume 2: 13.7 Foot problems

Th.M.E. Govaert formerly General Practitioner; formerly member of the Research Department of General Practice, University of Maastricht, Stein, The Netherlands
Volume 2: 16.9 Influenza

Sandra Gower Practice Manager and Executive Partner, Hemel Hempstead, UK
Volume 1: 12.5 Organization of services

Jan Grace Subspecialty Trainee in Reproductive Medicine, Guy's and St Thomas' Hospitals Trust, Assisted Conception Unit, Guy's Hospital, London, UK
Volume 2: 8.2 Sub-fertility

Roger Gray Consultant Ophthalmologist, Taunton and Somerset NHS Trust, Taunton and Somerset Hospital, Somerset, UK
Volume 2: 12.7 Eye trauma

Edward C. Green Senior Research Scientist, Harvard University, Center for Population and Development Studies, Boston, USA
Volume 1: 1.6 Traditional healers as health care providers: Africa as an example

Larry A. Green Professor and Director, The Robert Graham Center for Policy Studies in Family Practice and Primary Care, Washington DC, USA
Volume 1: 1.1 The nature of primary medical care

Sally Green Associate Professor, Monash Institute of Health Services Research, Monash University, Melbourne, Australia
Volume 2: 13.8 Tennis elbow

Trisha Greenhalgh Professor of Primary Health Care, University College London, London, UK
Volume 1: 13.3 Evidence-based medicine as a tool in quality improvement

R. Stephen Griffith Associate Professor & Chairman, University of Missouri Kansas City, Kansas City, Missouri, USA
Volume 2: 15.11 Bruising and purpura

Jeremy Grimshaw Professor and Director, Clinical Epidemiology Programme, Ottawa Health Research Institute, University of Ottawa, Canada
Volume 1: 13.4 Using and developing clinical guidelines
Volume 1: 13.5 Tools for quality improvement and change in practice

Peter P. Groenewegen Head of Research Department, Professor of Social and Geographical Aspects of Health and Health care, Utrecht University, NIVEL (The Netherlands Institute for Health Services Research), Utrecht, The Netherlands
Volume 1: 12.7 General practitioners' use of time and time management

Richard Grol Professor and Director, Centre for Quality of Care Research (WOK), Nijmegen University Medical Centre, Maastricht University, The Netherlands
Volume 1: 13.1 Principles and models for quality improvement
Volume 1: 13.6 Total quality management and continuous quality improvement
Volume 1: 13.7 The patient's role in improving quality

Stefan Grzybowski Children's and Women's Health Center of British Columbia, Vancouver, Canada
Volume 2: 8.1 Pre-conception care

Jane Gunn Associate Professor, University of Melbourne, Victoria, Australia
Volume 1: 14.3 Methods: quantitative

Allan C. Halpern Chief, Dermatology Service, Memorial Sloan-Kettering Cancer Center, New York, USA
Volume 2: 15.4 Pigmented skin lesions

Hilary Haman Fellow of The Chartered Institute of Personnel & Development, Organisational Management, Personnel Adviser, Cardiff, UK
Volume 1: 12.2 Staff

Philip Hannaford Grampian Health Board Professor of Primary Care, University of Aberdeen, Aberdeen, UK
Volume 1: 10.1 The individual and the population

Mark Harris Professor of General Practice, School of Public Health and Community Medicine, University of New South Wales, Sydney, Australia
Volume 1: 14.6 Outcomes

Susan Harris Head, Department of Family Practice, Children's and Women's Health Centre of British Columbia, Vancouver, Canada
Volume 2: 8.3 Contraception

Yvonne Hart Consultant Neurologist, Radcliffe Infirmary, Oxford, UK
Volume 2: 11.2 Epilepsy

M. Jawad Hashim Program Director, Primary Care Pakistan, Islamabad, Pakistan
Volume 1: 2.10 Primary care and general practice in Pakistan

Richard Hays Chair of General Practice and Rural Medicine, James Cook University, Queensland, Australia
Volume 1: 15.2 Vocational and postgraduate training

Jane Haywood Clinical Nurse Specialist, CLAS Team, Hurley Clinic, London, UK
Volume 2: 9.4 Drug misuse and dependence

M.S. Darrell Henderson Health Policy Analyst, American Academy of Family Physicians, Leawood, Kansas, USA
Volume 1: 2.12 Primary care and general practice in North America

John Henry Professor of Accident and Emergency Medicine, Imperial College Faculty of Medicine, St Mary's Hospital, London, UK
Volume 2: 14.7 Poisoning

John M. Hickner Professor of Family Practice, Michigan State University, Michigan, USA
Volume 2: 3.6 Acute sinusitis

Irene J. Higginson Professor and Head, Department of Palliative Care and Policy, King's College London, Weston Education Centre, London, UK
Volume 1: 7.8 Terminal and palliative care
Volume 2: 17.1 The dying patient and their family

Roger Higgs Professor of General Practice, Guy's, King's and St Thomas' School of Medicine, London, UK
Volume 1: 16.4 Confidentiality

Wolfgang Himmel Medical Sociologist, University of Göttingen, Göttingen, Germany
Volume 1: 7.1 Principles of patient management

Per Hjortdahl Professor of General Practice, University of Oslo, Oslo, Norway
Volume 1: 7.6 Continuity of care
Volume 1: 12.4 The office laboratory

Richard Hobbs Professor and Head of Primary Care and General Practice, Primary Care Clinical Sciences Building, University of Birmingham, Edgbaston, Birmingham, UK
Volume 2: 1.2 Heart failure
Volume 2: 1.11 Dyslipidaemia and cardiovascular disease

David B. Hogan Professor and Brenda Strafford Foundation Chair in Geriatric Medicine, University of Calgary Health Sciences Centre, Alberta, Canada
Volume 2: 16.5 Dementia

Mary P. Hogan Home Care and Office-based Nurse, Case Western University School of Medicine, Ohio, USA
Volume 1: 9.5 Working with families with chronic medical disorders

Tony Hope Professor of Medical Ethics, ETHOX (The Oxford Centre for Ethics and Communication in Health Care Practice), University of Oxford, Oxford, UK
Volume 1: 16.5 Ethics of research

Jan Lucas Hoving Senior Research Fellow, Monash University, Melbourne, Australia
Volume 2: 13.2 Neck pain

William Howlett Consultant Neurologist and Honorary Senior Lecturer in Neurology, King's College Hospital, London, UK
Volume 2: 11.8 Meningitis and CNS infections

Suber S. Huang Director, Vitreoretinal Diseases and Surgery, University Hospitals of Cleveland; Associate Professor of Ophthalmology, Case Western Reserve University, Cleveland, Ohio, USA
Volume 2: 12.6 Blindness

Pali Hungin Professor of Primary Care and General Practice, University of Durham, Durham, UK
Volume 1: 6.4 The therapeutic illusion: self-limiting illness
Volume 2: 4.7 Haematemesis and melaena

Brian Hurwitz D'Oyly Carte Professor of Medicine and the Arts, King's College, London, UK
Volume 1: 13.4 Using and developing clinical guidelines
Volume 1: 16.8 Medico-legal issues
Volume 2: 11.3 Movement disorders

Sally Irvine Haman and Irvine Associates, Morpeth, Northumberland, UK
Volume 1: 12.1 Practice structures

Neill Iscoe Toronto-Sunnybrook Regional Cancer Centre, Ontario, Canada
Volume 2: 6.11 Prostate cancer

D. Anna Jarvis Professor of Paediatrics, University of Toronto, The Hospital for Sick Children, Toronto, Canada
Volume 2: 14.8 Drowning and inhalations
Volume 2: 14.9 Electrical injuries

David Jewell Editor, British Journal of General Practice; Honorary Senior Lecturer in Primary Care, University of Bristol, Bristol, UK
Volume 1: 14.7 Publishing primary care research

Sandra Marchese Johnson Clinical Trials Unit Director, Dermatology, University of Arkansas, Arkansas, USA
Volume 2: 15.13 Photosensitivity

Roger Jones Wolfson Professor of General Practice and Primary Care, Guy's, King's and St Thomas' School of Medicine, London, UK
Volume 1: 1.4 Community primary care
Volume 1: 8.4 Clinical specialization
Volume 1: 12.3 Equipment and premises in general practice
Volume 1: 14.7 Publishing primary care research
Volume 2: 4.1 Dyspepsia

Norman B. Kahn Jr Vice-President, Science and Education, American Academy of Family Physicians, Leawood, USA
Volume 1: 2.12 Primary care and general practice in North America

Joe Kai Professor of Primary Care, School of Community Health Sciences, University of Nottingham, Nottingham, UK
Volume 2: 10.1 Approach to the sick infant

Victoria S. Kaprielian Clinical Professor, Duke University Medical Center, Durham, North Carolina, USA
Volume 1: 1.9 Management and leadership

Michael P. Kelly Director of Research and Information, Health Development Agency, London, UK
Volume 1: 5.4 Doctors' perceptions of their patients

Tony Kendrick Professor of Primary Medical Care, Director of Community Clinical Sciences Division, University of Southampton Medical School, Aldermoor Health Centre, Southampton, UK
Volume 1: 11.8 Anticipatory care of mental health problems
Volume 2: 9.1 Depression

Ngaire Kerse Senior Lecturer, University of Auckland, Auckland, New Zealand
Volume 1: 2.4 Primary care and general practice in Australia and New Zealand

Michael Richard Kidd Professor of General Practice, University of Sydney and President, Royal Australian College of General Practitioners, Sydney, Australia
Volume 1: 5.7 Computers in the consultation
Volume 2: 6.7 HIV/AIDS

George E. Kikano Chairman, Department of Family Medicine, Case Western Reserve University, Ohio, USA
Volume 2: 12.6 Blindness

Ann Louise Kinmonth Professor and Head, General Practice and Primary Care Research Unit, Institute of Public Health, University of Cambridge, Cambridge, UK
Volume 1: 5.1 The patient–doctor relationship
Volume 2: 5.2 Diabetes—Type 1 and Type 2

Colleen Kirkham Clinical Associate Professor, University of British Columbia, Vancouver, Canada
Volume 2: 8.1 Pre-conception care

Maarten Klomp General Practitioner, Center for Primary Care Achtse Barrier, Eindhoven, The Netherlands
Volume 2: 6.10 Benign prostate disorders

Arie Knuistingh Neven General Practitioner/Epidemiologist, Leiden University Medical Centre, Leiden, The Netherlands; Centre for Sleep Wake Disorders, MCH Westeinde Hospital, The Hague, The Netherlands
Volume 2: 9.9 Sleep disorders

Michael M. Kochen Professor of General Practice and Head, University of Göttingen, Germany
Volume 1: 7.1 Principles of patient management

Lakshmi Kolagotla Boston University Medical Center, Boston, Massachussetts, USA
Volume 2: 10.5 Failure to thrive

Eliana C. Korin Senior Associate and Director of Behavioral Science, Department of Family and Social Medicine, Montefiore Medical Center and Albert Einstein College of Medicine, New York, USA
Volume 1: 9.2 Families, health, and cultural diversity

Madelon W. Kroneman Researcher, International Health Care Systems, NIVEL (The Netherlands Institute for Health Services Research), Utrecht, The Netherlands
Volume 1: 2.1 Health care systems: understanding the stages of development

Phillipa M. Kyle Consultant in Maternal and Fetal Medicine, St Michael's Hospital, Bristol, UK
Volume 2: 8.8 Caring for women in labour

Toine Lagro-Janssen General Practitioner and Professor, Women's Studies Medicine University Medical Center, Nijmegen, The Netherlands
Volume 2: 7.6 Urinary incontinence
Volume 2: 16.6 Urinary incontinence

Henk Lamberts Professor of General/Family Practice, Division of Clinical Methods & Public Health, Academic Medical Center, University of Amsterdam, Amsterdam, The Netherlands
Volume 1: 4.3 Classification and the domain of family practice

Tim Lancaster Clinical Reader in General Practice, Department of Primary Health Care, Oxford University, Oxford, UK
Volume 1: 11.4 Changing behaviour: smoking
Volume 1: 14.5 Secondary research

Pekka Larivaara Professor in Systemic Family Medicine, University of Oulu, Finland
Volume 1: 9.1 Working with families in primary care

Hilary Lavender General Practitioner, London, UK
Volume 2: 1.12 Anaemia

Patricia Lebensohn Associate Professor of Clinical, Family and Community Medicine, Family Practice Residency Program, University of Arizona, Tucson, Arizona, USA
Volume 1: 9.2 Families, health, and cultural diversity

Barbara Lent Associate Professor, University of Western Ontario, London, Ontario, Canada
Volume 2: 7.13 Violence as a women's health issue

Alexander K.C. Leung Clinical Associate Professor of Paediatrics, The University of Calgary, Calgary, Canada
Volume 2: 12.2 Sticky eye

Morten Lindbak Associate Professor, Department of General Practice, University of Oslo, Oslo, Norway
Volume 2: 3.6 Acute sinusitis

Christos Lionis Associate Professor, University of Crete, Faculty of Medicine, Crete, Greece
Volume 2: 4.9 Jaundice

Verity Livingstone Associate Professor, University of British Columbia, Canada
Volume 2: 8.9 Breastfeeding

Irvine Loudon Medical historian (previously General Practitioner), Green College and Wellcome Unit for the History of Medicine, University of Oxford, UK
Volume 1: 1.2 From general practice to primary care, 1700–1980

Julie Lumeng Instructor of Pediatrics, Boston University School of Medicine, Boston, USA
Volume 2: 10.9 Developmental delay

Denise Mabey Consultant Ophthalmologist, St Thomas' Hospital, London, UK
Volume 2: 12.3 Loss of vision

Vincent E. MacDonald Grief Counselor, Private Practice, Nova Scotia, Canada
Volume 2: 17.4 Death of a child

Jane Macnaughton Centre for Arts and Humanities in Medicine, University of Durham, Durham, UK
Volume 1: 6.3 Clinical judgement

Antonio Maiques Primary Health Centre, Valencia, Spain
Volume 1: 11.7 Anticipatory care of established illness: vascular disease

David Mant Professor of General Practice, University of Oxford, UK
Volume 1: 11.1 Principles of prevention

Alon P.A. Margalit Atzmon Post Misgav, Israel
Volume 1: 9.3 Family interviewing and assessment

Ashfaq A. Marghoob Assistant Attending Physician, Memorial Sloan-Kettering Cancer Center, New York, USA
Volume 2: 15.4 Pigmented skin lesions

Marjukka Mäkelä Head, Finnish Office for Health Care Technology Assessment, Helsinki, Finland
Volume 1: 13.5 Tools for quality improvement and change in practice

Andrew K. Marsden Consultant Medical Director, Scottish Ambulance Service, Edinburgh, UK
Volume 2: 14.1 Out-of-hospital cardiac arrest

Martin Marshall Professor, National Primary Care Research and Development Centre, University of Manchester, Manchester, UK
Volume 1: 13.2 Measuring the quality of primary medical care

James Mason Professor of Health Economics, Centre for Health Services Research, University of Newcastle Upon Tyne, Newcastle upon Tyne, UK
Volume 1: 13.4 Using and developing clinical guidelines

Danielle Mazza Formerly Associate Professor, International Medical University, Kuala Lumpur, Malaysia
Volume 2: 7.4 Amenorrhoea
Volume 2: 7.9 Dyspareunia

Ronald McCoy General Practitioner and HIV Educator, Melbourne, Australia
Volume 2: 6.7 HIV/AIDS

Gary W. McEwen Associate Clinical Professor, Lee's Summit, Missouri, USA
Volume 2: 15.10 Skin infections

Ian R. McWhinney Emeritus Professor of Family Medicine, The University of Western Ontario, Centre for Studies in Family Medicine, London, Ontario, Canada
Foreword

Jack H. Medalie Dorothy Jones Weatherhead Professor Emeritus of Family Medicine, School of Medicine, Case Western Reserve University, Ohio, USA
Volume 1: 9.5 Working with families with chronic medical disorders

Villy Meineche-Schmidt General Practitioner, Copenhagen, Denmark
Volume 2: 4.11 Constipation

Juan Mendive La Mina Health Centre, Barcelona, Spain
Volume 1: 2.6 Primary care and general practice in Europe: West and South
Volume 2: 4.6 Nausea, vomiting, and loss of appetite

Job F.M. Metsemakers University of Maastricht, Maastricht, The Netherlands
Volume 1: 12.6 The medical record

Thomas M. Mettee Family Practitioner, Clinical Associate Professor, Case Western University School of Medicine, Ohio, USA
Volume 1: 9.5 Working with families with chronic medical disorders

Betty Meyboom-de Jong Professor and Chair, Department of General Practice, Groningen University, Groningen, The Netherlands
Volume 1: 4.4 Age and gender

Peter E. Mezciems Senior Staff Physician, Homewood Health Center, Guelph, Ontario, Canada
Volume 1: 15.7 Addictions and mental illness in physicians

Michael J. Michell Consultant Radiologist/Clinical Director, South East London Breast Screening Programme, King's Healthcare NHS Trust, King's College Hospital, London, UK
Volume 2: 7.11 Abnormal mammogram

J. Lloyd Michener Clinical Professor and Chairman, Duke University Medical Center, North Carolina, USA
Volume 1: 1.9 Management and leadership

William L. Miller Chair, Department of Family Medicine, Lehigh Valley Hospital, Allentown, Pennsylvania, USA
Volume 1: 14.2 Methods: qualitative

Louise M. Millward Research and Development Specialist, Health Development Agency, London, UK
Volume 1: 5.4 Doctors' perceptions of their patients

Rosie Moon General Practice Professorial Unit, University of Sydney, Manly Hospital, Manly, Australia
Volume 1: 2.4 Primary care and general practice in Australia and New Zealand

Charles Mouton Associate Professor and Associate Chief, Division of Community Geriatrics, University of Texas Health Science Center, Texas, USA
Volume 1: 9.6 Family violence

Robert D. Murray Research Fellow in Endocrinology, Christie Hospital, Manchester, UK
Volume 2: 5.7 Endocrine problems (calcium, water, and adrenal)

T. Jock Murray Professor of Medical Humanities, Tupper Link, Halifax, Canada
Volume 2: 11.6 Progressive neurological illnesses: multiple sclerosis and amyotrophic lateral sclerosis

John Murtagh Adjunct Professor of General Practice, Monash University, Melbourne, Australia
Volume 2: 11.1 Headache and facial pain

Lawrence Mynors-Wallis Consultant Psychiatrist, Dorset Healthcare NHS Trust, Alderney Community Hospital, Dorset, UK
Volume 2: 9.10 Psychological treatments for mental health problems

Irwin Nazareth Professor of Primary Care and Population Sciences, Royal Free and University College Medical School, London, UK
Volume 2: 11.4 Dizziness

John Newton Unit of Health Care Epidemiology, Institute of Health Sciences, Oxford, UK
Volume 1: 10.2 Defining the population: registration and record linkage

Richard A. Nicholas Denver, Colorado, USA
Volume 2: 15.9 Eczema and dermatitis

Mattijs E. Numans General Practitioner and Senior Staff Member, Julius Center for Health Sciences and Primary Care, University Medical Utrecht, Utrecht, The Netherlands
Volume 2: 4.4 Chronic abdominal pain

Natalie O'Dea Director, EdAct Pty. Ltd, Willoughby, Australia
Volume 1: 3.3 Health beliefs

Norma O'Flynn Lecturer in General Practice, Imperial College London, UK
Volume 2: 7.7 Menstrual disorders: menorrhagia
Volume 2: 7.8 Menstrual disorders: dysmenorrhoea

Karen S. Ogle Professor, Family Practice, Michigan State University, Michigan, USA
Volume 1: 16.7 End-of-life decisions

Inge M. Okkes Senior Researcher, Division of Clinical Methods & Public Health, Academic Medical Center, University of Amsterdam, Amsterdam, The Netherlands
Volume 1: 4.3 Classification and the domain of family practice

Frede Olesen Research Unit for General Practice, University of Aarhus, Aarhus C, Denmark
Volume 1: 2.8 General practice in Europe: Scandinavia
Volume 1: 8.3 Generalists in hospitals

Daniel J. Ostergaard Vice President, International and Interprofessional Activities, American Academy of Family Physicians, Kansas, USA
Volume 1: 2.12 Primary care and general practice in North America

Tim Overton Consultant Obstetrician and Gynaecologist, Norfolk and Norwich University Hospital, NHS Trust, Norfolk, UK
Volume 2: 8.7 Complications of pregnancy

Alan Owen Senior Research Fellow, Centre for Health Service Development, Faculty of Commerce, University of Wollongong, Australia
Volume 1: 1.8 First contact care in developing health care systems

James F. Pagel Assistant Clinical Professor, University of Colorado Medical School; Director, Sleep Disorders Center of Southern Colorado & Rocky Mt. Sleep Pueblo/Colorado Springs, Colorado, USA
Volume 2: 10.10 Sleep disorders in children

Claire Parker General Practitioner, Jericho Health Centre, Oxford, UK
Volume 1: 11.2 Immunization and vaccination

Steven Parker Associate Professor, Boston University School of Medicine, Boston Medical Center, Boston University, Boston, USA
Volume 2: 10.9 Developmental delay

Christopher Patterson Professor, Division of Geriatric Medicine, McMaster University, Hamilton, Ontario, Canada
Volume 2: 16.5 Dementia

Debra M. Phillips Professor, Family and Community Medicine, Southern Illinois University School of Medicine, Quincy, Illinois, USA
Volume 2: 10.12 School issues

William R. Phillips Clinical Professor, University of Washington, Seattle, Washington, USA
Volume 2: 10.3 Otitis media

Robert L. Phillips Jr Assistant Director, The Robert Graham Center: Policy Studies in Family Practice and Primary Care, Washington DC, USA
Volume 1: 1.1 The nature of primary medical care

Munir Pirmohamed Professor of Clinical Pharmacology and Consultant Physician, The University of Liverpool and the Royal Liverpool University Hospitals, Liverpool, UK
Volume 2: 16.8 Drugs in the elderly

Leon Piterman Professor of General Practice, Head of School of Primary Health Care, Monash University, Melbourne, Victoria, Australia
Volume 1: 7.2 Patient education, advice, and counselling
Volume 2: 1.1 Chest pain and myocardial infarction

Paul E. Plsek Consultant in Quality Management, Paul E. Plsek & Associates, Inc., Atlanta, Georgia, USA
Volume 1: 13.6 Total quality management and continuous quality improvement

Victor J. Pop Professor of Primary Health Care, Tilburg University, Tilburg, The Netherlands
Volume 2: 5.5 Thyroid disorders

David Portnoy Assistant Professor, McGill University, Montréal General Hospital, Montréal, Quebec, Canada
Volume 2: 6.5 Genital ulcers and warts
Volume 2: 6.6 Gonorrhoea and chlamydial infections

Jennifer Powell Consultant Dermatologist, Churchill Hospital, Oxford, UK
Volume 2: 15.1 Hair-related problems
Volume 2: 15.14 Genital disorders

David Price Assistant Professor, McMaster University, Stonechurch Family Health Centre, Ontario, Canada
Volume 2: 8.4 Normal pregnancy

Mike Pringle Professor of General Practice and Head of School of Community Health Sciences, Division of Primary Care, University of Nottingham, Newark, UK
Volume 1: 12.1 Practice structures

Luis E. Quiroga Medical School, UMSS, Cochabamba, Bolivia
Volume 2: 2.2 Lower respiratory tract infections

Anan S. Raghunath General Practitioner and Honorary Research Fellow, St Andrews Group Practice, Maramaduke Health Centre, University of Hull, UK
Volume 1: 2.9 Primary care and general practice in India

Alexander H. Rajput Associate Professor of Neurology, University of Saskatchewan, Royal University Hospital, Saskatoon, Canada
Volume 2: 16.2 Gait and movement disorders

Ali H. Rajput Professor Emeritus (Neurology), University of Saskatchewan, Royal University Hospital, Saskatoon, Canada
Volume 2: 16.2 Gait and movement disorders

A.S. Ramanujam Chief Medical Officer, Lal Bahadur Shastri Hospital, New Delhi, India
Volume 1: 2.9 Primary care and general practice in India

Victoria H. Raveis Associate Professor of Clinical Sociomedical Sciences, Columbia University, Mailman School of Public Health, New York, USA
Volume 2: 17.3 Bereavement and grief

Gerald M. Reaven Falk CVRC, Stanford Medical Center, Stanford, California, USA
Volume 2: 5.3 Insulin resistance/syndrome X

Shelley Rechner Assistant Clinical Professor, Faculty of Health Sciences, McMaster University, Southwest Family Health Centre, Hamilton, Ontario, Canada
Volume 2: 9.11 Adult survivors of sexual abuse

Graham J. Reid Assistant Professor, Bill and Anne Brock Family Professor in Child Health, Psychology and Family Medicine, University of Western Ontario, Ontario, Canada
Volume 2: 10.11 Behaviour problems in children

Melody Rhydderch Organisational Psychologist and NHS Research Training Fellow, Primary Care Group, The Clinical School, University of Wales Swansea, Swansea, UK
Volume 1: 5.5 Shared decision-making in clinical practice

David G. Riddell Clinical Professor of Pediatrics, University of British Columbia, Vancouver, Canada
Volume 2: 8.10 Feeding problems in infants and young children

Leone Ridsdale Senior Lecturer in Neurology and Reader in General Practice, Guy's, King's, and St Thomas' School of Medicine, King's College School of Medicine, London, UK
Volume 2: 9.8 Fatigue
Volume 2: 11.2 Epilepsy

Zoltan Rihmer National Institute for Psychiatry and Neurology, Budapest, Hungary
Volume 2: 9.3 Suicide and attempted suicide

Alan Riley Professor of Sexual Medicine, Cwmann, Wales, UK
Volume 2: 6.9 Female sexual dysfunction

Isabel Rodrigues Professeur adjoint de Clinique, Université de Montréal, CLSC-CHSLD du Marigot, Québec, Canada
Volume 2: 7.12 Screening for cancer in women

Anja Rogausch Psychologist, University of Göttingen, Göttingen, Germany
Volume 1: 7.1 Principles of patient management

Martin Roland Professor and Director, National Primary Care Research and Development Centre, University of Manchester, Manchester, UK
Volume 1: 8.2 The primary–secondary care interface
Volume 1: 13.2 Measuring the quality of primary medical care

Lewis C. Rose Associate Professor of Family Medicine, University of Texas Health Science Center, Texas, USA
Volume 2: 10.7 Disorders of growth

Peter Rose University Lecturer, University of Oxford, Institute of Health Sciences, Oxford, UK
Volume 1: 9.4 Assessment and management of genetic risk

Andrew Ross General Practitioner, Northfield Health Centre, Birmingham, UK
Volume 1: 10.3 Health surveillance

Walter W. Rosser Professor and Chair, Department of Family Medicine, Queens University, Kingston, Ontario, Canada
Volume 2: 10.4 Fever and common childhood infections
Volume 2: 10.6 Anticipatory guidance and prevention

James T.B. Rourke Assistant Dean, Rural and Regional Medicine, The University of Western Ontario, Director, Southwestern Ontario Rural Regional Medicine Education Research and Development Network, Canada
Volume 1: 1.7 Rural primary care

Greg Rubin Professor of Primary Care, University of Sunderland School of Sciences, Sunderland, UK
Volume 2: 4.10 Diarrhoea

Anthony G. Rudd Consultant Stroke Physician, Guy's and St Thomas' Hospital, London, UK
Volume 2: 1.7 Stroke and transient ischaemia

George Rust Professor of Family Medicine and Deputy Director, National Center for Primary Care at Morehouse School of Medicine, Atlanta, Georgia, USA
Volume 2: 10.2 Childhood respiratory infections

Jerry G. Ryan Associate Professor, University of Wisconsin–Madison, Madison, Wisconsin, USA
Volume 2: 13.3 Acute joint pain

Janice Rymer Senior Lecturer/Consultant in Obstetrics and Gynaecology, Guy's, King's and St Thomas' School of Medicine, Guy's and St Thomas' Hospital Trust, London, UK
Volume 2: 7.5 The menopause

Rebecca B. Saenz Associate Professor of Family Medicine, University of Mississippi Medical Center, Mississippi, USA
Volume 2: 7.2 Nipple discharge

Alena Salim Dermatologist, Royal Berkshire Hospital, Reading, UK
Volume 2: 15.14 Genital disorders

Robert B. Salter Professor Emeritus of Orthopaedic Surgery and Senior Scientist Emeritus, The Research Institute, The Hospital for Sick Children, Ontario, Canada
Volume 2: 10.8 The child with a limp

Deborah C. Saltman Professor of General Practice, University of Sydney, Australia
Volume 1: 2.4 Primary care and general practice in Australia and New Zealand
Volume 1: 3.3 Health beliefs

Sverre Sandberg Professor, NOKLUS, Division for General Practice and Laboratory of Clinical Biochemistry, Haukeland University Hospital, University of Bergen, Bergen, Norway
Volume 1: 12.4 The office laboratory

Kanwaljit Sandhu Specialist Registrar in Nephrology, St George's Hospital, London, UK
Volume 2: 6.2 Haematuria and proteinuria

Brenda Sawyer Adviser to the Institute of Healthcare Management; GP Tutor in South West and Mid Hampshire; Independent Management Consultant, UK
Volume 1: 12.7 General practitioners' use of time and time management

Arun Sayal Emergency Physician and Lecturer, North York General Hospital, University of Toronto, Toronto, Canada
Volume 2: 14.2 Fractures and limb trauma

François G. Schellevis Research Coordinator, NIVEL (The Netherlands Institute for Health Services Research), Utrecht, The Netherlands
Volume 1: 4.2 Physical and mental illness

H.J. Schers General Practitioner, University Medical Centre, St Radboud, Nijmegen, The Netherlands
Volume 1: 12.3 Equipment and premises in general practice

Theo Schofield Director of Communication, ETHOX (The Oxford Centre for Ethics and Communication in Health Care Practice), University of Oxford, Oxford, UK
Volume 1: 5.3 Communication skills

Knut Schroeder Clinical Lecturer, University of Bristol, Bristol, UK
Volume 2: 1.10 High blood pressure
Volume 2: 2.7 Haemoptysis

Brian Schwartz Assistant Professor, University of Toronto, Toronto, Ontario, Canada
Volume 2: 14.5 Non-accidental injuries

E. Robert Schwartz Professor and Chair, University of Miami, Miami, Florida, USA
Volume 2: 12.5 Visual disturbances

Martin Schwartz Consultant Neurologist, Atkinson Morley Hospital, London, UK
Volume 2: 11.5 Peripheral neuropathies

Roberta Schwartz Lecturer, Faculty of Medicine, University of Toronto, Toronto, Canada
Volume 2: 14.5 Non-accidental injuries

Gunjan Sharma Medicine/Pediatrics Resident, University of Massachusetts Medical Centre, Worcester, USA
Volume 2: 15.12 Lumps in and under the skin

Deborah J. Sharp Professor of Primary Health Care, University of Bristol, Bristol, UK
Volume 2: 9.13 Post-natal depression

Elizabeth Shaw McMaster University Medical Center, Hamilton, Ontario, Canada
Volume 2: 8.4 Normal pregnancy

Paul Shekelle Senior Research Associate, Veterans Affairs Health Services Research and Development Service, Greater Los Angeles Health Care System, California, USA
Volume 1: 13.4 Using and developing clinical guidelines

Andrew Shennan Professor of Obstetrics, St Thomas' Hospital, London, UK
Volume 2: 8.7 Complications of pregnancy

Pesach Shvartzman Chairman, Division of Community Health, Ben-Gurion University of the Negev, Beersheva, Israel
Volume 1: 2.11 Primary care and general practice in the Middle East

Bonnie Sibbald Professor, National Primary Care Research and Development Centre, The University of Manchester, Manchester, UK
Volume 1: 1.3 The health care team

Douglas E. Sinclair Chair of Emergency Medicine, Dalhousie University, Nova Scotia, Canada
Volume 2: 9.7 Psychiatric emergencies

Anne Slowther Research Fellow, ETHOX (Oxford Centre for Ethics and Communication in Health Care Practice), University of Oxford, Institute of Health Sciences, Oxford, UK
Volume 1: 16.5 Ethics of research

Gary Smith Research Assistant, The Surgery, Solihull, UK
Volume 2: 17.2 Pain concepts and pain control in palliative care

Gillian Smith Registrar, Department of Plastic Surgery, City General Hospital, Staffordshire, UK
Volume 2: 14.6 Burns

A. Patricia Smith Honorary Lecturer, Aberdeen Maternity Hospital, Aberdeen, UK
Volume 2: 7.10 Abnormal cervical smear

Leif I. Solberg Associate Medical Director for Care Improvement Research, HealthPartners Research Foundation, Minneapolis, USA
Volume 1: 8.6 Getting beyond disease-specific management
Volume 1: 13.6 Total quality management and continuous quality improvement

Peter Sonksen Emeritus Professor of Medicine, St Thomas' Hospital, London, UK
Volume 2: 5.6 Endocrine problems (pituitary and sex hormones)

Stephen J. Spann Professor and Chairman, Baylor College of Medicine, Texas, USA
Volume 1: 2.5 Primary care and general practice in Latin America

Bruce L.W. Sparks Faculty of Health Sciences, University of Witwatersrand, Johannesburg, South Africa
Volume 1: 2.2 Primary care and general practice in Africa

M.P. Springer General Practitioner; Professor of General Practice, Leiden University Medical Centre, Leiden, The Netherlands
Volume 2: 9.9 Sleep disorders

Yvonne Steinert Clinical Psychologist and Professor of Family Medicine, McGill University, Montréal, Canada
Volume 1: 15.6 Multi-professional education

Moira Stewart Professor and Director, Centre for Studies in Family Medicine, The University of Western Ontario, Ontario, Canada
Volume 1: 5.1 The patient–doctor relationship

Jelle Stoffers Associate Professor of General Practice, University of Maastricht, Public Health Research Institute (CAPHRI), Maastricht, The Netherlands
Volume 2: 1.5 Peripheral arterial disease

Tim Stokes Senior Lecturer in General Practice, University of Leicester, Leicester General Hospital, Leicester, UK
Volume 2: 7.3 Vaginal discharge

Nigel C.H. Stott Professor of General Practice, University of Wales College of Medicine, Cardiff, UK
Volume 1: 5.2 Consultation tasks

Derek Summerfield Honorary Senior Lecturer, Institute of Psychiatry, King's College, London, UK
Volume 2: 9.12 Post-traumatic stress disorder

Patricia Sunaert Assistant, Department of General Practice and Primary Health Care, Ghent University, Ghent, Belgium
Volume 2: 15.2 Nail disorders

Robert Sweet Assistant Professor Department of Otolaryngology, McGill University Health Centre, Montréal, Canada
Volume 2: 3.4 Hearing loss

Richard P. Swinson Morgan Firestone Chair in Psychiatry, McMaster University, Ontario, Canada
Volume 2: 9.2 Anxiety

Howard Tandeter Ben-Gurion University, Israel
Volume 1: 2.11 Primary care and general practice in the Middle East

Danny Tayar Family Physician, The Mifne Centre, Israel
Volume 1: 12.6 The medical record

Alison Taylor Consultant in Gynaecology and Reproductive Medicine, Assisted Conception Unit, Guy's and St Thomas' Hospitals Trust, London, UK
Volume 2: 8.2 Sub-fertility

Ted L. Tewfik Professor of Otolaryngology, McGill University; Director of Otolaryngology, Montréal Children's Hospital, Montréal, Quebec, Canada
Volume 2: 3.3 The discharging ear
Volume 2: 3.4 Hearing loss

Kate Thomas Deputy Director, Medical Care Research Unit, School of Health and Related Research, University of Sheffield, Sheffield, UK
Volume 1: 3.6 Alternative sources of advice: traditional and complementary medicine

Sharon Thomson The University of British Columbia Family Practice Centre, British Columbia, Canada
Volume 2: 8.3 Contraception

Geir Thue General Practitioner, NOKLUS, University of Bergen, Bergen, Norway
Volume 1: 12.4 The office laboratory

Arno Timmermans Executive Director, Dutch College of General Practitioners, Utrecht, The Netherlands
Volume 1: 2.6 Primary care and general practice in Europe: West and South

John M. Tomlinson Director, Men's Health Clinic, Royal Hampshire County Hospital, Winchester, UK
Volume 2: 6.8 Sexual dysfunction in men

Les Toop Pegasus Professor of General Practice, Christchurch School of Medicine, Christchurch, New Zealand
Volume 1: 7.4 Principles of drug prescribing

Simon Travis Consultant Gastroenterologist, John Radcliffe Hospital, Oxford, UK
Volume 2: 4.12 Perianal disease

Julian Tudor Hart Retired General Practitioner, Glyncorrwg, Swansea, Wales, UK
Volume 1: 10.4 Community interventions—physical health

André Tylee Professor of Primary Care Mental Health, Institute of Psychiatry, London, UK
Volume 2: 9.3 Suicide and attempted suicide

Martin Underwood Professor of General Practice, Barts and The London, Queen Mary's School of Medicine and Dentistry, Queen Mary University of London, London, UK
Volume 2: 5.4 Hyperuricaemia

Peter Underwood Professor of Public and International Health, Murdoch University, Murdoch, West Australia
Volume 1: 1.8 First contact care in developing health care systems

Richard P. Usatine Professor and Vice-Chair for Education, University of Texas Health Science Center, Texas, USA
Volume 2: 15.12 Lumps in and under the skin

Jaap J. van Binsbergen General Practitioner; Professor of Nutrition and Family Medicine, University Medical Centre Nijmegen, Nijmegen, The Netherlands
Volume 1: 11.5 Changing behaviour: diet and exercise

Eloy H. van de Lisdonk General Practitioner and Senior Lecturer, University of Nijmegen, Nijmegen, The Netherlands
Volume 1: 3.2 Illness behaviour
Volume 1: 14.4 Primary care research networks

Wil J.H.M. van den Bosch General Practitioner and Professor of General Practice, University Medical Centre, Nijmegen, The Netherlands
Volume 1: 8.1 Coordination and continuity of care
Volume 2: 13.4 Chronic joint pain

Pieter van den Hombergh Senior Research Assistant Working Party on Quality of Care Research (WOK), University of Nijmegen; Staff member, Dutch College of General Practitioners (NHG), Utrecht, The Netherlands
Volume 1: 12.2 Staff
Volume 1: 12.3 Equipment and premises in general practice

Willem Jan van der Veen Registratie Netwerk Groningen, Faculteit Medische Wetenschappen, Groningen, The Netherlands
Volume 1: 4.4 Age and gender

Danielle A.W.M. van der Windt Associate Professor, Department of General Practice, Institute for Research in Extramural Medicine, VU University Medical Centre, Amsterdam, The Netherlands
Volume 2: 13.5 Shoulder pain

Jouke van der Zee NIVEL (The Netherlands Institute for Health Services Research), Utrecht, The Netherlands
Volume 1: 2.1 Health care systems: understanding the stages of development

G.A. van Essen General Practitioner, Accredited to the Julius Centre for Health Sciences and Primary Care, University Medical Centre, Utrecht, The Netherlands
Volume 2: 16.9 Influenza

Peter van Hasselt Family Physician and Senior Lecturer, Utrecht University, The Netherlands
Volume 1: 2.7 Primary care and general practice in Europe: Central and East
Volume 1: 15.5 Reaccreditation and recertification

Eric van Hecke Professor of Dermatology, University Hospital Ghent, Belgium
Volume 2: 15.2 Nail disorders

Yvonne D. van Leeuwen Director of Postgraduate Training for General Practice, University of Maastricht, Maastricht, The Netherlands
Volume 1: 6.2 Clinical diagnosis: hypothetico-deductive reasoning and other theoretical frameworks
Volume 1: 8.4 Clinical specialization

Jan W. van Ree General Practitioner/Professor in General Practice, Maastricht University, Maastricht, The Netherlands
Volume 1: 1.10 The role of primary care in public health

Maurits W. van Tulder Senior Investigator Health Technology Assessment, Institute for Research in Extramural Medicine, VU University Medical Center, Amsterdam, The Netherlands
Volume 2: 13.1 Low back pain and sciatica

Chris van Weel Professor and Chairman, University Medical Center, Nijmegen, The Netherlands
Volume 1: 2.13 International organizations
Volume 1: 11.5 Changing behaviour: diet and exercise

Gregg K. VandeKieft Clinical Faculty, Providence St Peter Hospital Family Practice Residency Program, Olympia, USA
Volume 1: 16.7 End-of-life decisions

Theo J.M. Verheij Professor of General Practice, Julius Centre for Health Sciences and Primary Care, University Medical Centre Utrecht, Utrecht, The Netherlands
Volume 2: 2.1 Upper respiratory tract infections
Volume 2: 2.2 Lower respiratory tract infections

Myrra Vernooij-Dassen Coordinator, Alzheimer Centre, Nijmegen University; Senior Researcher, Centre for Quality of Care Research, Nijmegen, The Netherlands
Volume 1: 8.7 Collaboration between professional and lay care

Andrew Vickers Assistant Attending Research Methodologist, Integrative Medicine Service, Memorial Sloan–Kettering Cancer Center, New York, USA
Volume 1: 7.7 Complementary therapies

Paola Viterbori Unit of Clinical Epidemiology and Trials, National Cancer Institute, Genova, Italy
Volume 1: 7.8 Terminal and palliative care
Volume 2: 17.1 The dying patient and their family

Theo Voorn Professor of General Practice, University Medical Centre, Utrecht, The Netherlands
Volume 2: 12.1 Acute red eye

Patrick C.A.J. Vroomen Neurologist, Maastricht University Hospital, Maastricht, The Netherlands; Austin & Repatriation Medical Centre, Melbourne, Australia
Volume 2: 13.1 Low back pain and sciatica

Paul Wallace Professor of Primary Health Care, University College London, London, UK
Volume 1: 8.5 Interprofessional communication

Christopher Ward Professor of Rehabilitation Medicine, Head of the Division of Rehabilitation and Ageing, University of Nottingham Rehabilitation Research Unit, Derby City General Hospital, Derby, UK
Volume 2: 11.3 Movement disorders

Gary Ward Coventry and Warwickshire Hospital, Coventry, UK
Volume 2: 14.3 Control of haemorrhage

Helen Ward Clinical Senior Lecturer in Epidemiology and Public Health; Honorary Consultant in Genitourinary Medicine, Imperial College, London, UK
Volume 1: 11.6 Changing behaviour: promoting sexual health

John H. Wasson Dartmouth Medical School, New Hampshire, USA
Volume 1: 8.6 Getting beyond disease-specific management

Mary-Lynn Watson Assistant Professor, Dalhousie University, Halifax, Nova Scotia, Canada
Volume 2: 9.7 Psychiatric emergencies

David P. Weller Professor and Head, Department of General Practice, University of Edinburgh, Edinburgh, Scotland, UK
Volume 1: 14.3 Methods: quantitative
Volume 1: 14.4 Primary care research networks

Dennis Y. Wen Associate Professor, University of Missouri, Columbia, USA
Volume 2: 13.9 Hand and forearm problems

Michel Wensing Senior Researcher, University Medical Centre St Radboud, Nijmegen, The Netherlands
Volume 1: 3.7 Patients' expectations of treatment
Volume 1: 13.7 The patient's role in improving quality

W. Wayne Weston Byron Family Medicine Center, Ontario, Canada
Volume 1: 16.2 The doctor–patient relationship—ethical perspectives

Patrick White Senior Lecturer in General Practice, Guy's, King's and St Thomas' School of Medicine, King's College, London, UK
Volume 2: 1.4 Ankle swelling and breathlessness
Volume 2: 2.4 Asthma
Volume 2: 2.6 Chronic cough

Paula Whitty Senior Lecturer in Epidemiology and Public Health, Centre for Health Services Research, University of Newcastle, UK
Volume 1: 13.4 Using and developing clinical guidelines

Kimberley A. Widger Clinical Nurse Specialist, Pediatric Palliative Care Service, IWK Health Centre, Nova Scotia, Canada
Volume 2: 17.4 Death of a child

Ellen Wiebe Clinical Professor, University of British Columbia, Vancouver, British Columbia, Canada
Volume 2: 8.12 Unwanted pregnancy and termination of pregnancy

Tjerk Wiersma Senior Scientific Staff Member, Dutch College of General Practitioners, Utrecht, The Netherlands
Volume 2: 6.1 Urinary tract infections
Volume 2: 8.6 Vaginal bleeding in early pregnancy

Sara Willems Researcher, Department of General Practice and Primary Health Care, Ghent University, Belgium
Volume 1: 4.5 Socio-economic differences in health

Nefyn H. Williams Senior Clinical Fellow, University of Wales College of Medicine, Wrexham, Wales, UK
Volume 2: 13.2 Neck pain

Robert L. Williams Professor, University of New Mexico, Albuquerque, New Mexico, USA
Volume 1: 1.4 Community primary care

Adam Windak Head of Department of Family Medicine, Jagiellonian University Medical College, Krakow, Poland
Volume 1: 2.7 Primary care and general practice in Europe: Central and East
Volume 1: 15.5 Reaccreditation and recertification

Rena R. Wing Weight Control and Diabetes Center, Providence, Rhode Island, USA
Volume 2: 5.1 Obesity

Ron Winkens Associate Professor for Integrated Care Research, University Hospital Maastricht & Maastricht University, Maastricht, The Netherlands
Volume 1: 8.5 Interprofessional communication

Jan C. Winters General Practitioner, Department of Family Practice, University of Groningen, Groningen, The Netherlands
Volume 2: 13.5 Shoulder pain

Charles Wolfe Professor of Public Health Medicine, Guy's, King's, and St Thomas' School of Medicine, London, UK
Volume 2: 1.7 Stroke and transient ischaemia

Steven H. Woolf Virginia Commonwealth University, Virginia, USA
Volume 1: 13.4 Using and developing clinical guidelines

Robert F. Woollard Professor of Family Practice, Royal Canadian Legion Chair and Head, Department of Family Practice, University of British Columbia, Vancouver, Canada
Volume 1: 15.1 Medical education: the contribution of primary care

Lawrence R. Wu Medical Director, Marshall Pickens Family Medicine Center, Duke University, Durham, North Carolina, USA
Volume 1: 1.9 Management and leadership

Sally Wyke Professor and Director, Scottish School of Health Sciences, University of Edinburgh, Edinburgh, UK
Volume 1: 3.1 Use of health services

Michael Yelland Senior Lecturer in General Practice, Centre for General Practice, University of Queensland; Inala Health Centre General Practice, Queensland, Australia
Volume 2: 3.2 Ear pain in adults

Doris Young Professor and Head, Department of General Practice, University of Melbourne, Parkville, Australia
Volume 2: 9.6 Eating disorders

Catherine E. Zollman General Practitioner, Montpelier Health Centre, Bristol, UK
Volume 1: 7.7 Complementary therapies

Helen Zorbas Clinical Director, National Breast Cancer Centre, Camperdown, Australia
Volume 2: 7.1 Breast pain and lumps

Introduction—genomic medicine

Gordon Duff

The human genome project is a rare example of an international effort that reached its milestones inside budget and ahead of schedule. This success, based on vision and organization, has not yet had a significant impact on clinical medicine, but it will, and in time it will change everything. At the forefront of the new medicine the main exponent of human genomics is likely to be the primary care physician. This chapter is an attempt to scan the horizon of genomic medicine and to outline some of its current working hypotheses.

Genomic medicine is an emerging field that can be defined as the medical exploitation of the 'omics' databases of DNA (genomics), RNA (transcriptomics), and proteins (proteomics). The subject has stimulated keen interest in the media and the public, creating a heightened awareness of genomics, or 'the new genetics'. But public awareness of scientific advance is not synonymous with public understanding, and in between the ground is rich for misconstruction. Even within the profession, the level of information has not always been in step with the march of science. For example, there seems to remain vagueness about the difference between classical medical genetics and future genomic medicine. The first focused on diseases, mostly rare, with a predictable inheritance, while the second is essentially an expansion of fundamental biological principles to all branches of medicine.

Those who believe that biological knowledge is a key to increased quality and length of life should support genomics strongly. From a pragmatic point of view, health budgets probably cannot continue to rise as in the last century, to up to 14 per cent of gross domestic product in some industrialized countries. The aim of medicine in the twenty-first century should be to prevent the development of diseases, the common ailments of rich countries and the endemic infections of poor countries. Genomic medicine is one of the best routes to preventive medicine, and has the potential to redefine preventive medicine at the level of the individual. A period of intensive development is needed, within a regulatory framework that minimizes risk without unduly inhibiting medical progress.

Applications of genomics to health care

Genomic science will illuminate human physiology and pathology at a fundamental level, allowing improvements to many aspects of health care: optimal nutrition at different stages of life; the development of powerful diagnostics (applicable from pre-implantation to old age); new treatments for diseases, and strategies to prevent diseases. It should be possible to maintain mental and physical vigour for decades longer than is usual now. Applied to microbes, genomics promises effective vaccines, both therapeutic and prophylactic. Uses of vaccines against non-infectious diseases are likely, for example, against cancer or degenerative arterial disease. Genomics will bring many new biological medicines, proteins, and polypeptides with very specific mechanisms of action, treatments based on nucleic acids, and many safer and efficacious pharmaceutical medicines. Ultimately, the diagnosis and treatment of classical genetic diseases will be transformed by genomic science, but the greatest impact in the long term will be on the common, 'complex', or 'multifactor' diseases.

Evolutionary aspects of pathology

The genome does not replicate itself with 100 per cent fidelity: if it did we would not be here. Genomic instability, creating genetic diversity, is a prerequisite for evolution. Mutations in DNA occur at a predictable rate; those in somatic cells die with the individual, but mutations in germ-line cells are passed on to the next generation. If they contribute to reproductive advantage, their frequency in the population will increase, and are termed polymorphisms if the frequency reaches more than 1 per cent.

Polymorphisms can involve large stretches of DNA (e.g. deletions, insertions, or multiple repeat sequences) or a change in just one nucleotide base (single nucleotide polymorphisms or SNPs). The human genome sequence has 3 billion nucleotides, and SNPs are estimated to occur, on average, every 500–1000 bases, although they are not evenly distributed. There are, therefore, several million SNPs in the human genome and their locations, the 'SNP map', will become a major tool of genomic medicine. Another consequence of DNA polymorphism is that there is no standard human genome; each one (except in identical twins) is unique. Multifactor diseases can be thought of as products of necessary genomic diversity.

Many SNPs will be irrelevant or neutral in evolutionary terms, but some, undoubtedly, have been selected because they contributed a reproductive advantage at some time in the history of the species. The ability to survive microbial diseases in infancy, and reach sexual maturity, is a major contribution to reproductive advantage. Genes involved in defence against infection are especially polymorphic, reflecting the need to combat rapid microbial evolution that continuously throws up new pathogens. Diversity of defence mechanisms ensures species survival in a changing microbial environment, but the price of diversity in the modern world may be susceptibility to the chronic diseases that are now prevalent in industrialized countries.

Susceptibility to the chronic, multifactor diseases is based on gene polymorphisms transmitted from previous generations. We do not know the role in these diseases of somatic cell mutations accumulated over the lifetime of an individual. Such mutations are thought to be the basis of cancer, but inherited germ-line mutations, underlying familial cancer syndromes, can transmit a primary predisposition to cancer or a tendency to somatic mutations.

Multifactor diseases

Classical medical genetics was concerned with diseases that have a definable pattern of inheritance arising from defects in one or a few genes, but genomic medicine applies much more broadly. This is because genomics allows us to study complex genetic traits, those where the outcome is a product of environmental interaction with many genes. This, of course, takes place continuously from conception to death and is the basis of the common, multifactor diseases that burden health services across the developed world and, according to epidemiological trends, will accompany the economic development of all countries.

Genomic databases can be used to analyse susceptibility to diseases that occur in every family, like heart disease, asthma, Alzheimer's disease, diabetes, depression, arthritis, and cancer. These are examples of multifactor diseases where environmental variables are thought to interact with genetic make-up to cause disease. Defining the genetic susceptibility aspect of the disease will help us to identify the environmental triggers (Fig. 1).

An important difference between present-day medical genetics and genomic medicine is the nature of the information provided by genetic analysis of classical genetic diseases as opposed to multifactor diseases. In highly penetrant, monogenic diseases, genetic diagnosis can provide a quantitative risk assessment with a high degree of confidence, up to 100 per cent with pre-natal diagnosis in some diseases. With multifactor diseases, genetic diagnosis gives no such certainty because of the number of genes involved and the unmeasured component of risk that is environmental. In these diseases genetic diagnostics give an estimate of 'susceptibility'. Since many genes may contribute to the overall risk, the contribution of any individual gene may be relatively small, perhaps giving an odds ratio, or relative risk, of 2–3.

This information, however, can be valuable in medicine. We pay great attention to levels of cholesterol that carry a relative risk of around 2 for arterial disease. This is because arterial disease is a major public health problem and patients' cholesterol levels are relatively easy to change with diet and drugs. A relatively small risk factor, if it occurs at high frequency in the population, takes on a high attributable risk in the population and becomes significant in public health. Nevertheless, half of all first heart attacks occur in people with normal cholesterol, and with no other demonstrable risk factors, indicating how much there remains to learn.

As we discover more about individual gene risk, we will be able to define interactions between different genes, and between genetic and environmental risk factors. Multiple gene testing will occur using nanotechnologies such as small chips carrying arrays of many gene sequences known to contribute disease risk. First, there will be chips for specific conditions or processes, such as heart disease or inflammation; ultimately chip technology will allow the testing of the entire genome on one chip. There will be additive, multiplicative, and neutralizing effects in the interactions between genetic and environmental risk factors.

Defining the neutralizing effects of environmental manipulation on genetic risk offers a huge opportunity to arrest or prevent the development of multifactor diseases. A paradigm is provided in classical genetics by the way we manage the single gene disease, phenylketonuria, and an aim of genomic medicine is to explore the application of this approach to complex diseases. As the knowledge base expands, algorithms that calculate the environmental modifications needed to neutralize disease risk will capture information from diagnostic chips.

Gene diagnostics will have the capacity to indicate susceptibility to a disease and where, in the spectrum of disease, a particular individual might be placed. It will be possible to determine, for example, the clinical subset of multiple sclerosis, how destructive a case of rheumatoid arthritis is, or how rapidly progressive the complications of diabetes are likely to be, and so on. The ability to associate clinical phenotypes with distinct genetic patterns will lead to a new classification of diseases. We will be able to differentiate distinct disease entities that are now clumped together because they are defined in terms of clinical description.

Modifying genetic risk

It is not an easy proposition to alter the genome of an individual. Although advances in gene therapy offer the prospect of correcting single gene defects by gene replacement or gene repair, this is unlikely to be a practical option in multifactor diseases where many genes may contribute to susceptibility. But, as outlined above, if mutlifactor diseases arise from the interaction between specific genomes and the environment, the ability to estimate an individual's genetic risk factors also carries the potential to modify the risk by environmental manipulation. Risk modification in this way might take the form of pharmaceutical intervention, nutritional adjustments, choice of work environment, or relatively simple lifestyle changes. This approach, which might be called 'genetic ecology', places the individual, rather than the population, at the centre of medicine and increases peoples' ability to manage their own health in the light of their own risks (Fig. 2).

Genomics allows the possibility of defining at least one term in the gene/environment equation, the internal factors, and should help simplify the search for external factors. Attempting to analyse diseases in populations or individuals when both the internal and external factors are unknown is a more complex problem, where success so far has perhaps been less than spectacular.

Genetic analysis of treatment responses in individuals

The major impact of genomic medicine in practice probably lies many years away, but genetic diagnostics will affect the management of patients on a shorter timescale. Translating genomics into clinical benefits is an accelerating process which has already begun. Evidence of treatment responses linked with specific genotypes in cancer and other diseases is beginning to appear.

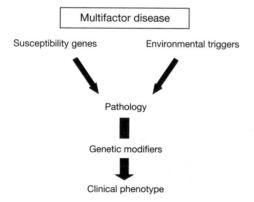

Fig. 1 This simple model of multifactor disease shows 'pathology' (adverse structural and functional changes in tissues) arising from an interaction between susceptibility genes and environmental factors. In the individual, different modifying influences will determine the clinical outcome of pathology, modifiers are shown as genetic in the model, but can also be environmental. The model is broadly applicable, for example, in infectious diseases; microbial pathogens would be the environmental trigger in genetically susceptible individuals, as would high-fat diet and cigarettes in vascular disease. In the chronic inflammatory and degenerative diseases, the environmental factors remain largely unknown.

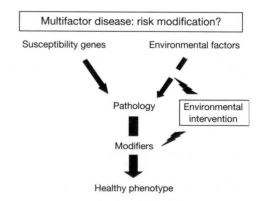

Fig. 2 Environmental modification is easier than genomic modification. This adaptation of the model in Fig. 1 shows the possibility of modifying environmental risk to negate or reduce genetic risk in multifactor diseases. After specific environmental modification, the risk interaction now leads to a healthy phenotype.

The response to a drug (or perhaps to any health intervention) is highly variable. The multifactor nature of disease and the genetic heterogeneity in the population, both in the systems that contribute to pathogenesis and the systems that control drug metabolism, would seem the most economical explanation of population variability in treatment responses. In other words, the drug response is, itself, a complex trait arising from genetic factors influencing both the pharmacodynamic and pharmacokinetic interactions between an individual and a drug or, indeed, any xenobiotic (Fig. 3).

In very general terms, leaving aside issues such as compliance, the same treatment will be beneficial in about one-third of patients, have little effect in another third and will be withdrawn because of intolerance in the remaining third. If, for example, we could develop ways to stratify populations into these three categories of drug response, we would have achieved great progress towards rational, safe, and cost-effective use of medicines (Fig. 4).

The new genome map

Very soon, a genome-wide SNP map covering every gene will be available (approximately 40 000 genes). This map will open up new and powerful approaches to the analysis of complex traits. Some SNPs will directly alter gene function or protein structure, and the map will become hierarchical, reflecting the hierarchical nature of the biochemical pathways that produce biological amplification.

Since SNPs are single base changes, they occur in two forms or 'alleles' (nucleotide A or nucleotide B at the defined position in the DNA sequence). SNPs are therefore binary, and an entire genome can be described in binary notation using SNP markers. The fact that DNA is inherited in chromosomal form means that polymorphisms in the same region tend to be inherited together at a frequency much greater than chance. The shorter the physical distance separating two polymorphisms, the smaller the likelihood of a chromosomal recombination event occurring at a point between them. This phenomenon (linkage disequilibrium) gives rise to patterns of polymorphisms that tend to recur in the same chromosomal regions of different individuals (haplotypes). Thus, one polymorphism can act as a marker for others with which it is in linkage disequilibrium. A linkage disequilibrium map simplifies whole genome scanning by using marker polymorphisms that are representative of chromosomal regions, rather than having to genotype every polymorphism in the genome. This facilitates direct comparison of genomes, for example, in patients with a certain disease compared with a matched population without the disease, or patients that respond to a drug compared with those that do not.

A linkage disequilibrium map, based on SNPs will, in principle, support association tests covering the entire genome. This has great potential importance for the analysis of any complex trait. While the statistical implications of testing thousands of alleles in a disease study seem daunting, the method is not implausible with available clinical resources.

For example, for a particular type of genetic analysis (the transmission disequilibrium test or TDT) where a unit of analysis is an affected individual and two parents (singleton), or an affected sibling pair and parents (asp), at a genotype relative risk of 2 and 80 per cent power, the number if units required can be calculated as:

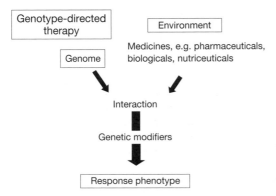

Fig. 3 In this version of the model, medicines are shown as an environmental variable, and the response to medicines is represented as a complex trait. The same model could apply to any xenobiotic, for example, toxins, allergens, etc. The use of pharmaceuticals may be directed by recipient genotype (pharmacogenomics) or they may be used prophylactically in healthy 'at risk' individuals (chemoprevention). This would apply equally to modern biological medicines such as cytokines and their inhibitors. Nutrients may be used in the same way for genetically directed risk modification (nutritional genomics). Some nutrients have biochemical effects that are as potent as pharmaceuticals (nutriceuticals); this is a very active area of current research.

Allele frequency	Units of analysis required	
	Singleton	asp
0.1	695	264
0.5	340	180

Clinical resources in this range are readily available through primary care or large hospital networks. Methods in genetic analysis are evolving fast and it is important that we plan ahead for clinical collections that are as comprehensive as possible since it is difficult to predict the best approaches, even in the near future. The collection and storage of DNA in clinical trials of drugs should also become a routine part of the protocol so we can begin to develop a database of drug response genetics.

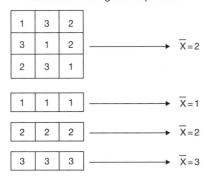

Subsets of biological responders

Fig. 4 In this model, the response to an environmental variable (e.g. drug) is divisible into categories: 1 = excellent benefit; 2 = marginal benefit; 3 = no benefit. The current approach (top box) is to accept a mean population response of 2, marginal benefit. The recipient population includes subsets with little likelihood of beneficial response and those in whom adverse drug reactions are likely. By stratifying the population genetically (lower three boxes), it is theoretically possible to define sub sets that will derive excellent benefit (1), marginal benefit (2), or no benefit (3). Those in category 1 should receive the drug. Those in categories 2 and 3 for a particular drug are likely to be in category 1 for another drug based on a different biological mechanism.

Social concerns

The previous sections described some of the concepts in genomic medicine in a deliberately upbeat way, taking no account of the financial, organizational, ethical, or social issues. There are, of course, many legitimate and serious social concerns over the use of, and access to, genetic information. Most of the difficult problems will occur in the early development of genomic medicine, before the full picture is available to us. In the long run, many of the problems we now foresee are likely to be self-resolving. For example, genome-based assessment of disease susceptibility may ultimately have no major effect on matters such as insurance or mortgages for at least two reasons: first, the same knowledge base that allows risk measurement will provide strategies for risk reduction; second, in common diseases, increased susceptibility to one disease will be balanced by decreased susceptibility to another.

In some ways we are, indeed, stepping into a different world, one where we have a deeper knowledge of our own biology. But genomic medicine is only a logical continuation of the attempt to understand health and disease in terms of biological mechanisms, an approach to medicine that is not new. In the last two centuries, clinical medicine has increasingly used biological markers of disease. Biochemical, histological, and haematological tests have become integral to the diagnosis and prognosis of disease, and to the monitoring of disease progression over time. Many of the diagnostics now commonplace in clinical practice can be regarded as indirect tests of the gene programme. Genomic medicine will test the gene programme directly and in a way that is specific to an individual. In this context, gene tests can be regarded as an extension of conventional clinical biochemistry

to the chemicals that make up genes. Ultimately, genomic medicine should allow people to take the right steps to preserve their health, and when disease does occur, to receive the treatment that is most likely to work on them.

In the future, will increasing self-determination in health matters create a demand for gene profiling in the supermarket, linked with advice on risk modification over the Internet? If so, will we have moved closer towards preventive medicine? If diseases become more preventable and treatable with effective remedies tailored to the individual, does it follow that there will be a better quality of life? Such questions must be answered so we know that the required investment in research is one that we want to make, probably not for our own benefit but for future generations (Fig. 5).

Further reading

Lander, E.S. et al. (2001). Initial sequencing and analysis of the human genome. *Nature* **409** (6822), 860–921.

Altman, R.B. and Klein, T.E. (2002). Challenges for biomedical informatics and pharmacogenomics. *Annual Reviews in Pharmacology* **42**, 113–33.

Duff, G.W. (2002). Genetic variation in cytokines and relevance to inflammation and disease. In *The Cytokine Network: Frontiers in Molecular Biology* (ed. F. Balkwill), pp. 152–73. Oxford: Oxford University Press.

Doerge, R.W. (2002). Mapping and analysis of quantitative trait loci in experimental populations. *Nature Reviews: Genetics* **3** (1), 43–52.

Schoolnik, G.K. (2002). Functional and comparative genomics of pathogenic bacteria. *Current Opinion in Microbiology* **5** (1), 20–6.

Weng, Z.P. and DeLisi, C. (2002). Protein therapeutics: promises and challenges for the 21st century. *Trends in Biotechnology* **20** (1), 29–35.

Gabrielson, E., Berg, K., and Anbazhagan, R. (2001). Functional genomics, gene arrays, and the future of pathology. *Modern Pathology* **14** (12), 1294–9.

Syvanen, A.C. (2001). Accessing genetic variation: genotyping single nucleotide polymorphisms. *Nature Reviews: Genetics* **2** (12), 930–42.

Cox, A., Camp, N.J., Nicklin, M.J.H., di Giovine, F.S., and Duff, G.W. (1998). An analysis of linkage disequilibrium in the interleukin-1 gene cluster using a novel method for grouping multi-allelic markers. *American Journal of Human Genetics* **62**, 1180–8.

Wilson, A.G., Symons, J.A., McDowell, T.L., McDevitt, H.O., and Duff, G.W. (1997). Effects of a polymorphism in the human tumor necrosis factor alpha promoter on transcriptional activation. *Proceedings of the National Academy of Science USA* **94** (7), 3195–9.

Zhang, H.P., Zhao, H.Y., and Merikangas, K. (1997). Strategies to identify genes for complex diseases. *Annals of Medicine* **29** (6), 493–8.

Nicklin, M.J.H., Weith, A., and Duff, G.W. (1994). A physical map of the region encompassing the human interleukin-1 alpha, beta and the interleukin-1 receptor antagonist genes. *Genomics* **19**, 382–4.

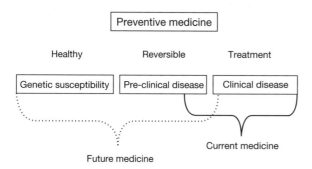

Fig. 5 If we believe that disease susceptibility is inherent, but is triggered by environmental factors, we can think of a human lifespan as a progression from susceptibility through pre-clinical disease to clinical disease. Much pre-clinical disease, before significant and permanent structural damage is done to essential tissues, will be reversible. Following structural damage and loss of function leading to clinical disease, some form of treatment is the only option. Currently, medicine concerns itself largely with the clinical disease phase, with some attempts to intervene at the pre-clinical stage (e.g. treatment based on prognostic markers such as cholesterol and hypertension as risk markers for myocardial infarction). In the future, biology-based medicine will increasingly engage the individual at the pre-clinical stage and earlier, perhaps ultimately aiming to modify risk in healthy, but genetically susceptible individuals.

1

Cardiovascular problems

1 Cardiovascular problems

1.1 Chest pain and myocardial infarction

Leon Piterman

Introduction: significance of chest pain as a presenting symptom

Few symptoms in clinical practice raise more concern in both patients and doctors than chest pain. Nevertheless, chest pain is not a common reason for encounter accounting for 1.3 per 100 patient encounters in the most recent Australian General Practice Morbidity Survey.[1] Community awareness of the significance of chest pain as a presenting symptom of cardiac disease is extremely high. Despite this, many patients (including medical practitioners) either deny or diminish the significance of their chest pain or attribute their chest pain to innocent causes, leading to delayed diagnosis or misdiagnosis, often with dire consequences. This not only applies to patients experiencing chest pain for the first time but also to those with known ischaemic heart disease who fail to respond with sufficient speed to an exacerbation of chest pain.

Correct diagnosis and management may also be delayed by the doctor's failure to recognize the important cues in the history, to misinterpret the significance of negative investigations, particularly negative resting electrocardiography, and to delay, or avoid altogether, appropriate referral.

Nowhere is history-taking more important than in the diagnosis of chest pain. However, history-taking is not undertaken in a clinical vacuum and is very much context driven and context determined. Medical students, young doctors and experienced clinicians, particularly general practitioners (GPs), will differ in their styles of history-taking,[2] the importance placed on critical cues,[3] knowledge of the patient, relevance of context, personal bias, and the nature of the doctor–patient relationship. Although medical practitioners are well aware of the traditional approach to exploring the symptom of pain, in this case chest pain, namely 'site, size, radiation, exacerbating and relieving factors, associated symptoms', the emphasis placed on each of these features and the responses given by the patients to direct questioning will be interpreted differently by different practitioners. For example, an experienced clinician may place more emphasis on chest pain 'brought on by exertion and relieved by rest' regardless of the site of the chest pain, than a medical student who expects cardiac pain to occur in the central part of the chest and radiate into the arms or neck. Unfortunately such typical chest pain only occurs in around 25 per cent of cases and up to 20 per cent of myocardial infarctions may be painless.[4]

Adopting a patient-centred approach to history-taking in general,[5] and to exploring chest pain in particular, is vitally important. Not only does it help fortify the doctor–patient relationship but it provides useful insights into the patient's health beliefs, fears, and anxieties, all of which can influence management outcomes. In the case of chest pain, this may simply require the doctor to ask the patient at the end of the routine history taking 'What

do you think might be causing the chest pain?' or 'What are your concerns regarding this chest pain?' and 'Why do you have these concerns?'.

As mentioned before, 'context' is vitally important in clinical decision-making. This is particularly so in the primary care setting, where an undifferentiated and unselected group of patients across a spectrum of age groups is seen. This is not the case in a coronary care unit or even in an emergency department of a hospital. Gastro-intestinal disorders, musculoskeletal problems, and somatic symptoms associated with psychological disorders are seen more frequently in general practice, whereas serious lung and cardiac conditions are encountered more often in hospital emergency departments.[6] The positive predictive value of cardiac investigations in the primary care setting is therefore likely to be less than in the hospital environment.

The following brief vignettes serve to illustrate the significance of 'context' in influencing clinical decision-making pathways. Readers should reflect on these vignettes and the approach they might take to history-taking, examination, investigation, diagnosis, and management in each case.

Vignette 1

A 17-year-old girl presents with a sudden onset of sharp, severe upper left-sided chest pain, made worse by breathing. She is also short of breath and appears distressed.

Vignette 2

A 23-year-old well-looking male athlete presents with a 3-day history of sharp central chest pains made worse by movement and deep breathing.

Vignette 3

A 35-year-old mother of three presents with sharp right-sided chest pain 8 days after giving birth by caesarian section to her third child. She was kept in hospital for 5 days due to wound infection. She has also had a cough and feels dyspnoeic with exertion.

Vignette 4

A 48-year-old obese male smoker presents with a history of tight chest pain on walking uphill or upstairs. His father died aged 55 of myocardial infarction. His mother is in her mid-70s and has hypertension and diabetes.

Vignette 5

A 38-year-old male presents with a 3-week history of recurrent episodes of chest tightness, palpitations, and difficulty breathing. These are worse when he is in crowded places.

These vignettes are considered later in the chapter.

Chest pain in primary care settings

Whilst chest pain is clearly an important potentially life-threatening symptom, most chest pain seen in primary care settings, particularly in general practice, is not of cardiac origin.

Faced with patients in whom there is a suspicion that their chest pain is of cardiac origin, the GP's course of action will usually be determined by the history and examination findings. If the history is suggestive of ischaemic heart disease and the patient appears well without any chest pain at the time of the consultation, the GP may carry out routine electrocardiography. If this proves negative and the pain was present in the past 24 h, routine electrocardiography (ECG) may be followed by rapid cardiac enzyme assays, usually creatinine kinase (CK-MB), and troponins (cardiac troponin I or T), which can provide results in a few hours; however, the CK-MB is non-specific and is likely to be superseded by other tests. When clinical findings and ECG are normal or equivocal these tests help decision-making in the clinically stable patient to the extent that acute hospital admission may be avoided. However, if there is still a strong clinical index of suspicion, referral to an emergency department is warranted. Indeed, many GPs may refer all suspicious, stable cases to an emergency department. Such referrals have created difficulties for these departments who are then left with the problem of sorting out those patients who need urgent admission from those who need further assessment and those whose pain is not of cardiac origin and can safely be discharged. Up to 30 per cent of emergency hospital admissions are due to acute chest pain[7] yet less than half of these will have a final diagnosis of acute myocardial infarction or unstable angina: as many as 50 per cent of emergency medical admissions with chest pain are non-cardiac.

This experience has led to the establishment of 'rapid assessment chest pain clinics'. These are designed to stratify patients into different levels of risk, which will influence admission rates as well as hospital budgets.

Davie et al.[8] described 317 patients in Edinburgh who were seen in such assessment clinics within 24 h. Of those only 18 per cent with acute coronary syndromes needed admission, the rest were sent home. These included 30 per cent with stable coronary heart disease and 49 per cent with non-cardiac chest pain. Psychosomatic chest pain was common in this group of patients. A 6-month follow-up of 90 per cent of the cohort showed high levels of satisfaction with the clinic and, importantly, no deaths. Similar results were reported by Newby et al.[9] in 1001 GP referrals, of which 60 per cent had non-cardiac chest pain.

The inadequacy and poor positive predictive value of routine ECG in assessment of recent onset chest pain in general practice[10] makes such clinics attractive, although their costs and benefits have yet to be systematically and widely evaluated.[11] However, from a general practice perspective, such clinics will not overcome the need to subsequently manage the large number of patients who have non-cardiac chest pain, in particular those with a psychological basis for the pain.

Diagnosis and management of non-cardiac causes of chest pain

Chest wall/musculo-skeletal pain

Chest wall pain may affect patients of all ages and includes the following conditions.

Costochondritis

Typically, this condition produces chest pain which is central, worse on breathing and movement with focal tenderness over several costochondral joints. Eliciting the tender spots is crucial for the diagnosis. It often affects young and otherwise fit and healthy persons (Vignette 2) who may feel alarmed by the presence of chest pain. Apart from explanation and reassurance topical anti-inflammatory gels or ointments and oral anti-inflammatory agents may be useful. In the absence of any history of trauma or strain the exact aetiology of this condition is unknown, although the minor outbreaks witnessed in clinical practice suggest a viral aetiology.

Disorders or dysfunction of the dorsal spine

Referred pain radiating to the anterior aspect of the chest may occur with disease of the intervertral joints or vertebral bodies. This is particularly so

for dysfunction of the lower cervical or upper thorax joints. Clinical assessment involves careful examination of the cervical spine and asking the patient to flex and rotate this region in the spine to reproduce the symptoms.

Radiological examination of the dorsal spine is essential to exclude osteoporotic compression fractures and pathological fractures related to metastatic disease, in elderly patients and those at risk of these conditions. However, X-ray examination is not particularly helpful in diagnosing intervertebral joint dysfunction. Treatment for this group may include physiotherapy and spinal mobilization, whereas fractures will require analgesia and treatment of the underlying cause.

Shingles

Herpes zoster virus affecting the upper thorax may produce chest pain which is difficult to diagnose prior to the onset of the rash. Once the rash has appeared, the use of an appropriate antiviral agent (acyclovir, famcyclovir, valaciclovir) within the first 72 h may reduce the severity of the rash and the likelihood of post-herpetic neuralgia in 6 months.[12] Topical treatment with 2 per cent phenol in calamine lotion may also alleviate the discomfort experienced by these patients. In the more severe cases, amitriptyline 50–75 mg nocte or carbamazepine 200 mg b.d. or t.d.s. may be helpful.

Digestive disorders

Gastro-oesophageal reflux disease, oesophageal spasm, and indigestion may all produce chest discomfort of various degrees of severity. The diagnosis is made more difficult when there is a known or suspected history of ischaemic heart disease (Vignette 4). Biliary disease may also produce pain in the lower part of the chest which may mimic inferior ischaemia or infarction. The presence of co-morbid ischaemia and digestive disorders often requires careful assessment. Therapeutic trials may be confusing as nitrates can relieve oesophageal spasm and although antacids relieve indigestion, patients may still have concurrent coronary ischaemia.

Gastro-oesophageal reflux disease and its management are discussed in Chapter 4.2.

Respiratory disorders

A number of respiratory conditions may present with acute chest pain. Diagnosis may be simple in young patients, or in those where there is an underlying respiratory condition or context for the development of an acute respiratory disorder, but becomes more difficult in older patients and in those with co-morbid disease.

Pneumothorax

The sudden onset of severe, sharp unilateral chest pain, with associated mild to moderate respiratory distress in an otherwise healthy often young individual should alert the physician to this possibility (Vignette 1). Radiological examination will confirm the diagnosis and the treatment will be determined by the size of the pneumothorax. Those occupying less than 10 per cent of the chest cavity may resolve spontaneously whereas larger ones may need drainage. Recurrence is common (around 30 per cent within 5 years) and pleurodesis may be required.[13]

Pulmonary embolism

This is unlikely to occur in the absence of a clinical context (Vignette 3) which suggests the development of deep vein thrombosis. Concerns have been raised regarding the risk of air travel in the aetiology of deep vein thrombosis and subsequent pulmonary embolism. In-flight leg exercises, intake of water, and avoidance of alcohol are generally recommended and other preventive measures such as compression stockings and low-dose aspirin are recommended for at-risk patients.

Pleurisy and pneumonia

Although these are causes of sharp unilateral chest pain, the diagnosis is made in the context of a febrile illness with cough, sputum, and systemic symptoms and is supported by positive radiological findings (see Section 2).

Psychological reasons

Patients with or without underlying ischaemic heart disease may experience chest pain which has a psychological basis. These patients are often thoroughly investigated, including angiography, and reassured about the absence of coronary artery disease. Where there is an underlying anxiety disorder (Vignette 5), depressive disorder or somatoform disorder merely excluding the presence the ischaemic heart disease may not be sufficient to alleviate the symptoms. As these patients are usually referred back to the GP following negative cardiological assessment, the onus is on the GP to ensure that appropriate psychological treatment is offered. GPs providing continuity of care will realize that in time some of these patients will develop ischaemic heart disease and monitoring their symptoms, together with risk factor management, is just as appropriate in this group of patients as it is in the rest of the community.

Cardiac causes of chest pain

Non-ischaemic causes of cardiac chest pain

Non-ischaemic causes of cardiac chest pain are pericarditis and aortic dissection.

Most of this section will be directed to discussion of chest pain of ischaemic origin. However, it is worth mentioning two important cardiac causes of chest pain which are not related to coronary artery disease.

Pericarditis

This is usually of viral origin although it may occur in a number of the connective tissue disorders such as systemic lupus erythematosis. Typically, the chest pain is relived by leaning forward and may be worse in inspiration. A friction rub may be audible on auscultation. Without the typical ECG changes (elevated concave ST segment) diagnosis may be difficult. Viral pericarditis is usually a self-limiting condition but careful monitoring for the possible development of pericardial effusion is essential.

Aortic dissection

This rare and often fatal disorder is usually characterized by hypertension with a tearing interscapular pain radiating into the interscapular region of the back. The pain is maximal from the time of onset and is unresponsive to nitrates or usual doses of morphine. A simple chest X-ray may not be helpful in diagnosing atherosclerosic aortic dissection, whereas it is helpful in diagnosing traumatic dissection.

Ischaemic heart disease

Aetiology

Ischaemic heart disease is caused by atherosclerosis of the coronary arteries. The underlying lesion is the atheromatous or fibro-fatty plaque. Plaques that extend into the lumen lead to obstruction of blood flow and can be visualized angiographically. Some extend externally into the arterial wall and do not impede blood flow. These may appear as minimal angiographic lesions. However, the majority of fatal infarcts result from thrombosis occurring on minimal lesions. The catastrophic event is rupture of the plaque leading to coronary thrombosis. Various coronary symptoms are related to the degree of stability of the plaque.

♦ *Stable plaque.* This has a thick fibrous cap and a lipid core not exposed to the lumen. It produces more luminal narrowing but has a low propensity to rupture and hence to cause myocardial infarction. It usually presents as stable angina.

♦ *Unstable plaque.* This has a thinner cap, is less flow limiting and less visible angiographically. Its lipid core is large with only a thin covering of smooth muscle and is more prone to rupture, accounting for 80–90 per cent of myocardial infarcts.

Recognition of the significance of plaque stability has therapeutic implications which will be discussed later in this chapter.

Prevalence of ischaemic heart disease

The impact of cardiovascular disease (CVD) on global health is enormous, with a rising prevalence in developing as well as developed economies. Overall, CVD is second only to infectious disease as the most common cause of death in the world today (14.8 million compared to 17.3 million per year).[14] By way of contrast, cancer was responsible for 6.2 million deaths in 1997. However, most cardiovascular deaths relate to just two conditions, namely coronary heart disease (CHD) and stroke, so that these disorders are the two leading causes of death in the world.[15] CVD is an even more important cause of illness in the United Kingdom than in many other countries: 110 000 people a year die from CVD in England, of whom more than 41 000 are under the age of 75. Over 1.4 million people in the United Kingdom suffer from angina and around 300 000 will have a heart attack each year. CHD accounts for around 3 per cent of all hospital admissions in England. Furthermore, CHD reinforces the health divide, with three times the rate of CHD deaths in lower compared to upper socio-economic groups and with major ethnic variations, particularly for people born in India or Pakistan, who have very high rates of CHD.

In 1995–1996, the incidence of coronary events, mainly myocardial infarctions, in Australia (population approximately 19 million), was estimated at 421 per 100 000 males aged 35–69 years and 137 per 100 000 females of the same age. Of these, about 65 per cent were non-fatal.[16]

Almost 156 000 hospital admissions were related to CHD, representing 3 per cent of all hospital admissions in 1996–1997. In about 25 per cent of cases, the first clinical manifestation of CHD is fatal. In 1996, CHD was the major cardiovascular cause of death, accounting for 23 per cent of all deaths. In Australian General Practice in 1999–2000,[17] cardiovascular conditions accounted for 11.1 per cent ($N = 153\,857$) of the problems managed or 16.3 per 100 encounters. This included hypertension (5.7 per cent), ischaemic heart disease (1.1 per cent), cardiac check-up (0.9 per cent), and heart failure (0.6 per cent).

This makes CVD the fourth commonest condition requiring GP management following respiratory (16.5 per cent), musculo-skeletal (11.6 per cent), and skin (11.6 per cent). This has changed since 1990–1991 when cardiovascular disease was the second commonest condition requiring management (12.6 per cent).

International comparisons for death rates from coronary heart disease are shown in Fig. 1.

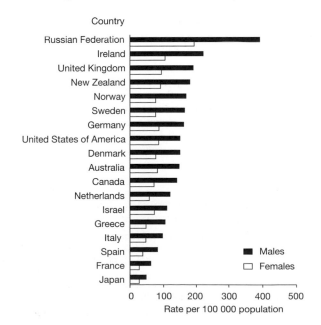

Fig. 1 Death rates from CHD for selected countries 1995–1996. (*Source:* WHO 2000, AIHW National Mortality Database.)
Note: Death rates have been standardized to the 2000 WHO standard population.

Risk factors

Increasing age, male gender, and a positive family history are risk factors which cannot be modified. Modifiable or manageable risk factors include tobacco smoking, hypertension, elevated blood lipids, physical inactivity, overweight and obesity, diabetes mellitus, and high alcohol consumption. Based on data gained in the Framingham study, the Multiple Risk Factor Intervention Study (MRFIT), and other large cohort studies, it is possible to calculate both the relative and absolute risk for an individual of having a myocardial infarct within a given time, usually 6–8 years. These studies have demonstrated the multiplier effect (rather than summative effect) of risk factors in determining global risk. Software packages are available for clinical use to assist in motivating and monitoring patients with risk factors for CVD.

In addition to these well-established risk factors, recent epidemiological and biomedical research has shed light on additional potential risk factors.[18] These include chronic infection with agents such as *Helicobacter pylori*, cytomegalovirus, and *Chlamydia pnueumoniae* (which may cause endothelial damage), fibrinogen and homocysteine.

Socio-economic factors and ethnicity influence risk factors and consequent cardiovascular morbidity and mortality. This is demonstrated in Tables 1 and 2.

Angina

Angina is the clinical manifestation of myocardial ischaemia and occurs when myocardial oxygen supply is insufficient to meet demand.

Stable angina

This is a clinical syndrome characterized by pain or discomfort over the chest, usually retrosternal or precordial, oppressive, tight or heavy in nature. The duration is minutes or longer but never momentary. The pain or discomfort may radiate to the left arm, neck, jaw, throat, shoulders, but also the right arm, face, and back.

It is usually precipitated by exertion, emotion, and factors that increase the heart rate. It is relieved by rest or nitrates. There may be associated features such as dyspnoea and sweating. Occasionally, dyspnoea without chest pain may be a manifestation of angina. Diabetic patients may suffer manifestations of ischaemia without experiencing pain. History is of paramount importance in establishing the diagnosis. Physical examination may be entirely normal, particularly if carried out whilst pain is absent. During angina, heart rate and blood pressure may increase, there may be a fourth heart sound, and a transient murmur of mitral regurgitation may be heard if there is papillary muscle dysfunction.

Investigations

In the general practice setting, investigation of angina is usually limited to resting ECG. This is helpful if positive but a negative ECG does not exclude significant underlying coronary artery disease. If the ECG is diagnostic, there is no need to proceed to exercise ECG.

Exercise ECG

◆ If resting ECG is normal, exercise testing should be performed in a properly equipped laboratory under supervision.

◆ If ischaemic changes occur at low workload, there is more likely to be widespread disease.

◆ False positive results may occur in 10 per cent of cases, false negatives in 30 per cent.

◆ False positive results are more common in females and in the young.

◆ The positive predictive value of exercise testing is enhanced if changes occur early, are of long duration, if there is a fall in BP and if there are dangerous arrhythmias.

Thallium stress test

◆ more sensitive and specific but much more expensive;

◆ useful in the presence of LBBB and if patient is unable to walk;

◆ can localize the area of ischaemia.

Coronary angiography

This remains the definitive test for diagnosing the presence and severity of coronary artery disease and is required before coronary angioplasty, stenting, or coronary bypass surgery are performed.

Table 1 Prevalence of risk factors for heart, stroke, and vascular disease by socio-economic status (SES), 1995

Risk factor	Males			Females		
	Low SES (%)	High SES (%)	Rate ratio	Low SES (%)	High SES (%)	Rate ratio
Hypertension	19.0	14.4	1.3	14.5	7.2	2.0
High cholesterol	20.4	19.2	1.1	18.9	13.9	1.4
Overweight (BMI >25)	49.8	50.3	1.0	40.2	31.4	1.3
Obese (BMI >30)	14.2	9.5	1.5	15.5	8.5	1.8
Smoking	35.9	18.5	1.9	27.5	15.1	1.8
At-risk alcohol intake	6.3	3.7	1.7	1.5	1.3	1.2
Physical inactivity	37.0	27.0	1.4	39.3	29.1	1.4

Source: Australia National Health Survey 1995 and NHF Risk Factor Prevalence Survey 1989, derived data.

Table 2 Death rates for heart, stroke, and vascular diseases by SES of area of residence, ages 25–64, 1991

Disease	Males			Females		
	Low SES	High SES	Rate ratio	Low SES	High SES	Rate ratio
Coronary heart disease	107.5	60.9	1.8	31.3	14.0	2.2
Stroke	22.0	8.5	2.6	13.8	7.3	1.9
Heart, stroke, and vascular disease	155.7	84.9	1.8	56.7	27.7	2.1

Source: AIHW National Mortality Database.

Table 3 Classification of patients according to risk

	% dead per year	% dead 5 years
Single-vessel disease		
LAD	2–4	10–20
RCA	1.2	2–8
CIRC	0.1	0–2
Two-vessel disease		
LAD + RCA or CIRC	7–10	35–50
RCA and CIRC	3–6	15–30
Three-vessel disease	10–12	50–60
Left main disease	15–25	70

Source: National Heart Foundation. Coronary Angioplasty Report
No. 10, Canberra: NHF, 1996.

Combined with assessment of left ventricular function, coronary angiography helps to classify patients according to risk. This is shown in Table 3.

Complication rates of coronary angiography (death, stroke, or heart attack) are around 3 per 1000.

Medical management of stable angina

1. Manage risk factors aggressively. This particularly includes the management of hypertension and hyperlipidaemia. Patients with ischaemic heart disease are increasingly advised to take statins if total cholesterol is above 4.0 mmol/l.[19]

2. Aspirin 75–150 mg/day.

3. Glyceryl trinitrate. Short-acting sublingual glyceryl trinitrate (anginine 600 μgm, nitro lingual spray 400 μgm, isosorbide dinitrate 5 mg).

4. Beta-blocking agents. Cardio-selective ones are preferable (metoprolol and atenolol), doses vary but usually 50–100 mg/day.

5. Long-acting nitrates. Isosorbide mononitrate orally 60–120 mg/day or glyceryl trinitrate dermal patches (5–10 mg/day) with an 8–12 h period free of patches to prevent tolerance.

6. Calcium channel blockers. Verapamil and diltiazem are negatively inotropic and chronotropic. Nifedipine and amlodipine do not affect contractility but may cause reflex tachycardia and can be used together with beta-blockers.

Unstable angina

This may have one or more of the following characteristics:

- angina of recent outset, at rest or crescendo, sudden decrease in exercise tolerance;

- increased frequency, severity, and duration;

- decreased effect of previously effective therapy;

- persisting longer than 20 min and refractory to GTN (suspect myocardial infarction);

- transient ECG changes without evidence of transmural (Q wave) infarction.

Unstable angina usually denotes complex atheromatous lesions with plaque rupture, platelet aggregation, thrombus formation, and coronary artery spasm. These patients are therefore at high risk of infarction.

Treatment of unstable angina

This begins with urgent medical treatment, which may be followed by percutaneous transluminal coronary angioplasty (PTCA) or surgery.

Urgent medical treatment consists of:

- admission to a coronary care unit;

- correction of precipitating factors, for example, arrhythmias, anaemia, infarction, thyrotoxicosis;

- increase nitrate dose orally, topically, or intravenously;

- anticoagulation with intravenous heparin;

- antiplatelet agents: aspirin 75–150 mg and continue long-term, clopidogrel or ticlopidine if intolerant to aspirin;

- calcium channel blockers: diltiazem, nifedipine, verapamil if associated vasospasm;

- beta-blockers.

If symptoms improve, medical therapy may be continued until elective coronary angiography is carried out with a view to PTCA/surgery. If symptoms are unchanged then urgent angiography and PTCA/surgery should be performed.

Acute myocardial infarction

This is usually caused by sudden thrombotic occlusion of a coronary artery at the site of an atheromatous plaque that has ruptured. Time from the onset of symptoms to arrival in hospital is critical for improving survival. Over 70 per cent of coronary deaths in males and 55 per cent in females occur before the victims reach hospital.[20] An Australian report showed that 50 per cent of heart attack patients delay seeking treatment by more than 6 h.[21] This delay is further compounded by delays in the administration of thrombolytic therapy, with a report showing that the proportion of patients with a heart attack seen within 10 min of arrival was only 26 per cent and that only 40 per cent received thrombolytic therapy within 1 h of arrival.[22]

The main thrombolytic therapies are streptokinase and tissue plasminogen activator (TPA)–alteplase. The efficacy and effectiveness of thrombolytic therapy in limiting the size of myocardial infarction and improving long-term survival is well established.[23] The main drawback is serious bleeding, particularly intracranial haemorrhage. Streptokinase is less costly than TPA but in the GUSTO study,[23] TPA was more effective than streptokinase.

Currently, coronary angioplasty with stenting is usually considered for patients who cannot be given thrombolytic therapy. However, there is an increasing tendency to use stenting in the acute treatment of heart attack based on studies showing improved outcomes with this technique.[24]

Acute management in the primary care setting

Patients with known ischaemic heart disease should be given clear instructions regarding requesting an ambulance in preference to waiting for a doctor. However, GPs in attendance should provide emergency care, stabilize and monitor patients with acute myocardial infarction until the ambulance with its expert resources arrive.

If the patient is unconscious, maintaining an airway and supporting the breathing and circulation (ABC) are essential. Many practices are equipped with a defibrillator and if the patient is connected to an ECG monitor and found to be in ventricular fibrillation, defibrillation should be carried out.

In the conscious patient, the following steps should be taken:

- administer oxygen (except in patients with severe chronic airways disease);

- give aspirin 300 mg unless contra-indicated;

- give sublingual glyceryl trinitrate;

- insert intravenous line, draw blood for tests (cardiac enzymes, troponin);

- administer morphine 2.5–5 mg intravenously and anti-emetic (metoclopramide 10 mg) provided there is no hypotension.

ECG changes in the acute phase

A number of changes may be apparent:

- ST segment changes, such as horizontal ST segment elevation, may occur within minutes and suggest infarction.

- ST depression, peaked T waves or deep symmetrical T wave inversion also suggest injury or ischaemia.

Table 4 Anatomical territory indicated by distribution of ECG abnormalities

ECG lead	Area	Artery
1, aVL, V4–6	Lateral	Circumflex
II, III, aVF	Inferior	Circumflex, right coronary
V1 (large R and ST↓)	Posterior	Right coronary
V2–4	Anterior	Left anterior descending

Source: Preisz, P. (1998). Myocardial infarction. In *Emergency Medicine: The Principles of Practice* 3rd edn. (ed. G. Fulde), Sydney: MacLennan and Petty.

- Pathological Q waves appear within hours and are associated with transmural infarction.
- Arrhythmias and increased ectopy may occur.
- Tachycardia is often related to sympathetic response, pain, and fear.
- Sinus bradycardia is common in those with inferior myocardial infarction.

The distribution of the ECG abnormalities indicates the anatomical territory involved (Table 4).

The role of the GP in primary and secondary prevention

As in primary prevention, GPs have an important role in secondary prevention, that is prevention of re-infarction or prevention of the long-term complications of established ischaemic heart disease, such as cardiac failure.

A considerable body of evidence now exists to support the following interventions following a myocardial infarct.[25]

Dietary advice
Lipid-lowering diets may be beneficial. The consumption of fatty fish rich in omega-3 fatty acids has been shown to reduce re-infarction and death.

Cardiac rehabilitation
Randomized trials of exercise-based rehabilitation have demonstrated a 20–25 per cent reduction in mortality after infarction.

Smoking
It is not ethically possible to conduct randomized post-infarction trials, but epidemiological studies demonstrate that risk declines rapidly after smoking cessation and may reach that of non-smokers within 3 years.

Lipid-lowering agents (statins)
The Scandinavia Simvastatin Survival Study (4S) showed a 34 per cent reduction in major coronary events and 37 per cent reduction in the need for re-vascularization within 5 years. Similar benefits have been shown in other trials using other statins. Some of the benefits are thought to be independent of the lipid-lowering effect of these drugs but rather related to their endothelial stabilizing properties (plaque stabilizing).

Aspirin
Low to medium dose (75–150 mg/day) aspirin has been shown to reduce re-infarction and death by 25 per cent. Similar benefits have been demonstrated with clopidogrel, which is more expensive than aspirin but may be used where aspirin is contra-indicated. Aspirin should be used life long following infarction.

Beta blockers
These drugs (with the exception of those with agonist activity) have been shown to reduce mortality and re-infarction by 20–25 per cent if given in the convalescent phase following myocardial infarction. This appears to be a class effect and has been documented with timolol, metoprolol and atenolol. Usual doses are 50 mg metoprolol or 25 mg atenolol daily. There is no similar evidence for calcium channel blockers.

Angiotensin converting enzyme (ACE) inhibitors
A number of trials have demonstrated the benefits of ACE inhibitors in reducing mortality. These trials have included captopril, ramipril, and zofenopril against placebo.[26] Patients with a large infarct and signs of cardiac failure are most likely to benefit. ACE inhibitors also reduce ischaemic events following myocardial infarction. Life-long therapy is recommended in all patients who have evidence of cardiac failure following infarction.

Key points

- Chest pain is usually an alarming symptom. Although most cases presenting in primary care are not cardiac in origin, assessment of patients with chest pain should always be thorough.

- Non-cardiac causes of chest pain may be musculoskeletal, digestive, respiratory, and psychological.

- Although deaths from ischaemic heart disease in most developed countries have declined over the past decade (due to improved detection and treatment), cardiovascular disease still remains the second commonest cause of death globally.

- Primary care physicians play a key role in the primary, secondary, and tertiary prevention and management of ischaemic heart disease. This involves patient education, screening individuals and populations for coronary risk factors and aggressive treatment including promoting lifestyle change, aspirin, lipid lowering agents, beta blockers and where indicated, calcium channel blockers, and ACE inhibitors.

- All primary care physicians should be able to administer emergency care to patients with myocardial infarction. This may include the administration of thrombolytic therapy in rural and remote areas.

References

1. **Britt, H.** et al. *General Practice Activity in Australia 1999–2000.* AIHW Cat. No. GEP5. Canberra: Australian Institute of Health and Welfare (General Practice Series No. 5), 2000.

2. **McWhinney, I.R.** (1976). Problem solving and decision making in family practice. *Canadian Family Physician* **25**, 1473–7.

3. **Elstein, A.S.** (1989). On the psychology of clinical decision making: what is a rational expectation? In *Learning in Medical School* Chapter 4 (ed. J.I. Balla, M. Gibson, and A.M. Chang), pp. 61–79. Hong Kong: Hong Kong University Press.

4. **Rass, R.S.** (1970). Ischaemic heart disease. In *Harrison's Principles of Internal Medicine* 6th edn. Chapter 271 (ed. Wintrobe et al.), pp. 1208–26. New York: McGraw Hill Publications.

5. **Weston, W.W.** and **Brown, J.B.** (1995). Overview of the patient-centred clinical method. In *Patient-Centred Medicine* Chapter 2 (ed. Stewart et al.), pp. 21–30. Thousand Oaks CA: Sage Publications.

6. **Buntinx, F.** et al. (2001). Chest pain in general practice or in the hospital emergency department: is it the same? *Family Practice* **18**, 586–9.

7. **Blatchford, O.** and **Capewell, S.** (1999). Emergency medical admissions in Glasgow: general practices vary despite adjustments for age, sex and deprivation. *British Journal of General Practice* **49**, 551–4.

8. **Davie, A.P.** et al. (1998). Outcome from a rapid assessment chest pain clinic: closing Pandora's box? *Quarterly Journal of Medicine* **1**, 339–43.

9. **Newby, D.E., Fox, K.A.A., Flint, L.L.,** and **Boon, N.A.** (1998). A 'same day' direct-access chest pain clinic: improved management and reduced hospitalisation. *Quarterly Journal of Medicine* **91**, 333–7.

10. **Norell, M.** et al. (1992). Limited value of the resting electrocardiogram in assessing patients with recent onset chest pain: lessons from a chest pain clinic. *British Heart Journal* **67**, 53–6.

11. **Capewell, S.** and **McMurray, J.** (2000). 'Chest pain—please admit': is there an alternative? *British Medical Journal* **320**, 951–2.

12. Jackson, J.L. et al. (1997). The effect of treating herpes zoster with oral aciclovir in preventing post herpetic neuralgia. A meta-analysis. *Archives of Internal Medicine* **157**, 989–92.

13. Lippert, H.L. et al. (1991). Independent risk factors for cumulative recurrence rate after first spontaneous pneumothorax. *European Respiratory Journal* **4**, 324–31.

14. Murray, C.J. and Lopez, A.D. (1998). The global burden of disease, 1990–2020. *Nature Medicine* **4**, 1241–3.

15. Murray, C.J. and Lopez, A.D. (1997). Mortality by cause for eight regions of the world: Global Burden of Disease Study. *Lancet* **349**, 1269–76.

16. Australian Institute of Health and Welfare. *Medical Care of Cardiovascular Disease in Australia.* Cardiovascular Disease Series No. 7. AIHN Cat. No. CVD4, Canberra: AIHN.

17. Britt, H. et al. *BEACH (Bettering the Evaluation and Care of Health) General Practice Activity in Australia 1999–2000.* Australian Institute of Health and Welfare. Cat. No. GEP5, Canberra, 2000.

18. Walker, J.M. (1999). Coronary artery disease: new epidemiological insights. *Journal of the Royal College of Physicians (London)* **33**, 8–12.

19. Lipid Management Guidelines (2001). *Medical Journal of Australia Supplement* **175**, S57–86.

20. Chambless, L. et al. (1997). Population versus clinical view of case fatality from acute coronary heart disease: results from the WHO MONICA PROJECT 1985–1990. Multinational Monitoring of Trends and Determinants in Cardiovascular Disease. *Circulation* **48**, 3849–59.

21. Dracup, K., McKinley, S.M., and Moser, D.K. (1997). Australian patients delay in response to heart attack symptoms. *Medical Journal of Australia* **166**, 228–9.

22. Palmer, D.J. et al. (1998). Factors associated with delay in giving thrombolytic therapy after arrival at hospital. *Medical Journal of Australia* **168**, 111–14.

23. GUSTO-1 Investigators (1996). One year results from the Global Utilization of Streptokinase and TPA for Occluded coronary arteries trial. *Circulation* **94**, 1233–8.

24. Suryapranta, H. et al. (1998). Randomised comparison of coronary stenting with balloon angioplasty in selected patients with acute myocardial infarction. *Circulation* **97**, 2502–5.

25. Secondary prevention of ischaemic cardiac events (2000). *Clinical Evidence. A Compendium of the Best Available Evidence for Effective Health Care* Issue 4, pp. 83–113. London: BMJ Publishing Group.

26. ACE Inhibitor MI Collaborative Group (1996). Evidence for early beneficial effect of ACE inhibitors started within the first day in patients with AMI: results of a systematic overview among about 100 000 patients. *Circulation* **94**, 1–90.

1.2 Heart failure

Richard Hobbs

Impact of disease

Heart failure is an increasingly major problem for primary care. The condition has become almost as common in adults as type II diabetes, occurring in around 2 per cent of the adult population,[1,2] rising to over 8 per cent of over 75-year-olds and 15 per cent of those over 85;[2] 3–4 per cent[2] of under 75-year-olds suffer left ventricular systolic dysfunction (LVSD), the commonest precursor for heart failure. Unlike most other cardiovascular diseases, which have declined in incidence in most developed economies over the last 20 years, the incidence of heart failure continues to rise, due in part to improved survival following acute myocardial infarction and an increasing elderly population.[3]

Symptomatic heart failure (all grades combined) has a worse prognosis than breast or prostate cancer and is only second to stroke in terms of health care utilization costs, mainly due to high rates of hospitalization.[4] The financial impact on the US health care system of heart failure is over US$ 8 billion per year. European health service burdens are of similar proportions, with 5 per cent of all admissions in the United Kingdom relating to heart failure.

In addition to facing a high risk of death or protracted hospitalization, patients with heart failure also suffer from a grossly impaired quality of life,[5] with symptoms ranging from dyspnoea, abdominal pain, cough, and fatigue to adverse renal function with fluid overload and exacerbation of existing oedema.[6] Heart failure symptoms may eventually become sufficiently serious to prevent patients performing the least taxing of activities.

Presentation and diagnosis of heart failure

Presentation of heart failure

Given the variable aetiology of heart failure and the fact that aetiologies often co-exist, the presentation of the syndrome may be varied and non-specific. The main causes include myocardial infarction, valve disease, arrhythmias (especially atrial fibrillation), or combinations of all three. For most patients onset is insidious, with increasing levels of symptoms, the commonest being shortness of breath, lethargy and exercise intolerance. Physical signs are predominantly fluid load related, for example, ankle swelling. Since these symptoms and signs are common and non-specific, diagnosis of heart failure is often delayed or incorrect (see Chapter 1.4).

Occasional patients will present acutely with decompensated (or congestive) heart failure, where symptoms may progress rapidly (within hours), with worsening shortness of breath (orthopnoea) or waking at night with frightening breathlessness (paroxysmal nocturnal dyspnoea). Such patients are likely to have clinical signs of fluid retention, namely crepitations in the basal lung fields and raised jugular venous pressure. Most acute presentations will be seen in patients who have recently suffered a major event (myocardial infarction or sudden onset arrhythmia) or have previously diagnosed heart failure.

Once confirmed, the stage of heart failure is most usefully assessed using the New York Heart Association (NYHA) breathlessness symptom score classification (Table 1).

Table 1 NYHA functional class (and definition) of subjects with heart failure due to LVSD (LVEF <40%) in the ECHOES cohort[2]

NYHA class	Definition of symptoms	No. of patients
I	No limitation; ordinary physical exercise does not cause dyspnoea	34 (47%)
II (s)	Slight limitation of physical activity; dyspnoea on walking more than 200 yards or on stairs	21 (29%)
II (m)	Moderate limitation; dyspnoea walking less than 200 yards	5 (7%)
III	Marked limitation of physical activity: comfortable at rest but dyspnoea washing and dressing or walking from room to room	5 (7%)
IV	Dyspnoea at rest, with increased symptoms with any level of physical activity	7 (10%)

Diagnosis of heart failure

Early and accurate diagnosis of heart failure is important since early treatment may modify disease progression and, once the cause and stage of heart failure is determined, there is a rich evidence base to guide overall management.

Unfortunately, as indicated earlier, heart failure is difficult to diagnose on clinical grounds. Studies exploring the validity of a clinical diagnosis of heart failure in primary care report high rates of misdiagnosis when patients are assessed against objective criteria (rates of 25–50 per cent accuracy reported in different series). Only 26 per cent of patients referred to a rapid access echocardiographic clinic with suspected heart failure were confirmed after investigation.[7] Clinical diagnosis by hospital physicians is just as poor.

To establish a diagnosis in primary care requires referral (in most situations) of the patient for cardiac imaging. Unfortunately, there is limited availability of this non-invasive test to primary care physicians in many countries. Are there alternatives in primary care to echocardiography? One is the electrocardiograph (ECG) since a normal recording will, in most cases, exclude left ventricular dysfunction.[8] However, changes may be subtle and the lack of ECG interpretation skills may still require referral for a specialist opinion. Another test often advocated, but with few supporting data, is the use of the chest X-ray (CXR). Both ECG and CXR are relatively expensive and can only act as 'rule-out-tests'.

A potential diagnostic aid for the future, of particular relevance to primary care settings, is the assessment of patients by brain natriuretic peptide (BNP) assays. Studies have demonstrated that BNP and NT proBNP have very high (99 per cent) negative predictive value for heart failure, but a lower positive predictive value (70 per cent) means the test is likely to be used as a pre-screening test to decide whom to refer for echocardiography.[9] Further indications for the assay may be confirmed for BNP-guided therapy,[10] analogous to glycosylated haemoglobin in diabetic follow-up.

The diagnosis of heart failure requires a combination of objective evidence of structural cardiac problems alongside careful clinical assessment. The primary care physician requires a structured approach to heart failure diagnosis, which involves the stratification of suspected cases into at-risk groups. For example, the prior probability of heart failure in patients with typical symptoms is significantly increased in those patients with a previous history of myocardial infarction (MI), with concurrent symptoms of ischaemic heart disease, with existing hypertension, or suffering diabetes (in descending order of likelihood). Patients must be assessed by objective tests, most appropriately echocardiography, preferably interpreted by a specialist.

Screening for left ventricular systemic dysfunction (LVSD) and heart failure

The most reliable data to inform this question arise from the ECHOES study.[2] Definite LVSD (an ejection fraction of <40 per cent) was found in 22 per cent of a randomly selected population of patients with previous MI, 8 per cent of those with angina, 6 per cent of those with diabetes, and 2 per cent of those with hypertension (which is the same rate as LVSD in the background population). In each group, around half of these patients were symptomatic with dyspnoea, and therefore had heart failure due to LVSD (Table 1).

Overall rates of heart failure, defined as symptoms of dyspnoea in association with objective evidence of any type of cardiac dysfunction (LVSD, atrial fibrillation, or significant valve disease) were 16 per cent in those with previous MI, 8 per cent in those with angina, 8 per cent in those with diabetes, and 3 per cent in those with hypertension (Table 2).

A high proportion of people with past histories of ischaemic heart disease and diabetes therefore have LVSD or heart failure. These data support the need for trials of targeted echocardiographic screening amongst these easily identifiable at-risk populations, to determine the feasibility and cost-effectiveness of screening.

Management of heart failure

Basic mechanisms for the development of heart failure and rationale for therapy

Left ventricular hypertrophy (LVH) is an important risk factor for heart failure, due to structural changes, or 'remodelling', of the heart caused by the stress of pressure and volume overload. Remodelling is characterized by a change in the dimensions of the left ventricle and the ventricular wall, with associated or subsequent myocardial fibrosis, myocyte hypertrophy, slippage, elongation and necrosis, and hypertrophy of coronary artery smooth muscle cells. LVH results in impaired cardiac function in addition to an increased risk of ventricular arrhythmia and coronary artery insufficiency due to increased myocardial oxygen demand. It has been suggested that remodelling is an adaptive response by local tissues stimulated by stretch receptors, which in turn mediate changes at the tissue level via angiotensin II. The reversal of these structural changes, known as 'cardioreparation', could be achieved by relief of the original causal stresses and inhibition of the renin angiotensin system.

Table 2 Rates of definite, probable, and total heart failure on defined criteria (exertional dyspnoea to NYHA functional class II or more, with objective evidence of structural cardiac abnormality) in the ECHOES cohort[2]

	Sinus rhythm with no valve disease	Atrial fibrillation	Valve disease	Atrial fibrillation and valve disease	Totals
Rates of patients with definite heart failure:					
EF <40%	30 (0.8%)	3 (0.1%)	5 (0.1%)	0	38 (1%)
EF 40–50%		8 (0.2%)	2 (0.1%)	2 (0.1%)	12 (0.3%)
EF >50%		22 (0.6%)	17 (0.4%)	3 (0.1%)	42 (1.1%)
Prevalence of total definite heart failure					92 (2.3%)
Rates of patients with probable heart failure:					
NYHA II or more functional class, plus EF 40–50% alone[2]					23 (0.6%)
Asymptomatic, EF <40%, on treatment, but previously symptomatic[3]					9 (0.3%)
Prevalence of total probable heart failure					32 (0.8%)
Combined prevalence of definite and probable heart failure					124 (3.1%)

Subjects were symptomatic on exertion except where indicated. EF = ejection fraction.

Guidelines for the management of heart failure

Guidelines for the evaluation and management of heart failure are established in the United States[11] and Europe.[12] Traditional therapy targeted the relief of the symptoms of congestion (pulmonary and peripheral oedema) or increasing cardiac contractility (e.g. with diuretics and digoxin, respectively). Current therapy strategies additionally modify the progression of heart failure and improve 'meaningful' survival. Within these guidelines angiotensin converting enzyme (ACE) inhibitors are confirmed as a mainstay of heart failure therapy.

ACE inhibitors as first-line treatment for heart failure

Guidelines recommend that all patients with heart failure due to systolic dysfunction, with or without symptoms, should receive an ACE inhibitor unless the patient is intolerant or the dong is contra-indicated. ACE inhibition in the treatment of heart failure improves haemodynamic parameters, symptoms, functional status, mortality, and progression. Further, ACE inhibitors significantly reduce risks of total mortality, primarily deaths due to progressive heart failure, [risk reduction (RR) 24 per cent, NNT 74] and reduce combined mortality and hospitalization for heart failure (Table 3).[13]

If fluid retention is present ACE inhibitors are used together with loop diuretics. Whilst side-effects occur early with ACE inhibitors, symptomatic improvement may not be seen until later. Furthermore, disease progression may be reduced even if symptoms are not relieved. Despite the evidence, the preference of physicians is to prescribe doses of ACE inhibitors in heart disease treatment lower than those demonstrated to be beneficial in mortality trials, possibly due to the common but unfounded assumption that ACE inhibitor side-effects are dose related.

In summary, ACE inhibitors are of proven clinical benefit in patients with symptomatic heart failure as well as asymptomatic patients with an ejection fraction of less than 35 per cent. These agents are well tolerated and not only reduce mortality but also improve functional status and reduce the risk of hospitalization for cardiac reasons.

β-Blockers in heart failure

Contrary to traditional teaching that this class of drugs was relatively contra-indicated in heart failure, recent studies and meta-analyses show significant mortality benefits following treatment of heart failure patients with certain β-blockers,[14] with a pooled mortality risk reduction of 35 per cent ($p < 0.001$), and with further significant reductions in hospitalization.

All patients with stable NYHA class II or III heart failure due to systolic dysfunction should receive a β-blocker unless the drug is contra-indicated or intolerant. β-Blockers are generally used together with diuretics and ACE inhibitors and are indicated for the long-term management of chronic heart failure. Side-effects may occur early but the drugs may reduce the risk of disease progression even in the absence of symptomatic improvement.

Diuretics and spironolactone in heart failure

Loop diuretics should be prescribed for all patients with symptoms of heart failure who have, or are predisposed to, fluid retention as they are the only means of controlling fluid overload. Importantly, diuretics may alter the efficacy and tolerability of other drugs used for the treatment of heart failure. Underdosing can lead to fluid retention which may diminish the response to an ACE inhibitor and increase risks of treatment with β-blockers. Overdosing can lead to increased occurence of hypotension and renal insufficiency with ACE inhibitors and other drugs.

It is especially important to monitor renal function (serum creatinine) in patients on diuretics who are commenced on an ACE inhibitor. Furthermore, because ACE inhibitors retain potassium, potassium-sparing

Table 3 Controlled clinical trials of ACE inhibitors and AT-II antagonists for patients with ventricular dysfunction

Drug class (study)	Drug treatment	Patients (n)	NYHA class/EF	Follow-up (months)	Outcome (RRR)	Comments
ACE inhibitors						
CONSENSUS	Enalapril 2.5–40 mg b.d.	253	IV	6	40% (6 months)	Due to reduction in heart failure deaths
V-HeFT II	Enalapril 20 mg b.d. versus H + I	804	I–III EF <45%	30	28% (2 years)	Largely reduction in sudden death
SOLVD (T)	Enalapril 2.5–20 mg b.d.	2569	II–III EF ≤35%	41	16%	Largely reduction in heart failure
SOLVD (P)	Enalapril 2.5–10 mg b.d.	4228	I–II EF <35%	37	29% (combined death/ heart failure development)	
MHEART FAILURET	Captopril 25 mg b.d. versus placebo	170	I–III (mean II)		Reduced progression heart failure	Largely due to reduction in heart failure
NETWORK	Enalapril 2.5, 5.0, or 10 mg b.d.		II–IV		Combined endpoint Rel Risk = 1.2	No dose response
ATLAS	Lisinopril 2.5–5.0 mg o.d. or 32.5–35 mg o.d	3165	II–IV (77% III)	46	8% RRR = 12%	Reduction combined endpoint: mortality and hospitalization
Angiotensin receptor antagonists						
ELITE	Losartan 50 mg o.d. or Captopril 50 mg t.i.d.	722	II = IV, EF <40%	48 weeks	Losartan (4.8%) mortality <Captopril (8.7%)	Largely reduction in sudden death
RESOLVD	Candesartan + Enalapril	769	Largely mild			Terminated due to increased mortality on candesartan
ELITE II	Losartan 50 mg o.d. or Captopril 50 mg t.i.d.	3152	>60, HF grades II–IV, EF <40%	2 years	Captopril/Losartan hazard ratio (95% CI): 0.88 (0.75, 1.05) $p = 0.16$	Losartan significantly better tolerated, with 9.4% withdrawals compared to 14.5% on Captopril, $p < 0.001$

RRR, risk reduction; EF, left ventricular ejection fraction.

diuretics should be avoided with their use. In severe heart failure patients with fluid retention despite loop diuretics, adding a thiazide has proven efficacy.

Spironolactone was previously contra-indicated in the treatment of heart failure patients already receiving an ACE inhibitor, due to fears of hyperkalaemia. However, spironolactone added to ACE inhibition and a loop diuretic in patients with moderate to severe heart failure was shown to reduce mortality by 27 per cent ($p = 0.0001$) compared to placebo, with a significant reduction in hospitalization.[15] Hyperkalaemia was not considered to be a problem, although 15 per cent of patients required dose reductions.

Digoxin in heart failure

Digoxin is recommended to improve the clinical status of patients with heart failure due to LVSD, used in conjunction with diuretics, ACE inhibitors, and β-blockers. Digoxin can improve symptoms and reduce hospitalizations, but has no effect on survival. It is generally well tolerated by most patients with heart failure, with a particular role in patients with rapid atrial fibrillation. However, since digoxin only limits resting heart rate, β-blockers may be advantageous in active atrial fibrillation because they further limit heart rate rises during exercise. Moreover, since effects on hospitalization are modest (6 per cent absolute risk reduction, 26.8 per cent versus 34.7 per cent RR 0.72, $p < 0.001$),[16] and there is no survival benefit, digoxin should only be used in patients in sinus rhythm after diuretics, ACE inhibitors and β-blockers have been initiated.

Angistensin receptor blockers in heart failure

Angiotensin receptor blockers (ARBs), the most recently developed major class of antihypertensives, are emerging as a possible therapeutic option in the treatment of heart failure. However, there is no evidence that ARBs are equivalent or superior to ACE inhibitors in the treatment of heart failure. Angiotensin receptor blockers for heart failure would therefore appear to be indicated only when ACE inhibition is contra-indicated or not tolerated.

Physician undermanagement of heart failure

The strong evidence base for the ACE inhibitors, allied with recommendations in key US and European guidelines, should have resulted in their widespread acceptance in the treatment of heart failure. However, in most countries, there is persisting evidence of physician underuse and underdosing of these effective drugs, in hospital and primary care practice.

Despite strong advice to prescribe ACE inhibitors to all patients with LVSD regardless of symptoms, many physicians have regarded ACE inhibitors as 'second-line' therapy in a role as an adjunct to diuretics.[17] The most recent information regarding perception and practice in European primary care physicians[18] reveals that most doctors believe there is strong evidence for the mortality benefits of ACE inhibitors (>90 per cent) and that although a larger majority claim to prescribe ACE inhibitors in heart failure, only between 47 per cent (Spain) and 62 per cent (Germany and Italy) actually do so.

Prescribing factors leading to undermanagement of heart failure

The underuse and underdosing of ACE inhibitors in heart failure may in part be due to a lack of familiarity on the part of physicians with this drug class and caution regarding known side-effects of this treatment. Those side-effects of most concern to physicians are largely first-dose hypotension, renal failure, and cough. However, clinical trial data show the incidence of first-dose hypotension is low and can be predicted by monitoring of systolic blood pressure. The risk can be further minimized by withholding diuretic administration several days prior to ACE inhibitor therapy, gradually titrating the ACE inhibitor dose up to an optimum level, and monitoring the patient for a short period after the first dose. Only in cases of renal

insufficiency is particular caution needed. In summary, if treatment is initiated as recommended, the incidence of such serious problems is low.

Cough is another side-effect associated with ACE inhibitors that concerns physicians, and is most commonly seen in the elderly and in Asian patients. Up to 20–30 per cent of heart failure patients on long-term ACE inhibitor therapy can develop cough, and half may need to be withdrawn from treatment. In many patients, cough has a delayed onset, with over 40 per cent of patients not affected until at least 6 months. Cough is regarded as a class effect and is only rarely resolved with a change in ACE inhibitor. However, before discontinuation, doctors should consider whether ACE inhibitor therapy or heart failure symptoms are the actual cause of cough. Patients should consider whether the inconvenience outweighs the mortality benefits of the ACE inhibitor, especially since spontaneous disappearance of cough is reported in over half of patients.

Diagnostic issues leading to underprescribing

Diagnoses of heart failure made in primary care are often not accurate, especially in the absence of echocardiography. Physicians may suspect that a proportion of patients labelled with heart failure on clinical grounds will be suffering less morbid conditions such as dependent oedema. This 'low-key' approach to heart failure management, whilst a pragmatic necessity to most primary care physicians with limited or no access to appropriate diagnostic tests, is unacceptable. Since accurate diagnosis and better categorization of patients is likely to improve prescribing in heart failure, widespread access to reliable echocardiography is essential.

Role of nurse-led structured care in heart failure management

There is generally positive evidence of the efficacy of nurse-led interventions in heart failure follow-up management. The involvement of trained nurses in pre-discharge patient education and home visiting, concentrating on adherence to treatment, and recognizing early signs of deterioration, has shown significant reductions in re-admission rates and patient quality of life, after either intensive[19] or minimal[20] follow-up. On current evidence, specialist nurses are not likely to positively impact on care outcomes if their role is essentially coordination of existing services, especially if such services are themselves of variable quality.[19] However, where the nurse has a well-defined role to deliver additional and specialized care to patients and their carers, especially medication monitoring, education about the signs of deteriorating disease, and specific advice on what follow-up is needed, their role would appear effective. Since all current studies of nurse-led packages of tailored care to patients with heart failure are small, further studies are needed to assess the effectiveness of clinical nurse specialists in each different role and setting, and in both clinical and cost terms.

Summary

Recent guidelines are based on the overwhelming evidence for treatment benefits in heart failure but recent surveys of practice in many fields show a low level of implementation. Responding to these data on underperformance requires positive action in a number of areas of physician practice. Enhanced access to diagnostic tests, especially echocardiography, is essential. However, there is an imperative that primary care physicians upgrade their perceptions of the importance of heart failure. Not only should they more actively suspect the disease in patients at most risk (post-MI, hypertension, diabetes), but once confirmed, the condition should be effectively managed. Treatment aims not only to improve symptoms but to reduce mortality. In heart failure patients with left ventricular dysfunction, treatment should include an ACE inhibitor at an adequate dose. If we re-interpreted heart failure as a condition with analogous prognosis to a serious malignancy, then our management might be more urgent and more appropriate.

Key points

1. Heart failure is a common condition affecting elderly adults, and is associated with poor prognosis, major symptoms, and high health care costs.

2. The commonest cause of heart failure is myocardial ischaemia, particularly following myocardial infarction.

3. Heart failure is difficult to diagnose and must be confirmed by objective investigation (using echocardiography).

4. Assay of pro-natriuretic peptide may become an important tool in improving diagnosis.

5. Heart failure has a substantial evidence base to guide management. Most patients are likely to benefit from ACE inhibitors, beta-blockers, with diuretics in cases of fluid overload.

6. Most heart failure has a poor prognosis so that palliative care is an important component of management

References

1. McDonagh, T.A. et al. (1997). Symptomatic and asymptomatic left ventricular systolic dysfunction in an urban population. *Lancet* **350**, 829–33.

2. Davies, M.K., Hobbs, F.D.R., Davis, R.C., Kenkre, J.E., Roalfe, A.K., Hare, R., Wosornu, D., and Lancashire, R.J. (2001). Prevalence of left ventricular systolic dysfunction and heart failure in the general population: main findings from the ECHOES (Echocardiographic Heart of England Screening) Study. *Lancet* **358**, 439–45.

3. Hobbs, F.D.R. (1999). Primary care physicians: champions of or an impediment to optimal care of the patient with heart failure? *European Journal of Heart Failure* **1** (1), 11–15.

4. Gillum, R.F. (1993). Heart and stroke facts. *American Heart Journal* **126**, 1042–7.

5. Hobbs, F.D.R., Kenkre, J.E., Roalfe, A.K., Davis, R.C., Hare, R., and Davies, M.K. (2002). Impact of heart failure and left ventricular systolic dysfunction on quality of life: a cross-sectional study comparing common chronic cardiac and medical disorders and a representative adult population. *European Heart Journal* **23**, 1867–76.

6. Rochow, S.B., Dalal, H.M., Karuana, M.P., and Mourant, A.J. (1997). Chronic heart failure in the community: a prospective general practice study. *British Journal of Cardiology* **4**, 33–7.

7. Cowie, M.J., Wood, D.A., Coasts, A., Thompson, S.G., Poole-Wilson, P.A., and Sutton, G.C. (1998). Incidence and aetiology of heart failure in the general population, abstract no. 20. In *Heart Failure Update 98*, Glasgow, Scotland, 25–27 June.

8. Davie, A.P., Francis, C.M., Love, M.P., Caruana, L., Starkey, I.R., Shaw, T.R.D., Sutherland, G.R., and McMurray, J.J.V. (1996). Value of an electrocardiogram in identifying heart failure due to left ventricular systolic dysfunction. *British Medical Journal* **312**, 222.

9. Cowie, M.R., Struthers, A.D., Wood, D.A., Coates, A.J.S., Thompson, S.G., Poole-Wilson, P.A., and Sutton, G.C. (1997). Value of natriuretic peptides in assessment with patients with possible new heart failure in primary care. *Lancet* **350**, 1349–53.

10. Murdoch, D.R., McDonagh, T.A., and Bryne, J. (1999). Titration of vasodilator therapy in chronic heart failure according to plasma brain natriuretic peptide concentration: randomised comparison of haemodynamic and neuroendocrine effects of tailored versus empirical therapy. *American Heart Journal* **138**, 1126–32.

11. American College of Cardiology/American Heart Association (1995). Guidelines for the evaluation and management of heart failure. Report of the American College of Cardiology/American Heart Association Task Force on Practice Guidelines (Committee on Evaluation and Management of Heart failure). *Circulation* **92**, 2764–84.

12. European Society of Cardiology. Task Force of the Working Group on Heart Failure of the European Society of Cardiology (1997). The treatment of heart failure. *European Heart Journal* **18**, 736–53.

13. Garg, R. and Yusuf, S. (1995). Overview of randomised trials of angiotensin-converting enzyme inhibitors on mortality and morbidity in patients with heart failure. *Journal of the American Medical Association* **273**, 1450–6.

14. Heidenreich, P.A., Lee, T.T., and Massie, B.M. (1997). Effect of beta-blockade on mortality in patients with heart failure: a meta-analysis of randomised trials. *Journal of the American College of Cardiology* **30**, 27–34.

15. RALES Investigators (1996). Effectiveness of spironolactone added to an angiotensin-converting enzyme inhibitor and a loop diuretic for severe chronic congestive heart failure [the Randomized Aldactone Evaluation Study (RALES)]. *American Journal of Cardiology* **78**, 902–7.

16. Kelly, R.A. and Smith, T.W. (1993). Digoxin in heart failure: implications of recent trials. *Journal of the American College of Cardiology* **22** (4 Suppl. A), 107–12A.

17. Hillis, G.S. et al. (1995). Angiotensin-converting-enzyme inhibitors in the management of cardiac failure: are we ignoring the evidence? *Quarterly Journal of Medicine* **89**, 145–50.

18. Hobbs, F.D.R. et al. (2001). European survey (EuroHEART FAILURE) of primary care physician perceptions and practice in heart failure diagnosis and management. *European Heart Journal* **21**, 1877–87.

19. Rich, M.W. et al. (1995). A multidisciplinary intervention to prevent the readmission of elderly patients with congestive heart failure. *New England Journal of Medicine* **333**, 1190–5.

20. Stewart, S. et al. (1998). Effects of home-based intervention on unplanned re-admissions and out-of-hospital deaths. *Journal of the American Geriatrics Society* **46**, 174–80.

1.3 Palpitations and silent arrhythmias

Kevin Barraclough

Introduction

Arrhythmias pose several problems in primary care. The patient presenting with palpitations, 'funny turns', or more rarely, collapse poses a problem of diagnosis. The patient with an established diagnosis of an arrhythmia may pose a problem of management. Both diagnosis and management may be carried out in primary care or, depending on the available resources, in combination with a specialist colleague. In developed countries, ischaemic heart disease will often form the background substrate of the arrhythmia, while in developing countries the prevalence of valvular disease will be higher.

Palpitations and 'funny turns' are common presentations in general practice. A proportion of these patients will have treatable, life-threatening arrhythmias. A missed diagnosis may result in an unexplained sudden death or a stroke.

Classification

Arrhythmias can be classified as symptomatic ectopic beats (extra-systoles), paroxysmal or sustained tachycardias [over 100 beats per minute (bpm)], and paroxysmal or sustained bradycardias (less than 60 bpm). Each of these can be further classified as supraventricular or ventricular.

The presentation and diagnosis of arrhythmias in primary care

The task for the primary care physician, as always, is to achieve the delicate balance between over- and under-investigation. The clues will lie in obtaining a precise history. The patient will present with either a history of palpitations or episodes of altered consciousness.

A 'palpitation' is an abnormal awareness of heart beat. However, patients may use the term to mean breathlessness or a feeling of panic.

Abnormal sensations

The physician should ask about coincident symptoms of hypoperfusion of the brain (dizziness), of the coronary arteries (chest pain), or of the lungs (breathlessness). If these are absent, serious disruption of arterial perfusion is unlikely, indicating a ventricular rate neither too fast nor too slow to maintain an adequate output, and a pattern of contraction of the ventricles (often disturbed in ventricular arrhythmias) sufficient to maintain pumping. It is often assumed that the absence of symptoms of hypoperfusion excludes a potentially malignant arrhythmia like ventricular tachycardia. While it may be reasonable to assume this in low risk patients (under the age of 35 without risk factors for ischaemic heart disease and with no family history of sudden premature death), it must be borne in mind that ventricular tachycardia can occur with relatively little haemodynamic disturbance and few symptoms.

It is extremely useful to ask the patient to tap out the rhythm of their heart beat on the desk. Often he or she will tap out a steady rate of 60 bpm but slap the desk hard indicating that the beats seemed 'strong'. This will normally have occurred at rest, often lying on the left side in bed, and is clearly benign. Sometimes, the rhythm will indicate a pattern of clear pauses ('I thought my heart had stopped') followed by a powerful beat. Here, the patient is usually describing an ectopic beat (of which they are unaware), and the compensatory pause, followed by a powerful beat because the heart has been filling in the prolonged diastole. If these symptomatic ectopics disappear on exercise then they are likely to be benign. A fast regular beat without haemodynamic disturbance in a young person is likely to be either a sinus tachycardia, which will slow gradually, or a paroxysmal supra ventricular tachycardia (SVT) which will stop abruptly and may be associated with subsequent polyuria if prolonged (possibly due to an effect on atrial natriuretic peptide). Consequently, it is useful to ask if the onset and offset was gradual or sudden. A highly irregular beat may suggest atrial fibrillation or frequent ectopics. Palpitations at rest are far more likely to be benign than palpitations occurring on exercise. The latter almost invariably signify a diseased heart struggling to produce the cardiac output required of exercise.

Changes in consciousness

Episodes of altered consciousness again require careful history taking. It is often most useful to question a witness. There will be pointers as to whether the cause is a faint, hypotension due to arrhythmias or hypotension due to other causes, such as epilepsy or transient cerebral ischaemia.

An episode of loss of consciousness will normally require investigation unless the features clearly indicate a faint. To make a persuasive diagnosis of a vaso-vagal syncope the patient should be young, fit, and at low risk of ischaemic heart disease (in developed countries) or valvular disease (in developing countries). There should be a warning period of hypotension—'greying' of vision (due to retinal hypoperfusion). The patient may have been sitting, more usually standing, but never lying. There may have been

a precipitant of emotion, pain, heat, or prolonged standing. If all of these features are clearly present, it is reasonable to make a diagnosis of a faint without further investigation. If the episode of loss of consciousness occurs without warning (a drop attack), it is not a faint and the most likely diagnoses are episodes of complete heart block (Stokes–Adams attacks) in the elderly, or primary generalized epilepsy. Complex or stereotypically similar auras point towards epilepsy. Brief episodes of unconsciousness without warning in the elderly are often erroneously ascribed to transient ischaemic attacks (TIAs)—see Chapter 1.7.[1] This is unlikely due to the anatomy of the blood supply and density of neurological structures in the brainstem. More likely causes are fits or arrhythmias (especially Stokes–Adams attacks).

Medical history

The medical history is clearly critical to stratifying risk in the patient with palpitations or 'funny turns'. Ventricular tachycardia can be relatively asymptomatic but is unlikely in a patient at low risk of ischaemic heart disease and without signs of heart disease. However, rare conditions occur in primary care and will be missed unless considered. The young, fit patient can have a viral myocarditis or cardiomyopathy of uncertain origin. A family history of sudden cardiac death may be due to a familial long QT syndrome or other rare condition, and would easily be missed.[2]

Drugs

Medications may be implicated in the arrhythmia. Drugs that increase AV node delay such as beta-blockers, calcium antagonists, or digoxin, can cause heart block. Drugs with anticholinergic effects can precipitate tachy-arrhythmias. Almost all antiarrhythmic drugs can be proarrhythmic.

Lifestyle

Lifestyle factors such as smoking, dietary, and exercise habits affect the risk of arterial disease. Alcohol consumption is frequently overlooked as a cause of atrial fibrillation and other arrhythmias. One study showed that 60 per cent of patients admitted with idiopathic atrial fibrillation were problem drinkers.[3] Another post mortem study showed that 26 per cent of men under 50 with sudden death had myocardial change compatible with chronic alcohol injury.[4] High alcohol consumption can cause patchy conduction delays in the myocardium leading to re-entrant tachy-arrhythmias (see below), and the hyperadrenergic state following alcohol withdrawal is also proarrhythmic.

Examination

Examination is usually less valuable than history but it can give some useful pointers. The pulse may show irregularities at rest. If these are still present after walking the patient briskly up and down the corridor this heightens suspicion that an arrhythmia is not benign. Hypertension dilates the atrial wall and may contribute to atrial fibrillation. Hypertensive left ventricular hypertrophy is proarrhythmic. A raised venous pressure may indicate heart failure which is proarrhythmic because of the damaged myocardium causing the failure, myocardial stretch, and the hyperadrenergic state. Fourth, and often third, heart sounds indicate a stiff, non-compliant myocardium and underlying disease. In developing countries, rheumatic valvular disease may contribute to volume or pressure overload of the heart chambers. In developed countries, mitral valve prolapse affects up to 5 per cent of the population and is associated with benign palpitations.[5] Examination may reveal causes of a sinus tachycardia—anaemia, thyrotoxicosis, hypovolaemia from over-diuresis, diabetes, or dehydration.

Investigations

In the primary care setting, a thorough history and examination will be all that is required in many cases to reassure both patient and physician that there is no serious underlying disease. However, a significant proportion of patients will require further investigation. The extent to which this is carried out in primary care or in secondary care will depend on the availability of resources, specialists, and the expertise of the primary care physician. Routine blood tests (including thyroid function tests and a full blood count) and a 12-lead electrocardiogram (ECG) will often be carried out in primary care. ECG interpretation can be helped (somewhat) by computerized reporting algorithms which over- rather than under-report abnormalities. However, interpreting ECGs is not as difficult as often believed and, since cardiac disease represents an increasing burden in an ageing world, to be unable to interpret an ECG is an increasing handicap in primary care. The rest of this chapter will assume the reader has a reasonable facility with ECG interpretation.

Investigations have become more widely available. The author now uses a patient event recording device which is the size of a matchbox, takes 5 min to fit, downloads onto a personal computer and records events continuously for up to 8 days. The cost of this device is around US$1500. The management of palpitations is easier and safer when a diagnosis has been made.

The significance and management of specific arrhythmias

Ectopic beats

Ectopic beats (extra-systoles) are either supraventricular (narrow complex) or ventricular (broad complex). Atrial extra-systoles are usually entirely benign. Doctors have been more ambivalent about ventricular extra-systoles. In the 1960s observation in coronary care units suggested that ventricular extra-systoles presaged ventricular tachycardia. Then, in 1969, the Tecumseh Community Study suggested that those adults in the 5000 studied who had frequent ventricular extra-systoles were at increased risk of sudden death.[6] We now know that the significance of frequent ventricular extra-systoles depends on the state of the underlying myocardium. In post-infarct patients or those with dilated or hypertrophic cardiomyopathy frequent ventricular extra-systoles at rest herald a poor prognosis. Ventricular extra-systoles that appear in exercise after an infarct are also associated with a poor prognosis. Suppressing these with flecainide in post-infarct patients increased mortality[7] but amiodarone has been shown to be beneficial.[8] However, ventricular ectopics usually have little significance in the healthy heart.[9]

Narrow complex tachycardias: 'SVTs'

Narrow complex tachy-arrhythmias have narrow QRS complexes because the ventricular depolarization travels rapidly on the specialized His–Purkinje conducting system. Consequently, they are necessarily supraventricular in nature. They can arise from the sinus node, ectopic foci in the atria, or from the AV node. They may be due to enhanced automaticity from one ectopic focus or to a self-sustaining re-entry mechanism (see below).

Sinus tachycardias are rarely faster than 150 bpm (slower in the elderly), have normal P wave morphology and a 1:1 correspondence with QRS complexes. They slow gradually with carotid sinus massage or on resolution of the precipitating trigger.

Atrial tachycardias are fast and regular with P waves of an abnormal morphology. They usually arises from an ectopic focus in the upper right atrium and so have similar polarity in the ECG leads to a sinus P wave. Occasionally, they are due to a re-entry circuit within the atria. The rate is usually 150–250 bpm, often with 2:1 or variable block. Digoxin toxicity commonly causes atrial tachycardia with some degree of AV nodal block. Other types of SVT can arise from re-entry circuits within the AV node (*nodal tachycardias*) or re-entry circuits with one limb through atrio-ventricular accessory pathways [as in *Wolff–Parkinson–White* (WPW) syndrome]. WPW has the characteristic ECG at rest showing a short PR interval (because the ventricle is depolarized prematurely by the accessory pathway that has no in built conduction delay like the AV node), a widened QRS (greater than 0.12 s or three small squares) and the characteristic delta wave. Nodal tachycardias are fast and regular and may have discernable retro-conducted P waves of abnormal morphology superimposed on the narrow QRS complex.

If SVTs are diagnosed in a young person, are infrequent and well tolerated, that treatment may not be required. Alternatively, episodes may be easily suppressed with a beta-blocker or calcium antagonist. However, poorly tolerated SVTs, and all SVTs with pre-excitation, should be referred to a specialist for consideration of radio-frequency ablation of the ectopic focus or the re-entrant pathway.[10]

Atrial fibrillation (AF) and flutter

These are the commonest arrhythmias. The population prevalence is 0.5 per cent but rises to 10 per cent in those over 75. These arrhythmias are associated with significant preventable morbidity and mortality (see Table 1).

Causes of atrial fibrillation and flutter

In sinus rhythm, the atria are depolarized by a coordinated wave that spreads over the surface of the atria. In AF, this single wavefront breaks up into multiple wandering wavelets. These may wander randomly or form re-entry circuits around obstacles such as pulmonary vein orifices. If the conduction time is short and the refractory period of the cells long, then the wandering wave will rapidly hit refractory tissue and die out (non-sustained AF) (Fig. 1). Three factors will favour continuing propagation of the fibrillating wavelets: slow atrial conduction time, shorter refractory period, and a greater surface area of atrium for the wavelets to wander through. Valvular disease, hypertension, and heart failure cause atrial dilatation and slower atrial conduction speeds. Atrial ischaemia, autonomic tone, and thyrotoxicosis slow conduction and reduce the refractory period. Alcohol slows conduction and increases adrenergic stimulation. These diseases create the myocardial substrate which allows a trigger, such as an ectopic depolarization from a focus adjacent to a pulmonary vein, to precipitate AF. With prolonged fibrillation the prospect of return to sinus rhythm reduces as maladaptive changes occur in the atrial tissue.

In about 15 per cent of patients with AF, no cause can be found. These patients are known as 'lone fibrillators', tend to be younger, often have paroxysmal symptoms, and seem to have a good prognosis. There is evidence that autonomic dysfunction plays a role in these patients. Thus some notice

Table 1 Percentage per annum risk of stroke with and without prophylaxis

Risk	No prophylaxis	Aspirin	Warfarin
High risk			
Previous stroke or TIA	12	10	4–5
Age >75, or other risk factors[a]	8	4–5	1–2
Moderate risk			
Age <65 plus other risk factors[a]	4	1–2	1–2
Or age 65–74			
Or age >75 and no other risk factors			
Low risk			
Age <65 and no risk factors	1	<1	<1

[a] For example: hypertension, diabetes mellitus, heart failure, LV function, or known coronary disease.

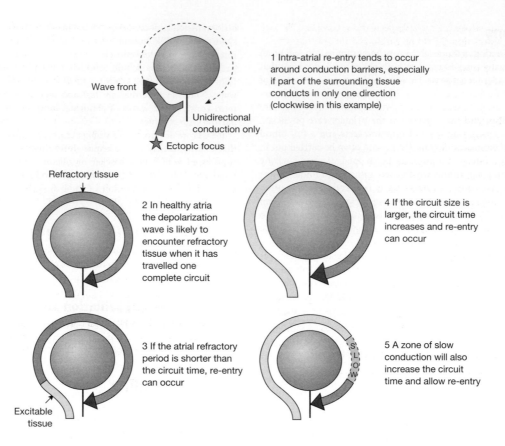

Fig. 1 Electrical re-entry, the mechanism responsible for initiating and maintaining atrial fibrillation. Illustration is from Grubb et al. (2001). *British Medical Journal* **322**, 777.

episodes of AF occur at times of high vagal tone—during sleep, after meals, or after exercise. These 'vagotonic' individuals may respond to drugs with anticholinergic properties like disopyramide. More rarely, AF is precipitated in lone fibrillators on exercise. These may respond to beta blockade.[11]

Atrial flutter seems to be a relatively pure form of a re-entrant circuit arrhythmia. There is evidence that it frequently arises with a specific circuit in the right atrium and thus is often associated with pulmonary disease, cor pulmonale, or sometimes vascular shunts. The sawtooth flutter waves at close to 300 bpm are often seen best in lead V_1 of the ECG. Atrial flutter should be considered whenever the ventricular rate is a divisor of 300 (150 in 2:1 block, 100 in 3:1, 75 in 4:1).

The 'sick sinus syndrome' refers to a sub-group of elderly patients with degenerative sinus node disease and a complex of brady- and tachy-arrhythmias, and AF.

Management of atrial fibrillation and flutter

Management focuses on treating the arrhythmia and preventing strokes.

Treating the arrhythmia

The arrhythmia is treated either by cardioversion (chemical or electrical) or by ventricular rate control. First consideration should always be given to treating any underlying disease that may have precipitated the arrhythmia such as a chest infection, myocardial infarction, or thyrotoxicosis.

A patient presenting with AF or flutter for the first time should be considered for cardioversion, especially if haemodynamically compromised. Underlying causes should be excluded. An echocardiogram will assess the valves, the presence of thrombus, and the size of the atria. Atrial enlargement makes successful cardioversion less likely and also increases the risk of thromboembolic stroke. If the duration of the AF is definitely less than 48 h,

many cardiologists will consider DC cardioversion immediately. Otherwise the patient is anticoagulated for at least 3 weeks before cardioversion. If cardioversion is successful, the patient will remain on warfarin for at least 6 weeks, or permanently if there is a high risk of re-occurrence. Cardioversion can sometimes be carried out chemically (under specialist supervision) using propafone, sotalol, or flecainide (all three can be proarrhythmic if LV function is impaired) or amiodarone. These drugs may also reduce the rates of recurrence but are not routinely used after a single episode of AF. Digoxin lowers the chance of spontaneous or successful electrical cardioversion.[11,12]

If cardioversion is not possible, then rate control is normally the management of choice. The aim should be to maintain the resting ventricular rate around 90 bpm. Digoxin is often the drug of first choice for resting rate control in AF. However, digoxin is poor at preventing exercise-induced tachycardias and is often combined with a beta-blocker or rate-limiting calcium channel blocker. It is helpful to check the heart rate after mild exercise in the surgery if the patient continues to suffer exertional breathlessness.

Radio-frequency ablation of ectopic foci, interruption of re-entrant circuits in the atria, AV nodal ablation with responsive dual chamber pacemakers, and overdrive atrial pacing are all techniques used increasingly frequently in specialist care.

Stroke prevention

Five major primary prevention trials through the 1980s into the 1990s have shown massive benefit in stroke reduction from anticoagulation of patients in chronic non-rheumatic atrial fibrillation. Individuals with paroxysmal AF seem to have a risk similar to chronic fibrillators and 30 per cent will progress to chronic AF in 2 years.[12] The consensus guidelines produced on the basis of this data are summarized in the Table 1. Individuals with chronic or paroxysmal AF over the age of 75, or under the age of 75 with previous stroke, diabetes, hypertension, coronary disease, heart failure, or LV dysfunction should be considered for anticoagulation with warfarin. The target INR range is 2.0–3.0. Those aged 65–75 with no other risk factors can be treated with either warfarin or aspirin. Patients under the age of 65 with no other risk factors can be treated with 300 mg aspirin daily.[13]

Broad complex tachycardia

In primary care, a broad complex tachycardia is normally ventricular tachycardia until proved otherwise and needs secondary care intervention. Sustained VT lasts more than 30 s. Non-sustained VT lasts from six beats to 29 s. Less than six beats is classified as repetitive ventricular beats. Monomorphic VT is a ventricular rate over 100 with constant morphology. Polymorphic VT changes QRS morphology, such as in torsade de pointes. Occurring in the weeks or months after a myocardial infraction, the broad complex tachycardia is very likely to be a monomorphic VT arising from the unstable myocardium on the edge of the infarct. All VT has the potential to degrade to ventricular fibrillation and needs urgent specialist assessment.

Brady-arrhythmias

Slow heart rates (less than 60 bpm) arise because of inhibition of the sino-atrial node, sino-atrial arrest, sino-atrial block, or atrio-ventricular block.

Inhibition of the sino-atrial node occurs because of high vagal tone during sleep, in the young, in athletes, during vaso-vagal syncope, excessive carotid sinus sensitivity, or inferior myocardial infarction. Drugs such as beta-blockers, calcium channel blockers, and amiodarone cause sinus bradycardia, as does hypothyroidism.

Sick sinus syndrome occurs in the elderly patient with idiopathic degeneration of the sino-atrial cells and is characterized by periods of sinus bradycardia or arrest that are often interrupted by a slower nodal escape rhythm. This may be accompanied by atrial tachycardias or AF.

Sino-atrial arrest or block maybe part of the sick sinus syndrome or, more rarely, is due to right coronary artery disease. Pauses maybe asymptomatic, cause near syncope or syncope.

Atrio-ventricular block is classified as first-degree block (a PR interval greater than 0.2 s, or five small squares), second-degree block (intermittent failure of conduction of atrial contractions to the ventricles), or third-degree block (complete heart block marked by atrial and ventricular disassociation). The cause is most frequently idiopathic fibrosis in the over seventies which is associated with sino-atrial disease in 25 per cent of cases. The block to conduction may occur within the node, in which case the escape rhythm will be narrow complex, or in the His–Purkinje system, in which case there will be wide complexes with bundle branch block. Drugs may potentiate the block (such as beta-blockers, calcium channel blockers, or digoxin). Intermittent episodes of complete heart block may present as Stokes–Adams attacks—drop attacks occurring without warning.

If treatment of a bradycardia is needed, ventricular pacing is usually employed.

Key points

1. A good history is essential to avoid over or under investigation.

2. Not all malignant arrhythmias cause haemodynamic disturbance.

3. The availability of patient event monitors means that conclusive diagnosis is now much easier to obtain.

4. Management of atrial fibrillation is important and a range of therapies can be used, including thromboembolic prophylaxis.

References

1. Patten, J. Neurological Differential Diagnosis, 2nd edn. Berlin: Springer, 1996.
2. Goodwin, J.F. (1997). Sudden cardiac death in the young. *British Medical Journal* 314, 843.
3. Beresford, T.P. et al. (1990). Comparison of CAGE questionnaire and computer assisted laboratory profiles in screening for covert alcoholism. *Lancet* 336, 482 5.
4. Vikhert, A. et al. (1986). Alcoholic cardiomyopathy and sudden cardiac death. *Journal of the American College of Cardiology* 8, 3–11A.
5. Alpert, M.A. (1993). Mitral valve prolapse. *British Medical Journal* 306, 943.
6. Chiang, B.N. et al. (1969). Relationship of premature systoles to coronary heart disease and sudden death in the Tecumseh epidemiologic study. *Annals of Internal Medicine* 70, 1159–66.
7. Garratt, C. et al. (1989). Lessons from the cardiac arrhythmia suppression trial. *British Medical Journal* 299, 806.
8. Amiodarone Trials Meta-Analysis Investigators (1997). Effect of prophylactic amiodarone on mortality after acute myocardial infarction and in congestive cardiac failure: meta-analysis of individual data from 6500 patients in randomised trials. *Lancet* 350, 1417–24.
9. Ventricular extrasystoles and the healthy heart—editorial. (1990). *Lancet* 335, 890.
10. Peters, N.S. (2000). Catheter ablation for cardiac arrhythmias. *British Medical Journal* 321, 716.
11. Narayan, S.M. et al. (1997). Atrial fibrillation. *Lancet* 350, 943–50.
12. Lip, G.Y., Beerers, D.G., and Coope, J.R. et al. (1996). ABC of atrial fibrillation. *British Medical Journal* 312, 175–8.
13. Cobbe, S.M., ed. (1999). Atrial fibrillation in hospital and general practice: The Sir James MacKenzie centenary consensus conference. Proceedings of the Royal College of Physicians (Edinburgh) 29 (Suppl. 6).

Further Reading

Bennett, D. *Cardiac Arrhythmias. Practical Notes on Interpretation and Treatment* 6th edn., 2002. (This is a simple and clear text aimed at the practicalities of diagnosis and treatment.)

Lip, G. and Beevers, G. *ABC of Atrial Fibrillation*. London: BMJ Publishing Group, 1996. (A very simple guide to this commonest of arrhythmias in general practice.)

Arrhythmia Octet. The Lancet 341, 1993. (A multi-author, authoritative summary of the state of electrophysiological knowledge on common arrhythmias.)

1.4 Ankle swelling and breathlessness

Patrick White

Introduction

The two symptoms of ankle swelling and breathlessness are extremely common. It is tempting to consider them as a connected duet, but even when the diagnosis seems beyond doubt at first sight, each must be considered separately, and on its own merits. In this chapter, ankle swelling and breathlessness will be examined individually as symptoms within the spectrum of cardiovascular diseases. Their connections to other system disorders will be made throughout the chapter, and cross-referenced to other chapters in the book.

Ankle swelling

Ankle swelling is common. It is a hazard in occupations involving hours of standing and often results also from prolonged sitting, especially in

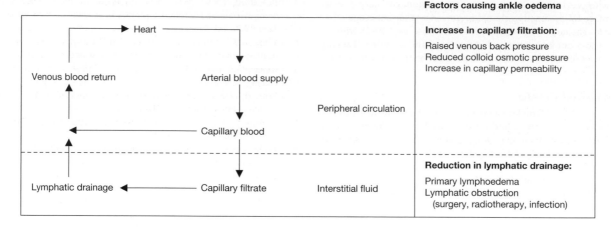

Fig. 1 Relationship between the circulation of the blood and the maintenance of the interstitial fluid.

long-distance air travel. The numerous causes of ankle swelling range from posture to secondary cancer of the pelvis, and include iatrogenic causes, such as the administration of calcium channel blocking drugs. A precise diagnosis is essential and since ankle swelling may be the first presentation of major disease there is no justification for treating it without first ruling out serious underlying causes.

Mechanisms of ankle oedema

The everyday experience of ankle oedema reflects precisely the mechanism which underlies ankle oedema as a pathological sign (Fig. 1). Oedema develops when the rate of capillary filtration exceeds the lymphatic drainage whether because of an increase in capillary filtration or because of a reduction in lymphatic drainage or both. Fluid filtered from capillaries is largely returned to the circulation through the lymphatic system with virtually no local re-entry into the vascular tree. In most cases, ankle oedema results from excess capillary filtration because of increased venous pressure, increased capillary permeability due to local inflammation, or hypoproteinaemia. In heart failure (Chapter 1.2), ankle oedema results from venous hypertension due to back pressure through the heart from the left ventricle (e.g. in ischaemic heart disease) or from the right ventricle in right heart failure due to chronic lung disease. Ankle oedema due to impaired lymphatic drainage is common in tropical countries where it is caused by filariasis. It is rare in temperate zones where it is due either to a primary disorder of the lymph system or to obstruction to lymph drainage such as sometimes follows cancer surgery or radiotherapy.

The assessment of ankle swelling

The assessment of ankle swelling (Fig. 2) is largely determined by the history: is it bilateral; is it acute; is it localized; is it influenced by posture or position; what is the associated medical history? The local examination consists of seeking evidence of pitting on pressure, evidence of superficial dilated or varicose veins, petechial haemorrhages, haemosiderin deposition, thickening or induration of the skin, and evidence of pelvic or groin swelling. The investigation of ankle swelling is determined by whether or not there is any associated systemic disease which might have caused it, or whether the cause is restricted to the leg. The task of investigation has been made easier by the development of precise techniques for assessing the venous and lymphatic systems in the legs and by the use of echocardiography for the assessment of heart failure.

Epidemiology

There are no precise figures for the prevalence of ankle oedema as a symptom of disease. The overlap between health and illness in the experience of

---

History
Unilateral or bilateral
Acute or chronic
Response to posture and position
Associated conditions:
   Varicose veins, previous deep vein thrombosis (DVT), heart disease, liver
   disease, kidney disease, COPD, malignant disease, pregnancy

Local examination
Evidence of pitting on pressure
Varicose veins
Dilated subcutaneous veins
Chronic venous leakage with haemosiderin staining
Thickening or induration of the skin
Pelvic or groin swelling
Petechial haemorrhages

Investigation
Haemoglobin (anaemia)
Serum sodium and creatinine (renal function)
Liver function tests (albumin, bilirubin, liver enzymes)
Urinalysis (blood or protein in the urine)
Chest X-ray (heart failure, hyperinflation in COPD)
Compression ultrasonography (DVT)
Venogram of the deep veins (DVT)
Impedance plethysmography (DVT)
Circulating D-dimer (DVT)
Lymphoscintigraphy (lymphoedema)
Lymphangiography (lymphoedema)
Electro- and echocardiography (heart disease, heart failure)

Fig. 2 The assessment of ankle oedema.

ankle oedema limit the usefulness of assessing its prevalence. There are many causes of ankle swelling and ankle oedema (Fig. 3). The main cause of ankle oedema as a symptom of disease is venous incompetence which affects more than a third of people over 35 years of age.[1] Venous incompetence does not always result in ankle oedema but it is likely to be present in most cases. Finding venous incompetence should only lead to naming it as the primary cause of ankle oedema in the absence of heart disease, and in the absence of venous obstruction in the groin or pelvis, lymphoedema, and hypoproteinaemia. Heart failure is a common cause of ankle oedema in the elderly affecting over 1 per cent of the population as a whole but more than 10 per cent of people over 80 years.[2] Heart failure is the commonest reason for hospital admission in the United States. Its detection should be a major priority within primary care services because of the striking reduction in its

Raised venous pressure in the lower limbs
Immobility with dependent limbs
Obesity
Venous incompetence
Varicose veins
Deep vein thrombosis
Compression of pelvic veins
Cardiac failure

Hypoproteinaemia
Liver disease
Nephrotic syndrome
Chronic renal failure with proteinuria
Nutritional deficiency of protein
Malabsorption
Protein-losing enteropathy

Lymphoedema
Congenital lymphatic hypoplasia
Lymphatic obstruction
    Surgery or radiotherapy
    Infection (e.g. filariasis)
    Trauma
    Local cancer

Tracking down of fluid from above
Ruptured gastrocnemius
Ruptured baker's cyst
Haemorrhage or haematoma in thigh or calf

Local tissue exudate
Insect bite
Systemic allergy (e.g. angioneurotic oedema)
Infection (e.g. cellulitis)
Local trauma (e.g. ankle sprain)
Joint effusion

Idiopathic
Idiopathic oedema of women

Fig. 3 Causes of ankle swelling.

mortality which can be achieved by modern treatment with ACE inhibitors, beta-blockers, and spironolactone (see Chapter 1.2). Ankle oedema is the commonest presenting symptom and sign of deep vein thrombosis (DVT) which has a prevalence of about 0.2 per cent in populations in Europe and North America. Hypo-proteinaemia is a less common cause of ankle oedema although it is an important factor among alcoholics and people at risk of liver disease (Chapter 4.9).

Venous stasis, varicose veins, and DVT

Chronic venous stasis causes aching in the feet and calves, itching in the skin, and heaviness and tension in the lower legs. It is usually associated with dilated superficial veins, varicose veins, peripheral oedema, and in more prolonged cases haemosiderin deposition leading to brown discoloration of the skin, petechial haemorrages, and thickening and hardening of the skin of the feet. Chronic venous ischaemia (due to stasis and oedema rather than arterial obstruction) leads to atrophy of the skin above the malleoli with ulceration, scarring, and atrophie blanche (white atrophic scarring). The treatment of chronic venous stasis is elevation of the limb, compression (hosiery or bandaging) and removal of varicose veins. Underlying causes such as obesity and immobility may be difficult to overcome but effective treatment of co-existing heart failure, anaemia, diabetes mellitus, and ischaemia may be crucial to successful management of the venous disease.[3] Where the pedal pulses are impalpable compression bandaging should not be applied unless the ankle-brachial pressure index is at least 0.8. The ankle-brachial pressure index is measured using a pencil doppler. The pressure at which the pedal pulse is obliterated is divided by that at

which the brachial pulse is obliterated. The goal of elevation of the limb and compression bandaging is to oppose the hydrostatic pressure of venous hypertension, and to force the stagnant interstitial fluid and venous blood out of the limb so that fresh arterial blood can restore oxygenation and nutrition. Infected ulcers will not respond to topical or systemic antibiotics while the floor of the wound is flooded with stagnant serous exudate.

Compression can be provided by elastic stockings (Class I, 12–17 mmHg at the ankle; Class II, 18–24 mmHg at the ankle; Class III, 25–35 mmHg at the ankle) or by the Charing Cross four layer bandaging regime.[4] Elastic stockings are removed at night when the patient is recumbent. Compression bandaging should be changed no more than twice a week.

Varicose veins are lengthened tortuous, dilated veins which arise spontaneously. They affect between 17 and 35 per cent of adults over 35 years. They are rarely due to other conditions such as DVT, pelvic tumours, or radiotherapy. The primary abnormality is a congenital weakness in the vein wall of the superficial veins or the perforating veins from the superficial to the deep venous systems. As the vein wall dilates the venous valve becomes incompetent and venous pressure in the lower superficial veins rises. Varicose veins are more common with increasing age. The Edinburgh vein study has shown that lifestyle factors do not figure prominently in venous reflux disease.[3] Previous pregnancy, use of oral contraception, and mobility while at work are predisposing factors in women. Increased height and straining at stool may be implicated in men.

The ideal test for varicose veins is colour duplex scanning which can identify incompetence between the deep and superficial systems and incompetence in superficial veins. Initial treatment with compression hosiery should control symptoms.[5] Injection sclerotherapy (obliteration of perforating veins with sclerosants such as microfoam, hypertonic saline, or liquid soap) has a high rate of recurrence within 5 years. Sapheno-femoral and sapheno-popliteal ligation with or without stripping of the long saphenous vein is more successful in the long-term but more than 20 per cent will recur after 10 years.

A more detailed discussion of varicose veins is provided in Chapter 1.8.

DVT occurs mainly in patients over 40 years. Risk factors include obesity, varicose veins, malignancy, personal or family history, combined contraceptive pill, hormone replacement therapy, pregnancy, immobility after major illness including surgery or myocardial infarction. The main clinical finding is pitting oedema of the lower leg which extends up to about six inches below the distal extent of the thrombosis. The most commonly used test is compression ultrasonography. This uses doppler ultrasound to show the presence of a non-compressible vein segment. Unsuccessful ultrasonography may lead to subsequent testing with a venogram, but measurement in the serum of one of the products of fibrin production, D-dimer, is a promising early diagnostic test with high negative predictive value especially in the absence of other acute illnesses. Patients in whom a DVT is suspected should be seen immediately in hospital for assessment using a clinical probability score with D-dimer testing and compression ultrasonography.[6] An algorithm for the diagnosis of DVT is shown in Fig. 4. This combines the use of compression ultrasonography with the clinical probability score of Wells and D-dimer testing. In this score, history and examination are used to provide a probability for the presence of DVT. The treatment of DVT requires early intravenous heparin with oral warfarin.[7] The heparin is continued for at least 5 days until warfarin anticoagulation is stabilized. Patients who can be safely managed at home can be treated with twice daily subcutaneous low molecular weight heparin which may be self-administered. In this case, anticoagulation monitoring is not continued.

Ankle oedema and hypoproteinaemia

Hypoproteinaemia is an uncommon cause of ankle oedema in primary care but should be considered where there is malnutrition, excessive alcohol use, or severe liver or kidney disease. Albumin accounts for most of the colloid osmotic pressure of plasma. Hypoproteinaemia or, more specifically, hypoalbuminaemia, leads to ankle oedema through a reduction in the colloid osmotic pressure which counters the hydrostatic pressure within the

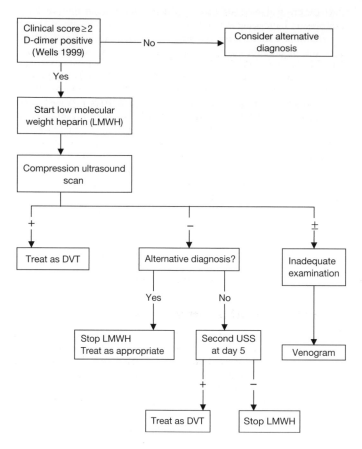

Fig. 4 Algorithm for clinical investigation of DVT. (Based on the clinical algorithm of the DVT clinic at Kings College Hospital NHS Trust, London.)

blood vessels. The liver is the only site of albumin synthesis producing about 15 g/day in a normal person. The body contains 3.5–5 g of albumin per kilogram of body weight of which about 38–45 per cent is in the intravascular space. Severe liver damage or dysfunction leads to hypoproteinaemia with ascites and peripheral oedema. Hypoproteinaemia also results from loss of protein in the urine in kidney disease. The oedema of nephrotic syndrome is not simply the result of protein loss. In nephrotic syndrome, the primary phenomenon leading to peripheral oedema is sodium retention due to increased sodium re-absorption in the collecting ducts with resultant fluid overload and venous hypertension. There may also be some increased capillary permeability due to the action of renin. Hypoproteinaemia which causes ankle oedema may also result from malabsorption, exudative skin diseases, protein-losing enteropathy, burns, and malignant disease.

Lymphoedema

Lymphoedema is a common disease in tropical countries where it is caused mainly by the thread-like, parasitic filarial worms *Wuchereria bancrofti* and *Brugia malayi* which are exclusive human pathogens. According to the World Health Organization it affects 120 million people worldwide in 73 tropical and sub-tropical countries.[8] The filarial worms lodge in the lymphatic system where they live for 4–5 years producing millions of larvae into the blood stream. The disease is spread from human to human by mosquitoes. The worms block the lymph vessels and can lead to massive lymphoedema of the limbs and genitals (elephantiasis).

Lymphoedema is an uncommon cause of ankle swelling in primary care in temperate countries where the prevalence is no more than 0.02 per cent.

It is usually the result of surgery or radiotherapy for malignant disease. Primary lymphoedema is rare.

The diagnosis of lymphoedema depends on the history, particularly the family history, the rate and time of onset, and the presence of predisposing conditions such as pelvic malignant disease. There are typical changes in the skin which becomes thick, making it impossible to pinch a fold of skin at the base of the second toe—Kaposi–Stemmer sign. Lymphoscintography is the best test for the diagnosis of lymphoedema. Radio-labelled protein is injected into the first web space of each foot and its passage into the lymph is monitored by a gamma camera. The diagnosis is determined by the speed of removal of the radioactive isotope and its appearance or retention outside the lymph vessels. Lymphoedema is extremely difficult to treat. Exercise to promote the movement of lymph, compression (hosiery, multilayer bandaging, massage, and pneumatic compression) to reduce capillary filtration and increase interstitial pressure, and elevation of the limb all help to minimize lymphoedema but are limited by the degree of the obstruction to lymph flow.

Other causes of ankle swelling

Ankle swelling may be the result of trauma to the thigh or calf either from the rupture of a muscle or from the accumulation of a large haematoma from both of which serum can ooze heavily. Insect bites or stings, systemic allergic reactions and infection act by increasing capillary permeability either through local chemical action or through the systemic release of inflammatory mediators. Effusion from joints due to inflammatory arthritis or injuries such as sprains commonly cause ankle oedema, but the diagnosis is usually obvious from the history. Idiopathic ankle oedema of women is poorly understood. It is most likely due to humoral mechanisms affecting capillary permeability. It is diagnosed by exclusion and should be treated in similar fashion to lymphoedema or venous stasis by increasing the pressure in the interstitium compared to the intravascular pressure.

Breathlessness and cardiovascular disease

Breathlessness is a universal experience, provoked by exercise or effort, relieved by rest. When breathlessness results from minor effort or comes on with no effort at all, it is frightening. If it is prolonged, breathlessness can lead to panic and the sensation of drowning or impending death. Breathlessness is a common symptom of disease. It is often described as dyspnoea which is the subjective experience of breathing discomfort.

The perception of breathlessness is complex.[9] The control of breathing is largely conducted in the brain stem in the respiratory centre of the medulla oblongata. Rate and depth of breathing are altered in response to changes in carbon dioxide (CO_2) or pH in the blood. This is augmented by peripheral monitoring of CO_2 and oxygen in the aortic and carotid bodies and by stimulation of chemical and physical receptors in the bronchial tree which are also associated with cough. Breathing is affected by emotional stimuli such as excitement, anxiety, and fear. The force of dyspnoea as a symptom is partly explained by the recent demonstration of the cortical representation of dyspnoea in the lingula and insula alongside sites associated with pain, hunger, and thirst.[10]

The perception of breathlessness varies between patients in their tolerance of and acclimatization to the symptom. In asthma, patients exhibit different thresholds of peak expiratory flow rate at which breathlessness is experienced.[11] Similarly in heart disease the perception of breathlessness and the experience of dyspnoea occur at different respiratory and cardiac rates in different patients. Furthermore, an individual's capacity to tolerate respiratory or cardiac impairment will be affected by physical training and by the co-existence of other diseases. Highly trained athletes who suffer major upper gastrointestinal haemorrhage may not experience symptoms of breathlessness at rest or tiredness until their haemoglobin level falls to 6 or 7 g/dl. On the other hand, minor changes in haemoglobin (1–2 g/dl) may provoke breathlessness in sedentary elderly people with poor cardiorespiratory reserves.

Mechanisms of breathlessness in heart disease

The symptom of breathlessness or dyspnoea results from a mismatch between the ventilation demanded and the ventilation achieved. This may be perceived by the patient as the failure to satisfy the demand for breath despite apparently effective breathing. Alternatively, it may be perceived as difficulty in the act of breathing itself either through obstruction to or restriction in the flow of air or through inadequacy of the muscles of breathing.

Although patients who are breathless often experience the sensation of not being able to get enough air, their urge to breathe is primarily the result of not being able to eliminate enough CO_2. The drive to breathe is largely dependent on CO_2 levels in the blood except where there is chronic CO_2 retention. In chronic obstructive pulmonary disease (COPD), the drive to breathe switches mainly to hypoxia because the breathing centre in the brain becomes insensitive to rising levels of CO_2.

In heart disease, breathlessness is most commonly the result of pump failure (Fig. 5). The heart is unable to pump enough blood to carry CO_2 from the tissues to the lungs. CO_2 is so easily diffusible across the alveolar wall in the lung that in heart failure whatever blood gets to the lung can usually exchange most of its CO_2 with the alveoli. The retention of CO_2 is made worse by the onset of pulmonary oedema due to heart failure. In acute pulmonary oedema, rising hydrostatic pressure in the pulmonary veins leads to rising hydrostatic pressure in the pulmonary capillaries with transport of fluid across the capillary wall into the pulmonary interstitium and the alveolar spaces. As the bronchioles swell and alveoli fill with fluid, there is less opportunity for the removal of CO_2 from the blood, arterial CO_2 rises and breathlessness increases.

A further factor in the breathlessness of heart disease is muscle fatigue. If breathlessness is prolonged, particularly in a patient with chronic heart disease who is unfit, fatigue reduces the efficiency of respiratory effort thereby increasing the breathlessness. Each component of breathlessness in heart disease may require a different therapeutic approach.

The breathlessness of heart disease is commonly complicated by other problems of advancing age including anaemia, muscle fatigue, impaired renal function, and COPD. Anaemia causes a compensatory tachycardia which can precipitate acute heart failure. Muscle fatigue reduces the efficiency of respiratory effort increasing breathlessness. There is good evidence of the efficacy of exercise programmes in heart failure both for the impact of improved fitness and for their direct humoral effects on the heart. Impaired renal function leads to both hyponatraemia and hypoproteinaemia causing cardiac irritability and worsening pulmonary and peripheral oedema respectively. COPD and ischaemic heart disease have smoking as a shared cause and frequently occur together, added to which COPD is the principal cause of cor pulmonale.

Epidemiology of breathlessness

Heart disease is not a common cause of breathlessness and breathlessness is a late symptom in heart disease, so its appearance is usually indicative of sustained heart damage. There are no good epidemiological data on the prevalence of breathlessness due to heart disease. Comparison with obstructive lung disease in the form of asthma whose prevalence is between 6 and 10 per cent or COPD which causes five deaths per 10 000 population helps to give some perspective on the place of breathlessness due to heart disease in primary care workload. Heart disease as a whole, of which ischaemic heart disease is the most common, affects between 2 and 3 per cent of the population in Europe and North America. Breathlessness is unlikely to be a prominent symptom in most of these as angina is the main limit to mobility in active ischaemic heart disease. Angina and tiredness are the principal symptoms of ischaemic heart disease so breathlessness may not be experienced until heart failure supervenes. Heart failure is almost invariably associated with breathlessness on exertion and is found among 0.8 per cent of populations in industrialized societies.[2,12]

Cardiac causes of breathlessness

The main causes of breathlessness in heart disease are listed in Fig. 5. Outflow obstruction leads initially to hypertrophy of the heart as it tries to overcome the resistance to flow. Breathlessness eventually ensues either because the cardiac output is inadequate or because pulmonary oedema results from back pressure into the pulmonary veins. Primary muscle pump failure results most often from chronic ischaemia in which the heart muscle is deprived of oxygen by coronary artery disease or from dilatation of the left ventricle due to infarction. In hypertensive heart disease, the ischaemia is exacerbated by left ventricular hypertrophy in response to chronic elevation of blood pressure. In cardiac arrhythmias breathlessness is usually due to a fall in cardiac output either because the heart rate is so low, for example, in complete heart block or because the heart rate is too fast to allow adequate ventricular filling during diastole. Mitral stenosis causes atrial enlargement, pulmonary venous hypertension and oedema. Supraventricular arrhythmias, of which atrial fibrillation is the commonest, often follow the atrial enlargement of mitral stenosis. Breathlessness is usually preceded by fatigue. Mitral incompetence is most often the result of ischaemia which causes papillary muscle infarction with scarring or rupture of the chordae tendineae or dilatation of the mitral ring due to left ventricular dilatation. Left ventricular output is reduced with regurgitation into the left atrium. Pulmonary venous hypertension follows and ultimately leads to pulmonary oedema.

Breathlessness and position

Severely breathless patients prefer to sit upright, leaning slightly forward resting on a table or the back of a chair. This position improves the efficiency of breathing by supporting the accessory muscles of respiration in the neck, by diverting excess interstitial fluid (oedema) into the lower body, by increasing the vertical dimension of the chest, and by maximizing the potential excursion of the diaphragm. In congestive heart failure with peripheral oedema, lying flat causes the excess fluid in the legs and lower trunk to move to the abdomen and chest. Pressure on the diaphragm increases, there is a build up of pulmonary oedema and a rise in pressure in the inferior vena cava. The breathlessness that results from lying flat is called orthopnoea and is characteristic of heart failure. Repeated awakening from sleep with breathlessness is called paroxysmal nocturnal dyspnoea. It may be associated with nocturia. Nocturia in heart failure is due to the reflex diuresis which results from lying flat. Fluid which was pooling in the lower limbs during the day returns to the trunk on lying down leading to an increase in the central vascular volume which is then reduced by the kidney causing nocturia.

Cardiac outflow obstruction
Aortic stenosis
Cardiomyopathy

Cardiac muscle pump failure
Ischaemic heart disease
Hypertensive heart disease
Cardiomyopathy

Cardiac arrhythmia
Bradyarrhythmia
    Heart block
    Drug effects
Tachyarrhythmia
    Supraventicular tachycardia
    Atrial fibrillation
    Ventricular tachycardia

Mitral valve disease
Rheumatic heart disease
Mitral incompetence

Fig. 5 Cardiac causes of breathlessness.

Extreme obesity can mimic heart failure. The pressure of abdominal obesity on the pelvic veins increases the venous pressure in the lower limbs leading to oedema. An extremely obese individual who lies flat will suffer immobilization (splinting) of the diaphragm and a return to the trunk of fluid which has been pooled in the lower limbs while the subject was sitting or standing. This will lead to paroxysmal nocturnal dyspnoea and nocturnal diuresis in otherwise fit people. A normal echocardiograph will rule out cardiac failure.

The assessment of breathlessness due to heart disease in primary care

Breathlessness is rarely the first presenting symptom of heart disease, but breathlessness and fatigue are common presenting symptoms of acute heart failure. Key aspects of the symptoms of breathlessness in heart disease are its speed of onset, its relation to rest and exercise, its frequency, its persistence, its time of onset, and the relationship it has to position (standing, sitting, or lying). Sometimes the description of breathlessness can point to the cause ('I get short of breath when I lie down'—pulmonary oedema) or ('I just can't get my breath in deep enough'—diaphragm spasm due to anxiety). A definitive diagnosis of breathlessness must always be sought (Fig. 6). In heart disease breathlessness invariably requires hospital investigation.[13] It is occasionally necessary to start the treatment of breathlessness due to heart disease solely on the basis of history and examination. The need for the primary care clinician to treat breathlessness in this relatively blind way will be determined by the speed of onset of breathlessness and its severity, and by the accessibility of specialist services.

If acute breathlessness is suspected to be the result of ischaemia, electrocardiograph (ECG) and cardiac enzymes should be arranged urgently with the local specialist medical team on call. Acute breathlessness with tachycardia, wheeze, and the absence of crepitations in a patient with a history of heart disease and asthma can prove difficult to diagnose. The diagnosis may be acute asthma or acute pulmonary oedema. Asthma can only be diagnosed by the response to treatment. Peak expiratory flow rate (PEFR) may be reduced in acute pulmonary oedema as well as in asthma or COPD due to oedema of small airways. A rapid response to high-dose inhaled bronchodilators may clarify the cause. The diagnosis of acute pulmonary oedema can be made on chest X-ray together with evidence of left ventricular strain on ECG. If the diagnosis depends on the response to treatment before both chest X-ray and ECG can be done, then it is preferable to start with the treatment of asthma. High-dose inhaled beta-agonists (e.g. salbutamol 100 μg × 4–8 doses, or terbutaline 500 μg × 4–8 doses) should be administered in a spacer device and the effect reviewed after 15–30 min. Alternatively, a nebulizer (salbutamol 5 mg) may be used. The beta-agonist may cause a minor increase in heart rate, but it is unlikely to adversely influence the outcome unless the patient's heart rate is already severely compromised (>110/min).

Breathlessness due to heart failure usually requires acute treatment with an intramuscular or intravenous loop diuretic, such as frusemide or bumetanide and the possible addition of an ACE inhibitor shortly afterwards. ACE inhibitors can be safely commenced in primary care with appropriate attention to their interaction with diuretics (hypotension within the first 12 h) and with monitoring of renal function (serum creatinine).

Anxiety is a common cause of breathlessness but the diagnosis should only be made by exclusion. Typically, patients with anxiety hyperventilation will be unaware of their tachypnoea but will present with paraesthesiae of the hands and face and a sensation of light headedness. Many patients who have anxiety-related breathlessness will complain of difficulty getting a deep enough breath and will engage a variety of manoeuvres including yawning to obtain a satisfactory breath. This symptom is probably due to diaphragmatic spasm. Most patients are relieved by the explanation of its cause, which allows clinician and patient to address the underlying anxiety.

The palliative care of breathlessness

Breathlessness is a common symptom in advanced cancer and the techniques which palliative care physicians use to treat it should be considered also for patients with advanced heart failure in whom treatment options may be limited.[14] Specific causes such as chronic anaemia may complicate terminal illness and may deserve treatment at least for symptomatic relief. With terminal disease the primary care clinician may request the services of the local hospice or palliative care team for advice on the use of:

♦ oxygen (should only be required by a small number of patients);[15]

♦ physiotherapy for advice on positioning patients in bed;

♦ high-dose corticosteroids;

♦ anxiolytics such as benzodiazepines;

♦ opioids such as codeine and morphine.

Drugs which are useful for breathlessness in terminal care include the first generation antihistamine promethazine which at a dose of 125 mg daily can reduce breathlessness and increase exercise tolerance in emphysema. Benzodiazepines reduce respiratory panic and improve sleep with no loss of ventilation at low doses. Opioids act on the respiratory centre in the medulla oblongata and alter sensitivity to CO_2. They also act as cortical sedatives and may also reduce hypersecretion in the respiratory tree. Morphine is the opiate of choice in terminal care. Methadone which has been used in the past should be avoided because of the risk of accumulation.

> **Breathlessness of acute onset**
> *Cardiac causes*
> Acute ischaemia
> Acute heart failure
> Acute bradycardia/tachycardia
>
> *Respiratory causes*
> Acute asthma
> Pneumothorax
> Pneumonia
> Pulmonary embolus
>
> *Other causes*
> Anaemia due to acute haemorrhage
> Anxiety with diaphragm spasm
> Hyperventilation
> Metabolic acidosis
> Acute malignant pleural effusion
>
> **Breathlessness of gradual onset**
> *Cardiac causes*
> Heart failure
> Valvular heart disease
> Aortic outflow obstruction
>
> *Respiratory causes*
> Asthma
> COPD
> Pulmonary fibrosis
>
> *Other causes*
> Chronic anemia
> Obesity
> Ascites in liver failure
> Malignant disease
>   Bronchial obstruction
>   Pleural effusion

Fig. 6 Breathlessness—differential diagnosis.

References

1. Franks, P.J. et al. (1992). Prevalence of venous disease: a community study in west London. *European Journal of Surgery* **158**, 143–7.

2. McMurray, J.J.V., Petrie, M.C., Murdoch, D.R., and Davie, A.P. (1998). Clinical epidemiology of heart failure: public and private health burden. *European Heart Journal* **19** (Suppl.), P9–16.

3. Fowes, F.G.R., Ler, A.S., Evans, C.J., Allen, P.C., Bradbury, A.W., and Ruckly, C.V. (2001). Lifestyle risk factors for lower limb reflux in the general population: Edinburgh Vein Study. *International Journal of Epidemiology* **30**, 846–52.

4. Fletcher, A., Cullum, N., and Sheldon, T.A. (1997). Systematic review of compression treatment for venous leg ulcers. *British Medical Journal* **315**, 576–80.

5. Task Force on Chronic Venous Disorders of the Leg (1999). The management of chronic venous disorders of the leg. *Phlebology* **14** (Suppl. 1).

6. Wells, P.S. and Anderson, D.R. (1999). Modern approach to diagnosis in patients with suspected deep vein thrombosis. *Haemostasis* **10** (Suppl. 1), 10–20.

7. Lensing, W.A., Prandone, P., Prins, M.H., and Buller, H.R. (1999). Deep vein thrombosis. *Lancet* **353**, 479–85.

8. Otteson, E.A., Duke, B.O.L., Karam, M., and Benbehani, K. (1997). Strategies for the control/elimination of lymphatic filariasis. *Bulletin of the World Health Organization* **75**, 491–503.

9. Harver, A., Mahler, D.A., Schwartzstein, R.M., and Baird, J.C. (2000). Descriptors of breathlessness in healthy individuals. Distinct and separable constructs. *Chest* **118**, 679–90.

10. Banzett, R.B., Mulnier, H.E., Murphy, K., Rosen, S.D., Wise, R.J.S., and Adams, L. (2000). Breathlessness in humans activates insular cortex. *Neuroreport* **11** (10), 2117–20.

11. Atherton, A., White, P.T., Hewett, G., and Howells, K. (1996). Relationship of daytime asthma symptom frequency to morning peak expiratory flow. *European Respiratory Journal* **9**, 232–6.

12. Davis, R.C., Hobbs, F.C.R., and Lip, G.Y.H. (2000). ABC of heart failure: history and epidemiology. *British Medical Journal* **320**, 39–42.

13. Task Force on Heart Failure of the European Society of Cardiology (1995). Guidelines for the diagnosis of heart failure. *European Heart Journal* **16**, 741–75.

14. Boyd, K. and Kelly, M. (1997). Oral morphine as symptomatic treatment of dyspnoea in patients with advanced cancer. *Palliative Medicine* **11**, 277–81.

15. Booth, S., Kelly, M., Cox, N., Adams, L., and Guz, A. (1996). Does oxygen help dyspnoea in patients with cancer? *American Journal of Respiratory and Critical Care Medicine* **153**, 1515–18.

Further reading

Packer, M. (1999). Consensus Recommendations for the management of chronic heart failure. *American Journal of Cardiology* **83** (2A), 1–37A. (This detailed review of chronic heart failure summarises the evidence for the modern treatment of heart failure and provides an exhaustive list of references.)

Donnelly, R. and London, N.J.M. *ABC of Arterial and Venous Diseases*. London: BMJ Books, 2000. [This book is a highly practical review of peripheral vascular disease. As the assessment and treatment of deep vein thrombosis is changing rapidly authoritative journals such as *Thrombosis and Haemostasis* (pub. Schattaeur) should be consulted for recent developments.]

Caruana-Montaldo, B., Gleeson, K., and Zwillich, C.W. (2000). The control of breathing in clinical practice. *Chest* **117** (1), 205–25. (A thorough review of the physiology of breathing and the control of breathing in disease.)

1.5 Peripheral arterial disease

Jelle Stoffers

General introduction

Definition

Peripheral arterial (occlusive) disease (PAD) is one of the terms used to describe the manifestation of atherosclerosis below the bifurcation of the abdominal aorta. Its clinical consequences are better described by the synonym 'chronic lower limb ischaemia'. PAD is the most common arterial disease of the elderly. There is a high association with other atherosclerotic diseases like coronary artery disease and cerebrovascular disease. PAD shares most of the well known cardiovascular risk factors with these diseases.

Description

The clinical course of the disorder can be described according to the four stages of Fontaine (Table 1).

The successive stages represent the advancing atherosclerotic process (stenosis, occlusion), leading to restriction of arterial blood flow and thus to increasing ischaemia in leg muscles and skin. Stage 1 is the asymptomatic or preclinical stage. Stage 2 is characterized by intermittent claudication. Stages 3 and 4 are generally referred to as 'critical ischaemia'.

Epidemiology

Epidemiological data on PAD come from various sources: cross-sectional and prospective studies in open populations from various countries, hospital-based studies as well as studies from primary care. Differences in diagnostic criteria used in these studies add to the variation in epidemiological data on prevalence, incidence, and prognosis of the disorder.

Prevalence

In epidemiological studies, the prevalence of PAD depends on diagnostic criteria, age, and sex distribution. Prevalence rises with age; above 65 years, figures vary from 6 to 27 per cent for women and from 10 to 27 per cent for men. The proportion of symptomatic cases is estimated at approximately 20 per cent. In primary care, probably a half to two-thirds of all patients are not known to have the disorder. In general practice morbidity studies, prevalence of registered intermittent claudication (symptomatic PAD) is reported to be around five per 1000 (age 65–74, 14 per thousand; 75+, 21 per thousand). In summary, per 1000 patients in primary care, there will be about 20–25 patients with PAD, of whom 16–20 are asymptomatic and 14–16 are not known.

Incidence

Epidemiological studies on PAD in primary care have reported figures between 11 and 23 new cases of PAD per 1000 person-years. For symptomatic

Table 1 Peripheral arterial disease: clinical stages according to Fontaine

Stage	Key feature	Symptoms	Associated ABPI
Fontaine 1	Diminished arterial flow	No complaints High risk for developing other cardiovascular diseases	ABPI <0.90
Fontaine 2	Arterial blood flow insufficient during exercise	Intermittent claudication	ABPI <0.80
Fontaine 3	Arterial blood flow insufficient at rest: 'threatened leg'	Rest pain Skin problems	ABPI <0.50 Ankle pressure <50 mmHg
Fontaine 4	Arterial blood flow insufficient at rest: 'threatened leg'	Ulcers, necrosis, gangrene, infection	ABPI ≪0.50

PAD, these figures are 1–3 per 1000 person-years. Morbidity registration studies also have reported incidence figures for intermittent claudication of around 3 per 1000 patients per year. The incidence rate of intermittent claudication in patients who are known to have asymptomatic PAD, is reported to be 90 per 1000 person-years.

Risk factors

Risk factors for PAD are similar to those of other cardiovascular diseases. Smoking inevitably is the most important risk factor for developing PAD. Other important risk factors are diabetes mellitus and hypertension. Although the role of hypercholesterolaemia (>5 mmol/l) for the development of atherosclerosis is well established, its role in PAD is less evident. A high HDL-cholesterol ratio appears to have a weak protective effect. There is growing evidence that a raised serum level of homocysteine (>15 μmol/l) is associated with cardiovascular disease, including PAD. However, the clinical relevance of this finding as yet remains unclear, given the absence of studies on the effect of lowering the homocysteine level with folic acid.

Prognosis and prognostic determinants

In most patients PAD in itself has a relatively benign course. Complaints of intermittent claudication can remain stable for many years. In referred patients with intermittent claudication, critical ischaemia develops in approximately 25 per cent. Eventually, 1.5–5 per cent of all referred patients require an amputation. A systematic review of population based studies showed that 4–10 per cent of patients with intermittent claudication experience symptom progression leading to specialist treatment including surgical intervention and amputation. Smoking and diabetes are the most important prognostic determinants of an unfavourable outcome.

Claudicants as well as asymptomatic PAD patients frequently have co-existing cardiovascular diseases or are at high risk of developing cardiovascular events, non-fatal or fatal. This leads to a reduction of life expectancy estimated at 10 years. A low ankle–brachial systolic pressure index is associated with a higher risk of fatal and non-fatal cardiovascular events.

In conclusion, although the prognosis of intermittent claudication for most patients will be good, life expectancy is reduced due to present or future cardiovascular co-morbidity. Also asymptomatic patients are at high risk of developing a cardiovascular event.

Quality of life

Research on the quality of life of patients with intermittent claudication is growing but is still limited and mostly concerns patients referred to a vascular clinic or an outpatient department. Patients with intermittent claudication perceive their overall general health and quality of life as significantly reduced compared to persons without intermittent claudication. The most important determinants of the reduced quality of life are pain and reduced physical mobility. Patients also report more loss of energy, more emotional reactions, more sleep disturbances, and more social dysfunction. Severity of the disease is positively associated with physical immobility, pain, sleep disturbances, loss of energy, and social dysfunction.

Presentation in primary care

Many patients with PAD do not present themselves to a doctor. Some patients regard intermittent claudication as a normal symptom of ageing. Many adapt their lifestyle by walking less or for a shorter time or at a slower speed. In some patients, other disorders restrict their walking capacity, for example, heart disease, chronic pulmonary disease, or osteoarthrosis. In these patients, symptoms of PAD are masked by lack of mobility. In primary care, most patients with PAD will present with complaints associated with Fontaine stage 2, intermittent claudication. Intermittent claudication typically is characterized by the following features: the patient experiences pain or other discomfort in a leg, usually in the calf, but buttock or thigh

claudication is also possible—after walking a certain distance. The pain quickly (<10 min) diminishes when resting, but reappears when approximately the same distance is covered. The pain arises sooner or gets worse when the patient is in a hurry, is walking uphill or carrying a load. There are no complaints on sitting or standing.

The top three reasons for encounter (ICPC) in a Dutch morbidity registration project (Amsterdam) consisted of 'symptoms of leg or thigh' (27 per cent), 'symptoms of foot or toes' (11 per cent), and 'pain attributed to the circulation' (10 per cent). After questioning the patient, often a more or less typical pattern of intermittent claudication becomes apparent (Table 3). Patients mostly (>90 per cent) are above 40 years old. The majority (75–90 per cent) of patients with PAD are or have been smokers. Although in epidemiological studies the prevalence among men and women is almost equal, men more often have symptomatic disease and concomitant cardiovascular disorders. Therefore, the diagnosis 'PAD' more often is made in men. Most patients with PAD are treated in primary care. It can be estimated that 25–50 per cent of all patients are referred to a vascular specialist.

The most frequent concomitant chronic diseases of patients with PAD are hypertension (±20 per cent), diabetes mellitus (±14 per cent), chronic ischaemic heart disease (±10 per cent), congestive heart failure (±10 per cent), and osteoarthrosis (±10 per cent).

Diagnosis

Medical history and physical examination

Table 2 summarizes the most relevant differential diagnostic options. Guidelines for history taking and physical examination with regard to PAD are given in the Tables 3 and 4.

Evaluation

In Table 5—adapted from a study among primary care PAD patients, comparing clinical diagnostic features with non-invasive testing—the diagnostic values of the most important clinical diagnostic features are summarized.

The clinical relevance of a thorough physical examination is illustrated by the relatively high odds ratios for almost all examination features. If a patient has good arterial foot pulses, the diagnosis 'PAD' can virtually be excluded. The following 10 features independently contributed to the diagnosis (in order of decreasing odds ratio):

1. abnormal arterial foot pulses;

2. history of intermittent claudication;

3. male sex;

4. femoral bruit;

5. lower skin temperature on palpation of one foot;

6. age above 60;

7. smoking;

8. history of coronary artery disease;

9. history of diabetes mellitus;

10. blood pressure above 165/95 mmHg.

The more of these features are present, the higher the probability that PAD is present. Conversely, each feature that scores negative reduces the probability of PAD being present. Thus, in many patients that present with leg complaints on walking, the general practitioner will be able to exclude PAD with a high certainty. However, only in a small number of patients he will be able to establish the diagnosis of PAD with enough certainty. In many cases additional investigations will be needed:

♦ to establish the diagnosis, if it is ambiguous on clinical grounds;

♦ to assess the location and severity of stenoses, when the diagnosis has been established but specialist intervention is being considered.

Table 2 Differential diagnosis

Diagnosis	Different from PAD	Worse/relieved	Other
Spinal stenosis (pseudoclaudication, Verbiest's syndrome)	Pain on walking, not on cycling Paraesthesia rather than pain	Pain usually increases on: standing, carrying heavy object Pain decreases on: sitting down, leaning against wall, bending back	Severity of complaints on walking are variable, i.e. not reproducible: 'good' and 'bad' days
Sciatic pain, lumbar disc prolapse	Backache Radiation into the leg	Complaints worsened by coughing, sneezing, exerting pressure (LDP)	
Peripheral neuropathies	Distal pain Loss of sensation, paraesthesia, hyperaesthesia Loss of power		Association with diabetes
Osteoarthrosis	Pain at rest (sitting, standing) Joints: knee, hip, lumbar region Stiffness with inactivity: pain already on start of walking	Complaints usually worst in the morning After some walking: pain decreases After long walk: pain increases Then standing still: pain decreases only slowly or not at all	Not reproducible: 'good' and 'bad' days
Chronic venous insufficiency	History of varicose veins Standing occupation Tired, heavy, dull, painful sensation in the (lower) legs, also at rest Nocturnal cramps in the calves Itch (secondary to dermatitis) Swollen ankles	More complaints at night than in the morning Standing: complaints usually increase Walking: complaints often decrease Leg elevation: complaints often decrease	Not reproducible: 'good' and 'bad' days
Nocturnal leg cramps			Especially in the elderly Also occurring in chronic venous insufficiency Usually no PAD
Restless legs			Neurovegetative lability? Iron deficiency? Usually no PAD
Thromboangiitis obliterans (Bürger's disease) Entrapment of the popliteal artery Anterior tibial artery syndrome			Especially in young people

Investigations

If the diagnosis of PAD cannot be rejected, non-invasive testing is appropriate. In most cases measurement of the ankle–brachial systolic pressure index (ABPI) is sufficient. Sometimes an additional exercise test is necessary. Specialist investigations to assess the severity of PAD, that is, to motivate the choice of invasive treatment decisions, are duplex scanning, angiography, and magnetic resonance angiography.

Investigations to establish the diagnosis of PAD

Measurement of the *ABPI at rest* is a fairly simple technique that can be done in primary care in 10–15 min. To guarantee reproducibility, sufficient experience should be maintained, which will be easier in group practices, health centres, or primary care diagnostic centres. While the patient is lying flat, systolic pressures are taken at both arms (brachial artery) and ankles (posterior tibial or dorsalis pedis artery) using a hand-held Doppler stethoscope and a manometer. ABPI is defined as the ankle pressure divided by the highest arm pressure. In a healthy arterial system, the ankle pressure is higher than the brachial pressure (ABPI >1.0). PAD is considered present when the ABPI is below 0.9. In general, patients with intermittent claudication seen in primary care have ABPI values between 0.5 and 0.8. A validation study in general practice comparing the ABPI with more sophisticated non-invasive testing, yielded the following rules of thumb for primary care:

- PAD can be excluded (predicted probability ≥99 per cent) if the ABPI measured once is above 1.1 or if the mean of three measurements is above 1.0.

- PAD is most probably present (predicted probability ≥95 per cent) if the ABPI measured once is below 0.8 or if the mean of three measurements is below 0.9.

Some patients with diabetes mellitus have hardly compressible arterial walls (Mönckenberg's sclerosis). In such cases, the ABPI cannot be assessed accurately.

An *exercise test* can further reduce the number of false negative test results. The ABPI is measured at rest and then several times after exercise (walking on a treadmill). A drop in the ABPI by more than 30 per cent of the initial resting index or an absolute drop of more than 20 mmHg indicates PAD. This procedure can be carried out in larger diagnostic centres or in vascular function departments of general hospitals.

Specialist investigations to assess the severity of PAD

Duplex scanning is a non-invasive technique, combining pulsed-Doppler signal analysis and B-mode ultrasound (video screen). Site, size, and degree of arterial obstructions can be assessed in a patient friendly manner. On the basis of its results in most cases a treatment decision—angioplasty or bypass surgery—can be made.

Table 3 History

Are there symptoms of intermittent claudication?	
Ischaemic nature of complaints?	Pain or other discomfort in leg
	Induced by exercise (walking)
	Quickly relieved (<10 min) in rest
	Worse when walking uphill or in a hurry or carrying a load
	No complaints on sitting or standing
Location?	Calf, buttock, thigh
	One/both legs
Reproducible pattern?	Similar complaints after same walking distance
Impaired maximum walking distance	</>100 m
Are there symptoms associated with the development of critical ischaemia?	
Pain at rest?	At night? Relieved when suspending the leg over the edge of the bed or by getting up briefly?
	At rest?
Location?	Forefoot, toes
Colour of skin?	Dusky red hue on dependency, pallor on elevation
Skin or nail problems?	Irregular growing nails
	Badly healing wounds, ulcers (heel, toes)
Does the patient feel impaired by his/her complaints?	
Less physical activity?	
Restrictions in daily life?	Work, home, shopping, hobbies, sleep
	Social life
	Holidays
Are there other clinically relevant issues?	
Presence of cardiovascular risk factors	Smoking
	Family history (event in first-degree relative before age 60)
	Diabetes
	Hypertension
	Hypercholesterolaemia
Co-occurence of cardiovascular diseases	
Use of vaso-active medication	Ergotamine, beta-blocking agents
Impaired mobility due to other chronic conditions	COPD, congestive heart failure, osteoarthrosis, rheumatoid arthritis

Angiography has long been the 'gold standard' for the detection of arterial obstructions. After puncture of the common femoral artery, a small catheter is introduced, contrast agent is injected and X-ray pictures are taken. Digital subtraction techniques strongly improve contrast resolution, allowing a smaller amount of contrast fluid to be used. In many cases the choice between angioplasty and surgical intervention can be made by duplex scanning. When bypass surgery appears to be the preferred treatment option, additional angiography may be necessary. During angioplasty, supplementary angiography sometimes is required.

Magnetic resonance angiography (MRA) is a rapidly evolving technique for the assessment of PAD. Neither X-rays nor catheterization is necessary. Recent meta-analyses conclude that MRA is highly accurate for the detection of relevant stenoses or occlusions in the entire lower extremity arterial tree.

Management

PAD: cardiovascular risk management

Since patients with PAD, regardless of their complaints or symptoms, form a patient category with a high risk of cardiovascular morbidity and mortality, the basic treatment strategy for all PAD patients is cardiovascular risk management. In asymptomatic PAD patients, a cardiovascular risk chart—for example, the joint British societies chart, the joint European societies chart, the New Zealand tables—can be used for individualized cardiovascular risk calculation. Risk factors that can be influenced are smoking, diabetes mellitus, hypertension, hypercholesterolaemia, overweight, and hyperhomocysteinaemia. Risk factors that cannot be influenced are male sex, ageing, and family predisposition.

Smoking cessation

Smoking is the most important risk factor for the development of intermittent claudication, worsening of the condition, and the occurrence of complications. In contrast to patients with a myocardial infarction, of whom around 50 per cent stop smoking permanently, the number of patients with PAD who actually stop smoking is low, about 10 per cent. In general, the effectiveness of strategies for giving up smoking is disappointing. The success rate varies from 5 per cent (advised once) to 26 per cent (intensive support programme including nicotine patches). In general practice, the maximum success rate is around 20 per cent. The best way to motivate patients to give up smoking probably is to keep repeating the message of (on smoking cessation) what can be achieved by giving up smoking and explaining the possible consequences of not giving up smoking, in personal conversations between doctor and patient. Examples are given in Table 6. See also Chapter 11.1 in Vol. 1.

Control of hypertension

Treating hypertension reduces the incidence of stroke and coronary heart disease. The literature on the treatment of hypertension in patients with PAD is mostly limited to the effectiveness of drugs and their side-effects. Most attention is focused on beta-blocking agents. These drugs have scarcely any effect on symptoms or on walking distance. However, patients do report being disturbed by cold feet, as is often the case with beta-blockers. So, other antihypertensives like diuretics and ACE inhibitors, could be considered for PAD patients presenting with hypertension for the first time.

Control of diabetes mellitus

Intensive treatment and support of patients with insulin-dependent diabetes mellitus results mainly in a reduction of microvascular complications. One can probably extrapolate from this to patients with diabetes mellitus type II. The effects of good control on the course of macrovascular complications are less clear.

Control of lipids

The introduction of statins has allowed an effective reduction in cholesterol concentration. Although an extreme reduction of the serum cholesterol concentration in experimental studies does result in angiographic regression of atherosclerosis, the clinical relevance for the treatment of PAD has not been established. However, most current guidelines on secondary cardiovascular prevention advocate the use of a statin in patients with intermittent claudication and a raised cholesterol level to reduce the risk of myocardial infarction and stroke. In patients with asymptomatic PAD (ABPI <0.90), prescribing a statin could be considered in those cases in whom other cardiovascular risk factors are present.

Reduction of overweight

Theoretically, excess weight limits walking distance. One study reported that each added extra kilogram reduced the claudication distance by 10 m. Weight control by a calorie-controlled diet and encouraging exercise should form part of the secondary prevention of vascular disease.

Reducing hyperhomocysteinaemia

Administering folic acid reduces the homocysteine level. It is unknown yet whether this also results in clinical relevant reduction of (cardio)vascular disease. Several trials are currently being conducted.

Table 4 Examination

Vascular physical examination		
Inspection of skin, nails, hair of feet and lower legs	Trophic disturbances? Colour?	Left–right difference?
Palpation of skin temperature of feet and lower legs	Cold? Left and right	Left–right difference?
Palpation of arterial pulses of feet and legs	Dorsalis pedis artery, left and right	Present/weak/absent
if there are no pulsations in both foot arteries	Posterior tibial artery, left and right	Present/weak/absent
Auscultation	Femoral artery, left and right	Present/weak/absent
Elevation-dependency test	Popliteal artery, left and right	Present/weak/absent
	Femoral artery, left and right	Present/weak/absent
	Left and right. Elevation: quickly appearing pallor?	Left–right difference?
	Dependency: slowly becoming rosy/red, finally dusky red hue?	
General cardiovascular examination		
Blood pressure		
Body mass index		
Stigmata of hypercholesterolaemia	Arcus lipoides, xanthelasmata, xanthomas of triceps and achilles tendon	
After diagnosis PAD has been established		
Auscultation	Heart, carotid arteries, abdominal aorta	
Palpation	Abdominal aorta	
Laboratory	Fasting glucose level, cholesterol (total, HDL)	

Table 5 Diagnostic value of signs and symptoms associated with PAD

Variable	Categories	Odds ratio	95% Confidence interval	Sensitivity (%)	Specificity (%)	Predictive value+ (%)	Predictive value− (%)
Patient record							
Gender	Female, male	1.8	(1.4–2.4)	59	56	12	93
Age group	40 ≤60, 60 ≤80 years	4.1	(3.0–5.7)	77	55	15	96
Ischaemic heart disease	No, yes	3.5	(2.6–4.6)	48	79	19	94
Cerebrovascular disease	No, yes	3.8	(2.5–5.9)	14	96	26	92
Hypercholesterolaemia	No, yes	1.9	(1.3–2.7)	19	89	15	92
Diabetes mellitus	No, yes	2.5	(1.7–3.5)	20	91	18	92
History							
Intermittent claudication	No, yes	5.6	(4.2–8.1)	31	93	30/45[a]	93
Smoking	No/stop >5 years, yes/stop <5 years	1.8	(1.3–2.4)	71	42	11	94
Examination							
Wounds or sores toes/foot	No, yes	6.0	(1.8–19.3)	2	99.7	38	91
Colour of foot/leg	Normal, abnormal[b]	3.8	(2.8–5.1)	35	87	22	93
Unilateral lower skin temperature	No, yes	6.4	(3.9–12.3)	10	98	36	92
Posterior tibial and dorsalis pedis pulse	Normal, abnormal[c]	30.4	(20.2–45.8)	73	92	41	98
	Normal, doubt	8.6	(5.8–12.9)	69	80	17	98
Femoral artery pulse	Strong, absent	6.1	(2.9–13.0)	7	99	31	93
	Strong, weak	3.7	(2.7–5.0)	33	67	21	93
Femoral artery bruit	No, yes	7.8	(5.4–10.9)	29	95	37	93
Body mass index	≤30, >30	0.6	(0.39–0.86)	13	79	6	90
Blood pressure	Normal, high[d]	1.8	(1.4–2.4)	51	63	12	93

[a] PV+ = 45% if criteria for 'typical' intermittent claudication are met.

[b] Abnormal = pale, red, or blue.

[c] Normal combinations = strong/strong or strong/weak, abnormal = absent/absent or absent/weak.

[d] High = systolic >160 mmHg or diastolic ≥95 mmHg.

PAD: ABPI <0.90, present in 9% of all legs, 12% of all individuals; n = 4910 legs of 1340 women and 1115 men, aged 40–78.

Adapted from: Stoffers, H.E.J.H. et al. (1997). Diagnostic value of signs and symptoms associated with peripheral arterial occlusive disease seen in general practice. *Medical Decision Making* **17**, 61–70.

Table 6 The benefits of giving up smoking for PAD patients

Benefit	Evidence
Better life expectancy	Non-smokers with PAD live 8–10 years longer than smokers
Longer walking with less pain	Walking distance improves in many patients (85%) who have stopped smoking compared with 20% among those who did not stop
Less progression of symptoms; less surgery and amputation	Compared to non-smokers and patients who have stopped smoking, patients who continue smoking are more likely to experience a worsening of symptoms, particularly rest pain, and to require surgical intervention or even amputation
Less re-occlusions after bypass surgery	Among non-smokers or patients who have stopped smoking, the number of re-occlusions after peripheral bypass surgery is three to four times as low as among smokers
Less fatal heart attacks	People with PAD are two to three times as likely as the rest of the population to die of ischaemic heart disease within 5 years. Stopping smoking cuts this risk by half

Intermittent claudication: conservative treatment

The issue of smoking cessation has been discussed earlier.

Walking exercise

Conservative therapy of intermittent claudication includes the advice to perform daily walking exercises to improve functioning in daily life. Compared to percutaneous transluminal angioplasty (PTA) walking exercise possibly has better results after 6 months. Recent meta-analyses and reviews showed that pain free and maximum walking distance of patients with intermittent claudication both improve. There is no conclusive evidence yet on improvement of functional status or quality of life.

Many exercise protocols exist; important factors for success appear to be: duration more than 6 months, a frequency more than or equal to three sessions per week, not less than 30 min per session, and supervision of any kind. Walking until near maximum pain has better results than other forms of exercise. Until supervised programmes become more widely available, the role of exercise supervisor might be taken up by the general practitioner and perhaps also by a trained practice nurse or physiotherapist.

Foot care

Even when the PAD patient does not suffer from diabetes as well, good foot care is important to prevent damage to the skin. Some advice:

- Do not walk barefoot; wear good-fitting, low shoes with a wide toe; wear good-fitting socks or stockings and use a fresh pair every day.
- Wash your feet daily in warm (not hot) water; dry gently without fierce rubbing; use oil to prevent a dry skin.
- Do not cut your toenails but use a nail file.
- Callosity and corns should be removed by a chiropodist.
- In case of a wound or a fungal infection see your doctor.
- In case of foot deformations, specially made or orthopaedic shoes should be worn.

Medical treatment of PAD

Antithrombotic drugs

The combination of aspirin and dipyridamole was studied in patients with moderate to severe PAD in a hospital population. A positive effect of aspirin on the degree of obstruction measured angiographically could be demonstrated. These results have not been confirmed in clinical studies on PAD (claudication symptoms, walking distance, specialist interventions).

The benefits of aspirin in the secondary prevention of myocardial infarction and stroke have been convincingly shown in several larger studies. Recent reviews on the use of aspirin as secondary prophylaxis for vascular disease recommend that patients with intermittent claudication who have additional cardiovascular risk factors should be treated with aspirin. Other reviews indicate that new platelet inhibitors like ticlopidine and clopidogrel could reduce clinically important vascular events in patients with intermittent

claudication even better than aspirin, but there is some uncertainty about the size of the additional benefit. Both agents are associated with less gastrointestinal haemorrhage and other upper gastrointestinal upset than aspirin. They can be prescribed to patients who are intolerant of aspirin. More experience in general practice is required before a definite judgement on large-scale application of these drugs can be given.

Other drugs

Vasodilators (sympathicolytics, calcium antagonists, nicotinic acid derivatives, cyclandelate) are neither effective in reducing atherosclerotic narrowing, nor beneficial with regard to claudication symptoms or walking distance. They often produce side-effects such as orthostatic dizziness, flushing, throbbing headaches, oedema of the ankles and palpitations, including reflex tachycardia. Also for buflomedil, the evidence for clinical efficacy in intermittent claudication is lacking.

The positive effect of pentoxifylline on peripheral blood flow, particularly in the microcirculation, is primarily attributed to the increased plasticity of the erythrocytes. Reviews of placebo-controlled studies concluded that treatment with pentoxifylline can lead to a moderate improvement in walking distance. If the effect is unsatisfactory after 3 months, there is no point in continuing.

Specialist interventions

Referral

An absolute indication for referral is the subacute development of critical ischaemia (arterial thrombosis) in patients with intermittent claudication. This condition requires thrombolyis followed by endovascular or surgical intervention.

Patients with intermittent claudication should be referred to a vascular specialist if symptoms deteriorate—increasing pain or decreasing walking distance or a progressive drop of the ABPI. Also when the patient complains of stable claudication interfering with his daily life (work, hobbies, social life), and not improving by regular walking exercise, a visit to the specialist to discuss the potential benefit of an invasive intervention is warranted.

Specialist interventions for chronic PAD

Percutaneous transluminal angioplasty (PTA) with or without stent may be appropriate for patients with intermittent claudication or critical ischaemia. The treatment goal is better quality of life through better walking capacity and less pain. *Bypass surgery* at various levels, using autologous venous or synthetic grafts may be appropriate in patients with serious, disabling intermittent claudication or critical ischaemia. The treatment goal in these patients is limb salvage. *Amputation* can be applied at various levels, from toe to upper leg, and is appropriate in cases of critical limb ischaemia when limb salvage is no longer possible. The chances of good wound healing (proximal vascularization) and rehabilitation capacity of the patient guide the choice of the level of amputation.

The choice of endovascular or surgical procedure depends on the site of the arterial lesion (aorta, iliac, femoropopliteal; uni- versus bilateral; mono- versus multilevel), its size (stenosis or occlusion, long or short) and the general medical condition of the patient. Treatment decisions are best made in a multidisciplinary vascular team. When amputation is considered, a rehabilitation specialist should be consulted, preferably before the intervention.

Long-term and continuing care

PAD is a manifestation of a systemic disease, atherosclerosis, and is a chronic condition. This implies that the patient, the general practitioner, and the vascular specialist have to collaborate. Once the diagnosis has been established it is the responsibility of the general practitioner to plan regular follow-up meetings with the patient. The general practitioner's tasks can be described as follows:

- Monitoring the course of the disease (symptoms, vascular status, ABPI, functional status), including the patient's cardiovascular risk profile, and treating medical conditions appropriately.

- Guiding and supervising necessary lifestyle changes. Stopping smoking, doing exercise, following a diet, or losing weight is nearly impossible merely by prescription only. It requires an active, voluntary collaborative involvement of both patient and supervisor. Various methods exist to support the patient's behavioural change: health counselling, stages of change, minimal intervention strategy. The role of 'lifestyle counsellor' could be taken up by the general practitioner but also by other personnel such as trained practice nurses, physiotherapists, and dieticians.

- Being an intermediate between patient and vascular specialists: interventional radiologist, vascular surgeon, and rehabilitation physician, the general practitioner not only keeps the medical record of his patient, but is also familiar with his/her psychosocial context. Both perspectives are crucial in medical decision-making regarding specialist interventions.

Key points on differential diagnosis and management

- The key to the clinical diagnosis of PAD is a thorough vascular physical examination.

- Measurement of the ankle–brachial systolic pressure index (ABPI) is a valid diagnostic technique to confirm the diagnosis of PAD in primary care.

- A reduced ABPI is associated with an increased risk of cardiovascular morbidity and mortality.

- Conservative treatment of patients with PAD is aimed at increasing walking distance and improving functional capacity.

- A patient with PAD belongs to a cardiovascular high-risk group and one of the main objectives of treatment is optimizing the cardiovascular risk profile to prevent future ischaemic heart disease or stroke.

- Patients should be encouraged to stop smoking, keep walking, and take the medication prescribed for hypertension, diabetes, hypercholesterolaemia, and atherothrombosis.

Further reading

Stoffers, H.E.J.H., Kaiser, V., Kester, A.D.M., Rinkens, P.E.L.M., and Knottnerus, J.A. (1997). Diagnostic value of signs and symptoms associated with peripheral arterial occlusive disease seen in general practice: a multi-variable approach. *Medical Decision Making* **17** (1), 61–70. (A cross-sectional study among 2455 individuals with leg complaints, from 18 general practice centres. Signs and symptoms were compared with the results of non-invasive testing. The resulting multivariable model can be used as a diagnostic checklist.)

Stoffers, H.E.J.H., Kester, A.D.M., Kaiser, V., Rinkens, P.E.L.M., Kitslaar, P.J.E.H.M., and Knottnerus, J.A. (1996). The diagnostic value of the measurement of the ankle-brachial systolic pressure index in primary health care. *Journal of Clinical Epidemiology* **49** (12), 1401–5. (A study among 117 subjects from three general practice centres. The ABPI measured in primary care is validated against more sophisticated non-invasive tests. The authors provide a rule of thumb for the interpretation of ABPI results in primary care.)

Hooi, J.D., Stoffers, H.E.J.H., Knottnerus, J.A., and van Ree, J.W. (1999). The prognosis of non-critical limb ischaemia: a systematic review of population-based evidence. *British Journal of General Practice* **49**, 49–55. (A criteria-based review of population-based studies on the prognosis of symptomatic and asymptomatic PAD with regard to PAD symptom progression, cardiovascular morbidity, and mortality.)

Hirsch, A.T. et al. (2001). Peripheral arterial disease detection, awareness, and treatment in primary care. *Journal of the American Medical Association* **286** (11), 1317–24. (A comprehensive multicentre study on diagnosis, treatment, and prevention in primary care among 6979 patients from 350 primary care practices. Main message: primary care physicians can perform better!)

Antithrombotic Trialists' Collaboration (2002). Collaborative meta-analysis of randomized trials of antiplatelet therapy for prevention of death, myocardial infarction and stroke in high risk patients. *British Medical Journal* **324**, 71–86. (The latest update on antithrombotic drugs. In the same issue critical comments on pages 59–60 by M. Reilly and G.A. FitzGerald and on the pages 103–5 by J.G.F. Cleland.)

Leng, G.C., Fowler, B., and Ernst, E. (2002). Exercise for intermittent claudication (Cochrane Review). In *The Cochrane Library* Issue 1. Oxford: Update Software. (A criteria-based review of randomized trials of exercise regimens in patients with intermittent claudication.)

Hankey, G.J., Sudlow, C.L.M., and Dunbabin, D.W. (2002). Thienopyridine derivatives (ticlopidine, clopidogrel) versus aspirin for preventing stroke and other serious vascular events in high vascular risk patients (Cochrane Review). In *The Cochrane Library* Issue 1. Oxford: Update Software. (A critical review of four trials among vascular high-risk patients.)

Leng, G.C., Price, J.F., and Jepson, R.G. (2002). Lipid-lowering for lower limb atherosclerosis (Cochrane Review). In *The Cochrane Library* Issue 1. Oxford: Update Software. (A review of seven trials involving 698 participants from seven different countries. Lipid-lowering therapy produced a marked but non-significant reduction in mortality but little change in non-fatal events.)

Donelly, R. and London, N.J.M. *ABC of Arterial and Venous Disease.* London: BMJ Books, 2000. (This guide is the book version of the series of articles in the *British Medical Journal*. It provides up-to-date coverage of the diagnosis and investigation of the diseases, as well as clinical management chapters and strategies for complication prevention. The book is very well illustrated.)

Wood, D. et al. *Clinician's Manual on Total Risk Management. A Guide to Prevention of Coronary Heart Disease.* London: Science Press, 2000. (This guide is written by members of the 'Joint European Societies Task Force on Coronary Prevention'. It contains chapters on the use of coronary risk charts, behavioural change, and lifestyle modification.)

The Cochrane Library (www.update-software.com/cochrane/) contains regularly updated databases on intermittent claudication, for example systematic reviews, controlled trials, health technology assessment and economic evaluations of healthcare interventions. Some reviews are cited above.

1.6 Thrombosis and thromboembolism

David A. Fitzmaurice

Introduction

Venous thromboembolic disease consists of two clinical entities, deep vein thrombosis (DVT) and pulmonary embolism (PE), which are different manifestations of the same disease process. The principal manifestation of arterial thromboembolism is stroke although arterial thrombosis and emboli can occur throughout the arterial tree.

The challenge for primary care lies mainly in diagnosis although more recently there have been developments in preventative strategies especially based on the identification of patients with either acquired or congenital thrombophilia. This chapter describes the diagnosis and management of venous and arterial thromboembolic disease from a primary care perspective.

Venous thromboembolic disease

Venous thromboembolism is a major cause of morbidity and mortality worldwide, although routine data collection for these conditions is unreliable. US data suggest that there are around 250 000 hospital admissions, with around 50 000 deaths, for either DVT or PE, per year.[1] The fatality rate from acute PE appears not to have altered since the 1970s.

Deep vein thrombosis

The typical presentation of DVT is as an acutely painful, red swollen calf. It can be defined as a radiologically confirmed partial or total occlusion of the deep venous system of the leg sufficient to produce symptoms of pain or swelling.[2] DVT is associated with pregnancy, contraceptive pill use, immobility, surgery, malignancy, advancing age, smoking, and certain clotting disorders.[3] Both proximal and isolated calf vein thromboses can cause post-thrombotic syndrome, recurrent venous thrombosis and pulmonary embolus, with associated morbidity and mortality.

Anticoagulation, in terms of early intervention with heparin and warfarin and with prolonged warfarin treatment, has been demonstrated to reduce sequelae associated with DVT, particularly PE.[4] Since anticoagulation therapy carries a risk of haemorrhagic complications it is important that a diagnosis of DVT is objectively confirmed before starting treatment. The treatment of below-knee DVT remains controversial but there is evidence that when calf thrombi are symptomatic anticoagulation treatment is of benefit.[5]

Diagnosis and investigation

The clinical diagnosis of DVT is generally made on the basis of pain, swelling, venous distension, and pain on forced dorsiflexion of the foot (Homan's sign).[6] The differential diagnosis includes musculo-skeletal pain and popliteal inflammatory cysts (Baker's cysts).[6] It has traditionally been taught that the clinical diagnosis of DVT is unreliable.[7]

The gold standard for diagnosis is venography, but this is an invasive test which is inconvenient, painful, and can be associated with allergic and other side-effects.[7]

Although light reflection rheography is an effective non-invasive technique for screening patients with suspected DVT,[8] the method of choice is ultrasonography, whilst D-dimer tests can be used as a pre-screening tool before ultrasound. The sensitivity and specificity of ultrasound has been reported as 78 and 98 per cent, respectively.[7] D-dimer tests indicate active fibrinolysis and hence provide a screening technique for DVT. Whilst not specific to DVT, D-dimer has a high (>95 per cent) negative predictive value and is a reliable method for the exclusion of DVT in symptomatic patients.[9]

Prevention

One of the most useful advances in the area of thromboembolic disease has been preventative therapy, particularly pre-operatively. For patients who are at high risk or for high-risk operations, there are a variety of options to reduce the incidence of DVT. These include formal anticoagulation, use of compression stockings, intraoperative pressure devices, and use of low-molecular weight heparin (LMWH). There are reports of newer agents such as oral thrombin inhibitors which appear to be as effective as warfarin in both treatment and prevention of thromboembolism, but these remain to be confirmed.

A significant risk factor for DVT is the use of female hormones, either as hormone replacement therapy (HRT) or as oral contraception. The increased risk is very small, however, and particularly in the case of oral contraception, the overall health risk of not taking therapy outweighs the risk of taking it. The absolute risk of venous thrombosis in healthy young women is around 1 per 10 000 person-years, rising to 3–4 per 10 000 person-years during the time oral contraceptives are being used.[10] Pregnancy, however, is itself a risk factor for DVT. Pregnant patients at high risk or with a previous history of thrombosis should be treated with LMWH. Warfarin is contra-indicated in pregnancy as it is teratogenic.

Various conditions predispose to a clotting tendency. These are generally congenital (e.g. Factor V Leiden, protein C deficiency) but may be acquired (e.g. lupus anticoagulant antiphospholipid syndrome). These are generally not problematic and are only investigated if a patient presents with an unusual thrombotic history or recurrent miscarriage.

An increasing problem encountered in primary care is what to do with patients who have a history of thrombosis and wish to travel by air. The risk of thrombosis appears to be greatest when there is travel of over 6 h and the patient is confined to a particular position (usually sitting). Traveller's thrombosis has been reported from air, car, and bus travel. If there is any suggestion of an association between long-distance travel and thrombosis or there is a strong family history of thrombosis, then specialist referral is indicated. The risk of prolonged travel, either by air or other means, is probably overstated, with patients suffering an event being predisposed to thromboembolism anyway. The principal risk factor for traveller's thrombosis appears to be previous history of a clot. The main preventive measures are the use of full-length graduated compression stockings,[11] or prophylactic LMWH. In flight measures should include exercise and the avoidance of dehydration.

Treatment

The goals of treatment of DVT are prevention of PE with the restoration of venous patency and valvular function.[12,13] Standard management for these patients remains emergency referral to hospital for diagnostic confirmation, bed rest, and commencement of anticoagulation. Anticoagulation typically involves a hospital inpatient stay of around 7 days for intravenous heparin administration with daily partial thromboplastin time (PTT) estimation, together with warfarin for approximately 3 months (with monitoring).[6] Recent studies and a meta-analysis have shown that subcutaneous administration of LMWH is as safe and effective as traditional intravenous therapy with less complications and the advantage that PTT monitoring is not required.[14] Dosing schedules for LMWH are based solely on body weight. Secondary care data suggested that LMWH can be cost effective due to the reduced cost of monitoring and reduced hospital stay.[15] These studies also highlighted the possibility of home treatment, with patients either self-dosing or receiving injections from a nurse or a relative.[16]

Whilst oral anticoagulation is established in the treatment of patients with DVT, the duration of therapy remains debatable. Two prospective randomized studies of treatment of proximal DVT, comparing 4 weeks with 3 months[17] and 6 weeks with 6 months warfarin therapy,[18] have gone some way to resolving the issue. Whilst there are problems in comparing studies due to difficulties in standardizing diagnostic criteria, these studies showed recurrence rates after 2 years of 8.6 per cent in the 4-week group compared with 0.9 per cent in the 3-month group (odds ratio = 10.1,

95 per cent confidence interval 1.3–81.4), and 18.1 per cent in the 6-week group compared to 9.5 per cent in the 6-month group (odds ratio = 2.1, 95 per cent confidence interval 1.4–3.1).

Debate continues over the treatment of distal DVT where thrombus is limited to the calf veins only. However, evidence for treatment is strong. Untreated symptomatic calf vein thrombosis in non-surgical patients has a recurrence rate of over 25 per cent, with an attendant risk of proximal extension and pulmonary embolization. This risk is reduced to 7.6 per cent with treatment aiming for an INR of 2.0–3.0 for 3 months, which compares with rates of 12.4 per cent with 4 weeks, 11.8 per cent with 6 weeks, and 5.8 per cent with 6 months oral anticoagulant therapy.[18]

Recommendations for DVT

Treatment of idiopathic proximal DVT should be continued for 6 months. For patients with isolated DVT without continuing risk factors, 6 weeks oral anticoagulation therapy is sufficient. The evidence for patients with idiopathic symptomatic isolated calf vein thrombosis supports treatment aimed at a target INR of 2.5 for 3 months. For post-operative calf-vein thrombosis, however, 6 weeks therapy is as effective as treatment for 3 months. The guidelines for recurrent thrombosis whilst off treatment recommend lifelong therapy, and for recurrence whilst on treatment lifelong therapy at a higher therapeutic intensity.

Pulmonary embolism

Pulmonary emboli usually arise from veins in the pelvis and leg. The risk factors are the same as for DVT. Up to 50 per cent of those with fatal PE have no warning signs. The clinical presentation depends upon the size of the emboli with small emboli remaining asymptomatic. Large non-fatal emboli cause acute pleuritic chest pain associated with shortness of breath, tachycardia, and pyrexia. Associated features include haemoptysis, pleural effusion, hypotension, cyanosis, and shock. All cases of suspected PE need to be treated as medical emergencies with admission to hospital arranged if possible. The mainstay of diagnosis remains the ventilation/perfusion scan although a spiral CT scan is now regarded as the gold standard for diagnosis.

Treatment

The management of PE includes haemodynamic stabilization and thrombolysis, followed by anticoagulate in exactly the same manner as for DVT. This remains essentially the same today although advances in the use of LMWH for DVT have prompted investigations into the use of LMWH for the home management of PE.[19] Whilst this may be suitable for a small number of stable patients, the main priority from a primary care perspective is to arrange for hospital admission for assessment, stabilization and confirmation of the diagnosis.

No studies have looked specifically at the intensity of oral anticoagulation therapy for the treatment of pulmonary embolus. The current UK recommendation for patients diagnosed with a first pulmonary embolus is to aim for an INR of 2.5. These recommendations are based on results of studies primarily investigating the treatment of proximal DVT where the occurrence of a pulmonary embolus was taken as an endpoint in interventional studies.

Data are available which show that fatal recurrence of pulmonary embolus following DVT is extremely rare when treated, with heparin initially, followed by a longer period of warfarin therapy.[20] The range of INR between 2.0 and 3.0 was chosen as it gives the lowest recurrence and bleeding rates in treatment of proximal deep vein thrombosis.[21]

Recommendations for pulmonary embolus

The clinical decision as to whether or not to anticoagulate patients with suspected PE will be dependent upon the strength of the clinical suspicion (pre-test probability) combined with the results of ventilation perfusion scanning.[22] Patients with a normal or low probability scan should not be treated.[23]

Arterial thromboembolic disease

The most serious manifestation of arterial thromboembolism is stroke. In this case, emboli arise from the left side of the heart (e.g. mural thrombus following myocardial infarction, atrial fibrillation, mitral valve disease) or the carotid arteries. Formal anticoagulation with warfarin is recommended for patients with a demonstrable ischaemic stroke when either a left-sided heart lesion or atrial fibrillation is found. This should not be commenced until at least 14 days after the initial event.

Short-term warfarin is effective in preventing reocclusion in peripheral arterial reconstructive surgery. Antiplatelet therapy (usually aspirin) should be the first line treatment in all other situations. Warfarin may have a role as a therapeutic adjunct but no evidence exists on this subject at present.

Warfarin has not been evaluated in the immediate post-operative period for vein graft occlusion, although it is known that this is invariably due to thrombosis. Aspirin reduces thrombotic risk by up to 30 per cent and should be first line therapy.

Aspirin and heparin reduce the risk of acute occlusion following angioplasty. There are currently no data for warfarin in either angioplasty or for patients with coronary artery stents. Aspirin is recommended as first line treatment.

References

1. Anderson, F.A. Jr. et al. (1991). A population-based perspective of the hospital incidence and case-fatality rates of venous thrombosis and pulmonary embolism: The Worcester DVT study. *Archives of Internal Medicine* **151**, 933–8.

2. Fitzmaurice, D. and Hobbs, F. (1999). Thromboembolism. *Clinical Evidence* Issue 2, 130–5.

3. Hirsh, J. and Hoak, J. (1996). Management of deep vein thrombosis and pulmonary embolism. *Circulation* **93**, 2212–45.

4. Lensing, A.W.A., Prandoni, P., Prins, M.H., and Buller, H.R. (1999). Deep vein thrombosis. *Lancet* **353**, 470–84.

5. Giannoukas, A.D., Labropoulos, N., Burke, P., Katsamouris, A., and Nicolaides, A.N. (1995). Calf deep venous thrombosis: a review of the literature. *European Journal of Vascular and Endovascular Surgery* **10**, 398–404.

6. Weinman, E.E. and Salzman, E.W. (1994). Deep-vein thrombosis. *New England Journal of Medicine* **331**, 1630–44.

7. Wells, P.S. et al. (1995). Accuracy of clinical assessment of deep-vein thrombosis. *Lancet* **1**, 1326–30.

8. Thomas, P.R.S., Butler, C.M., Bowman, J., Grieve, N.W.T., Bennett, C.E., Taylor, R.S., and Thomas, M.H. (1991). Light reflection rheography: an effective non-invasive technique for screening patients with suspected deep venous thrombosis. *British Journal of Surgery* **78**, 207–9.

9. Turkstra, F., van Beek, J.R., ten Cate, J.W., and Buller, H.R. (1998). Reliable rapid blood test for the exclusion of venous thromboembolism in symptomatic outpatients. *Thrombosis and Haemostasis* **79**, 32–7.

10. Vandenbroucke, J.P., Rosing, J., Blomenkamp, K.W.M., Middeldorp, S., Helmerhorst, F.M., Bouma, B.N., and Rosendaal, F.R. (2001). Oral contraceptives and risk of venous thrombosis. *New England Journal of Medicine* **344**, 1527–35.

11. Scurr, J.H., Machin, S.J., Bailey-King, S., Mackie, I.J., McDonald, S., and Smith, P.D. (2001). Frequency and prevention of symptomless deep-vein thrombosis in long-haul flights: a randomised trial. *Lancet* **357**, 1485–9.

12. Lagerstedt, C.I., Olsson, C.G., Fagher, B.O., Oqvist, B.W., and Albrechtsson, P. (1985). Need for long term anticoagulant treatment in symptomatic calf vein thrombosis. *Lancet* **ii**, 515–18.

13. Kakkar, V.V. et al. (1969). Natural history of post-operative deep-vein thrombosis. *Lancet* **2**, 230–2.

14. Hull, R. et al. (1992). Subcutaneous low-molecular-weight heparin compared with continuous intravenous heparin in the treatment of proximal vein thrombosis. *New England Journal of Medicine* **326**, 975–82.

15. Gould, M.K., Dembitzer, A.D., Sanders, G.D., and Garber, A.M. (1999). Low-molecular-weight heparins compared with unfractionated heparin for

treatment of acute deep venous thrombosis. A cost-effectiveness analysis. *Annals of Internal Medicine* **130** (10), 789–99.

16. **Wells, P.S., Kovacs, M.J., Bormanis, J., Forgie, M.A., Goudie, D., Morrow, B., and Kovacs, J.** (1998). Expanding eligibility for outpatient treatment of deep venous thrombosis and pulmonary embolism with low-molecular-weight heparin: a comparison of patient self-injection with homecare injection. *Archives of Internal Medicine* **158** (16), 1809–12.

17. **Levine, M.N.** et al. (1995). Optimal duration of oral anticoagulant therapy: a randomized trial comparing four weeks with three months of warfarin in patients with proximal deep vein thrombosis. *Thrombosis and Haemostasis* **74**, 606–11.

18. **Schulman, S.** et al. (1995). A comparison of six weeks with six months of oral anticoagulant therapy after a first episode of venous thromboembolism. *New England Journal of Medicine* **332**, 1661–5.

19. **Simonneau, G.** et al. (1997). A comparison of low-molecular-weight heparin with unfractionated heparin for acute pulmonary embolism. The THESEE Study Group. Tinzaparine ou Heparine Standard: Evaluations dans l'Embolie Pulmonaire. *New England Journal of Medicine* **337**, 663–9.

20. **Carson, J.** et al. (1992). The clinical course of pulmonary embolism. *New England Journal of Medicine* **326**, 1240–5.

21. **Hull, R., Hirsh, J., and Jay, R.** (1982). Different intensities of oral anticoagulation therapy in the treatment of proximal vein thrombosis. *New England Journal of Medicine* **307**, 1676–81.

22. **Fennerty, T.** (1997). The diagnosis of pulmonary embolism. *British Medical Journal* **314**, 425–9.

23. **PIOPED Investigators** (1990). Value of ventilation/perfusion scan in acute pulmonary embolism. *Journal of the American Medical Association* **263**, 2753–9.

1.7 Stroke and transient ischaemia

Charles Wolfe and Anthony G. Rudd

The disease

Stroke (or brain attack) is a clinical diagnosis defined as a syndrome characterized by rapidly developing clinical symptoms and/or signs of focal loss of cerebral function with symptoms lasting more than 24 h or leading to death, with no apparent cause other than that of vascular origin. *Transient ischaemic attack* (TIA) is defined in the same way as stroke but with the deficit lasting less than 24 h. Amaurosis fugax is a TIA affecting the retinal artery producing transient loss of vision in one eye. The pathogenesis of stroke and TIA are the same and should be managed with equal vigour. Stroke can be classified according to the underlying cause [Table 1 (adapted from the TOAST classification[1]) or the affected territory within the brain (Table 2)[2]].

Epidemiology

The impact of stroke is detailed in Tables 3 and 4.

Global picture

It is estimated there are 5.45 million deaths a year from stroke in the world and over 9 million stroke survivors.[3] Sixty-five per cent of these deaths

Table 1 Aetiological classification of stroke[5]

Ischaemic
Cardioembolic, for example
　Atrial fibrillation
　Mural thrombus
　Paradoxical embolism through patent foramen ovale
　Embolism from infective endocarditis
Atherothromboembolic, for example
　Carotid atheroma
　Vertebral atheroma
　Cerebral artery occlusion
　Carotid dissection
Small vessel disease, for example
　Hypertensive arterial disease
　Diabetic vasculopathy
　Vasculitis
Other examples
　Venous thrombosis
Unknown

Haemorrhage
Sub-arachnoid
　Arteriovenous malformation
　Aneurysm
Parenchymal haemorrhage, for example
　Hypertensive arterial disease
　Amyloid angiopathy

Table 2 Clinical classification of stroke[2]

Total anterior circulation strokes (TACS): all of
Contralateral hemiplegia or hemiparesis
Contralateral hemisensory loss
New disturbance of higher cerebral function, for example dysphasia, visuo-spatial disturbance

Partial anterior circulation strokes (PACS): any of
Motor/sensory deficit and hemianopia
Motor/sensory deficit and new higher cortical dysfunction
New higher cortical dysfunction and hemianopia
New higher cortical dysfunction alone
Pure motor deficit less extensive than for LACS, for example monoparesis

Lacunar strokes (occlusion of single deep perforating artery)
Maximum deficit from a single vascular event
No visual field deficit, no new higher cortical dysfunction, no signs of brainstem disturbance

Posterior circulation strokes: any of
Ipsilateral cranial nerve palsy with contra-lateral long tract signs
Bilateral motor and/or sensory deficit
Disorder of conjugate eye movements
Cerebellar dysfunction
Isolated hemianopia or cortical blindness

occur in the developing world. Stroke accounts for nearly 5 million disability adjusted life years lost in the world. The pattern of this impact varies with highest rates in parts of Europe, SE Asia, and the Western Pacific. One in four men and nearly one in five women aged 45 can expect to have a stroke if they live to their 85th year.

There are differences in the standardized mortality ratios (SMRs) for stroke (i.e. mortality rates adjusted for age and sex) between regions of the world, with the highest rates in Eastern Europe and the former Soviet Union (309 and 156 per 100 000 per year among men and 222 and 101 per 100 000 per year among women).[4] Countries with the lowest stroke mortality, such as the United States, Canada, Switzerland, and Australia, experienced the steepest decline.

Table 3 Acute (0–7 days), 3-week and 6-month impairment/disability rates

Phenomenon	Acute[a] (%)	3 weeks (%)	6 months (%)
Impairments			
Initial loss/depression of consciousness	5	—	—
Not oriented (or unable to talk)	55	36	27
Marked communication problems (aphasia)	52	29	15
Motor loss (partial or complete)	80	70	53
Disabilities			
Incontinent of faeces	31	13	7
Incontinent of urine	44	24	11
Needs help grooming (teeth, face, hair)	56	27	13
Needs help with toilet/commode	68	39	20
Needs help with feeding	68	38	33
Needs help moving from bed to chair	70	42	19
Unable to walk independently indoors	73	40	15
Needs help dressing	79	51	31
Needs help bathing	86	65	49
Very severely dependent	38	13	4
Severely dependent	20	13	5
Moderately dependent	15	15	12
Mildly dependent	12	28	32
Physically independent	12	31	47

These data relate only to survivors.

[a] The 'acute' figures are of limited accuracy as many patients were not assessed within the first week; many of these were very ill and probably very dependent. Consequently, the figures relating to acute disability are minimum estimates.

From: Wade, D. (1994). Stroke (acute cerebrovascular disease). In *Health Care Needs Assessment* Vol. 1 (ed. A. Stevens and J. Raftery), pp. 111–255. Oxford: Radcliffe Medical Press.

Table 4 Some figures per 100 000 population (per year where relevant)[6]

General—SAH, TIAs, stroke—diagnosed	
Cases SAH per year	14
New cases TIA per year	42
Carotid territory TIAs	34
First strokes per year	200
All acute strokes per year	240
Stroke survivors alive in community	600
Presenting for diagnosis	Not known
Impairment/disability—presentation (i.e. need acute care), all stroke	
With reduced consciousness	84
Severely dependent	140
Incontinent of urine	106
Disoriented/unable to communicate	132
Unable to get out of bed unaided	168
Impairment/disability—at 3 weeks (i.e. need rehabilitation), all stroke	
Needs help dressing	86
Needs help walking	67
Needs help with toilet	66
Communication problems	49
Impairment/disability—at 6 months (i.e. need long-term support)	
Needs help bathing	71
Needs help walking	22
Needs help dressing	45
Difficulty communicating (aphasia)	22
Confused/demented (or severe aphasia)	39
Severely disabled (Barthel <10/20)	13
Services—at 6 months	
Needs long-term institutional care	23
Possibly needs speech therapy	24

Note: This assumes: all stroke, first and recurrent (2.4 per 1000 per year); 30% die by 3 weeks; 40% die by 6 months; minimal contribution from SAH to care and rehabilitation needs.

Incidence

The incidence of ischaemic stroke doubles with each decade over the age of 55, with an overall rate 0.2 per 1000 in those aged 45–54 and 10 per 1000 in those aged over 85 years.[5,6] As the number of elderly people is increasing worldwide, the burden of stroke on individual families and on the health services is unlikely to fall rapidly. It has been estimated that between 1983 and 2023 there will be an absolute increase in the number of patients experiencing a first stroke of about 30 per cent.

Men have a 25–30 per cent increased chance of having a stroke. African-Caribbean and African men and women have approximately double the risk of stroke compared to the Caucasian population. People in the lowest social class have a 60 per cent increased chance of having a stroke compared to those in the highest social class.[5,6]

Case fatality and recurrence

The risk of death is about 30 per cent by 3 months, but varies according to sub-type. The cumulative risk of recurrence over 5 years is high, ranging from 15 to 42 per cent in community studies and the pathological subtype of recurrence is the same as the index stroke in 88 per cent of cases.[5,6]

Prevalence of stroke

The overall prevalence of stroke is estimated to be 47 per 10 000 and as such is the most common cause of adult physical disability. Cognitive impairment (33 per cent), problems with lower limbs (30 per cent) and speech difficulties (27 per cent) are the most common residual impairments.[5,6]

Needs of families and carers

Carers needs are frequently unrecognized and morbidity amongst carers is high.[7] Carers need information, skills training, emotional support, regular respite, advice about services, and easy access to aids and equipment. Morbidity results from depression and anxiety, physical illness, financial hardship, and social isolation.

Current service provision for stroke

Currently, preventive and therapeutic services for stroke vary considerably within and between countries. Major differences include the structuring and responsibility of primary care for prevention and rehabilitation. Primary care is involved to a varying extent in the acute diagnosis, but where there is involvement prior to emergency care treatment is markedly delayed.

It is estimated that stroke services accounted for at least 4–6 per cent of the NHS budget in the United Kingdom, but these figures do not take into account social service and carer costs. Similar proportions of budgets have been estimated elsewhere.

Primary care

The morbidity survey in general practice in the United Kingdom estimates that circulatory diseases account for 9 per cent of consultations, 36 per cent of which are 'serious' with the most common reason being for essential hypertension. Specific stroke surveys in the United Kingdom over the last 15 years indicate poor follow-up of patients once discharged. Under half of patients were followed up by their GPs, less than a third by community nurses, and less than 20 per cent had access to other services.

Secondary care

Secondary care services for stroke management span many specialties and there are very different patterns of care within and between countries. The outcomes in European hospitals using more resources tend to be better in terms of survival and disability.[8] In an audit of stroke care in the United Kingdom in 1999, only 18 per cent of patients spent over half their stay in a stroke unit which contrasts with surveys in Finland where the majority of patients are managed on a stroke unit.

What are the risks after stroke and how is stroke managed as a chronic disease?

Stroke survivors have a 15-fold increased risk of recurrence. This can be reduced by appropriate risk factor management.[5,6]

The evidence for secondary prevention of stroke

In a population of 1 million, around 2400 will present each year with a first (1800) or recurrent (600) stroke and another 500 with transient ischaemic attack.[9] There will be around 1300 deaths or dependent survivors who may have benefited from appropriate secondary prevention in the United Kingdom. The national clinical guidelines for stroke have been drawn up by a multidisciplinary working party and grade the evidence and make suggestions as to their adaptation for local guidelines[9,10] (Table 5).

Hypertension

The major risk factor for stroke is hypertension. Current trial data, although limited, suggest that lowering blood pressure by 5–6 mmHg diastolic and 10–12 mmHg systolic for 2–3 years should reduce annual risk of stroke from 7 to 4.8 per cent with 45 patients needed to be treated (NNT) to avoid one stroke per year. The PROGRESS trial[11] suggests that treatment with perindopril and indapamide, producing a mean reduction in systolic blood pressure of 9/4 mmHg, reduces the risk of recurrence by 28 per cent (95 per cent CI 17–38, $p < 0.0001$), in both hypertensive and normotensive patients.

Smoking

Smoking increases the risk of stroke by around 50 per cent and reduction by nicotine replacement patches, behavioural modification, combined with advice and social skills training, and encouragement and brief advice given by well-trained GPs or other health professionals during routine

Table 5 Guidelines for secondary prevention applicable to all patients, even those not admitted to hospital[10]

All patients should have their blood pressure checked, and hypertension persisting for over 1 month should be treated (A)
All patients, not on anticoagulation, should be taking aspirin (50–300 mg) daily (A), or low-dose aspirin and dipyridamole modified release (MR). Where patients are aspirin intolerant clopidogrel 75 mg daily or dipyridamole MR 200 mg twice daily should be used (A)
Anticoagulation should be started in every patient in atrial fibrillation unless contraindicated (A)
Anticoagulation should be considered for all patients who have ischaemic stroke associated with mitral valve disease, prosthetic heart valves, or within 3 months of myocardial infarction (C)
Anticoagulation should not be started until brain imaging has excluded haemorrhage, and 14 days have passed from the onset of an acute ischaemic stroke (A)
Anticoagulation should not be used after transient ischaemic attacks or minor strokes unless cardiac embolism is suspected (A)
Any patient with a carotid artery stroke, and minor or absent residual disability should be considered for carotid endarterectomy (A)
Carotid ultrasound should be performed on all patients who would be considered for carotid endarterectomy (C)
Carotid endarterectomy should only be undertaken by a specialist surgeon with a proven low complication rate, and only if the stenosis is measured at greater than 70 per cent (A)
All patients should be assessed for other vascular risk factors and be treated or advised appropriately (B)
All patients should be given appropriate advice on lifestyle factors (C)
Therapy with a statin should be considered for patients with a history of myocardial infarction and a cholesterol above 5 mmol/L following stroke (A)

A, meta-analysis or RCT evidence; B, at least one well-designed controlled, quasi-experimental, or descriptive study; C, expert committee report or respected authority report.

consultations are all effective. The number needed to quit smoking is 43 to avoid one stroke per year.

Cholesterol reduction

The association between raised cholesterol and stroke sub-type is not clear cut. There have been no formal trials of cholesterol lowering in TIA/stroke but there is indirect evidence that cholesterol reduction using statins reduces the risk of stroke risk by around 24 per cent. Sub-group analysis suggests that the NNT for statin therapy would be 59 to avoid one stroke per year.

Antiplatelet drugs

Giving aspirin to patients who have had an ischaemic stroke in doses above 75 mg daily reduces the risk of stroke by around 13 per cent and the NNT is 100. Aspirin is appropriate for around three-quarters of stroke patients and is cheap. Clopidogrel is more effective than aspirin with an NNT of 62. The combination of dipyridamole and aspirin is again more effective (NNT 53) than aspirin. The other, much more expensive, antiplatelet agents should only be considered where aspirin is contraindicated.

Anticoagulation

With the ageing of the population, the prevalence of atrial fibrillation is set to increase dramatically and management with aspirin or warfarin is effective at reducing recurrence. Warfarin is more effective (NNT 12), although management is often difficult; side-effects are not inconsiderable and aspirin should be considered if treatment with warfarin is not possible. Warfarin has been shown to be superior to aspirin in mild to moderate strokes.

Carotid endarterectomy

The trial evidence would suggest an NNT of 26 for severe stenosis but this is an expensive surgical procedure.

Other behavioural risk factors

Being overweight, leading a sedentary lifestyle, excessive alcohol intake, and having a poor diet all contribute to cardiovascular risk. Generally the evidence base for interventions here is poor.

How to establish the diagnosis

Clinical features (Table 2)

Stroke usually occurs without warning. Occasionally, there may be preceding headache especially with intracerebral or sub-arachnoid haemorrhage. Neurological symptoms most often develop rapidly, within a few minutes, although can develop in a stuttering fashion over several hours. Classically, haemorrhage develops rapidly and is associated with headache, vomiting, and sometimes clouding of consciousness. With the increasing use of brain imaging in the early stages of stroke it is being realized that haemorrhage frequently presents in ways that are indistinguishable from infarction.

Many conditions can mimic stroke. Space-occupying lesions such as cerebral neoplasm or abscess may have presented with a more gradual onset, although tumours may remain silent until they haemorrhage thus presenting in an identical way to stroke. Subdural haematoma more commonly presents with clouding of consciousness or confusion and only minor focal signs. A history of head injury is only obtained in about 50 per cent of cases of subdural haematoma. Epilepsy can leave a patient with residual focal neurological symptoms and signs for some days after a fit. There may be a history of previous events to provide a clue. Migraine is itself a cause of stroke, particularly in younger patients, but can present with focal neurological symptoms such as hemianopia, dysphasia, or hemiparesis. The onset is usually less abrupt than stroke and unilateral headache and a past history will help establish the diagnosis. It is always essential to exclude hypoglycaemia. Multiple sclerosis only very rarely presents with hemiparesis, although cerebellar or brainstem signs resulting from demyelination can be difficult to distinguish from stroke.

TIA is one of the most over-diagnosed syndromes, being falsely implicated in to a wide range of symptoms from vertigo, confusion, dizzy episodes, and loss of consciousness.

Immediate management for the primary care physician

Stroke is a medical emergency. Early access to treatment, usually only available in hospital, may affect the outcome. Patients require immediate hospital admission unless the symptoms of TIA or stroke have fully resolved by the time they are seen or unless prior knowledge about the patient would indicate that only palliative care should be given. The TIA and fully resolved stroke patients should be seen in a neurovascular clinic, preferably within 7 days.[11] If the patient or their carer contacts by phone with symptoms suggestive of stroke they should be instructed to call an ambulance rather than waiting to be attended at home.

Oxygen should be given, the blood glucose checked, and the patient's regular medication sent with the patient. Dysphagia is present in about 35 per cent of patients, and the patient should be advised not to eat or drink until their swallowing status has been checked. Aspirin should not be given until a brain scan is performed to exclude haemorrhage, although when the patient is unlikely to receive a scan within 48 h, it is reasonable to give aspirin immediately unless haemorrhage is clinically suspected. Hypertension should not be treated acutely. For patients already on antihypertensive medication, it is reasonable to stop it for a couple of days and then restart at original doses. Careful control of hydration, blood glucose, oxygenation, temperature, nutrition, and blood pressure are all important during the early phase of acute cerebral ischaemia.

Investigations

All patients need brain imaging, preferably within 48 h. Immediate scanning is required where hydrocephalus is suspected, for example, in patients with rapid onset cerebellar symptoms, where the patient is taking anticoagulants or where there is a suspicion of subdural haematoma or other space-occupying lesion. Immediate scanning is also required if thrombolysis is being considered. Electrocardiography is required to exclude atrial fibrillation or recent myocardial infarction. Full blood count looking for anaemia, thrombocytosis, polycythaemia, or white cell abnormalities, a clotting screen and electrolytes and creatinine need to be checked. Thrombophilia and immunological screening will be needed for some patients. In areas where malaria is prevalent this should be excluded.

Carotid duplex scanning should be performed in any patient where carotid endarterectomy would be considered. Surgery is appropriate where the artery is between 70 and 99 per cent occluded. Lesser degrees of stenosis are better managed using antithrombotic drugs.

Acute stroke treatment

In two trials, aspirin given within 48 h (150–300 mg) to patients with cerebral infarction reduced the long-term mortality and disability[5] although the effect was small (NNT 77). Heparin should not be used.

Thrombolysis using recombinant thrombin platelet activator (rTPA) has been shown to be effective when given to selected patients within 3 and possibly as long as 6 h after the onset of symptoms (NNT 7). It carries a high risk of intracerebral haemorrhage and should be administered in centres with the appropriate expertise. Anticoagulation is not recommended after ischaemic stroke because although it does reduce the risk of deep venous thrombosis, it also increases the risk of haemorrhage into the infarct causing higher levels of morbidity and mortality overall.

Prevention of complications in patients managed at home

Deep venous thrombosis (DVT) is common (up to 50 per cent) in the hemiparetic leg. Pulmonary embolism remains one of the commonest causes of death acutely after stroke. Heparin, even in low doses, is contra-indicated, but aspirin may help to reduce the incidence of DVT. Current recommendations, although not evidence based, are to use antiembolism stockings and encourage early mobilization.

Aspiration pneumonia in patients with dysphagia should be avoided by prompt recognition of those patients at risk. Testing the gag reflex is insufficient. A protocol to test the safety of the swallow should be used and an expert therapist should review any patient where there is doubt.

Malnutrition secondary to dysphagia, loss of appetite after acute illness, or difficulty in self-feeding, while not definitively having been shown to affect outcome, is unlikely to be beneficial. Supplementary enteral nutrition should be considered, either using nasogastric or gastrostomy tubes.

Depression occurs in up to 40 per cent of hospitalized stroke patients. Antidepressant treatment has not been shown to be beneficial.

Pressure sores are almost always avoidable and yet occur frequently. Recognizing risk, through the use of validated tools such as the Waterlow score and acting upon the findings rapidly through good-quality nursing and use of pressure-relieving mattresses and cushions, will prevent a costly and distressing complication.

Urinary tract infections are frequent, especially in women. Avoiding catheterization wherever possible is essential. Incontinence in the early stages of stroke is present in over 50 per cent of patients, but is not an indication for catheterization. Accurate diagnosis and appropriate treatment will result in the majority resolving.

Constipation can be managed with regular toileting and judicious use of aperients. Faecal incontinence can result from large strokes, especially those involving the frontal lobes. Faecal impaction with overflow is the commonest cause of incontinence.

Shoulder pain, as a result of damage to the capsule of the joint, may result from poor handling and lifting techniques or inappropriate positioning, particularly where the paretic arm is flaccid or the patient has sensory impairment or neglect of the affected side.

Rehabilitation: hospital or home?

Meta-analysis has shown that patients managed on a specialist stroke unit have lower death rates and improved long-term function when compared to patients cared for in other settings (NNT 12). The assessment and investigation necessary for the patient is complex and would be difficult and costly to organize in the patient's own home. However, there will always be some patients who refuse admission or for whom it is considered inappropriate.

Trials comparing early hospital discharge with rehabilitation at home against conventional hospital-based care have shown that outcomes are not compromised and that there can be some resource savings, provided that discharge is to a specialist stroke rehabilitation team. Use of routine services has been shown to result in higher mortality and morbidity compared with those who continued care in the inpatient stroke unit.

Rehabilitation after stroke needs to begin immediately, and should not wait until the patient is deemed to be medically 'stable'. The key components are:[10]

- involvement of the appropriate specialist staff who may include physiotherapists, occupational therapists, speech and language therapists, psychologists, dietitians, nurses, social workers, physicians, and psychiatrists;

- using evidence-based guidelines to inform the decision making process;

- using a clear framework and assessment measures to structure the therapy process;

- regular (at least weekly) team meetings to coordinate treatment and set achievable objectives for the patient;

- involvement of the patient and carer in the rehabilitation process;

- regular audit of the effectiveness of treatment being provided by the service.

Discharge from hospital

The hospital stroke service should maintain close working relationships with the primary care teams to ensure seamless care between hospital and home. One of the most common complaints from patients and their carers is not knowing where support is available. Individual needs assessments should be performed, to identify what the requirements after discharge are likely to be. The components of successful discharge will include:

- detailed and rapid information exchange between hospital and primary care;

- prior assessment of the home environment, with all necessary aids and adaptations having been made prior to discharge;

- identification of the key individuals and clear routes of access to them, for support and treatment after discharge;

- education and training given to the patient and their carers about living with the consequences of their stroke;

- a secondary prevention strategy;

- recognition of the burden stroke places on the carers, both psychologically and physically, with a plan in place to support them.

Longer-term management

In a population-based survey in south London one-third of survivors were severely or moderately disabled and two-fifths of survivors were more disabled than they had been at 3 months after their stroke.[7] Recovery of impairments after stroke can continue for many months after the acute

event. Language, sensory, and higher cognitive deficits are often slower to recover than motor deficits. Specific issues that the primary care physician may need to consider will be:

- *Driving.* Regulations will vary but absolute contraindications to driving will include persistent visual field defects, inattention or neglect, uncontrolled epilepsy, significant higher cognitive deficits, and problems with arousal.

- *Work.* The decision as to whether the patient should return to work will depend on the residual impairments and the employment they are in. Wherever possible, patients should be encouraged to return to their pre-morbid activities.

- *Leisure.* Individualized assessment of function, combined with the patients personal goals should enable a realistic plan for resuming leisure acitivities to be developed. There is rarely, if ever, a contra-indication to resuming normal sexual activity, although erectile failure is not uncommon after stroke. Reviewing medication to exclude this as a side-effect of treatment, and reassuring the patient as to the safety of sexual activity, may be sufficient. Sildafenil may be considered for use late after stroke.

- *Post-stroke pain.* Shoulder pain and central post-stroke pain are the two most frequent causes of pain. No effective treatments have been identified for treating established shoulder pain. Central post-stroke pain, previously called thalamic pain, needs early and aggressive treatment. Many cases will respond to adequate doses of tricyclic antidepressants, for example, amitryptiline or maprotilene. Gabapentin and mexilitine have proved effective for some patients.

- *Epilepsy.* Approximately 5 per cent of stroke patients develop epilepsy following stroke. Referral for investigation and treatment to a neurologist is appropriate. Phenytoin remains the most widely used drug and is successful in most cases.

Key points

- One in four men and one in five women over the age of 45 will have a stroke.

- Specialist care after stroke saves lives.

- Specialist interdisciplinary rehabilitation reduces long-term disability.

- Active surveillance and management of risk factors reduces recurrence.

- Effective treatment will save resources and reduce morbidity in carers.

References

1. Madden, K., Karanjia, P., Marshfield, W.I., Adams, H., Clarke, W., and the TOAST Investigators (1994). Accuracy of initial stroke subtype diagnosis in the TOAST trial. *Neurology* **44** (Suppl. 2), A271.

2. Bamford, J., Sandercock, P., Dennsi, M., Burn, J., and Warlow, C. (1991). Classification and natural history of clinically identifiable subtypes of cerebral infarction. *Lancet* **337**, 1521–6.

3. World Health Organization. *The World Health Report 2000, Health Systems: Improving Performance.* Geneva: WHO, 2000.

4. Sarti, C., Rastenyte, D., Cepaites, Z., and Tuomilehto, J. (2000). International trends in mortality from stroke 1968 to 1994. *Stroke* **31**, 1588–601.

5. Warlow, C.P., Dennis, M.S., van Gijn, J., Hankey, G.J., Sandercock, P.A.G., Bamford, J.M., and Wardlaw, J. *Stroke: A Practical Guide to Management.* Oxford: Blackwell Science Ltd, 2000. (A textbook of stroke covering aetiology, epidemiology, prevention, and management which has extensive bibliography.)

6. Wade, D. (1994). Stroke (acute cerebrovascular disease). In *Health Care Needs Assessments* Vol. 1 (ed. A. Stevens and J. Raftery), pp. 111–255. Oxford:

Radcliffe Medical Press. (An epidemiological overview of stroke with details of rates, outcomes, and evidence of effectiveness.)

7. **Wolfe, C., Rudd, T., and Beech, R.** *Stroke Services and Research.* London: Stroke Association, 1996. (An overview of the epidemiology, health services impact, and management of stroke.)

8. **Grieve, R.** et al. (2001). A comparison of the costs and survival of hospital-admitted stroke patients across Europe. *Stroke* **32**, 1684–91.

9. **Hankey, G.J. and Warlow, C.P.** (1999). Treatment and secondary prevention of stroke: evidence, costs, and effects on individuals and populations. *Lancet* **354**, 1457–63. (A systematic review of the literature on secondary prevention.)

10. **Royal College of Physicians of London.** *National Clinical Guidelines for Stroke.* London, 2000. (Evidence-based guidelines developed by a multidisciplinary working group in a national context.)

11. **PROGRESS Collaborative Group** (2001). Randomised trial of a perindopril-based blood-pressure-lowering regimen among 6105 individuals with previous stroke or transient ischaemic attack. *Lancet* **358**, 1033–41.

1.8 Varicose veins

Denise Findlay

Introduction

The venous system comprises the superficial veins within the skin and subcutaneous tissue, the deep veins in the muscle compartment within the deep fascia, and the perforating or communicating veins which, with the exception of those in the foot, direct unilateral flow from the superficial veins into the deep system. The deep venous system returns about 90 per cent of all lower limb blood. The venous valves have an important role in directing blood flow and venous return relies on negative intrathoracic pressure generation during inspiration, the competence of the valves and adequate calf muscle function.

Varicose veins are dilated, tortuous, or lengthened veins, and may be:

- truncal—varicosities in the line of the long or short superficial saphenous vein;

- reticular—dilated, tortuous, subcutaneous veins;

- telangiectasia—intradermal venules (often called spider veins, thread veins).

Varicose veins were thought to occur because of valve failure which then led to reflux and vein dilation, but it is now believed that the vein wall is inherently weak, resulting in dilatation of the vein and separation of the valve cusps resulting in venous incompetence and reflux.

Incidence

There are few studies on the incidence of varicose veins but the Framingham study found a 2-year incidence of 39.4 per 1000 for males and 51.9 per 1000 for females. A prevalence study in the United Kingdom in 1992 found the prevalence of varicose veins to be 17 per cent in males and 31 per cent in females.[?]

Presentation in primary care

Patients with varicose veins may present in primary care because of:

- *Cosmetic* concerns due to the varicose veins appearance.

- *Symptoms.* Symptoms usually associated with varicose veins include lower limb heaviness or tension, swelling, aching, restless legs, cramps, itching, and tingling. However, a UK cross-sectional population study (1999)[1] found that in men only itching was significantly related to the presence and severity of truncal varices. In women, there was a significant relationship between truncal varices and the symptoms of heaviness or tension, aching, and itching. There was no association between reticular varices and symptoms. This study suggests that even in the presence of truncal varices most lower limb symptoms probably have a non-venous cause.

- *Complications.* Complications associated with varicose veins include haemorrhage, thrombophlebitis, and changes related to venous insufficiency—oedema, skin pigmentation (haemosiderin deposits), eczema, atrophie blanche, lipodermatosclerosis, and venous ulceration. There is no evidence that primary varicose veins are a risk factor for spontaneous deep venous thrombosis.

Diagnosis

History and examination may identify secondary causes for the development of varicose veins such as previous deep vein thrombosis, occlusive pelvic tumours, or arteriovenous fistulae. The majority of varicose veins however are primary. Risk factors associated with the development of primary varicose veins include increasing age and parity, occupations which require a lot of standing and obesity in women.

Clinical examination with the patient standing allows identification of the distribution of the varicose veins and any secondary skin changes associated with long-standing venous insufficiency. The presence of varicose veins can be missed in the obese patient or in an oedematous limb. Examination can also distinguish between incompetence of the perforating and junctional venous system. Using the Brodie–Trendelenburg technique, the superficial venous system is emptied with the patient lying supine and a superficial venous occlusion tourniquet is applied. When the patient stands, the superficial veins fill slowly from below and tourniquet release does not alter this. In the presence of incompetence of the sapheno-femoral junction, rapid filling occurs from above when the tourniquet is released. If rapid filling occurs with the tourniquet in situ this suggests incompetence of the perforating veins and the level can be determined by placing further tourniquets along the limb and removing distal tourniquets sequentially.

Investigations

A number of non-invasive tests can be used to determine the patency and competence of the superficial and deep venous system.

- A hand-held continuous wave Doppler can test for reflux. With the patient standing, the doppler probe is placed over the vein and reflux is identified by a prolonged audible retrograde flow using the tourniquet. This technique is not usually accurate for localizing perforator incompetence.

- Colour flow duplex ultrasonography is the investigation of choice, and provides both anatomical detail and flow data and is valuable in assessing perforator and junction reflux before surgery. It is of particular benefit in localizing deep and superficial reflux and when assessing the cause of recurrent varicose veins.

- Photoplethysmography and light reflective rheography are non-invasive methods used to assess venous refilling times.

- Plethysmography (gravimetric or volumetric) provides quantitative information on reflux and calf muscle pump function.

- Ambulatory venous pressure measurement is an invasive technique which is sometimes used to identify the presence and site of reflux.

Management of varicose veins

A number of management options are available.

Reassurance

Some patients present with symptoms which may or may not be associated with their varicose veins. They may be concerned about possible complications or worsening of the varicosities. Provided there is no evidence of skin changes suggestive of venous insufficiency, reassurance may be all these patients require.

Compression hosiery

Compression hosiery can provide symptomatic relief, although patients will need to replace their stockings every 6–8 months and wear them for the remainder of their life. Generally, compression hosiery providing 15–20 mmHg at the ankle is suggested for symptomatic mild varicosities, increasing to 20–30 or 30–40 mmHg for moderate and pronounced varicosities, respectively. If symptoms respond to compression this suggests that other surgical interventions may be beneficial.

Surgery

Surgery for truncal varices removes the underlying abnormality. Commonly, this involves ligation at the sapheno-popliteal or sapheno-femoral junction and stripping of the long saphenous vein with multiple avulsions. In most cases, surgery is a day procedure and compression bandages are used immediately post-operatively. Depending on the patient's occupation, they usually return to work within 1–3 weeks.

Complications include: temporary saphenous or sural nerve neuralgia (about 17 per cent); recurrent varicose veins—some 20–30 per cent of patients develop recurrence within 10 years[1]—this may be due to inadequate primary surgery or the development of new sites of reflux; deep venous thrombosis and possible pulmonary embolus; arterial injury; or permanent nerve injury. The latter three more serious complications occur in less than 1 per cent of cases.

Sub-fascial endoscopic surgical techniques are currently being used for perforator surgery. Reconstructive surgery of the deep venous system is also being undertaken and includes valvuloplasty, venous segmental transposition and transplantation.

Reticular varices can be treated by surgical avulsion through small stab wounds and it is the standard treatment for veins greater than 4 mm in diameter.

Sclerotherapy

In sclerotherapy, a sterile irritant solution is injected into the vein lumen to produce irreversible mural denaturation and subsequent resorption of the vein. This technique can be used for truncal varices. Reticular varices and telangiectasia can be treated with microinjections. Duplex ultrasound guided sclerotherapy is a newer technique.

The effectiveness of sclerotherapy is dependent on: injection into an empty vein (to avoid sclerosant dilution); the amount and concentration of sclerosant used; application of adequate post-treatment compression (both the degree and duration of compression); and prior treatment of reflux or larger feeding veins.

Complications of sclerotherapy include: skin staining; ulceration and scarring due to extravascular necrosis; symptomatic superficial thrombophlebitis; telangiectatic matting; allergic reaction; deep venous thrombosis (very rare); or recurrent varicose veins. (This can occur due to inadequate technique, but can also be the result of the development of new varicosities.)

Laser

Laser therapy is proving effective in clearing leg telangiectasia and reticular veins. It is considered the first line of treatment for isolated, superficial, fine-calibre, non-arborizing telangiectasia (usually <3 mm) and post-sclerotherapy telangiectatic matting. It is also of benefit to patients who are afraid of needles or where there has been a poor response to sclerotherapy. Complications are usually transient. Epidermal erythema, itching, and crusting resolve over a few days, while hyperpigmentation

(about one-third) and hypopigmentation (12–20 per cent) changes resolve over a few months.

Complications of varicose veins

Superficial thrombophlebitis

Superficial thrombophlebitis usually presents as severe pain, with erythema, pigmentation, and tenderness over the hardened vein. In varicose veins, this is usually the result of stasis. Management consists of compression and in some cases local application of heparinoid. The natural history is of resolution over 1–2 weeks and there is no indication for antibiotics. Groups at high risk of developing deep venous thrombosis in association with superficial thrombophlebitis include:

◆ previous history of deep vein thrombosis;

◆ older patients;

◆ bilateral thrombophlebitis;

◆ thrombophlebitis in the absence of varicose veins.

In patients with thrombophlebitis extending proximally up the long saphenous vein, some surgeons advise duplex scanning and emergency ligation at the sapheno-femoral junction to avoid the extension of the thrombosis into the femoral vein and the associated risk of pulmonary embolus.

Haemorrhage from varicose veins

Haemorrhage is usually the result of trauma and can be a dramatic event for the patient. Management consists of limb elevation and local compression to stop the bleeding. On rare occasions a suture may be needed. To avoid recurrence, correction of the underlying problem is required.

Chronic venous insufficiency

Long-standing varicose veins and reflux (chronic venous insufficiency) can result in a number of skin changes—red/brown pigmentation (haemosiderin deposits), eczema, lipodermatosclerosis, atrophie blanche, and venous ulceration (Fig. 1). These changes occur with isolated superficial

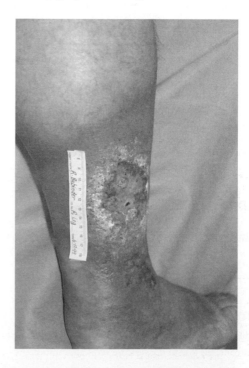

Fig. 1 Chronic venous insufficiency with haemosiderin staining, early lipodermatofibrosis, and ulceration in the 'gaiter' region.

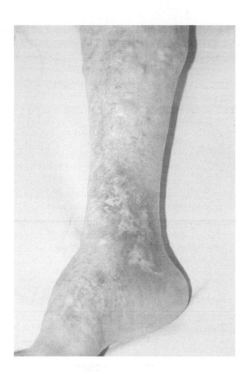

Fig. 2 Atrophie blanche with evidence of varicose veins. Distal area of atrophy blanche acutely painful.

vein incompetence but are almost inevitable if there is deep venous incompetence with perforator incompetence.

Lipodermatosclerosis is a result of fat necrosis, chronic inflammatory induration, fibrosis, and scarring. It results in a woody induration of the skin and is usually found on the lower medial side of the leg. The associated fibrosis is responsible for the characteristic inverted 'champagne bottle' deformity described in chronic venous insufficiency.

Atrophie blanche appears as small grey-white fibrous areas. Although frequently found in venous disease, it can occur in other circumstances. These can remain static for years but can also become acutely painful and ulcerate. It is believed that atrophie blanche is the result of thrombosis and obliteration of capillaries in the middle and deep dermis (Fig. 2).

Implications of the problem

While there are a number of effective treatments for varicose veins, their high prevalence has implications for health care expenditure. Patients with truncal varices and skin changes are at risk of long-term sequelae and in terms of a cost–benefit analysis, are a high priority for treatment. Conversely treatment for patients with asymptomatic reticular varicose veins or telangiectasia is a low priority. The long-term risks for patients with truncal varicose veins and no skin changes are not clear and therefore the cost–benefit of treatment is also unclear. Treatment of this group is probably a moderate priority.

Key points

1. The majority of varicose veins are primary in origin.

2. Even in the presence of truncal varices, most lower limb symptoms probably have a non-venous cause.

3. There is no evidence that primary varicose veins are a risk factor for spontaneous deep vein thrombosis.

4. Complications of varicose veins include haemorrhage, thrombophlebitis and skin changes, and ulceration due to chronic venous insufficiency.

5. Colour flow duplex ultrasonography is the investigation of choice to identify the patency and competence of the superficial and deep venous system.

6. Varicose vein treatment options include reassurance, compression hosiery, surgery, sclerotherapy, and laser therapy.

Reference

1. **London, N.J.M. and Nash, R.** (2000). ABC of arterial and venous disease. Varicose veins. *British Medical Journal* **320**, 1391–4. (Review of varicose veins and their management.)

1.9 Leg ulcers

Denise Findlay

Incidence

Excluding foot ulcers, the point prevalence of active leg ulceration in Western populations (including Europe, United Kingdom, United States, and Australia) has been estimated at 1.5–3 per 1000. This increases with age—6.3 per 1000 in the over 65 years age group. The period prevalence is 0.39 per 1000.

Presentation in primary care

The conditions which can cause leg ulcers are numerous. In primary care in the Western population, the major causes of leg ulcers seen are venous insufficiency (70 per cent), arterial insufficiency (6 per cent), mixed arterial and venous insufficiency (20 per cent), with other causes accounting for the remainder e.g. malignancy, pressure, lymphoedema, vasculitis, pyoderma gangrenosum, etc.

Diagnosis

Although trauma is probably the commonest initiating cause of leg ulcers, it should not be considered a diagnosis for chronic leg ulceration. Most acute leg wounds heal with appropriate management. Poor healing is not usually due to the initial trauma but rather the presence of other factors inhibiting healing.

In primary care, a number of studies have demonstrated that in up to 50 per cent of patients with chronic leg ulceration a formal diagnosis of the cause of the ulcer is not made.

A careful history and examination will help determine the cause of the ulceration and involves assessment of the whole patient as well as the ulcer. Specific symptoms, relevant past history, examination including palpation of peripheral pulses and the overall appearance of the ulcer, its site, size and shape, and location can provide a guide to ulcer diagnosis.

In addition to identifying the cause of the ulcer, it is also important to identify any other factors which may be affecting healing. These include: ageing, nutritional status, systemic illness, medications, infection, presence of a foreign body, the local wound environment, and radiation therapy.

Investigations

Investigations are directed by the clinical findings and may include:

- *Ankle–brachial pressure index (ABPI).* This is a simple non-invasive investigation and can identify the presence of arterial disease. Using a hand-held Doppler ultrasound with an 8 mHz probe brachial and ankle systolic pressures are measured. The ABPI is calculated by dividing the highest ankle pressure by the highest brachial pressure. The clinical implications are summarized in Table 1. The accuracy of the ABPI measurement is variable and dependent on operator technique, the presence of severe limb oedema and the presence of arterial wall calcification.
- *Colour duplex ultrasonography* to identify patients with venous ulcers who would benefit from surgical intervention. It is also a useful non-invasive investigation for the presence of arterial insufficiency.
- *Photoplethysmography (PPG).* This non-invasive test can provide objective evidence of venous insufficiency and is also being considered as a screening tool for early detection of venous insufficiency in high-risk groups.
- *Biopsy.* Wound biopsy is a simple and effective investigation to diagnose the presence of malignancy or other more unusual causes of ulceration, for example, vasculitis, pyoderma gangrenosum, *Mycobacterium ulcerans*.
- *Wound swabs.* A wound swab for microbiology and culture may be useful where there is clinical evidence of infection. There is, however, little value in routinely swabbing leg ulcers as they are often colonized with organisms and the presence of these organisms has no effect on the treatment or prognosis.

Table 1 The clinical significance of the ABPI

ABI	Significance	Clinical issues
>1.2	Arterial calcification	Commonly occurs in diabetic patients and the elderly
		Index provides little information about intraluminal flow
		A Doppler waveform or toe pressures will serve as an indication of the presence or absence of arterial occlusion
0.9–1.1	Normal	Graduated compression can be used
<0.8	Arterial insufficiency	
	0.7–0.8	A history of intermittent claudication is likely with indices less than 0.8
		Vascular assessment recommended (particularly if indices <0.7)
		Ulcer may be mixed venous–arterial in origin. Light graduated compression may be tolerated
	0.5–0.7	Ulcer may be mixed venous-arterial in origin, but the arterial component is more significant
		Compression is best avoided and is usually not tolerated
	<0.5	A history of rest pain is frequently associated with indices less than 0.5
		Healing of ulcers by conservative means is less likely
		Compression is contraindicated

Reproduced from: *The Australian Family Physician*, December 1996.

- *Other tests.* Other investigations may need to be considered if clinically indicated—haemoglobin, full blood examination, ESR, blood glucose, urea and electrolytes, rheumatoid factor, and antinuclear antibodies.

Management

The aims of management of leg ulceration are firstly to heal the ulcer, and then to maintain the healed skin to prevent further recurrences. In a minority of cases, where it may not be possible to heal the ulcer, the aim of treatment is to minimize the morbidity caused by the ulcer.

The main principles of management include:

1. Eliminate or control the major aetiological factors and any other factors affecting healing.
2. Choose an appropriate wound dressing. The ideal dressing is one which provides a moist wound environment but removes excess exudate, and maintains a slightly acidic pH and an optimal wound temperature (37°C) at the wound.
3. Plan a regime that is appropriate for the patient's context.
4. Monitor progress, including:
   (i) Measurement of the size of the wound using a tape measure, or by tracing the margin.
   (ii) approximation of the degree of necrotic tissue, slough, granulation tissue, and epithelial tissue. for example, 70 per cent slough with 30 per cent granulation.
   (iii) Estimation of degree of exudate. This may be assessed by identifying the amount of 'strike-through' of exudate or the frequency of dressing change required. A increase in exudate level alerts the practitioner to the possibility of infection.
   (iv) Measurement of the smallest ankle dimension (above the malleoli) and largest calf dimension to assess the degree of oedema control achieved when using compression bandaging.
5. Maintain healed skin.

Specific leg ulcer conditions

Venous leg ulcers

The diagnosis of venous ulceration can usually be made clinically. Table 2 outlines the typical features of venous ulceration, not all of which will be present; some patients have significant pain with venous ulceration that is not due to infection nor the presence of arterial disease. Figures 1 and 2 in Chapter 1.8 demonstrate some of the typical appearances of venous ulceration.

Management

The mainstay of treatment is the control of the venous insufficiency and venous hypertension using compression, exercise to encourage calf muscle pump activity, and elevation.

Compression

The application of graduated compression is a fundamental component of the management of venous ulceration. High compression is more effective than low compression and multilayered systems are more effective than single-layered systems. A high-compression system should provide at least 25 mmHg at the ankle, preferably 30–45 mmHg.

One significant problem with compression bandaging is the potential for inappropriate and variable pressures because of variations in application technique and operator experience level. High compression stockings, on the other hand, offer consistent pressures, relatively unaffected by operator application technique. They can, however, be difficult to apply over dressings and can appear costly at initial purchase. Also as the limb size reduces with compression a stocking may need to be replaced with a smaller size, while bandages readily adapt to these size changes.

Table 2 Classic features of arterial and venous leg ulceration

	Arterial ulcers	Venous ulcers
History	Intermittent claudication Rest pain Bypass Sympathectomy Diabetes Evidence of other vascular problems, for example, AMI, CVA, etc. Smoker	Previous DVT or pulmonary embolus Recurrent ulceration Limb oedema Previous 'vein stripping' May have history of failed skin grafts Obesity
Pain	Usually moderate to severe	Usually nil to mild pain
Oedema	Usually absent (unless as a result of keeping the leg dependent)	Usually present
Ulcer site	Distal to ankle Upper two-thirds of leg	Around the ankle and lower one-third of the leg, especially above the medial malleolus 'gaiter region'
Ulcer features	'Punched out' appearance Often deep, involving deep fascia	'Ragged' edge Usually superficial Usually moderate to heavily exudating
Associated limb features	'Cool' extremities Shiny, pale, hairless skin Postural colour change (Buerger's sign)	Evidence of varicosities Varicose eczema Haemosiderin deposits (brown staining) Atrophy blanche Lipodermatofibrosis Evidence of previous ulceration
Pedal pulses	Diminished or absent pedal pulses	Normal pedal pulses

Reproduced and adapted from: *The Australian Family Physician*, September and October 1996.

Where no other significant conditions are present to inhibit healing the use of high compression results in approximately 75 per cent of venous ulcers healing at 12 weeks and 84 per cent at 24 weeks.

High-compression systems should not be used if there is evidence of concomitant arterial disease nor should they be applied to ankles with a circumference of less than 18 cm because of the increased risk of pressure ulceration.

Exercise
Patients should be encouraged to walk to improve calf muscle pump activity and venous return. Patients with a limited range of ankle movement (e.g. arthritis, the elderly) appear to respond more slowly to compression because of the lack of calf muscle pump action.

Elevation
Elevation can be helpful to improve gravitational drainage of the affected limb. To achieve this, the ulcer/limb must be elevated to a level higher than the heart—vertical leg drainage. Bed blocks can also be a useful addition. However, 'resting' can result in reduced mobility and increased joint stiffness reducing calf muscle pump action. It is therefore a technique to be used in conjunction with compression and ambulation, and not on its own.

Dressings
Dressings play a secondary role to adequate compression and many different dressings can be used. Zinc-impregnated paste bandages can be useful where venous eczema is also present. Patch testing may be performed before use, to exclude an allergic response. Topical corticosteroids can also be applied up to the ulcer margin to control venous eczema, without any adverse effect on ulcer healing.

Surgery
There is currently no conclusive evidence that surgery or injection sclerotherapy alone improves the healing of venous ulceration, particularly if deep venous incompetence is present. Skin grafting has been used, but there is currently insufficient evidence that autografts alone (e.g. split skin grafts) increase the healing of venous ulcers.

Pharmacological treatments
Oedema associated with venous ulceration is usually readily controlled by compression and there is little need for diuretics, which are ineffective alone.

Antibiotics should only be used in venous ulceration where there is evidence of clinical infection. There is no evidence to support the routine use of oral zinc supplementation. Oxypentifylline appears to be an effective adjunct to compression bandaging (particularly if used for longer than 24 weeks) but cost may mitigate against its routine use. There is little evidence to support the routine use of agents such as stanazol, aspirin, or cinnarizine in treating venous ulceration.

Other therapies
New treatments, for which there are limited data, include a combination of HeNe laser and infrared light; vacuum assisted therapy and warming therapy; growth factors, such as transforming growth factor β (TGFβ), epidermal growth factor (EGF), and plasminogen activator inhibitor 2 (PAI-2); and human skin equivalents, such as human dermal replacement (Dermagraft) and bilayered skin equivalent (Apligraft).

Maintenance of healed skin
Once the ulcer is healed, the patient should be encouraged to wear graduated compression stockings for life to reduce the risk of ulcer recurrence, unless corrective surgery is possible. Patients should be encouraged to use the highest compression that they can tolerate and are able to apply.

Venous surgery is beneficial for ulcer prevention in the presence of isolated superficial venous reflux where there is no deep vein disease (about one third to one half of patients with venous leg ulceration). Likewise, surgery to communicating veins appears to be beneficial but only if associated with obliteration of the superficial veins (in patients with normal deep veins).

Arterial ulcers

Table 2 outlines the typical features of arterial ulceration, also illustrated in Fig. 1.

The mainstay of treatment in patients with arterial ulceration is vascular assessment with a view to surgical intervention. Investigations such as the ABPI (ABPI <0.8) and arterial duplex scans further confirm the diagnosis, whereas angiography is required to determine the technique of reconstruction.

Surgical intervention (angioplasty, stent, bypass graft) with re-establishment of good arterial blood flow will, in most cases, result in the ulcer healing. However, for some patients surgery is delayed, is considered inappropriate because of other medical problems, or is simply not possible (with amputation the only remaining surgical option). In these situations, despite significant ischaemia, it may be possible to heal some of these arterial ulcers with an appropriate conservative management regime. This requires assessment and control of any other contributing problems including improving diabetic control, cessation of medications such as β blockers, ensuring adequate nutrition, together with adequate pain relief, and the use of an appropriate wound dressing to aid healing and reduce the risk of infection.

Mixed arterial–venous disease

Elements of both venous and arterial disease in the history and examination suggest the presence of mixed arterial–venous disease (Fig. 2). The ABPI may help confirm clinical suspicions. The mainstay of management initially consists of vascular assessment and surgery to improve the arterial insufficiency wherever possible. Once the arterial disease is corrected, the venous component may become more apparent and appropriate compression, which was previously contraindicated because of the presence of arterial disease, often needs to be reinstated.

Malignancy

Factors indicating malignancy

Malignancy should be considered if:

♦ the ulceration is long-standing and has failed to heal despite appropriate treatment

♦ the ulceration is in an unusual area

♦ the edge has a 'rolled' appearance

♦ firm hypergranulation is present and persistent

♦ regular bleeding occurs despite the use of appropriate moist wound products

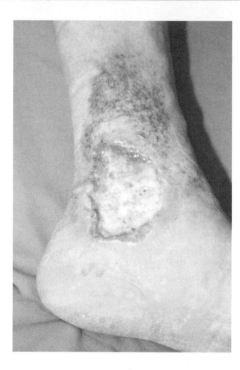

Fig. 2 Mixed venous ischaemic ulcer. Past history of recurrent venous ulceration, on examination poor palpable pedal pulses and unable to tolerate compression. (See Plate 2.)

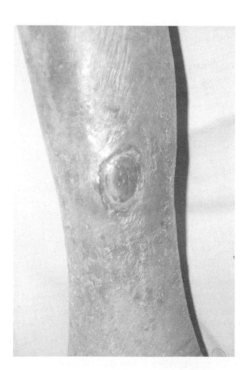

Fig. 1 Arterial leg ulcer with 'punched out' appearance and muscle in the base. (See Plate 1.)

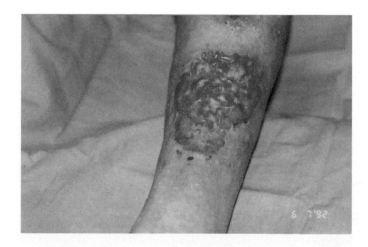

Fig. 3 Large hypergranulating ulcer present for over 2 years. Biopsy revealed squamous cell carcinoma. (See Plate 3.)

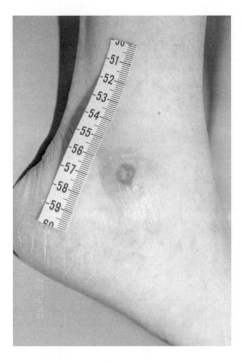

Fig. 4 Classical lateral malleolus pressure ulcer. (See Plate 4.)

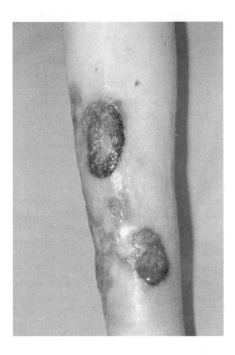

Fig. 5 Painful vasculitic ulcer with rapidly extending necrotic border and evidence of palpable purpura. (See Plate 5.)

Biopsy will confirm the diagnosis, usually either a squamous cell or basal cell carcinoma (Fig. 3). In many cases, the carcinoma was initially misdiagnosed and unsuccessfully treated as an 'ulcer'. In other cases, however, long-standing leg ulceration (usually venous) can undergo malignant change to a squamous cell carcinoma—a Marjolin's ulcer (originally described in chronic burns). Treatment consists of excision with or without skin grafting.

Pressure ulceration

Pressure ulcers in the leg usually occur over bony prominences, for example, the malleoli (Fig. 4). The presence of concomitant arterial insufficiency increasing the risk of pressure ulceration should be considered. Treatment involves redistribution of pressure away from the ulcer site by using pressure relieving dressings, adhesive compressed felt doughnuts, or foot pressure relieving booties.

Vasculitis

Factors indicating vasculitis

Factors suggestive of vasculitis as a cause of leg ulceration include:

- history of rheumatoid arthritis, systemic lupus erythematosus, hypergammaglobulinaemia, other connective tissue diseases, lymphoma, leukaemia, Hodgkin's disease, myelodysplasias

- medications which can cause vasculitis, for example, allopurinol, aminosalicylic acid, ampicillin, captopril, cimetidine, frusemide, methotrexate, sulfonamides and warfarin.

- ulceration preceded by palpable purpura

- clinical appearance of an arterial ulcer with or without necrosis and associated with good pedal pulses (Fig. 5)

- severe pain and rapidly worsening ulceration in the absence of infection

Investigations may include a diagnostic screen for underlying autoimmune disorder or other conditions as outlined above. Other small vessel organ damage needs to be assessed. Diagnosis in the early stages may be confirmed by biopsy (fresh, no formalin) examined with immunofluorescence.

Treatment is symptomatic, including removal of the initial cause if possible, pain relief, appropriate wound dressings, bed rest, and in some cases hospitalization. While there is a tendency for gradual remission systemic corticosteroids should be commenced if the ulceration is worsening. Occasionally, if control is poor with corticosteroids, azothiaprine, cyclophosphamide, dapsone, or hydroxychloroquine may be used.

Lymphoedema

Lymphoedema is the result of poor lymphatic flow and drainage due to obstruction, destruction, or agenesis of lymphatic vessels. It presents as swollen oedematous legs which in the initial stages may 'pit'. As the condition becomes chronic skin fibrosis develops and non-pitting oedema occurs. Impairment of the lymphatic drainage also predisposes the affected area to recurrent cellulitis, often as the result of a minor abrasion or interdigital tinea.

Lymphoedema can be primary (commonly familial) or secondary, caused by obstruction from a space-occupying lesion, surgical removal of lymph nodes, radiotherapy to lymph nodes, neoplastic infiltration or infection (e.g. filiariasis, recurrent acute bacterial infection). It can cause general skin exudation with little evidence of ulceration to frank ulceration which can have the appearance of venous ulceration.

The principles of management include:

- prevention of injury;

- prevention of infection (and aggressive treatment if infection is present);

- control of oedema

  - very high compression bandage systems (often >40 mmHg);

  - lymphoedema massage.

High-compression full limb stockings are usually required for maintenance. Generally patients should be referred to specialist lymphoedema units.

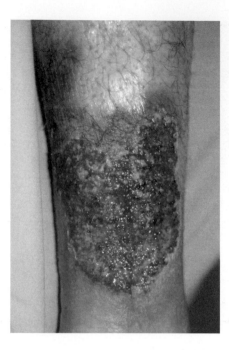

Fig. 6 Pyoderma gangrenosum. One of four bilateral painful ulcers. All healed rapidly with oral corticosteroids. (See Plate 6.)

Pyoderma gangrenosum

Pyoderma gangrenosum is a rapidly developing painful ulcerative condition. The ulcer often has a distinctive blue, raised border (Fig. 6). During active phases there may be a zone of erythema surrounding the ulcer which can be confused with an infective cause. Approximately 10–30 per cent of pyoderma gangrenosum is idiopathic and the remainder is associated with systemic disease, for example, ulcerative colitis, inflammatory arthritis, and blood dyscrasias (monoclonal gammopathy, myeloproliferative disease, leukaemia). The activity of the pyoderma does not always follow the activity of the underlying condition. New lesions can occur with minor trauma.

Investigations include screening for associated conditions and biopsy for histopathology (lymphocytic vasculitis). Unfortunately, biopsy often only reveals non-specific changes and diagnosis must then be made on clinical grounds and response to treatment.

The principles of management include provision of adequate pain relief, appropriate wound dressings, treatment of the underlying condition, and the use of immunosuppressive agents including topical, intralesional, and/or oral corticosteroids. Second line options include azothiaprine, dapsone, colchicine, or minocycline. In some cases, hospitalization for pulsed corticosteroids or agents such as cyclosporin is required.

Mycobacterium ulcerans

Infection by *Mycobacterium ulcerans* commonly begins as a papule on the leg, thigh, or arm with no history of injury. The papule enlarges, ulcerates, and continues to expand resulting in an ulcer that is undermined and extends into the subcutaneous fat (necrotic fat may be seen at the ulcer base). It is relatively painless. It is usually diagnosed by swab or biopsy for microbiology and culture. Surgical excision is the treatment of choice. Untreated, it can heal with deep scarring and contractures.

Implications of leg ulceration

Leg ulcers are common. They impact on patient's quality of life particularly because of pain, sleep disturbance, and impaired mobility. Anger,

depression, fear, and poor self-esteem are also common sequelae. Employment can be affected—in the United States, it is estimated that 2 million workdays are lost annually because of leg ulcers. In 1992, 1.3 per cent of the total health care budget in the United Kingdom was used for the treatment of venous ulcers.

Establishment of community leg ulcer clinics is one strategy for the effective management of leg ulcers. However, much can be achieved in primary care by a careful and accurate assessment of both the patient and the leg ulcer. Appropriate management initiated at this early stage has the potential to reduce the overall incidence of chronic leg ulceration. Assessment and regular reassessment of the patient presenting with a chronic leg ulcer can result in improved leg ulcer healing rates because appropriate management (based on a clear diagnosis) can be instituted.

As the majority of chronic leg ulcers are venous in origin, learning when and how to appropriately apply high-compression systems and then using this skill in the primary care setting is essential. This is a simple step primary care practitioners can take towards reducing the overall burden chronic leg ulceration places on the patient, their family, and the community.

Key points

1. Assess the whole patient not just the leg ulcer.

2. The primary principle of ulcer management is the control or elimination of factors inhibiting healing (both the major aetiological cause and other contributing factors).

3. The majority of chronic leg ulcers are due to chronic venous insufficiency.

4. The mainstay of treatment of venous ulceration is the application of high compression, exercise, and elevation.

Further reading

Carville, K. *Wound Care Manual*. Western Australia: Silver Chain Nursing Association, 1995. (Extensive, easy to read practical book providing an overview of assessment and management of wounds including leg ulcers. Reviews wound dressing products.)

Callum, N., Nelson, E.A., Fletcher, A.W., and Dheldon, T.A. (2000). Compression bandages and stockings for venous leg ulcers (Cochrane Review). In *The Cochrane Library*. Oxford: Update Software. (Systematic review of compression for venous leg ulcers.)

Thomas, S. and Nelson, A. (1998). The science of compression bandaging. *Journal of Wound Care* (Supplement September). (Series of three articles outlining the principles of compression and the types and selection of bandages.)

Stubbing, N.J., Bailey, P., and Poole, M. (1997). Protocol for accurate assessment of ABPI in patients with leg ulcers. *Journal of Wound Care* **6** (9), 417–18. (Protocol for performing an ABPI.)

1.10 **High blood pressure**

Tom Fahey and Knut Schroeder

Epidemiology

High blood pressure has a positive, continuous, and independent association with cardiovascular disease (stroke, myocardial infarction, congestive heart failure, peripheral vascular disease), renal failure, cognitive decline, and all-cause mortality.[1–3] Systematic reviews of randomized controlled trials (RCTs) of antihypertensive drugs have shown that blood pressure lowering (5–6 mmHg diastolic blood pressure) is associated with a reduction of stroke (fatal and non-fatal) by 38 per cent and coronary heart disease (fatal and non-fatal) by 18 per cent.[4] The overall relative risk reduction of antihypertensive drug therapy is estimated to be 30 per cent (range 20–40 per cent) for cardiovascular disease and 10 per cent (range 5–20 per cent) for all-cause mortality.[1] Associations between blood pressure and cardiovascular disease are stronger for systolic blood pressure, particularly in the elderly.

Absolute risk of cardiovascular disease is strongly modified by the presence of additional risk factors, evidence of target organ damage, and increasing age.[1–3] Blood pressure is a normally distributed characteristic in a population. The estimated prevalence of hypertension depends on the blood pressure level used to define the condition, which is arbitrary.[1,4] Overall, 15 per cent of the UK population take antihypertenive drugs to lower their blood pressure, the prevalence increasing sharply in the elderly to up to 30 per cent. In the United States, over half the population aged more than or equal to 60 years have high blood pressure when a criterion of more than or equal to 140/90 mmHg is used.[3] There is some evidence to suggest that detection, treatment, and control has improved over the last 25 years in the United States.[3] However, in European countries control of blood pressure has remained inadequate: even when a liberal criterion of 160/95 mmHg is used, 40–50 per cent of individuals with high blood pressure taking antihypertensive drugs remain inadequately controlled.

How common is this presentation in primary care?

Treatment of high blood pressure is one of the commonest reasons to visit a family physician. In the United States, management of high blood pressure accounts for about 8 per cent of all office encounters. In the United Kingdom, 16 per cent of people aged 65–74 and 14 per cent of people aged between 75 and 84 visit their family physician with high blood pressure. Females are more commonly affected than males with the male to female ratio changing from 0.9 at age 45–74 to 0.7 at age more than or equal to 75.

Possible causes of high blood pressure

The cause of high blood pressure is not usually identified in most patients presenting to their family physician. The term 'essential' hypertension has been attributed to those individuals in whom blood pressure is judged to be harmful. As blood pressure is a normally distributed characteristic in populations, the definition of high blood pressure or 'essential' hypertension is arbitrary.[4] National guidelines have all adopted different thresholds above which treatment is recommended. For most individuals with high blood pressure, the cause is attributed to an interaction of genetic and environmental factors.

In a minority of individuals an underlying cause is found. These people suffer from secondary hypertension. The frequency of secondary hypertension in primary care settings is uncertain but probably low, with estimates ranging between 1 and 5 per cent.[1] The common causes of secondary hypertension that family physicians might encounter include:

♦ Renovascular disorders—usually atherosclerotic renal artery stenosis.

♦ Renal parenchymal disease—resulting from acute or chronic renal failure.

♦ Adrenal disorders—most often Cushing's syndrome.

♦ Renin secreting tumours—lung, pancreas, kidney.

♦ Vascular disease—coarctation of the aorta (commonest cause in children).

Because of its low prior probability, uncovering secondary hypertension presents a diagnostic challenge to the family physician. There is no agreed diagnostic approach or suitable clinical prediction rule to aid in the diagnosis of secondary hypertension. Consensus guidelines recommend referral if clinical suspicion is raised by the history, physical examination, or selected laboratory studies. Clinical features that increase the probability of secondary hypertension include:

♦ Onset of high blood pressure before age 30.

♦ Documented sudden onset or worsening high blood pressure in middle age.

♦ Malignant hypertension (WHO criteria: diastolic blood pressure >130 mmHg with bilateral retinal haemorrhage and exudates).

♦ High blood pressure resistant to more than three drug regimen.

♦ Renal impairment of unknown cause.

♦ Generalized peripheral vascular disease (particularly abdominal bruits) or severe generalized atherosclerotic disease.

♦ Recurrent pulmonary oedema or heart failure with no obvious cause.

How to make a diagnosis of high blood pressure

High blood pressure is an asymptomatic condition and is usually detected by case finding by health professionals. Very rarely, patients may present to their family physician with symptoms of malignant hypertension. In such patients, the commonest symptoms are headache, visual disturbance, dyspnoea due to heart failure, and gastrointestinal symptoms such as anorexia, nausea, and vomiting.[4]

When assessing a patient with suspected high blood pressure, the objective is to simultaneously evaluate cardiovascular risk, end-organ damage, and likely contributory factors. The following should be specifically asked about:

History

♦ Age and sex.

♦ Review of systems: chest pain; shortness of breath; episodic dizziness; blurred vision; slurred speech; memory loss; cognitive impairment; leg pain.

♦ Past history: myocardial infarct; angina; stroke; transient ischaemic attack (TIA); dementia; left ventricular hypertrophy; heart failure; coronary angioplasty or bypass surgery; diabetes; renal disease.

♦ Family history: premature cardiovascular disease (first-degree male relatives with CVD before 55 years, female relatives before 65 years); renal disease; diabetes.

♦ Social history: smoking status; alcohol intake; exercise taken; diet.

♦ Medication history: corticosteroids; non-steroidal anti-inflammatory drugs (NSAIDs); amphetamines (appetite suppressants); caffeine; liquorice, sympathomimetics (nasal decongestants or bronchodilators); oral contraceptives; sodium containing medications (antacids).

Examination

♦ Assessment of height and weight (calculate body mass index).

♦ Assessment of end-organ damage: fundal haemorrhages or exudates; evidence of heart failure or left ventricular hypertrophy; abdominal bruits.

Investigations

1. Urinalysis checking for proteinuria and glycosuria.

2. Blood tests: urea, electrolytes, and creatinine levels; total cholesterol/HDL cholesterol.

The accuracy and reliability of many of the elements of the history, examination, and investigations undertaken when assessing patients with high blood pressure is unknown, for example, grading of hypertensive retinopathy.[1]

Blood pressure measurement

Careful attention to blood pressure measurement technique is necessary so that the accuracy and reliability of this diagnostic test is maximized.[1,2,5] When taking a patient's blood pressure consensus guidelines recommend that:

- The patient is seated in a quiet environment with an arm resting on a support that places the midpoint of the upper arm at the level of the heart.

- Measure sitting blood pressure routinely; standing blood pressure in elderly and diabetic patients.

- Use a cuff of appropriate size (bladder should encircle ≥80 per cent of the arm and lower edge of cuff should be 2 cm above antecubital fossa).

- Inflate cuff rapidly to 70 mmHg and then inflate by 10 mmHg increments palpating radial pulse until pulse disappears. Note pressure at which pulse disappears and subsequently reappears during deflation.

- Place the low-frequency bell over the brachial artery pulsation.

- Inflate bladder 20 mmHg above level previously determined by palpation. Deflate bladder by 2 mmHg per second. Note the blood pressure level with the appearance of repetitive sounds (Korotkoff phase 1) and measure diastolic at the disappearance of sounds (Korotkoff phase 5). Systolic and diastolic pressure readings should be rounded to the nearest 2 mmHg.

- Take two measurements at each visit, at least more than 30 s apart.

- Use the average for several visits (≥3) when estimating sustained blood pressure reading.

Family physicians should be aware of the patient, health professional, and instrument factors that lead to inaccurate blood pressure measurement.[1,5] The commonest reasons include: use of an inappropriately small cuff; deflating the cuff too quickly; failing to palpate maximal systolic blood pressure before auscultation; and inaccurate 'rounding' errors when recording blood pressure reading.

Mercury sphygmomanometers are likely to be phased out for health and safety reasons. There will be increasing use of alternative devices to measure blood pressure including aneroid, semi-automated, and automated devices. There is substantial evidence that some of these alternative devices are inaccurate when subjected to validation. Prior to purchasing alternatives to a mercury sphygmomanometer, care should be taken to buy a device that accords to validated standards (e.g. the British Hypertension Society standards protocol). Regular calibration of devices, particularly anaeroid sphygmomanometers is required.[2]

Ambulatory blood pressure monitoring (ABPM)

Ambulatory blood pressure monitoring permits repeated non-invasive measurement of blood pressure over a prolonged period of time, reducing variability and measurement error of blood pressure readings.[6] Firm evidence concerning the value of ABPM is limited but it has been shown to correlate better with end-organ damage when compared to clinic blood pressure measurement. ABPM may be indicated in the following situations:

- When blood pressure shows unusual variability, particularly episodic hypertension.

- Apparent drug resistance (blood pressure >150/90 mmHg after taking more than three drugs).

- When symptoms suggest the possibility of hypotension when taking antihypertensive therapy.

- Suspected autonomic dysfunction.

- In the diagnosis of white-coat hypertension. This is the phenomenon whereby blood pressure measured by medical personnel is elevated when

compared to ABPM readings (present only when clinic ABPM difference exceeds the population average difference).

ABPM is not indicated for all patients with high blood pressure, particularly those at high levels of cardiovascular risk (>15 per cent over 10 years) or those with end-organ damage. Of note, average daytime blood pressure should be used for treatment decisions when using ABPM. ABPM readings are systematically lower than clinic measurement and treatment targets need to be adjusted accordingly (on average by 12/7 mmHg).[2]

Role of home self-measurement

This technique is becoming increasingly popular with patients. Evidence concerning the role of self-measurement is less extensive than ABPM but the same considerations about validated devices and blood pressure recordings apply.

Risk stratification and calculation of cardiovascular risk

High blood pressure should be managed in the context of overall cardiovascular risk. Cardiovascular risk calculation requires assessment of age, sex, history of diabetes, smoking status, serum lipids, family history, and past history of cardiovascular disease. Health professionals' intuitive estimates of absolute risk are inaccurate. All national guidelines now recommend cardiovascular risk estimation and some provide charts to facilitate accurate estimation (Table 1). Risk estimation can now be undertaken via the Internet using either the Framingham risk equation or the risk equation developed from data derived from RCTs of antihypertensive therapy (see websites).[7] Patients with high blood pressure often disagree with guidelines and health professionals over the level of cardiovascular risk they are prepared to accept as either safe or hazardous. Similarly, different blood pressure thresholds have been recommended by different consensus guidelines above which blood pressure treatment is recommended (Table 1). We feel that cardiovascular risk assessment and blood pressure level should be viewed as the starting point when discussing the risks and benefits of blood pressure treatment with patients and not an end in itself. Patients' preferences are as important an element as cardiovascular risk when deciding on whether antihypertensive treatment is necessary.

Educational interventions and written materials have been shown to improve patients' understanding and knowledge of blood pressure and may facilitate shared decision making between patient and health professional.

Detection of high blood pressure

Controlled trial evidence of interventions aimed at improving coverage of the population and detection of hypertension are inconclusive.[8] Screening programmes aimed at reaching disadvantaged groups do not appear to be effective. In countries with well-developed primary care services, case finding appears to be an effective way of identifying patients with high blood pressure, particularly when linked to training of primary care staff, adherence to protocols, and reminders to record blood pressure aimed at health professionals and patients.[8]

Principles of management

The principal objectives when treating high blood pressure in patients is to:[1]

1. Decrease their cardiovascular risk associated with hypertension.

2. Decrease the risk of any other co-existing cardiovascular risk factors.

3. Select antihypertensive drugs that are likely to do more good than harm for each individual's mix of co-existing medical conditions, risk factors, preferences, and social circumstances.

4. Minimize the adverse effects and inconvenience of antihypertensive drugs.[1]

Table 1 Recommended treatment thresholds and treatment targets in the current WHO (International Society of Hypertension), US, and UK hypertension guidelines

National guideline	Threshold recommendation	Treatment target
WHO-ISH	Recommend that hypertension should not be based on level of BP alone but on cardiovascular risk level (fatal and non-fatal stroke and myocardial infarction from Framingham risk equation) Cardiovascular risk should be stratified according to blood pressure level: ◆ Grade 1 (SBP 140–159, DBP 90–99) ◆ Grade 2 (SBP 160–179, DBP 100–109) ◆ Grade 3 (SBP ≥ 180, DBP ≥ 110) and presence of: ◆ Cardiovascular risk factors ◆ Target-organ damage ◆ Associated clinical conditions Patients then stratified by absolute level of cardiovascular risk: ◆ Low (<15%)—begin treatment/monitor depends on BP level ◆ Medium (15–20%)—begin treatment /monitor depends on BP level ◆ High (20–30%)—treat immediately ◆ Very high (≥30%)—treat immediately * Diabetics with SBP 130–139/85–89 mmHg should be considered for drug treatment	<140/90 mmHg
US	Risk stratification based on level of BP and risk group status, target-organ damage (TOD), clinical cardiovascular disease (CCD) and risk factor status, presented as a table Cardiovascular risk stratified according to blood pressure level: ◆ High-normal (SBP 130–139 or DBP 85–89) ◆ Hypertension stage 1 (SBP 140–159 or DBP 90–99) ◆ Hypertension stage 2 (SBP 160–179 or DBP 100–109)—start treatment irrespective of risk group status ◆ Hypertension stage 3 (SBP ≥180 or DBP ≥110)—start treatment irrespective of risk group status and presence of: ◆ Risk group A—no risk factors, no TOD, no CCD ◆ Risk group B—at least one risk factor, not including diabetes, TOD or CCD ◆ Risk group C—TOD/CCD and/or diabetes, with or without other risk factors Lifestyle modification or drug treatment recommended according to combination of BP level and risk group status	<140/90 mmHg
UK	Initial blood pressure measurement: BP levels ≥160/≥100—start treatment BP levels 140–159/90–99—stratify cardiovascular risk Target organ damage or CVS complication or 10-year CHD risk ≥15%—start drug treatment For diabetics, BP threshold for starting treatment is ≥140/90	Optimal <140/85 mmHg <140/80 mmHg (diabetes) Audit standard <150/90 mmHg <140/85 mmHg (diabetes)
New Zealand	Patients divided into: (1) high-risk patients for whom risk table assessment is deemed unnecessary: ◆ Clinically proven coronary heart disease ◆ Angioplasty or coronary artery bypass grafts ◆ Ischaemic stroke or atherosclerotic TIAs ◆ Proven intermittent claudication from peripheral vascular disease ◆ Patients with genetic lipid disorders ◆ Patients with diabetic nephropathy (albuminuria >300 mg/day) (2) Lower cardiovascular risk patients in whom risk table assessment is carried out: ◆ Patients cardiovascular risk assessed by means of cardiovascular risk table taking into account: age, sex, diabetic status, smoking status, total cholesterol/HDL ratio, and blood pressure level ◆ Patient then classified into one of eight cardiovascular risk categories (>30%, 25–30%, 20–25%, 15–20%, 10–15%, 5–10%, 2.5–5%, <2.5%) ◆ Treatment recommended if cardiovascular risk >10–15% over 5 years ◆ Some flexibility for patients with high cholesterol (>8.5–9 mmol/l) or blood pressure (>about 170/100 mmHg). Risk equations may underestimate their true risk. Therefore, it is recommended that treatment be considered at lower absolute CVD risks than in other patients	No explicit treatment goal mentioned but BP reduction of 12/6 mmHg in patients with BP >140–150/90 is the underlying assumption of guideline so can be assumed to be minimum treatment goal

Non-pharmacological treatment

Risk factor modification is frequently recommended as an initial alternative to drug treatment. The magnitude of blood pressure reduction for most interventions is modest. The respective mean reduction in systolic blood pressure (95 per cent confidence interval) for the following interventions is as follows: salt restriction, -2.9 mmHg (-5.8, 0.0); weight loss, -5.2 mmHg (-8.3, -2.0); stress control, -1.0 (-2.3, 0.3); exercise, -0.8 mmHg (-5.9, 4.2). More recent evidence in the elderly suggests that non-pharmacological treatment, particularly salt restriction and weight reduction, may be a feasible alternative to drug treatment.

Pharmacological treatment

There has been a move away from the 'stepped care' approach of drug treatment, that is, starting with a thiazide or beta-blocker and then adding in other classes of antihypertensive drugs. A 'tailored care' approach is now favoured: individualizing drug therapy to the patient's risk factor and co-morbid profile. Table 2 summarizes the indications, contra-indications, and side-effects of antihypertensive drugs.

Case control, cohort, and randomized studies suggest that short and intermediate acting dihydropyridine calcium channel blockers such as nifedipine and isradipine may increase cardiovascular morbidity and mortality.[9] Calcium channel blockers are a heterogeneous class of drugs with different postulated mechanisms of action (slowing atrioventricular node conduction, reducing contractility and peripheral vasodilatation). They are unlikely to have a similar class effect for patients with high blood pressure.[1] The issue of safety of calcium channel blockers compared to other antihypertensive drugs is not fully resolved.[9,10] Ongoing prospective trials are likely to provide more definitive answers about the possible harms of calcium channel blockers. Until then, caution is required with short and intermediate acting agents when treating patients with a past history of myocardial infarct or heart failure.[10]

Aspirin has been shown to reduce the risk of cardiovascular events. However, the risks of bleeding may outweight cardiovascular benefits in patients whose cardiovascular risk is less than 1–1.5 per cent per year. Low-dose aspirin (75 mg/day) is recommended for patients with well controlled blood pressure ($<150/90$ mmHg) who have no contraindications to aspirin and who fall into the following categories:

♦ History of previous cardiovascular disease.

♦ Cardiovascular risk greater than 20 per cent over 10 years.

♦ Presence of target organ damage (left ventricular hypertrophy, renal impairment, or proteinuria).

♦ Type 2 diabetes mellitus.

Specific groups of patients are considered in the following sections.

Coronary heart disease and myocardial infarction

Beta-blockers without intrinsic sympathomimetic activity are recommended first-line agents. Calcium channel blockers can be used for patients with angina in whom beta-blockers are contra-indicated or if anginal symptoms are uncontrolled. Calcium channel blockers should be avoided in

Table 2 Indications, contra-indications, and side-effects of the major antihypertensive drugs

Drug class	Indications	Contra-indications	Common side-effects
Thiazide diuretics	Elderly Diabetes (type 2) African-Caribbean ethnic groups	Gout Dyslipidaemia Urinary incontinence	Hypokalaemia Hyponatraemia Sexual dysfunction Gout Glucose intolerance
Beta-blockers	Myocardial infarction Angina Heart failure Migraine	Asthma/COPD Heart block PVD Dyslipidaemia	Fatigue Insomnia Cold peripheries Bradycardia
ACE inhibitors	Diabetes Myocardial infarction Angina Heart failure Chronic renal disease[a]	Pregnancy Renovascular disease PVD[b]	Cough First dose hypotension Taste disturbance Angio-oedema
Calcium channel blockers	Elderly Angina Pregnancy African-Caribbean ethnic groups	Myocardial infarction[c] Heart failure[c]	Constipation Peripheral oedema Flushing Headache
Alpha blockers	Prostatism	Heart failure Urinary incontinence Postural hypotension	Nasal stuffiness Dizziness Postural hypotension
Central agents (methyldopa)	Pregnancy	Postural hypotension	Depression Haemolytic anaemia
ACE II antagonists	Intolerance to other drugs Heart failure	Pregnancy Renovascular disease PVD	Angio-oedema

[a] ACE inhibitors need to be used with caution in chronic renal disease as they may precipitate renal failure; they require regular supervision and specialist advice in these patients.

[b] PVD frequently associated with renovascular disease.

[c] Amlodipine (long-acting dihydropyridine) can be used, other calcium channel blockers are best avoided.

COPD, chronic obstructive pulmonary disease; PVD, peripheral vascular disease.

patients with a previous history of myocardial infarction and left ventricular dysfunction. ACE inhibitors can be considered for patients with angina and are of proven benefit after myocardial infarction, particularly in those patients with left ventricular systolic dysfunction.[1]

Heart failure

ACE inhibitors (in addition to diuretic therapy) and beta-blockers are known to reduce mortality in patients with heart failure due to left ventricular systolic dysfunction and can be recommended in routine practice. Current evidence suggests that calcium channel blockers and alpha-blockers may worsen clinical outcomes and should be avoided.

Diabetes

Aggressive blood pressure control is warranted in all diabetic patients. Patients with diabetes are at high risk of cardiovascular disease. Aspirin should be offered to all patients with evidence of end-organ damage, previous cardiovascular disease, or cardiovascular risk exceeding 5 per cent over 5 years. Total cholesterol should be measured in all diabetic patients and treated with statins in those patients in whom readings exceed 5 mmol/l.

The threshold for treatment is above 140/90 mmHg. There is good evidence that intensive blood pressure control (<80 mmHg diastolic) is better than less intensive control. Blood pressure lowering and ACE-inhibitor treatment slow the rate of decline of renal function in diabetic nephropathy and delay progression from the microalbuminuric phase to overt nephropathy.[2] ACE inhibitors may have specific renoprotective effects, over and above their blood pressure lowering effects, and are recommended first-line therapy for patients with incipient or overt nephropathy. Diabetic patients with persistent microalbuminuria or proteinuria who have blood pressure readings with the 'normal' range may also benefit from ACE inhibition titrated to the maximum recommended dosage. In type 2 diabetes, ACE inhibitors, beta-blockers, and low-dose thiazide diuretics are all effective agents.

Renal disease

High blood pressure in patients with chronic renal failure accelerates the rate of loss of renal function. Randomized trials have shown that ACE inhibitors reduce the risk of progression to end-stage renal failure compared to placebo and other antihypertensive drugs (beta-blockers or calcium channel blockers).[1,2] ACE inhibitors are considered to be first-line agents for patients with mild to moderate renal impairment and high blood pressure. The threshold for treatment is not less than 140/90 mmHg.[2] Patients with renal failure are at high risk of cardiovascular disease and require aspirin and statin treatment in addition to non-pharmacological measures in their management. Specialist referral is often warranted so that appropriate investigation as to the cause of their renal failure can take place and appropriate management started.

Elderly

Systolic blood pressure rises with age resulting in a higher prevalence of high blood pressure in people aged more than 60 years. Low-dose thiazide diuretics are the drugs of choice in the elderly, for both isolated systolic hypertension and systolic and diastolic hypertension. Dihydropyridine calcium channel blockers are suitable alternatives when thiazides are contra-indicated or poorly tolerated.[2]

Pregnancy

When high blood pressure is discovered in a pregnant woman, three possible diagnostic possibilities exist. Firstly, she suffers from chronic high blood pressure (defined as blood pressure ≥140/90 mmHg before 20 weeks' gestation or if high blood pressure persists more than 6 weeks after delivery). This can be diagnosed prior to, during, or after pregnancy. Secondly, she may develop pregnancy-induced high blood pressure (pre-eclampsia). Lastly, pregnancy-induced high blood pressure may be superimposed on existing chronic high blood pressure. Consensus definitions of hypertension are 'moderate' if blood pressure is more than or equal to 140/90 mmHg and 'severe' if more than or equal to 170/110 mmHg.

Chronic high blood pressure is associated with a modest increase in risk to both the mother and baby. Potential complications include stillbirth, placental abruption, superimposed pre-eclampsia, foetal growth restriction, pre-term delivery, and maternal mortality.[1]

Current consensus is that severe high blood pressure in pregnancy (≥170/110 mmHg) warrants drug treatment. Treatment of moderate high blood pressure (≥140/90 mmHg) is less certain in terms of benefit to the mother and may affect foetal growth.[1,2] Evidence underpinning the choice of antihypertensive in pregnancy is limited. Methyldopa is regarded as the first-line agent for pregnancy-induced and chronic high blood pressure associated with pregnancy because of its long and extensive use without reports of serious side-effects on the foetus.[1,2] Calcium channel blockers (particularly nifedepine) and the beta-blocker labetalol are commonly used as second-line agents. ACE inhibitors are associated with adverse foetal effects when used in the second and third trimesters and they should be avoided.

Long-term and continuing care

Principles

The underlying principles of long-term care can be summarized as follows:

- ensure that blood pressure is at target level;
- treat relevant co-morbid conditions.

Goals of treatment

Intensive lowering of blood pressure has been shown to reduce cardiovascular disease. Randomized trials that compare aggressive versus less aggressive lowering of blood pressure report no adverse J-shaped relationship (too great a lowering of blood pressure leading to an increase in cardiovascular events). The optimal target blood pressure has been proposed as less than 140/85 mmHg for non-diabetic patients and less than 140/80 mmHg for diabetic patients.

Problem of uncontrolled hypertension

The care that patients with high blood pressure receive is often variable and incomplete. The consequence is that in many countries a large proportion (usually in the range of 40–50 per cent, depending on the blood pressure level used to define target blood pressure) of patients taking antihypertensive drugs have not reached target blood pressure goals.[8] These individuals are said to have 'uncontrolled' high blood pressure. Common reasons and proposed solutions why individuals do not reach target blood pressure include:

- Inaccurate blood pressure measurement.
- White-coat hypertension—ask other health workers to measure patients' blood pressure at other times; if still raised, try self-monitoring or referral for ABPM.
- Disease progression—can only be attributed to disease progression after excluding other possible causes.
- Sub-optimal treatment—at least half the patients with high blood pressure will require two or more classes of antihypertensive drugs to ensure adequate blood pressure control.
- Non-adherence to antihypertensive drugs—has been reported to occur in at least 50 per cent of patients with high blood pressure. Clinical judgement of adherence is poor but non-threatening direct questioning is worthwhile in those patients in whom non-adherence is suspected. There is some evidence that adherence can be enhanced by educating and discussing adherence issues with patients and by involving other members in the primary health care team.[8]

◆ Concurrent use of antagonizing drugs—several drugs raise blood pressure and these should be specifically asked about when taking a history. Of particular note, NSAIDs are commonly prescribed, particularly in the elderly. It is estimated that they increase blood pressure by about 3–5 mmHg in hypertensive individuals.

◆ Co-existing conditions—includes excessive alcohol use, obesity, anxiety, hyperinsulinism with insulin resistance, sleep apnoea, and current smokers.

◆ Secondary hypertension—requires further investigation and specialist referral.

There is inadequate evidence to recommend the optimal timing for patient review, self-management strategies (including self-monitoring by patients), and the value of dedicated hypertension clinics. There is evidence that involvement of the primary health care team, particularly practice nurses, structured care, characterized by registration of patients, recall, and regular review improves both blood pressure control and prevents cardiovascular disease. The cost effectiveness of such an intensive approach to long-term care is less certain.

Implications of the problem

Quality of life and side-effects from treatment

There is some evidence of a 'labelling' effect on patients diagnosed as having high blood pressure. Knowledge that a person has high blood pressure has been found to increase their absenteeism from work and produce a negative impact on self-reported psychological well-being. However, the overall impact of high blood pressure on quality of life is not thought to be substantial.[1]

Symptomatic adverse effects vary by drug class and by agents within classes. Overall, 10–18 per cent of individuals receiving antihypertensive treatment report side-effects.[1] However, in some groups of patients side-effects can be more common, for instance, over a quarter of elderly people who received a calcium channel blocker report ankle oedema. Family physicians should be aware of the common side-effects from the major classes of antihypertensive drugs summarized in Table 2.

Further research

The following research areas are likely to produce research evidence that may alter management recommendations in the near future:

◆ The role of ABPM versus clinic blood pressures in monitoring response to drug treatment.

◆ The role of aspirin in primary prevention, particularly in post-menopausal women.

◆ The efficacy and safety of treatment drug regimens based on different classes of antihypertensive drugs.

◆ Impact of adherence-enhancing strategies on adherence to drugs and blood pressure control.

◆ The role of patients' preferences in treatment choice and subsequent impact on adherence.

References

1. **Mulrow, C.D.**, ed. *Evidence-based Hypertension*. London: BMJ Books, 2001.

2. **Ramsay, L.E.** et al. (1999). Guidelines for the management of hypertension: report of the third working party of the British Hypertension Society. *Journal of Human Hypertension* **13**, 569–92.

3. **Joint National Committee**. *The Sixth Report of the Joint National Committee on Prevention, Detection, Evaluation and Treatment of High Blood Pressure*. Bethesda MD: National Institutes of Health, 1997.

4. **Swales, J.D.**, ed. *Textbook of Hypertension*. Oxford: Blackwell Scientific Publications, 1994.

Key points

◆ High blood pressure is an independent risk factor for cardiovascular disease, renal failure, cognitive decline, and all-cause mortality.

◆ Measurement of blood pressure requires adherence to recommended blood pressure measurement techniques to ensure a valid and reliable record.

◆ Assessment of high blood pressure should be viewed in the context of overall cardiovascular risk and formal risk estimation is recommended for all patients.

◆ Treatment with antihypertensive drugs has been shown to reduce cardiovascular events by 30 per cent.

◆ Drug treatment should be 'tailored' to each patient's co-morbid and risk factor profile. Complete blood pressure control requires two or more classes of antihypertensive drugs for the majority of patients.

◆ Long-term management requires regular recall and review. Family physicians should be alert to the common reasons why patients do not attain treatment goals.

5. **Reeves, R.** (1995). Does this patient have hypertension? How to measure blood pressure. *Journal of the American Medical Association* **273**, 1211–18.

6. **Beevers, G., Lip, G.Y.H.**, and **O'Brien, E.** *ABC of Hypertension*. London: BMJ Books, 2001.

7. **Pocock, S.J.** et al. (2001). A score for predicting risk of death from cardiovascular disease in adults with raised blood pressure, based on individual patient data from randomised controlled trials. *British Medical Journal* **323**, 75–81.

8. **Ebrahim, S.** (1998). Detection, adherence and control of hypertension for the prevention of stroke: a systematic review. *Health Technology Assessment* **2**, 11.

9. **Pahor, M.** et al. (2000). Health outcomes associated with calcium antagonists compared with other first-line antihypertensive therapies: a meta-analysis of randomised controlled trials. *Lancet* **356**, 1949–54.

10. **Blood Pressure Lowering Treatment Trialists' Collaboration** (2000). Effects of ACE inhibitors, calcium antagonists, and other blood pressure lowering drugs: results of prospectively designed overviews of randomised trials. *Lancet* **356**, 1955–64.

Websites

New Zealand cardiovascular risk charts (based on the Framingham risk equation)—http://www.nzgg.org.nz/library/gl_complete/bloodpressure/table1.cfm.

Cardiovascular risk score (based on individual patient data from randomised trials)—http://www.riskscore.org.uk/.

British Hypertension Society—www.hyp.ac.uk/bhs.

US guidelines, 1997—http://www.nhlbi.nih.gov/guidelines/hypertension/jncintro.htm.

WHO guidelines, 1999—http://www.who.int/ncd/cvd/ht-guide.html.

1.11 Dyslipidaemia and cardiovascular disease

Richard Hobbs

The principal manifestations of cardiovascular diseases, namely coronary heart disease (CHD) and stroke, represent the two most common causes of death in the world today.[1] Cardiovascular diseases result in the highest health care utilization costs in most countries, for the treatment of stroke and heart failure.[2,3]

Although more than 200 risk factors for CHD have now been identified, the single most powerful predictor of CHD risk is abnormal blood lipid levels.[4] To reduce the rates of cardiovascular disease, both primary and secondary prevention strategies are essential. Unfortunately, there is considerable evidence of under-management of patients with elevated cholesterol and cardiovascular risk who are eligible for secondary prevention. Better recognition of patients at increased risk, but without established disease (primary prevention), will require greater familiarity with the clinical use of CHD risk scoring systems, most of which are based upon the Framingham equation. Primary prevention is at least partly justified by the fact that one in five coronary deaths present with sudden death as the first and only symptom.

One factor in the current under-performance by physicians in cardiovascular disease prevention is likely to be gaps in knowledge[5] or confusion over recommendations, such as the selection of patients for primary or secondary prevention, the use of CHD risk equations,[6,7] and target levels for lipid fractions during treatment.[8]

Lipids and cardiovascular disease risk

A number of modifiable predisposing factors has been shown to predict the development of coronary disease, long in advance of symptoms (Table 1). The primary risk factors of hyperlipidaemia, hypertension, smoking, and impaired glucose tolerance appear to promote CHD by accelerating the pace of atherosclerotic change. Other important predisposing factors include diet, physical inactivity, obesity, and genetic influences.

A strong positive and graded relationship with death due to CHD has been documented for total cholesterol (TC) levels above 4.63 mmol/l (180 mg/dl).[8] Moreover, studies have also demonstrated that the individual lipid fractions, namely low-density lipoprotein cholesterol (LDL-C), high-density lipoprotein cholesterol (HDL-C), and triglycerides (TG), are independent risk factors, with LDL-C emerging as the most significant predictor of individual CHD risk.

Table 1 Risk factors for CHD and recommended European target goals

Non-modifiable	
Age	Men: ≥45 years
	Women: >55 years
Personal history of CHD	
Family history of CHD	

Modifiable	Target goals
High TC	<5.0 mmol/l (<190 mg/dl)
High LDL-C	<3.0 mmol/l (<115 mg/dl)
Low HDL-C	>1.1 mmol/l (>40 mg/dl)
High TG	<1.2 mmol/l (<150 mg/dl)
Hypertension	<140/90 mmHg
Diabetes mellitus	Normalize glucose levels
Current tobacco use	Smoking cessation
Obesity	Body mass index <25
Sedentary lifestyle	Exercise daily

LDL-C as the primary risk factor for CHD

In addition to the positive correlation between LDL-C and CHD (Table 2), primary[9,10] and secondary[11,12] prevention trials have demonstrated that therapeutic interventions to lower LDL-C to target levels are associated with a significant reduction in CHD morbidity and mortality. There was initial concern over possible risks of long-term aggressive lipid-lowering interventions, but four large trials have confirmed that all-cause mortality was reduced 22–30 per cent with no increase in death from non-CHD causes in patients receiving lipid-lowering therapy.

High LDL-C may also be a modifiable risk factor for cerebrovascular atherosclerosis and stroke. Ultrasound studies of carotid atherosclerosis have shown that reduction of LDL-C levels can slow progression of atherosclerotic disease.

The role of HDL-C and TG as risk factors for CHD

In contrast to the adverse influence of other lipid fractions, epidemiological studies have established a powerful protective relationship between HDL-C and the incidence of CHD.[13] Individuals with low HDL-C levels [<1.04 mmol/l (≤40 mg/dl)] and average TC levels [<5.2 mmol/l (≤200 mg/dl)] have the same CHD risk as individuals with high TC levels [6.7 mmol/l (≥260 mg/dl)]. Observational epidemiological studies project a 2–3 per cent reduction in CHD risk for every 0.02 mmol/l (1 mg/dl) incremental increase in HDL-C.[14]

Although established as an independent risk factor for CHD, the degree of cardio-protection provided by raising HDL-C levels in most patients at risk for CHD requires further elucidation in trials. Currently, therefore, HDL-C remains secondary to LDL-C as a target for predicting and preventing CHD risk.

Plasma TG concentration is an independent risk factor for CHD in both men and women.[15] A meta-analysis of 17 prospective population-based studies determined that for men the overall relative risk is 1.32, which correlates with a 30 per cent increase in risk for a 1 mmol/l increase in TG level. TG levels are an even more powerful risk factor in women, with an overall relative risk of 1.76. Although these observational data are highly suggestive of a causal association, the effect of reduction in plasma TG and the risk of CHD has yet to be demonstrated.

Multifactorial risk assessment for primary prevention of CHD

Although high LDL-C levels may be the most important individual risk factor for CHD, cardiovascular disease is multifactorial in origin and CHD risk factors appear multiplicative in nature. Estimation of an individual's actual risk for future CHD events, or the need for primary prevention, must take into account all other coexistent CHD risk factors. Indeed, risk associated with any level of cholesterol is markedly influenced by coexistent risk factors. LDL-C acts as an accelerator of risk; as baseline LDL-C increases, the CHD risk impact of other risk factors increases at a faster rate. Therefore, an individual with a number of modest risk factors may be at considerably greater risk for CHD than a person with one very high risk factor.

These risk factor interactions provide the rationale for determining patient eligibility for primary prevention treatments on the basis of formal CHD risk scoring. European[16,17] and US guidelines[18] for CHD risk assessment use gender, age, smoking status, systolic blood pressure, presence of left ventricular hypertrophy, and TC to assess 10-year risk for CHD (Figs 1 and 2). Individual risk is determined by using one of the various algorithms available, based upon the Framingham equation.[19] These tools include the third edition of the *Sheffield Risk Tables*,[20] the European Coronary Risk Chart (Fig. 1),[21] or the New Zealand Risk Assessments Tool.[22] In addition to these colour charts which classify risk, a number of computer-based programs[23] are available.

In most countries, individuals are considered to be at sufficiently high risk for an adverse outcome to warrant lipid-lowering treatment if they have an

Table 2 Major statin trials demonstrating efficacy of lipid lowering in reducing CHD

	WOSCOPS[9]	AFCAPS/TexCAPS[10]	4S[26]	CARE[11]	LIPID[12]
Study characteristics					
N (% women)	6596 (0)	6605 (15)	4444 (19)	4159 (14)	9014 (17)
Duration	4.9	5.2	5.4	5	6.1
Intervention	Pravastatin 40 mg/day	Lovastatin 20–40 mg/day	Simvastatin 20a–40 mg/day	Pravastatin 40 mg/day	Pravastatin 40 mg/day
% Lipid changes (mg/dl)					
TC	−20	−19	−26	−20	−18
LDL-C	−26	−26	−36	−28	−25
HDL-C	+5	+5	+7	+5	+5
TG	−12	−13	−17	−14	−11
Endpoints (% change in risk), treatment versus placebo					
Non-fatal MI/CHD death	−31	−25	−34	−24	−24
Fatal/non-fatal MI	NR	−40	−42	−25	−29
Acute major coronary events	NR	−37	NR	NR	NR
Total mortality	−22	+3 (NS)	−30	−9 (NS)	−22
CHD mortality	−28	Too few	−42	−20	−24
Revascularization	−37	−33	−37	−27	−20
Stroke	−11 (NS)	NR	−30	−31	−19
Confidence intervals	95%	95%	95%	95%	95%

a Two patients were titrated down to 10 mg/day.

WOSCOPS, West of Scotland Coronary Prevention Study; AFCAPS/TexCAPS, Air Force/Texas Coronary Atherosclerosis Prevention Study; 4S, Scandinavian Simvastatin Survival Study; CARE, Cholesterol and Recurrent Events; CHD, coronary heart disease; HDL-C, high-density lipoprotein cholesterol; LDL-C, low-density lipoprotein cholesterol; LIPID, Long-Term Intervention with Pravastatin in Ischaemic Disease; MI, myocardial infarction; NS, non-significant; NR, not reported; TC, total cholesterol; TG, triglyceride.

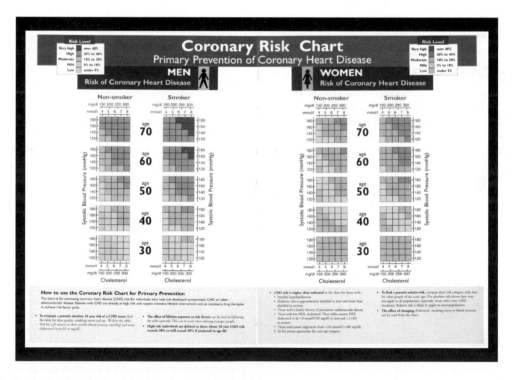

Fig. 1 European CHD risk calculator for primary prevention of coronary heart disease.

absolute 10-year CHD risk, or a CHD risk projected at age 60, of 20 per cent or greater. However, economic considerations are used in some countries, including the United Kingdom, for setting thresholds for therapy determined by a 10-year CHD risk score of 30 per cent rather than 20 per cent.

Secondary prevention of CHD

Importantly, and many physicians remain confused by this distinction, patients with established CHD (angina or myocardial infarction) or CHD equivalents (peripheral vascular disease, stroke, and, in the United States, diabetes) have effectively selected themselves as being at very high risk for future cardiovascular events. Therefore, since they already have a greater than 30 per cent 10-year CHD risk, treatment decisions (secondary prevention) should not be determined by CHD risk calculation. In these patients, lifestyle changes and pharmacologic therapy should therefore be aggressively pursued to bring cholesterol to below target levels, regardless of risk score.

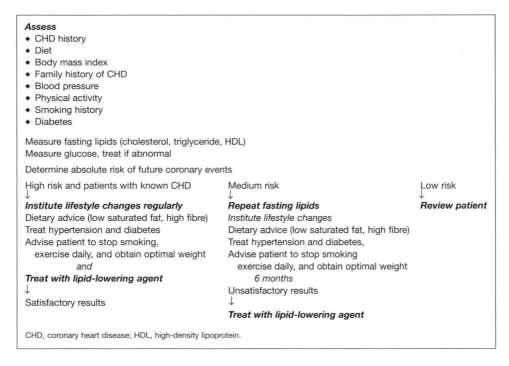

Assess
- ◆ CHD history
- ◆ Diet
- ◆ Body mass index
- ◆ Family history of CHD
- ◆ Blood pressure
- ◆ Physical activity
- ◆ Smoking history
- ◆ Diabetes

Measure fasting lipids (cholesterol, triglyceride, HDL)
Measure glucose, treat if abnormal

Determine absolute risk of future coronary events

High risk and patients with known CHD	Medium risk	Low risk
↓	↓	↓
Institute lifestyle changes regularly	*Repeat fasting lipids*	*Review patient*
Dietary advice (low saturated fat, high fibre)	*Institute lifestyle changes*	
Treat hypertension and diabetes	Dietary advice (low saturated fat, high fibre)	
Advise patient to stop smoking, exercise daily, and obtain optimal weight	Treat hypertension and diabetes,	
and	Advise patient to stop smoking exercise daily, and obtain optimal weight	
Treat with lipid-lowering agent	*6 months*	
↓	Unsatisfactory results	
Satisfactory results	↓	
	Treat with lipid-lowering agent	

CHD, coronary heart disease; HDL, high-density lipoprotein.

Fig. 2 Risk assessment based management of CHD.

Identifying patients with dyslipidaemia

In order to reduce the incidence of CHD, patients at risk must first be identified. European guidelines emphasize the importance of incorporating regular CHD risk factor assessment into clinical practice. All adults are potentially eligible for cardiovascular screening, but in practice it is reasonable to focus on adults from age 40 onwards and on the basis of formally risk-scoring anyone with a single CHD risk factor such as having hypertension or being a current smoker. However, anyone with premature CHD (established CHD before 55 in men and 65 in women) in a first-degree relative should be screened as early as practical, to exclude familial hyper-cholesterolaemia.

Initial CHD risk assessment should begin with questions regarding life-style (smoking status, physical activity level, alcohol use/abuse, oral contraception use) and family history (relatives with premature CHD, hypertension, or diabetes). Body mass index and blood pressure should also be measured. Lipid levels (TC and LDL as a minimum) should also be assessed in any individual with a risk factor such as elevated blood pressure, obesity, family history, or diabetes. Other markers, such as HDL-C [<1.0 mmol/l (≤40 mg/dl)] and fasting TG [>2.0 mmol/l (≥180 mg/dl)] should preferably be used for identifying individuals at increased coronary risk, but suffer from the requirement to collect a fasting blood sample.

In patients 40–69 years, metabolic risk factors (i.e. hypertension, diabetes, dyslipidaemia) become more prevalent. For middle-aged women, premature menopause is an additional risk factor for CHD. The largest proportion of high-risk individuals will be found in the older population (≥70 years). Hypertension, smoking, and hyperlipidaemia are the three most important modifiable risk factors in this population.

Physicians should advise patients of their global risk of CHD, review the individual risk factors, and discuss interventions that will target and normalize each risk factor. All physician practice surveys, however, point to serious under-management problems. In the United States, only 37 per cent of hypercholesterolaemic patients reached the LDL-C goals set by the clinical guidelines[24] and only 18 per cent of CHD patients met the LDL-C goal of 100 mg/dl. Treatment levels are not much better in Europe, even in specialist settings.[25]

Treatment of dyslipidaemia

Lowering LDL-C is the primary focus of treatment for dyslipidaemia. Treatment will require lifestyle interventions and often pharmacotherapy to achieve recommended goals (Fig. 2). In low- and moderate-risk individuals, guidelines advocate an initial management strategy of dietary adjustment [reduced intake of total fats, reduced intake of saturated fats, increased intake of fresh fruits and vegetables (five portions daily), reduced salt intake (<1 g/day)], reduced alcohol use, increased physical activity, and weight reduction, if needed.

For some, lifestyle counselling may be the only intervention required to lower CHD risk status. Moderate-risk patients who do not achieve target LDL-C levels with lifestyle modifications and patients in the highest-risk category should be considered for pharmaceutical intervention. Patients with established CHD (secondary prevention patients) should always be offered lipid-lowering therapy if their lipid levels are above target.

Current European recommendations suggest a target LDL-C level of not more than 3 mmol/l (≤115 mg/dl), regardless of degree of individual risk. However, a threshold level below which LDL-C lowering no longer provides additional reduction in CHD risk has not been identified and debate surrounds the question of what the minimal LDL-C target should be. Indeed, there is accumulating evidence for lowering lipid levels to below the currently recommended targets. In the United States, lipid targets are slightly more complicated, with less than 100 mg/dl (<2.6 mmol/l) for secondary prevention, less than 130 mg/dl (<3 mmol/l) for primary prevention with two risk factors, and less than 160 mg/dl (<3.4 mmol/l) for primary prevention when there is only one risk factor.

Although there is insufficient evidence to justify absolute treatment goals for TG or HDL-C, US and European guidelines suggest that modifying HDL-C to above 1 mmol/l and TG to below 300 mmol/l in addition to

LDL-C targets is an important part of risk factor modification for secondary prevention of CHD.

Where therapy is necessary, four classes of lipid-lowering agents are currently available: bile acid sequestrants, niacin, fibrates, and 3-hydroxy-3-methylglutaryl coenzyme A (HMG-CoA) reductase inhibitors ('statins'). The guidelines state that preference should be given to statin monotherapy due to the strong evidence supporting their efficacy in reducing coronary morbidity, mortality, and prolonging survival in CHD patients and those at risk for CHD (Table 2). All of the statins are well tolerated and have good long-term safety records. There are differences between statins in their effectiveness at LDL-C lowering at comparable doses and their duration of action. Shorter-acting statins must be taken at night. If the target LDL-C goal is not reached within a reasonable time period, the statin dose should be increased.

Summary

European and US guidelines emphasize the importance of identifying and treating hypercholesterolaemia in individuals with CHD or at high risk of developing CHD. Although tools that can aid the identification and treatment of individuals at risk of CHD are available, substantial numbers of opportunities to reduce morbidity and mortality are being missed. Elevated LDL-C is an important risk factor and, when managed aggressively, is associated with a significant reduction in CHD.

Unfortunately, despite compelling evidence that lowering LDL-C reduces CHD events, many patients with CHD are not receiving lipid-lowering treatment, and those receiving treatment do not achieve target levels. If the substantial global toll of CHD is to be reduced, preventive cardiology for individuals at risk for CHD must become a medical priority. Identification of at-risk individuals and the institution of a regimen of aggressive risk factor modification needs to become standard practice, in compliance with international treatment guidelines.

Key points

1. Coronary heart disease (CHD) and stroke represent the two most common causes of death in the world and result in the highest health care utilization costs.

2. CHD is a multi-factorial disease, though the single most powerful predictor of CHD risk is abnormal blood lipid levels, especially low density lipoprotein (LDL).

3. To reduce the rates of cardiovascular disease, both primary (absence of disease) and secondary (established disease), prevention strategies are needed.

4. For primary CHD prevention, eligibility for treatments are based upon formal CHD risk assessment, usually determined using a risk score based upon the Framingham equation. Individuals are at sufficiently high risk to warrant lipid-lowering treatment if they have an absolute 10-year CHD risk, or a CHD risk projected at age 60, of 20 per cent or greater.

5. Patients with established CHD (angina or myocardial infarction) or CHD equivalents (peripheral vascular disease, stroke, and in the United States, diabetes), have over 30 per cent, 10-year CHD risk and treatment decisions (secondary prevention) should be instituted automatically.

6. Lowering LDL-C is the primary treatment focus for dyslipidaemia. Treatment will require lifestyle interventions and usually hydroxy-3-methylglutaryl coenzyme A (HMG-CoA) reductase inhibitors (statin) therapy to achieve lipid targets.

References

1. Murray, C.J. and Lopez, A.D. (1998). The global burden of disease, 1990–2020. *Nature Medicine* **4** (11), 1241–3.

2. Gillum, R.F. (1993). Heart and stroke facts. *American Heart Journal* **126**, 1042–7.

3. O'Connell, J.B. and Bristow, M.R. (1994). Economic impact of heart failure in the United States: time for a different approach. *The Journal of Heart and Lung Transplantation* **13** (Suppl. 4), S107–12.

4. Castelli, W.P. (1996). Lipids, risk factors and ischaemic heart disease. *Atherosclerosis* **124** (Suppl.), S1–9.

5. Hobbs, F.D.R. and Erhardt, L. (2000). Reassessing European Attitudes about Cardiovascular Treatment (REACT) survey: physician perceptions and attitudes towards cholesterol guidelines. *European Journal of Cardiology*.

6. Peters, T.J., Montgomery, A.A., and Fahey, T. (1999). How accurately do primary health care professionals use cardiovascular risk tables in the management of hypertension? *British Journal of General Practice* **49**, 987–8.

7. Grover, S.A., Lowensteyn, I., Esrey, K.L., Steinert, Y., Joseph, L., and Abrahamowicz, M. (1995). Do doctors accurately assess coronary risk in their patients? Preliminary results of the coronary health assessment study. *British Medical Journal* **310**, 975–8.

8. Neaton, J.D. et al. (1992). Serum cholesterol level and mortality findings for men screened in the Multiple Risk Factor Intervention Trial. Multiple Risk Factor Intervention Trial Research Group. *Archives of Internal Medicine* **152** (7), 1490–500.

9. Shepherd, J. et al. (1995). Prevention of coronary heart disease with pravastatin in men with hypercholesterolemia. West of Scotland Coronary Prevention Study Group. *New England Journal of Medicine* **333** (20), 1301–7.

10. Downs, J.R. et al. (1998). Primary prevention of acute coronary events with lovastatin in men and women with average cholesterol levels: results of AFCAPS/TexCAPS. Air Force/Texas Coronary Atherosclerosis Prevention Study. *Journal of the American Medical Association* **279** (20), 1615–22.

11. Sacks, F.M. et al. (1996). The effect of pravastatin on coronary events after myocardial infarction in patients with average cholesterol levels. The Cholesterol and Recurrent Events Trial (CARE) investigators. *New England Journal of Medicine* **335** (14), 1001–9.

12. LIPID Study Group (1998). Prevention of cardiovascular events and death with pravastatin in patients with coronary heart disease and a broad range of initial cholesterol levels. The Long-Term Intervention with Pravastatin in Ischaemic Disease (LIPID) Study Group. *New England Journal of Medicine* **339** (19), 1349–57.

13. Kannel, W.B. (1990). Contribution of the Framingham Study to preventive cardiology. *Journal of the American College of Cardiology* **15**, 206–11.

14. Gordon, D.J. et al. (1989). High-density lipoprotein cholesterol and cardiovascular disease. Four prospective American studies. *Circulation* **79** (1), 8–15.

15. Austin, M.A. (1998). Plasma triglyceride as a risk factor for cardiovascular disease. *Canadian Journal of Cardiology* **14** (Suppl. B), 14B–17B.

16. Second Joint Task Force (1998). Prevention of coronary heart disease in clinical practice. Recommendations of the Second Joint Task Force of European and other Societies on coronary prevention. *European Heart Journal* **19** (10), 1434–503.

17. Wood, D., De Backer, G., Faergeman, O., Graham, I., Mancia, G., and Pyorala, K. (1998). Prevention of coronary heart disease in clinical practice: recommendations of the Second Joint Task Force of European and other Societies on Coronary Prevention. *Atherosclerosis* **140** (2), 199–270.

18. National Cholesterol Education Program (NCEP) (1994). Second report of the Expert Panel on Detection, Evaluation, and Treatment of High Blood Cholesterol in Adults (Adult Treatment Panel II). *Circulation* **89** (3), 1333–445.

19. Anderson, K.M., Odell, P.M., Wilson, P.W.F., and Kannel, W.E. (1990). Cardiovascular disease risk profiles. *American Heart Journal* **121**, 293–8.

20. Wallace, E.J. et al. (2000). Coronary and cardiovascular risk estimation for primary prevention: population validation of a new Sheffield table in the 1995 Scottish health survey population. *British Medical Journal* **11**, 671–6.

21. Wood, D. et al. for the Second Joint Task Force of European and other Societies of Coronary Prevention (1998). Prevention of coronary heart disease in clinical practice. *European Heart Journal* **19**, 1434–503.

22. Jackson, R. Absolute, five year risk of a cardiovascular event (newly diagnosed angina, MI, CHD, death, stroke or TIA). http:\\cebm.jr2.ox.ac.uk\docs\prognosis.html

23. Ramsay, L.E. et al. (1999). Guidelines for management of hypertension: report of the third working party of the British Hypertension Society, *Journal of Human Hypertension* **13**, 569–92.

24. Pearson, T.A., Laurora, I., Chu, H., and Kafonek, S. (2000). The lipid treatment assessment project (L-TAP): a multicenter survey to evaluate the percentages of dyslipidemic patients receiving lipid-lowering therapy and achieving low-density lipoprotein cholesterol goals. *Archives of Internal Medicine* **160** (4), 459–67.

25. EUROASPIRE I and II Group (2001). Clinical reality of coronary prevention guidelines: a comparison of EUROASPIRE I and II in nine countries. *Lancet* **357**, 995–1001.

26. Scandinavian Simvastatin Survival Group. Randomised trial of cholesterol lowering in 4444 patients with coronary heart disease: the Scandinavian Simvastatin Survival Study (4S).

1.12 Anaemia

Hilary Lavender

Anaemia (defined in Table 1) causes massive morbidity and mortality throughout the world, but especially in the tropics. In impoverished communities, about half of all pregnant women and pre-school children are anaemic.[1] Adults with anaemia are less productive: for example, in Guatemalan labourers, maximal work capability dropped by a half in those whose haemoglobin was 7–9 g/dl compared with those whose haemoglobin was 13–15 g/dl.[2] In childhood, anaemia is associated with delayed development.[3]

With the migration of peoples throughout the world, the primary care worker will meet a variety of anaemias, inherited or acquired (Table 2).

Symptoms and signs of anaemia

The symptoms and signs vary according to the acuteness of onset and severity of the anaemia.

In acute blood loss, signs are collapse, dyspnoea, tachycardia, poor pulse volume, and low blood pressure.

When the onset of anaemia is slow, there is time for the body to compensate:

As anaemia develops, cardiac output increases. There may be lassitude, and pallor, especially of the mucous membranes and nail beds.

When the haemoglobin falls below about 7 g/dl, cardiac output increases more. Symptoms include worsening fatigue, breathlessness at rest, palpitations, headache, throbbing in the head and ears, tinnitus, dim vision, cramps, and feeling cold. Signs include a rapid, bounding pulse and ejection systolic murmur.

When the haemoglobin approaches 3 g/dl, the oxygen supply to the myocardium is insufficient, and high-output cardiac failure develops with symptoms of severe fatigue and breathlessness. Signs include cardiomegaly, raised jugular venous pressure, crackles in the lungs, hepatomegaly, ascites, and oedema of the legs.

In patients with atherosclerosis, the first symptoms of anaemia may be worsening angina, claudication of the legs or myocardial infarction.

Table 1 The World Health Organization's definition of anaemia[4]

Haemoglobin	
Men	<13 g/dl
Women	<12 g/dl
Children	
6 months to 6 years	<11 g/dl
6–14 years	<12 g/dl

Table 2 Important causes of anaemia

Blood loss
Acute: Trauma, childbirth
Chronic: Menstruation, worm infestations, other gastrointestinal and renal losses

Defective red cell production in the bone marrow
Nutritional: Iron, folate, vitamin B_{12}, other vitamins and minerals
Anaemia of chronic disease: Infections (TB, HIV), inflammation (connective tissue diseases), cancer, hypothyroidism
Low erythropoetin: Chronic renal failure
Infiltration: Leukaemia, lymphoma, secondary carcinoma, myelofibrosis
Aplastic anaemia: Drugs, chemicals, radiation, idiopathic
Thalassaemias: Alpha (α) and beta (β)

Shortened red cell survival
Congenital red cell defects: Sickle cell disease, G6PD deficiency, spherocytosis
Acquired red cell defects: Burns, drugs, chemicals, toxins, disseminated cancer, malaria
Immune mechanisms: Auto-immune haemolytic anaemia, haemolytic disease of the newborn

Investigating anaemia

If you suspect anaemia, get a full blood count. If anaemia is confirmed, a film can give useful information. Then ask

- What is the mean corpuscular volume (MCV)?
  - microcytic: MCV less than 80 fl;
  - normocytic: MCV 80–98 fl;
  - macrocytic: MCV over 98 fl.
- Are there any clues on the film?

Table 3 covers some of the terms used to describe blood films, and Figs 1–3 provide diagnostic algorithms.

Common anaemias and their management

Iron-deficiency anaemia

Iron deficiency is the commonest cause of anaemia. About 51 per cent of people in poorer countries versus about 8 per cent in richer countries suffer from iron-deficiency anaemia.[5] Prevalence is particularly high in young children and women around childbirth.

The consequences of iron deficiency are

- *In infants and children:* impaired motor and language development, poor achievement at school, behavioural problems, and fatigue.
- *In adults of both sexes:* decreased physical work and earning capacity.
- *In pregnant women:* increased maternal and infant morbidity and mortality, premature delivery, and low birth weight.

Table 3 Interpretation of abnormal blood films

Term	Meaning	Possible significance
Microcytosis	The red cells are small. The MCV is low	Iron deficiency, thalassaemia
Macrocytosis	The red cells are large. The MCV is high	Alcohol, liver disease, B_{12} and folate deficiency, hypothyroidism
Hypochromia	The red cells are pale, because they contain less haemoglobin	Iron deficiency, thalassaemia
Polychromasia	Red cells with a bluish tinge on Romanowsky stain, due to many young red cells: a 'reticulocytosis'	Haemolysis, bleeding, haematinic therapy
Punctate basophilia	Blue dots on Romanowsky staining of young red cells	Severe anaemia, β thalassaemia, chronic lead poisoning
Poikilocytosis	The red cells are different shapes	Various anaemias
Anisocytosis	The red cells are different sizes	Various anaemias, especially megaloblastic anaemias
Elliptocytosis	The red cells are elliptical or oval	Iron deficiency, hereditary elliptocytosis
Spherocytosis	The red cells are spherical due to an abnormal red cell membrane	Hereditary spherocytosis, immune haemolysis
Target cells	Flat red cells with a ring of pallor between the centre and outer part	Liver disease, hyposplenism, haemoglobinopathies
Howell–Jolly bodies	Remnants of the red cell nucleus	Non-functioning or absent spleen, megaloblastic anaemia
Nucleated red cells	Very young red cells from vigorous erythropoesis, or marrow irritation	Severe anaemia (except aplastic), leukaemia, infiltration by secondary tumour
Sickle cells	The red cells are shaped like sickles	Sickle cell anaemias

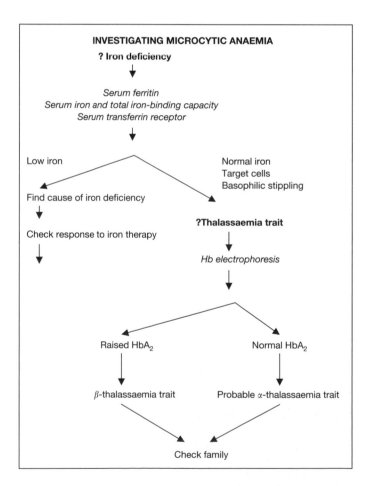

Fig. 1 Investigating microcytic anaemia.

Causes of iron deficiency

◆ *Poor diet:* foods low in animal protein, foods high in substances that inhibit iron absorption, such as phytates in cereals, polyphenols in nuts and legumes, tannin in tea, soy protein, and fibre.

◆ *Loss of iron due to bleeding:* Hookworm, schistosome, and whipworm infestations are very important in the tropics. Gastrointestinal losses (oesophageal varices, hiatus hernia, peptic ulcer, carcinoma of the stomach, colon, or rectum, colitis, angiodysplasia, diverticulitis), haematuria, menorrhagia, childbirth.

◆ *Increased demands:* Prematurity, adolescent growth spurt, pregnancy.

◆ *Malabsorption:* Coeliac disease, gastrectomy.

Clinical features of iron deficiency

The symptoms and signs of iron deficiency are mainly those of anaemia (see section on 'Symptoms and signs of anaemia'). However, patients may also have angular stomatitis, glossitis, loss of skin pigmentation, brittle fingernails, and sometimes flattening or concavity of the fingernails (koilonychia). Dysphagia is rare, and pica (the eating of strange items) happens occasionally.

Investigations for iron-deficiency anaemia

Investigate according to the history, examination, age, sex, and circumstances of the patient.

◆ *Full blood count:* Low MCV (<80 fl), low mean corpuscular haemoglobin (MCH) (<26 pg) and low mean corpuscular haemoglobin concentration (MCHC) (<30 g/dl).

◆ *Blood film:* Microcytic, hypochromic red cells with poikilocytosis (pencil shapes), anisocytosis and target cells.

◆ *Serum ferritin:* (Normal 15–300 µg/l.) Iron is normally stored in the body as ferritin. The concentration of serum ferritin is normally directly related to tissue stores of iron. However, serum ferritin is raised in acute and chronic illnesses, such as liver disease, inflammation, malignancy, and infections such as malaria.

◆ *Serum iron:* (Normal 10–30 µmol/l.) The serum iron is subject to diurnal variation and low levels are found in inflammation and infection.

◆ *Serum total iron binding capacity (TIBC):* (Normal 16–60 per cent.) A low serum iron associated with a high TIBC is much more specific for iron deficiency. However, the TIBC may be reduced by poor nutrition.

◆ *Serum transferrin receptor:* (Normal 2.8–8.5 mg/l.) Serum transferrin receptor is raised in iron deficiency anaemia, but is normal or only slightly raised in the anaemia of chronic disease.

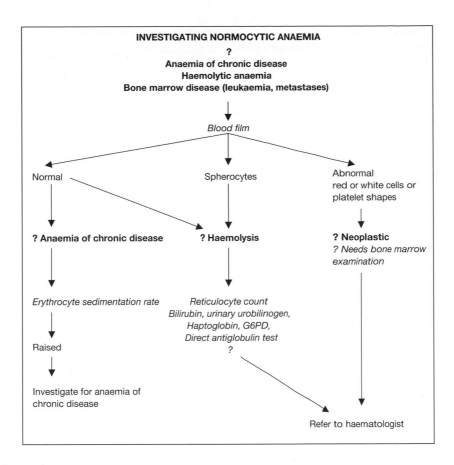

Fig. 2 Investigating normocytic anaemia.

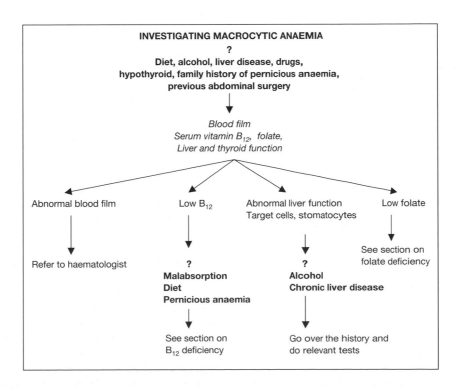

Fig. 3 Investigating macrocytic anaemia.

What is the cause of the iron deficiency?

Search for the cause of the iron deficiency, so that important pathology is not missed. Gastrointestinal causes can be missed easily. So, even when a non-gastrointestinal cause for the anaemia is assumed, do faecal occult bloods, and, in patients from the tropics, stool examination for ova and parasites.

Management of iron deficiency anaemia

◆ Treat the underlying cause if possible.

◆ Give iron replacement: The cheapest effective treatment for adults and adolescents is ferrous sulphate 200 mg tablets (60 mg of elemental iron) three times a day. For infants and children, give liquid preparations in divided doses to provide 5 mg of elemental iron per kilogram body weight per day. Iron should be continued for at least 3 months after the haemoglobin has returned to normal, in order to replenish iron stores.

Children are more susceptible to malaria during the response to iron therapy. Where malaria is endemic, give an initial curative antimalarial course followed by a prophylactic for 3 weeks.

Intramuscular iron should only be given if oral therapy has failed. There is a risk of anaphylactic reactions, and so it should be given where there are resuscitation facilities, preferably in hospital.

Prevention of iron-deficiency anaemia

In countries where iron deficiency is prevalent, consider

◆ Prophylactic iron for high-risk groups: pregnant women, pre-school children, and adolescent girls.

◆ Antihelminthics for children.

◆ Local fortification of food with iron and encouraging high ascorbic acid intake to enhance the absorption of iron.

Folate deficiency

Minor degrees of folate deficiency are frequent in most countries. Pregnancy is a risk factor for severe folate deficiency. In early pregnancy, folate deficiency is associated with an increased incidence of neural tube defects in the baby.

Causes of folate deficiency

◆ *Poor diet:* Folates are found in a wide variety of both animal and vegetable foods.

■ good sources: liver, green vegetables, tubers (e.g. yams and sweet potatoes), mangoes, peppers, eggs, cheese, and yeast products;

■ moderately good sources: red meat and poultry;

■ poor sources: rice, maize, sorghum, millet, cassava root, non-green vegetables, boiled milk and goats' milk.

◆ *Cooking:* Folates are heat labile and water soluble, so that prolonged cooking, or boiling in large volumes of water can greatly reduce folate intake.

◆ *Malabsorption:* Gluten-sensitive enteropathy, tropical sprue, partial gastrectomy, jejunal resection, inflammatory bowel disease.

◆ *Increased demand:*

■ pregnancy, prematurity, and infancy;

■ haemolytic anaemia, especially sickle cell disease and thalassaemia major;

■ malignancies;

■ inflammatory: tuberculosis, malaria, Crohn's disease, psoriasis, rheumatoid.

◆ *Drugs:* Cholestyramine, sulphasalazine, methotrexate, pyrimethamine, anticonvulsants, and others.

Clinical features of folate deficiency

The clinical features are those of anaemia and also of the underlying disease.

Investigations for folate deficiency

◆ *Full blood count:* macrocytic anaemia (MCV >98 fl);

◆ *Fasting serum folate:* less than 3 μg/l (normal 3–20 μg/l);

◆ *Red cell folate:* less than 160 μg/l (normal 160–640 μg/l) red cell folate may be normal if folate deficiency is of recent onset.

Management of folate deficiency

Treat with folic acid 5 mg daily for 4 months to replace stores. For maintenance, give 5 mg once a week. It is very important to make sure there is no vitamin B_{12} deficiency before treating with folic acid, because treatment with folic acid can bring on the neurological manifestations of B_{12} deficiency.

Prevention of folate deficiency

◆ *To prevent neural tube defects:* Give folic acid 400 μg for 3 months both before and 3 months after conception.

◆ *Premature infants and babies with diarrhoea:* Folic acid 50 μg/day.

◆ *Thalassaemia, sickle cell disease, and other chronic haemolytic anaemias:* 5 mg/day.

◆ *In populations with a high prevalence of folic acid deficiency:* Fortification of the staple diet with folic acid. For example, in the United States there is mandatory fortification of cereal grains at 1.4 mg/kg.

Vitamin B_{12} deficiency

Iron and folate deficiencies are much more common than vitamin B_{12} deficiency. Vitamin B_{12} is found in animal foods, including milk and eggs, but not in vegetables. When vitamin B_{12} is eaten, it combines in the stomach with intrinsic factor, which is secreted by the gastric parietal cells. The vitamin B_{12}–intrinsic factor complex is taken up by special receptor sites in the terminal ileum, where the B_{12} is absorbed. Up to 3-years' supply is stored in the liver. As well as causing anaemia, vitamin B_{12} deficiency can cause severe damage to the nervous system.

Causes of vitamin B_{12} deficiency

◆ *Nutritional:* Vegans (people who eat no animal products at all).

◆ *Malabsorption due to intrinsic factor deficiency:* Either from gastrectomy, or Addisonian pernicious anaemia. Addisonian pernicious anaemia is the commonest cause of vitamin B_{12} deficiency in Caucasians. The incidence is about 13 per 10 000 and it is rare under aged 40. Pernicious anaemia is an autoimmune disease, which causes gastric atrophy, so that intrinsic factor is no longer secreted by the stomach. About 50 per cent of patients have serum antibodies to intrinsic factor and 90 per cent have antibodies to parietal cells. Pernicious anaemia may be associated with other autoimmune diseases such as vitiligo, Hashimoto's thyroiditis, and Addison's disease.

◆ *Malabsorption from other causes:* Crohn's disease of the terminal ileum, fistulae, strictures, blind loops, HIV disease (B_{12} deficiency reported in 23 per cent patients with HIV), ileocaecal TB, tropical sprue, fish tapeworm, the antidiabetic drug metformin.

Clinical features of vitamin B_{12} deficiency

The clinical features are those of anaemia and sometimes of neuropathy and dementia. Loss of mental and physical drive, numbness, paraesthesiae or difficulty in walking suggest neuropathy. Vitamin B_{12} deficiency may present with neurological symptoms in the absence of anaemia.

Investigations for vitamin B_{12} deficiency

Full blood count: Macrocytic anaemia (MCV >98 fl).
Serum vitamin B_{12}: less than 160 ng/l (normal 160–760 ng/l).
Serum intrinsic factor and parietal cell antibodies.
The Schilling test finds out how well B_{12} is absorbed from the gut.

Management of vitamin B_{12} deficiency

If the anaemia is severe, refer the patient to hospital. Inject hydroxycobalamin 1000 μg every 3–4 days for six doses to replenish body stores, and then inject 1000 μg every 3 months.

Prevention of vitamin B$_{12}$ deficiency

After total gastrectomy or ileal resection, give prophylactic vitamin B$_{12}$ injections 1000 μg every 3 months.

Glucose-6-phosphate dehydrogenase (G6PD) deficiency

G6PD deficiency particularly affects people from Sub-Saharan Africa (7–26 per cent), the Middle East (0.5–26 per cent), South East Asia (0.5–14.9 per cent), and the Mediterranean (0.5–9.9 per cent).[6] The severity of the deficiency varies. People with G6PD deficiency can develop haemolysis in response to the following:

♦ *Infection:* viral or bacterial.

♦ *Food:* fava beans.

♦ *Drugs:*

 ▪ Definite risk: Dapsone and other sulphones, methylene blue, niradazole, nitrofurantoin, pamaquin, primaquine, quinolones, sulfonamides.

 ▪ Possible risk: Aspirin, chloroquine (acceptable in acute malaria), menadione, probenicid, quinidine and quinine (acceptable in acute malaria).

♦ *Other:* mothballs containing naphthalene.

If haemolysis occurs, maintain a high urine output to prevent renal failure, and refer to hospital.

Sickle-cell disease (sickle-cell anaemia)

Sickle-cell anaemia is an autosomal recessive genetic disease. In tropical Africa, 30 per cent of the population carry the gene, but it is also found in populations in India, the Arabian peninsula, Turkey, Greece, and southern Italy. The sickle-cell gene is also common where there have been migrations of people from Africa: for example, the prevalence of the gene in the west Indian population is about 10 per cent.

A normal haemoglobin molecule (HbA) is made up of two α and two β globin chains. Sickle haemoglobin (HbS) has a defect in the β chain. The defect is caused by a single gene mutation. As sickle-cell anaemia is an autosomal recessive disease, the sufferer has to inherit the sickle-cell gene from both parents in order for the disease to show itself (HbSS). In sickle-cell trait, the sickle-cell gene has been inherited from one parent, and the normal gene for HbA has been inherited from the other parent. So the person has a mixture of HbA and HbS (HbAS). Sickle-cell trait does not cause illness unless there is severe hypoxia. Actually, sickle-cell trait has a survival advantage, because the trait gives some protection against falciparum malaria.

There are other variants of the haemoglobin chain, such as haemoglobin C, D, and E, and the β thalassaemias which, when inherited with haemoglobin S, can also cause sickle-cell disease (e.g. SC disease, SD disease, S-β thalassaemia).

In sickle-cell disease, the solubility of haemoglobin is decreased, especially in acidosis and hypoxia. The insoluble haemoglobin damages the red cell membrane, causing the characteristic sickle-cell shape. These sickle cells may block small blood vessels, causing infarction or pooling (sequestration) of blood depending on which blood vessels are involved. Sickle cells have a very short life, and so the bone marrow is overactive trying to keep up blood production. These pathological processes lead to the clinical manifestations of the disease.

Clinical features of sickle-cell disease

Sickle-cell disease has an extremely variable clinical course, ranging from a crippling anaemia with frequent acute exacerbations known as 'crises' (see Table 4), to a mild disorder found by screening test. The damage to organs caused by crises accumulates, leading to chronic ill-health.

Sickle-cell disease in infancy and childhood

During the first few months of life, foetal haemoglobin (HbF) is gradually replaced by HbS, so that by about the age of 4–6 months there is enough

Table 4 Crises in sickle-cell disease

Occlusive: precipitated by infection, dehydration, exposure to cold, hypoxia
Bones: infarction causes severe pain
Abdomen: distension, rigidity, and quiet bowel sounds
Lung syndrome: dyspnoea and pleuritic pain
Brain syndromes: usually in childhood—fits, transient neurological symptoms, strokes

Haemolytic: sudden worsening haemolysis causing dangerous anaemia—often during a painful crisis

Aplastic: transient bone marrow aplasia, often from intercurrent infection, especially from parvovirus

Sequestration: rapid pooling of blood in the spleen or liver: mainly in babies and young children, but hepatic sequestration can occur in adults. Death can occur from severe anaemia

HbS to cause problems:

♦ *In babies:* painful swelling of the fingers and feet, due to infarctions in the small bones: 'hand–foot syndrome'.

♦ *Anaemia:* haemoglobin 6–8 g/dl with a reticulocyte count of 10–20 per cent.

♦ *Splenomegaly:* from increased splenic activity, and also during sequestration crises. Splenomegaly usually resolves due to repeated splenic infarctions, eventually causing hyposplenism. Hyposplenism causes susceptibility to infection, especially with pneumococcus, meningococcus, haemophilus, salmonella, and malaria.

♦ *Chronic mild jaundice:* due to haemolysis. The increased red cell production leads to folic acid deficiency.

Chronic complications of sickle-cell disease

The chronic complications of sickle-cell anaemia result largely from repeated episodes of vascular occlusion. Almost any organ can be involved, but common problems are:

♦ joint destruction, especially from aseptic necrosis of the heads of the femur and humerus;

♦ osteomyelitis in the bone infarcts, Salmonella infection is a common culprit;

♦ progressive renal dysfunction;

♦ chronic leg ulceration;

♦ progressive visual loss;

♦ gallstones occur in over 30 per cent of children by the age of 15 years.

Lifespan is usually shortened. The most common cause of death at all ages, is acute infection. Renal failure is becoming a more frequent cause of death, as people survive longer.

Investigations for sickle-cell disease

Sickle-cell trait:
Sickling test: positive;
Hb electrophoresis: both HbA and HbS are present.

Sickle-cell disease: positive sickling test.
Full blood count: Hb 6–8 g/dl;
Blood film: sickled erythrocytes, reticulocyte count (10–20 per cent);
Hb electrophoresis: mostly HbS, absent HbA, and HbF in small quantities.

Management of sickle-cell disease

The principles of management are:

1. screening for the trait and the disease;

2. prevention of complications;

3. treatment of complications.

Screening for the trait and the disease

Offer counselling and screening to at risk groups especially

- before general anaesthesia;
- before conception;
- at diagnosis of pregnancy;
- for the neonate;
- to the sexual partner of a person with sickle-cell trait or diseases if a baby is planned;
- to relatives.

Primary care prevention of complications

- refer to a *specialist sickle-cell service*, if one is available, for education, monitoring, and treatment of crises. Develop shared care protocols between the sickle-cell service and primary care.
- Give *pneumococcal vaccine* as soon as possible after diagnosis.
- Start lifelong oral *penicillin prophylaxis* to prevent pneumococcal disease. Pneumococcal vaccine does not give complete protection.
    - 3 months to 1 year: Penicillin V 62.5 mg twice a day;
    - 1–5 years: Penicillin V 125 mg twice a day;
    - 5 years onwards: Penicillin V 250 mg twice a day;
    - if allergic to penicillin, prescribe erythromycin.
- Give *folic acid:* up to 1 year: 500 μg/kg daily; over 1 year—5 mg daily.
- Give *haemophilus influenzae* and *meningococcal vaccines*.
- Give annual influenza vaccine.
- Give continuous *antimalarial prophylaxis* where malaria is endemic.
- *Avoid cold, fatigue, and dehydration.*

Primary care treatment of complications

Painful crises

- Use the 'analgesic ladder' according to the severity of the pain. The analgesic ladder starts with paracetamol, then codeine and the non-steroidal anti-inflammatory drugs. If the patient needs morphine, admit to hospital.
- Keep well hydrated and warm.

Indications for referral to hospital in sickle-cell disease

Pain uncontrolled by non-opiate analgesia
Central nervous system deficit including vision problems
Swollen painful joints (infection or ischaemia)
Chest pain or breathlessness (acute sickle chest syndrome or pneumonia)
Symptoms and signs of an acute abdomen (mesenteric sickling or bowel ischaemia)
Sudden enlargement of the spleen or liver (sequestration)
Renal colic or haematuria (renal papillary necrosis)
Priapism

Future developments

Bone marrow transplantation offers the opportunity for cure. Research is needed to find optimal regimes for the treatment of sickle cell crises in the community.

The thalassaemias

The thalassaemias are found mainly in people from the Mediterranean, Middle East, India, and South East Asia. They are a group of inherited anaemias characterized by decreased or absent synthesis of either the α or the β-globin chains of the haemoglobin molecule. Normal haemoglobin is made up of a haem molecule attached to two pairs of α globin ($\alpha\alpha$) chains and two pairs of β globin ($\beta\beta$) chains (Table 5).

Each person has two genes for β-globin and four genes for α globin, which are inherited co-dominantly. In β-thalassaemia trait, the person has one abnormal and one normal gene. In α-thalassaemia trait, the person has one or two abnormal genes out of the four α-globin genes.

Clinical features of the thalassaemias

The thalassaemias cause anaemia because of haemolysis and defective haemopoesis. They range in severity from death in utero due to hydrops foetalis, to extremely mild, symptomless hypochromic anaemias (see Table 6).

Thalassaemia major

- *Failure to thrive* at 3–6 months of age, when haemoglobin changes from foetal to adult.
- *Hepatosplenomegaly* due to haemolysis and extramedullary erythropoesis.
- *Bone expansion* due to bone marrow hyperplasia. There are prominent frontal, parietal, and malar bones.
- *Infections*, especially bacterial.
- *Haemosiderosis* due to repeated transfusions.

Thalassaemia intermedia

The clinical features are less severe than in thalassaemia major.

Thalassaemia minor

Symptoms are absent or minimal. There is a mild, microcytic, hypochromic anaemia.

Investigating the thalassaemias

- *Hypochromic, microcytic anaemia* often with target cells. In thalassaemia trait, the diagnosis is often only made when a patient does not respond to iron therapy.

Table 5 Normal haemoglobins

Foetal haemoglobin	
HbF: $\alpha\alpha\gamma\gamma$	
Adult haemoglobins	
HbA: $\alpha\alpha\beta\beta$ = over 95% of haemoglobin	
HbA$_2$: $\alpha\alpha\delta\delta$ = less than 3.6% of haemoglobin	

Table 6 Classification of the thalassaemias according to clinical severity

Hydrops foetalis	Fatal α thalassaemia	All four α chains deleted
Thalassaemia major	Severe transfusion-dependent anaemia	Both β chains deleted
Thalassaemia intermedia	Anaemia and splenomegaly	α Thalassaemia with three α chains deleted (Hb H disease) or β Thalassaemia with defective production of β chains from both genes
Thalassaemia minor	Symptomless carrier state	α Thalassaemia trait β Thalassaemia trait

• *Haemoglobin electrophoresis:* in β thalassaemia, HbA$_2$ and HbF are raised to compensate for the inability to make β chains.

Management of thalassaemia in primary care

Patients with thalassaemia major and intermedia should be managed in secondary care, especially if transfusion and iron chelation are needed. Patients with hypersplenism may be treated with splenectomy, but this is delayed if possible until after aged 5 years, because of the risk of overwhelming infection.

In primary care the following can usefully be done:

• immunization against pneumococcus, haemophilus, meningococcus, hepatitis B, and influenza;

• penicillin prophylaxis as with sickle-cell disease;

• folic acid supplements;

• prophylactic antimalarials in endemic areas;

• information for families about thalassaemia;

• teaching families the signs of infection.

Prevention of thalassaemia

Screening for carriers with genetic counselling before conception is ideal. If termination of pregnancy is an option, prenatal diagnosis by globin-chain synthesis studies can be done on foetal blood samples obtained by fetoscopy.

Future developments

Bone marrow transplantation has been successful for selected patients. Gene therapy is a possible future development, but it is still a long way off.

Key points

In anaemia

• try to find the cause of anaemia;

• classifying anaemias into microcytic, normocytic, and macrocytic categories is a useful tool for diagnosis.

In the haemoglobinopathies

• protect against infection by

 ◾ immunization against pneumococcus, meningococcus, and haemophilus influenzae;

 ◾ prescribe prophylactic penicillin;

• genetic counselling is the key to prevention.

References

1. **World Health Organization.** *Battling Iron Deficiency Anaemia.* Geneva: WHO, 2001. http://www.who.int/nut/ida.htm.

2. **Viteri, F.E. and Torun, B.** (1974). Anaemia and physical work capacity. *Clinical Haematology* **3**, 609–26.

3. **Nokes, C., Van Den Bosch, C., and Bundy, D.** The effects of iron deficiency and anaemia on mental and motor performance. International Nutritional Anaemia Consultative Group, 1998.

4. **World Health Organization.** *Nutritional Anaemias.* WHO Technical Report Series **503**. WHO: Geneva, 1972.

5. **Cook, J.D., Skikne, B.S., and Baynes, R.D.** (1994). Iron deficiency: the global perspective. *Advances in Experimental Medicine and Biology* **356**, 21928.

6. **World Health Organization Working Group** (1989). Glucose-6-phosphate dehydrogenase deficiency. *Bulletin of the World Health Organization* **67**, 601–11.

Further reading

APoGI at University College, London. http://www.chime.ucl.ac.uk/ApoGI/data/html/hb/menu/htm. (Information for counsellors on haemoglobin disorders.)

Ledingham, J.G.G. and Warrell, D.A., ed. *Concise Oxford Textbook of Medicine.* Oxford: Oxford University Press, 2000. (Comprehensive section on haematology.)

Cook, G.C., ed. *Manson's Tropical Diseases.* London: Saunders, 1996. (Practical and detailed approach to haematology in the tropics.)

2

Respiratory problems

2 Respiratory problems

2.1 Upper respiratory tract infections

Theo J.M. Verheij

Introduction

Upper respiratory tract infections are very common syndromes which are taken to include all respiratory infections above the vocal chords: acute otitis media, acute sinusitis, rhinitis, common cold, pharyngitis, and tonsillitis. In this chapter, only the common cold and acute sore throat, including pharyngitis and tonsillitis, will be discussed. The other upper respiratory tract infections are described in Chapter 3.

Common cold

Incidence and natural history

Almost everybody has a common cold or coryza yearly. On average, young children have six episodes per year, adults have one to two per year. Elderly people do not have colds more often than young adults, but their colds are complicated more frequently by a lower respiratory tract infection. Most cases present during the winter season, probably due to crowding and staying indoors. The well-known symptoms of the common cold are rhinorrhoea, sneezing, a sore throat, coughing, feeling ill, and sometimes fever and myalgia. Coryza also can give sinusitis-like complaints, such as headache and maxillary pain. It is very likely that every rhinitis is accompanied by some, usually mild, inflammation in the adjacent sinuses. The term acute sinusitis is used for the more severe forms of sinusitis with pronounced mucosal swelling and fluid levels within one or more sinuses.

The average duration of symptoms is between 1 and 2 weeks. Common complications of the common cold are otitis media, sinusitis, and acute bronchitis. These complications are almost always self-limiting and symptoms last up to 1 week for otitis media and 1–2 weeks for sinusitis and bronchitis. In some cases, an upper respiratory tract infection like coryza can give rise to a more serious lower respiratory tract infection. In addition, an upper respiratory tract infection can cause asthmatic symptoms in the lower respiratory tract of susceptible patients. Infection with the measles virus, a paramyxovirus, also starts with a rhinopharyngitis and can produce, among others, symptoms of a common cold.

Aetiology

In 50–80 per cent of persons with a common cold, a viral pathogen can be detected. The most important viruses involved are rhinovirus and influenza virus, but also para-influenza, corona virus, adenovirus, respiratory syncytial, and enterovirus are frequent. Bacterial pathogens like *Streptococcus*

pneumoniae, Haemophilus influenzae (in the beginning of the last century the supposed cause of influenza!), *Mycoplasma* and *Chlamydia pneumoniae* can also be found in some patients. Most infections are acquired by direct contact with infected subjects, for instance, hand–hand contact, and through very small air-borne droplets. Because the pathogens involved are very common and the infected persons very contagious, everybody in the society will be infected frequently. Whether a clinical infection will develop depends on individual resistance.

Diagnosis

The diagnosis is made on clinical signs and symptoms. Most patients make the diagnosis themselves. During influenza epidemics, the presence of respiratory tract symptoms like rhinorrhoea, sore throat, and coughing, combined with fever and myalgia gives a chance of 60 per cent that the patient suffers from influenza. Additional examinations are not indicated, unless complications are suspected that need treatment, like pneumonia or exacerbations of asthma. Diagnosis and treatment of these complications are discussed elsewhere.

Management

There are not many diseases for which so many different treatments are advocated as the common cold. Most of them do not have clinically relevant beneficial effects. Treatment is hampered by the fact that common cold is a predominantly viral illness, in which viral replication peaks in the first 1–2 days of the clinical stage, whereas most patients, understandably, seek advice only after a few days.

Having said this, it is not surprising that studies on the effects of antibiotics did not show clear differences between antibiotics and placebo apart from more side-effects in patients on antibiotic treatment.[1] The benefits of oral treatment with zinc for the common cold are under discussion. There is some evidence that zinc reduces the duration and severity of symptoms, but other studies fail to confirm these findings. The exact mechanism through which zinc would affect coryza is not clarified. Because the taste of zinc lozenges is bad and other side-effects such as nausea are common, this treatment is therefore not indicated.[2] Whether local intranasal treatment with zinc is effective is still not clear.

Treatment with antihistamines, both locally and orally anticholinergics, vitamin C, steam inhalation, and topical corticosteroids have shown to have a small but not clinically relevant effect on rhinorrhoea and sneezing. Treatment with nasal sprays containing adrenergic agonists has proven to have a pronounced decongestive effect on the nasal mucosa and thus are an effective treatment to alleviate symptoms that accompany rhinitis.

During influenza epidemics, adult patients with common cold symptoms, fever, and myalgia can obtain a small benefit from treatment with one of the new neuraminidase inhibitors. When started within 2 days after onset of symptoms, treatment can shorten symptoms with about 1 day. More pronounced effect (1.5–2 days) can be expected when treatment is started within 1 day of the onset of illness. Until now, the studies on these new drugs have included almost exclusively healthy young adults. Whether these effects also apply to patients at risk for complications such as the elderly and patients with chronic diseases such as asthma is still unknown.[3]

Long-term care and prevention

Long-term care is only relevant if a patient suffers from very frequent episodes of common cold. Further examinations to rule out allergic rhinitis or chronic sinusitis are indicated in such cases. Prevention is only possible for common cold symptoms caused by influenza. Vaccination is advocated for patients with chronic diseases like diabetes, chronic lung diseases, chronic heart failure, kidney diseases, for the elderly, and in some countries, for health care workers. Vaccination is given 1–2 months before the winter season starts and each year its composition is based on the global forecast for predominant strains for that particular season. In a vaccinated population, 60 per cent less cases of influenza occur, compared with an unvaccinated population. Continuous use of a neuraminidase inhibitor during an epidemic has shown to prevent 70 per cent of cases of influenza.

Acute sore throat

Incidence and natural history

It is estimated that during a 3-month period, 5–10 per cent of the population suffers from a sore throat, but only a small percentage of these patients with a sore throat contact their general practitioner to ask for advice or treatment. The main cause of an acute sore throat is acute pharyngitis and/or tonsillitis. The reported overall incidence of acute pharyngitis/tonsillitis in general practice is 20 per 1000 persons per year. In children and young adults, the incidence is higher than average.

Symptoms accompanying pharyngitis, that is, a sore throat, general malaise, and painful swallowing, last on average for 5–7 days. Throat infections caused by the Epstein–Barr virus (kissing disease) can give complaints for 14 days or even longer. Complications are relatively rare. In untreated patients, peritonsillair abscess or quinsy occurs in roughly 1–2 per cent. The incidence of acute rheumatic fever, once a feared complication with high morbidity and mortality, has declined enormously in the last century, now being only 0.5–1 per 100 000 persons per year. Better hygiene and nutrition is thought to be an important reason for this decreasing occurrence. Acute glomerulonephritis has also become a very rare complication of streptococcal infections with an incidence of one in 30 000 persons per year. In patients with toxic shock syndrome, pharyngitis is the porte d'entrée in only a very small sub-group.

In children, a throat infection with beta-haemolytic streptococci can cause scarlet fever. Nowadays, scarlet fever almost always runs a benign, self-limiting course with mild symptoms.

Aetiology

Acute throat infections are caused by either viral or bacterial infections which are acquired by droplet spread. Most throat infections are viral, caused by rhinoviruses, corona viruses, influenza A and B, and para influenza viruses, sometimes by the Epstein–Barr virus, herpes simplex, Coxsackie A, and cytomegalovirus. Around 30–60 per cent of patients with an acute sore throat, depending on the clinical picture, have a positive bacterial throat culture. The main bacterial pathogen involved is group A beta-haemolytic streptococcus, but group B, C, F, and G can also play a role. However, a positive throat culture does not mean that the cultured bacteria are the main cause of the illness. Bacterial carriage can cause overestimation of the role of bacteria in this respect. In healthy children, beta-haemolytic streptococci are found in 10–20 per cent of cases and in healthy adults this percentage is between 5 and 10.

Rarely, sexually transmitted diseases, like gonorrhoea and syphilis can cause throat infections, usually accompanied by characteristic signs and symptoms. In non-Western countries, infections with *Corynebacterium diphteriae* should be kept in mind. Diphtheria is usually characterized by severe malaise, vomiting, tachycardia, and a pseudomembraneous exudate in the pharynx. Diagnosis and treatment of these rare causes of throat infections will not be discussed in this chapter.

Diagnosis

Patients usually present with a sore throat, painful swallowing, fever, and feeling generally unwell. On physical examination, patients have pharyngeal erythema, sometimes with exudates, a swollen uvula, and, if present, reddened swollen tonsils with exudate. Tender enlarged anterior cervical nodes are often present. In some cases, petechiae on the palate may be seen and the papillae of the tongue can also be swollen and red, the so-called strawberry tongue.

In children, streptococcal throat infections can be accompanied by scarlet fever, with a typical diffuse rash on body, arms, legs and face, except the area around the nose and mouth.

Several studies have shown that the so-called Centor criteria have predictive value for the presence of a streptococcal infections, especially in adults. If all four Centor criteria are present, that is, fever, tonsillar exudate, enlarged cervical nodes and absence of cough, the chance that a streptococcal infection is present is approximately 55 per cent.[4]

The value of additional examination is under discussion. In some countries, rapid tests, which bind antigens of group A beta-haemolytic streptococci and give a visual colour change in the test material are used. If these rapid tests are positive, the chance that the patient has a streptococcal infection is between 80 and 90 per cent. In patients with a negative test result, the chance that the throat culture is negative is in the same range, between 80 and 90 per cent.[5] Cultures are expensive, adequate laboratory facilities in the vicinity are necessary and results are only available after 48 h. Several blood tests are available that are said to have some value in distinguishing between viral and bacterial infections. Although in some countries the use of some of these blood tests, notably measuring C-reactive protein, is advocated to detect bacterial infections, their diagnostic value is uncertain.

Last but not least, it should be mentioned that the value of detecting potential bacterial pathogens, either by rapid tests or cultures, is also undermined by the limited benefits of antibiotic treatment (see below) and possible carriership.

In patients with symptoms lasting longer than seven days, tiredness and enlarged cervical nodes, serologic testing for Epstein–Barr infection (glandular fever) should be considered.

Management

The main question is whether to give antibiotics to patients with an acute throat infections or not. Generally speaking, the beneficial effects of antibiotic treatment on complaints are modest: treatment will shorten the duration of complaints from 7 to 6 days.[6] In patients with a positive throat culture for streptococci, the beneficial effects are somewhat more marked, shortening the duration of complaints by 2–3 days.[7] Antibiotic treatment has a clear beneficial effect on the occurrence of quinsy: in untreated patients the incidence of this complication is approximately 2 per cent, in patients treated with antibiotics the incidence is less than 0.5 per cent. However, adequate patient education and monitoring to detect the onset of a peritonsillar abscess is usually sufficient to ensure a timely referral of the patient to an ENT surgeon who can assess the necessity of surgical treatment. Other complications like rheumatic fever are very rare and the effects of antibiotic treatment on preventing them uncertain.

Besides beneficial effects antibiotic treatment also have side-effects: one in five patients on treatment will have, usually mild, nausea and diarrhoea.

Appreciation of these beneficial and adverse effects of antimicrobial treatment in deciding whether to treat or wait and see, will of course depend on the doctor and the patient. Assessing the presence of the so-called Centor criteria and performing a rapid test for the presence or absence of group A streptococci can help in that respect. Next to the Centor criteria and test results, impaired immunity or a history of rheumatic fever are relative indications for antibiotic treatment. Presence of artificial joints or other artificial material in a patient with a pharyngitis or tonsillitis is in itself no reason for antibiotics.

Since beta-haemolytic streptococci are always susceptible to penicillin, this should be the drug of first choice. In adults a narrow-spectrum penicillin like feneticillin three times 500 mg daily for 7 days is sufficient. If there is intolerance to penicillin, treatment with a macrolide like azithromycin, or clarithromycin is a good alternative.

Patients with upper respiratory tract infections may obtain relief from a range of remedies, including anti-pyretic analgesics (paracetamol, aspirin and non-steroidal anti-inflammatory drugs), steam inhalations, iced water, gargles and a wide range of proprietary, over-the-counter preparations.

Long-term care and prevention

In children with frequent recurrent tonsillitis, with at least three episodes in the last 3 years or seven in the last year, tonsillectomy has proven to reduce the incidence of throat infections.

Antibiotic treatment of patients with acute throat infections has never clearly proved to prevent spread of streptococcal infections in the community. Improvement of nutrition and hygiene and changing virulence of circulating types of streptococci are probably the main reasons for the declining incidence of complications of acute throat infections.

In Western countries, diphtheria is very effectively prevented by vaccination in young children (see Chapter 11.2 in Vol. 1).

References

1. **Arroll, B. and Kenealy, T.** Antibiotics for the common cold. *Cochrane Database of Systematic Reviews: CD000247.* Oxford: Update Software, 2000. (Recent systematic review on this subject in which the data from seven trials with 2056 subjects were reviewed.)

2. **Marshall, I.** Zinc for the common cold. *Cochrane Database of Systematic Reviews: CD001364.* Oxford: Update Software, 2000. (Recent systematic review on this subject reviewing seven trials involving 754 patients.)

3. **McNicholl, I.R. and McNicholl, J.J.** (2001). Neuramidase inhibitors: zanamivir and oseltamivir. *Annals of Pharmacotherapy* **35**, 57–70. (Recent systematic review on the pharmacology and efficacy of zanamavir and oseltamivir for the prophylaxis and treatment of influenza.)

4. **Centor, R.M.** et al. (1981). The diagnosis of strep throat in adults in the emergency room. *Medical Decision Making* **1**, 239–46. (The classic study on the predictive value of signs and symptoms for the presence of a streptococcal throat infection.)

5. **Dagnelie, C.F.** et al. (1998). Towards a better diagnosis of throat infections with group A beta-haemolytic streptococcus in general practice. *British Journal of General Practice* **48**, 959–62. (Recent study on the diagnostic value of a rapid streptococcus antigen test.)

6. **Del Mar, C.B. and Glasziou, P.P.** Antibiotics for the symptoms and complications of sore throat. *The Cochrane Library.* Oxford: Update Software, 1998. (Systematic review of trials in this field comprising data on 10 484 cases of acute sore throat.)

7. **Zwart, S.** et al. (2000). Penicillin for acute sore throat: randomised double blind trial of seven days versus three days treatment or placebo in adults. *British Medical Journal* **320**, 150–4. [Recent clinical trial on this subject not included in the Cochrane review (ref. 6).]

2.2 Lower respiratory tract infections

Luis E. Quiroga and Theo J.M. Verheij

Lower respiratory tract infections (LRTIs) are among the most common diseases encountered in primary care and comprise acute (tracheo) bronchitis and pneumonia. Differential diagnosis between these two entities in daily practice is difficult and underlying chronic lung conditions like asthma and chronic obstructive lung disease (COPD) should be acknowledged.

Mild cases of LRTIs are self-limiting and antibiotic treatment is of limited use. Pneumonia, however, is associated with serious complications and mortality both in children (discussed in detail in Chapter 10.2) and the elderly. This chapter will deal with the most common forms of LRTI. The management of pneumonia caused by legionella and by other pathogens in immunocompromised patients need special attention and expertise that may not be within the scope of the average general practitioner and is mentioned briefly. The management of pulmonary tuberculosis is discussed in detail in Chapter 2.5.

Epidemiology

Acute tracheobronchitis, usually reffered to as acute bronchitis, has an incidence of about 50 per 1000 patients per year. Pneumonia is much less common with an estimated average incidence of 5–10 cases per 1000.[1] Pneumonia is diagnosed more frequently in young children and the elderly. In patients over 75 years of age, for instance, the estimated annual incidence is about 20 per 1000. Reported mortality rates of community-acquired pneumonia (CAP) vary considerably among countries from 10 to 50 per 100 000 inhabitants,[2] with much higher mortality rates in some developing countries. Worldwide, tuberculosis is still a major cause of death.

The pathogens of LRTIs are usually spread by small droplets in the air and direct contact between human beings. Most of these infections occur more often in winter than in summer seasons. The incidence of several of them, like influenza and *Mycoplasma pneumoniae*, show a epidemic pattern. This phenomenon is due to immunological changes in pathogens to whom the population has to develop resistance each time.

The natural course of acute bronchitis can take from 5 days up to 3–4 weeks and is usually self-limiting. Since pneumonia is nowadays seldomly studied without treatment, one can only say that even under proper treatment it will take an average patient with CAP at least 2 weeks to recover. General malaise and cough may take several weeks to resolve. The average mortality among patients with CAP in Western societies is around 2 per cent.

Aetiology

There are few studies on the aetiology of LRTIs outside hospital. Acute bronchitis is mostly caused by viruses, mainly influenza A and B, respiratory syncytial virus, parainfluenza, and adenoviruses. Several studies have shown that in about 30 per cent of patients a possible bacterial pathogen can be found. *Streptococcus pneumoniae* is the most frequent bacterial pathogen, next to *Haemophilus influenza* (originally named so because it was suspected of being the cause of the flu) and *Moraxella cattaralis*. *Mycoplasma pneumoniae* can be a relevant pathogen during epidemics, mainly in children and young adults. Somewhat under-rated in adults with an LRTI is the incidence of infections with *Bordetella pertussis*. Several studies have shown that 10–20 per cent of adults, and especially, elderly with prolonged cough lasting more than 2 weeks in fact have whooping cough.[3]

Concerning the aetiology of CAP, bacterial pathogens are more predominant than in acute bronchitis: with modern techniques bacterial pathogens can be detected in two-thirds of the patients. *S. pneumoniae* is by far the most common pathogen. Other important pathogens are *H. influenza* (more frequent in patients with COPD) and viruses. *M. pneumoniae* infections also occur in small epidemics. In 25 per cent of pneumonia cases, no defined cause can be identified. It is not known whether this is due to undiscovered pathogens, insensitivity of diagnostic techniques, or noninfectious causes of the pneumonia clinical syndrome.

A severe acute respiratory syndrome (SARS), thought to be due largely to coronavirus infection, has recently been described in southeast Asia, with spread to Canada, and has been associated with high case fatality rates in debilitated and elderly patients.

Diagnosis

Two key features of the differential diagnosis include the discrimination between acute bronchitis and pneumonia and the recognition of significant underlying pathology such as asthma and COPD.

A patient usually presents with an acute cough with or without accompanying symptoms like fever, dyspnoea, etc. The majority will have a self-limiting LRTI but to detect the small number of patients with pneumonia within this group is not easy in daily practice. Fever, dyspnoea, tachypnoea, and localized chest signs do have predictive value for the presence of pneumonia.[4] The main problem is that absence of one of these symptoms or signs does not mean that a pneumonia can be ruled out. Additional tests such as a chest X-ray improve the diagnostic certainty considerably but a strategy in which this is done in every patient with an acute cough is not cost-effective. Chest X-rays should therefore only be obtained in those patients in whom pneumonia is suspected on clinical grounds. Testing for C-reactive protein in patients suspected of having pneumonia can support the diagnosis; levels of C-reactive protein above 50 mg/l are said to be associated with a 50 per cent chance that pneumonia is present.

It should be noted that the clinical syndrome does not allow discrimination between viral and bacterial LRTI or prediction of the kind of bacteria causing a pneumonia as suggested by terms like 'atypical pneumonia'. Additional tests like gram stains or sputum cultures are not feasible in primary care and have poor test characteristics. A major problem in this respect is the difficulty of discriminating between real pathogenity and carriership.

In patients with lower respiratory tract symptoms lasting longer than 14 days, asthma or COPD should be suspected and will be present in about 40 per cent of these patients. This proportion is higher in female patients, those with wheeze, (ex-)smokers, and in patients with symptoms related to allergens.[5]

Symptoms suggestive of LRTIs can also be caused by other diseases such as pulmonary embolism, cardiac failure, and pneumothorax (see subsequent chapters in this section).

Management

Acute bronchitis

The average patient with acute bronchitis needs no antibiotic treatment. All available meta-analyses show that adult immunocompetent patients do not benefit from antimicrobial therapy and that side-effects develop in approximately 20 per cent of cases.[6] There is uncertainty about the effects of antibiotics in the elderly and in patients with co-morbidity such as COPD or cardiac failure. In the treatment of acute bronchitis in patients with COPD, the present opinion is that mild forms of acute bronchitis in patients under 65 years of age do not benefit from antibiotics and should be managed by temporarily adjusting their chronic lung medication. In elderly patients with COPD with increased dyspnoea, increased sputum volume and sputum purulence, antibiotic treatment has beneficial effects.[7]

The choice of antibiotic depends on local bacterial resistance patterns. The frequency of bacterial resistance in the community is usually much lower than in hospitals. Unless there is clear evidence that *S. pneumoniae* and *H. influenzae* in the open population have a high resistance against penicillin or tetracylines, amoxycillin and doxycycline should be regarded as drugs of first choice. These antibiotics are cheap and when used prudently do not cause high bacterial resistance rates. More expensive newer drugs which can cause significant bacterial resistance rather quickly, such as the new macrolides and quinolones, should be reserved for second- or third-line therapy. When there is bacterial resistance or intolerance to the drug of

first choice, one of the new macrolides, such as clarithromycin or azithromycin should be used. Macrolides are also the agents of first choice when a patient has whooping cough. The general practitioner should note that antimicrobial treatment of whooping cough is only useful in the first 2 weeks after clinical symptoms appeared.

Although used by some general practitioners, there is still insufficient evidence to support the use of either bronchodilators or anti-inflammatory drugs in patients with uncomplicated acute bronchitis.

An important issue is the management of underlying chronic diseases when a LRTI is present. In patients with COPD or asthma, chronic lung medication should be temporarily intensified and a short course of oral steroids can significantly improve symptoms. In patients with cardiac failure and diabetes, extra support for the underlying disorder is required.

There are few other symptoms for which so many symptomatic drugs are available as cough. The only drugs that can possibly alleviate the inconvenience caused by cough are cough suppressants such as codeine, pholcodeine, and dextramethorphan. However, cough is a useful mechanism for removing sputum from the respiratory tract and these agents should not be used when there is considerable production of sputum. In addition, codeine should not be used in small children because some studies have suggested a relation between codeine and cot death.

Pneumonia

Although a proportion of pneumonias are in fact caused by viruses, there is no doubt that every patient suspected of having pneumonia should be treated with an antibiotic. As explained earlier the bacterial pathogens that can cause CAP are the same as in bacterial acute bronchitis. This means that amoxycillin and doxycycline are the drugs of first choice unless local bacterial resistance in the community is such that these antibiotics should be replaced by one of the newer macrolides. As in acute bronchitis, quinolones should only be used if first- and second-choice treatment is contraindicated because of local bacterial resistance against both penicillin, tetracyclines, and macrolides, or in the case of side-effects or intolerance against these drugs.[8]

When to refer to hospital?

The decision to refer a patient with a pneumonia to hospital should be based on: (a) assessment of the risk of complications; and (b) treatment failure.

In Table 1, the main risk factors for complications in patients with CAP are mentioned.[9] Presence of these risk factors should guide the general practitioner towards the decision to admit a patient with pneumonia. When a patient does not respond clinically to initial treatment within 2–4 days, hospital referral should also be considered.

Long-term care and prevention

The main two options to prevent LRTIs are vaccination against influenza and against pneumococcal infections.

Influenza vaccination is advocated for patients with chronic diseases such as diabetes, chronic lung diseases, chronic heart failure, kidney diseases, for the elderly, and in some countries, for health care workers.

Table 1 Risk factors for complications of CAP

Underlying chronic disease: COPD, chronic heart failure, neoplasia
Altered mental state
Pulse rate >125 beats per minute
Respiratory rate >30 per minute
Systolic blood pressure <90 mmHg
Temperature <35 or >40°C
Age >75 or <1 year(s)

Vaccination is given 1–2 months before the winter season starts and each subsequent year. Its composition is based on the global forecast for predominant strains for that particular season. In a vaccinated population, 60 per cent less cases of influenza occur, compared with an unvaccinated population.

Pneumococcal vaccination is advocated in many countries in certain risk-groups such as young children and the elderly. The currently used 23-valent vaccine is given as a single dose and should be repeated every 5 years. The new conjugate vaccine produces a better antibody response than the older vaccine, especially in children. Both vaccination with the 23-valent vaccine and with the conjugate vaccine has shown to protect against serious invasive pneumococcal disease[10] and to some extent against pneumonia. Whether pneumococcal vaccination has relevant additional value to influenza vaccination is still uncertain. There is still little evidence on the preventive impact of the effective management of chronic diseases such as COPD, cardiac failure, or diabetes mellitus on the occurrence of LRTIs in these patients.

Implications of the problem

LRTIs have a considerable impact on quality of life in daily activities. Uncomplicated acute bronchitis causes bothersome symptoms lasting between 5 and 21 days and patients will stop their daily activities for on average 3–5 days. Patients with pneumonia are not able to perform their daily activities for at least 2–3 weeks. Since LRTIs have such a high incidence and lead to many GP consultations and hospital admissions they incur considerable costs. For instance, in the United Kingdom, respiratory tract infections account for 6 per cent of all consultations in health care and 4 per cent of all hospital admissions. LRTIs remain a significant cause of death in both developed and developing countries.

More research, especially on improving diagnostic strategies and accurate indications for treatment and preventive measures, is required.

Key points

1. Discriminating between viral and bacterial LRTIs by assessing signs and symptoms is not possible.

2. Acute bronchitis is usually a mild self-limiting disease that does not require antibiotic treatment.

3. When indicated in both acute bronchitis or community-acquired preumonia, antibiotic drugs of first choice are doxycycline, amoxycillin or, in certain situations, macrolides. Only if local bacterial resistance in the community or intolerance of the patient exclude the use of these antibiotics, other antibiotics should be used.

References

1. van de Lisdonk, E.H., van den Bosch, W.H.J.M., Huygen, F.J.A., and Lagro-Janssen, A.L.M., ed. *Ziekten in de Huisartspraktijk* 3rd edn. Maarssen: Elsevier/Bunge, 1999.

2. Huchon, G. and Woodhead, M. (1998). Management of adult community-acquired respiratory tract infections. *European Respiratory Reviews* 8, 391–426. (European guidelines on LRTIs with a high quality description of management in primary care. An update will be published in 2004.)

3. Nennig, M.E., Shinefield, H.R., Edwards, K.M., Black, S.B., and Fireman, B.H. (1996). Prevalence and incidence of adult pertussis in an urban population. *Journal of the American Medical Association* 275, 1672–4. (Good study on the incidence of pertussis in adults with an acute cough.)

4. Metlay, J.P., Kapoor, W.N., and Fine, M.J. (1997). Does this patient have community-acquired pneumonia? Diagnosing pneumonia by history and physical examination. *Journal of the American Medical Association* 278, 1440–5. (Important study on the value of history and physical examination for the detection of pneumonia.)

5. Thiadens, H.A., de Bock, G.H., Dekker, F.W., Huysman, J.A.N., van Houwelingen, J.C., Springer, M.P., and Postma, D.S. (1998). Identifying asthma and chronic obstructive pulmonary disease in patients with persistent cough presenting to general practitioners: descriptive study. *British Medical Journal* 316, 1286–90. (Important diagnostic study on the detection of chronic lung disease in patients with persistent cough.)

6. Smucny, J., Fahey, T., Becker, L., Glazier, R., and McIsaac, W. (2000). Antibiotics for acute bronchitis. In *Cochrane Database Systematic Reviews* 4, CD000245.

7. Sachs, A.P.E., Koeter, G.H., Groenier, G.H., van der Waay, D., Schiphuis, J., and Meyboom de Jong, B. (1995). Changes in symptoms, peak expiratory flow and sputum flora during treatment with antibiotics in exacerbations in patients with chronic obstructive lung disease in general practice. *Thorax* 50, 758–63. (High-quality randomised trial in general practice showing no additional effects of antibiotic in mild exacerbations of COPD.)

8. BTS Standards of Care Committee. BTS guidelines for the management of community-acquired pneumonia in adults. *Thorax* 56 (Suppl. 4), IV, 1–64, 2001. (Recent guidelines in this field with a good description of management of pneumonia outside hospital.)

9. Fine, M.J. et al. (1997). A prediction rule to identify low risk patients with community-acquired pneumonia. *New England Journal of Medicine* 336, 243–50. (Important study on the prediction of complications in CAP.)

10. Fine, M.J., Smith, M.A., Carson, C.A., Meffe, F., Sankey, S.S., Weissfeld, L.A., Detsky, A.S., and Kapoor, W.N. (1994). Efficacy of pneumococcal vaccination in adults. A meta-analysis of randomised trials. *Archives of Internal Medicine* 154, 2666–77.

2.3 Acute non-infective respiratory disorders

Justin Beilby

Introduction

In this chapter on acute non-infective respiratory disorders (excluding asthma), four conditions are discussed:

- pulmonary embolus;
- hypersensitivity pneumonitis (or extrinsic allergic alveolitis);
- pneumothorax;
- aspiration of a foreign body;

These are not common in primary care but occur often enough to require a primary care physician to have an understanding of the epidemiology, how they may present, current clinical management and areas where more evidence is required.

Pulmonary embolus

It is well known that the classic Virchow triad of local trauma to the vessel wall, hypercoagulability and stasis predispose to venous thrombosis and, at times pulmonary embolism (PE). There is now evidence that some patients with underlying genetic predisposition, when exposed to certain circumstances, such as prolonged immobility, will be at even higher risk of venous embolism. The most common genetic predisposition is a resistance to the endogenous anticoagulant protein, activated protein C-designated Factor V Leiden.[1] Other known inherited hypercoagulable states include deficiencies in protein S, antithrombin III, and disorders of plasminogen.

Epidemiology

Within the United States, a state-wide study, examining trauma patients admitted to hospital found that the incidence of PE was 0.3 per cent but the mortality was 26 per cent.[2] A study completed in 1992 found that in the United States one to two patients per year will present to a family physician with a deep vein thrombosis (DVT).[3] In Holland, the incidence of those who present to general practitioners has been reported as 0.4 (men) and 0.5 (women) per 1000 conditions (as diagnosed by the treating general practitioners).[4] If half have a PE,[5] then a family physician will probably see one patient a year with this condition.

Leclerc argues that, globally, thromboembolic venous disease is the third most important cardiovascular disease.[6]

It is rare in young people and becomes more common with advancing age.[7]

Presentation in primary care

A number of clinical situations predispose to a pulmonary embolus. These include:

- surgery and trauma;
- obesity;
- oral contraceptives, pregnancy and the post-partum period;
- cancer and those patients receiving cancer chemotherapy;
- immobilization, for example, after a stroke, long-haul air travel;
- indwelling central venous catheter.

Possible causes

The sources of a pulmonary embolus can be seperated into two groups—venous and non-thrombosis related. In the former, venous thrombi dislodge from an established thrombus in the deep veins of the legs or pelvis and travel to the lungs. About half of these patients with leg or pelvic thrombi will have a proven PE.[5] They can either embolise to the pulmonary artery or paradoxically travel to the arterial circulation through a patent foramen ovale.

Non-thrombotic emboli include fat embolism from long bone fractures and blunt trauma, injected causes such as hair or talc (IV drug users) and amniotic fluid (associated with pregnancy).

The presence of a proven PE requires a careful search for the cause. It is important to localize the embolus and, in those with recurrent thromboembolism, to identify any risk factors for the development of the condition and importantly exclude occult malignancy and thrombophilic abnormalities.

Diagnosis

The most frequent symptom is dyspnoea and the most frequent sign is tachypnoea. The presentation may vary from massive PE with dyspnoea, hypotension, syncope, and/or cyanosis to a small PE with pleuritic pain, cough, or haemoptysis. The diagnosis can be difficult at times and PE has been called the great masquerader. Apart from these signs and symptoms other unusual presentations can occur—a young person with anxiety and an older person with vague chest discomfort.

The differential diagnosis will include:

- myocardial infarct;
- unstable angina;
- pneumonia;
- chronic obstructive pulmonary disease (COPD) exacerbation;
- congestive heart failure;
- asthma;
- pericarditis;
- primary pulmonary hypertension;
- rib fracture and pneumothorax;
- costochondritis;
- musculo-skeletal pain;
- anxiety.

At times, a PE may co-present with some of these conditions and non-resolution of a condition such as pneumonia, after appropriate management would suggest a search for a PE.

The diagnostic work up initially consists of an ECG and chest X-ray (CXR) to exclude other cardiac and pulmonary causes. The ECG with a patient with a PE may reveal sinus tachycardia, newly established atrial fibrillation, and some other non-specific signs of a S wave in lead 1, Q wave in lead V3, and an inverted T wave in lead V3. The CXR may be normal but subtle signs may include a peripheral wedge-shaped density above the diaphragm. Neither investigation has high sensitivity or specificity for the definitive diagnosis of pulmonary embolism.

Definitive diagnosis requires the use of the more sophisticated investigations including radionuclide imaging in the form of ventilation/perfusions scan and computed tomography angiography.[8] The former technique is more accurate if there is no history of a previous PE, no history of chronic obstructive pulmonary disease or grossly abnormal CXR. The measurement of D-dimers is emerging as a promising diagnostic test for thromboembolism.

If there is no history of the conditions discussed above, the patient with a suspected PE will require a ventilation/perfusion scan. If this is positive, the patient will be considered to have a PE and be anticoagulated. If it is equivocal, the patient should go on to have computed tomography pulmonary angiography. If there is a past history of the conditions described above, then the patient should go directly to computed tomography pulmonary angiography.[8]

Principles of management

There is a need to stratify people suffering with a PE according to risk. The above investigations will allow differentiation of patients into those who are normotensive and have normal right ventricular function and those who are hypotensive, and have right ventricular hypokinesis. The former can usually be safely managed with anticoagulation (e.g. heparin) and warfarin, whereas the latter group will be candidates for urgent intervention. If less than 30 per cent of the lung is affected by the PE, then right ventricular function is seldom affected[1] and good outcomes can be expected with anti-coagulation. In the group requiring urgent intervention, options include catheter based treatment, principally thrombolysis but also including suction embolectomy and fragmentation with distal dispersion, as well as surgical approaches (acute embolectomy), which are usually reserved for life-threatening circumstances. Other adjunctive measures include pain relief and oxygenation and inotropic agents such as dobutamine, where there is right heart failure and cardiogenic shock.

There are two current approaches to management. The traditional approach uses an initial dose of intravenous unfractionated heparin in a bolus of 5000–10 000 units followed by a continuous infusion of 1000–1500 units/h. Warfarin is initiated with a dose of 7–10 mg. This may need to be adjusted to a patient's weight and level of nourishment.[1] There is usually a 5-day overlap period as the warfarin is stabilized and heparin reduced. Treatment continues for 3 months for a patient with no previous history of a PE, but for those people with a recurrence of the condition, anticoagulation may continue for life.

Recent research suggests that low-molecular-weight heparin (LMWH), as an alternative management strategy has a place in the treatment in venous thromboembolism, particularly those ambulatory patients with deep vein thrombosis. Although a number of well-designed randomized controlled trials have suggested that LMWH is safe and efficacious for patients with acute DVT, the evidence for patients with pulmonary emboli is less clear. A small number of patients with a PE and who are stable have been treated with LMWH, but not enough to suggest this is current accepted practice.[9]

Long-term management

Schulman et al. have found that there is a two year recurrence rate of 14 per cent of patients who have had PE.[10] The recurrence rate is higher in those who have cancer, massive obesity and if the course of anticoagulation was less than 6 weeks.

Other issues

Prevention of PE is crucial and where there is an increased risk of venous thromboembolism (VTE), techniques such as compression stockings and LMWH are used.[11]

There has been recent controversy regarding the risk of VTE on long plane flights.[12] Hirsh and O'Donnell argue that there is still not enough rigorous evidence to confirm an association with long distance air travel with VTE but that it is appropriate to suggest that 'regular isometric muscle contraction and adequate hydration' be instigated for all patients.[12] High-risk patients (see above) and those with previous VTE need personal management.[12]

Key points

- The presentation may vary from massive PE with dyspnoea, hypotension, syncope and/or cyanosis to a small PE with pleuritic pain, cough, or haemoptysis.

- The diagnosis can be difficult at times and PE has been called the great masquerader. Apart from these signs and symptoms other unusual presentations can occur—a young person with anxiety and an older person with vague chest discomfort.

- The presence of a proven PE requires a careful search for the cause. It is important to localize the PE, identify any risk factors for the development of a PE and importantly exclude occult malignancy and thrombophilic abnormalities.

Hypersensitivity pneumonitis (or extrinsic allergic alveolitis)

This condition is an immunologically-induced inflammatory lung disease which follows the repeated inhalation of a number of agents in a susceptible host.[13,14] The disease may present acutely, subacutely and as a chronic condition. The immunological response involves immune complex and T-cell mediated responses.[13]

Epidemiology

The prevalence of the condition is unknown and varies with the local environmental exposure to an antigen. In one cohort study that followed a group of 1500 dairy farmers for 10–15 years, the prevalence of farmer's lung disease was 4.2 per 1000 farmers per year.[15] Among Dutch general practice attendees, the incidence has been reported as less than 0.1 per 1000 conditions.[4]

Presentation in primary care

This is an uncommon presentation in primary care. In the acute phase the patient may present within 4–6 h of exposure to the antigens, commonly with cough, dyspnoea, wheeze, myalgia, and fever and chills.[14]

Possible causes

The common antigens that precipitate this condition are listed in Table 1. Other antigens that have been implicated include mouldy cheese, coffee beans, fish meal, mouldy barley, cork dust, mould on tobacco or wine, and oak and maple trees.[16] The key to the correct identification is a careful social and occupational history to identify the possible causative antigen.

Diagnosis

The diagnosis requires the drawing together of a number of suggestive elements within a patient:

- history of exposure to the antigen;
- symptom as outlined above;
- signs such as wheeze and dyspnoea;
- blood picture: neutrophilia and lymphopaenia, raised C-reactive protein, and erythrocyte sedimentation rate, and a search for serum precipitans to the suspected antigens;
- radiological findings; there are no specific signs on CXR, but at times in the acute phase there may be 'poorly defined, patchy or diffuse infiltrates or with discrete, nodular infiltrates'.[16] CT scan can be helpful and in thin section approximately half of the patients will reveal nodular opacities and a centri-lobular ground glass appearance;
- pulmonary function tests usually reveal restrictive pattern with decrease in lung volume and impaired diffusion capacity;
- occasionally lung biopsy or bronchoalveolar lavage will be required.

Principles of management

The key step is avoidance of the antigen and its source.[13] Due consideration must be given to the fact that this may affect a person's livelihood and living environment. Visits to a patient's home or work setting may be required to clarify the cause. The use of respiratory protective techniques (e.g. pollen masks, personal dust respirators) may be useful.

Table 1 Common causes of hypersensitivity pneumonitis

Disease	Exposure source	Antigen
Farmer lung	Mouldy hay	Mienopolyspora faeni
Humidifier lung	Contaminated humidifier and air-conditioning systems	Thermoactinomyces vulgaris
Bird fancier lung	Bird droppings and feathers	Avian proteins
Mushroom worker lung	Mushroom compost	Thermophillic actinomycetes
Malt worker lung	Mouldy malt	Aspergillus clavatus
Wood pulp worker's lung	Mouldy wood dust	Altemania tenuis
Bagassosis	Mouldy sugar cane	Thermoactive myces sacchari
Wheat weevil lung	Contaminated wheat	Sitophilus grananus
Tobacco worker disease	Mould on tobacco	Arpergillus sp.
Coffee worker lung	Coffee beans	Coffee bean dust

In the acute phase, prompt and aggressive treatment is required, particularly where marked respiratory impairment has occurred. The treatment of choice is corticosteroids, adjusted to the patient's clinical state.

Long-term management

Avoidance of the antigen will be required.

Key point

♦ Although this is uncommon in primary care, the diagnosis should be considered in people who work in these environments and present with a non-specific and recurring acute non-infective respiratory condition.

Pneumothorax

A pneumothorax occurs when there is gas in the pleural space. The gas can come from an opening in the chest wall or from an internal cause such as a defect in the lung itself. There are three main types:

♦ *Spontaneous*, where no prior chest trauma precedes the condition. This is further separated into primary and secondary. Primary describes the situation where no underlying lung disease is present and secondary where underlying disease is present with chronic obstructive pulmonary disease (COPD) being the principle condition.[17]

♦ *Traumatic*, where the condition results from penetrating or non-penetrating chest injury.

♦ *Tension* refers to the situation where the pressure is positive throughout the respiratory cycle.

Epidemiology

Pneumothorax is a relatively uncommon occurrence in primary care except in communities where chest injuries, either penetrating or non-penetrating, occur frequently. In the United States, 20 000 new cases of spontaneous pneumothoraces occur each year.[16] Among Dutch general practice attendees, the condition has a reported incidence of 0.3 (men) and 0.1 (women) per 1000 conditions.[4] Pneumothorax occurs more commonly in aesthenic (tall and thin) individuals.

Presentation in primary care

The presentation varies with the different types. A primary spontaneous pneumothorax occurs after the rupture of an apical pleural bleb, usually in smokers. Patients may present with dyspnoea and pleuritic chest pain. The commonest group of patients who present with secondary spontaneous pneumothoraces are those with chronic obstructive airways disease, although all lung diseases can precipitate this condition. With this group, careful assessment is required because a pneumothorax may compromise an already reduced pulmonary reserve. Pneumothorax should be considered in all patients who suffer chest trauma.

Diagnosis

A CXR is mandatory where pneumothorax is suspected, but physical examination may also provide strong diagnostic clues. Typically, there will be reduced or absent breath sounds on the side of a pneumothorax, combined with respiratory distress. Hypotension, distended neck veins, tracheal deviation, and hyporesonance on the affected side of the chest may be found. There may be no physical signs with small pneumothoraces. In the case of a tension pneumothorax, collapse of the opposite lung may occur

due to pressure of expanding gas. In this situation, breath sounds may be decreased over the collapsed lung.

Principles of management

Small primary spontaneous pneumothoraces can be monitored with oxygen supplementation, regular clinical review, and CXR. Oxygen supplementation should be at 3 l/min via nasal cannula or high-flow mask. Simple aspiration may be required at times using an intravenous catheter or comparable device. Some patients with small pneumothoraces can safely be followed up as outpatients.

Secondary spontaneous pneumothoraces often need more active approaches. The potential to further compromise a patient with COPD with the development of a pneumothorax requires the use of a large-bore chest tube.[17]

Chest tubes will be required where there is respiratory compromise or traumatic pneumothorax. Baumann recommends at least a 28F chest tube where significant air leaks are possible (e.g. in a mechanically ventilated patient) but smaller tubes may be used where the chances of air leaks are small.[17]

Secondary and recurring primary pneumothoraces may need the instillation into the chest cavity of sclerosing agents such as talc and doxycycline. Surgical interventions (e.g. pleurectomy and bullectomy) offer the best option to prevent recurrence.[17]

A tension pneumothorax is life-threatening and occurs usually during mechanical ventilation or efforts to resuscitate patients or as a result of trauma. The positive pleural pressure can be transmitted to the mediastinum, decreasing venous return to the heart and reducing cardiac output. A large-bore needle should be immediately inserted into the chest via the second anterior intercostal space and remain in place until a chest tube can be inserted.

Traumatic pneumothoraces can be caused by both penetrating and non-penetrating injuries, such as those caused by knives and vehicle accidents, and also by iatrogenic events such as transthoracic aspiration and insertion of central venous catheters.

Long-term management

It is important to note that approximately 50 per cent of the primary spontaneous pneumothorax group will have a recurrence.

Key points

♦ The diagnosis of pneumothorax should be considered with people presenting with acute dyspnoea and pleuritic chest pain, for which no obvious cause can be identified.

♦ A pneumothorax should be excluded in all situations where significant chest trauma has occurred.

♦ Tension pneumothorax is an emergency and may require a large bore needle be inserted into the chest via the second anterior intercostal space until a chest tube is inserted.

Aspiration of a foreign body

Epidemiology

The ingestion of foreign bodies by children under 5 is still a problem in both developed and underdeveloped countries, with the condition being recorded as the fourth cause of death in this group in the United States.[18] Among Dutch general practice attendees, foreign bodies (not exclusively but predominantly in the respiratory tract) have a reported incidence of 18 (men) and 7 (women) per 1000 conditions.[4] Inhaled foreign body is a known factor in anoxic brain damage in children. Most of these occur in children under 3[19,20] with a peak incidence of 61.9 per cent in this age group[20] and a male:female ratio of 2:1.[20]

Presentation in primary care

A toddler will be brought to a primary care physician with a history of a choking spell, often while eating or playing. Associated symptoms will include coughing (73.9 per cent in one series[19]), wheezing (69.5 per cent[20]), dyspnoea, and fever. Over 75 per cent present from 1 day to 1 week[18,20] although some infrequent cases can present after longer periods, for example, 2 months[20] and even 20 months.[18]

In a series of 20 children, Bodart et al. found that the clinical signs were variable.[18] Three out of 20 had normal findings; four had localized end expiratory wheeze; six generalized wheeze; and 11 asymmetrical reduced air entry.

Significant hypoxaemia can occur in a small number of children, requiring oxygen supplementation.

Possible causes

The commonest cause is peanuts,[20] but any foreign body which is small and firm can lodge in the tracheobronchial tree. Other foreign bodies include beads, grapes, walnuts and parts of children's toys.

Diagnosis

The diagnosis rests on a careful clinical history and the appropriate use of radiological investigations. If a child presents with a history of choking or ingestion of a foreign body then two possible scenarios will develop. In the first, the physical examination will be abnormal (see above) and a CXR will be abnormal. If there is a suspicion of a foreign body ingestion, then inspiratory and expiratory radiographs are required. In 5–15 per cent, a radio-opaque foreign body will be seen,[19,20] but otherwise indirect signs will be sought. These include air-trapping, expiratory mediastinal shift, atelectasis, and pneumonia.[19]

In the second group of patients who present with a suggestive history, physical examination may be normal. If the radiological examination is suggestive, then management should follow normal management protocols (see below). If the radiological examination is normal then re-examination of the patient in 24 h is appropriate.[19] It is important to note that a normal radiograph does not exclude the diagnosis of an inhaled foreign body.[19]

Principles of management

Children with a definitive history and radiological signs should move immediately to bronchoscopic evaluation and removal of the foreign body. The children with suggestive history should also be considered for bronchoscopy.

Long-term management

The long-term complication rate is low and dependent on the length of time the foreign body has been in the chest. About 5–15 per cent suffer from mild complications such as bronchospasm and atelectasis.

Key points

- For toddlers under 3, who present with the classic history discussed in this section, ingestion of a foreign body should be excluded as a cause.

- The diagnosis is often complicated by the lack of history and physical findings and inconclusive radiographs.

Acute respiratory failure

This condition occurs when there is an inability to adequately ventilate or oxygenate a patient.

Epidemiology

This is uncommon in primary care.

Presentation in primary care

The patient with a background of the predisposing condition will present with increasing dyspnoea and distress. With increasing compromise, the dyspnoea will worsen. The patient will become tachypnoeic and if appropriate management is not instigated cyanotic.

Possible causes

The causes are separated into two main groups:[21]

- *Hypoxic respiratory failure.* This condition usually results from an insult to the pulmonary tissues and common conditions include pneumonia (community acquired or nosocomial), acute respiratory distress syndrome, cardiogenic pulmonary haemorrhage, and pulmonary contusion.

- *Hypercarbic respiratory failure.* This occurs when conditions cause a reduction in minute volume or an increase in physiological dead space. Common causes include respiratory muscle fatigue due to extra workload, COPD, asthma, and exacerbation of underlying neuromuscular diseases.

Diagnosis

- *Hypoxic respiratory failure.* This state is diagnosed when the arterial oxygen saturation is below 90 per cent, with an inspired oxygen fraction of greater than 0.6.

- *Hypercarbic respiratory failure.* This state is diagnosed when the P_{CO_2} values exceed 50 mmHg and the arterial pH is below 7.30.

Principles of management

Mechanical ventilation is used in both situations,[21] although a number of systematic reviews have suggested that non-invasive positive pressure ventilation[22,23] may have a role in some situations where acute respiratory failure has occurred. This is principally where the patients have COPD and is complemented by appropriate disease specific management aimed at alleviating the underlying cause.

References

1. **Goldhaber, S.** (2000). Pulmonary thromboembolism. In *Harrison's Principles of Internal Medicine* 14th edn., Chapter 261 (ed. A. Fauci, E. Braunwald, K. Isselbacher, J. Wilson, J. Martin, D. Kasper, S. Hauser, and D. Longo), pp. 1469–72. New York: McGraw-Hill.

2. **Tuttle-Newball, J.** et al. (1997). Statewide, population-based, time-series analysis of the frequency and outcome of pulmonary embolus in 318 554 trauma patients. *Journal of Trauma: Injury, Infection and Critical Care* **42** (1) 90–9.

3. **Anderson, F.** et al. (1991). A population based perspective of the hospital incidence and case-fatality rate of deep vein thrombosis and pulmonary embolism: The Worcester DVT Study. *Archives of Internal Medicine* **151**, 933–8.

4. **Van de Lisdonk, E.H., van den Bosch, W.H.J.M., Huygen, F.J.A., and Lagro-Janssen, A.L.M.** *Ziekten in de Huisartspraktijk*. Maarssen: Elsevier/Bunge, 1999.

5. Meigan, M. et al. (2000). Systemic lung scans reveal a high frequency of silent pulmonary embolism in patients with proximal deep venous thrombosis. *Archives of Internal Medicine* **160**, 159–65.

6. Lellerc, J. (1999). Strategies de prevention de l'embolic pulmonaire au decours des chirurgies a risqué et en milieu medical. *Revue des Maladies Respiratoires* **16**, 939–48.

7. Lensing, A. (1999). Deep vein thrombosis. *Lancet* **353**, 479–85.

8. Lau, L. *Imaging Guidelines* 4th edn. The Royal Australian and New Zealand College of Radiologists, 2001. ISBN 0959285415.

9. Elliot, G. Concise review: low-molecular-weight heparin in the treatment of acute pulmonary embolism. http://www.harrisonsonline.com/serverjava/ Arknoid/harrisons/1096-7133/Updates/Editorials/?Up=edl1908.

10. Schulman, S. et al. (1995). A comparison of six weeks with six months of oral anticoagulant therapy after a first episode of venous thromboembolism. *New England Journal of Medicine* **332**, 1601–5.

11. Amarigiri, S. and Lees, T.A. (2001). Elastic compression stockings for prevention of deep vein thrombosis (Cochrane Review). In *The Cochrane Library* Issue 2. Oxford: Update Software.

12. Hirsh, J. and O'Donnell, M. Venous thromboembolism after long flights: are airlines to blame? http://www.theLancet.com/journal/vol357 . . . N357.9267.editorial_and_review.16253.1.

13. Masayuki, A., Montaku, S., and Kohngi, H. (1999). A new look at hypersensitivities pneumonitis. *Current Opinion in Pulmonary Medicine* **5**, 299–304.

14. Matar, L., Page McAdams, H., and Sporn, T. (2000). Hypersensitivity pneumonitis. *American Journal of Roentgenology* **174**, 1001–66.

15. Marx, J. et al. (1990). Cohort studies of immunological lung disease among Wisconsin dairy farmers. *American Journal of Industrial Medicine* **18**, 263–8.

16. Hunningsake, G. and Richerson, H. (2000). Hypersensitivity pneumonitis and eosinophilic pneumonias. In *Harrison's Principles of Internal Medicine* 14 edn., Chapter 253 (ed. A. Fauci, E. Braunwald, K. Isselbacher, J. Wilson, J. Martin, D. Kasper, S. Hauser, and D. Longo), pp. 1426–9. New York: McGraw-Hill.

17. Baumann, M. Concise review to Chapter 262: Disorders of the pleura, mediastinum and diaphragm. Contemporary management of spontaneous pneumothorax. http://www.harrisonsonline.com/server-java/Arknoid/ harrisons/1096-7133/Updates/Editorials/?Up=edl1908.

18. Bodart, E., Bilderling, G., Tuerlinckx, D., and Gillet, J. (1999). Foreign body aspiration in childhood: management algorithm. *European Journal of Emergency Medicine* **6**, 21–5.

19. Messner, A. (1998). Pitfalls in the diagnosis of aerodigestive tract foreign bodies. *Clinical Pediatrics* **37**, 359–66.

20. Carluccio, F. and Romeo, R. (1997). L'inalazione di corpi estranei: dati epidemiologici e considerazioni cliniche alla luce di una revisione statistica su 92 casi. *Acta Otorhinolaryngologica Italica* **17**, 45–51.

2.4 Asthma

Ian Charlton and Patrick White

Introduction

Asthma is treated mainly in primary care. In systems where primary medical care is the point of first contact with health services, 85 per cent of asthma patients are treated exclusively by their family doctors. In a primary care setting, asthma is very different to the asthma seen in secondary care. It is usually less severe, so patients who have not experienced an acute severe attack or hospital admission may be less willing to accept the diagnosis and the implications it might have for treatment. The decision to treat asthma with drugs, the involvement of the patient in self-management (needing regular inhaled steroids and a peak flow meter), and the invitation to attend the doctor's office for regular review may all be greeted with scepticism. In primary care, patients with such asthma may be reluctant to include themselves in the broad class of asthmatics because they see asthmatics as ill and by definition different.

Of course, all asthmatics may be the patients of family doctors, so primary care physicians must be as competent in treating acute severe asthma as they are in negotiating a management plan with patients who see asthma as a minor inconvenience. In this chapter, the epidemiology, diagnosis, and management of asthma will be considered from a primary care perspective.

Epidemiology

Asthma is the commonest respiratory condition requiring the attention of general practitioners (GPs) and ranks as the second most commonly managed chronic problem in general practice after hypertension. Asthma accounts for 2–3 per cent of GP consultations.[1]

The prevalence of asthma in both adults and children varies around the world. Australia, New Zealand, the United Kingdom, and the Republic of Ireland have the highest rates of asthma, with prevalence rates of 30 per cent in children and 8 per cent in adults.[2] Russia and Taiwan, with an overall prevalence of 3 per cent, are among the countries with the lowest prevalence rates. As yet there is no convincing explanation for this variation, nor are there any clear reasons why there has been at least a doubling in the prevalence of asthma over the last 30 years.

The prevalence of asthma is difficult to calculate because the definition of asthma requires subjects to have lung function assessed on more than one occasion. To overcome this obstacle, epidemiologists have used symptom prevalence questionnaires whose validity and repeatability have been tested against doctor-based diagnosis. In the UK arm of the ISAAC study, the national 12-month prevalences in 12–14-year-old children of any wheezing, speech limiting wheeze, four or more attacks of wheeze, and frequent night waking with wheeze were 33.3, 8.8, 9.6, and 3.7 per cent, respectively.[3] The prevalence of ever having had a diagnosis of asthma was 20.9 per cent. In total, 19.8 per cent of pupils reported treatment with antiasthma drugs in the past year, but, of pupils reporting frequent nocturnal wheeze in the past year, 33.8 per cent had no diagnosis of asthma and 38.6 per cent denied receiving or using inhaler therapy.

The level of affluence in a population is linked to the prevalence of asthma. This has been demonstrated in studies examining the changes in societal structure associated with the unification of East and West Germany. East Germany had a relatively low asthma prevalence prior to unification but its rate is now similar to West Germany and other developed countries. This may be due to changes in housing, resulting in greater exposure to house dust mite and moulds. Alternatively, the increased use of antibiotics and disinfectants may have reduced exposure to important infections that may play a role in maturation of the immune system in childhood and the protection of children from developing asthma (the hygiene hypothesis).[4]

Asthma mortality also varies greatly between countries. In the United Kingdom, the mortality rate from asthma has been relatively constant in the past 20 years at approximately 0.32 per 100 000 per year.[5] UK GPs, therefore, are likely to see a patient die from asthma less than once in 20 years. With the United Kingdom at the top of the asthma prevalence league table, deaths from asthma may be even less common in the experience of primary care physicians in other countries. Hospital admissions for asthma are much commoner events than death, but likely to be dependant somewhat on the availability of and access to hospital facilities. In developed countries, hospital admission rates for asthma vary between 0.5 and 4 per 1000 population per year.

The diagnosis of asthma

Asthma is reversible airways obstruction. It is characterized by recurrent or continuous breathlessness, wheeze, cough, and night waking or any combination of these, although breathlessness is by far the commonest. It usually responds immediately to inhaled beta-adrenergic stimulants such as salbutamol or terbutaline, but in some cases, the diagnosis may depend on the response to high-dose oral steroids over a period of 2 weeks. The obstruction may be reversible either spontaneously or in response to drugs. It can be measured either as peak expiratory flow rate (PEFR) using the Mini-Wright peak flow meter or as forced expiratory volume in the first second (FEV_1) using a bellows or an electronic spirometer. A difference between two readings on separate occasions of at least 15 per cent more than the lowest reading in either of these parameters confirms the diagnosis. The diagnosis is not always easy to make especially in children under 6 years in whom it may be difficult to measure expiratory lung function. It may rest in these cases on the history and on the response to treatment where it has not been possible to demonstrate the diagnostic criteria in lung function testing. The treatment of asthma is safe, so a trial of treatment to determine the diagnosis is usually justifiable even in very young children. Symptomatic improvement in response to bronchodilators followed by deterioration on their withdrawal is diagnostic. Making a clinical distinction between asthma, respiratory syncytial viral bronchiolitis, and the so-called wheezy bronchitis is largely theoretical. Relief or abolition of symptoms by bronchodilators or steroids justifies continuing their use until the condition has cleared and holding them ready for the next episode.

Additional support for the diagnosis may come from a family history of atopy or a personal history of eczema or hay fever. If one parent has asthma, eczema, or hay fever, then the child has a 40 per cent chance of inheriting some form of allergic disease. If both parents are atopic, then there is an 80 per cent chance of the tendency being inherited.

The pathophysiology of asthma is little different between children and adults and it can be argued there is little value in the current trend to produce different sets of guidelines for these groups. This argument is given added impetus now that the role of cromoglycate in children is less prominent and the impact of steroids on children's growth is thought to be temporary and to represent less of a problem than the consequences of uncontrolled asthma.

Lung function measurement in asthma

Peak expiratory flow is the simplest method of confirming the diagnosis of asthma. PEFR meters are cheap, robust, and highly reliable.[6] Due to the variable orifice mouthpiece, PEFR meters tend to overestimate PEFR at flow rates less than 100 l/min and to underestimate PEFR at flow rates more than 600 l/min. In recognition of these inaccuracies, the American Thoracic Society (ATS) has produced a graduated scale that takes them into account and provides a highly accurate measurement. Spirometry has not been shown to have any advantage over PEFR in the diagnosis and treatment of asthma.[7] It is superior to PEFR in the diagnosis and assessment of severity in COPD and should be the test of choice where the diagnosis is in dispute between asthma and COPD. The relationship between PEFR and FEV_1 is discussed in more detail in Chapter 2.6 (Chronic cough).

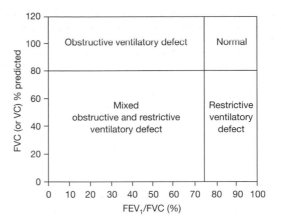

Fig. 1 The interpretation of spirometry as a function of VC (FVC) as percentage predicted and the FEV_1/FVC per cent ratio. The vertical line represents the lower limit of normal FEV_1/FVC per cent (varies with age and sex) and the horizontal line is an estimate of the lower limit of normal for VC or FVC.

Asthma does not commonly cause significant or permanent lung damage itself (unlike COPD), and the Forced Vital Capacity (FVC) in asthma is usually close to normal. The airways, however, are narrowed and constricted and so the FEV_1 is reduced. A convenient way to assimilate this information is by using the Clarkson quadrant (see Fig. 1).

PEFR is also used to record in diary form variation in lung function in asthma in order to make the diagnosis, to assess the degree of diurnal variation, and to assess the response to treatment.[8] PEFR diaries are especially useful if patients report symptoms that vary at different times of the day or in different circumstances, or have symptoms that seem to correlate poorly with lung function.[9] The diaries can provide a baseline record against which treatment is measured and an indication of the lability of the airways in the recovery from an acute episode.

The differential diagnosis of asthma is usually straightforward in a young adult. Two important possibilities to keep in mind are acute pneumonia and pneumothorax. In smokers over 35 years COPD may be an additional problem and in patients with a history of heart disease asthma may be difficult to distinguish from acute left ventricular failure. In all of these cases, a trial of treatment may be worth undertaking while more definitive investigations such as chest X-ray or echocardiography are awaited.

Vocal cord dysfunction is uncommon but should be suspected in patients when a 'wheeze' is refractory to therapy. Characteristically, it is associated with women between 20 and 40 who have a past history of anxiety, depression, or somatization. The tendency to an inspiratory wheeze helps differentiate it from the expiratory ronchi of asthma. The wheeze is most audible over the larynx and not well transmitted to the chest. The diagnosis of asthma is excluded by failing to show an improvement in PEFR after prolonged oral or inhaled steroid use.

Pathogenesis

Asthma is an inflammatory disorder mediated largely by granulated white cells.[10] Bronchial inflammation in response to allergy or other stimuli such as infection leads to excessive adherent mucous, acute inflammatory infiltration, and swelling and bronchial muscle spasm. There are two principal models for the inflammatory reaction that leads to asthma (Fig. 2). Atopy, the first model, involves stimulation by allergen of antigen presenting cells leading to mast cell de-granulation with the release of histamine, prostaglandins, and leukotrienes. This causes acute airways obstruction. The second mechanism, which is the late-inflammatory response, involves recruitment and activation of eosinophils, basophils, neutrophils, and macrophages. The role of the eosinophil is predominant. Between 50 and 100 mediators have been identified in the pathogenesis of asthma. The roles of

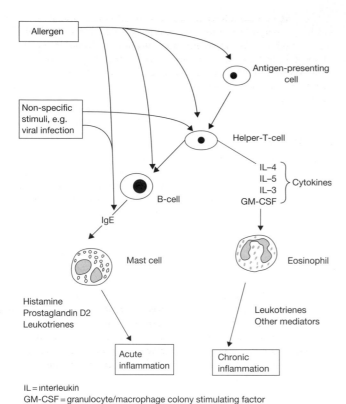

IL = interleukin
GM-CSF = granulocyte/macrophage colony stimulating factor

Fig. 2 Schematic representation of the inflammatory response in asthma.

most of these remain uncertain, but much research is focused on remedies to inhibit their production or block their action. Mediators are involved in broncho-constriction, airways secretion, plasma exudation, neural effects, chemotaxis, and airway hyper-responsiveness. Most of the structural cells of the lung are also involved in producing asthma mediators. Some of these mediators lead to long-standing structural change or a remodelling of the airways. Specific remedies have been devised to block the role of IgE and the leukotrienes, and current research is developing new compounds to block the cytokines IL 3, 4, 5 and GM-CSF among others.

Natural history of asthma

Asthma can present for the first time at any age and patients may develop recurrent asthma symptoms after an interval of many months or years. Typically, patients present with asthma after an upper respiratory tract infection or exposure to a specific allergen. Since the overall population prevalence of asthma is relatively constant, the same proportion of patients who are suffering a recurrence of symptoms is matched by those whose symptoms are in remission. The coming and going of asthma symptoms, both in frequency and severity, is one of the main characteristics of the disease.

The natural history of asthma is variable and in many patients symptoms and signs resolve or disappear over time. However, various degrees of airflow obstruction may persist and, in the long-term, may become moderately or completely irreversible. An unfavourable course, including severe irreversible airflow obstruction, can occur in the absence of other risk factors such as smoking and environmental insults, despite apparently appropriate therapy. Studies examining subjects with persistent asthma show a progressive decline in lung function, compared with normal subjects.

- ◆ Factors that adversely impact on the outcome in adult asthma include:
  - female gender,
  - environmental tobacco smoke exposure in childhood,

- personal tobacco smoking in adolescence and adulthood,
- late onset of symptoms,
- severity of childhood asthma,
- duration of asthma,
- severity of lung function abnormality in childhood,
- low bronchodilator reversibility,
- degree of airway hyper-responsiveness,
- delay in initiating anti-inflammatory therapy.

- ◆ Remission among adult asthmatics is uncommon, and is associated with:
  - better initial lung function,
  - young age,
  - male gender,
  - lesser degrees of airway responsiveness.

- ◆ Conversely, risk factors for death from asthma include:
  - older age,
  - smoking,
  - atopy,
  - impaired lung function,
  - moderate to high reversibility,
  - under-use of inhaled steroids,
  - late presentation for treatment.

Treatment can improve lung function, reduce airway hyper-responsiveness, and improve quality of life. The overall effect of treatment on the natural history of the disease is not yet clear, despite significant short-term improvements from effective anti-inflammatory therapy.

Late onset asthma represents another variation and characteristically begins in the mid-50s. It affects 4–8 per cent of patients over 65. This form of asthma tends not to be associated with IgE allergy and is more likely to progress to fixed airways disease and become resistant to treatment. Whilst it has the same pathophysiological processes as childhood asthma, the aetiology of this form of asthma is less well understood.

Principles of management

The main aim of therapy is to reduce the impact of the disease on the patient's life and retain lung function as close to normal as possible. In the majority of cases, it is possible to achieve good control of symptoms and near normal airflow. For most patients, asthma is a symptomatic disease only. There is little evidence that vigorous treatment of mild disease has any long-term benefits. The decision to use medication is, therefore, dependent on the patient's perception of the benefits of the drugs being greater than their inconvenience. Patients with asthma make up a broad spectrum from the highly compliant 'accepters' to the poorly compliant 'deniers'.[11] It is important, therefore, to understand where the individual patient fits in this spectrum and to negotiate a treatment plan that acknowledges and respects the patient's position.

Careful involvement of the patient in decisions about asthma treatment is essential to guarantee an optimal outcome. There are three key elements to this process: the respective roles of relieving and preventing medications; the most suitable delivery devices; and action to be taken if asthma gets worse. These elements should be the basis of self-management in asthma. For patients with mild asthma responsive to treatment, self-management is simply a matter of taking the inhalers when symptoms occur and stopping when symptoms remit. For patients who suffer acute severe attacks or have continuing symptoms, the role of steroids may be complex and demand careful monitoring. In patients where symptoms are perceived late in an acute attack, self-monitoring with a PEFR meter may be required.

Drugs in asthma management

Asthma drugs have been conceptually divided into relievers and preventers in order to emphasize both the immediate action of the adrenergic and anticholinergic bronchodilators and the delayed action of inhaled steroids. A wide variety of treatments is now available and it is apparent that no one agent has the ability to completely control the disease process for all patients. Different chemical pathways are responsible for driving the inflammatory process and combinations of therapy may be required to satisfactorily manage the asthma.

Inhaled bronchodilators

Inhaled bronchodilators are either short-acting adrenergic (e.g. salbutamol, terbutaline), long-acting adrenergic (e.g. salmeterol, eformoterol), short-acting anticholinergic (ipratropium), or long-acting anticholinergic (oxytropium, tiotropium) compounds. These drugs are locally acting equivalents of adrenaline and atropine. They are delivered in such small doses that systemic effects are rare. They were originally thought to be purely muscle relaxants, but their concomitant anti-inflammatory action has now been established. This explains the dramatic relief from the acute inflammatory response achieved by high-dose inhaled or parenteral adrenergics such as salbutamol or terbutaline. These remain the mainstay of the treatment of the acute attack. Salbutamol and terbutaline have an onset of action within 5 min and their peak activity is achieved after 20 min. The onset of action of ipratorpium is 20 min and its peak action is achieved after 40 min.

Long-acting bronchodilators were developed from short-acting bronchodilator molecules with long side chains that bind to the beta receptors for up to 12 h. Their role is in reducing the patient's need to use short-acting inhalers frequently and in reducing their reliance on high-dose steroids. Combination inhalers offer long-acting bronchodilators and inhaled steroids together. The margin of advantage is small and the high cost of these inhalers demand that their use should be justified by objective evidence of improvement in lung function.

Inhaled steroids

Inhaled steroids have long-term inflammatory actions and offer the most effective approach for the majority of patients with daily symptoms. Corticosteroids prevent the development of airways inflammation, but have limitations. They are not effective in all patients and studies in viral-induced wheeze have been disappointing. They should be taken twice daily although studies with budesonide have indicated reasonable control with once daily regimes. Some patients suffer recurrent pharyngeal thrush and often hoarseness due to irritation of the vocal cords. There is little to separate beclomethasone, budesonide, and fluticasone in terms of clinical efficacy, although fluticasone may have a faster onset of action. Beclomethasone may have a greater influence on child growth but it appears that this effect is temporary. One large multi-centre study found that budesonide 200 µg/day produced 1.1 cm less growth in the first year of treatment, but at the end of 5 years there was no difference in height. Patients on budesonide had a better quality of life than those on placebo or nedocromil sodium. High-dose inhaled steroids (eight doses of 250 µg fluticasone aerosol) have been found to be as effective as 30 mg oral steroids in controlling asthma exacerbation and may cause less suppression of the pituitary adrenal axis.

Cromolyns

Sodium cromoglycate was the original anti-inflammatory agent derived from a herbal soup used by Egyptian women for the treatment of colds. Whilst recognized to be effective, it has a short half-life and is fully excreted in the urine after 6 hours, so it has to be administered four times daily.

Nedocromil sodium is reported to be more effective than sodium cromoglycate and equivalent to 400 µg of inhaled steroids. It is taken ideally four times a day but it has been used successfully twice daily. Nedocromil has an inhibitory effect on upper airway sensory nerve endings (C fibres) and as such may be more effective than inhaled steroids or sodium cromoglycate in managing cough. Approximately 17 per cent of patients find the taste intolerable.

Xanthines

Xanthines (aminophylline and theophylline) are oral bronchodilators. Their half-lives are about 3–4 h, but in sustained release preparations they can be active for up to 12 h. They also have a vasodilator action and can reduce cardiac pre-load and after-load, making them useful in elderly patients who have a combination of airways disease and cardiac failure. Xanthines have had a chequered career in asthma, finding themselves in and out of fashion over the last 50 years. More recently, it has been suggested that xanthines may have an anti-inflammatory role and are more effective if the dosage is adjusted to allow peaks and troughs rather than maintain constant levels.

Unfortunately, xanthines have a narrow therapeutic window, making the dose range between efficacy and side-effects relatively small. They affect sleep and school performance in children. Xanthines are available over the counter in many countries including the United Kingdom. Overdosage and side-effects are significant risks if intravenous xanthines are prescribed in an acute attack for patients who have already been taking the oral form without the knowledge of their doctor.

Leukotriene inhibitors

Leukotrienes are the most recently developed drugs in the management of asthma. Their role is still being evaluated. Leukotriene inhibitors are oral agents with anti-inflammatory activity. They inhibit the LTD4 receptor on bronchial and vascular smooth muscle and are effective in up to 60 per cent of patients. The onset of action is within 4–6 days and their effectiveness can be gauged after 2 weeks of therapy. They can have an effect comparable to a daily dose of 400 µg of beclomethasone and may be valuable in managing asthma in children. However, results from clinical trials have been relatively disappointing with only a small additional improvement in lung function when added to inhaled bronchodilators and steroids. They can be extraordinarily effective in patients with aspirin- or salicylate-sensitive asthma. Montelukast is taken once daily and zafirlukast twice daily.

Other treatment strategies in asthma

Up to 70 per cent of asthma patients have associated nasal congestion. Nasal congestion has been linked to worsening of asthma. Treating the nasal pathology is generally felt to enhance the symptom control of patients with asthma not only by correcting post-nasal drip but also improving the performance of the nose to warm and clean the air. However, documentary evidence of the benefits of treating the nose are limited. Improvement of nasal performance also enhances night-time oxygenation and, therefore, may reduce daytime fatigue in asthma patients.

Exercise induced asthma

Exercise-induced bronchoconstriction (EIB) is a fall of at least 15 per cent in FEV_1 or PEFR following vigorous exercise, usually of 6 min duration. Eighty per cent of asthma patients will demonstrate some EIB. It is thought to be due to a change in the osmolality of bronchial mucosal fluid that occurs with drying of the mucosal lining on the sudden increase in ventilation in exercise. It occurs more readily on exposure to cold air. It leads to immediate and late responses that are very similar to those caused by allergy. Most patients will respond to a standard dose (200 µg) of salbutamol or equivalent 10–15 min before exercise is taken. Inhaled asthma remedies are allowed by the International Olympic Committee but oral and systemic bronchodilators and steroids are prohibited.

Allergen avoidance

Avoidance of potential triggers in asthma is the hallmark of many asthma guidelines. Unfortunately, this is much easier said than done and research examining the success of this approach is either very limited or conflicting. The house dust mite produces in its faeces one of the most highly allergenic materials. Attempts to minimize its impact with housing modification, mattress covers, cleaning techniques, and pesticides have had variable outcomes. This is summarized in two meta-analyses on dust mite prevention that came to opposite conclusions.[12,13]

Regardless of these controversies, there may still be a role for skin prick testing in general practice. If a patient is found to have allergy then they are more able to make a choice regarding lifestyle changes such as removal of the cat or maintaining regular prophylaxis. Alternatively, if testing is negative the patient is more able to appreciate that viruses or temperature change are their triggers, not so easily avoided, and better managed with regular therapy. To this end skin prick testing may be more useful in encouraging compliance than directing allergy avoidance.

Drug delivery in asthma

One of the vital components in asthma management is the delivery of the drug to the airways efficiently and effectively. Failure to ensure the drug is delivered effectively is probably the commonest reason patients fail to respond to medication. Patients need regular instruction and supervision of the appropriate technique. The key issues in choice of inhaler are ease of use, acceptability to the patient, and cost. Metered dose inhalers (MDIs) revolutionized the treatment of asthma in the 1960s and are still the most frequently prescribed form of asthma treatment. On their own, they remain the most difficult of all to use effectively. With the advent of other suitable methods of inhalation, continued use of simple MDIs is a matter of judgement with individual patients unless used with spacer devices (Aerochamber, Fisonair, Nebuhaler, Volumatic), or a breath-actuated device (autohalers and easibreathes). The problem with simple MDIs is that it is difficult for most people and almost impossible for many to coordinate the actuation of the inhaler with their breathing. The result is that the aerosol is either discharged into the air or around the face or is deposited uselessly on the lining of the mouth and throat. With an MDI alone about 18 per cent of the available drug is delivered to the lung compared to 32 per cent with an MDI and spacer (Fig. 3). The remainder of the dose is delivered to the stomach.

Before the advent of large spacers and breath-actuated devices, a variety of powder inhalers were introduced. All of these can result in a rate of drug delivery that matches both the MDI and spacer and the breath-actuated MDI. All are far easier to use than MDIs alone. However, they do involve extra cost. The additional costs of these devices should be considered against the hidden costs of inadequately treated asthma that might result from poorly used MDIs. Powder inhalers are not dependent on coordination for effective use. There are two main types. The turbohaler is used for delivering terbutaline, budesonide, and formotorol. This is a low-volume device that leaves no taste and little or any inspiratory sensation. For some patients the lack of a positive sensation is a drawback whereas for others it is an advantage. High-volume powder devices (spinhaler, rotahaler, diskhaler, accuhaler) are used for delivering cromoglycate, salbutamol, beclomethasone, fluticasone, and salmeterol. They leave a powdery taste in the mouth, which confirms that they have been used but which may be unacceptably unpleasant for some people.

Inspiratory flow rate determines the effectiveness of drug delivery from each device. High rates of inspiratory flow increase the deposition of drug on the pharynx. At lower flow rates, the drug particles are accelerated enough to get them suspended in the air but not so fast that they hit the pharynx when the inspiratory flow turns a right angle to enter the trachea. Desirable flow rates vary between devices depending on particle size and mass. Inspiratory flow can be measured using the Clement Clarke

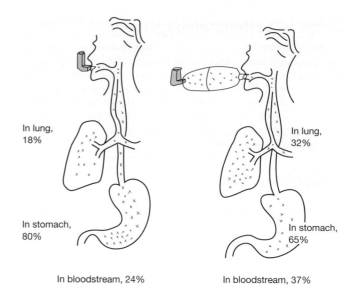

Fig. 3 Distribution of inhaled beta-agonist from an MDI alone and from an MDI with large volume spacer.

Inspiratory Flow Meter. This can help train patients in achieving the most efficient flow rate. Ideal inspiratory flow rates are between 20 and 60 l/min for the easibreathe breath-actuated inhaler and metered dose inhalers, between 30 and 60 l/min for the autohaler, 30–90 l/min for the accuhaler. Inspiratory flow is important to consider for the very young, very old, and very sick who may not be able to develop sufficient inspiratory effort to extract the medicine from the device particularly when they are unwell.

Doses delivered by inhalation are relatively small. The standard dose delivered by salbutamol MDI is 100 µg. This is one-twentieth of a small salbutamol tablet formerly used in children. It is one-fifth of the standard salbutamol injection, and one-fiftieth of the standard nebulizer dose. Much of the drug discharged into the mouth is absorbed into the blood stream irrespective of whether or not it is inhaled to the lungs. However, the size of the dose absorbed is small and when distributed throughout the body has little or no side-effects although some patients do report tremulousness, irritability, and palpitations after high doses of inhaled bronchodilators. Bronchodilators are absorbed into the blood stream largely via the lungs. Little is absorbed through the gastrointestinal tract. Inhaled steroids are well absorbed from the gut and poorly absorbed from the lungs. The significance of these findings is that most side-effects from these drugs are the result of systemic absorption. By achieving the best possible technique and using the lowest effective dose the side-effects of the drugs can be avoided.

Despite the difference in the size of the dose used, the spacer device is as effective as a nebulizer in acute severe asthma. Ten puffs of salbutamol via a spacer device has been found to have the same effect as a nebulizer. The suitability of the spacer is dependent on the patient having adequate inspiratory flow. Where patients are exhausted and can only achieve very low inspiratory flow rates the nebulizer should be used in acute asthma. The addition of a face mask to a spacer device can ensure that even the very young can derive benefit from a spacer (Table 1).

Managing the acute attack

Acute asthma presents with breathlessness, chest tightness, wheeze, and cough. If possible, peak expiratory flow should be measured at the beginning of the assessment. If the diagnosis is clear then the first line of treatment is high-dose inhaled beta-adrenergic agonists. This may be adequately provided using the patient's own relievers. Frequently, the patient will report a poor response from their own drugs. In most cases, adequate doses of beta-adrenergic agonists can be delivered using an MDI with a spacer (e.g. salbutamol 100 µg). Usually up to 10 separate actuations (1000 µg) of

Table 1 Advantages and disadvantages of commonly available inhaler devices

Inhaler device	Advantages	Disadvantages
Metered dose inhaler (MDI)	Cheap, transportable, and available for most asthma medications Newer smaller particle size CFC inhalers are of greater efficiency and require reduced dosages	50% of patients cannot use well Due to the relative inefficiency of the device there is a large amount of oropharyngeal deposition Up to 15% of patients gag or cough when the aerosol hits the throat, making the inhalation unreliable
Metered dose inhaler with large volume spacer device	For many patients the most reliable method of delivery 10 puffs, ideally delivered one at a time, is as effective as a nebulizer dosage 32% of drug will find its way to the lung Less oropharyngeal deposition	Not very portable. Small volume spacers have yet to be evaluated Requires rinsing once a week in warm soapy water to prevent the build up of electrostatic charge that reduces efficiency Internal scouring reduces device efficiency
Breath-activated Autohaler and Easibreathe	Much more effective than standard MDI for most people. Operates at an inspiratory flow of 20–60 l/min	Not easy to tell when empty
Breath-activated Turbohaler	Portable and easy to use Good range of therapies Dose-counter alerts patients to empty device	Needs an inspiratory effort of 60 l/min, which is not always achievable by children, the elderly, or patients when they are unwell Needs to be loaded in upright position Susceptible to humidity and wetting
Breath-activated Accuhaler and diskhaler and Clickhaler	Operates at flow rates of 30–90 l/min Has a counter to warn when device is empty	Susceptible to humidity
Breath-activated Aerolizer	Easy to determine dosage has been taken	Cumbersome to load by comparison to self-contained devices Limited availability of drug choices
Nebulizer therapy	Delivers a big dose relatively easily The preferred method for patients too ill to use other devices Newer ultrasonic devices overcome the portability and efficiency issues	Expensive, noisy, requires electricity, and 10–15 min to deliver dosage Require regular servicing of filters Large volume spacers are clinically as effective as nebulizers

an MDI in the spacer will suffice. Each actuation should be inspired deeply and then repeated after 20–30 s or as soon as the patient is able to do the manoeuvre comfortably. Patients who are very breathless may find a nebulizer more comfortable. The dose to be used in acute asthma is 5 mg salbutamol in adults and 2.5 mg salbutamol in children.

Patients who remain breathless at rest or on minimal exertion after the treatment should be transferred immediately to hospital. Patients whose symptoms are relieved and who experience an immediate improvement in PEFR of at least 50 per cent of the initial level should be considered for a short course of high-dose oral steroids (40 mg/day in adults, 20 mg/day in children under 12 years). In all patients who suffer acute severe asthma, inhaled steroids should be initiated immediately. Patients should be reviewed in 2 weeks if initial recovery is satisfactory. At follow-up, PEFR, symptom level, and inhaler technique should be reassessed and advice given on action to be taken in the event of a further exacerbation.

Long-term management

Acute asthma in which a distressed patient needs urgent treatment is rewarding to treat as patients generally respond rapidly. Far more challenging is the long-term management of asthma with the need to monitor progress, maximize lung function, minimize lifestyle intrusions, and provide medicines that are cost-effective and with minimal side-effects. Perhaps the greatest challenge is communicating management strategies to our patients so that they can take control of the disease themselves. An understanding of the processes that occur in an asthma attack from the patient's perspective may allow many of the barriers to effective management to be overcome.

Active asthma is usually marked by continuing symptoms, but key indicators of poor asthma control over time should include hospital admission, requirement for rescue courses of oral steroids, and high use of short-acting inhaled beta-agonists.

The stepped approach of the British Guidelines on Asthma Management for the management of chronic asthma in adults and children offers a skeleton

upon which the long-term management of asthma can be based (Forms 1 and 2). For every 8 action plans written by a GP, one after-hours asthma visit will be prevented. For every 20 plans written, one hospital admission will be prevented.[14] In primary care, long-term management of asthma is helped by the establishment of an effective partnership with the patient. Asthma is typically a relapsing disease, so for optimal treatment the patient should feel confident not only about every day management but also about what to do in an acute attack. In the early stages of an asthma attack (see Fig. 4), few symptoms other than tightness may occur. It may not be until a patient is at 60 per cent capacity that wheeze and cough becomes evident to the parent or a wheeze may be heard on auscultation. At 50 per cent capacity the patient may be waking at night. It is not uncommon for patients to leave it until they are at 40 per cent capacity before they seek medical attention and then require high dose bronchodilators, oral steroids and even hospital admission.[15]

Unfortunately, many patients (and doctors) mistake the yellow eosinophil-enriched allergic sputum for purulent infected sputum and antibiotics are prescribed as well.

As the patient recovers, their sleep improves, they lose their wheeze and cough and at the 80 per cent level feel they no longer need their medications.

This causes two problems. Firstly, the patient continues at the 80 per cent level, performing well below their best. Secondly, at the beginning of the attack it may take relatively high doses of allergen to trigger an episode. In the fragile recovery phase, it only takes small doses of allergen to trigger further episodes. During the recovery phase in a typical asthma attack it takes two weeks for symptoms to resolve, 12 weeks for spirometry and peak flow readings to recover, 18 weeks for the need for bronchodilator treatment to cease but up to 18 months before airway hyper-responsiveness as measured by histamine challenge testing, abates.[16]

With patients naturally reluctant to take long-term medication beyond their own obvious symptoms and the bronchial hyper-reactivity lasting upto 18 months, they never fully recover and roll from one asthma attack to another. Typically patients have a 'winter of discontent'.

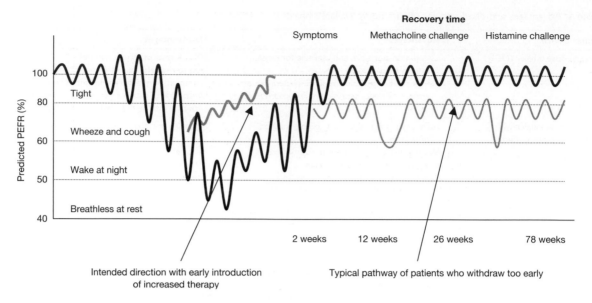

Fig. 4 Variation in lung function following an acute exacerbation of asthma.

Asthma action plan

When well Preventer medication .... Use .... Times per day .... Use .... Times per day Reliever medication .... Use .... Times per day .... Use .... Times per day Before exercise use .... Use			Peak flow ....
When not well or first sign of a cold Preventer medication .... Use .... Times per day .... Use .... Times per day Reliever medication .... Use .... Times per day .... Use .... Times per day When your symptoms are better return to the doses in the grey zone			Peak flow between .... and ....
If symptoms get worse. PHONE YOUR DOCTOR Take Prednisolone tablets/syrup .... For ....days Take Reliever medication up to .... puffs every .... hours			Peak flow between .... and ....
If you follow this plan but your symptoms get worse, <div align="center">Call an ambulance. 000</div>			Peak flow below
I have participated in the construction of the above management plan and feel that it meets my needs. Patient............ Nurse............ Doctor............			

Form 1

Using a peak flow meter and diary can help patients identify where they are in their recovery phase, and establish the role of inhaled steroids in restoring normal lung function.

As symptoms improve and the patient is able to return to normal activities the temptation is to stop treatment. The underlying inflammatory process may not have resolved, so the need for continuing long-term inhaled steroids may not be evident. It is difficult to be certain when inhaled steroids should be stopped, but if the patient can continue for at least 6 months after the return of PEFR to normal the chances of a relapse are minimized. The evidence for the effectiveness of prolonged inhaled steroid use in preventing relapses in asymptomatic patients after an acute attack is uncertain. It may take up to 18 months before bronchial

---

When well
You will
    Be free of regular night-time wheeze or cough or chest tightness
    Have no regular wheeze or cough or chest tightness on waking or during the day
    Be able to take part in normal physical activity without getting asthma symptoms
    Need reliever medication less than three times a week (except if it is used before exercise)

When not well
You will
    Have increasing night-time wheeze or cough or chest tightness
    Have symptoms regularly in the morning when you wake up
    Have a need for extra doses of reliever medication
    Have symptoms that interfere with exercise

If symptoms get worse, this is an acute attack
You will
    Have one or more of the following: wheeze, cough, chest tightness, or shortness of breath
    Need to use your reliever medication at least once every 3 h or more often

Danger signs
    Your symptoms get worse very quickly
    Wheeze or chest tightness or shortness of breath continue after using reliever medication
    Or return within minutes of taking reliever medication
    Severe shortness of breath, inability to speak comfortably, blueness of lips

IMMEDIATE ACTION IS NEEDED: CALL AN AMBULANCE

Take this action plan with you when you visit your doctor

Form 2

hyper-reactivity settles and the airways can be classified as 'healed'. Some patients will have continuing symptoms and lower than expected lung function despite maximal therapy.[17] In these patients, vulnerability to acute exacerbations is even greater, so the role of inhaled steroids and the action to be taken in an acute attack should be written down. Underlying all these approaches should be an annual review of device choice, inhaler technique, and the overall management plan.

Despite effective treatments, under-treatment is still common. In general practice, the concept of classifying asthma severity into mild, moderate, and severe, episodic or frequent, is difficult to operationalize. Features overlap so much and individuals move over time between the categories. Children who have so-called 'episodic viral induced asthma', common during the winter months, have sometimes been found to have constant asthma although their symptoms only become apparent to parents (and doctors) during exacerbations induced by viruses. Preventive, anti-inflammatory therapy remains the cornerstone of treatment for such patients.

Structured care

Structured care of asthma enables primary care teams to apply the principles of long-term management to the population of patients under their care. Structured care requires a register of patients at risk, a system of recall for those who do not attend, and a systematic assessment of patients who attend for review. Priority in providing structured care should be given to patients who have had a hospital admission or a rescue course of oral steroids in the previous 12 months, and to patients who request repeat prescriptions for more than 200 doses of inhaled beta-agonists each month.

Identifying patients suitable for ongoing asthma care

It is now recognized that not all patients are willing to accept they have asthma or desire the help of doctors and nurses to manage it. Understanding

Patients asthma streams[18]
1. Those patients that are anonymous to the system. These patients deny they have a problem and tolerate considerable disability in preference to seeing a doctor or taking medications.
2. Those patients isolated from the system. These patients see the doctor or nurse as just a supplier of what they need and a hurdle to getting what medications they feel are appropriate to their condition whether they be antibiotics, short-acting bronchodilators or oral steroids.
3. Patients who are ambivalent. These patients often have a good relationship with their doctor although they are unwilling to engage completely in a shared care arrangement and are excessively reliant on bronchodilators.
4. Patients who are optimally managed, motivated, well informed and have a good working relationship with their doctor or nurse and work in a partnership to minimize the impact of the asthma on their lives.

Goal is to move patients into stream 4

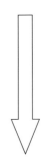

Fig. 5 The four groups into which asthma patients can be divided.

at what stage a patient is at and how ready they are to embrace long-term asthma care is important in determining the long-term success of any management programme.

Patients can be divided into 4 groups. Each group comprises about 25 per cent of patients. See Fig. 5.

One of the most significant events which helps patients move from groups 1, 2, and 3 into group 4 is that at some point a practitioner 'engages' the patient. This process involves the practitioner alerting the patient to the deficiency in their care and offering the time to sort out the asthma or organize the appropriate referral. It seems that when patients are confronted by a caring individual who is prepared to make an effort on their behalf, the patient is more likely to make the necessary changes to their own lives and take on some responsibility to improve matters.

References

1. McCormick, A., Fleming, D., and Charlton, J. *Morbidity Statistics from General Practice. Fourth National Survey 1991–1992*. Royal College of General Practitioners, Office of Population Censensus and Surveys, Department of Health. London: HMSO, 1994.

2. **International Study of Asthma and Allergies in Childhood (ISAAC)** (1998). World wide variation in prevalence of symptoms of asthma, allergic rhino-conjuctivitis and atopic eczema. *Lancet* **351**, 1225–32.

3. **Kaur, B., Anderson, H.R., and Austin, J.** (1998). Prevalence of asthma symptoms, diagnosis, and treatment in 12–14 year old children across Great Britain (international study of asthma and allergies in childhood, ISAAC UK). *British Medical Journal* **316**, 118–24.

4. **Von Hertzen, L.C.** (2000). Puzzling associations between childhood infections and the later occurrence of asthma and atopy. *Annals of Medicine* **32**, 397–400.

5. **Campbell, M.J., Holgate, S.T., and Johnston, S.L.** (1997). Trends in asthma mortality. *British Medical Journal* **315**, 1012–1012.

6. **Miller, M.** (2000). Peak expiratory flow meters. *Eur Respir Buyers* **3**, 12–14.

7. **Leroyer, C.** et al. (1998). Comparison of serial monitoring of peak expiratory flow and FEV_1 in the diagnosis of occupational asthma. *American Journal of Respiratory and Critical Care Medicine* **158**, 827–32.

8. **Charlton, I., Charlton, G., Broomfield, J., and Mullee, M.A.** (1990). Evaluation of peak flow and symptoms only self management plans for control of asthma in general practice. *British Medical Journal* **301**, 1355–9.

9. **Atherton, A., White, P.T., Hewett, G., and Howells, K.** (1996). Relationship of daytime asthma symptom frequency to morning peak expiratory flow. *European Respiratory Journal* **9**, 232–6.

10. **Saetta, M. and Turato, G.** (2001). Airway pathology in asthma. *European Respiratory Journal* **18** (Suppl. 34), 18s–23s.

11. **Adams, S., Pill, R., and Jones, A.** (1997). Medication, chronic illness and identity: the perspective of people with asthma. *Social Science and Medicine* **45**, 189–202.

12. **Gotzsche, P.C., Johansen, H.K., Burr, M.L., and Hammarquist, C.** (2001). House dust mite control measures for asthma. *Cochrane Database Syst. Rev.* **3**.

13. **Custovic, A., Simpson, A., Chapman, M.D., and Woodcock, A.** (1998). Allergen avoidance in the treatment of asthma and atopic disorders. *Thorax* **53**, 63–72.

14. **Gibson, P.G., Powell, H., Coughlan, J., Wilson, A.J., Hensley, M.J., Abramson, M., Bauman, A., and Walters, E.H.** (2002). Related articles: Patient education programs for adults with asthma (review). *Cochrane Database Systems Review* (2), CD001005.

15. **Gibson, P.G., Wong, B.J., Hepperle, M.J., Kline, P.A., Girgis-Gabardo, A., Guyatt, G., Dolovich. J., Denburg, J.A., Ramsdale, E.H., and Hargreave, F.E.** (1992). A research method to induce and examine a mild exacerbation of asthma by withdrawal of inhaled corticosteroid. *Clinical and Experimental Allergy* **22** (5), 525–32.

16. **Woolcock** (2001). *Clinical and Experimental Allergy* **1** (2), 62–4.

17. **Nolan, D. and White, P.T.** (2002). Symptomatic asthma: attendance and prescribing in general practice. *Respiratory Medicine* **96**, 102–9.

18. **Harris, G.S. and Shearer, A.G.** (2001). Beliefs that support the behavior of people with asthma: a qualitative investigation. *Journal of Asthma* **38** (5), 427–34.

Further reading

Two comprehensive guideline publications which summarize much of the research background to the current treatment of asthma:

British Thoracic Society, General Practitioners in Asthma Group, British Paediatric Society, British Association of Accident and Emergency. British Guidelines on Asthma Management. 1995 Review and Position Statement. *Thorax* 1997 **57**, S1–20.

National Asthma Education and Prevention Program. *Guidelines for the Diagnosis and the Management of Asthma*. Expert panel report 2. NIH no 97-4051. Bethesda MD: National Institutes of Health, 1997.

2.5 Chronic lower respiratory disorders

An de Sutter and Marc De Meyere

Apart from chronic airway disorders (asthma, COPD), there exists a large number of relatively rare chronic pulmonary diseases with many divergent causes: infections, genetic disorders, auto-immune processes, exposure to certain materials, drugs, poison, radiation, etc. Often, the aetiology is unknown.

These conditions are mainly managed in secondary care. For the general practitioner, it is important to identify the population at risk, to recognize early symptoms, and to supervise the patients and their treatment at home.

In this chapter, we will mainly focus on tuberculosis because of its globally high and rising incidence, and cystic fibrosis because of the particular aspects of home care. Other conditions will be briefly reviewed.

Tuberculosis

Epidemiology

Tuberculosis (TB) remains one of the deadliest diseases in the world. The WHO estimates that each year more than 8 million new cases of TB occur and approximateley 3 million persons die from the disease. Ninety-five per cent of tuberculosis cases occur in developing countries. In terms of numbers of cases, the biggest burden of TB is in South-East Asia. In many countries, incidence is now rising again after a long period of steady decline. Factors contributing to the rise in TB are firstly HIV. This infection weakens the immune system and someone who is HIV-positive and infected with TB is many times more likely to become sick with TB. In Africa, HIV is the single most important factor determining the increased incidence of TB in the last 10 years. Global trade, the number of people travelling in airplanes, and migration of people have all increased dramatically over the last 40 years and this movement also helps to spread TB. In many industrialized countries, at least one-half of TB cases are among foreign-born people. Further, the number of refugees and displaced people in the world is constantly growing. Untreated TB spreads quickly in crowded refugee camps and shelters and is difficult to treat as treatment takes at least 6 months. As many as 50 per cent of the world's refugees may be infected with TB and as they move, they may spread the infection.

TB in general practice

In spite of the high incidence of TB worldwide, in most industrialized countries TB is a rare disease in general practice. In the Netherlands, for example, the incidence in general practice is about three per 10 000 patients per year, which means that a GP taking care of 2500 patients sees less than one new case of TB each year.

This is a consequence of the low incidence of TB in these countries (except for some specific risk populations) and of the fact that in the most countries screening and management of TB is organized centrally by the health authorities and general practitioners are thus not directly involved. Yet, because of the changing epidemiology and worldwide rising incidence, GPs will probably be confronted more and more with patients who might be at risk of TB infection or disease.

Aetiology and pathogenesis

Tuberculosis is caused by infection with *Mycobacterium tuberculosis*. This infection spreads through the air by droplet nuclei produced when persons with pulmonary TB cough, sneeze, speak, or sing. A droplet nucleus is so small, containing only two or three organisms, that it can—when inhaled—reach the alveoli. It, thus, implants in a respiratory bronchiole or alveolus where the bacilli then can multiply within the alveolar macrophage. The bacilli may also spread via the lymphatics to other parts of the body. After 2–12 weeks, they reach a sufficient number to elicit a cellular immune response. This immunologic reaction arrests further proliferation. The whole process is usually clinically and radiographically inapparent. Most commonly, a positive tuberculin skin test result is the only indication that infection with *M. tuberculosis* has taken place.

Individuals with a latent TB infection but no active disease are not infectious and thus cannot transmit the organism.

If not given preventive therapy, about 10 per cent of individuals who acquire tuberculosis infection will eventually develop active TB. The risk is highest in the first 2 years after infection, when half the cases will occur. In children and patients with chronic diseases, the ability of the host to respond to the organism is reduced, and thus the likelihood of developing TB disease increased.

In a person with intact cell-mediated immunity, the response to infection with the tubercle bacillus usually provides protection against reinfection.

Diagnosis

Diagnosis of latent tuberculosis infection (LTBI): tuberculin skin test

The tuberculin skin test is primarily intended to identify infections with *M. tuberculosis* in persons who do not currently exhibit signs and symptoms of clinical disease but who require preventive therapy.

Immunologic basis and administration

Infection with *M. tuberculosis* produces a delayed-type hypersensitivity reaction to certain antigenic components (tuberculins) that are contained in extracts of culture filtrate of the organism. For skin testing 0.1 ml containing 5 TU (Tuberculin Unit) of purified protein derivative (PPD) tuberculin is used. This is injected intracutaneously in the volar or dorsal aspect of the forearm. If correctly injected just beneath the skin, a small wheal, 6–10 mm across, will form. Delayed hypersensitivity reactions usually begin 5–6 h after the injection, reach a maximum at 48–72 h and subside over a period of a few days (although positive reactions can persist for up to 1 week).

Specificity and sensitivity of the tuberculin test

Specificity of the tuberculin test is 99 per cent in populations that have no other mycobacteria exposure or BCG vaccination. A false positive skin test response can, however, occur after exposure to other mycobacteria including BCG vaccination. In these population specificity is lower (95 per cent). Yet, these cross-reactions tend to result in smaller amounts of induration and specificity can thus be improved by progressively increasing the cut point for positivity.

In any population, the likelihood that a positive test represents a true infection is influenced by the prevalence of infections with *M. tuberculosis* in the population. At the moment prevalence in people in industrialized countries without known exposure to TB is so low that screening of groups without a known or likely exposure is not recommended as a false positive result is more likely than a true positive.

Sensitivity of the tuberculin test is virtually 100 per cent in patients with a normal immunoresponse. False negative results can, however, occur, namely in patients with recent or overwhelming *M. tuberculosis* or with immunosuppression caused by medications, chronic diseases, malignancy, HIV infection, or vaccination with live-attenuated virus. If false negative reactions are suspected, specialist advise should be obtained. A list of factors causing false negative tuberculin skin tests are summarized in Table 1.

Tuberculin skin test interpretation

To increase specificity, three cut-off levels have been recommended for defining a positive tuberculin reaction. For individuals at great risk of developing tuberculosis disease if they become infected with *M. tuberculosis* a cut point of not less than 5 mm is advised (Table 2). A cut point of not less than 10 mm is suggested for individuals with a high likelihood of being infected

Table 1 Causes of false negative results for PPD tuberculin skin tests[1]

Inaccurate reading of induration
Patient age greater than 45 years
Acquired immunodeficiency syndrome
Alcoholism
Haematologic or lymphoreticular disorders
Intestinal bypass or gastrectomy
Malnutrition
Renal failure
Sarcoidosis
Systemic viral, bacterial, and fungal infections
Use of corticosteroids or other immunosuppressive drugs
Zinc deficiency
Live virus vaccines: measles–mumps–rubella, poliovirus

Table 2 Interpretation of the PPD tuberculin skin test[1]

I An induration of 5 mm or more is classified as positive in persons with any of the following: (a) Human immunodeficiency virus infection   (b) Recent close contact with persons who have active tuberculosis   (c) Chest radiographs showing fibrosis (consistent with healed tuberculosis)
II An induration of 10 mm or more is classified as positive in all persons who do not meet any of the criteria in section I but have other risk factors for tuberculosis
III An induration of 15 mm or more is positive in persons who do not meet any of the criteria from sections I or II
IV Recent tuberculin skin test conversion is defined as an increase in induration of 10 mm or more within a two-year period, regardless of age
V In health care workers, the recommendations in Sections I, II, and III generally should be followed. In facilities where tuberculosis patients frequently receive care, the optimal cut-off point for health care workers with no other risk factors may be an induration of 10 mm or greater

but without other risk factors that would increase their likelihood of developing active disease (Table 2). Persons who are not likely to be infected should generally not be tuberculin tested since the predictive value of a positive test in low-prevalence populations is poor. If tested, a cut point of not less than 15 mm is suggested (Table 2).

A tuberculin skin test conversion is defined as an increase in reaction size of 10 mm or more within a period of 2 years and should be considered as indicative for recent *M. tuberculosis* infection.

Indications for tuberculin testing

Tuberculin testing for LTBI is to identify persons at high risk for developing TB who would benefit by treatment of LTBI, if detected. Persons with increased risk of developing TB include those who have recent infection with *M. tuberculosis* and those who have clinical conditions that are associated with an increased risk for progression of LTBI to active TB.

These risks are: (a) close contact with persons with infectious pulmonary TB; (b) immigrants from areas of the world with high rates of TB; (c) homeless persons; (d) HIV-infected persons or persons at risk of HIV infection and serostatus unknown; (e) injection drugs users; (f) residents or people employed in institutions with persons at risk of TB (hospitals, homeless shelters, correctional facilities, nursing homes, residential homes for patients with AIDS); (g) patients with medical conditions that increase the risk of TB (e.g. diabetes, silicosis, lymphoma, chronic renal failure, etc.); (h) children exposed to adults belonging to high-risk groups.

Mandatory skin-testing programmes (e.g. among teachers, foodhandlers) are not recommended unless the targeted groups contain substantial proportions of persons at high risk.

Boosted reactions and serial tuberculin testing

Although PPD skin sensitivity persists throughout life, over time the size of the skin reaction may decrease or even disappear. If PPD is administered to infected individuals whose skin tests have waned, the reaction of the initial test may be small or absent. However, there may be an accentuation of response on repeated testing. This 'booster' effect can be misinterpreted as a skin test conversion. If repeated tuberculin testing is anticipated, as in health care workers, for example, a two-step method is recommended: those who have a negative or doubtful initial PPD skin test undergo a second tuberculin test 1–3 weeks after the first. The results from the second test should be considered to be the 'correct' result.

Previous vaccination with BCG

In more than 70 per cent of countries worldwide, BCG vaccine is still commonly used. There is ample evidence that it protects against disseminated TB and TB meningitis in children, yet protection against pulmonary TB, both in children and adults, is unproven.

BCG vaccination presents a dilemma in screening for TB, because it is not possible to distinguish a positive tuberculin reaction after vaccination from one caused by infection. Guidelines recommend consideration of a positive tuberculin reaction as indicating infection regardless of previous BCG vaccination, especially among persons from countries with a high prevalence of tuberculosis. Reasons for this approach are: (a) tuberculin test conversion rates after vaccination may be much less than 100 per cent; (b) the mean reaction size among persons who have received BCG is often less than 10 mm; (c) tuberculin sensitivity tends to wane over time—although it can be boosted by serial testing.

Diagnosis of active TB

A patient with a positive tuberculin test should always be further investigated for active TB. Active TB should also be considered in any patient with symptoms possibly indicating TB, such as chronic cough, weight loss, night sweats, haemoptysis, fever, and malaise. In patients with active disease, a tuberculin skin test may be negative in 10–20 per cent of cases.

The first step is a chest X-ray examination as active pulmonary TB nearly always causes abnormalities on the chest film.

If abnormalities are suggestive of TB, the patient should be investigated with at least three sputum or gastric aspirate examinations for acid fast bacilli. Collection of these specimens must be performed very carefully, and

is thus best supervised by experienced personnel. Often, this will mean a referral to a specialized centre. Demonstration of acid fast bacilli in sputum provides a quick first confirmation of the clinical diagnosis of TB (results can be obtained within 24 h) and the number of demonstrated bacilli is also indicative of the infectiousness of the patient. Sensitivity of three acid fast smears for identifying active TB is, however, only 70 per cent. Therefore, all specimens suspected of containing mycobacteria should also be cultured: cultures are more sensitive and allow species identification drug susceptibility testing. Their disadvantage is a delay of several weeks before results are available. In the future, sensitivity of direct examination of clinical specimens—and consequently early treatment decisions—will be greatly improved by molecular amplification methods.

In non-HIV-infected patients, active TB is in 85 per cent limited to the lungs. In patients with HIV, extra-pulmonary TB is more frequent. Extra-pulmonary TB may be associated with many symptoms, including altered mental status, back pain, and abdominal pain. It involves relatively inaccessible sites and, because of the nature of the sites involved, fewer bacilli can cause much greater damage. The combination of small numbers of bacilli and inaccessible sites makes bacteriologic confirmation of a diagnosis more difficult, and invasive procedures are frequently required to establish a diagnosis. The most common types of extrapulmonary TB, in descending order of frequency, are pleural, lymphatic, bone and joint disease, genitourinary tract and miliary disease, meningitis, and peritonitis.

Management

Management of latent TB infection

All patients with a positive skin test and a *high risk of TB* infection (see indications for tuberculin testing) but without findings of active TB should be treated in order to prevent the development of active TB disease. A history of BCG vaccination should not influence this decision.

The preferred regimen for adults is *isoniazid* 300 mg daily during 9 months. Randomized trials have shown an efficacy of 54–88 per cent in reducing incidence of TB disease (depending largely on compliance with medication). Isoniazid is bactericidal, relatively non-toxic, easily administered, and inexpensive. The most severe toxic effect is hepatitis. In Table 3, dose, toxicity, and monitoring requirements of isoniazid therapy are summarized.

In children at high risk of TB, treatment of LTBI is even more important. Infants and children (less than 5 years) with LTBI have always been infected recently and are at high risk of progressive disease. They are also more likely to develop life-threatening forms of TB, especially meningitis and disseminated TB. Isoniazid treatment of LTBI appears to be more effective in children than in adults (70–90 per cent prevention of active TB); risk of

Table 3 Isoniazid to treat latent tuberculosis infection[2]

Drug	Oral dose (mg/kg) (maximum dose)				Adverse reactions	Monitoring	Comments
	Daily		Twice weekly				
	Adults	Children	Adults	Children			
Isoniazide	5 (300 mg)	10–20 (300 mg)	15 (900 mg)	20–40 (900 mg)	Rash Hepatic enzyme elevation Peripheral neuropathy Mild central nervous system effects Drug interactions resulting in increased phenytoin (Dilantin) or Disulphiram (Antabuse) levels	Clinical monitoring monthly Liver function tests at baseline in selected cases and repeat measurements if: baseline results are abnormal Patient is pregnant, in the immediate postpartum period, or at high risk for adverse reactions Patient has symptoms of adverse reactions	Hepatitis risk increases with age and alcohol consumption Pyridoxine (vitamin B_6, 10–25 mg/day) may prevent peripheral neuropathy and central nervous system effects

toxicity is minimal and children generally tolerate the drug better than adults. The dose in children is 10–20 mg/kg/day during 9 months. Even children with negative tuberculin skin test but who are contacts of patients with TB should be best treated until 8–12 weeks after the contact has ended and then tested again. If the tuberculin test remains negative, treatment can then be stopped.

Patients with a *low risk* of developing TB should, in general, not receive tuberculin skin tests as positive reactions are more likely to be false positive than true positive. If tested anyway, and the result is positive, then possible advantages of treatment must be weighted carefully against risk of toxicity. Is there a high likelihood of TB transmission to vulnerable contacts (e.g. children or HIV infected patients) if treatment was not given and the patients were to develop active TB? Is there a high likelihood of drug toxicity? Treatment is only appropriate if the anticipated benefit exceeds the assessed risk of drug toxicity.

Treatment success largely depends on compliance. If compliance is doubtful, directly observed therapy (DOT) of isoniazid 900 mg (20–40 mg/kg in children) twice weekly during 9 months is preferred.

For some patients with LTBI, other medications and treatment regimens are advised and consultation with a TB specialist is necessary. These are, for example, patients who cannot tolerate isoniazid, HIV-infected persons taking AIDS medications, patients with a positive skin test and old fibrotic lesions on chest X-ray, pregnant or lactating women with LTBI, and patients who are contacts of isoniazid-patients resistant TB.

Management of active TB infection

In general, initial treatment of active TB consists of 2 months of a four-drug regimen of isoniazid, rifampicin, pyrazinamide, and ethambutol. After this treatment, to which initial isolates were sensitive, patients continue treatment with isoniazid and rifampicin alone if repeat sputum cultures are negative and the patient has improved clinically. Patients continue these two medications for another 4 months, at which time treatment may be discontinued if sputum cultures remain negative. There are several options for initial treatment: daily treatment, daily treatment for 2 weeks, followed by twice weekly treatment or thrice weekly treatment. Compliance with treatment is crucial but often a problem because of the complexity and duration of the therapy, because symptoms disappear quickly after beginning of therapy and because of medication side-effects. Non-compliance can cause multidrug resistance, disease progression, or relapse. As it is difficult to predict non-compliance in advance, directly observed therapy is recommended for all patients. This is usually offered by local health departments.

In special groups, deviation of this basic four-drug treatment will be necessary, namely in children, pregnant or lactating women, HIV-infected persons, and persons with drug restistance or drug intolerance.

Patients under treatment should be evaluated monthly by a physician and sputum acid fast smears and cultures should be performed.

Apart from treating patients, all measures to prevent nosocomial transmission must be adequately taken as long as the patients is (suspected) infective. Also, contact of patients must be localized and offered tuberculin test and treatment of LTBI if necessary.

The GP and TB in low-incidence countries: alertness and support

In most countries with established market economies the incidence of TB is very low with the consequence that doctors and society as a whole have little experience with TB. Yet, the GP will often be the first to be consulted by a symptomatic patient, and must be alert to the possibility of TB. Delay in diagnosis must be avoided since it increases the risk of disease progression for the patients and of the spread to others. The GP should also be alert for an increased risk of TB infection in asymptomatic people and check if they are adequately screened. In patients with a history of active TB, he/she must keep the possibility of reactivation of the disease in mind. In most of the low-incidence countries, TB prevention and control is organized centrally by the public health authorities. This systematic approach has been very succeful in decreasing incidence, morbidity, and mortality of TB. The practical organization differs between countries and every GP should know how the system functions. These organizations can be responsible for targeted screening, for source and contact tracing; they also can provide facilities for diagnosis, treatment, and follow-up of LTBI or active TB and offer directly observed treatment. The GP mainly plays a complementary part to these organizations by identifying, screening—and if necessary treating LTBI—in patients who are at increased risk of TB but are not included in a screening programme. If active TB is suspected, for example, on chest X-ray, the patient will usually be referred for treatment to these specialized centres or to secondary care. The GP is generally not directly involved in the management of active TB, but will usually give information, support, encouragement, and motivation.

TB in high-incidence countries: the DOTS strategy

In contrast with these countries, TB is a big and growing problem in many parts of the world. Reasons include the breakdown of health service (e.g. Eastern Europe), the spread of HIV/AIDS (e.g. Africa), and of the emergence of multidrug resistant TB (e.g. the former Soviet Union).

Stopping the TB epidemic is now one of the top priorities of the WHO. The strategy to achieve this is called DOTS or Directly Observed Therapy Short-course.

This strategy has five key components: political commitment to sustained TB control, case detection and diagnosis by direct sputum examination, standardized short-course chemotherapy with direct observation of drug intake, sufficient and regular drug supply, recording and reporting of patient progress and treatment oucome. DOTS is a highly effective strategy: it produces cure rates of up to 95 per cent, prevents further spread of infection, prevents the development of multidrug resistant TB (MDR-TB), and is relatively cheap. In 1999, about 24 per cent of all TB patients were treated through the DOTS strategy.

Drug resistance

One important aim of DOTS is prevention of emerging of drug-resistant TB. Drug-resistant TB is caused by inconsistent or partial treatment, when patients do not take all their drugs regularly for the required period because they start to feel better, doctors and health workers prescribe the wrong treatment regimens, or the drug supply is unreliable. From a public health perspective, poorly supervised or incomplete treatment of TB is worse than no treatment at all. Failure to complete standard treatment regimens or prescribing the wrong treatment results in bacilli developing resistance to anti-TB drugs. Those infected will consequently also have drug-resistant TB. A particularly dangerous form of drug-resistant TB is MDR-TB, with resistance against at least isoniazid and rifampicin—the two most effective anti-TB drugs. MDR-TB is rising at alarming rates in some countries, especially in the former Soviet Union, and threatens global TB control. While drug-resistant TB is (usually) treatable, it requires extensive and very expensive chemotherapy, which is also more toxic to patiens. 'DOTS plus' is the WHO strategy to control MDR-TB.

Key points

1. TB is one of the deadliest diseases in the world. Ninety-five per cent of cases occur in developing countries. In industrialized countries, TB is limited to immigrants and disadvantaged populations.

2. Targeted tuberculin testing is used to identify infected persons at high risk of TB. Screening of groups without known or likely exposure to *M. tuberculosis* is not recommended as a false positive result is more likely than a true positive.

3. Treatment of latent TB infection aims to prevent progression of LTBI to active TB. Treatment of active TB cures the patient and prevents spread of TB to other people.

4. Compliance is crucial for successful therapy. Directly observed therapy is recommended when non-compliance is anticipated. Incomplete treatment may lead to incomplete cure and to emergence and spread of drug-resistant bacilli. From a public health point of view no treatment at all is better than an incomplete treatment.

5. In low-incidence countries, TB prevention and control is usually organized centrally by public health organizations. The GP's part is in detecting and timely referral of patients with active TB and by screening patients at risk who have not been screened elsewhere.

6. In countries with high or rising TB incidence, the WHO uses the DOTS (Directly Observed Therapy Short-course) strategy to control the TB epidemic.

Table 4 Presenting features of more than 20 000 cystic fibrosis patients in the United States[a]

Feature	%
Acute or persistent respiratory symptoms	50.5
Failure to thrive, malnutrition	42.9
Abnormal stools	35.0
Meconium ileus, intestinal obstruction	18.8
Family history	16.8
Electrolyte, acid base abnormality	5.4
Rectal prolapse	3.4
Nasal polyps, sinus disease	2.0
Hepatobiliary disease	0.9
Other[b]	1.0–2.0

[a] Data from the patient registry. Cystic Fibrosis Foundation, Bethesda, MD.

[b] Includes pseudotumour cerebri, azoospermia, acrodermatitis-like rash, vitamin deficiency states, hypoproteinaemic oedema, hypoprothrombinaemia with bleeding, meconium plug syndrome.

Cystic fibrosis

Epidemiology

Cystic fibrosis (CF) occurs in approximately 1 per 3500 white live births and 1 per 17 000 black infants in the United States. The median age of survival is 28 years. Seventy per cent of patients are diagnosed in the first year of life, 80 per cent by age 4 years, and 90 per cent by age 12 years. Pulmonary disease is the most common cause of morbidity and mortality.

CF in primary care

CF is the major cause of severe chronic lung disease in children and is responsible for most exocrine pancreatic insufficiency during early life. It is also responsible for many cases of salt depletion, nasal polyposis, pansinusitis, rectal prolapse, pancreatitis, cholelithiasis, and insulin-dependent hyperglycaemia. CF may present as failure to thrive and occasionally as cirrhosis or other forms of hepatic dysfunction. Therefore, this disorder enters into the differential diagnosis of many paediatric conditions.

Pathogenesis

The *CF gene* was cloned in 1989 and is located on the *long arm of chromosome 7*. The protein product, the CF transmembrane conductance regulator (CFTR), consists of 1480 amino acids. Approximately 150 different mutations have been found. The most common mutation in patients from Northern European ancestry is the deletion of phenylalanine at codon 508 of the CF gene.

Four long-standing observations are of fundamental pathophysiologic importance: failure to clear mucous secretions, a paucity of water in mucous secretions, an elevated salt content of sweat and other serous secretions, and chronic infections in the respiratory tract.

How to make a diagnosis

Typical clinical features

The list of presenting signs and symptoms is lengthy, although recurrent upper respiratory tract infections and gastrointestinal presentations predominate (Table 4).

Diagnosis

Standard diagnosis: sweat test

The diagnosis of CF has been based for many years on a positive quantitative sweat test ($Cl^- \geq 60$ mEq/l) in conjunction with one or more of the following: typical chronic obstructive pulmonary disease, documented exocrine pancreatic insufficiency, or a positive family history.

Heterozygote detection and prenatal diagnosis Mutation analysis should be fully informative when testing potential carriers or a foetus provided that mutations within the family have been previously identified. Testing a spouse of a carrier with a standard panel of probes is approximately 90 per cent sensitive. The rational for pre-natal detection of risk and termination of pregnancy is currently a matter of considerable discussion.

Newborn screening Most newborns with CF can be identified by determination of immunoreactive trypsinogen in blood spots, coupled with confirmatory sweat or DNA testing. This screening test is at best only 95 per cent sensitive. There is no evidence that early diagnosis improves long-term outcome. The case for routine newborn screening is open for debate.

Management

General principles

- A period of hospitalization for accurate diagnosis, baseline assessment, initiation of treatment, clearing of pulmonary involvement, and education of the patient and parents is recommended.

- Immunoprophylaxis specifically against measles, pertussis, and influenza is essential.

- A nurse, respiratory therapist, social worker, dietitian, and psychologist should participate in the care programme.

- Home treatment programmes have advantages (see section on CF home care).

- The goal of the therapy is to maintain a stable condition. This can be accomplished for most patients by interval evaluation and adjustment of the home treatment programme. However, some children have episodic acute or low-grade chronic lung infection that progresses. For these patients, 2 weeks or more of intensive inhalation and physical therapy and i.v. antibiotics are indicated.

Specific therapy

The major components of the care are pulmonary and nutritional therapy.

Pulmonary therapy

The objective is to clear secretions from airways and to control infection.

- *Aerosol therapy* is used to deliver medications and to the lower respiratory tract. The basic aerosol solution is 0.45–0.9 per cent saline.

β-*Agonists* can be added when the airway pathogens are resistant to oral antibiotics or when the infection is difficult to control at home.

◆ *Chest physical therapy (PT)*. This treatment usually consists of chest percussion combined with postural drainage.

◆ *Antibiotic therapy*. Antibiotics are the mainstay of therapy designed to control progression of lung infection. The goal is to reduce the intensity of endobronchial infection and to delay progressive lung damage. The usual signs of acute chest infections, such as fever, tachypnoea, or chest pain, are often absent. Consequently, all aspects of the patients history and examination must be a guide. Indication, choice and duration of antibiotic therapy are made by the hospital or home care team. Whenever possible, the choice of antibiotics should be guided by in vitro sensitivity test.

Nutritional therapy

◆ With the advent of improved pancreatic enzyme products, *normal amounts of fat* in the diet are usually tolerated and preferred.

◆ Extracts of animal pancreas (*pancreatic enzymes*) reduce but do not fully correct stool fat and nitrogen losses. Several (1–3 per day) enteric-coated, pH-sensitive enzyme microspheres are prescribed, containing 20 000 IU of lipase units/capsules. Infants may need only one-half capsule or may prefer pancreatic powder.

◆ Because pancreatic insufficiency results in malabsorption of fat-soluble vitamins (A, D, E, K), *vitamin supplementation* is recommended.

◆ Sweat salt losses can be high especially in warm climates. Children should have *free access to salt*. Regimented salt supplements are no longer prescribed.

CF home care

The *advantages* of home care include reduced hospital admissions on patient's length of stay. Many aspects of treatment, for example, i.v. antibiotics, can be administered at home as effectively as in hospital.

Nurses undertaking home care are part of a hospital-based multidisciplinary team including the CF specialists, a social worker, a nutritionist, a physical therapist, and a geneticist. The key to successfull care in the community is effective communication and liaison between all involved with the patients. Good liaison between the hospital CF specialists and the GP is essential.

The nurse should be able to monitor weight, lung function, and oxygen saturation. She should be able to educate, counsel, and advise the patient on every aspect of the disease or know where to seek advice.

Specific aspects of home care of CF patients are numerous.

For the newly diagnosed patient, patient/carer information and education is vital. There is often a psychosocial transition, by which the family moves from seeing themselves as a healthy family to accepting the reality of a long-term health problem. The home care team can help in this proccess by enabling the family.

A child or adult with a chronic illness seriously affects the entire family. By providing home care, it reduces the emotional trauma to the whole family, by minimizing the separation of the child from family and home. Parents are less anxious, have a greater sense of being in control, and an increased capacity for learning new care skills.

In conclusion, CF home care has many advantages for selected patients. In the interests of patients we must ensure that the flexibility for treatment is maintained and that change in health care is not just cost driven. Home care is here to stay on the grounds of patient preference and convenience.

Perspective

◆ *Lung transplantation* is a final option for patients who have end-stage pulmonary disease.

◆ *New therapeutics:* approaches include stimulation of alternative chloride transport mechanisms, pharmocologic upregulation of mutated CFTR, and gene therapy.

◆ *Prognosis:* CF remains a life-limiting disorder, although survival has improved during the last 40 years. Life table data now indicate a median cumulative survival of 30 years. With appropriate medical and psycho-social support children and adolescents with CF generally cope well. Achievement of an independent and productive adulthood is a realistic goal for many.

Key points

◆ CF occurs in approximately 1 per 3500 *white live* births and 1 per 17 000 black infants.

◆ CF is the major *cause* of severe chronic lung disease in children and is responsible for most exocrine pancreatic insufficiency during early life.

◆ CF is also *responsible for* many cases of salt depletion, nasal polyposis, pansinusitis, rectal prolapse, pancreatitis, cholelithiasis, and insulin-dependent hyperglycaemia. CF may present as failure to thrive and occasionally as cirrhosis or other forms of hepatic dysfunction.

◆ The *diagnosis* of CF is based on a positive sweat test (Cl$^-$ ≥60 mEq/l) in conjunction with one or more of the following: typical chronic obstructive pulmonary disease, documented exocrine pancreatic insufficiency, or a positive family history.

◆ The major components of the *therapy* are pulmonary and nutritional therapy. Antibiotic therapy, if possible by aerosol, chest physical therapy, and bronchodilatators are standard drugs. Pancreatic enzymes and fat-soluble vitamins are recommended.

◆ The *advantages of a home care team* include reduced hospital admissions and, therefore, hospital-acquired infections. The ability to attend school and work avoids disruption to normal daily activities. Home care reduces the emotional trauma to the whole family.

Chronic interstitial lung diseases

Interstitial lung diseases (ILDs) are caused by a variety of disease processes. The most frequent causes are sarcoidosis, cryptogenic fibrosing alveolitis, allergic alveolitis, and fibrotic-vascular diseases, for example, RA, SLE. In total, there are about 150 different disease entities of which about 35 per cent have a known cause (see Tables 5 and 6).

The incidence of ILD is low: in the Netherlands, for example, about 1.16 per cent of clinically treated lung patients suffer from an ILD and registrations in New Mexico show an incidence of 58 per 10^5 per year.

In ILDs the pathological process is initiated by damage to the alveolar epithelium by an inhaled or blood-borne stimulus, by damage due to infiltration of the pulmonary interstitium, or by damage to the vascular endothelium. This initial damage is followed by an active toxic or immunologic alveolitis, which leads to disturbance and reform of the pulmonary parenchyma. The further course may be: complete recovery, recovery with fibrotic scars, or (rapid or slow) progression to 'end-stage' lungs with complete loss of functional alveolocapillar structures and a honeycomb image on radiology.

The differential diagnosis between the different ILDs is difficult due to the wide variety of pathologies involved, the large number of causes and the relative rarity of most of the diseases.

Table 5 Diffuse lung disease: known causes

Organic dusts
Avian, e.g., pigeon antigens, buderigar
Fungal, e.g., *Aspergillus* sp.
Chemical, e.g., diisocyanates

Pneumoconiosis
Fibrogenic inorganic dusts, e.g.
   Beryllium
   Asbestos
   Silica
   Hard metal alloy
Inert inorganic dusts

Infection
Viruses, e.g., cytomegalovirus, adenovirus, respiratory syncytial virus
Bacteria, e.g., tuberculosis
Fungi, e.g., histoplasmosis, *Pneumocystis* sp.
Protozoa, e.g., toxoplasma
Helminths, e.g., ascaris, filaria
HIV

Drugs
Producing lung injury, e.g., cytotoxic/chemotherapeutic, opiate abuse
Producing immunogenic lung injury, e.g., anti-inflammatory, cardiovascular
Causing eosinophilia, e.g., antibiotics; anti-inflammatory, anticonvulsant, cytoxic
Systemic lupus erythematosus-like responses, e.g., hydralazine
Organizing pneumonia, e.g., acebutalol, gold, sulfasalazine

Neoplasia
Lymphangitis carcinomatosa
Lymphoma
Alveolar cell carcinoma

Miscellaneous
Radiotherapy
Gases, e.g., mercury vapour, high O_2 concentrations, NO_2
Chemical, e.g., paraquat
Associated with chronically elevated left atrial pressure, uraemia
Multiple emboli, e.g., fat emboli
Post-adult respiratory distress syndrome
Trauma with haemorrhage
Lipoid pneumonias

Table 6 Diffuse lung disease: unknown causes

With interstitial fibrosis
Cryptogenic fibrosing alveolitis
Systemic sclerosis
Polymyositis
Sjögren's syndrome
Rheumatoid arthritis
Systemic lupus erythematosus (SLE)

With granulomata
Sarcoidosis
Wegener's granulomatosis
Langerhans' cell histiocytosis
Eosinophilic granulomatosis (Churg–Strauss syndrome)
Lymphomatoid granulomatosis
Bronchocentric granulomatosis

Inherited disorders
Tuberous sclerosis
Neurofibromatosis
Hermansky–Pudlak syndrome
Lipid storage disorders
Familial fibrosing alveolitis

With vasculitis
Wegener's granulomatosis
Microscopic polyarteritis
Rheumatic disease, e.g., SLE, rheumatoid arthritis
Hypersensitivity vasculitis, e.g., response to drugs
Goodpasture's syndrome

Individual pathology
Cryptogenic pulmonary eosinophilia
Allergic bronchopulmonary aspergillosis
Idiopathic pulmonary haemosiderosis
Pulmonary veno-occlusive disease
Lymphangioleiomyomatosis
Lymphoid interstitial pneumonia
Other lymphoproliferative disorders
Cryptogenic organizing pneumonia ('BOOP' in the USA)
Alveolar proteinosis
Alveolar microlithiasis
Amyloidosis
Behçet's syndrome
Tuberous sclerosis
Panbronchiolitis

For the GP, it is important to recognize the first symptoms, and to timely refer patients for further diagnosis and treatment. Table 5 shows which previous exposures (e.g. pigeon antigens, asbestos, certain drugs, etc.) can lead to ILDs and thus which patients may be at risk.

The most frequent presenting symptom is progressively increasing shortness of breath. Sometimes, chronic cough or fatigue are also present. In the more acute forms, patients may suffer from fever, joint inflammations, or erythema nodosum. On chest examination, the most frequent findings are bilateral basal inspiratory crepitations. Spirometric examination will show a restrictive or mixed restrictive–obstructive disorder.

In general, management of patients with ILD consists of four main steps: (a) Establishment of a certain diagnosis. This includes extensive history-taking to detect possible causative exposures, chest X-ray examination, blood count, specific antibody detection, sputum examination (in particular, bronchio-alveolair lavage), CT-scan, lung biopsy. (b) Ascertainment of the progression rate, which is important to predict the possible effect of immunosuppressive therapy. (c) Ascertainment of seriousness, which indicates the urgency of starting treatment with potentially damaging immunosuppressive therapy. (d) Close follow-up with accurate documentation and co-ordination of different therapies, results, complications, etc. All this will mainly take place in secondary care and the primary task of the GP will be to support these patients through a serious, chronic pulmonary disease and difficult treatments.

References

1. Jerant, A.F., Bannon, M., and Rittenhouse, S. (2000). Identification and management of tuberculosis. *American Family Physician* **61**, 2667–78, 2681–2.

2. Targeted tuberculin testing and treatment of latent tuberculosis infection. Official statement of the American Thoracic Society and Centers for Disease Control and Prevention. *American Journal of Respiratory and Critical Care Medicine* 2000 **161**, S221–47.

Further reading

Diagnostic standards and classification of tuberculosis in adults and children. Official statement of the American Thoracic Society and the Centers for Disease Control and Prevention. *American Journal of Respiratory and Critical Care Medicine* 2000 **161**, 1376–95.

Remington, J.S. and Hollingworth, G.R. (1995). New tuberculosis epidemic. Controversies in screening and preventive therapy. *Canadian Family Physician* **41**, 1014–23.

WHO. Tuberculosis: strategy and operations (http://www.who.int/inf/gtb).

Hoeckelman, R., Friedman, S., and Nelson, N. *Primary Pediatric Care* 3rd edn. St. Louis: Mosby, 1997, pp. 416–22.

Bernstein. D. and Shelov, S. *Pediatrics*. Baltimore: Williams and Wilkins, 1996, pp. 540–3.

Behrman, R., Kliegman, R., and Jenson, H. *Nelson's Textbook of Pediatrics* 16th edn. Philadelphia: WB Saunders Company, 2000, pp. 1315–27.

Hodson, M. and Geddes, D. *Cystic Fibrosis* 2nd edn. London: Arnold, 2000.

Demedts, M., Dijkman, J.H., Hilvering, C., and Postma, D.S., ed. *Longziekten*. Leuven: Van Gorcum, Assen. Universitaire pers, 1999.

Brewis, R., Corrin, B., Geddes, D.M., and Gibson, G.J., ed. *Respiratory Medicine* 2nd edn. London: WB Saunders Company Ltd, 1995.

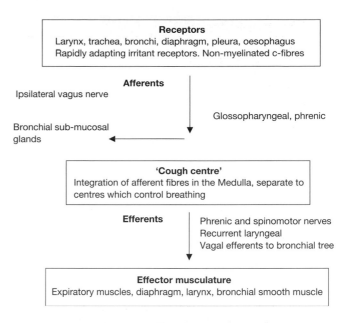

Fig. 1 Anatomy of the cough reflex.[1] (Reproduced with permission, Elsevier Science.)

2.6 Chronic cough

Patrick White and Helena Elkington

What is chronic cough?

Chronic cough affects more than half of those who smoke and may affect more than 10 per cent of non-smoking adults. The main cause of chronic cough is smoking and a significant respiratory impact of smoking is chronic obstructive pulmonary disease (COPD). COPD is considered separately in this chapter. In non-smokers, the main causes of chronic cough are likely to be post-nasal drip syndrome (PNDS), asthma, or gastro-oesophageal reflux disease (GORD). The diagnosis of each of these three conditions is often by therapeutic trial and in more than 90 per cent of cases an effective treatment can be found.

Cough is universal. It may be laden with ominous meaning in societies devastated by tuberculosis (TB). It may recall nights of terror for parents of children with croup or weeks of exhaustion from whooping cough. For others, persistent cough may have been the first sign of lung cancer.

In developed countries, chronic cough is no longer linked to TB but is a sign of lifelong smoking. Although the prevalence of smoking has fallen by more than half among men in Western countries since 1970, the worldwide prevalence of smoking has hardly changed and smoking among women continues to increase. The continued popularity of smoking means that COPD and lung cancer will remain among the commonest causes of death and disability for the next 30 years at least.

Cough is the most common symptom for which patients seek medical care. It is a defensive reflex designed to remove mucus and inhaled irritants from the lower respiratory tract involving forced expiration against a closed glottis, which achieves sudden and high flows of air with raised intra-thoracic pressures. It may be voluntary or involuntary.

The cough reflex

Cough is initiated by stimulation of irritant receptors in the respiratory tract, in the pharynx, larynx, trachea, and major bronchi. There are also cough receptors in the diaphragm, pleura, and oesophagus. Cough requires synchronization of the respiratory muscles and the larynx with central coordination. Stimuli causing cough include mechanical irritation by excessive mucus, dust or foreign material, and chemical irritation by toxic gases and fumes. Irritant impulses are carried to the cough centre by the vagus nerve, and the glossopharyngeal and phrenic nerves. The cough reflex is then orchestrated in the cough centre and executed by the respiratory

muscles, the diaphragm, the larynx, and bronchial smooth muscle. The anatomy of the cough reflex is shown in Fig. 1.[1]

Complications of cough

Coughing causes strain not only on the intrathoracic organs but also on the abdomen and chest wall and high pressures are transmitted to the head and neck. Cough commonly causes headache, petechial haemorrhages on the cheeks and soft palate, sub-conjunctival haemorrhage, tearing of respiratory muscles, and urinary incontinence and may even cause rib fractures. Figure 2 gives a list of the effects of cough that lead to patients presenting to their doctor. Irwin et al. have examined the perception of chronic cough and its impact on the quality of life.[2,3] Patients sought medical care because they needed reassurance that nothing was seriously wrong (77 per cent), because they were concerned something was wrong (72 per cent), because of specific symptoms (55 per cent), or because of interference with everyday life (53 per cent). Chronic cough was associated with insomnia (45 per cent), pain (45 per cent), and incontinence (39 per cent).

When is chronic cough chronic?

The prevalence of chronic cough is uncertain because the definition of chronic cough is arbitrary.[4] The definition is neither pathological nor epidemiological. The definition of chronic cough as a cough which continues for longer than 3 weeks provides a framework for investigation and management. In the setting of primary care, the management of chronic cough is likely to remain partly intuitive, at least initially. This means that the decision to investigate or to consider a trial of treatment for a putative cause will depend on the severity of the cough, the interference by the cough in the daily life of the patient, and the patient's general condition. It is unlikely that the decision to investigate or treat will simply be a matter of the duration of the symptom. Irwin, who has been at the forefront of cough research for the last 20 years, has suggested an intermediate stage of sub-acute cough from 3 to 8 weeks, and a definition of chronic cough as cough of more than 8 weeks duration.[5] This approach to defining chronic cough will make more sense to primary care clinicians, especially in health care systems where they operate as the gate keepers to secondary care.

Impacts on self-perception
Embarrassment
Self-consciousness
Fear of serious disease
Need for reassurance

Neurological
Headache
Epilepsy
Transient ischaemic attack
Stroke

Cardiovascular
Cough syncope
Arrhythmias
Rupture of subcutaneous and nasal vessels

Gastrointestinal
Gastro-oesophageal reflux
Inguinal hernia
Rectal prolapse

Genitourinary
Urinary incontinence
Genital prolapse

Musculoskeletal
Muscle tearing in chest and abdomen
Rib fractures

Respiratory
Pneumothorax
Subcutaneous emphysema
Laryngeal injury
Trachoobronchial injury
Acute asthma

Fig. 2 The effects of cough.

Chronic cough is rarely the sole indicator symptom of serious underlying disease with the exception of COPD and cancer. If cough is associated with weight loss, or with haemoptysis, or with recurrent fever, or with night sweats, then the need to investigate may be urgent. In these instances, it is not the symptom of chronic cough that is the primary motive for investigation. In the absence of other significant symptoms, the investigation of chronic cough is aimed firstly at the relief of symptoms and secondly at the identification of their cause.

Chronic obstructive pulmonary disease

COPD is mainly caused by smoking. It is usually the result of smoking at least one pack of 20 cigarettes for 20 years (20 pack years). In susceptible people, cigarette smoking leads to an inflammatory response which ultimately causes both irreversible narrowing of the small airways and destruction of the architecture of the lung. The pathological changes of COPD are irreversible, but in smokers the progressive decline in lung function can be halted by stopping smoking.

COPD may lead to repeated infective exacerbations before the patient is diagnosed. Diagnostic lung function testing can be instrumental in getting the patient to stop smoking. From diagnosis onwards careful integration of primary and secondary care services using the skills of doctors, nurses, physiotherapists, pharmacists, and lung function technicians is essential to optimizing the outcome for COPD patients. The efforts of primary care teams should be focused on: early identification of and intervention with smokers, active treatment of the reversible component of airways obstruction, pulmonary rehabilitation in established disease, long-term oxygen therapy (LTOT) for patients at risk of or with cor pulmonale, and the coordination of services for advanced disease as patients approach the end of

life. There is considerable argument both about the role of drugs in COPD and about how the impact of drugs should be assessed. These two controversies are discussed in this section and possible routes to their resolution are described.

Epidemiology

COPD affects 10–20 per cent of people who have smoked 20 cigarettes a day for 20 years. It results from the inflammatory response of the lung to cigarette smoke and other gases and particles and in rare cases (less than 0.1 per cent) results from an inherited enzyme deficiency—α_1 antitrypsin deficiency. The fact that less than a fifth of smokers are likely to get COPD suggests that there are genetic or environmental elements in its pathogenesis which are critical to its development.

The prevalence of COPD is difficult to assess accurately because it is dependent on performing lung function tests in large populations. Even in moderate COPD, patients may be relatively asymptomatic and may not present to health professionals. Nonetheless, the burden of COPD is huge. In the United Kingdom, COPD primary care consultation rates are 64 per 10 000 patient years at risk in 45–64-year-olds (a patient year at risk takes into account the proportion of a year that a patient remains registered with a GP).[6] In 75–84 year olds, the consultation rates in primary care for COPD rise to 184 per 10 000 patient years at risk. COPD causes about 3.4 admissions per 1000 population in the United Kingdom in 2000–2001.[7] This is equivalent to six to seven admissions per GP per year. The death rate from COPD in the United Kingdom in 2000 was about 0.6 per 1000 population. Twenty-three thousand five hundred people died from COPD in England and Wales in that year, a figure approaching the number of deaths from lung cancer.

Pathogenesis

Chronic airway inflammation is found in both asthma and COPD but there are key differences between them. Eosinophils, mast cells, T_2 helper lymphocytes, and macrophages predominate in asthma, whereas in COPD the inflammatory cells consist mainly of neutrophils, CD8 lymphocytes, and macrophages. Smoking generates an inflammatory response which is characterized by more structural damage, and more intense and permanent remodelling of the airways. Above all, the inflammatory response to smoking is largely resistant to steroids.

Asthma and COPD often exist together. As COPD progresses, the permanent structural changes of COPD outweigh the reversible elements of asthma and the initial responsiveness of the airway obstruction is gradually lost. In an acute exacerbation, steroids and bronchodilators may play a temporary role in managing a patient who is usually unresponsive to treatment.

Diagnosis

The diagnosis of COPD is made from a combination of spirometric findings—a forced expiratory volume in the first second (FEV_1) of less than 80 per cent with an FEV_1/FVC ratio of less than 70 per cent (FVC is the forced vital capacity). COPD has been defined by both the British Thoracic Society (BTS) and the Global Initiative for Obstructive Lung Disease (GOLD) which is based in the United States. Each give slightly different parameters. Both values are given here.

Classification of COPD	% predicted	
	BTS	**GOLD**
Mild COPD	FEV_1 60–79%	$FEV_1 \geq 80\%$
Moderate COPD	FEV_1 40–59%	$30\% \leq FEV_1 < 80\%$
Severe COPD	$FEV_1 < 40\%$	$FEV_1 < 30\%$

The diagnosis of COPD can only be made with confidence using spirometry. A history of smoking usually precedes the onset of symptoms. Asymptomatic patients may be picked up through screening of smokers or occupational surveillance programmes. Examination of patients with mild disease may be normal. With increasing severity of disease may come hyperinflation, expiratory wheeze, central cyanosis, and peripheral oedema.

The differential diagnosis of COPD should include asthma, congestive heart failure, bronchiectasis, tuberculosis, obliterative bronchiolitis, and diffuse panbronchiolitis. The latter two are primarily diseases of young non-smokers. Asthma, congestive heart failure, and bronchiectasis often occur alongside COPD.

Investigations in COPD

Chest X-ray is valuable in the differential diagnosis of COPD, in out-ruling complications such as pneumonia and pleurisy, and in picking up concomitant lung cancer.

Haemoglobin should be assessed in advanced disease to identify polycythaemia of chronic hypoxia.

Lung function testing in COPD is a matter of controversy in primary care. Spirometry is essential for the diagnosis but the role of spirometry in routine management is less clear. FEV_1 may fall to a greater extent than peak expiratory flow rate (PEFR) in severe COPD due to the destruction of lung tissue and the loss of support for the small airways. Collapse of the small airways occurs after peak expiratory flow has been reached (0.1 s) curtailing FEV_1 (expiration continuing up to 1 s) while PEFR remains less affected. The significance of this finding for management is doubtful. Therapeutic interventions in COPD cannot undo the damage done by smoking. The drugs are designed to improve airway calibre which can be measured by PEFR as well as it can by FEV_1. So PEFR may be as suitable for assessing the effect of drugs in COPD as FEV_1. Interest has been expressed in the role of relaxed vital capacity (RVC) in COPD treatment but as yet there has been little research to support its use. At the time of writing, spirometry has been generally advocated in the continuing management of COPD. For primary care teams, PEFR is a measurement in daily use whereas spirometry is not widely used. Until more conclusive research has been published, the precise role of spirometry in primary care should be held in question. Reliable and repeatable use of spirometers requires staff training, maintenance of expertise by regular operation, and regular calibration of the equipment. All of these may be beyond the resources of average primary care teams.

Blood gas estimation (paO_2 and $paCO_2$) may be useful in acute exacerbations of COPD in patients attending A&E to assess the degree of hypoxia and hypercapnia especially in patients who are drowsy or exhausted. Blood gases are also indicated for patients with severe COPD in assessing the need for long-term oxygen therapy. This decision should be made by a respiratory physician. Respiratory failure is indicated by a paO_2 less than 8 kPa with or without hypercapnia while breathing air at sea level.

Treatment

There are three interventions that alter the natural history and life expectancy in COPD: smoking cessation, long-term oxygen therapy in advanced COPD, and appropriate treatment of acute exacerbations. All other treatments are used for symptom relief and improvement of quality of life. COPD causes severe morbidity through impaired lung function, social isolation, and loss of the capacity to undertake the activities of daily living. As a result, in the latter stages of the disease the symptoms of cough, breathlessness, and fatigue are complicated by loneliness and psychological morbidity such as depression and anxiety.

In patients with COPD who continue to smoke the disease is likely to progress. A key challenge at each point of trying a new drug in COPD is to assess the effectiveness of the drugs prescribed against some agreed criterion of outcome. Without setting a standard against which the drug effect is measured, drugs will be prescribed with little evidence of their effectiveness. Potential costs are enormous. Once a patient starts a drug in COPD it may be difficult to withdraw it, especially if it is inhaled. Inhaled drugs cause few side-effects and the impact of physically administering a compound into the pulmonary system which is itself so impaired may be psychologically rewarding. Against this reservation it must be remembered that patients with COPD often have a reversible element to their disease (an asthmatic component) which should be treated as fully as possible.

The British Thoracic Society Guidelines for the management of COPD (1997) described a COPD treatment 'escalator' which summarizes the stages of COPD in symptoms and offers a range of treatments to be considered at each stage (Fig. 3).

The Global Initiative for Obstructive Lung Disease (GOLD) published 4 years later in 2001, uses a table of stages based on (FEV_1) with a recommended treatment list for each stage. The treatment stages in both guidelines are almost identical. They begin with smoking cessation and move

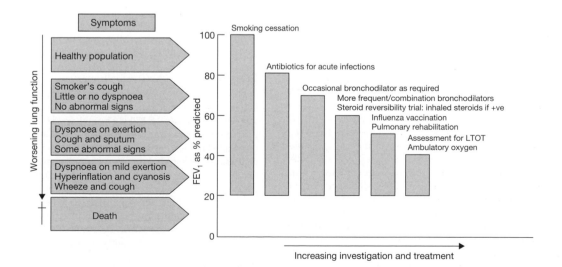

Fig. 3 The COPD escalator. Summary of the principal components of a management plan for COPD. Note that, as disease severity increases, symptoms and signs become more obvious whilst the number of treatments used rises. [Reproduced with permission from: British Thoracic Society (1997). Guidelines for the management of chronic obstructive pulmonary disease. *Thorax* **52** (Suppl. 5), S1–28, BMJ publications.]

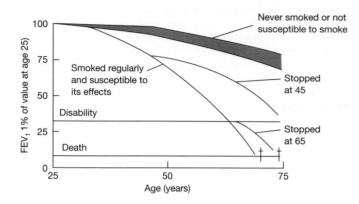

Fig. 4 Model of annual decline in FEV$_1$ with accelerated decline in susceptible smokers. On stopping smoking, subsequent deterioration is similar to that in healthy non-smokers. [Reproduced with permission from: British Thoracic Society (1997). Guidelines for the management of chronic obstructive pulmonary disease. *Thorax* **52** (Suppl. 5), S1–28, BMJ publications.]

through trials of asthma treatment, treatment of acute exacerbations, influenza vaccination, pulmonary rehabilitation, long-term oxygen therapy, and surgical removal of redundant emphysematous bullae.

Smoking cessation

Smoking cessation is the single most important intervention in COPD and arrests the decline in lung function[8] (Fig. 4).

Simple and brief advice from health care professionals can increase smoking cessation rates.[9] Members of the primary health care team should ask about smoking at every opportunity, advise and assist smokers to stop and arrange follow-up. Nicotine replacement therapy (NRT) doubles cessation rates in primary care from 5 to 10 per cent. All four NRT products (patch, gum, nasal spray, inhalator) have similar success rates, and there is no evidence to favour one product over another. Bupropion is another effective aid to smoking cessation. Evidence of its effectiveness is limited to smokers who are receiving motivational support in addition to medication.

Drugs in COPD

The asthma drugs which should be tried in COPD are described in the chapter on asthma and will not be described in detail here. Objective measures of improvement should be sought when these are prescribed. Although the severity of COPD is best assessed with FEV$_1$, PEFR may be as effective in assessing the lung function response to inhaled bronchodilators and steroids, as described above. Inhaled anticholinergics (ipratropium, oxytropium, and tiotropium) have theoretical advantages in COPD because of their potential to reduce bronchial secretions. Evidence of their effectiveness is limited, but they should be tried using the criterion of improved FEV$_1$ or PEFR to justify their sustained use. Other measures to assess the impact of asthma drugs in COPD include exercise testing such as the shuttle walk test but these are impractical in primary care. The role of *N*-acetyl-cysteine in COPD is uncertain. *N*-acetyl-cysteine is an antioxidant which has been shown to reduce the frequency of exacerbations in COPD. Its place in the general treatment of COPD requires more definitive research although it may be useful in patients who suffer frequent acute exacerbations. Nebulizers are often prescribed in advanced COPD without proof of effectiveness. They can deliver drugs more easily to patients who are breathless at rest but they can take between 15 and 30 min to use each time and drugs for nebulization are expensive.

Specialist referral

Specialist referral may be needed to confirm the diagnosis of COPD and to exclude other pathology, to assess patients with severe disease for home oxygen, nebulizers or oral corticosteroids, and to manage complications such as cor pulmonale.

Acute exacerbations

Antibiotics are the mainstay of the treatment of acute exacerbations of COPD. Broad spectrum antibiotics (e.g. amoxycillin, oxytetracycline, or erythromycin) should be prescribed if two of the following three criteria are present:

- increasing volume of sputum;
- productive cough with purulent sputum;
- increasing breathlessness.

Can exacerbations of COPD be managed at home? In selected patients, hospital at home care appears to be a practical alternative to hospital admission. In one study, patients were assessed in the emergency room and if randomized to hospital at home care, went home with a specialist nurse, and received nebulized ipratropium bromide and salbutamol, oral prednisolone, and antibiotics.[10] Nurses visited the patients morning and evening for 3 days and thereafter at their discretion. The primary care physician was notified and social support was immediately available if required. Patients were followed up for 3 months and no differences were found between the two groups in mortality, admission rates, or health status.

Oxygen

Long-term oxygen therapy (LTOT) in severe COPD improves survival.[11] It is indicated for patients with paO$_2$ less than 7.3 kPa when breathing air during a period of clinical stability. It can also be prescribed to patients with clinically stable paO$_2$ between 7.3 and 8 kPa when one of the following is present: secondary polycythaemia, nocturnal hypoxaemia, peripheral oedema, or evidence of pulmonary hypertension. Arterial blood gases should be measured on two occasions not less than 3 weeks apart to ensure clinical stability. Blood gas tensions should also be checked with supplemental oxygen to ensure that the set flow is achieving a paO$_2$ greater than 8 kPa without an unacceptable rise in paCO$_2$. Ideally LTOT is delivered via an oxygen concentrator which should be regularly checked three monthly.

Pulmonary rehabilitation

Pulmonary rehabilitation defined by the American Thoracic Society as a 'multi-disciplinary program of care for patients with chronic respiratory impairment that is individually tailored' includes exercise training and may also have a role in education and psychological support.[12] Pulmonary rehabilitation improves patients' exercise capacity, functional ability, and quality of life even though lung function does not change.[13] It is widely endorsed for patients with moderate and severe disease.

Vaccination

Annual vaccination against influenza should be offered to all patients with COPD. Pneumococcal vaccination may also be provided but evidence of its effectiveness in COPD is lacking.

Depression

van Ede et al. performed a systematic review to address the question 'Do patients with COPD show a higher than normal prevalence of depression?'.[14] Ten studies fulfilled the authors' review criteria and reported prevalence rates of depression ranging from 6 to 42 per cent. The instruments used to measure depression varied, as did the cut-off score to detect depression. Four studies were case controlled, two of which showed a statistically increased rate of depression among COPD patients compared to controls. Of the remaining six studies three showed a higher than normal prevalence of depression among COPD patients but these studies were methodically less robust and the results therefore less reliable. Isolation and depression are major problems in advanced COPD and formal treatment of depression with antidepressants may be required.

Multidisciplinary issues

Patients with COPD often have diverse needs, and various health care professionals and agencies may be involved in service provision. The patient may be in contact with services in primary care—the GP, the practice nurse, the district/community nurse, the pharmacist—and in secondary care—the respiratory specialist. Respiratory nurse specialists may liaise with primary and secondary care. Other health professionals involved may include physiotherapists (e.g. as part of a pulmonary rehabilitation programme), occupational therapists, psychologists and palliative care specialists (to advise on symptom control and end of life care). Benefits advisers may be able to assist patients and their families in applying for statutory allowances.

COPD at the end of life

COPD causes considerable morbidity and mortality. For patients with severe disease, management focuses on symptom control and optimizing quality of life, palliation as opposed to cure. Patients are often severely disabled by breathlessness, and may be dependent on LTOT, suffering with co-morbid illness and with very limited mobility. Meeting the needs of these patients presents a challenge to primary care. Palliative care, increasingly recognized to have a role in non-cancer disease, may be able to assist in end of life care in COPD. Respiratory nurse specialists who can liaise with primary and secondary care may provide a vital link to patients who are often housebound and isolated, and for whom physicians have no further active interventions to offer.

Chronic cough in non-smokers

The 1998 Consensus Panel Report of the American College of Chest Physicians—'Managing cough as a defense mechanism and as a symptom'—provided guidance for the management of chronic cough in non-smokers

Nasal/pharyngeal/laryngeal causes
Chronic rhinitis
Allergic rhinitis
Sinusitis
Polyposis
Smoking
Common cold
Mediastinal mass
Chronic laryngitis
Post-nasal drip syndrome

Tracheobronchial causes
Asthma
Chronic obstructive pulmonary disease
Smoking
Bronchiectasis
Chronic lung infection (TB, HIV, Pertussis)

Oesophageal causes
Gastro-oesophageal reflux disease (GORD)
Tracheo-oesophageal fistula

Parenchymal causes
Cryptogenic fibrosing alveolitis
Secondary alveolitis/interstitial lung disease
Chronic haemosiderosis
Pulmonary embolism

Pleural causes
Pleural effusion
Pleurisy
Mesothelioma

Muscular causes
Sub-phrenic infection

Other causes
Left ventricular failure
Angiotensin converting enzyme inhibitors
Beta-blockers

Fig. 5 The causes of chronic cough.

which has been unequalled in its detail and analysis.[4] However, the advice in this report to undertake the investigation of cough after 3 weeks is unlikely to receive approval from primary care physicians for the reasons mentioned above. The concept of sub-acute cough proposed by Irwin was designed to highlight cough which follows a respiratory infection.[5] The cause of this is likely to be post-infectious cough, bacterial sinusitis, or asthma. Of course chronic cough is included in this definition but the clinician may feel justified in dealing mainly with the possibilities of sinusitis and asthma at this stage. The causes of chronic cough can be considered before 8 weeks and the urgency of investigation may be set by other symptoms or findings.

A list of the possible causes of chronic cough in non-smokers is presented in Fig. 5. In the absence of symptoms and signs pointing to a specific cause unexplained chronic cough is likely to be the result of one of the following:

- angiotensin converting enzyme inhibitors (ACEIs);
- post-infectious cough;
- post-nasal drip syndrome;
- asthma;
- gastro-oesophageal reflux disease (GORD).*

Angiotensin converting enzyme inhibitors

Cough resulting from the use of ACEIs can present for the first time more than 2 months after commencing the drug, although it is usually experienced in the first 2 or 3 weeks.[15] The effect is not dose related, appears to be a class effect, and is equally likely to occur with all drugs in the class. Cough is not a side-effect of angiotensin II receptor antagonists. The treatment of ACEI-induced cough is withdrawal of the drug. The cough usually subsides within 4 weeks. Where the use of ACEI is considered essential, the cough may be relieved by inhaled sodium cromoglycate, nifedipine, or non-steroidal anti-inflammatory drugs (NSAIDS) such as indomethacin. Cough is a rare side-effect of other drugs among which beta-blockers are the next most common group.

Post-infectious cough

Cough which follows a respiratory infection, in which the chest X-ray is normal, and which does not respond to treatment, is often referred to as post-infectious cough. The classic post-infectious cough is the whooping cough of *Bordetella pertussis* which can continue for 3 months. With high rates of pertussis immunization in many countries, whooping cough is less common. Whooping cough is rarely seen in countries where rates of immunization of children under 1 year exceed 80 per cent. Chronic cough may follow repeated respiratory infections. Specific infection with *Mycoplasma pneumoniae*, *Chlamydia pneumoniae*, or the respiratory viruses, *parainfluenza* and *respiratory syncytial virus* have all been associated with chronic cough. The mechanism is likely to be persistent tracheal or bronchial inflammation. It invariably resolves spontaneously.

Post-nasal drip syndrome

PNDS is a less precise diagnosis than it sounds. The diagnosis is made by any combination of symptoms including post-nasal drip, a need to clear the throat, a tickle in the throat, nasal congestion, nasal discharge, and hoarseness and signs including mucus drainage in the posterior pharynx, nasal discharge, cobblestone pharyngeal mucosa, and swollen inferior turbinates. The diagnosis is confirmed by the response to treatment with first generation antihistamine (e.g. chlorpheniramine), oral decongestants (pseudoephedrine), and/or local sprays of ipratropium bromide or inhaled steroids such as beclomethasone, budesonide, and fluticasone.

The quality of evidence in support of the treatment of PNDS is not high and does not include randomized controlled trials. However, these are safe

* Gastro-oesophageal reflux disease (GORD) is known as GERD or gastro-esophageal reflux disease in North America.

medications and in patients with prolonged symptoms a trial of treatment is indicated. The differential diagnosis of PNDS should include seasonal allergic rhinitis (e.g. hay fever), non-allergic non-perennial rhinitis, vasomotor rhinitis, and rhinitis medicamentosa.

Asthma

Cough is a prominent symptom of asthma with more than 40 per cent of patients with symptomatic asthma reporting cough at least once a week.[16] Undiagnosed and unrecognized asthma is a common cause of chronic cough. The diagnosis is important because of the implications for treatment. In primary care, a 2-week diary of peak expiratory flow (PEF) readings should reveal the diagnosis if PEF is normal during a surgery consultation or there is no response to inhaled salbutamol when PEF is low. If a methacholine challenge is available in the local lung function laboratory, a normal methacholine test outrules the diagnosis of asthma. Clinical response to a trial of high dose oral steroids does not necessarily confirm the diagnosis of asthma, unless lung function objectively improves by at least 15 per cent, because oral steroids are also effective in treating eosinophilic bronchitis.

Eosinophilic bronchitis is characterized by cough with sputum eosinophilia but without evidence of airway obstruction.[17] The condition is defined by the finding of at least 3 per cent eosinophils in the sputum cell count. There should be no evidence of airway hyper-responsiveness after methacholine challenge. Treatment is with inhaled or oral steroids.

Gastro-oesophageal reflux disease

GORD is an interesting cause of cough because it is asymptomatic from a gastrointestinal point of view in up to 75 per cent of cases of chronic cough in which it is the cause.[18] The diagnosis is complex and outside specialist centres is best made by therapeutic trial. If the initial therapeutic trial fails, stronger and longer courses of treatment are recommended before the diagnosis is outruled.

GORD is due to the reflux of stomach contents into the oesophagus. It commonly results in heartburn and epigastric or retrosternal pain or discomfort. It is probably due to ineffective lower-oesophageal sphincter tone, or transient lower-oesophageal sphincter relaxation. GORD is not always associated with evidence of oesophageal inflammation. The cough reflex may be mediated solely by cough receptors in the oesophagus with no evidence of overspill of gastric contents into the larynx, but GORD may cause chronic cough due to gross aspiration of stomach contents, microaspiration of stomach contents, and complex vagally mediated oesophageal and tracheobronchial reflex mechanisms.

GORD has been identified as the cause in more than 20 per cent of adults with chronic cough and up to 15 per cent of children. The diagnosis of GORD as the cause of chronic cough can only be made with certainty when the cough disappears with specific anti-GORD therapy. Twenty-four-hour ambulatory oesophageal pH testing is the most sensitive and specific test of GORD. The temporal relationship of oesophageal pH to cough can be assessed further confirming the diagnosis.

Conservative measures should be tried first—weight reduction, high-protein and low-fat diet, elevation of the head of the bed, avoidance of coffee, and smoking. H_2 antagonists are likely to be successful. Recent studies of the effect of proton pump inhibitors on chronic cough due to GORD have shown them to be more rapidly effective than H_2 antagonists.[19] Twenty-four-hour ambulatory oesophageal pH testing can be performed to confirm the appropriateness of treatment. Prokinetic agents such as domperidone and cisapride, which promote gastric emptying and the onward passage of the stomach contents have been effective in cohort studies, but cisapride is associated with unacceptable cardiac side-effects. Overall, the treatment may not lead to the abolition of cough until it has been taken for at least 2 months.

Multiple causes

Chronic cough is due to more than one cause in between 20 and 90 per cent of cases. A partial response to treatment should not lead to that treatment being abandoned. It may be necessary to use two or three treatments together to completely relieve the cough.

The assessment and treatment of chronic cough in primary care

A step-wise approach to the management of chronic cough in non-smokers (excluding COPD) is presented in Fig. 6.

Non-smokers who are not using ACEIs, who develop cough lasting more than 3 weeks, are likely to have had a recent respiratory infection. In people with cough for more than 8 weeks, the diagnosis is likely to be PNDS, asthma, or GORD. PNDS symptoms and signs should be treated with a first generation antihistamine and decongestant. At the same time, PEFR should be measured followed by a trial of salbutamol if the PEFR is low. A chest X-ray should be considered and if the diagnosis of PNDS seems unlikely a 2-week diary of PEFR should be commenced. Only when PNDS and asthma have been sought and outruled should a trial of GORD treatment be started.

By the time acid suppressing drugs have been started, the diagnosis of PNDS should be very unlikely, and that of asthma should have been ruled out or else its treatment started. H_2 antagonists or proton pump inhibitors should be prescribed at full dosage for at least one month and a cough diary kept at the same time. At this point referral for a specialist opinion should be considered. This can be best provided by a chest physician or a gastroenterologist, but a telephone consultation with the specialist will identify the most useful source of advice.

Symptomatic treatment of chronic cough should not prevent the systematic search for a cause which can nearly always be found. If symptoms are temporarily relieved, it will be more difficult to seek the actual cause with the same determination.

The treatment of cough in palliative care

Cough can be a prominent problem in terminal lung cancer and to a lesser extent in cancers of the nose and throat. All opiates have antitussive effects

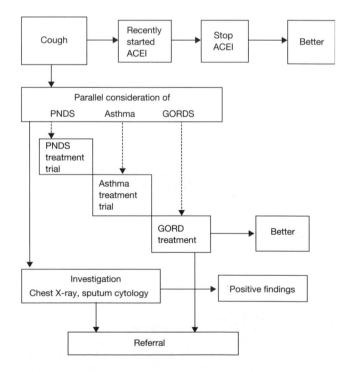

Fig. 6 Algorithm for the management of chronic cough in primary care.

and this is why codeine linctus and its derivative pholcodine linctus are used as antitussives in acute cough. In terminal care, it is important to control symptoms quickly and effectively and so morphine should be the drug of choice for the suppression of cough. Methadone has been used in the past but should be avoided because of the risk of accumulation.

References

1. Ing, A.J. (1997). Cough and gastroesophageal reflux. *American Journal of Medicine* **103**, 91S–6S.
2. French, C.L., Irwin, R.S., Curley, F.J., and Krikorian, C.J. (1998). Impact of chronic cough on quality of life. *Archives of Internal Medicine* **158**, 1657–61.
3. Irwin, R.S. and Curley, F.J. (1991). The treatment of cough: a comprehensive review. *Chest* **99**, 1477–84.
4. A Consensus Panel Report of the American College of Chest Physicians (1998). Managing cough as a defense mechanism and as a symptom. *Chest* **114**, 133S–81S.
5. Irwin, R.S. and Madison, J.M. (2000). The diagnosis and treatment of cough. *New England Journal of Medicine* **343**, 1715–21.
6. Morbidity Statistics from General Practice, 4th National Study, 1991–1992, Series MB5 No. 3, London: ONS © Crown Copyright 1995.
7. **Department of Health Hospital In-patient data** 2000/2001, www.doh.gov.uk/hes/.
8. Raw, M., McNeill, A., and West, R. (1998). Smoking cessation guidelines for health professionals. A guide to effective smoking cessation interventions for the health care system. *Thorax* **53** (Suppl. 5, Pt 1), S1–S19.
9. West, R., McNeill, A., and Raw, M. (2000). Smoking cessation guidelines for health professionals: an update. *Thorax* **55**, 987–99.
10. Davies, L., Wilkinson, M., Bonner, S., Calverley, P.M.A., and Angus, R.M. (2000). 'Hospital at home' versus hospital care in patients with exacerbations of chronic obstructive pulmonary disease: prospective randomised controlled trial. *British Medical Journal* **321**, 1265–8.
11. **Working Party on Domiciliary Oxygen Services.** *Domiciliary Oxygen Therapy Services. Clinical Guidelines and Advice for Prescribers.* A report of the Royal College of Physicians. London: RCP, 1999.
12. **American Thoracic Society** (1999). Pulmonary rehabilitation—1999. *American Journal of Respiratory and Critical Care Medicine* **159**, 1666–82.
13. Goldstein, R.S., Gort, E.H., Avendano, M.A., and Guyatt, G.H. (1994). Randomised controlled trial of respiratory rehabilitation. *Lancet* **344**, 1394–7.
14. van Ede, L., Yzermans, C.J., and Brouwer, H.J. (1999). Prevalence of depression in patients with chronic obstructive pulmonary disease: a systematic review. *Thorax* **54**, 688–92.
15. Sebastian, J.L., McKinney, W.P., Kaufmann, J., and Young, M.J. (1991). Angiotensin converting enzyme inhibitors and cough prevalence in an outpatient medical clinic population. *Chest* **99**, 36–9.
16. White, P.T., Atherton, H.A., Hewett, G., and Howells, K. (1995). Using information from asthma—a trial of information feedback in primary care. *British Medical Journal* **311**, 1065–9.
17. Brightling, C.E., Ward, R., Goh, K.L., Wardlaw, A.J., and Pavord, I.D. (1999). Eosinophilic bronchitis is an important cause of chronic cough. *American Journal of Respiratory and Critical Care Medicine* **160**, 406–10.
18. Irwin, R.S., French, C.L., Curley, F.J., Zawacki, J.K., and Bennet, F.M. (1993). Chronic cough due to gastroesophageal reflux. Clinical diagnostic and pathogenetic aspects. *Chest* **104**, 1511–17.
19. Ours, T.M., Kavuru, M.S., Schilz, R.J., and Richter, J.E. (1999). A prospective evaluation of esophageal testing and a double-blind, randomized study of omeprazole in a diagnostic and therapeutic algorithm for chronic cough. *The American Journal of Gastroenterology* **94**, 3131–8.

Further reading

A Consensus Panel Report of the American College of Chest Physicians (1998). Managing cough as a defense mechanism and as a symptom. *Chest* **114**, 133S–81S. (This is a detailed treatise on chronic cough from a secondary care perspective with an exhaustive list of references.)

British Thoracic Society (1997). Guidelines for the management of chronic obstructive pulmonary disease. *Thorax* **52** (Suppl. 5), S1–S28.

Pauwels, R.A., Buist, A.S., Calverley, P.M.A., Jenkins, C.R., and Hurd, S.S. (2001). Global strategy for the diagnosis, management, and prevention of chronic obstructive pulmonary disease. NHLBI/ WHO Global Initiative for Chronic Obstructive Lung Disease (GOLD) Workshop Summary. *American Journal of Respiratory and Critical Care Medicine* **163**, 1256–76.

These last two are authoritative guidelines on the management of COPD with a comprehensive list of references on all aspects of COPD.

2.7 Haemoptysis

Knut Schroeder and Tom Fahey

Definition

The term haemoptysis describes the coughing up of blood or blood-stained sputum from the respiratory tract below the larynx. Bleeding from other sites such as the oropharyngeal cavity or the gastrointestinal tract can sometimes resemble haemoptysis and is referred to as pseudohaemoptysis. Haemoptysis is often classified by its severity into mild (less than 15–20 ml in 24 h), moderate (less than 600 ml in 24 h), or massive blood loss (more than 600 ml in 24 h), although accurate clinical estimation of the amount of blood loss is often impossible.[1]

Importance

Haemoptysis poses an important diagnostic and management problem in primary care. The main challenge for the primary care practitioner is to evaluate the likelihood of a serious and potentially treatable underlying cause and to make the decision whether and when to refer to hospital for further investigation and treatment.

Consultation rates

Consultation rates for haemoptysis in primary care are likely to vary in different parts of the world, but reliable data are not available. Patients usually regard coughing up blood as a potentially serious symptom and will often seek medical advice quickly. They may present with an acute episode of blood-stained sputum due to respiratory tract infection that may not have any special significance. But if chronic and recurrent—or even massive—it can be a marker of severe and possibly unsuspected underlying disease such as bronchial carcinoma. Detecting and managing the underlying condition is important for determining long-term prognosis and survival. Because of the need for investigation, most patients will need to be referred to hospital, although admission will not always be necessary.[2]

Causes

The main causes for haemoptysis arise from the respiratory tract, but also include cardiovascular and systemic conditions. Often no obvious cause may be found for an episode of haemoptysis (Tables 1 and 2).

Table 1 Possible causes of haemoptysis

System	Cause for haemoptysis
Respiratory	Bronchial carcinoma
	Bronchial adenoma
	Metastatic disease (rare)
	Bronchitis
	Bronchiectasis
	Lung abscess
	Tuberculosis
	Necrotizing pneumonia
	Ruptured bronchus (traumatic, iatrogenic)
	Iatrogenic after bronchoscopy, Swan–Ganz-catheterization or lung biopsy
Cardiovascular	Pulmonary embolism
	Left ventricular failure
	Mitral stenosis
	Atrioventricular fistula
	Pulmonary hypertension
Haematologic	Coagulopathy
	Disseminated intravascular coagulation
	Platelet dysfunction
	Thrombocytopaenia
Systemic disease	Goodpasture's syndrome
	Systemic lupus erythematosus
	Wegener's granulomatosis
	Osler–Weber–Rendu disease (hereditary haemorrhagic telangiectasia)

Table 2 Approximate frequencies for selected causes of haemoptysis

Severity	Underlying condition	Approximate frequency (%)[a]
Mild	Bronchitis	40
	Bronchogenic carcinoma	40
	Other	20
Moderate	Bronchiectasis	30
	Bronchogenic carcinoma	15
	Bronchitis/pneumonia	15
	Tuberculosis	15
	Other	25
Massive	Chronic cavitary tuberculosis	50
	Bronchogenic carcinoma	10
	Other	40
Patients with HIV infection	Bacterial pneumonia	60
	Kaposi sarcoma	15
	Pulmonary embolus	10
	Bronchogenic carcinoma	10
	Other	5

[a] Frequencies are approximate and may vary substantially depending on the clinical setting and the population.[3,4]

Diagnosis and differential diagnosis

Making a diagnosis

A carefully taken history and thorough examination should allow the primary care physician to rank the likely causes for the haemoptysis, depending on the clinical setting.[3,5] Reaching a helpful working diagnosis to direct further management will also depend on other factors such as personal experience, knowledge of clinical presentations and acquaintance with the precision and accuracy of test results.[6–8]

Taking the history

Background

Age is an important factor in the diagnosis of haemoptysis. In children and previously healthy young adults, the cause of haemoptysis may be unusual (e.g. inhalation of foreign body, arteriovenous malformation, bronchial adenoma). Patients over 40 years of age are at higher risk of malignancy, which should be excluded if haemoptysis is present for longer than a week. The likelihood of a diagnosis such as tuberculosis depends on its prevalence in a population, and it is therefore important to know from which area of the world a patient originates, or if they have recently returned from an area where the prevalence of HIV or tuberculosis infection is high.

Source and severity of bleeding

It is important to find out if the patient's haemoptysis is truly the coughing up of blood from the lower respiratory tract, differentiating between haemoptysis and pseudohaemoptysis. Haematemesis and haemoptysis are sometimes difficult to distinguish, and dyspepsia, heartburn, abdominal pain, and other gastrointestinal symptoms point towards a bleeding source in the gastrointestinal tract. Because blood can be swallowed and then regurgitated, coffee grounds vomit along with haemoptysis does not guarantee that the bleeding is gastrointestinal in origin.

Association with respiratory symptoms

As haemoptysis is most commonly due to underlying lung disease, it is important to ask about other respiratory symptoms such as cough, shortness of breath, wheeze, chest pain, and sputum production. Acute onset of coughing up small amounts of blood together with symptoms and signs of upper respiratory infection make infection a likely cause. The absence of respiratory symptoms does not exclude bleeding from the lower respiratory tract. Pleuritic chest pain increases the likelihood of pulmonary infarction. The presence and characteristics of acute or chronic sputum production and whether it is tinged with blood or purulent may also give important clues (Table 3).

Other symptoms

A history of frequent nose bleeds with symptoms worse in the supine position indicate bleeding from the nasopharynx. A painful throat, tongue, or mouth or the recent onset of hoarseness or dysphonia suggest that the haemoptysis arises from the oropharynx or larynx. General symptoms such as weight loss, fever, night sweats, lymphadenopathy, or bleeding into other sites such as skin or bowels are suggestive of systemic disease including bronchogenic carcinoma or chronic infection. Rarely, associated haematuria may be due to Wegener's granulomatosis or Goodpasture syndrome.

Medical history

Chest problems from childhood associated with recurrent cough and sputum suggest a diagnosis of bronchiectasis, which can result in bleeding at any age. Any history of lung diseases such as tuberculosis, chronic bronchitis, recurrent pneumonia, or cancer can play a role in the development of haemoptysis. A number of heart conditions can cause recurrent haemoptysis such as mitral stenosis or left ventricular failure. A past history of venous thrombosis or pulmonary embolism is important. Risk factors such as a recent injury or operation, any form of immobilization, childbirth, or taking the contraceptive pill are therefore of clinical significance. Finally, medication usage should be documented, particularly the use of anticoagulant drugs.

Family history

It is worth enquiring about a diagnosis or symptoms of tuberculosis in the close family or a close associate. A familial bleeding tendency such as haemorrhagic telangiectasia or a defect of coagulation may also lead to haemoptysis.

Occupational and social history

Past or current history of cigarette smoking should be documented. Occupational exposures must be considered as risk factors for lung diseases

Table 3 Indicators for selected causes of haemoptysis

Potential causes	Clues			
	History	Symptoms and signs	Sputum	Chest X-ray

Bronchogenic carcinoma	Age >40 years
	Smoking history
	Asbestos exposure
		Constitutional
		  symptoms and signs
		Lymphadenopathy
		Clubbing
			Frankly bloody,
			  blood streaking
				Peripheral or
				  central mass
				Fibrocavitary
				  lesion
				Lobar atelectasis

Tuberculosis	Exposure to silica	Constitutional
		  symptoms and signs
			Frankly bloody,
			  blood streaking
				Apical lesions
				Fibrocavitary
				  disease

Bronchiectasis	Recurrent chest
	  problems
		Clubbing	Bloody,
			  mucopurulent
				Thickened
				  bronchi

Pulmonary oedema	Heart disease	Symptoms and signs
		  of left ventricular
		  failure
			Pink, frothy	Oedema

that can lead to haemoptysis. For example, asbestos is a risk factor for bronchial carcinoma, whereas silica exposure may predispose to the development of tuberculosis.

Physical examination

Immediate assessment

The initial examination should record the vital signs of pulse, respiratory rate, blood pressure, and temperature to provide an objective measure of general physical health. These records may provide valuable baseline measurements when subsequently monitoring the patient. Patients presenting with massive haemoptysis are a medical emergency. In such cases it is necessary to follow the basic ABC (assessment of *Airways*, *Breathing*, *Circulation*) of resuscitation.

General physical examination

General wasting may suggest a serious disease such as disseminated malignancy. A malar flush may be present with mitral stenosis. Oedema and swelling of the neck may be due to mediastinal obstruction caused by carcinoma of the bronchus. Inspection of the skin may reveal purpura as a result of a generalized bleeding disorder. Clubbing of the fingers is not specific but may be a warning sign in chronic suppurative lung disease or bronchial carcinoma and can sometimes be seen in advanced pulmonary tuberculosis. Scurvy is an important possible diagnosis to consider, especially in an elderly person with a poor diet.

Respiratory system

Although the most important signs are likely to be found in the chest, it is prudent to start with the examination of the nose, mouth and gums. Localized tenderness of the chest wall may suggest a rib fracture, particularly if the pain is made worse on external pressure. The typical signs of bronchitis, pneumonia, or bronchiectasis may be present. Diffuse fine crepitations may be suggestive of interstitial lung disease. A collapsed lobe or whole lung in a child suggests an inhaled foreign body, whereas in adults this sign is more often due to carcinoma or adenoma. In cases of bronchial obstruction, delayed unilateral expiration on the affected side may be present with or without a localized wheeze over the area. A pleural rub can be a feature of pneumonia but is also common in pulmonary infarction.

Sputum

Blood coughed up from the respiratory tract is usually bright red and frothy, but its consistency and appearance can vary. Thick, purulent sputum mixed with blood indicates an underlying infection, whereas spitting up blood without any pus may be due to cancer, tuberculosis, or pulmonary infarction. If blood is foul-smelling, it might originate from a pulmonary abscess. Pink and frothy sputum is commonly due to pulmonary oedema. An alkaline pH of the sputum is highly suggestive of a pulmonary cause for the bleeding, whereas an acidic pH indicates haematemesis.

Cardiovascular system

A sinus tachycardia may simply be due to anxiety but is often an important early sign of pulmonary embolus. The pulse may be irregular and small in atrial fibrillation due to mitral stenosis. Main cardiac features to look out for are the signs of mitral stenosis or other causes of left ventricular failure, although in tight mitral stenosis the murmur may be absent. The legs must be examined thoroughly for evidence of deep venous thrombosis.

Investigation

The history and physical examination usually provide enough information to form a differential diagnosis. Before arranging further tests, it should be possible to rank the likely causes and estimate the prior probability for the relevant diagnoses which will depend on the underlying prevalence in the population (Table 2). Basic parameters such as sex, age, and the main symptoms alter these probabilities, which are further modified by the findings from the history, examination and simple tests readily available in primary care.[9] The patient's views about treatment, the availability of treatment and the implications of an underlying condition all have be taken into account when deciding about further investigations. Many of the tests are not available in primary care, and early specialist referral is indicated. All investigations have false positive and negative rates that should be taken into account when forming a differential diagnosis and considering specialist referral.

Diagnostic imaging

Chest radiography

A plain chest radiograph (postero-anterior and lateral) is the single most useful investigation, although its diagnostic utility for many common causes of haemoptysis is not known.[4] It is often readily available, relatively inexpensive, and should be the first test to evaluate the lungs and heart.[10] It can often reveal unsuspected respiratory or cardiac diseases as an explanation for haemoptysis. Conditions such as pneumonia, lung abscess, carcinoma, or tuberculosis may sometimes be obvious. Fractured ribs may also be seen, although sometimes only with considerable difficulty. Any pleural effusion needs to be aspirated and the pleura biopsied to search for malignancy or tuberculosis involving the pleura. A localized reduced vascularity in a portion of the lung (oligaemia) can be a sign of pulmonary infarction. If pulmonary embolus is suspected, a radioisotope ventilation/perfusion scan should be arranged together with non-invasive investigation for deep venous thrombosis. The characteristic feature of a mycetoma is the appearance of a solid ball within a cavity surrounded by an air shadow in the shape of a crescent. However, in up to 30 per cent of cases, the chest X-ray may be normal. Because chest radiography can produce false negative results, a common strategy is to repeat the chest X-ray after 4–5 weeks if an intrathoracic cause is suspected. The cardiac outline may indicate mitral stenosis, or there may be general enlargement of the heart due to left ventricular failure from any cause. If heart disease is suspected then echocardiography is a suitable next step.

Computerized tomography (CT) or magnetic resonance imaging (MRI)

CT is not readily available in many settings and is much more expensive than plain radiography. If the diagnosis is uncertain, it does have the advantage of being able to detect small lung cancers within the tracheobronchial tree and the lung parenchyma and can be useful for indentifying bronchiectasis and interstitial lung disease.

Fibreoptic bronchoscopy

The direct visualization of the tracheobronchial tree via fibreoptic bronchoscopy is a useful procedure if lung cancer is suspected. It has the advantage that small cancers may be diagnosed and biopsied. Bronchial secretions can be aspirated for microbiological investigation and cytology. Foreign bodies can be detected and removed.

Other investigations

Sputum

Any sputum should be examined and cultured for tubercle as a routine in all cases of haemoptysis where tuberculosis is suspected from the chest X-ray. Except for the diagnosis of Klebsiella pneumonia, routine microscopy and culture of sputum is otherwise rarely of value for investigation of haemoptysis. Sputum cytology is of great value in the diagnosis of bronchial carcinoma and may allow a diagnosis to be made even in the absence of radiological abnormalities.

Electrocardiogram (ECG)

A sinus tachycardia or right heart strain on the ECG may occasionally suggest pulmonary hypertension or infarction. Rarely, atrial fibrillation may lead to clot formation and result in pulmonary infarction with haemoptysis.

Blood tests

Simple blood tests may aid in the investigation of haemoptysis. A full blood count is useful in that it may reveal anaemia due to chronic disease or malignancy. A raised white cell count may be due to infection, and coagulopathies are sometimes associated with thrombocytopaenia. Checking the electrolytes may reveal hyponatraemia which can be due to paraneoplastic syndromes as well as infections.

Upper gastrointestinal tract endoscopy

If there is doubt about whether blood is coughed up or vomited, upper gastrointestinal endoscopy may be considered to exclude bleeding lesions in the oesophagus, stomach, or duodenum.

Principles of management

Management of haemoptysis depends on the severity of the bleeding and whether the cause for haemoptysis is known. The main three aims of treatment are prevention of asphyxiation, to stop any acute bleeding and to treat the primary disease.[11]

Acute and life-threatening bleeding

Tachycardia and later arterial hypotension together with pale and cool skin may indicate life-threatening shock, and a large intravenous cannula should

be inserted and fluid replacement started. Oxygen should be given where available, and urgent hospitalization is mandatory for treatment, investigation, and monitoring in intensive care. Most deaths are caused by asphyxiation rather than exsanguination, and patients should be positioned in such a way that the involved lung is in the dependent position. Careful airway protection is very important in those patients with massive haemoptysis.

Mild haemoptysis

If mild haemoptysis is suspected to be due to infectious or inflammatory lung disease, treatment with appropriate antibiotics and antitussives may be appropriate.[4] Close follow-up is advised and should lead to further investigations if the haemoptysis does not subside after treatment.

Moderate haemoptysis

If haemoptysis is moderate, admission to hospital for further investigation, observation and treatment is recommended.

Implications

Haemoptysis is a symptom that has to be taken seriously because of potential immediate danger to the patient and the possibility of serious underlying disease. Although investigations in primary care are limited, a careful assessment is necessary to make decisions about further investigations and the urgency of specialist referral. Using a systematic and focused approach, this should be possible to achieve in most primary care settings.

Key points

- Haemoptysis can be acute or chronic and may be caused by trivial or serious underlying disease.

- Haemoptysis needs to be distinguished from bleeding arising from other systems, particularly local bleeding and haemorrhage in the gastrointestinal tract.

- The likely cause of haemoptysis is influenced by the patient's age, ethnic status, past medical and social history, and associated respiratory symptoms.

- Completion of a full history and clinical examination is the most appropriate diagnostic strategy for primary care physicians, so that likely causes can be ranked and investigated appropriately.

- Chest radiography is the most accessible and useful investigation in primary care; referral to secondary care is usually necessary if further diagnostic investigation is required.

References

1. Sarinas, P. and Raffin, T.A. (1985). Diagnosis: the patient with hemoptysis. A chest film is the single most helpful diagnostic tool. *Hospital Medicine* 21, 166–83.

2. Hirshberg, B. et al. (1997). Hemoptysis: etiology, evaluation and outcome in a tertiary referral hospital. *Chest* 112, 440–4.

3. Lewis, M.M. and Read, C.A. (2000). Hemoptysis, part 1: identifying the cause. *Journal of Respiratory Diseases* 21, 335–41.

4. Boyars, M. (1999). Current strategies for diagnosing and managing hemoptysis. *Journal of Critical Illness* 14, 148–56.

5. Lenner, R., Almenoff, P.L., and Lesser, M. (1999). A systematic approach to hemoptysis. *Patient Care* 33, 49–56.

6. Richardson, W.S. et al. (2000). Users' guides to the medical literature. XXIV: how to use an article on the clinical manifestations of disease. *Journal of the American Medical Association* 284, 875.

7. **Richardson, W.S.** et al. (1999). Users' guides to the medical literature. XV: how to use an article about disease probability for differential diagnosis. *Journal of the American Medical Association* **281**, 1214–19.

8. **McGinn, T.G.** et al. (2000). Users' guides to the medical literature. XXII: how to use articles about clincial decision rules. *Journal of the American Medical Association* **284**, 84.

9. **Dileo, M.D. and Gianoli, G.J.** (1994). Diagnosis and management of hemoptysis. *Journal of the Lousiana State Medical Society* **146**, 115–18.

10. **Colice, G.** (1996). Hemoptysis—three questions that can direct management. *Postgraduate Medicine* **100**, 227–36.

11. **Lewis, M.M. and Read, C.A.** (2000). Hemoptysis, part 2: treatment options. *Journal of Respiratory Diseases* **21**, 392–4.

Further reading

Black, E.R., Bordley, D.R., Tape, T.G., and Panzer, R.J. *Diagnostic Strategies for Common Medical Problems*. Philadelphia: American College of Physicians, 1999. (Textbook providing estimates of pre-test probability of disease and likelihood ratios for symptoms, signs, and diagnostic tests for specific conditions.)

3

Ear, nose, and throat problems

3 Ear, nose, and throat problems

3.1 Epistaxis

Francoise P. Chagnon

Epistaxis is usually a minor event that does not require medical intervention. However, epistaxis can be a source of major blood loss or the harbinger of sinonasal or systemic disease. Primary care physicians are expected to be proficient in controlling nasal haemorrhage and initiating treatment.

Epistaxis affects all age groups and those suffering from allergies or sinus disease are at increased risk of being affected. The incidence of epistaxis is higher in cold winter months and in association with upper respiratory tract infections. In adults with multiple medical problems, epistaxis can be a manifestation of multiple systemic and local factors. While symptomatic treatment of the bleeding is essential, management of underlying disorders is just as important.

Epistaxis is commonly characterized into anterior and posterior, in reference to the site of origin in the nasal cavity. Anterior epistaxis arises from the anterior nasal septum, the nasal vestibule (the entrance to the nasal cavities from which emanate the nasal hairs), and the lateral wall of the nose proximal to the inferior turbinate. Posterior epistaxis arises from the posterior septum and the lateral nasal wall.

Most epistaxis originate from the anterior part of the nose, in particular, the anterior nasal septum. Osteocartilaginous spurs from a deviated nasal septum and the edges of septal perforations are also sites of predilection. Epistaxis commonly results from nose picking, forceful nose blowing, or dry inspired air. It is the most frequent adverse effect of nasal steroid sprays. Mucosal inflammation from infection, allergies, or exposure to irritants presents as blood-tinged rhinorrhea. In children, foreign bodies in the nose might go undetected until epistaxis occurs.

Determining the site of origin of epistaxis is often difficult because of a deviated nasal septum or turbinate hypertrophy. It is often assumed that the bleeding site is posterior when it cannot be readily identified on the anterior septum. Posterior epistaxis is most often seen in adults with hypertension, arteriosclerosis, and blood dyscrasias.

Anterior epistaxis is usually minor and recurrent, while profuse bleeding is more likely to occur from the lateral and posterior nose. When seeing patients with an epistaxis, the physician should not assume that spontaneous resolution will occur. All cases warrant examination of the nasal cavities in search of clues.

Nasal tumours do not commonly present with epistaxis. Nevertheless, epistaxis associated with nasal obstruction and unilateral rhinorrhea might signal nasal tumours such as juvenile angiofibromas in adolescent males or nasopharyngeal carcinomas in adults.

Hereditary haemorrhagic telangiectasia (Osler–Weber–Rendu disease) is a rare autosomal dominant disease presenting with telangiectasias in the mucosa of the digestive and respiratory tracts. Epistaxis is recurrent and troublesome. Telangiectasias covered with friable mucosa are visible on the anterior septum and turbinate, oral cavity, and lips.

Management

The initial management of epistaxis is aimed at controlling the bleeding while simultaneously addressing any cardiovascular compromise or coagulopathy that might exist. Since most epistaxis occurs from the anterior septum, patients should be instructed to blow their noses and apply direct pressure to the septum by pinching the nose for 5 min. This should be sufficient to at least temporarily control the bleeding. Inserting a gauze pack under the upper lip and applying pressure towards the root of the nose is another technique that can reduce bleeding from the anterior septum. The application of ice packs to the nose and forehead is of no benefit.

Successful examination of the nasal cavity depends on good illumination and instrumentation (see Fig. 1). Topical vasoconstriction of the nasal turbinates using cotton strips soaked in topical phenylephrine 0.5–1 per cent or adrenaline chloride solution (1 : 1000), or oxymetazoline hydrochloride allows visualization of the nasal septum for potential sites of bleeding. Inactive mucosal bleeding sites appear as a tiny mucosal excrescence. Such excrescenses can be triggered to bleed by gently stroking the septum and the turbinates with a cotton tip swab. Once identified, the bleeding point is cauterized by applying a silver nitrate stick for 30 seconds. If there is no bleeding at the site to be cauterized, the silver nitrate should be activated by dipping it briefly in water prior to application. Profuse bleeding is arrested by compression with a cotton-tipped applicator that is only released an instant before the silver nitrate is applied. For this procedure, cocaine solutions provide excellent analgesia but lidocaine 4 per cent topical solutions are sufficient and safer.

While some concern has been raised that silver nitrate cauterization could be carcinogenic, it seems highly unlikely that the minute doses applied would in fact be harmful. Topical vasoconstriction alone with agents such as oxymetazoline can be effective in some cases but is not the ideal definitive treatment.

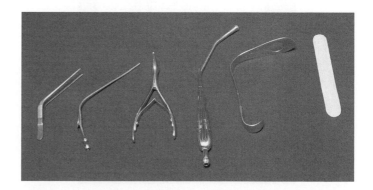

Fig. 1 Epistaxis tray instruments. (From left to right: Bayonet forceps, Frazier tip nasal suction, nasal speculum, Yankauer pharyngeal suction, Sweetheart tongue retractor, tongue depressor.)

Alternative techniques for the control of anterior epistaxis are:

♦ When bleeding from the anterior nose cannot be controlled by topical vasoconstriction, the anterior septum can be injected with 2 ml of 1 per cent lidocaine hydrochloride with epinephrine.

♦ Properly applied anterior nasal packing using petrolatum or antibiotic-coated gauze strip will apply pressure on the septum. The packing from the floor of the nasal cavity to the upper recesses of the nose is layered and anchored in the nose by making sure each layer extends deeply into the bony aperture of the nose. The packing can remain in place for 24–48 h.

Patients with epistaxis often fail to receive adequate treatment because they are not actively bleeding at the time of presentation. If the history indicates that profuse bleeding has occurred, prophylactic anterior nasal packing and close observation often is warranted.

Once an anterior epistaxis has been arrested, precautions should be instituted for the next week to allow undisrupted healing of the nasal mucosa. Humidification of inspired air, insufflation of normal saline into the nose two or three times a day, the application of nasal lubricants such as petrolatum gel or propylene glycol gel to the anterior nasal cavity three times a day with a cotton-tip applicator and, where indicated, the avoidance of airborne dust and other pollutants by wearing masks are all preventative measures. Epistaxis in the presence of rhinitis or sinusitis requires antibiotics.

Profuse epistaxis (which often originates in the posterior nasal cavity) calls for additional interventions:

♦ Establishing rapport with the patient. Epistaxis is a frightening event and patients need to be reassured as their collaboration is essential for intranasal interventions. Both the patient and the physician should wear protective clothing. It will be difficult to achieve intranasal anaesthesia and the physician must work expeditiously.

♦ Assessing the degree of blood loss and cardiovascular compromise and instituting immediate fluid resuscitation.

♦ Clearing the oropharyngeal and nasal airway of blood clots (using Yankauer and Frazier tip suctions) to establish the site of origin of the bleeding. The epistaxis can appear bilateral at first because of retrograde bleeding from the nasopharynx.

♦ Protecting the lower airway by the insertion of a number 16 or 18 Foley catheter balloon through the anterior naris so that the tip lies in the nasopharynx. The balloon is inflated with 15–30 ml of air (depending on the size of the nasal cavity) and the catheter is pulled back into the nose until a slight resistance is felt (overinflation of the balloon will displace the soft palate and obstruct breathing). The catheter is secured to the cheek (see Fig. 2).

♦ Packing of the nasal cavity with 1-in. petrolatum or antibiotic-coated strip gauze as described above (see Fig. 2). Packing of the opposite nasal cavity may be added for counter-pressure.

Alternative techniques to be considered are listed below in order of ease of use:

♦ Insertion of a commercially made double-balloon epistaxis management catheter.

♦ Commercially made non-absorbable nasal packing are easy to insert and very efficient since they swell as they absorb blood.

♦ Absorbable surgical packing such as oxidized cellulose, gelatin sponge, or microfibrillar collagen packing do not require removal and are particularly useful in cases of epistaxis due to blood dyscrasias.

♦ Commercially made vaginal tampons can be trimmed to size to fit into the nasal cavity.

♦ The traditional gauze roll posterior pack. Two-inch gauze is rolled and fastened with two long strings. Alternatively, a tonsil gauze pack or dental roll may be used (see Figs 3a and b).

Special considerations apply to epistaxis resulting from trauma:

♦ Epistaxis resulting from nasal fractures is usually self-limiting. When displacement of the nasal pyramid is evident, manual reduction of the nasal fractures will resolve refractory cases of epistaxis.

♦ Epistaxis resulting from basilar skull injuries requires endotracheal intubation and oropharyngeal packing. Caution is warranted in blindly inserting catheters into the nose, which could enter the cranial cavity.

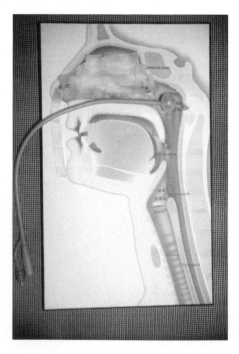

Fig. 2 Combined anterior gauze and posterior Foley catheter packing. (The packing gauze is layered from the floor of the nose upwards. The packing is inserted well beyond the nasal valve and bony nasal aperture. The Foley catheter is secured to the patient's cheek or knotted to abut onto the nasal packing at the nostril.)

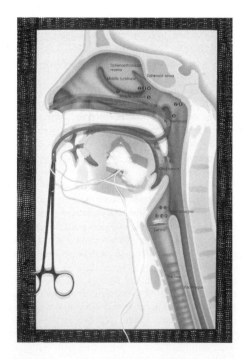

Fig. 3a Traditional posterior nasal packing. (The catheter is inserted into the side of the nose that is actively bleeding. The catheter is pulled from the mouth. The long string of the gauze roll packing is tied to the end of the catheter. The catheter is withdrawn through the nose and the packing is guided into the nasopharynx. The string is detached from the catheter.)

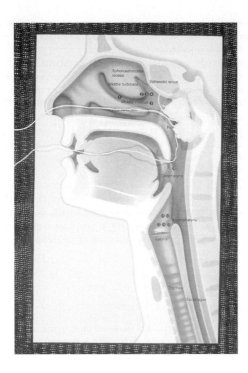

Fig. 3b Traditional posterior nasal packing. (The gauze roll packing is guided into the nasopharynx. Tension is maintained on the long string while anterior nasal packing is inserted. Note the additional safety string, which exits from the mouth. The strings are secured to the anterior nose or cheek. Attention is given not to exert pressure necrosis to the nasal alae or palate.)

Combined anterior and posterior nasal packing may be kept in place for 48 h but consideration should be given after 24 h to deflating the posterior balloon catheter to avoid pressure necrosis of the nose and palate. Such packings are uncomfortable to the patient and have high rates of complications. Nasal obstruction leads to hypoventilation, hypoxemia, and cardiac arrhythmia. Patients should be hospitalized, receive supplemental oxygen and humidified air by mask, and be closely monitored. Prophylactic antibiotics are customary to prevent sinusitis and otitis.

Intractable posterior epistaxis (persistent or recurrent bleeding despite nasal packing, or magnitude of bleeding sufficient to require blood transfusion) often requires surgical ligation of the ethmoidal and maxillary arteries or transarterial embolization.

Conclusion

Treatment options vary according to the aetiology and the severity of the bleeding. Minor anterior bleeding is usually controlled by pinching the nose or by silver nitrate cautery of anterior septal bleeding sites. Most other patients can be managed with nasal packing and supportive care in an ambulatory care setting. Those with posterior epistaxis and underlying systemic disease require hospitalization for monitoring and consideration for surgical or radiological interruption of the affected blood supply.

Key points

- Do not expect spontaneous resolution of epistaxis.
- Successful examination of the nose requires good illumination and instrumentation.
- Preparation of an epistaxis instrument tray and use of readily available materials assures expedient management.

Further reading

Maceri, D.R. (1993). Epistaxis and nasal trauma. In *Otolaryngology—Head and Neck Surgery* (ed. C.W. Cummings and J.M. Frederickson), pp. 723–36. St Louis: Mosby-Year Book Inc.

Chin, K.N. and Kennedy, D.W. (1995). *Epistaxis*. Slide Lecture Series. American Academy of Otolaryngology—Head and Neck Surgery Foundation, Inc. (A comprehensive and practical review of epistaxis management.)

3.2 Ear pain in adults

Chris Del Mar and Michael Yelland

Causes of ear pain

Perhaps with the exception of the abdomen, few parts of the body present such a confusing array of causes for pain as the ear. Of course, earache is usually attributable to ear structures. However, pathology in structures adjacent to the ear commonly and confusingly can cause earache. This can lead to medical disasters: the primary care doctor must be aware of these possibilities and ensure that dangerous causes are not missed when an adult presents with earache.

The reason for the confusion arises because of complicated embryology. Structures within the ear and nearby are evolved from ancient gill arches. They, therefore, carry with them their nerve supplies. This means that sensory innervation of the ear and temporomandibular joint can be perceived as coming from the same site, as can input from the throat/pharynx. One must, therefore, think of the pharynx, base of the tongue, and temporomandibular joint as well as the middle and outer ear itself, when an adult complains of earache.

In particular, persistent earache in an adult is a common presentation of malignancies of the tongue, jaw, fauces, and pharynx.

A diagnostic approach to ear pain[1]

'What is the most likely cause of earache in an adult?'

The most likely causes are otitis media and otitis externa. These are discussed in more detail below.

A clue to the diagnosis is often contained in the history: in otitis media, the classical history is of earache sensitive to pressure changes (flying, sneezing, or even bending forward), which is associated with a recent upper respiratory infection. Unfortunately, the association of symptoms of upper respiratory infection and the supposed aetiological connection to middle ear infection, is diagnostically unhelpful: symptoms of cough and rhinitis are equally likely to be found in a child with otitis media as without.[2]

The diagnosis is made on the appearance and mobility of the ear drum: if the tympanic membrane is bulging and red, the diagnosis is straightforward. A diagnostic study of nearly 12 000 consultations for ear problems in children subjected them to the gold standard of aspirating the middle ear for pus. It found that 'redness' of the tympanic membrane is much less predictive of middle ear infection than expected: less than half the cases of children with ear drum 'redness' (or 'definite redness') had inflammatory material in the middle ear. On the other hand, bulging of the drum is very strongly predictive of infective material in the middle ear space (the likelihood ratio was in the range of 10–20).[2] This information is only available for children, so we have to extrapolate these findings to adults.

In otitis externa, there is usually recent exposure to moisture in the external ear canal—swimming (particularly in bacteria-rich water such as rivers and the sea) or people washing their ears with detergent (shampoo). It is more common in hot, humid weather.

'What diagnoses must not be missed?'

Because cancers of the head and neck are potentially fatal, and since many are amenable to curative treatment, early diagnosis is paramount. Establishing the absence of cancer may be very difficult, and involves the search of many parts of the oral cavity, throat, and base of the tongue. Bi-digital palpation of the floor of the mouth may detect secondary lymph nodes of metastatic cancers not otherwise detectable.

'Common pitfalls'

A common pitfall is temporomandibular joint pain (see below): it is often forgotten as a cause of earache. It should be suspected if the pain is related to eating, yawning, or recent dental procedures. Tenderness and crepitus over the joint are often found.

Commonly missed lesions in the external ear include simple boils (furunculosis) of the ear canal. They may be confused with otitis externa as both cause tenderness of the pinna and tragus. Examination of the canal may show localized tenderness only in the early stages and localized erythema and swelling as the boil enlarges. In otitis externa, the canal erythema and swelling are more generalized. Less difficult to diagnose are local lesions such as impacted wax, foreign bodies, and squamous cell carcinomas that can present in the skin of the ear meatus.

Conditions referring pain to the ear include dental problems such as dental caries and abscesses. Any lesion, infective or neoplastic, of the pharynx (such as pharyngitis, peritonsillar abscess, or carcinoma) or tongue (carcinomas of the base of the tongue often being difficult to diagnose) can produce ear pain. So also can dysfunction of the upper cervical spine, where pain may be related to specific neck movements or postures and is often felt just behind the ear. Neck pain and headache may also point towards this diagnosis.

'The masquerades'

Masquerades are common conditions that lead to misdiagnosis. One of these is depression, which should be considered in any patient with a pain syndrome that does not immediately fall into any straightforward diagnostic category.

Other relevant conditions to consider include nerve root pain (e.g. herpes zoster may present with pain before the tell-tale vesicles appear in the skin of the relevant nerve root), alcohol or other drug misuse, and migraine.

Acute middle ear infection (otitis media)

Epidemiology

Middle ear infections are less common in adults than in children. The reasons for this are not known, but may be related to: the decreased uncomplicated acute respiratory infection rate in adults (the antecedent to most cases); the fact that the Eustachian tube (which, as we will see, is crucial to understanding the mechanism of otitis media), is so much larger than in children; or possibly because the immune system is better armed for dealing with newly encountered organisms.

Middle ear infections are also the most common suppurative complication of acute respiratory infection. The incidence is increased in adults with cleft palate and Down syndrome.

Pathophysiology

The mechanism of otitis media is thought to begin with an infection arising from the upper respiratory tract via the Eustachian tube, and secondarily infecting the middle ear air space. Perhaps the mucosal swelling causes the Eustachian tube to obstruct, thereby causing the failure of the discharge of the contents of the middle ear into the pharynx.

The microbiology of acute otitis media is discussed in Chapter 10.3. Whatever the cause of the infection, the final common pathway is established. Infected mucus, trapped in the middle ear by the secondarily blocked Eustachian tube, sets up an inflammatory process. This has two effects. First, the tympanic membrane bulges out (laterally) under pressure, stimulating stretch receptors in the membrane. This in effect constitutes an abscess of the middle ear. Systemic symptoms are often associated with this element of the illness, including spiking fevers, very severe pain in the affected ear, malaise, and vomiting.

Secondly, the replacement of air by fluid in the middle ear means that hearing acuity is compromised: transmission of sound vibrations from the tympanic membrane is dampened by the fluid and vibrations reach the inner ear with decreased amplitude. Low-frequency hearing in particular is lost. Very rarely the infection can extend into the mastoid space.

Clinical features

Symptoms

The typical story is of a patient with a non-specific upper respiratory infection whose illness suddenly takes a turn for the worse. The patient develops pain and systemic illness with an increase in fever, and malaise.

The pain and associated symptoms (mostly systemic) are generally short-lived. Among children about 60 per cent are resolved within 24 h of presenting to the doctor. The same is probably true in adults. Resolution can occur in one of several ways: the infected material can discharge through the tympanic membrane (which is usually accompanied by immediate relief of pain, and pus or even blood, in the external ear canal); the contents can discharge through the Eustachian tube; or the inflammation gradually settles without discharge.

Deafness often accompanies the pain and may persist long after the acute inflammatory phase has settled, with about a quarter of patients still suffering decreased hearing acuity 1 month later. If this persists beyond about 3 months it is called 'glue ear' (see section on Complications).

Signs

As discussed above, the diagnosis is focussed on the appearance of the tympanic membrane. If the eardrum is bulging towards the observer and is bright red, the diagnosis is straightforward.

However, the diagnosis is sometimes difficult. Deciding whether there is a bulging drum can be difficult. Similarly, deciding whether the colour is red from inflammation behind it rather than from the flush of pyrexia can be difficult. Empirical studies in children have shown that the best predictors of infection of the middle ear are bulging of the tympanic membrane and loss of its transparency (becoming 'cloudy'). However, there are no very good signs for ruling it out. That is to say that the absence of bulging of the tympanic membrane for ruling out acute otitis media is not useful, with a negative likelihood ratio of about 0.5.

On the other hand, impaired mobility of the tympanic membrane is useful. This is elicited by use of the pneumatic auroscope. Air can be 'puffed' into the auroscope by means of a rubber bulb. If there is a good airtight fit between speculum and ear canal, altering the pressure externally with the rubber bulb allows an estimate of the mobility of the ear drum. Impaired tympanic membrane mobility has a positive likelihood ratio of 3–5 and a negative ratio of 0.03–0.08 for the diagnosis of otitis media. Tympanometry will show a flattened (type B) tracing. The main areas of confusion are with serous otitis media (glue ear), where there is also cloudiness of the tympanic membrane and impaired movement of the ear drum.[2]

Treatment

There are several approaches to treatment. These are curiously different in different cultures (see also Chapter 10.3).

To some, a middle ear infection represents a small abscess. There is pus that should be drained. This is not difficult in theory: there is access via the tympanic membrane. In the hands of a skilled operator, a small knife can safely make a small incision in the lower part of the tympanic membrane, releasing the pus, and effecting resolution. Unfortunately, this requires considerable skill and is alarming to many patients.

To others, the illness is an infection with a spectrum of microorganisms that may be susceptible to common antibiotics. Indeed, otitis media is one of the most common single reason for prescribing antibiotics in the West. Evidence comes from randomized trials only in children, which suggest that the benefits of antibiotics for middle ear infections are only modest. They make no difference to the resolution of deafness. Nor do antibiotics influence the resolution of illness for the majority (60 per cent) whose pain resolves within 24 h of seeing the doctor. However, they do make a difference to the others whose pain will not resolve within a day: here there is a 30 per cent reduction.[3] This translates into a number needed to treat with antibiotics of 20 to reduce the duration of pain in otitis media. To treat the rare complication of mastoiditis in adults would require treating astronomical numbers to prevent one case.

This means that many people are beginning to use these empirical data to withhold antibiotics as routine initial treatment for this condition. This has been, in fact, normal practice in many parts of Northern Europe, especially Holland and Scandinavia.

Adequate analgesia is, therefore, required, and it has been shown that simple analgesics are effective in the control of the pain of otitis media in adults.[4]

Other medications for which there is unknown evidence of benefit include steroids and other treatments aimed at preventing inflammation and allergic processes.

Complications

The most common complication is the persistence of the original illness (particularly discharging suppuration and deafness), or the development of a new locus of infection as in acute mastoiditis. Chronic otitis media is covered in Chapter 3.3.

Glue ear (persistent deafness)

This is also called *otitis media with effusion* (OME) and *chronic secretory otitis media*. The inflammatory processes largely settles, leaving a liquid material within the middle ear. This is rarely painful (although discomfort may be a feature) but the prominent problem is deafness.

Prevention

In theory, at least, prescribing antibiotics might prevent the complications of middle ear infections. This can be quantified in meta-analyses.[5] Treating sore throats with antibiotics does appear to prevent the complication of middle ear infections. However, the number of adults with sore throat who must be treated with antibiotics is high (about 150 to prevent one case of acute otitis media).

Use of pneumococcal vaccine has been trialled, with modest benefits in terms of reducing episodes of otitis media. On the other hand, influenza vaccine has been shown in randomized controlled trials to reduce by about 25 per cent the number of primary acute respiratory infections. Some of these will include, or give rise to, acute otitis media. Therefore, one can by extrapolation assume that influenza vaccine is an effective prophylactic. How this operates is unclear: our model for the effectiveness of influenza vaccine is that the vaccine is only specific for a limited range of influenza virus varieties.[7]

External ear infection (otitis externa)

Pathophysiology

Otitis externa is a cause of earache seen more commonly in the warmer months when water sports are popular.[8] Its common synonyms ('tropical ear' and 'swimmer's ear') relate to the major aetiological factors of heat and moisture, which lead to an overgrowth of organisms. Trauma to the ear canal and partial obstruction due to wax, foreign bodies, or exostoses may also encourage infection. Many varieties of otitis externa have been described but over 90 per cent of cases are due to acute bacterial and fungal infections. The most common organism isolated is *Pseudomonas* sp.[9] Other common bacterial pathogens include *Staphylococcus aureus*, *Escherichia coli, and Acinetobacter calcoaceticus.* The common fungal pathogens are *Candida* sp. and *Aspergillus* sp. A fuller discussion of ear discharge is provided in the next chapter.

Clinical features

Symptoms of acute otitis externa include earache (often severe), itching in the ear canal, and discharge from the canal. Hearing loss may occur if canal obstruction or tympanic membrane thickening is present, but it is usually mild.

Signs include tenderness on moving the tragus, pinna or jaw, canal erythema, and discharge. The discharge may be tinged green with *Pseudomonas*, pale cream 'wet blotting paper' with *Candida albicans*, or may occasionally show black spores with *Aspergillus niger*. In more severe cases, canal oedema may be present to the extent that it may occlude the canal or extend onto the pinna.

Acute otitis media may have more prominent constitutional disturbance, greater hearing loss, and less tragal tenderness and canal oedema. Although rarely indicated, tympanometry is flattened (type B tracings) in otitis media but normal (type A tracings) in otitis externa.[10]

Treatment

The aims of treatment include pain relief, eradication of infection, reduction of oedema, and prevention of recurrence. The pain of otitis externa can be excruciating and may require strong analgesics. When associated with marked oedema, pain may be reduced more rapidly by adding oral corticosteroids.

Meticulous ear toilet is generally regarded as the keystone of successful therapy, as it not only removes the culture medium of the pathogens but also allows access of topical medications to the infected skin. Methods include suction under magnification, cotton wool mopping, small wire loops, or gentle syringing. A dilute solution (one part to six parts water) of white vinegar can be used to restore the canal's protective acid mantle and should be followed by careful drying with cotton wool mops or a hair dryer.

Once the canal is clean, topical agents can be applied. The choice of agent and its vehicle depends on the severity of the condition. The more severe cases of bacterial otitis externa with oedema respond best to a combined antibiotic/corticosteroid cream or ointment applied on a gauze wick. The antibiotic should be effective against *Pseudomonas* sp. and *S. aureus*. The wick is carefully packed with forceps into the canal, placing it as close to the drum as possible. There is no need to pack it under pressure, as this will only increase the patient's suffering. Simply filling the ear with the cream or ointment can be as effective as using a wick.[10] The wick is removed after 2 days, by which time most of the oedema and pain will have gone, and treatment can proceed as for mild to moderate cases. If there has been no improvement, the adequacy of aural toilet and the choice of topical agent should be reviewed and a swab taken for culture. For mild to moderate cases, the same cream can be applied to the canal on a cotton wool mop every 2 days until symptoms have disappeared, or the patient can use a similar preparation in drop form three to four times daily until 2 days after symptoms have resolved. Wicks that expand on contact with liquid are a useful adjunct to ensure the effective application of drops.

If the otitis externa does not resolve with careful adherence to this treatment, or if there are clinical features of fungal infection, a topical antifungal agent such as clotrimoxazole, nystatin, or amphotericin B should be used.[11] In fungal infections, meticulous aural toilet is even more important, as the fungi are often quite adherent to the canal skin.

Oral antibiotics have a limited role in the treatment of otitis externa seen in the primary care setting, as nearly all cases will resolve with the above regimen.[9] They may play a role in furunculosis, acute exacerbations of chronic otitis externa, and malignant otitis externa (a condition of the elderly, diabetic, and immuno-compromised, where the infection invades the temporal bone and in which antibiotics effective against *Pseudomonas*, such as ciprofloxacin, are effective).[12,13]

Prevention

People who have suffered otitis externa often ask about prevention. The use of earplugs during swimming and the use of acetic acid and alcohol drops after swimming is recommended, but without evidence of effectiveness. Trauma to the ear canal from scratching with fingernails or sharp objects should be avoided, as should 'cleaning' with almost any foreign object.

Temporomandibular joint disorder

In over 10 per cent of cases, pain from the temporomandibular joint (TMJ) disorders is felt in the ear. TMJ pain may arise after any activity that alters the balance of chewing, such as a toothache, or a visit to the dentist with prolonged extension of the jaw for a procedure. The joint forms the anterior part of the ear canal. Therefore, tenderness anterior to the ear suggests the joint is a source of pain. Failing this, asymmetrical tenderness and clicking with pressure over the joint while the patient opens and closes the mouth is suggestive. A more provocative test is to ask the patient to chew in a rotatory fashion (like a cow chewing cud) while pressure is applied to the joint. If all these tests are negative, the joint is unlikely to be the source of pain. Associations with pain referred from the TMJ include tinnitus, symptoms of stress, bruxism, and, in men, neck pain.

Signs of TMJ disorder include tenderness over the TMJ and in the masseter and temporalis muscles, restricted opening of the jaw, and joint crepitus. When the problem is unilateral, the jaw may deviate towards the painful, restricted side on opening. The teeth may appear unusually worn. X-rays of the mandible may show osteoarthritic changes in the TMJ, but normal X-rays do not exclude the TMJ as a source of pain.

Treatment may include local heat, simple analgesics, and non-steroidal anti-inflammatory drugs. There is some evidence for the effectiveness of occlusal splints, EMG biofeedback, and physical therapy. The effectiveness of physical therapy seems to be proportional to the amount of therapy given. In some clinical trials, it has been no more effective than placebo therapy, although placebo therapy is more effective than no treatment. There is no evidence that ultrasound is useful.

References

1. Murtagh, J. (1990). Common problems: a safe diagnostic strategy. *Australian Family Physician* **19**, 733–40.
2. Pirozzo, S. and Del Mar, C. (2000). Otitis media. In *Evidence Based Pediatrics and Child Health* (ed. V.A. Moyer), Chapter 27, pp. 238–47. London: BMJ Books.
3. Glasziou, P.P., Del Mar, C.B., Hayem, M., and Sanders, S.L. *Antibiotics for Acute Otitis Media in Children (Cochrane Review)* Issue 4, 2000. Oxford: Update Software.
4. Godlee, F., ed. *Clinical Evidence. A Compendium of the Best Available Evidence for Effective Health Care* 5th edn. London: BMJ, 2001, p. 599.
5. Del Mar, C.B., Glasziou, P.P., and Spinks, A.B. *Antibiotics for Sore Throat (Cochrane Review)* Issue 4, 2000. Oxford: Update Software.
6. Eskola, J., Kilpi, T., Palmu, A., Jokinen, J., Haapakoski, J., Herva, E., Takala, A., Kayhty, H., Karma, P., Kohberger, R., Siber, G., and Makela, P.H. (2001). Efficacy of a pneumococcal conjugate vaccine against acute otitis media. *New England Journal of Medicine* **344**, 403–9.
7. Nichol, K.L., Lind, A., Margolis, K.L., Murdoch, M., McFadden, R., Hauge, M., Magnan, S., and Drake, M. (1995). The effectiveness of vaccination against influenza in healthy, working adults. *New England Journal of Medicine* **333**, 889–93.
8. Strauss, M.B. (1987). Otitis externa associated with aquatic activities (swimmer's ear). *Clinical Dermatology* **5**, 103–11.
9. Yelland, M.J. (1993). Efficacy of oral cotrimoxazole in the treatment of otitis externa in general practice. *Medical Journal of Australia* **158**, 697–9.
10. Barr, G.D. and al-Khabori, M. (1991). A randomized prospective comparison of two methods of administering topical treatment in otitis externa. *Clinical Otolaryngology* **16** (6), 547–8.
11. El-Gothamy, M.A.B. and El-Gothamy, Z. (1977). Otomycosis—a new line of treatment. *Castellania* **5**, 215–16.
12. Fombeur, J.P., Barrault, S., Koubbi, G., Laurier, J.N., Ebbo, D., Lecomte, F., Sorrel, N., and Dobler, S. (1994). Study of the efficacy and safety of ciprofloxacin in the treatment of chronic otitis. *Chemotherapy* **40** (Suppl. 1), 29–34.
13. Lang, R., Gashen, S., Kitzes Cohen, R., and Sadse, J. (1990). Successful treatment of malignant otitis externa with oral ciprofloxacin: report of experience with 23 patients. *Journal of Infectious Diseases* **161**, 537–40.

3.3 The discharging ear

Ted L. Tewfik

Otorrhoea or discharge from the ear is a sign of ear disease. The treating physician must determine the source of the discharge in order to establish the diagnosis. Differences in amount, colour, clarity, and odour may provide important clues. The causes of otorrhoea may be infectious or non-infectious. The infectious causes may originate from the external auditory canal (EAC), the middle ear, or the mastoid cavity. The non-infectious causes include cerebrospinal fluid leak, which might occur after head trauma. Tables 1–3 summarize the possible causes of otorrhoea according to certain physical characteristics of the discharge.[1,2] A few important examples of otorrhoea have been selected and will be discussed.

Otitis externa

Bacterial otitis externa

Bacterial otitis externa is an infection of the EAC. The typical patient will present with symptoms of otalgia and itching. A sensation of ear fullness may also be present. On physical examination, erythema and oedema of the EAC will be noted. These signs may extend to the pinna. On otoscopic examination, clear or purulent secretions associated with debris may be seen in the EAC, and manipulation of the auricle, particularly the tragus, will elicit pain, which can be severe. Otitis externa can be divided into pre-inflammatory, acute inflammatory, and chronic inflammatory stages.

In the pre-inflammatory phase, there is oedema of the canal skin and obstruction of the drainage ducts of apocrine glands in the external ear canal. In this stage, the main complaint is pruritus and fullness of the ear. The patient begins to relieve the itch by scratching. The itch/scratch cycle further damages the protective lipid coat and introduces bacteria. In the acute inflammatory stage, scratching of the ear disrupts the epithelial layer and allows bacterial invasion, which leads to pain and tenderness.[3]

Table 1 Causes of serous, mucoid, and purulent otorrhoea

Congenital
First branchial cleft fistula (usually presents at birth or shortly after)

Inflammatory
External ear
  Foreign bodies
  Otitis externa (bacterial, fungal, NEO[a])
  Bullous myringitis (viral or mycoplasmal, causing painful lesions on the
    drumhead)
  Herpes simplex
  Herpes zoster oticus   } of the EAC[b]
  Seborrheic dermatitis
  Neurodermatitis
Middle ear
  Acute otitis media (suppurative, necrotizing)
  Acute mastoiditis
  Chronic otitis media
  Tuberculous otitis media
  Langerhan's cell histiocytosis (LCH[c])
  Iatrogenic (post-tympanostomy tube insertion)

Neoplastic
External ear
  Benign
  Malignant
Middle ear
  Benign (adenoma, neurofibroma, glomus jugulare)
  Malignant (squamous cell, metastatic)

[a] Necrotizing external otitis.

[b] External auditory canal.

[c] Previously known as Histiocytosis X, 50 per cent of cases are diagnosed before the age of
5 years. Eosinophilic granuloma is the most common form of LCH. Other forms include
Hand–Schuller–Christian disease and Letterer–Siwe disease.

Table 2 Causes of bloody otorrhoea

Congenital
  Vascular conditions, presenting in infancy or early childhood

Inflammatory
  Otitis externa
  Otitis media (acute, chronic)

Traumatic
  Temporal bone fracture
  Foreign body
  Iatrogenic (tympanic tube, cerumen removal)

Coagulation defects

Neoplastic

Examination of the ear canal will reveal erythema and mild oedema
accompanied by a small amount of clear or cloudy secretions.

As the disease progresses to the stage of moderate inflammation, the
pruritus, pain, and auricular tenderness increase in intensity. The exudate
becomes thicker and the EAC oedema is more impressive but the canal
remains patent. Should the disease remain untreated, it will attain the stage
of severe inflammation, characterized by intolerable pain, intensified by
chewing, or movement of the surrounding skin or soft tissues. The oedema
will obliterate the lumen of the EAC, which now contains profuse,
greenish, and purulent discharge.

Chronic otitis externa results from repeated low-grade infections that
have been incompletely treated.

Table 3 Causes of clear otorrhoea

Congenital
Isolated foot plate fistula
Associated with defect of temporal bone
  Mondini dysplasia
  Klippel Feil anomaly
  Pendred syndrome
  Craniosynostosis
  Wide cochlear aqueduct

Acquired
Post-stapedectomy fistula
Penetrating wounds in ear
Barotrauma
Erosion of bone
  Luetic
  Cholesteatoma
  Neoplastic

The treatment of acute otitis externa is guided by the following four
fundamental principles:

1. frequent and thorough cleansing of the EAC;

2. judicious use of antibiotics;

3. treatment of associated pain;

4. prevention of future infection.

Meticulous cleaning of the EAC is as important, if not more important,
than antibiotic treatment. The canal should be freed of exfoliated debris,
cerumen, and purulent secretions. This is best accomplished with a microscope but can be performed adequately with an otoscope and ear curette or
suction. If the canal is cleaned by irrigation, it must be dried completely
with suction or a cotton swab.[5] (For more details on bacterial otis externa,
the reader is referred to Chapter 3.2.)

Fungal otitis externa

Fungal otitis externa accounts for 10–30 per cent of all cases of otitis
externa. Fungi have three basic growth requirements: moisture, warmth,
and darkness. It becomes evident that the predisposing factors for fungal
otitis externa are similar to those for bacterial otitis externa. Note that moisture also plays a key role in the aetiology and is the only modifiable factor.
Diabetes or immunocompromised status are predisposing factors.
Aspergillus accounts for 80–90 per cent of otomycosis and *Candida* species
account for the remaining 10–20 per cent of cases. Other organisms such as
Phycomycetes, *Rhizopus*, and *Actinomyces* might be involved but play
a minor role. Fungal otitis externa presents with itching and otorrhoea. On
otoscopic examination, the EAC often contains black, grey, yellow, greenish,
or white debris. The treatment of fungal otitis externa is similar to that of
bacterial otitis externa in that thorough cleaning is required. Antifungal otic
drops are indicated. One that is readily available is a combination of the
topical corticosteroid flumethasone and the antifungal clioquinol
(Locorten Vioform).[3,4]

Necrotizing external otitis

Necrotizing external otitis (NEO), previously known as malignant otitis
externa, is a serious and potentially life-threatening complication of otitis
externa. In NEO, the infection that began in the EAC spreads to the surrounding soft tissues and bone. This can lead to osteomyelitis of the temporal bone. If the infection spreads further to the skull base and involves the
cranial nerves, the prognosis becomes dismal. This disease usually occurs in
the elderly diabetic. It also occurs in the immunocompromised, including
patients with diabetic renal failure, the acutely ill, or chronically debilitated
patient. The patient has a history of a long-standing (more than 1 month)
otitis externa with severe pain and aural discharge. Physical examination

reveals purulent secretions in the EAC accompanied by granulation tissue. All cranial nerves must be examined carefully to rule out any neuropathy. Particular attention should be paid to cranial nerves VII, X, and XI as they are the most commonly involved.

Plain X-rays are of little use in the diagnosis of NEO. CT scanning with contrast is the imaging test of choice and often demonstrates soft tissue thickening, clouding of the mastoid air cells, erosion of the anterior wall of the EAC, or erosion of the skull base. Magnetic resonance imaging (MRI) with gadolinium enhancement can be helpful in evaluating cerebral involvement. Bone and gallium scans are useful baseline studies as they will normalize with resolution of the infection.

NEO is mentioned to alert the physician to the potential severity of otitis externa and the importance of adequate treatment and follow-up. Should the clinician suspect NEO, the patient should, if possible, be immediately referred to an otolaryngologist in a tertiary care institution for treatment. As the cause of NEO is almost always *P. aeruginosa*, the treatment consists of intravenous antipseudomonal antibiotics for a minimum duration of 6 weeks, accompanied by thorough and frequent cleaning of the EAC. Surgical treatment, which consists of wide debridement of infected tissues and bone, should only be used as a last resort.[3]

Otitis media

Otitis media is the most common cause of purulent otorrhoea. In 1990, a survey conducted by the Centers for Disease Control and Prevention in Atlanta, Georgia, estimated 24.5 million doctor's visits related to otitis media in the United States. Various types of otitis media that cause discharge from the ear are discussed in this section.

Suppurative otitis media

In this type of infection, there is a copious amount of fluid, which may be haemorrhagic, serosanguinous, or mucopurulent. Perforation of the tympanic membrane occurs in the pars tensa, which is the lower third of the drumhead. Otalgia is usually relieved as soon as the perforation occurs. The drainage will continue until the middle ear inflammation settles. If the infection spreads to the mastoid cavity, the discharge will persist. In general, otorrhoea becomes more profuse and foul-smelling when mastoiditis occur.[6]

Otorrhoea associated with tympanostomy tubes

The most common complication of tympanostomy tubes is otorrhoea. The reported incidence of occurrence varies between 15 and 50 per cent depending on the population studied and the type of tube (grommet) used. The discharge is usually purulent and the patient usually does not complain of pain. Cleaning of the ear may be accomplished with a cotton swab or suction. In most cases, antibiotic drops are sufficient to treat the condition. If otalgia is present, an oral broad-spectrum antibiotic should be administered for 7–10 days. If the discharge persists, adjustment of the antibiotic, possibly guided by culture of the discharge, is usually required. The formation of granulation tissue or polyp around the tympanostomy tube may lead to persistent purulent or blood-tinged otorrhoea. This usually responds to topical therapy. Removal of the persistent granulation polyp might be needed if the discharge continues.[6] In resistant cases, the grommet may have to be extracted, since it acts as a foreign body. [For more details on bacterial otitis media, the reader is referred to Chapter 3.2 (Ear pain in adults) and Chapter 10.3 (Otitis media in children)].

Chronic persistent otitis media

Otorrhoea associated with chronic otitis is usually painless and is accompanied with hearing loss. The onset of this condition is often insidious. If the acute perforation of the drumhead fails to heal after 3 months, it is labelled chronic. The patient might not seek medical attention until complications develop. Associated otalgia indicates complications. Examination of the ear reveals a persistent tympanic membrane perforation. The margins of the perforation are usually covered with intact epithelium. The persistent mucoid or mucopurulent discharge becomes profuse when the patient has concomitant upper respiratory tract infection. If the discharge persists and becomes malodorous, suspect the presence of cholesteatoma—see below.

Mastoiditis

Mastoiditis can be acute, subacute, or chronic. In the acute phase, infection spreads to the periosteum and tenderness occurs over the post-auricular area.[6] At this stage, oral or intravenous antibiotics are required to prevent abscess formation. The development of a mastoid abscess will be manifested by loss of the post-auricular crease, swelling of the external canal, and possibly fluctuation in the post-auricular region. This will necessitate surgical drainage.

Cholesteatoma

Acquired cholesteatoma occurs in the majority of cases with chronic otitis media. It is to be differentiated from congenital cholesteatoma, which occurs behind an intact tympanic membrane, and will not be discussed in this chapter.

The acquired or most common variety of cholesteatoma is divided into stages according to the involvement of the ossicular chain, and extension beyond the middle ear and temporal bone. The condition starts when stratified squamous keratinizing epithelium accumulates in the middle ear and spreads to the pneumatized spaces of the mastoid bone. A retraction pocket in the superior part of the tympanic membrane (membrana flaccida) is an early sign of cholesteatoma that progresses to perforation, usually with otorrhoea. The perforation in this anatomic location should be differentiated from perforation in the lower part of the tympanic membrane, the membrana tensa. Many otologists refer to the ear with discharge and perforation of the superior part (membrana flaccida) as a dangerous ear, since cholesteatoma may erode the ossicles and spread to the intracranial cavity. Surgical treatment is indicated when cholesteatoma is diagnosed. A modified radical or radical mastoidectomy with or without tympanoplasty is required.

In summary, otorrhoea is an important sign of ear disease. The examining physician should be able to determine the aetiology of the drainage. When the condition persists or recurs frequently, one must search for resistant organisms or unusual causes for otorrhoea.

Key points

- The treatment of acute otitis externa should include frequent and thorough cleansing of the external auditory canal, judicious use of antibiotics, treatment of associated pain, and prevention of future infection.

- Moisture plays a key role in the aetiology of fungal otitis and is the only modifiable factor. Diabetes or immunocompromised status are predisposing factors. *Aspergillus* accounts for 80–90% of otomycosis.

- Necrotizing external otitis (NEO), formerly known as malignant otitis externa, is a serious and potentially life-threatening complication of otitis externa.

- Cholesteatoma starts when stratified squamous keratinizing epithelium accumulates in the middle ear and spreads to the pneumatized spaces of the mastoid bone. A retraction pocket in the superior part of the tympanic membrane (membrana flaccida) is an early sign of cholesteatoma that progresses to perforation, usually with otorrhoea.

- The most common complication of tympanostomy tubes is otorrhoea.

- Otitis media is the most common cause of purulent otorrhoea.

References

1. **Schloss, M.D. and Pearl, A.J.** (1996). Otorrhea. In *Pediatric Otolaryngology* 3rd edn. (ed. C. Bluestone, S. Stool, and M. Kenna), pp. 243–8. Philadelphia: WB Saunders. (An excellent chapter on the differential diagnosis of otorrhoea.)

2. **Tewfik, T.L., Teebi, A.S., and Der Kaloustian, V.M.** (1997). Selected syndromes and conditions. In *Congenital Anomalies of the Ear, Nose, and Throat* (ed. T.L. Tewfik and V.M. Der Kaloustian), pp. 441–545. New York: Oxford University Press.

3. **Bojrab, D.I., Bruderly, T., and Abdulrazzak, Y.** (1996). Otitis externa. *Otolaryngologic Clinics of North America* **29**, 761–82.

4. **Kimmelman, C.P.** (1992). Office management of the draining ear. *Otolaryngologic Clinics of North America* **25**, 739. (Comprehensive chapter on the aetiology and treatment of otitis externa.)

5. **Marshall, K.G. and Attia, E.L.** *Disorders of the Ear.* Boston: John Wright, PSG Inc, 1983, pp. 73–5.

6. **Bluestone, C.D. and Klein, J.O.** *Otitis Media in Infants and Children* 3rd edn. Philadelphia: WB Saunders, 2001, pp. 58–78. (Most recent book on otitis media written by leaders of paediatric otology.)

3.4 Hearing loss

Robert Sweet and Ted L. Tewfik

Introduction

Helen Keller said, 'Blindness separates people from things. Deafness separates people from people'. However, thanks to the work of people like her, services for the hard-of-hearing have increased, integration of the deaf into mainstream society has improved, and a deaf culture has developed within which there is no stigma to being deaf. For those who wish to hear better, reconstructive surgery, hearing aids, assistive listening devices, and cochlear implants are constantly being improved.

This chapter is divided into four parts: *screening* for hearing loss in those who do not complain of it, the *diagnosis* of hearing loss in those who do, *treatment*, and *prevention*.

Definitions

Deaf: inability to hear and understand speech through the ear alone; primary mode of communication may be sign language, especially for prelingual hearing loss.

Hard-of-hearing: reduced ability to hear and understand speech through the ear alone; primary mode of communication is speech.

Hearing loss (HL) or impairment: measurable limitation of the ability to hear.

Conductive HL: HL due to conditions of the middle and/or external ear.

Perceptive or neurosensory HL (NSHL): HL due to conditions of the cochlea and/or eighth cranial nerve (VIII).

Mixed HL: HL due to a combination of conductive and NSHL.

Retrocochlear HL: HL due to a condition proximal to the cochlea, involving VIII and/or central nervous system.

Pre-lingual/post-lingual: occurring before/after the acquisition of speech.

Decibel (dB): a measure of sound intensity.

dBA: dB scale weighted to account for the human ear's greater sensitivity to some frequencies.

Hearing handicap: degree of subjective disadvantage in communication due to HL.

Disability: the actual or presumed inability to remain employed at full wages.

Screening for hearing loss

Scope of the problem

About one child per 1000 is born deaf. The incidence of congenital HL of moderate severity or greater is double that. The most critical period for speech and language development is from birth to 3 years of age, and hearing plays a vital role. The goal of universal newborn screening is to identify children by 3 months and intervene by 6 months.

Overall, about 10 per cent of the general population is hard-of-hearing and about 0.6 per cent is deaf. Twenty-five per cent of people at age 65 are hard-of-hearing and 50 per cent at age 75. Despite the fact that hearing aids can improve the quality of life significantly, they are under-utilized.

Newborn

In some jurisdictions, all infants are screened with otoacoustic emissions, or automated auditory brainstem responses (ABR), prior to discharge from the newborn nursery. Where universal screening is not available, newborns are selected for screening tests based upon the presence of risk factors. However, this may miss up to 50 per cent of children with HL. Some of the more important risk factors are a family history of HL, maternal TORCH infections during pregnancy (toxoplasmosis, rubella, cytomegalovirus, herpes), syphilis, craniofacial malformations, birthweight less than 1500 g, kernicterus, birth asphyxia, and meningitis.

Paediatric and geriatric

Screening for HL should be part of the routine paediatric evaluation even if the child passed newborn screening, because of the possible development of serous otitis media and delayed onset NSHL. Pay special attention to the abovementioned risk factors, and check the milestones for speech and hearing: under 3 months, startled by loud sounds and calmed by familiar voices; by 6 months, able to localize sounds; at 9 months, responds to name and mimics environmental sounds; and by 1 year expresses first meaningful words. Ask the parents whether they suspect a hearing problem and how their child's speech is developing. Note the following points: Is it difficult to get the child's attention? Does the child prefer the television loud? Is there a behaviour problem? How is the child doing at school?

To screen for HL in the geriatric population, ask the patient or a relative whether he/she has difficulty carrying on a conversation, complains that others mumble, or fails to hear the telephone ring. Bear in mind that withdrawn individuals may have HL.

Diagnosis of hearing loss

History

Events associated with the onset of HL are often useful in pointing to a diagnosis if the onset is sudden or relatively rapid—upper respiratory tract infection, air travel, swimming, occupational or recreational noise exposure, or open heart surgery (cochlear hypoxia).

Check whether the patient uses cotton-tipped applicators as they can push wax into the canal and occlude it. Ask about the cardinal ear symptoms of vertigo, tinnitus, otalgia, otorrhoea, and facial paralysis. Ask the patient specifically if there was a past history of HL or treatment for ear disease as some patients will not volunteer the information of prior hearing aid use or even ear surgery. Ask whether there is a family history of HL or a history of exposure to noise or ototoxic medication.

Physical examination

General

Note the articulation and volume of the patient's speech. Poor articulation may indicate a pre-lingual HL. Loud speech suggests NSHL and quiet speech conductive HL. The person who dominates the interview might be hiding a HL.

If it is difficult to converse with the patient, the physician should quantify his/her impression by whispering five words at two and ten feet (0.5 and 3 m) with the mouth covered so that the patient cannot lipread. What percentage is detected and what percentage correctly repeated? Test each ear separately by covering the non-test ear.

Wax and foreign-body removal

With a headlight or otoscope, check the ear canals for wax and foreign bodies. The most common cause of sudden hearing loss is to be found here.

Wax can be removed by syringe, curette, forceps, or suction. In the presence of infection, if a drum perforation is suspected, or if the foreign body is vegetable material that can swell with water, syringing is inadvisable. However, for the majority of patients, syringing is the method of first choice. A specially made metal ear syringe is widely available and produces an effective jet of water, but a disposable 10-cc syringe with a soft intravenous catheter can also be used. If syringing is unsuccessful, instruct the patient to use mineral oil, if the wax is hard, or 3 per cent peroxide, if the wax is soft, twice a day and return in a week for repeat syringing. For those with eczema, give antibiotic drops for a few days after syringing to prevent bacterial otitis externa. Curettage works best for dry wax in the outer part of the canal. Hard foreign bodies are removed by passing a small angled curette or blunt hook beyond the object and extracting it. Insects in the canal can be killed with 70 per cent isopropyl alcohol and removed with alligator forceps. The young child might need a general anaesthetic for foreign-body removal.

Ear drum

Pneumatic otoscopy is covered in the paediatric section.

Tuning fork evaluation

Equipment

The most useful tuning fork for testing hearing is the 512-Hz fork. One low-frequency fork, 125 Hz, and one high-frequency fork, 4096 Hz, can give helpful additional information: low-frequency NSHL is seen in Meniere's disease and high-frequency NSHL is seen in presbycusis and noise-induced NSHL.

Air conduction comparison

Position the vibrating 512-Hz fork in a consistent orientation and distance from each of the patient's ears in turn, asking the patient to compare the loudness between the right and left ears. Repeat the procedure with the low- and high-frequency forks.

Weber test

Set the 512-Hz fork vibrating and wrap gauze around the stem for hygiene. Ask the patient to bite the fork with the central incisors and indicate the direction from which the sound appears to be coming. In the edentulous patient, press the fork firmly in the midline of the mandible or forehead. The sound tends to lateralize toward an ear with a conductive loss and away from a neurosensory loss.

Rinne test

The stem of the vibrating 512-Hz fork is placed firmly on the skull behind the auricle and the patient asked to listen to this bone conduction (BC) sound. Then, change the position of the fork to the usual one for air conduction (AC) and ask the patient to compare the loudness. Normally, or for moderate NSHL, AC is louder than BC. For a conductive HL more than 15 dB, BC is louder than AC.

Cranial nerves

Symptoms of facial weakness and nystagmus are checked.

Nose and throat

Persistent serous otitis media in the adult necessitates evaluation for cancer of the nasopharynx by direct visualization of that area and examination of the neck for adenopathy.

Audiological evaluation

Hearing can be evaluated at any age. This will determine the presence of HL, the degree of HL, and the proportions of conductive and NSHL. For NSHL, a distinction between cochlear and retrocochlear site-of-lesion can be made.

The standard audiological evaluation as performed by an audiologist consists of three parts:

- *Pure tone threshold audiogram:* a graph of the patient's hearing sensitivity in decibels for frequencies ranging from 250 to 8000 Hz is generated with an air curve and a bone curve for each ear. In conductive HL, there is a gap between the curves; in NSHL, the curves overlie each other. Some configurations are diagnostic. Thresholds of 0–20 dB are classified as normal, while 20–40 dB indicate a mild HL, 40–60 dB a moderate, 60–80 dB moderately-severe, 80–100 dB severe, and over 100 dB a profound HL.

- *Speech audiometry:* words are presented at a comfortable volume, and the percentage correctly repeated, the speech discrimination score, is a measure of the clarity of hearing. Low scores suggest retrocochlear involvement and poor hearing aid candidacy.

- *Impedance tympanometry:* a probe is positioned firmly in the ear canal and the machine performs the test automatically in a few seconds, generating a graph of eardrum mobility versus middle ear pressure.

For babies, young children, and adults who cannot cooperate or who have a decreased level of consciousness, special techniques and the following automated tests can be performed:

- *Auditory brainstem responses (ABR):* repetitive click stimuli evoke central nervous system potentials, which are recorded by scalp electrodes and computer-averaged to reveal a waveform.

- *Otoacoustic emissions:* an ear canal probe is used to record very faint sound emissions originating from the outer hair cells of the cochlea, thus providing a measure of cochlear integrity.

Differential diagnosis

Conductive hearing loss

- Except for wax, the most common cause of conductive HL or mixed HL is *otitis media*, including serous otitis media, perforations, cholesteatoma, and tympanosclerosis. This is covered in another chapter.

- If the eardrum is normal, the most likely cause is *otosclerosis*. Typically, it causes fixation of the footplate of the stapes with mixed HL. Stapedectomy is highly effective.

- *Head trauma* may cause haemotympanum and ossicular chain dislocation.

Neurosensory hearing loss

- The most common cause of NSHL is aging (*presbycusis*).

- The second most frequent cause is *noise exposure*, both occupational and recreational (see section on Prevention).

- *Head trauma* can cause all degrees of NSHL.

- *Infections*, in particular, in utero TORCH infections, meningitis, otitis media, and spirochetal infections.

- Some drugs, in particular the aminoglycoside antibiotics and some antineoplastic agents (especially cisplatin), can produce permanent NSHL (see section on Prevention).

- *Meniere's disease* is an inner ear dysfunction diagnosed by the triad of episodic vertigo, fluctuating low-frequency NSHL, and tinnitus.

Classically, the severe whirling vertigo attacks last about 30 min and are separated by intervals of days to months of calm. The examination is normal (except for the NSHL) between attacks. With time, the HL progresses to a permanent, moderate-to-severe NSHL, across all frequencies and the vertigo lessens. It becomes bilateral in 20 per cent of patients. The aetiology is unknown. Systemic illnesses should be ruled out, and ABR or imaging is done to exclude acoustic neuroma. Treatment is empirical and begins with: management of any stress or systemic illness identified; a low sodium diet; and avoidance of caffeine, alcohol, tobacco, or any other trigger the patient identifies. If symptoms persist to an unacceptable degree, a daily diuretic is started. If control is still inadequate, betahistine 8–16 mg bid-qid is tried before considering chemical or surgical labyrinthectomy.

◆ *Idiopathic sudden NSHL* occurs over a period of minutes to hours and is thought to be a cochlear event caused by viral infection, vascular insufficiency, or rupture of an inner ear membrane. Prognosis for recovery of hearing is worse if the patient is elderly, if there is vertigo, or if the degree of HL is severe. Empirical treatment with steroids and antiviral medications may be started while blood tests and imaging are done to rule out systemic illnesses and acoustic neuroma.

◆ *Acoustic neuroma* is, in fact, a schwannoma of the vestibular portion of VIII and should be considered in any patient with unilateral (or asymmetrical) NSHL. The gold standard for diagnosis is magnetic resonance imaging. Alternatives are contrast-enhanced CT of the cerebellopontine angles and ABR. Excision is desirable, but radiotherapy and watchful waiting are also employed.

◆ *Genetic* hearing loss may be present at birth or appear later in life; also, genetic factors probably play a role in most forms of HL.

Treatment

The child with permanent childhood hearing impairment will require thorough evaluation, amplification, and possibly cochlear implantation. Hearing aids can be fitted to infants as young as 2 months; cochlear implantation has been performed successfully at 7 months. Parental counselling and special education for the child may be desirable depending on the degree of HL. Sign language, oral communication, or a combination may be used as a basis for education. In general, conductive HL is surgically correctable but NSHL is not.

Hearing aids provide amplification and are especially successful for conductive HL and NSHL with good discrimination. They are considered desirable when the hearing loss reaches about 30 dB. Some hearing aids are small enough to fit in the ear canal; newer digital aids provide improved intelligibility, but consumer dissatisfaction is still high. Therefore, middle ear implantable hearing aids are being developed.

Assistive listening devices include a diverse range of products designed for specific problems. Examples include microphone-and-headset systems for the classroom or church, captioned television programmes, and visual alerting systems for the doorbell.

Cochlear implants involve the placement of a wire into the scala tympani of the cochlea, to enable electrical stimulation of the cochlear nerve endings by sound. They are not widely available in most countries. Most implants have been for bilateral, profound, post-lingual hearing loss, when there was no benefit from hearing aids. Recently, indications have been extended to include lesser degrees of hearing loss, as well as very young (prelingual) children who seem to derive the most benefit of all. However, the deaf community has expressed strong opposition to implantation in children.

Prevention

Noise-induced NSHL

Noise reduction in the workplace is a public health initiative that can have a great impact on HL. Safe doses of steady noise (90 dBA for 8 h) and impact noise have been determined, but can be costly for industry to achieve. Earmuffs provide more protection (40 dB attenuation) than earplugs (20 dB); in very noisy environments, workers should use both. Legislation should require industries with noise levels above 85 dBA to implement hearing conservation programmes consisting of audiometric monitoring, personal hearing protection, and otologic referral if HL is identified.

NSHL from recreational noise is commonly seen in those who use firearms, power tools, and chain saws, and occasionally in those who listen to loud music. Education and recommendation of ear protectors can help many avoid the permanent sequelae of NSHL and tinnitus.

Ototoxicity

Although salicylates, quinines, and loop diuretics can produce tinnitus and (usually temporary) NSHL, it is the aminoglycoside antibiotics (e.g. streptomycin, gentamicin, neomycin), cisplatin and erythromycin, which are the most important ototoxic agents the primary care physician may need to regulate. For aminoglycosides, the dose is calculated based on weight and renal function, the serum peak and trough levels monitored, administered for as short a time as possible, and the concurrent use of loop diuretics avoided. Several eardrop preparations contain aminoglycosides and should not be given in the presence of a perforated eardrum. Question patients receiving ototoxic drugs about audiovestibular symptoms, and arrange audiologic monitoring for those on prolonged courses of aminoglycosides and all patients on cisplatin.

Key points

1. Screening for hearing loss should be part of routine paediatric and geriatric examinations.

2. Audiologists can evaluate infants suspected of having hearing loss. There is no need to wait for the child to get older.

3. Sudden neurosensory hearing loss may benefit from immediate evaluation and treatment.

4. Unilateral, or asymmetric, neurosensory hearing loss warrants an investigation for acoustic neuroma.

5. Persistent, unilateral serous otitis media in the adult is nasopharyngeal carcinoma until proven otherwise.

6. Prevention of noise-induced neurosensory hearing loss and ototoxicity is more effective than treatment.

Further reading

Cummings, C. et al., ed. *Otolaryngology—Head and Neck Surgery* 3rd edn. St Louis: Mosby, 1998.

Alberti, P.W. and Ruben, R.J., ed. *Otologic Medicine and Surgery*. New York: Churchill Livingstone, 1988.

Grundfast, K.M. (1996). Hearing loss. In *Pediatric Otolaryngology* 3rd edn (ed. C. Bluestone, S. Stool, and M. Kenna). Philadelphia: WB Saunders Company.

American Academy of Otolaryngology: www.entnet.org.

Canadian Hard of Hearing Association: www.chha.ca.

Horn, K.L. and McDaniel, S.L., ed. (December 1999). Early identification and intervention of hearing-impaired infants. *The Otolaryngologic Clinics of North America* **32** (6).

Doyle, K.J., ed. (October 2000). Audiology. In *Current Opinion in Otolaryngology & Head and Neck Surgery* (ed. P. Donald and J. Gluckman) **8** (5), 403–40.

3.5 Hoarseness and voice change

Francoise P. Chagnon

Voice disorders are ubiquitous and usually temporary. Everyone has experienced the hoarseness of laryngitis or vocal fatigue after a long day of talking. Persistent hoarseness, however, will bring the patient to medical attention because it alters vocal identity or impairs vocal performance.

For many reasons, women with voice disorders (dysphonia) are more likely to consult than are men. Diseases of the vocal cords readily alter the acoustics of the female voice and the occupational demands on women's voices may exceed the physiological output of the female larynx. The female larynx is also exposed to hormonal fluctuations and changes in the voice during the pre-menstrual period do occur and can be troublesome for singers.

Childhood voice disorders are the result of congenital or early acquired malformations of the larynx and vocal cords. In school-age children, particularly boys, dysphonias are the result of excessive voice use during play.

Detecting anomalies in the voice requires an attentive ear and gives full meaning to the adage that physicians should listen to their patients. Voice changes are often interpreted as signs of fatigue or stress while the possibility of an organic vocal pathology can be too easily dismissed. Many systemic disorders have laryngological manifestations of which hoarseness is an early symptom.

A basic knowledge of the mechanics of phonation (the production of sound by the larynx) is helpful in the understanding of voice disorders. Voicing is the result of volitional control of expiration, vocal cord approximation, and the fine-tuning of the vocal musculature and vocal tract. The sound that emanates from the lips is the result of sound produced at the glottis and modulated in the resonant oropharynx. Diseases may impair phonation by decreasing expiratory flow or by distorting the surface cover of the vocal cord. Diseases affecting the vocal musculature or the integrity of the crico-arytenoid joint interfere with vocal cord mobility. The innervation of the larynx makes it susceptible to lesions impinging on the course of the laryngeal nerves in the neck and mediastinum.

The diagnosis of voice disorders

History

Most voice disorders develop slowly and are not accompanied by significant disability or discomfort. It is only when the dysphonia becomes obvious (as a change in vocal identity) to the listener or connotes ill health that patients feel pressured to seek medical care.

It is important to determine if symptoms are restricted to voicing or if other laryngeal functions, such as swallowing and coughing, are affected as well.

The term hoarseness is used to describe a variety of vocal symptoms. It usually refers to a coarse or scratchy sound. Habitual clearing of the throat in attempts to restore voice quality is commonly associated. Alterations in the intensity of the voice are described as breathiness or weakness. Vocal fatigue is a subjective feeling of effortful phonation and difficulty in sustaining the quality of the voice. Patients may refer to throat feelings of dryness, tightness or choking, and painful voicing.

Singers are aware of discrete perceptual changes in vocal quality and provide detailed and accurate description of the nature of their vocal ailments. They will refer to a loss of vocal range (especially in the high notes), pitch breaks (momentary loss of sound), and difficulties in the transition between 'chest voice' (low vocal range) and 'head voice' (high vocal range).

Certain features of the medical history point to specific aetiological possibilities:

- Sudden onset of dysphonia or aphonia is a rare event in the absence of trauma. Sustained phonation at high intensity (yelling and screaming)

can traumatize the delicate surface on the vocal cords. Indeed, the most common lesions on the vocal cords (nodules and polyps) are benign and the result of acute or repeated trauma during phonation. Endotracheal and nasogastric intubations can injure vocal cords and the crico-arytenoid joints. Traumatic life event can lead to psychogenic aphonia and patients with this may not volunteer such occurrences; history-taking must explore possible causal links.

- A rapidly developing dysphonia typically occurs with acute inflammatory conditions such as allergic or infectious laryngitis.

- Intermittent dysphonia can be linked to patterns of voice use or environmental factors. The occupational and social history must be explored.

- Chronic dysphonias are usually the result of chronic inflammatory disorders of the larynx such as smoker's laryngitis. Inquiries into smoking habits should not omit the smoking of marijuana or hashish in addition to tobacco. Alterations in the habitual hoarseness of a smoker may herald laryngeal cancer. If chronic neurological disorders such as multiple sclerosis or amyotrophic lateral sclerosis lead to difficulty in swallowing, the voice is also invariably affected.

Common diseases affecting the voice

Frequently encountered disease entities affecting the voice include the following:

- *Gastroesophageal reflux laryngitis:* the dysphonia is typically worse upon arising from sleep as reflux occurred in the supine position. The voice is low pitch and the throat must be repeatedly cleared of secretions. There is a constant feeling of dryness and irritation of the throat.

- *Laryngeal nerve paralysis:* surgery to the neck, thyroid, chest, and mediastinum are a frequent cause of unilateral vocal cord paralysis. Idiopathic causes are thought to be viral neuropathies of the recurrent laryngeal nerve (similar to Bell's palsy). Pulmonary and mediastinal malignancies can involve the recurrent laryngeal nerve.

- *Other neurological disorders:* conditions such as amyotrophic lateral sclerosis, multiple sclerosis, or myasthenia gravis can lead to weakness of the voice or a spasmodic and strained voice. Difficulties in swallowing and speech as well as other neurological signs will usually be present. The exception is spasmodic dysphonia or laryngeal dystonia, a condition which primarily affects women and is commonly mistaken for psychogenic dysphonia (see below).

- *Respiratory disorders:* conditions that result in respiratory dysfunction, such as asthma and chronic obstructive pulmonary disease, tend to reduce vocal output and cause vocal fatigue.

- *Endocrine disorders:* advanced hypothyroidism leads to swelling of the vocal cords, hoarseness, and vocal fatigue. Changes in the voice during the pre-menstrual period do occur and can be troublesome for singers.

- *Psychological disorders:* the voice manifests anxiety and emotional stress. The larynx does so by inappropriate tension of the laryngeal muscles on phonation. The voice is either strained (effortful phonation) or strangled (a choking sound) in hyperfunctional dysphonias or very weak in hypofunctional dysphonias.

- *Laryngeal cancer:* cancer of the larynx most commonly arises from the surface epithelium of the vocal cords. Cancers of the larynx arising from other sites may go undetected until such times as they obstruct the airway and before obvious voice changes occur.

- *Adverse drug effects:* many medications adversely affect the voice and do so by drying the vocal tract, affecting neuromuscular control, or by hormonal influences. Some of the worst offenders are antihistamines, anxiolytics, tricyclic antidepressants, and hormonal replacement therapies.

Physical examination

Before attention is given to the larynx, a complete examination of the ears, nose, throat, and neck is necessary when looking for evidence of infectious or allergic sinonasal conditions or cervical masses.

The diagnosis of voice disorders cannot be made by the perception of the voice alone as vocal pathologies do not have characteristic acoustic patterns. The acoustics are determined by the location of the lesion on the vocal cord, its effects on vocal cord approximation, and compensatory laryngeal behaviours. Nevertheless, it is safe to assume that diplophonia (hearing two pitches on phonation) is caused by asymmetries in vocal cord mass and tension while breathiness or aphonia results from incomplete vocal cord approximation.

The severity of the dysphonia is not always a predictor of the severity of the vocal pathology. For example, acute viral laryngitis leads to aphonia from mild vocal cord oedema, while patients with laryngeal cancers may have a normal voice.

Patients with dysphonia should be put through simple vocal tasks to evaluate the essential laryngeal functions of breathing, deep inspiration and expiration through an open glottis, coughing (is the cough strong?), swallowing (witness swallowing of water and check for aspiration or coughing), and phonation (take a deep breath and sustain a vowel; sing up and down the scale).

Laryngoscopy

Indirect mirror laryngoscopy visualizes the vocal cords and surrounding structures of the larynx and pharynx. Diminishing the gag reflex with topical anaesthesia of the pharynx with lidocaine 10 per cent spray is very helpful.

Indirect mirror *examination* addresses two important questions:

◆ *Are the vocal cords mobile?* Vocal cord mobility is assessed during quiet breathing (the glottis should assume a triangular shape), during forced inspiration and expiration (the glottis will assume a pentagonal shape), and during phonation of the vowel 'e' (both vocal cords should meet in the midline). Failure of one vocal cord to adduct towards the midline during phonation will allow the escape of air through the glottis (with a resulting breathy voice and weak cough) while allowing aspiration during deglutition. Failure of both vocal cords to abduct still permits good phonation but biphasic stridor will be elicited on deep respiration. Involuntary movements of the cords during quiet breathing are signs of neurological disorders such as tremor or dystonia.

◆ *Are there obvious laryngeal lesions?* Swelling of the larynx or obvious tumour masses may impair the glottic airway. Pedunculated tissue may flop in and out of the glottic airway causing breaks in phonation or intermittently obstructing the airway. Having the patient vary the rate and depth of respiration may bring such lesions into view.

Inflammatory lesions are the most frequent conditions found during laryngoscopy. In acute bacterial or viral laryngitis, the larynx is diffusely erythematous and the vocal cords oedematous. Allergic laryngitis causes vocal oedema. Typical whitish deposits scattered throughout the larynx are seen in fungal laryngitis, while tuberculous granulomas have a predilection for the posterior glottis. Gastroesophageal reflux laryngitis will appear with swelling, erythema, and mucosal changes (pachydermia) of the posterior glottis.

Benign traumatic lesions on the vocal cords appear as localized sub-epithelial swellings and haemorrhages. Vocal nodules (singer's nodules) are bilateral localized sub-mucosal excrescences due to swelling, situated in the middle third of the free edge of the vocal cords. Vocal polyps are sessile or pedunculated and usually unilateral. The exception is the diffuse polypoidal degeneration of both vocal cords typically seen in female smokers.

Cancer of the vocal cords presents initially as white keratinous patches. More advanced cancers will appear as a fungating mass impairing vocal cord mobility.

There are pitfalls to indirect mirror laryngoscopy.

A variety of glottic lesions may not be visible on indirect mirror laryngoscopy and, therefore, a 'negative' examination does not necessarily rule out significant disease. When further assessment is clinically indicated, the technique of choice for a rapid and easily performed examination of the upper airway is the flexible fibreoptic naso-pharyngo-laryngoscopy. Coupled with stroboscopic examination of the vibratory surface of the vocal cords, this technique can define subtle vocal disorders.

Investigations

In the case of unilateral vocal cord immobility due to laryngeal nerve paralysis, radiological imaging of the chest, neck, or cranium is often indicated. Computerized tomography of the larynx is ancillary in the diagnosis of laryngeal cancers or thyroid tumours affecting the larynx. Barium oesophagram findings might support the diagnosis of gastroesophageal reflux.

Treatment

Since voice disorders are most often multifactorial, treatments aimed at concomitant disorders are essential. In particular, treatment of allergic and bacterial sinonasal and pharyngotonsillar infections is needed.

Some otolaryngologists use systemic corticosteroids in the treatment of mild acute inflammatory vocal oedema when it is essential for the patient to use the voice in the immediate future. Such treatment is usually reserved for professional singers obliged to perform and is given only after full disclosure of the potential side-effects of the drugs.

Topical analgesics to the laryngeal and pharyngeal structures should be avoided as they encourage forceful phonation. Lozenges and throat gargles are of little direct benefit in the treatment of inflammatory vocal lesions but may prove soothing and help clear tenacious secretions from the vocal cords.

If no obvious vocal lesions are identified on indirect laryngoscopy, general principles of vocal hygiene that can be instituted while awaiting clarification of the diagnosis from an otolaryngologist include the following:

◆ *Voice rest:* voice rest is of benefit to most vocal ailments but social needs make it difficult to maintain complete silence beyond 2 days. Whispering should be avoided as it induces vocal tension. Rather, a confidential tone of voice can be used. Patterns of abuse (such as prolonged talking) or misuse (such as speaking loudly) of the voice should be avoided and frequent breaks in talking should be scheduled during the workday. Teachers and public speakers should be encouraged to use voice amplification devices.

◆ *Hydration:* increased daily intake of water and inspiration of water or saline through a vaporizer or steam generator are very helpful.

◆ *Antireflux measures:* elevation of the head of the bed; avoidance of eating 3 h before going to sleep; antacids.

◆ *Smoking cessation.*

Most patients with voice disorders will benefit from the expertise of a speech–language pathologist. Voice therapy is particularly useful in acquiring efficient phonation behaviours and preventing further vocal trauma. It is the treatment of choice for vocal nodules. Psychogenic voice disorders may prove recalcitrant to treatment and a source of prolonged vocal disability. Psychotherapeutic interventions combined, when indicated, with antidepressants are often necessary.

The primary care physician may be asked to assess the ability of a singer to perform with an acute vocal ailment. The presence of an acute vocal haemorrhage would be a contra-indication to singing. If the dysphonia is mild, the singer might be able to adapt the repertoire to a limited vocal range. When in doubt, it is better to prevent singing and recommend strict voice rest for 24 h. Professional singers with voice disorders should receive prompt attention from an otolaryngologist since early intervention can prevent permanent disabilities of the singing voice.

Conclusion

Basic knowledge of the mechanics of phonation and the ability to perform indirect laryngoscopy are a prerequisite to understanding voice disorders.

Combined with the information obtained from a detailed medical history, most disorders affecting the voice can be identified.

The primary care physician plays a significant role in the prevention and detection of voice disorders. Since most voice disorders are the result of trauma to the vocal cords from the overuse of the voice, high-risk individuals are easily identified and benefit from a referral to an otolaryngologist and speech–language pathologist.

Key points

♦ Voice disorders are multifactorial.

♦ Mirror laryngoscopy may miss discrete vocal lesions.

♦ Most vocal lesions are benign and the result of phonotrauma.

Further reading

Simpson, C.B. and Fleming, D.J. (2000). Medical and vocal history in the evaluation of dysphonia. *The Otolaryngology Clinics of North America. Voice Disorders and Phonosurgery I.* (ed. C.A. Rosen and T. Murray) **33** (4), 719–29. WB Saunders Company.

Sataloff, R.T. (1988). Professional singers: the art and science of clinical care. In *Instructional Courses* (ed. J.T. Johnson, A. Blitzer, R.H. Ossof, and J.R. Thomas), pp. 299–327. The American Academy of Otolaryngology and Head and Neck Surgery. St Louis: The C.V. Mosby Company. (An excellent review for those involved in the care of professional voice users.)

3.6 Acute sinusitis

Morten Lindbak and John M. Hickner

Epidemiology of acute sinusitis

The incidence of sinusitis-like illness severe enough to prompt a visit to the doctor is between 1.6 and 3.5 episodes per 100 adults per year in Western developed countries.[1,2] A Norwegian study found an incidence of 3.5 cases per 100 adults per year. Seven per cent of the patients had two episodes and 0.5 per cent had three or more episodes during a 12-month period.[1] There was seasonal variation with the highest frequency in the winter and lowest in the summer and autumn. In a Swedish study, acute sinusitis constituted 2 per cent of all primary care consultations.[3] We know little about how frequently sinusitis occurs in tropical areas and in people who do not seek medical care. In a phone survey in Canada, during a 2-week period, only 15 per cent of people with acute respiratory infection symptoms sought medical care.[4] From community-based studies in the United States, it has been estimated that adults have two or three common colds each year and that 0.5–2 per cent of these result in acute bacterial sinusitis.[5]

Gender differences in acute sinusitis

Acute sinusitis is diagnosed more often in women than in men. In a large Norwegian study of 250 000 patients in primary care, 68 per cent of those with acute sinusitis were women compared to 58 per cent for other acute respiratory illnesses.[6] The higher frequency in women may be due to differences in health-care seeking behaviour, greater exposure to upper respiratory infections from child care duties, and increased mucosal thickening due to oestrogen exposure leading to a greater likelihood of ostial obstruction and subsequent sinus infection.[1]

Frequency of acute sinusitis in children

The incidence of acute bacterial sinusitis in children is unknown. Children experience several viral respiratory infections per year and 7–10 per cent of these are complicated by acute bacterial sinusitis.[7] In a study of children in primary care practice, acute sinusitis accounted for 9.3 per cent of all visits and 17.3 per cent of visits for patients with cold and cough symptoms.[8] The bacteria causing acute sinusitis in children are the same as in adults.

Pathogenesis, aetiology, and definitions

Sinusitis means inflammation of the mucosa of the paranasal sinuses irrespective of the cause. Some prefer the term rhinosinusitis because isolated inflammation of the sinuses is uncommon. By definition, acute sinusitis lasts less than 30 days, subacute sinusitis lasts from 1 to 3 months, and chronic sinusitis lasts longer than 3 months.[9] Most cases of sinusitis involve more than one of the paranasal sinuses, most commonly the maxillary and ethmoid sinuses. In a study of acute bacterial sinusitis diagnosed by CT scan (a positive test was either a fluid level or total opacification), two-thirds of the patients had involvement of the maxillary sinuses, frequently in combination with the ethmoid sinuses. One-third had involvement of the ethmoid, sphenoid, or frontal sinuses without involvement of the maxillary sinuses.[10]

Predisposing factors

The most common predisposing factor is a viral upper respiratory infection. Allergic rhinitis is assumed to be a predisposing factor, but research data are conflicting.[5] Viral upper respiratory infections and allergic rhinitis can lead to mucosa oedema, ostial narrowing, increased secretion, and decreased mucociliary activity. A dysfunctional mucociliary system, anatomic malformations, polyps, septal deviation, foreign bodies, and tumours may cause ostial obstruction leading to sinusitis.[11] In some cases, sinusitis is caused by upper tooth infections that spread directly to the maxillary sinus.[5]

Viral (serous) sinusitis

Viral infections cause mucosal thickening that may narrow or close the ostium causing decreased oxygen concentration, increased carbon dioxide concentration, and formation of a serous secretion in the sinus.[12] This condition is called *serous sinusitis* and may give modest symptoms of facial pressure. Most of these cases resolve spontaneously.[13]

Bacterial (purulent) sinusitis

Acute bacterial sinusitis is usually a secondary infection resulting from sinus ostia obstruction and/or impaired mucus clearance mechanisms caused by an acute viral upper respiratory tract infection.[5] When bacteria enter via the ostium and serous secretions and good growth conditions are present, bacteria grow rapidly. The body responds with an inflammatory reaction, and polymorphonuclear leucocytes are mobilized resulting in pus formation, or *acute mucopurulent sinusitis*. The finding of mucopurulent pus usually means a good prognosis. But occasionally the inflammatory system of the body does not limit bacterial growth. The infection progresses and the pus becomes thinner, homogenous, and foul smelling. When this occurs, there is greater risk of irreversible damage to the sinus mucosa and complications.

Microbiology

The most common bacterial pathogens are *Streptococcus pneumoniae* and *Hæmophilus influenzae*, accounting for about 50 per cent of infections.[5,14]

Moraxella catarrhalis and Group A streptococci are the next most common pathogens. Anaerobic bacteria, most of them beta-lactamase producing, occasionally cause sinusitis. Fungal sinusitis is uncommon but should be considered in immunocompromised patients.

Diagnosis of acute bacterial sinusitis

For most primary care patients, the diagnosis of sinusitis can be made based on the clinical history and examination without any supportive laboratory or imaging studies. Four studies from primary care provide useful information on symptoms, signs, and blood tests that help discriminate bacterial sinusitis from viral sinusitis and viral upper respiratory infections.[2,14–16] Purulent rhinorrhoea as a symptom was associated with bacterial sinusitis in three of the four studies. The finding of purulent secretions in the nasal cavity and tooth pain was associated with bacterial infection in two. Other findings are less consistent predictors of bacterial sinusitis. A biphasic history with worsening following initial improvement and lack of effect of decongestants were associated with bacterial infection in one study each and were not investigated in the others. An erythrocyte sedimentation rate (ESR) greater than 10 for men and greater than 20 for women was associated in the two studies where it was investigated, while C-reactive protein (CRP) greater than 10 was associated in one, but not in the other where it was investigated. However, all these studies are limited by use of imperfect diagnostic standards. (The best diagnostic standard is sinus puncture and aspiration of purulent fluid growing greater than 10^4 organisms per millilitre.) No single sign or symptom had strong diagnostic value in any of these studies.

A number of clinical signs and symptoms presented in clinical guidelines have not been proven to be of value in primary care studies. These are: illness starting with an upper respiratory tract infection, pain on bending forward, unilateral or bilateral pain over the maxillary sinuses, pain over the frontal sinuses, headache, allergy, malaise, cough, foul taste and foul smell, nasal congestion, fever greater than 38°C, tenderness over the maxillary and frontal sinuses, purulent pharyngeal discharge, swelling over the maxillary sinuses, and a prior diagnosis of sinusitis. Although many of these factors occur frequently with acute sinusitis, they are not good predictors of bacterial sinusitis because these symptoms are equally common with viral upper respiratory tract infections.[15,16]

Because acute bacterial sinusitis usually develops as a complication of viral upper respiratory tract infections, experts have proposed that duration of illness of less than 7 days be used as a negative diagnostic criterion. In clinical trials of diagnosis and treatment of sinusitis, duration of illness alone did not reliably distinguish prolonged viral infection from bacterial sinusitis. However, in two studies by Lindbaek, 80 per cent of patients with CT-confirmed sinusitis were symptomatic for more than 7 days, while 70 per cent of patients with similar symptoms but without CT-confirmed sinusitis were symptomatic for more than 7 days.[16,17] The difference in duration between patients was statistically significant ($p = 0.03$), but this difference is small from a clinical standpoint.

Use of radiography and ultrasound in the diagnosis of acute bacterial sinusitis

The value of plain sinus X-rays in the diagnosis of bacterial sinusitis is limited. When using fluid level or opacity as the criteria for bacterial sinusitis, the sensitivity and specificity of X-ray is 76 and 79 per cent, respectively.[18] When mucosal thickening more than 5 mm is included as a positive test, the specificity is much lower. The test characteristics of ultrasonography are unstable and unsatisfactory.[19] The average specificity is low, 69 per cent, giving a high proportion of false positive cases. However, a normal plain X-ray or ultrasound is good evidence against bacterial infection. Sinus CT has a high specificity, about 90 per cent, when using presence of a fluid level or total opacification as the diagnostic criteria for acute bacterial sinusitis. CT has the advantage of giving a good evaluation of the frontal, sphenoid, and ethmoid sinuses, which are frequently affected, especially the ethmoid sinuses. The disadvantages of CT are expense and lack of general availability.

Differential diagnosis

A severe common cold is the condition most often confused with acute bacterial sinusitis.[5] A number of recurring pain conditions such as atypical migraine, tension headache, trigeminal neuralgia, and dysfunction of the temporal–mandibular joint must be considered, as these conditions can mimic bacterial sinusitis.[20] Recurrent episodes of facial pain without purulent nasal secretions suggest a non-infectious cause. A negative X-ray or ultrasonography will exclude sinusitis in these cases. A combination of a painful condition and a common cold can be difficult to distinguish from bacterial sinusitis.

Diagnosis in children

Accurate diagnosis of acute bacterial sinusitis in children is difficult, but should be based on the clinical presentation rather than imaging studies. Bacterial sinusitis should be suspected in children with persistent or severe sinusitis-like symptoms lasting greater than 10–14 days.[21] Unfortunately, symptoms in children include even less specific than in adults. Symptoms suggesting bacterial sinusitis include persistent nasal or post-nasal discharge of any quality and persistent daytime cough not explained by asthma or allergic disease. Facial pain and tenderness are not common findings in children with bacterial sinusitis.[21] A symptom-free period during a prolonged respiratory infection suggests a second viral infection rather than bacterial sinusitis. High fever for 3–4 days accompanied by facial pain and/or purulent nasal discharge suggests severe sinusitis that needs urgent management.[21]

Imaging studies are not often helpful in children with sinusitis-like complaints. In a study of children aged 2–16, positive bacterial cultures were obtained on sinus puncture in 70–75 per cent of children with persistent or severe sinusitis-like symptoms and abnormal sinus radiographs (complete opacification, mucosal thickening of at least 4 mm or an air-fluid level).[22] However, persistent unimproved symptoms for longer than 10 days predict abnormal sinus radiographs in 80 per cent of cases, so radiographs add little predictive value to diagnosis over clinical presentation. As in adults, a completely normal sinus radiograph is strong evidence against bacterial sinusitis.

Treatment of acute sinusitis

Symptomatic treatment

Topically or orally administered alpha-adrenergic agents (decongestants), proteolytic enzymes, nasal irrigation with salt water, mucolytic agents, antihistamines, and corticosteroids have been used for symptom relief in acute sinusitis. Though none of these are of proven value, they may be offered for symptom relief. The results of eight randomized trials of various symptomatic treatments in adults have been summarized.[23] Theoretically, agents that encourage drainage of sinus secretions may be of value. Pain control is always worthwhile.[16,24]

Antibiotic treatment

Patients presenting with less than 7 days of mild to moderate symptoms consistent with acute sinusitis should be given symptomatic treatment only. Most of these cases of sinusitis are caused by viruses or mild bacterial infections that will resolve without antibiotic treatment. Antibiotic treatment should be reserved for patients with moderately severe symptoms of bacterial sinusitis of greater than 7 days duration and for those with severe sinusitis symptoms (severe pain or fever greater than 39°C) regardless of duration of illness.

Five randomized double-blind clinical trials, using valid methods, have compared antibiotic with placebo treatment of acute sinusitis in adults.[17,25–28] One used clinical findings for diagnosis,[28] three used plain radiographs,[25–27] and one used computed tomography criteria.[17] When considered in aggregate, 47 per cent of the antibiotic-treated subjects and 32 per cent of the control subjects were considered cured at 10–14 days follow-up, while 81 per cent of antibiotic-treated patients and 66 per cent of controls were responders (with clinical findings of either cure or improvement).[29] This is an absolute benefit of 15 per cent, giving a number needed to treat of seven.

However, two of these placebo-controlled trials failed to find a significant effect of antibiotic treatment. Stalman studied the effectiveness of doxycycline compared to placebo in general practice patients with symptoms of bacterial sinusitis.[28] There was no significant difference in time to resolution of facial pain and return to normal activities between the treatment and control groups. Using radiographs for the diagnostic standard with total opacity, fluid level or mucosal thickening greater than 5 mm, van Buchem found no significant advantage of a 7-day course of amoxicillin over placebo at 14 days.[27] Symptoms were substantially improved or resolved in 83 per cent of patients on amoxicillin and 77 per cent of patients on placebo. These two primary care studies suggest that the overall effect of antibiotic treatment of sinusitis is small for patients diagnosed by signs and symptoms or X-ray because many of these patients have viral infections that will resolve as rapidly without antibiotic treatment. Using more accurate diagnostic criteria, air-fluid level or complete opacification on CT scan, Lindbaek showed a positive treatment effect for amoxicillin and penicillin.[17] At day 10 of treatment, 56 per cent of patients treated with placebo, 82 per cent of those treated with penicillin, and 89 per cent of those treated with amoxicillin were substantially better.

A recent randomized placebo-controlled trial from Denmark included 133 patients from general practice with suspected acute sinusitis who had sinus pain and an elevated ESR and/or CRP.[30] After 10 days, 71 per cent were cured with penicillin versus 37 per cent with placebo. In summary, antibiotics do hasten the resolution of symptoms in patients with bacterial sinusitis, but it is difficult to identify which patients have bacterial infection rather than viral infection.

Three recent meta-analyses have concluded that newer and broad-spectrum antibiotics are not significantly more effective than narrow-spectrum agents.[18,29,31] Initial treatment should be with the narrow spectrum agent that is most active against the likely pathogens, *S. pneumoniae* and *H. influenzae*. However, due to the rapid increase in antibiotic resistance of *S. pneumoniae* and *H. influenzae*, treatment must take into account current local recommendations for treating infections due to these organisms. Knowledge of local antibiotic resistance patterns should guide anti-biotic selection, although amoxicillin is considered the drug of choice in most countries and erythromycin or sulfamethoxazole for patients allergic to penicillin. Failure to improve in 48–72 h suggests either an incorrect diagnosis such as viral infection, a facial pain syndrome, or bacterial resistance.

Sinus puncture

The indication for puncture and irrigation of the sinuses is sinus empyema when antibiotic treatment has produced no improvement. In these cases, antibiotics have low penetration and the mucosal concentration does not reach bactericidal levels, even with high dosages. However, the need for puncture in the treatment of acute bacterial sinusitis seems to be rare. In two studies of antibiotic treatment of sinusitis where the need for puncture was reported, only 1–2 per cent of the patients needed puncture to resolve their symptoms.[1,27]

Complications

Serious complications of sinusitis include brain abscess, orbital cellulitis, subdural empyema, and meningitis. There is no mention of such complications among more than 2700 patients in 27 clinical trials of sinusitis treatment. Large referral hospitals rarely report such complications. Among the studies on diagnosis and treatment that have been performed in general practice, only one case of serious complication was reported: a case of meningitis secondary to a bacterial sinusitis.[1]

Another important complication is the development of chronic sinusitis from inadequately treated acute sinusitis. From the studies of van Buchem and Lindbaek, one may conclude that 1–2 per cent of the patients with acute sinusitis may develop chronic sinusitis.[1,27]

Recurrent sinusitis

Patients with recurrent sinusitis constitute 7–9 per cent of all patients with acute sinusitis.[1,2] They may have an underlying physiologic or anatomic abnormality. The most common is allergic rhinitis, which may respond well to a variety of treatments, and the first choice should be a topical steroid.[9] If allergic rhinitis is not present, other predisposing factors should be considered such as immune compromise or an underlying anatomic abnormality. Nasal polyps or abnormalities in the osteomeatal complex may cause reduced drainage of the sinuses. A specialist should evaluate patients with more than three episodes of acute sinusitis per year.

Chronic sinusitis

Chronic sinusitis is sinusitis with symptoms for at least 12 weeks. Chronic sinusitis differs in many ways from acute sinusitis. In acute sinusitis, the trigger is usually a viral upper respiratory infection. Chronic sinusitis, however, is associated with allergic rhinitis, asthma, anatomic abnormalities of the nasal cavity, immunocompromised states such as acquired immune deficiency syndrome (AIDS) and diabetes mellitus, and a number of underlying diseases—most notably cystic fibrosis.[32,33] Chronic sinusitis may also result from untreated or insufficiently treated acute bacterial sinusitis.

Histologically, chronic sinusitis is a proliferative process with fibrosis of the lamina propria. There is infiltration with lymphocytes, plasma cells, and eosinophils. Bony changes may occur. There may be polyp formation and granulomas. Chronic smouldering bacterial or fungal infection may be present. Acute exacerbations may be due to a flare up of infection and usually require prolonged courses of the appropriate antimicrobial agent.[33]

Patients with chronic sinusitis are often infected with the same bacterial pathogens as those with acute sinusitis, but *Pseudomonas aeruginosa*, group A streptococcus, *Staph aureus*, and anaerobes may be involved. *Aspergillus* sp. are the organisms most often associated with fungal sinusitis in immunocompetent and immunocompromised individuals.[34] Patients with diabetes mellitus, leukaemia, solid malignancies, those on high-dose steroid therapy, and patients with severe impaired cell-mediated immunity are those most likely to get fungal sinusitis.

Treatment of chronic sinusitis requires recognition and treatment of underlying predisposing factors and diseases.[32,35] Nasal cytology to diagnose allergic disorders, sweat chloride to test for cystic fibrosis, and tests for immunodeficiency, such as quantitative immunoglobulins, antibody tests, serum IgE and complement components, may be helpful if an underlying immunodeficiency is suspected. Patients with chronic sinusitis usually benefit from consultation with an otorhinolaryngologist for a more detailed anatomic and histological evaluation than is feasible in primary care. An allergy referral may be of benefit as well.

Treatment of chronic sinusitis is directed at control of infection, reduction of tissue oedema, and facilitation of the drainage of sinus secretions. Both medical and surgical therapies, including functional endoscopic surgery, are used to treat chronic sinusitis, but selection of the optimal treatment strategy is difficult because of lack of controlled trials comparing treatments.[35]

Treatment of acute sinusitis in children

Antibiotic treatment is generally recommended to hasten symptom resolution for children with persistent symptoms of bacterial sinusitis, but results of placebo-controlled trials are inconsistent. One double-blind placebo controlled trial of children with acute sinusitis diagnosed by clinical and radiographic findings demonstrated improved recovery at 3 and 10 days with amoxicillin and amoxicillin-clavulanic acid compared to placebo.[36]

On the third day, 83 per cent of children on the antibiotics were cured or improved compared to 51 per cent in the placebo group. At day 10, 79 per cent treated with an antibiotic and 60 per cent receiving placebo were cured or improved. However, in a recent study of children with clinically diagnosed acute sinusitis, neither amoxycillin nor amoxycillin-clavulanate was beneficial compared to placebo.[37]

When antibiotic treatment is needed, amoxycillin is the drug of choice in 2001, but this may change due to increasing bacterial resistance to penicillins and other narrow-spectrum agents. Antibiotic therapy must be guided by local resistance patterns and patient response to treatment.

Allergic rhinitis

Epidemiology

Allergic rhinitis most often starts before age 7, and 10–20 per cent of the population suffers from it. Intensity of symptoms is highest in school-age children. The condition includes seasonal allergic rhinitis (hay fever) and perennial allergic rhinitis.[38] The frequency of allergy varies considerably between various countries and regions of the world due to the great variation in allergens.[39] The prevalence of allergic rhinitis as well as other atopic diseases is increasing, especially in the Western countries.[40]

Allergic rhinitis is an atopic disease, defined as increased production of IgE as a response to allergens. There is a higher risk of getting the disease if one of the parents has an atopic condition. The risk is over 50 per cent if both parents have allergies.[38] Allergy to pollen and animal hair is the most common cause. Dust mite is a common allergen as well. Half of patients with allergic rhinitis have pollen allergy, but most patients have symptoms at other times of the year, too.

History and physical findings

The typical symptoms are nasal congestion, serous nasal secretion, and sneezing. The diagnosis is often obvious when the symptoms appear in the pollen season. Conjunctivitis with itching and tearing increases the probability of allergic origin of the rhinitis. However, allergic rhinitis can appear without conjunctivitis, especially in allergy to house dust mite. The presence of another atopic disease such as eczema or asthma increases the probability of allergic rhinitis.

At anterior rhinoscopy a varying degree of mucosal oedema, rubor, and watery secretion is found. In some patients nasal polyps are present. Increased tearing and bilateral red conjunctiva may be present.

Sometimes, the patient is aware of what is causing the allergic symptoms. When the allergic reaction appears in spring or summer, pollen allergy is the most likely cause, and the time of symptom onset suggests which pollen is the allergen. For example, birch in May and grass pollen in June–July in northern climates.

Laboratory investigation

If the allergic rhinitis is seasonal in spring, summer, or fall, it is not always necessary to perform further investigations. In perennial allergic disease it may be helpful to identify the specific allergens with blood or skin testing. Allergic patients may have elevated levels of IgE and specific antibodies to allergens like pollen, house dust mite, and animal hair from horse, cat and dog, and fungi. The specific antibody tests have a high sensitivity and specificity of 90 per cent.[38] Skin prick testing is an alternative to blood tests.

Treatment

The most important treatment principle is to identify the agent that causes the allergic reaction in order to avoid or reduce the exposure. Patients with pollen allergy should avoid areas with high pollen concentrations and stay indoors at the worst times. To reduce exposure to house dust mite, regular and thorough cleaning and dust removal is important. In allergy to animal hair, contact with all animals of that kind should be avoided. This is even more important if the patient has asthma. In general, it is important to avoid allergens as much as possible since this is an important predictor of development of further atopic disease such as asthma.

Five classes of medication can be used in the treatment of allergic rhinitis: antihistamines, steroids, cromoglycates, adrenergics, and antileucotriens.[41] In most patients antihistamines and/or topical nasal steroids provide excellent symptom relief. Antihistamines and topical steroids are the most commonly used medication for adults and children over 12 years.[41] Topical steroids give the best symptom relief and are especially effective against nasal congestion. Newer non-sedating antihistamines have far less side-effects than the older antihistamines.[41] Use of medications varies from country to country because of tradition and medication availability. In some countries most medications for allergic rhinitis can be purchased without a prescription. Desensitization injections are effective but are used less frequently now because of the excellent symptomatic medications that are available.

Treatment of allergic rhinitis in children under 12 years is still debated. Topical antihistamines and cromoglycate are still the drugs of choice. Growth retardation has been reported in children using topical steroids for prolonged periods,[42] so prescribing the minimum effective dose and regular growth monitoring is necessary.

Key points

1. The clinical diagnosis of acute bacterial sinusitis is difficult in primary care practice. A history of purulent rhinorrhoea, purulent secretions in the nasal cavity on examination, tooth pain, worsening of symptoms following initial improvement, and lack of effect of decongestants are supportive evidence of bacterial infection. Patients with symptoms for less than 7 days are not as likely to have bacterial infection.

2. Sinus imaging studies are not recommended in routine diagnosis but may be helpful in selected cases.

3. Most cases of acute sinusitis are initiated by viral infections and resolve without antibiotic treatment.

4. Antibiotic treatment of acute sinusitis is indicated only for patients with severe symptoms of sinusitis or for patients with moderate symptoms for longer than 7 days.

5. Other than pain medication, symptomatic treatments are unproven.

References

1. Lindbaek, M., Hjortdahl, P., and Holth, V. (1997). Acute sinusitis in Norwegian general practice—incidence, complications, referral to ear–nose–throat specialist and economic costs. *European Journal of General Practice* 3, 7–11.

2. van Duijn, N.P., Brouwer, H.J., and Lamberts, H. (1992). Use of symptoms and signs to diagnose maxillary sinusitis in general practice: comparison with ultrasonography (see comments). *British Medical Journal* 305 (6855), 684–7.

3. Hovelius, B. and Widäng, K. (1986). Common cold or sinusitis. In *Infektioner i primärvård* (ed. P.H. Mårdh), pp. 75–9. Stockholm: Almquist & Wiksell.

4. McIsaac, W.J., Levine, N., and Goel, V. (1998). Visits by adults to family physicians for the common cold. *Journal of Family Practice* 47 (5), 366–9.

5. Gwaltney, J.M., Jr. (1996). Acute community-acquired sinusitis. *Clinical Infectious Diseases* 23 (6), 1209–23; quiz 1224–5.

6. Mellbye, H. *Lunger og luftveier.* (*Lungs and Airways.*) Oslo: Gyldendal-Ad Notam, 1997.

7. Wald, E.R. (1994). Sinusitis in children. *Israel Journal of Medical Sciences* **30** (5–6), 403–7.

8. Aitken, M. and Taylor, J.A. (1998). Prevalence of clinical sinusitis in young children followed up by primary care pediatricians. *Archives of Pediatrics & Adolescent Medicine* **152** (3), 244–8.

9. Willett, L.R., Carson, J.L., and Williams, J.W., Jr. (1994). Current diagnosis and management of sinusitis. *Journal of General Internal Medicine* **9** (1), 38–45.

10. Lindbaek, M. et al. (1996). CT findings in general practice patients with suspected acute sinusitis. *Acta Radiologica* **37** (5), 708–13.

11. Low, D.E. et al. (1997). A practical guide for the diagnosis and treatment of acute sinusitis (see comments). *Canadian Medical Association Journal* **156** (Suppl. 6), S1–14.

12. Carenfelt, C., Lundberg, C., Nord, C.E., and Wretlind, B. (1978). Bacteriology of maxillary sinusitis in relation to quality of the retained secretion. *Acta Oto-Laryngologica* **86** (3–4), 298–302.

13. Lindbaek, M., Kaastad, E., Dolvik, S., Johnsen, U., Laerum, E., and Hjortdahl, P. (1998). Antibiotic treatment of patients with mucosal thickening in the paranasal sinuses, and validation of cut-off points in sinus CT. *Rhinology* **36** (1), 7–11.

14. Hansen, J.G., Schmidt, H., Rosborg, J., and Lund, E. (1995). Predicting acute maxillary sinusitis in a general practice population (see comments). *British Medical Journal* **311** (6999), 233–6.

15. Williams, J.W., Jr., Simel, D.L., Roberts, L., and Samsa, G.P. (1992). Clinical evaluation for sinusitis. Making the diagnosis by history and physical examination (see comments). *Annals of Internal Medicine* **117** (9), 705–10.

16. Lindbaek, M., Hjortdahl, P., and Johnsen, U.L. (1996). Use of symptoms, signs, and blood tests to diagnose acute sinus infections in primary care: comparison with computed tomography. *Family Medicine* **28** (3), 183–8.

17. Lindbaek, M., Hjortdahl, P., and Johnsen, U.L. (1996). Randomised, double blind, placebo controlled trial of penicillin V and amoxycillin in treatment of acute sinus infections in adults (see comments). *British Medical Journal* **313** (7053), 325–9.

18. Benninger, M.S., Sedory Holzer, S.E., and Lau, J. (2000). Diagnosis and treatment of uncomplicated acute bacterial rhinosinusitis: summary of the Agency for Health Care Policy and Research evidence-based report. *Otolaryngology—Head & Neck Surgery* **122** (1), 1–7.

19. Laine, K., Maatta, T., Varonen, H., and Makela, M. (1998). Diagnosing acute maxillary sinusitis in primary care: a comparison of ultrasound, clinical examination and radiography. *Rhinology* **36** (1), 2–6.

20. Engquist, S. and Lundberg, C. (1986). Akut sinuit—nar, hur och av vem bor den behandlas? (Acute sinusitis—when, how and by whom should it be treated?) *Lakartidningen* **83** (38), 3112–14.

21. Wald, E.R. (1996). Diagnosis and management of sinusitis in children. *Advances in Pediatric Infectious Diseases* **12**, 1–20.

22. Wald, E.R. et al. (1984). Treatment of acute maxillary sinusitis in childhood: a comparative study of amoxicillin and cefaclor. *Journal of Pediatrics* **104** (2), 297–302.

23. Hickner, J.M. (2001). Acute rhinosinusitis: a diagnostic and therapeutic challenge (letter; comment). *Journal of Family Practice* **50** (1), 38–40.

24. Hansen, J.G., Schmidt, H., Rosborg, J., and Lund, E. (1995). Predicting acute maxillary sinusitis in a general practice population (see comments). *British Medical Journal* **311** (6999), 233–6.

25. Axelsson, A., Chidekel, N., Grebelius, N., and Jensen, C. (1970). Treatment of acute maxillary sinusitis. A comparison of four different methods. *Acta Oto-Laryngologica* **70** (1), 71–6.

26. Gananca, M. and Trabulsi, L.R. (1973). The therapeutic effects of cyclacillin in acute sinusitis: *in vitro* and *in vivo* correlations in a placebo-controlled study. *Current Medical Research & Opinion* **1** (6), 362–8.

27. van Buchem, F.L., Knottnerus, J.A., Schrijnemaekers, V.J., and Peeters, M.F. (1997). Primary-care-based randomised placebo-controlled trial of antibiotic treatment in acute maxillary sinusitis (see comments). *Lancet* **349** (9053), 683–7.

28. Stalman, W., van Essen, G.A., van der Graaf, Y., and de Melker, R.A. (1997). The end of antibiotic treatment in adults with acute sinusitis-like complaints in general practice? A placebo-controlled double-blind randomized doxycycline trial (see comments). *British Journal of General Practice* **47** (425), 794–9.

29. Williams, J.W., Jr. et al. (2000). Antibiotics for acute maxillary sinusitis. *Cochrane Database of Systematic Reviews* (computer file), Issue 2, 2000 (2), CD000243.

30. Hansen, J.G., Schmidt, H., and Grinsted, P. (2000). Randomised, double blind, placebo controlled trial of penicillin V in the treatment of acute maxillary sinusitis in adults in general practice. *Scandinavian Journal of Primary Health Care* **18** (1), 44–7.

31. de Bock, G.H., Dekker, F.W., Stolk, J., Springer, M.P., Kievit, J., and van Houwelingen, J.C. (1997). Antimicrobial treatment in acute maxillary sinusitis: a meta-analysis. *Journal of Clinical Epidemiology* **50** (8), 881–90.

32. Evans, K.L. (1994). Diagnosis and management of sinusitis (see comments). *British Medical Journal* **309** (6966), 1415–22.

33. Lanza, D.C. and Kennedy, D.W. (1997). Adult rhinosinusitis defined. *Otolaryngology—Head & Neck Surgery* **117** (3 Pt 2), S1–7.

34. Cody, D.T., II, Neel, H.B., III, Ferreiro, J.A., and Roberts, G.D. (1994). Allergic fungal sinusitis: the Mayo Clinic experience. *Laryngoscope* **104** (9), 1074–9.

35. Mirza, N. and Lanza, D.C. (2000). Diagnosis and management of rhinosinusitis before scheduled immunosuppression: a schematic approach to the prevention of acute fungal rhinosinusitis. *Otolaryngologic Clinics of North America* **33** (2), 313–21.

36. Wald, E.R., Chiponis, D., and Ledesma-Medina, J. (1986). Comparative effectiveness of amoxicillin and amoxicillin-clavulanate potassium in acute paranasal sinus infections in children: a double-blind, placebo-controlled trial. *Pediatrics* **77** (6), 795–800.

37. Garbutt, J., Goldstein, M., Gellman, E., Shannon, W., and Littenberg, B. (2001). A randomized, placebo-controlled trial of antimicrobial treatment for children with clinically diagnosed acute sinusitis. *Pediatrics* **107** (4), 619–25.

38. Anonymous (1994). International Consensus Report on the diagnosis and management of rhinitis. International Rhinitis Management Working Group. *Allergy* **49** (Suppl. 19), 1–34.

39. Strachan, D. et al. (1997). Worldwide variations in prevalence of symptoms of allergic rhinoconjunctivitis in children: the International Study of Asthma and Allergies in Childhood (ISAAC). *Pediatric Allergy & Immunology* **8** (4), 161–76.

40. Ross, A.M. and Fleming, D.M. (1994). Incidence of allergic rhinitis in general practice, 1981–92. *British Medical Journal* **308** (6933), 897–900.

41. Weiner, J.M., Abramson, M.J., and Puy, R.M. (1998). Intranasal corticosteroids versus oral H1 receptor antagonists in allergic rhinitis: systematic review of randomised controlled trials. *British Medical Journal* **317** (7173), 1624–9.

42. Findlay, C.A., Macdonald, J.F., Wallace, A.M., Geddes, N., and Donaldson, M.D. (1998). Childhood Cushing's syndrome induced by betamethasone nose drops, and repeat prescriptions (see comments). *British Medical Journal* **317** (7160), 739–40.

4

Digestive problems

4 Digestive problems

4.1 Dyspepsia

Roger Jones

Dyspepsia is a common problem for patients and doctors. It can signal a range of underlying disorders, from the trivial to the life-threatening. Its epidemiology and natural history are well documented in Western societies and the Antipodes, but less information is available for many other societies, particularly Africa, the Middle East, and Central Asia. The management of dyspepsia remains controversial, not least because of the changing epidemiology of conditions such as peptic ulcer disease, oesophageal adenocarcinoma, *Helicobacter pylori* (HP) infection and gastro-oesophageal reflux disease (GORD). Dyspepsia has a significant impact on health care resources, and although costs and strategic approaches to management vary from country to country, it is now possible to provide reasonably evidence-based guidance on clinically appropriate and cost-effective management.

Dyspepsia is defined, for the purposes of this chapter, as pain and discomfort experienced in the upper abdomen or chest, sometimes accompanied by heartburn or other gastrointestinal (GI) symptoms, and often related to eating or drinking. Although there is a move to separate predominant reflux-like symptoms from other forms of dyspepsia, in order to provide an overview in this chapter all dyspepsia sub-groups will be considered—reflux-like, ulcer-like, and dysmotility-like. There is considerable overlap between these dyspepsia sub-types and patients frequently present in primary care with a mixture of, for example, ulcer-like and reflux-like symptoms. There is also considerable overlap between functional lower bowel disorders and the experience of upper GI symptoms, predominantly gastro-oesophageal reflux.

Epidemiology and natural history

Dyspepsia is a common symptom in Western societies, and in countries such as the United Kingdom, Australia, North America, and Sweden between 15 and 40 per cent of the population will experience significant dyspeptic symptoms in any 1-year period. Most community-based surveys indicate that the prevalence of dyspeptic symptoms is reasonably consistent internationally, and has remained stable over time, but there is evidence of more notable international differences in the prevalence of reflux-like symptoms and also a steady increase in the experience of reflux symptoms and the diagnosis of GORD, particularly in Asian countries. There are also interesting within-country variations in dyspepsia prevalence, possibly related to factors such as socio-economic deprivation, heavy cigarette smoking, and alcohol abuse and rates of HP infection which vary considerably within and between developed and developing countries. Interestingly, there is an inconsistent relationship between HP infection and the prevalence of peptic ulcer disease and gastric cancer. Although long-term community-based studies are few, the available information suggests that the majority of patients reporting one particular sub-type of dyspepsia continue to do so over time, although a significant minority of patients move between dyspepsia sub-types, including dysmotility-like symptoms.

Consultation for dyspepsia

Dyspepsia is also common in primary care. Around 10 per cent of all consultations in Western primary care systems are related to GI disorders, and about half of these are for upper GI problems, predominantly dyspepsia. As with many other common symptoms, the patients encountered in primary care represent only a proportion of the 'symptom iceberg'; around 75 per cent of people reporting dyspepsia in community-based surveys never seek medical attention for their symptoms. The decision to consult a primary care physician is partly related to symptom severity, but consultation behaviour is more strongly predicted by patients' health beliefs and concerns about their symptoms, including worries that dyspepsia might represent a serious or potentially fatal condition and, more specifically, about the possibility of underlying heart disease or cancer. In one survey in the United Kingdom, over 50 per cent of people consulting their general practitioners with dyspepsia harboured concerns about cancer.

The impact of dyspepsia on service use is considerable, because of the range of possible underlying causes, the investigations required to explore these and the increasing costs of acid-suppressing drugs, amounting to around 10 per cent of primary care prescribing in many Western countries.

Causes of dyspepsia

Causes range from self-limiting disorders to serious and potentially life-threatening conditions, and these are summarized in Table 1. This information is derived from the endoscopic diagnoses made in patients referred for upper GI endoscopy. The majority of patients in an

Table 1 Causes of dyspepsia

	Prevalence at open access endoscopy (%)
Common	
Acute gastritis	
NSAID and other drug side-effects	10–20
Dietary indiscretions, including alcohol abuse	
Gastro-oesophageal reflux disease	10–20
Non-ulcer dyspepsia	20–40
Duodenal ulcer	5–10
Gastric ulcer	
Uncommon	
Gastric cancer	2–3
Biliary tract disease, including cholelithiasis	
Rare	
Adenocarcinoma and squamous cell carcinoma of the oesophagus	
Pancreatic cancer	1–2
Small bowel and colon cancer	
Mesenteric ischaemia	

otherwise unselected series of patients with persistent dyspepsia will have normal findings at endoscopy (non-ulcer or functional dyspepsia), and in most surveys peptic ulcer disease (duodenal and gastric ulcer) represent around 10 per cent of the total, with a further 10–20 per cent of patients having oesophaghitis. Gastric cancer is found in 1–2 per cent of patients with persistent dyspepsia, but whether the dyspeptic symptoms for which the endoscopy is performed are related to the cancer remains controversial.

For most primary care physicians in Western health care systems, the early identification and adequate treatment of patients with significant, organic lesions, essentially peptic ulcer disease and cancer, is the priority; for the majority of patients without the alarm signals mentioned below, more timely investigation can proceed, using time as a diagnostic tool and, in cases of continuing uncertainty, specialist referral.

Diagnosis

Diagnosis in dyspepsia is dependent on a carefully taken history, an appreciation of the patients' psycho-social milieu and the factors leading to this particular consultation, a focused physical examination, and a limited number of investigations. Endoscopy and other more invasive investigations may well be available to primary care physicians, but in many countries require specialist referral. Endoscopy is likely to be required as part of the initial evaluation in perhaps 10–20 per cent of patients, but will be undertaken in 50–60 per cent of those with persistent symptoms.

History

The history is important, and indeed the initial 'triage' of patients into the minority, in whom urgent investigation is mandatory, and the majority, in whom significant illness is unlikely, is based on a response to a set of factors in the clinical history, described as *alarm symptoms* which are summarized in Table 2. These symptoms, based on a number of studies in which regression analyses have been conducted to identify factors predictive of a final diagnosis of ulcer disease or cancer, still represent a somewhat qualitative approach to diagnosis. It is difficult to make a firm diagnosis based on history alone, and indeed the positive predictive value of symptoms for ulcer disease or cancer, based on various scoring systems using selections of these factors, remains disappointing. It has also been pointed out that some of these symptoms, although important, are merely evidence of inoperability in malignant disease.

The role of the physical examination, in terms of adding to diagnostic precision, is limited, although from the patient's point of view it is important. Rarely, the physician will encounter a patient with obvious weight loss, anaemia/cachexia or other signs of advanced disease or may find an abdominal mass or notable tenderness or organomegaly, but in most patients with dyspepsia general physical and abdominal examination yield few additional clues.

Table 2 Alarm symptoms in dyspepsia

Previous history of peptic ulcer disease
New symptoms in a patient aged over 50–55 years
Persistent pain
Weight loss
Evidence of bleeding
Evidence of systemic illness
Male sex
Smoking
Anaemia

Helicobacter pylori

HP infection has had a huge impact on the initial evaluation of patients with dyspepsia. This organism, a gram-negative flagellated spiral rod, has been shown to be an important causative factor in duodenal ulcer disease and, to a lesser extent, in gastric ulcer disease. It is the principal cause of the rare mucous associated lymphatic tissue (MALT) lymphoma, and has been classified by the WHO as a Class 1 risk factor for gastric cancer. Its immunological sub-types—CagA and CagB—differ in their virulence for peptic ulcer disease and also in their carcinogenicity. The role of HP in non-ulcer dyspepsia (NUD) remains controversial, and the organism does not have a direct effect on the initiation or maintenance of mucosal damage in GORD. However, testing for HP infection in patients presenting in primary care with persistent dyspepsia is likely to be helpful, especially in countries with a high prevalence of both peptic ulcer disease and HP infection. There is now persuasive evidence that a 'test and treat' strategy, as described below, in patients with dyspepsia provides a cost-effective and clinically appropriate approach to management.

In practice, HP testing can be performed in a number of ways, including office-based whole blood finger-prick tests, based on an antibody assay, although at present the test characteristics of these kits (positive and negative predictive values) are barely acceptable as a basis for guiding management. A hospital electro-immunological sorbent assay (ELISA) test, performed on whole blood, is cheaper and more accurate, with sensitivity and specificity values of around 92–95 per cent. The most accurate investigation is a urea breath test (UBT), employing either ^{13}C- or ^{14}C-labelled urea, which is drunk by the patient and split by the urease produced by HP to liberate labelled CO_2, which is then measured. The UBT is much more useful for determining the success of HP eradication than the serological tests because the latter can only confirm successful eradication after 3–6 months have elapsed, and antibody levels have fallen. Stool antigen tests are now being developed, which may provide better sensitivity and specificity, although their acceptability is variable. The gold standard for diagnosing HP infection is the histological analysis or culture of gastric mucosa obtained at an endoscopic biopsy.

Upper gastrointestinal endoscopy

This technique is widely used in the investigation of dyspepsia and for many years our understanding of dyspepsia and peptic ulcer disease depended almost entirely on visualization of the gastric and duodenal mucosa. Modern narrow-bore endoscopes permit inspection of the oesophagus, stomach, and duodenum with only the minimum of sedation and, therefore, of side-effects, although sedation may be required in certain patients. Not only is endoscopy more accurate than barium radiology in the diagnosis of upper GI lesions, but it is also more acceptable to elderly patients, who may find the contortions of a barium meal difficult. Patients with compromised cardiopulmonary function should be carefully evaluated before endoscopy. Upper GI endoscopy is frequently carried out in primary care settings in many countries, and some general practitioners are involved in community- and hospital-based endoscopy services. In many countries, however, radiology remains the predominant investigation because of shortage of endoscopic facilities. Other investigations in dyspepsia make a much smaller contribution to diagnosis and management. The routine haematological and biochemical investigations available to general practitioners are likely to add little to diagnostic precision, although unexpected results may make us re-think our differential diagnoses, such as the discovery of disordered liver function tests or of iron-deficiency anaemia. Further investigations may follow, such as a cholecystogram or biliary ultrasound when biliary tract disease appears a possibility, although these would not be seen as a 'routine' part of the dyspepsia work-up.

For most primary care physicians, investigations beyond this level will be the domain of the specialist gastroenterologist. Further investigations in dyspepsia include oesophageal manometry, oesophageal pH-metry, pancreatic function tests, measurements of GI motility, and advanced imaging techniques.

Management

Management of dyspepsia depends initially on symptom-based triage, as described earlier, which includes the identification of patients at high risk of serious, organic disease, and their rapid investigation or referral, and the more timely investigation and diagnostic approach to patients at low risk. The availability of investigations, the prevalence of disease and of HP infection, the costs of procedures and drugs, and local practice will all influence the choice of management strategies in different countries; four approaches may be followed and each can be both clinically appropriate and cost-effective in particular circumstances.

1. *Early endoscopy.* If patients have persistent dyspepsia there are persuasive arguments for making an early diagnosis on which to base management and, particularly when the endoscopy is negative, on which to base patient reassurance. When endoscopy is costly, this represents an expensive option, because most patients will have negative endoscopies, but there may be a long-term gain in terms of rational management and resolution of patients' concerns.

2. *Empirical drug treatment.* This means the prescription of acid-suppressing medication in patients who have not been investigated. Clearly, if a previous diagnosis of, for example, GORD has been established, and symptoms have not changed, early investigation may be inappropriate and drug therapy can be prescribed immediately. More commonly, empirical therapy refers to the 'experimental' prescription of a course of full-dose acid suppression, either using a histamine 2 receptor antagonist (H2RA) or, more commonly in recent years, a proton pump inhibitor (PPI). Response to therapy, irrespective of the placebo effect, is taken to imply the presence of an acid-related disorder, and abolition of symptoms may represent temporary cure of a mucosal lesion. However, the physician is left without a diagnosis, peptic ulcer symptoms will recur, as will those of GORD, and there are weakly supported suggestions that gastric cancer symptoms may be masked, delaying diagnosis. On the other hand, empirical therapy will be an effective first approach to management in the majority of patients. For GORD patients (30 per cent of the total) acid suppression is effective while, for the majority with functional dyspepsia, favourable outcomes are more likely to be linked to the good prognosis of the condition than to the effect of treatment.

3. *Test and endoscope.* This refers to the performance of an HP test, chosen according to local availability from the list above, and the onward referral of patients testing positive for endoscopy. Patients testing negative are regarded as having non-ulcer dyspepsia (or possibly GORD), whilst of those testing positive a significant proportion will have peptic ulcer disease, which will be picked up at endoscopy. Although this has never been a popular strategy, it reduces the number of endoscopies required in a dyspeptic population by around one-quarter.

4. *Test and treat.* This refers to the early establishment of a patients' HP status, using an office- or hospital-based test, and providing HP eradication therapy to all patients testing positive. Whilst acknowledging that many patients with non-ulcer dyspepsia and other conditions will receive 'unnecessary' HP eradication therapy, there is accumulating evidence that this approach is both safe and cost-effective, especially where the prevalence of peptic ulcer disease and HP infection are both high.

Patients found, at endoscopy, to have peptic ulcer disease, or patients with a proven history of peptic ulcer disease and recurrence of typical symptoms, should be offered HP eradication therapy. It has been shown conclusively that HP eradication produces a virtual cure of peptic ulcer disease, with extremely low recurrence rates at follow-up. Eradication therapy is usually prescribed as a 1-week course of triple therapy, typically a PPI with two antibiotics. The combination varies from country to country, depending on factors including antibiotic resistance and costs, but typical combinations would include omeprazole, amoxycillin, and clarithromycin or omeprazole, amoxycillin, and metronidazole or amoxycillin, metronidazole, and clarithromycin, each given twice daily for 1 week, although many physicians prefer to continue the PPI for a further 3 weeks, to ensure symptom suppression while gastro-duodenal healing is taking place.

Patients investigated by endoscopy who have persistent dyspeptic symptoms but normal endoscopic findings are likely to fall into two important groups, those with endoscopy-negative reflux disease (ENRD) and those with NUD. Patients with ENRD respond well to acid suppression, and a PPI test—the prescription of 2 weeks of double dose PPI, with symptom assessment at the end of the course—is a useful diagnostic approach if ENRD is suspected. The management of NUD is much more difficult because few approaches, including HP eradication, have been shown to produce substantial improvement. Acid suppression seems to help a minority of NUD patients (possibly where NUD is a misdiagnosis for ENRD), and HP eradication also provides relief in a subset of patients, but the number needed to treat (NNT) for HP eradication is in the region of 15, and therapeutic gain over placebo is only about 9 per cent.

Specialist referral, apart from the necessity of investigating undiagnosed, persistent dyspepsia, is needed in patients in whom significant lesions, such as gastric or oesophageal cancer, are found, and these patients will require appropriate surgical management.

Long-term care

Long term care in dyspepsia principally relates to the long-term management of GORD. Primary care physicians need to be aware that GORD can lead to troublesome complications and also that acid reflux now appears to be a risk factor for the development of adenocarcinoma of the oesophagus, a cancer with the most rapidly rising incidence rates worldwide. Effective acid suppression in reflux disease is likely to be important, and PPIs represent the therapy of choice, although H2RAs may be used when these drugs are not available. There is some evidence that a 'step-down' approach to therapy, beginning with maximum therapy and reducing dosage to a level at which symptoms are controlled, is most appropriate, although the long-term cost-effectiveness of this approach remains to be determined. Many patients with intermittent symptoms can be cost-effectively managed by the use of on-demand therapy, in which medication is taken in response to symptoms. The need for follow-up endoscopy to look for Barrett's oesophagus and subsequent surveillance of Barrett's, is discussed in Chapter 4.2, although recommendations still remain controversial because of a paucity of good-quality follow-up data.

Opportunities for preventive measures and patient education in dyspepsia are relatively limited, although the importance of lifestyle modification in reducing risk, in common with many other clinical areas in primary care, should be taken, including attention to patients' smoking and alcohol drinking habits and their approach to weight control, diet, and exercise. The public health issues related to dyspepsia include the carcinogenicity of HP infection and the increasing incidence of oesophageal adenocarcinoma. Interestingly, HP infection rates are falling in Western societies, possibly due to a cohort effect in which acquisition of the infection was related to earlier, poor socio-economic conditions and to poor hygiene. The possible protective effect against oesophageal cancer of HP infection is still debated, and the epidemiology of all these conditions demonstrates a number of international differences. For example, in Africa HP infection is common in the community, but both gastric cancer and peptic ulcer disease are rare whilst, in Japan, gastric cancer has a much higher community prevalence, to the extent that screening programmes have been instituted, but its relationship to HP infection is also less clear.

Health services implications

Health services implications of dyspepsia are extensive, as described earlier, particularly in relation to the costs of investigation and treatment. Because of its ubiquity, dyspepsia has a substantial impact on health care systems and on patients' quality of life, so that effective therapy is important.

Peptic ulcer disease and the upper GI cancers remain causes of high levels of morbidity and mortality, and their early diagnosis and management will continue to be important. Primary care research needs to focus on the long-term outcomes, including health economic analyses, of the various dyspepsia management strategies, in order to better define the role of different investigative modalities in different countries and the appropriate use of expensive medication.

Key points

1. Dyspepsia is common and can represent a range of disorders, from the trivial and self-limiting to the serious and life-threatening.

2. Patients with dyspepsia may have significant concerns about the seriousness of their disease and the possibility of heart disease and cancer.

3. A range of management strategies is available, the choice depending on individual health care systems, and include early endoscopy, empirical drug therapy, a *Helicobacter pylori* 'test and endoscope' strategy and a *Helicobacter pylori* 'test and treat' strategy.

4. *Helicobacter pylori* should be eradicated in all patients with peptic ulcer disease.

5. The role of *Helicobacter pylori* in non-ulcer dyspepsia and in relation to gastro-oesophageal reflux disease remains unclear.

6. Whilst *Helicobacter pylori* infection and gastric cancer rates are falling, oesophageal adenocarcinoma rates are rising, and may be related to oesophageal acid exposure.

Further reading

Lydeard, S. and Jones, R.H. (1989). Factors affecting the decision to consult with dyspepsia: comparison of consulters and non-consulters. *Journal of the Royal College of General Practitioners* **39**, 495–8.

Delaney, B. et al. (2000). The management of dyspepsia: a systematic review. *Health Technology Assessment (Rockville, MD)* **4** (39) iii–v, 1–189.

Dent, J., Jones, R., Kahrilas, P., and Talley, N. (2001). Clinical review: management of gastro-oesophageal reflux disease in general practice. *British Medical Journal* **322**, 344–7.

Agreus, L. and Talley, N. (1997). Challenges in managing dyspepsia in general practice. *British Medical Journal* **315**, 1284–8.

Moayyedi, P. et al. (2000). Systematic review and economic evaluation of *Helicobacter pylori* eradication treatment for non-ulcer dyspepsia. *British Medical Journal* **321**, 659–64.

4.2 Dysphagia

John M. Galloway

Dysphagia means literally, 'difficult eating', but to most doctors is the term used to describe difficulty swallowing food or liquids and may be associated with either a sensation of 'something sticking' or pain on swallowing—*odynophagia.*

Since all anatomy beyond the fauces relating to swallowing is inaccessible to physical examination, most useful information is obtained from a carefully taken history to discover whether the patient really has dysphagia and

where the cause is likely to be situated. Dysphagia is a symptom to be taken seriously and merits investigation unless the cause is obvious, such as acute tonsillitis.

Differential diagnosis of dysphagia

- ◆ Pharyngeal causes
  - Tonsillitis
  - Muscular dystrophy
  - Myasthenia gravis
  - Polymyositis, dermatomyositis
  - Brainstem cerebrovascular accident
  - Parkinson's disease
  - Motor neuron disease
  - Multiple sclerosis
  - Mucosal webs
  - Carcinoma of the pharynx/larynx
  - Pharyngeal pouch
- ◆ Stricturing lesions of the oesophagus
  - Peptic stricture/erosive oesophagitis
  - Caustic stricture caused by ingestion of caustic or hot substances
  - Carcinoma
  - Shatzki ring
- ◆ Motility disorders of oesophagus
  - Achalasia
  - Diffuse spasm
  - Scleroderma
- ◆ Extrinsic causes
  - Carcinoma of the bronchus
  - Retrosternal goitre
  - Aortic arch lesions
  - Mitral stenosis—giant left atrium
- ◆ Acute onset
  - Impaction of foreign body
  - Impaction of food bolus
  - Candida infection of oesophagus
  - Acute ulceration—drug induced
  - Intramural haematoma
  - Radiotherapy to mediastinum

Epidemiology

With such a wide range of causes, it is not possible to cover the epidemiology of every aspect of dysphagia. There is an increasing incidence of oesophagitis in the Western world as evidenced by the high prescription rates for proton pump inhibitors. Factors such as diet, obesity, and smoking are thought to be relevant. Chronic reflux is believed to be the cause of Barrett's columnar lined oesophagus,[1,2] which is associated with 30–125-fold increased risk of developing adenocarcinoma of the oesophagus. Gastro-oesophageal reflux is becoming increasingly common and is associated with obesity, increasing age, high-fat diets, and smoking. Interestingly, patients who have had *Helicobacter pylori* induced gastritis often develop gastro-oesophageal reflux after eradication of the infection. It is thought that the gastritis induces a hypergastrinaemia, which causes a rebound hypersecretion of acid after the gastritis has been healed with eradication therapy.[3,4] The excess acid refluxes into the oesophagus where it causes oesophagitis.

Oesophageal cancer shows greater geographical variation in worldwide incidence than any other cancer. Striking differences are found both between local areas of the same region and between different ethnic groups within regions. These differences suggest that environment and lifestyle factors play crucial parts in the aetiology of these cancers.

In developed countries, oesophageal cancer is strongly associated with alcohol and tobacco consumption. These both increase risk independently and act synergistically, accounting for an estimated 90 per cent of oesophageal cancers in developing countries. The relative risk of developing oesophageal cancers in high alcohol consumers who are non-smokers is 18 compared with 5.5 for non-drinking smokers and 44.4 for heavy alcohol and tobacco users. There are weaker links with diet but high fruit and vegetables intake seems to reduce risk.

There are two distinct types of oesophageal cancer—sqamous cell cancer and adenocarcinoma. Squamous cell cancers arise from the true oesophageal mucosa and arise in the upper or middle part of the oesophagus and are most closely associated with tobacco and alcohol intake. The incidence of adenocarcinoma of the oesophagus is on the increase in many Western parts of the world and the incidence has now increased beyond that of sqamous cell cancers. The death rates from cancers of the oesophagus and gastro-oesophageal junction, adjusted for age, have risen steadily since the early 1970s (from 3 to 6 per 100 000 and from 1.5 to 3 per 100 000 population in the United Kingdom, respectively). These figures are comparable to those in northern Europe and the United States. The incidence of adenocarcinoma in the United States[1,5] has increased from 0.3 per 100 000 to 2.3 per 100 000 over the past three decades. Many of these cancers are of the cardia and may be classified as gastric cancers but present as dysphagia because of their position.

Adenocarcinoma of the oesophagus arises from metaplastic change in the oesophageal mucosa as a result of chronic gastro-oesophageal reflux— Barrett's oesophagus (Fig. 1). This condition is very common, affecting 8 per cent of patients examined with endoscopy and 2 per cent of the population. Interestingly, patients who have developed Barrett's changes experience less in the way of oesophageal pain from their chronic reflux. Both types of cancer are rare in people under the age of 40 but the incidence rises steeply over the age of 55. The main presenting symptoms are dysphagia and odynophagia (painful swallowing). A UK general practitioner with responsibility for 2000 patients can expect to see one patient with oesophageal cancer every 2–3 years. The 1-year survival rate in the United Kingdom is 27 per cent compared with 33 per cent in Europe, but at 5 years there is little difference at 10 per cent.[6]

Clues to the diagnosis from history

Stricture of the pharynx

Lesions which constrict the pharynx cause a sensation of food sticking at the moment of swallowing, often accompanied by the prompt return of food into the mouth. As the constriction gets worse liquids have to be sipped rather than gulped. This type of dysphagia, which is fairly uncommon, is seen in patients with carcinomas of the hypopharynx and cervical oesophagus and benign mucosal webs. Malignant lesions usually have a short progressive history of a few months whilst benign lesions give intermittent symptoms over a long period of time.

Strictures of the oesophagus

Benign and malignant strictures are the commonest cause of dysphagia. The benign peptic stricture occurring at or near the gastro-oesophageal junction is particularly common (Fig. 2). The patient is usually middle aged or elderly and often female. There is often a history of long-standing gastro-oesophageal reflux. Some patients give a history of painful dysphagia but on investigation have no sign of stricturing. Ingestion of corrosive agents taken accidentally or in an attempt at self-harm can lead to oesophageal stricturing. Gastro-oesophageal reflux as a result of dysmotility due to systemic sclerosis can also result in a peptic stricture.

Malignant strictures are the second most common cause of oesophageal dysphagia.

Whether benign or malignant, the patient will complain of a sensation of food sticking several seconds after swallowing and will often localize the point of sticking anywhere between the hyoid bone and the epigastrium, but this sign is less useful than the time interval of dysphagia after swallowing for localizing the site of the stricture. Initially, the dysphagia is for solids, particularly bulky materials such as meat and dry bread and dysphagia for liquids rarely occurs until the oesophagus is narrowed virtually to a pinhole. This helps to distinguish mechanical obstruction from motility disorders.

Benign lesions are usually slow in evolution with symptoms sometimes being intermittent for up to a year before presenting. Oesophagitis will have often caused pain after hot drinks or alcohol. Benign lesions are not usually associated with weight loss, as patients can maintain their calorie intake with sloppy liquid diets.

Malignant lesions usually present with a history of weeks, rather than months, of dysphagia and the symptoms are rapidly progressive and are associated with weight loss.

Some patients with a hiatus hernia develop a fibromuscular ring above the mucosal junction, the so-called Shatzki ring (Fig. 3). These rings are often asymptomatic until complete obstruction occurs due to impaction of a bolus of particularly solid food.

Neuromuscular disorders causing a bulbar or pseudobulbar palsy will lead to difficulty in *initiating swallowing* both solids and liquids. Often the

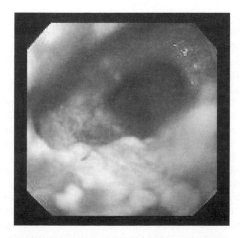

Fig. 1 Adenocarcinoma arising in Barrett's epithelium. (See Plate 7.)

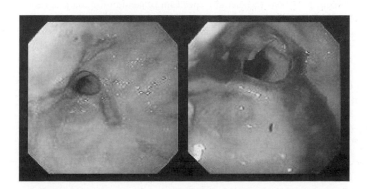

Fig. 2 Benign stricture before and after dilatation. (See Plate 8.)

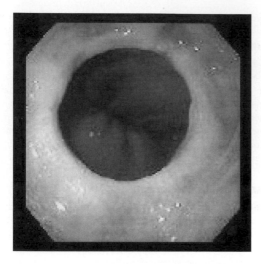

Fig. 3 Shatzki ring. (See Plate 9.)

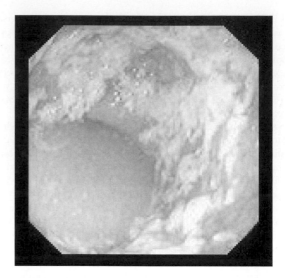

Fig. 4 Achalasia showing dilated oesophagus with fluid level. (See Plate 10.)

problem becomes worse when the patient is embarrassed or stressed and several attempts to swallow food may be followed by regurgitation of fluid through the nose due to failure of closure of the nasopharynx or coughing due to failure to close the epiglottis. Diagnosis of the cause of the dysphagia is rarely a difficult problem as there will be other signs of stroke, motor neuron disease, multiple sclerosis, or Parkinson's disease.

Lesions of the pharynx leading to constriction cause food to stick immediately and prompt regurgitation of the food bolus into the mouth.

A pharyngeal pouch may cause intermittent dysphagia, the patient describing immediate return of food or liquid into the mouth on swallowing. Some regurgitation may occur hours after a meal, particularly when the patient is lying down. A characteristic feature of this disorder is that when drinking, the patient may experience a gurgling swelling in the neck.

Pharyngeal and post-cricoid carcinomas usually have a short history, starting with a feeling of something being stuck in the throat, whereas benign causes such as webs and pouches have a longer intermittent history. Pharyngeal webs are frequently accompanied by iron-deficient anaemia, which may disappear with iron therapy (Plummer–Vinson syndrome), but there is an increased malignant potential. Most of these causes are rare.

Motility disorders of the oesophagus

These can be divided into primary and secondary disorders. Primary disorders include achalasia, diffuse oesophageal spasm, and non-specific or intermediate type motility disorders. The non-specific category includes the hypertensive lower oesophageal sphincter syndrome (nutcracker or super-squeezer oesophagus). Achalasia and diffuse oesophageal spasm are thought to be two variants in a spectrum of conditions, and progression from diffuse oesophageal spasm to achalasia has been described. In diffuse oesophageal spasm, gross muscular hypertrophy of the oesophagus is the main pathological finding with some pre- and post-ganglionic nerve degeneration. Segmenting, non-propulsive high-pressure contractions develop in the lower oesophagus and a high pressure is maintained in the lower oesophageal sphincter.

In achalasia, there is degeneration of the post-ganglionic nerve fibres (Auerbach's plexus) in the oesophageal muscle leading to a dilated atonic oesophagus with a hypertensive lower oesophageal sphincter. The dilated oesophagus becomes filled with saliva and food debris, which may be regurgitated or aspirated when the patient become recumbent (Fig. 4).

Diffuse oesophageal spasm is often associated with odynophagia followed by dysphagia whereas achalasia is mostly characterized by dysphagia soon after swallowing. Some achalasia sufferers describe a sudden relief of dysphagia if they stand up, as this can lead to gravity overcoming the

hypertensive lower oesophageal sphincter. Both conditions are made worse if the patient eats quickly.

The incidence of achalasia is rare at 1 in 100 000 in Western countries with an equal sex distribution in most countries and can occur throughout life but is very uncommon in children under the age of 5.

Secondary motility disorders are either part of a systemic disease or of inflammatory or malignant processes involving the oesophageal wall. This group includes conditions such as scleroderma, dermatomyositis, diabetes, amyloid, alcoholic neuropathy, and infection with *Trypanosoma cruzi* (Chagas' disease). The latter is rare and most commonly occurs in South America. It usually takes about 30 years to develop after the initial infection and the clinical features are very similar to achalasia.

Extrinsic lesions

The commonest culprit is carcinoma of the bronchus, due either to local spread of the tumour or enlargement of nodes pressing on the oesophagus as it passes through the mediastinum. Again timing of dysphagia after swallowing is the most valuable symptom in determining the site of obstruction.

Other less common causes include large cervical osteophytes from cervical spondylosis and retropharyngeal abscess or tumour.

In the mediastinum a retrosternal goitre, an aneurysmal aortic arch or an enlarged left atrium due to mitral stenosis are uncommon causes of dysphagia.

Sudden onset dysphagia

Complete and sudden onset of dysphagia is usually due to the impaction of a bolus of poorly chewed food on an oesophageal abnormality such as a stricture or diverticulum.

Oesophageal candidiasis (Fig. 5) can cause a fairly sudden onset of dysphagia and odynophagia and is common in debilitated and immuno-compromised patients. In particular, oesophageal candidiasis is seen in AIDS sufferers or in patients on antibiotics, steroids, and cytotoxic drugs. Asthmatics using inhaled steroids may develop oesophageal candidiasis. A clue to the diagnosis would be concurrent oral candida.

During mediastinum radiotherapy, oesophageal radiation damage can lead to an acute dysphagia and odynophagia.

Certain drugs, such as doxycycline, emepromium bromide, slow-release potassium, and aspirin can cause acute oesophageal ulceration if taken dry and not washed down with adequate fluids. The onset of odynophagia and dysphagia is sudden, but can be persistent if stricturing occurs subsequent to ulceration.

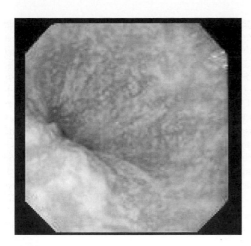

Fig. 5 Oesophageal candida. (See Plate 11.)

Motility disorders such as achalasia are helped by disrupting the hypertensive lower oesophageal sphincter, either by cardiomyotomy or pneumatic oesophageal dilatation at endoscopy. These procedures often lead to an incompetent antireflux mechanism and the resulting oesophagitis requires long-term proton pump inhibitors.

Oral candidiasis usually responds to oral nystatin or amphotericin, although occasionally a systemic anti-fungal such as itraconazole is required.

Patients with neurological disorders such as stroke and motor neuron disease can be helped by liquidizing food initially but ultimately will require nasogastric or percutaneous gastrostomy feeding tubes.

Although most primary care physicians would not be involved in the initiation of these treatments, they will be involved in their long-term management at home afterwards and many patients will want to discuss the treatment options with their doctor before they are initiated. Primary care physicians will need to enrol the help of other professionals including dieticians and nurses.

Pseudodysphagias

Patients suffering with anorexia, dementia, depression may complain of a difficulty in swallowing but the cause is due to a failure to initiate swallowing with food being chewed, moved around the mouth and eventually spat out.

Globus hystericus is due to somatisation in anxiety states. The patient complains of food sticking in the mouth but further questioning often reveals the symptom to be a sensation of tightness or lumpiness in the throat, which actually diminishes on swallowing.

The feeling of a crumb being stuck in the throat merits early ENT referral as it can signify the presence of an early pharyngeal tumour. It is mentioned here to highlight the danger of diagnosing globus too readily.

Investigation of dysphagia

Clues to the diagnosis are often found from the history, age of the patient, and mode of onset. A clinical examination may reveal neurological abnormalities in motor neuron disease such as a wasted fasciculating tongue, dysarthria of Parkinson's disease, or of a pseudobulbar palsy. Oral candida may be associated with oesophageal candida. A pharyngeal pouch may be accompanied by a gurgling sensation in the neck on swallowing. Goitre may be present. Enlarged cervical lymph nodes may suggest deposits from pharyngeal, oesophageal, gastric, or lung malignancies.

The mainstay of investigation is the barium swallow and endoscopy. These investigations are complementary rather than exclusive. A barium swallow will provide information about pharyngeal webs and pouches and oesophageal motility disorders that are difficult to appreciate at endoscopy. It is easier to distinguish a peptic stricture at endoscopy than by radiology. A peptic stricture is usually central and has oesophagitis above it and normal gastric mucosa below, often with a hiatus hernia. Malignant strictures are irregular and usually have normal oesophageal mucosa above.

Treatment available for dysphagia

Oesophageal cancers can only be cured if diagnosed early, before metastatic spread, and are amenable to oesophagectomy. Squamous cancers are more sensitive to radiotherapy and adenocarcinoma is often treated with adjuvant chemotherapy.

Cancer not amenable to surgery can be palliated with the placement of an oesophageal stent and can be locally ablated with alcohol injection and laser therapy.

Pharyngeal pouches can be stapled and excised. Oesophageal peptic strictures can be dilated at endoscopy with tapered dilators. Oesophagitis is most effectively treated with long-term proton pump therapy.

Key points

Dysphagia has many causes. The most common in the Western world is oesophagitis caused by gastro-oesophageal reflux. This is related to lifestyle—obesity,[7] diet, and smoking. Oesophageal cancer is showing a marked change in incidence with adenocarcinoma assuming the dominant type. This is again thought to be related to reflux and Barrett's oesophagus.[1,5]

At present there is no consensus as to whether endoscopic surveillance of Barrett's oesophagus is effective as a screening test for early oesophageal cancer as most cancers arising in Barrett's sufferers are found as a result of the development of new symptoms rather than in the screened population. It is likely that surveillance of Barrett's is more likely to be driven by medico legal considerations than evidence of efficacy.

There is no evidence that treatment of Barrett's mucosa with proton pump inhibitors causes regression of the condition or that treatment of oesophagitis with the same prevents Barrett's.[8]

Most other causes of dysphagia are rare and many practitioners may not see cases in their medical careers.

Acknowledgements

Acknowledgements to The Online Atlas of Gastrointestinal Endoscopy, www.mmdspring.com/~dmmmd/atlas_1.html for the use of endoscopic pictures.

References

1. Jankowski, J.A., Harrison, R.F., and Perry, I. (2000). Gastro-oesophageal cancer: death at the junction. *British Medical Journal* **321**, 463–4 (editorial).

2. Lagergren, J. et al. (1999). Symptomatic gastroesophageal reflux as a risk factor for esophageal adenocarcinoma. *New England Journal of Medicine* **340** (11), 825–31.

3. Haruma, K. et al. (1999). Eradication of *Helicobacter pylori* increases gastric acidity in patients with atrophic gastritis of the corpus—evaluation of 24-h pH monitoring. *Alimentary Pharmacology & Therapeutics* **13**, 155–62.

4. Dent, J. et al. (1999). An evidence based appraisal of reflux disease management—the Genval workshop report. *Gut* **44** (Suppl. 2), S1–16.

5. Devesa, S.S., Blot, W.J., and Fraumeni, J.K., Jr. (1998). Changing patterns in the incidence of esophageal and gastric carcinoma in the United States. *Cancer* **83** (10), 2049–53.

6. Survival rates among patients with upper gastro-intestinal cancers (England and Wales, age standardized). Office for National Statistics, 1999.

7. **Brown, L.M., Swanson, C.A., Gridley, G. Swanson, G.M., Shoenberg, J.B., Greenberg, R.S., Silverman, D.T., Pottern, L.M., Hayes, R.B., Schwartz, A.G., Liff, J.M., Fraumeni, J.F., Jr., and Hoover, R.N.** (1995). Adenocarcinoma of the esophagus: role of obesity and diet. *Journal of the National Cancer Institute* **87**, 104–9.

8. **Sharma, P., Sampliner, R.E., and Carmargo, E.** (1997). Normalization of oesophageal pH with high dose omeprazole proton pump inhibitor therapy does not result in regression of Barrett's esophagus. *American Journal of Gastroenterology* **92**, 582–5.

Further reading on the Internet

EUCAN—European Cancer Registry on www.encr.com.fr.
GLOBOCAN—Global Cancer Registry on www.iacr.com.fr.
WHO Mortality Statistics on www.who.int/whois/mort/.

4.3 Acute abdominal pain

Niek J. de Wit

Introduction

For many reasons, the management of acute abdominal pain is a major challenge for primary care physicians. Acute abdominal syndromes may be life-threatening, requiring urgent surgical intervention. Patients are aware of that, and the patient's perception of abdominal pain is often 'acute', and as such not a reliable indicator of a true abdominal emergency.

Not all patients with acute abdominal pain require immediate surgery; after proper assessment, many are relieved with adequate analgesics. The general practitioner (GP) has the difficult task of making this distinction.

Diagnostic tools for this task in primary care are limited: history and physical examination will usually have to suffice to reach the correct diagnosis. The primary care physicians can use the typical primary care instruments to come to the proper diagnosis: knowledge of the patients' history, risk assessment, and knowledge of prior probabilities.

Proper management of the acute abdomen does not usually need complicated investigations. However, circumstances are often not optimal: late-night assessment of the abdomen of a crying child in a sagging bed at home requires much skill. Though signs and symptoms are highly sensitive for acute appendicitis or ruptured aneurysm, they are often less typical in children or in the elderly.

In this chapter, we will review the epidemiological features of acute abdominal symptoms, the differential diagnosis and the value of signs and symptoms for effective management in primary care.

Acute abdominal pain; incidence in the community

There are hardly any data available on the incidence of acute abdominal signs and symptoms in the community. Given the fact that most patients with acute complaints will usually present to the GP, population and primary care data are less likely to be as divergent as in other conditions, where consultation bias is much more prominent.

In the Western world, acute appendicitis is the most frequent cause of acute abdominal pain in all age groups. The lifetime risk of developing appendicitis is estimated at 7 per cent, occuring in most patients before 30 years. The mortality of appendicitis is generally low, (less than 0.2 per cent), but higher in patients under 2 and over 60 years. One-third of the patients with gallbladder disease present as an emergency. Cholecystitis is the second ranking cause of acute abdominal complaints in adults, and even more frequent in the elderly. In many parts of the world, rupture of ectopic pregnancy is a leading cause of maternal deaths. One in every 200 pregnancies gestates outside the uterine endometrium. Risk factors are prior infection or surgery of the adenexae, and the presence of an intra-uterine contraceptive device.

In the Netherlands, the number of hospital admissions for appendicitis is 114 per 100 000, that for nephrolithiasis 78 per 100 000 annually. Intestinal haemorrhage and diverticulitis are rare conditions (22 and 29 admissions per 100 000); more than 50 per cent of these patients are older than 65 years.

Consultation for acute abdominal pain

The incidence of generalized abdominal pain in general practice varies from 11 to 13 per 1000 patients per year. The incidence of acute appendicitis in primary care registration networks in the Western world varies from 0.7 to 1.6 per 1000 per year. Gallstones and cholecystitis are also prevalent (1–2.4 per 1000 patients annually) but pancreatitis is rare (0.2 per 1000 patients a year).

Data on diagnosis in over 10 000 patients presenting with acute abdominal pain reveal that inflammation of appendix and gallbladder represent the majority of the acute abdominal problems referred to the surgeon, and that in one-third of the patients no specific cause for the complaints can be found (Table 1).

More than half of the children referred for an acute abdomen have non-specific abdominal pain while appendicitis represents one-third of the patients (Table 1). Urinary tract infection (2 per cent) and intussusception (1 per cent) are rare. In the elderly patient, the spectrum is different: cholecystitis is the most common cause, while obstruction and cancer are three times more frequent than in the younger age groups (Table 1).

In summary, in a primary care practice of 3000 patients, on average three to four patients present with acute abdominal complaints every month. Annually, 25 patients are referred to secondary care; in eight of these patients no cause can be found; three to five of these patients have acute appendicitis, five to six have gallbladder related problems, and two to three have nephrolithiasis. Vascular emergencies, obstruction, and pancreatitis are rare causes.

Table 1 Diagnosis in acute abdominal patients referred to 26 surgical departments in 17 countries

Diagnosis	% of all patients (n = 10 320)	% children (n = 1020)	% patients >50 (n = 2406)
Non-specific abdominal pain	34	62	16
Appendicitis	28	32	15
Cholecystitis	10		21
Small bowel obstruction	4	2	12
Acute gynaecological disease	4		
Acute pancreatitis	3		7
Renal colic	3	0.5	
Ulcer perforation	3		
Cancer	2		4
Diverticulitis	2		6
Miscellaneous	8		

Differential diagnosis

The differential diagnosis of acute abdominal pain covers a broad spectrum of potential causes. Classification can be made in several ways, guided by onset, pathophysiological background, localization, organ, or specialism. In primary care, a classification combining background, cause, and location is most useful (Table 2).

A number of diagnoses in patients presenting with acute abdominal symptoms do not reflect an acute abdominal syndrome. Examples are abdominal wall muscle pain, abdominal lymphadenitis, gastroenteritis, acute food poisoning, and urinary tract infections.

The cause of the acute pain may be extra-abdominal: especially pneumonia, but even otitis media in children may present as acute abdominal pain. Epigastric pain may be the first and only sign of a (inferior) myocardial infarction in the elderly, while a strangulated femoral hernia may cause pain in the groin or the upper leg.

There are a number of exceptional causes of acute abdominal pain syndromes that every primary care physician will encounter once or twice in his/her professional career. Amongst these are Mediterranean fever, acute porphyrias, hereditary angio-oedema, lead or mushroom intoxication, typhoid fever, herpes zoster before the rash, and abdominal tuberculosis or syphilis. These diagnoses may often be hard to establish.

Making a diagnosis in primary care

Risk assessment for the patient with acute abdominal pain in primary care is based on two questions: (a) does the patient have an acute abdominal syndrome? and (b) does the patient need urgent surgical intervention?

Appropriate history taking and physical examination can answer both questions.

History

The *age* of the patient is an important factor in the differential diagnosis in acute abdominal symptoms. In *children*, appendicitis, lymphadenitis, and (in very young children) intussusception are the most frequent causes. In *adolescents*, appendicitis and (in women) gynaecological conditions are the most frequent. With ageing, the chance of gallbladder disease rises,

and in the *elderly* the chance of vascular disease, diverticulitis or bowel obstruction due to a malignant process is much higher.

The medical *history* of the patient plays an important role: in those who have had abdominal surgery in the past ileus due to herniation or adhesions should be considered. Patients with a history of vascular disease are at risk for an abdominal aneurysm or mesenteric thrombosis.

The use of *medication* is important. Frequent use of non-steroidal anti-inflammatory drugs (NSAIDs), especially in the elderly, is an important risk factor for a peptic ulcer, perforation or bleeding. The use of anti-coagulants might cause a rectus haematoma, intra-abdominal bleeding or complicate an existing peptic ulcer.

In women, the recent *menstrual history* is helpful in assessing the possibility of a gynaecological cause of the acute abdominal syndrome. A missed menstrual period, combined with sudden pain and vaginal blood loss are the main clinical features of ectopic pregnancy. However, less than half of the patients have subjective pregnancy sensations.

Symptoms

Pain is the most important symptom in acute abdominal syndromes.

Sudden *onset* of pain occurs in the case of perforation of a peptic ulcer, cysts, or vascular obstruction. A gradual onset of pain is more typical for an infectious cause; the pain intensity rises quickly in the case of mesenteric thrombosis, bowel obstruction, or pancreatitis.

The *character* of the pain is important. Colicky pain that comes and goes is typical for the spasms with which the ureter or cystic duct tries to expel a stone. The upper abdominal pain in the case of a perforated peptic ulcer or acute pancreatitis is sharp, knife-like. The rupture of an ectopic pregnancy causes acute severe pain, often referred to the shoulder. Patients should be asked to indicate the *location* of the pain in the abdomen (with one finger), as this is often an important clue to the diagnosis (Table 3). Pain caused by irritation of the visceral peritoneum leads to general abdominal pain, which is often difficult to localize (gastroenteritis, colitis, and bowel obstruction). Once the parietal peritoneum gets involved, the pain is localized in the upper or lower abdomen. The transit from visceral to parietal pain is illustrated by the typical history of the patient with appendicitis: the pain starts as a vague feeling of discomfort in the umbilical region, and migrates to the right lower abdomen, while getting more intense.

Finally, the *radiation* of the pain is an important feature. Colicky pain starting in the back and migrating to the pelvic area is indicative of urolithiasis. Referral to the back is typical for retroperitoneal causes of pain (pancreatitis, ruptured aneurysm), while referral to the right shoulder might be a sign of a sub-diaphragmatic cause of the acute abdomen.

The patient may present other symptoms. The early occurrence of *fever* in combination with acute abdomen is suggestive of an infectious cause. The fever in appendicitis is usually mild, not exceeding 38.5°C. Half of all patients with pelvic inflammatory disease and the majority of those with cholecystitis present with fever. *Nausea* and *loss of appetite* often occur, but are not very discriminatory. Vomiting occurs usually early in case of a high bowel obstruction, but only late in case of obstruction in the colonic area. Massive blood loss in the gastrointestinal tract (*melaena* and *haematemesis*)

Table 2 Differential diagnosis in acute abdominal pain

Location	Cause	Diagnosis
Intra-abdominal	Peritonitis	Appendicitis
		Cholecystitis
		Diverticulitis
		Salpingitis
	Perforation	Peptic ulcer
		Extra-uterine pregnancy
		Ovarian cyst
	Bowel obstruction	Volvulus
		Hernia
		Intussusception
	Vascular emergency	Mesenterial thrombosis
		Aneurysm
		Torsion of the testis
	Colic	Nephrolithiasis
		Cholelithiasis
	Traumatic	Ruptured spleen
		Kidney contusion
		Bowel perforation
Extra-abdominal	Myocardial infarction	Myocardial infarction
	Oesophagus	Cramps
	Pulmonary	Pneumonia

Table 3 Localization of pain in relation to potential causes

Area	Potential causes
Right upper abdomen	Cholecystitis, hepatitis, liver abcess
Epigastrium	Ulcer, pancreatitis, myocardial infarction, aneurysm
Left upper abdomen	Spleen infarction or rupture, pneumonia
Right lower abdomen	Appendicitis, hernia, extra-uterine pregnancy, ovarian cyst, diverticulitis, ureteric stone
Left lower abdomen	Nonspecific, hernia, extra-uterine pregnancy, ovarian cyst, diverticulitis, ureteric stone
Back	Kidney stone, pyelitis, retro-peritoneal bleeding

is highly suggestive of a bleeding peptic ulcer or mesenteric thrombosis (see Chapter 4.7); jaundice suggests cystic duct obstruction. Recent *change in stool pattern* may be a clue to a (malignant) bowel obstruction.

Physical examination

In the classic surgical approach, the abdomen should first be inspected, then auscultated, percussed, and finally, be palpated.

Inspection of the abdomen does usually not add much information, except for the presence of scars of previous surgery, missed in the history. It could probably be better replaced by inspection of the patient at a distance: are there any signs of a stress reaction (sweating, pale face) is the patient in real pain, avoiding coughing and lying still to prevent pain provocation. In established obstruction, abdominal distension may occur, and bowel movements may even become visible. Inspection of the groins and scrotum might reveal possible swelling.

Bowel sounds may be completely absent in cases of peritonitis (silent abdomen). If the bowel passage is locally disturbed due to a paralytic ileus or an obstructing lesion high-pitched bowel sounds may be found as a sign of partial intestinal obstruction.

Percussion may be helpful in demonstrating enlargement of the liver or spleen or bladder distension.

Palpation of the abdomen provides the most useful information (Box 1). It helps the physician to discriminate between peritoneal irritation/ peritonitis and the extraperitoneal abdominal conditions. However, it requires skill, and conditions should be optimal.

Guarding (passive muscle resistance) is the crucial sign to look for: a locally increased tone of the abdominal wall muscles due to irritation of the peritoneum. If present, it is highly indicative of peritonitis (83 per cent specificity), but it is not so useful to rule out peritonitis (sensitivity of 59 per cent). In contrast, *local tenderness* and the more painful *rebound pain* are useful to rule out peritonitis, but not so good to identify it (sensitivity 91 per cent, specificity 60 per cent). In case of appendicitis, there is often local peritonitis in the right lower abdomen, McBurney's point. Patients may complain of pain on active movement of the hip (the so-called psoas sign). Patients with acute cholecystitis demonstrate guarding in the right upper abdomen. Liver and spleen enlargement should be detected on palpation; intra-abdominal tumours can be palpated depending on size and adiposity. A pulsating swelling of the aorta may support the diagnosis of an aneurysm.

For *rectal examination*, many advocate routine digital examination in the acute abdominal patient. Its additional value should be considered in every primary care patient, and weighed against the discomfort it causes. It might detect low bowel cancer, obstruction or abscesses of the pouch of Douglas. A painful rectal examination supports the suspicion of peritonitis, but does not usually identify it. The empty rectum confirms, but does not exclusively diagnose, the obstructed bowel.

On suspicion of gynaecological disease, it should be replaced by a *vaginal examination*, which provides an impression of the size and condition of uterus and adnexae. Painful swelling in the pelvis may, combined with information about the menstrual cycle, reveal an ectopic pregnancy or an ovarian cyst. Pain on subtle manipulation of the cervix may be a sign of a local peritonitis caused by pelvic inflammatory disease or a ruptured extra-uterine pregnancy.

Box 1 Palpation technique

> The patient should be on a firm flat bed or couch, avoiding the abdomen from withdrawing under the palpating hand. This hand should—especially in children—not be too cold, to avoid any adverse body movements. The legs can be bent at the knees to relax the rectus muscle as much as possible. Above all, the child should be put at ease; abdominal examination of a crying child is a lost mission. Slowly rocking the pelvis, while looking for any facial reaction of pain is a good way to start the abdominal palpation.

Investigations

The management of acute abdominal pain in primary care is based on history and physical examination. In most cases, a diagnosis and subsequent risk assessment can be made, sufficient for the decision to either refer the patient for surgery or treat and review the patient in primary care.

Routine additional testing is not required but may be useful where there is doubt. Testing in primary care requires time, and should not cause unnecessary diagnostic delay. Tests are most helpful in the grey zone of the diagnostic process (between 20 and 80 per cent prior chance of disease). Both at a very low and at a high prior chance of disease most tests have limited additional value to detect or rule out a specific cause, and the risk of false positive and negative results is high.

Laboratory techniques

The erythrocyte sedimentation rate (ESR) is raised in cases of infection, but only if this has been present for more than 24 h. In the acute onset of complaints, the ESR does not have additional diagnostic value, but it can be helpful in diagnosing abscess (appendicular or pelvic abcess). The C-reactive protein (CRP) is generally elevated in cases of infection, as is the white blood count (WBC). Both may assist in diagnosing an abdominal emergency (positive predictive value of 79 and 75 per cent, respectively) but they are not very helpful in excluding this (negative predictive value of 64 and 42 per cent respectively). However, a normal CRP and WBC almost rules out appendicitis.

The differential WBC might reveal a lymphocytosis in case of a viral gastrointestinal infection or a granulocytosis in case of a bacterial cause explaining the abdominal symptoms. *Urinalysis* can detect a urinary tract infection. Haematuria can be the clue to the diagnosis of urolithiasis. Finally, serum *amylase* may be helpful in the diagnosis of pancreatitis. Abnormal liver function tests may give a clue to the diagnosis in case of right-sided abdominal pain. GGT and bilirubin may be high in many hepatic conditions. AP is more specific for cystic duct obstruction (due to gallstone or tumour), and ALT and AST are disturbed in parenchymal liver disease (see Chapter 4.9). A pregnancy test may be helpful in acute pain in women, as a negative test almost excludes ectopic pregnancy.

Diagnostic imaging

Diagnostic imaging of the patient most often requires referral to the hospital. However, there may be circumstances in which the primary care physician can use imaging techniques (ultrasound available in the practice, open access facility). In case of diagnostic doubt, it is often more efficient to refer the patient directly to the surgical department.

Ultrasonography has proved to be very helpful in the diagnosis of right-sided abdominal pain in children or young women. Pooled sensitivity and specificity of ultrasound for diagnosing appendicitis is 85 per cent and 92 per cent, respectively. However, it hardly contributes in the case of a classical appendicitis, and should only be used in the case of atypical presentation. Ultrasound will demonstrate 90 per cent of gallstones, and though it may miss some urinary stones, is very sensitive in demonstrating hydronephrosis.

Plain abdominal X-ray is the examination of choice when there is a suspicion of perforation (air under the diaphragm) or bowel obstruction (fluid levels). Plain X-rays miss the majority of gallstones, as only 15 per cent are calcified. In contrast, the majority of urinary calculi are radio-opaque and are demonstrated on plain X-ray films.

When there is persisting diagnostic doubt, *computer axial tomography* (CAT) or *magnetic resonance imaging* (MRI) of the abdomen may reveal the underlying pathology.

Management of acute abdominal pain in primary care

Less than half the patients with acute abdominal pain are referred to hospital, and half of the referred group undergo surgery.

Box 2 Management of acute abdominal complaints

◆ The *first step* is to rule out an acute life-threatening disorder: if the patient is haemodynamically unstable, resuscitation and prompt referral to the hospital is required.

◆ If the patient is stable, the *second step* is to assess whether there is abdominal rigidity as a sign of peritonitis. Most patients with peritonitis will need surgical intervention. The localization of the pain, history, and additional symptoms often lead to the diagnosis, and the patient will usually be referred urgently.

◆ For patients who are not critically ill and who have no signs of peritonitis, there is no need for urgent referral. In *step three*, primary care management takes place. In cases of a clear colic attack due to a ureteric stone, the pain may be relieved appropriately. It may often be difficult to identify the cause of the symptoms immediately. Re-assessment in a later stage or the use of additional diagnostic tests may be appropriate.

Management of the patient with acute abdominal complaints in primary care is based primarily on clinical assessment, and consists of three steps (Box 2).

Children with acute abdominal complaints require a different approach. Information on symptoms and history can sometimes only be given by the parents. The clinical presentation is far less typical than in adults: pain is often not localized but referred to the umbilical region and fever may be absent. Persisting pain in the abdominal periphery is often a sign of local pathology.

Under 2 years appendicitis is uncommon, but once it is found it is usually perforated. The safe surgical management of suspected appendicitis includes the removal of up to 10 per cent normal appendices. Bowel colic occur in many children in the first 3 months, but a number of congenital causes should be ruled out (inguinal herniation, intussusception, gastric outlet obstruction, Meckel's diverticulum, or a toxic megacolon). Urinary tract and ENT infections may cause abdominal complaints.

Acute abdominal complaints in the elderly have a different morbidity (Table 1). Appendicitis is relatively less frequent, while the incidence of cholecystitis rises with age. Above 60 years, bowel obstruction due to cancer and vascular causes of acute abdomen are more frequent. Comorbidity and declining cerebral functions may confuse the clinical presentation, causing serious patients' and doctors' delay in the diagnosis. The risk of surgery, morbidity, and mortality is also higher in elderly patients and this should be considered in management. Mortality rates for acute cholecystectomy and appendectomy may reach up to almost 10 per cent in patients above 65 years.

Key points

◆ Appendicitis is the most frequent cause of acute abdominal pain and should always be in the top two of the differential diagnosis.

◆ Clinical features in young children and elderly patients may be atypical; therefore broad confidence intervals should be used in management.

◆ The main diagnostic tools in evaluating acute abdominal pain are history and physical examination.

◆ Guarding is a vital sign demonstrating peritonitis.

◆ Re-evaluation after a few hours is a safe policy in the primary care management of acute abdominal pain.

◆ Diagnostic tests are of limited value in the primary care management of acute abdominal pain; clinical impression should always prevail.

Further reading

Epidemiology and differential diagnosis

Wormgoor, B.F. (1985). Acute abdomen in the Netherlands. *Nederlands Tijdschrift Voor Geneeskunde* **129** (11), 495–9.

Roy, S. and Weimerscheimer, P. (1997). Nonoperative causes of abdominal pain. *The Surgical Clinics of North America* **77** (6), 1433–54.

de Dombal, F.T. (1988). The OMGE acute abdominal pain survey. *Scandinavian Journal of Gastroenterology Supplement* **144**, 35–42.

Telfer, S., Fenyo, G., Holt, P.R., and de Dombal, F.T. (1988). Acute abdominal pain in patients over 50 years of age. *Scandinavian Journal of Gastroenterology Supplement* **144**, 47–50.

Hawthorn, I.E. (1992). Abdominal pain as a cause of acute admission to hospital. *Journal of the Royal College of Surgeons of Edinburgh* **37** (6), 389–93.

Dickson, J.A., Jones, A., Telfer, S., and de Dombal, F.T. (1988). Acute abdominal pain in children. *Scandinavian Journal of Gastroenterology Supplement* **144**, 43–6.

Kizer, K.W. and Vassar, M.J. (1998). Emergency department diagnosis of abdominal disorders in the elderly. *American Journal of Emergency Medicine* **16** (4), 357–62.

de Dombal, F.T. (1994). Acute abdominal pain in the elderly. *Journal of Clinical Gastroenterology* **19** (4), 331–5.

Purcell, T.B. (1989). Nonsurgical and extraperitoneal causes of abdominal pain. *Emergency Medical Clinics of North America* **7** (3), 721–40.

Hoffman, S.H. (1989). Tropical medicine and the acute abdomen. *Emergency Medical Clinics of North America* **7** (3), 591–609.

History and physical examination

Bemelman, W.A. and Kievit, J. (1999). Physical examination—rebound tenderness. *Nederlands Tijdschrift Voor Geneeskunde* **143** (6), 300–3.

Festen, C. (1999). 'Acute abdomen' in children. *Nederlands Tijdschrift Voor Geneeskunde* **143** (4), 182–5.

Williams, N.M., Johnstone, J.M., and Everson, N.W. (1998). The diagnostic value of symptoms and signs in childhood abdominal pain. *Journal of the Royal College of Surgeons of Edinburgh* **43** (6), 390–2.

Laboratory testing and imaging

Mendelson, R.M. and Kelsey, P.J. (1995). Abdominal ultrasound. An overview for general practitioners. *Australian Family Physician* **24** (4), 585–6, 588–9, 592–3.

Chi, C.H., Shiesh, S.C., Chen, K.W., Wu, M.H., and Lin, X.Z. (1996). C-reactive protein for the evaluation of acute abdominal pain. *American Journal of Emergency Medicine* **14** (3), 254–6.

Schwartz, M.Z. and Bulas, D. (1997). Acute abdomen. Laboratory evaluation and imaging. *Seminars in Pediatric Surgery* **6** (2), 65–73.

Nordback, I. and Harju, E. (1988). Inflammation parameters in the diagnosis of acute appendicitis. *Acta Chirurgica Scandinavica* **154** (1), 43–8.

Bank, S. (1990). Serum amylase values in the acute abdomen. *Journal of Clinical Gastroenterology* **12** (1), 121–2.

Patrick, G.L., Stewart, R.J., and Isbister, W.H. (1985). Patients with acute abdominal pain: white cell and neutrophil counts as predictors of the surgical acute abdomen. *The New Zealand Medical Journal* **98** (778), 324–6.

Gupta, H. and Dupuy, D.E. (1997). Advances in imaging of the acute abdomen. *Surgical Clinics of North America* **77** (6), 1245–63.

General management

Farber, M.S. and Abrams, J.H. (1997). Antibiotics for the acute abdomen. *Surgical Clinics of North America* **77** (6), 1395–417.

Martin, R.F. and Rossi, R.L. (1997). The acute abdomen. An overview and algorithms. *Surgical Clinics of North America* **77** (6), 1227–43.

Simpson, E.T. and Smith, A. (1996). The management of acute abdominal pain in children. *Journal of Paediatrics and Child Health* **32** (2), 110–12.

Bender, J.S. (1989). Approach to the acute abdomen. *Medical Clinics of North America* **73** (6), 1413–22.

Specific disease management

Walker, J.S. and Dire, D.J. (1996). Vascular abdominal emergencies. *Emergency Medical Clinics of North America* **14** (3), 571–92.

Richards, W.O. and Williams, L.F., Jr. (1988). Obstruction of the large and small intestine. *Surgical Clinics of North America* **68** (2), 355–76.

Williams, L.F., Jr. (1988). Mesenteric ischemia. *Surgical Clinics of North America* **68** (2), 331–53.

Jordan, P.H., Jr. and Morrow, C. (1988). Perforated peptic ulcer. *Surgical Clinics of North America* **68** (2), 315–29.

Chappuis, C.W. and Cohn, I., Jr. (1988). Acute colonic diverticulitis. *Surgical Clinics of North America* **68** (2), 301–13.

Koch, M.O. and McDougal, W.S. (1988). Urologic causes of the acute abdomen. *Surgical Clinics of North America* **68** (2), 399–413.

Burnett, L.S. (1988). Gynecologic causes of the acute abdomen. *Surgical Clinics of North America* **68** (2), 385–98.

Potts, J.R., III. (1988). Acute pancreatitis. *Surgical Clinics of North America* **68** (2), 281–99.

Sharp, K.W. (1988). Acute cholecystitis. *Surgical Clinics of North America* **68** (2), 269–79.

4.4 Chronic abdominal pain

Mattijs E. Numans

Epidemiology

Chronic abdominal pain is defined as pain in the abdomen occurring continuously for at least 12 weeks in the past 12 months, and can be caused either by organic or functional disorders.[1] Open survey and population studies have shown that around 20 per cent of the adult population suffers from these complaints. In the United Kingdom and the United States, the male/female ratio among patients with chronic abdominal pain ranges from 0.3 to 0.9.[2,3]

Consultation rates

Less than half of people with chronic abdominal pain consult their physician. In general practice in the United Kingdom and the Netherlands, approaching 10 per cent of all consultations concern gastrointestinal (GI) disorders, and half of these are for chronic abdominal pain. The majority of patients presenting their complaint in primary care suffer from functional disorders, so that irritable bowel syndrome (IBS) is one of the most frequent GI disorders seen in primary care in Western societies.[4] Male patients consult less often than women, but once they do, the risk of finding serious disease is slightly higher.

Causes of chronic abdominal pain

In the West, the majority of complaints of chronic abdominal pain have no organic origin and are considered to be functional. However, with increasing age, a history of one or more surgical interventions for other reasons and an increase of exposure to infections, the risk of organic causes increases. Because of population differences the range of differential diagnoses is unlikely to be the same in every primary care practice. In general, however, the primary care physician confronted with chronic abdominal pain should consider IBS, non-ulcer dyspepsia, constipation, inflammatory bowel disease (IBD), chronic GI infection, peptic ulcer disease, lactose intolerance, gallstone disease, intermittent herniation in intra-abdominal scars, diverticular disease, and diseases in other organ systems, including abdominal aortic aneurysms, renal, ovarian, and uterine causes. Many of these are discussed in other chapters of this textbook. Rarer conditions, which may underlie chronic abdominal pain, include chronic hepatobiliary and pancreatic disorders; chronic amoebiasis and other parasitic infections should be considered in tropical and sub-tropical areas and slowly developing malignant disease must also be borne in mind.

Diagnosis

History

Consultations in primary care for chronic abdominal pain need to pay careful attention to the patients' history in order to establish the basis for consultation on which the physician may discriminate organic from functional complaints. Although few specific symptoms have been found to predict organic disease, alarm symptoms and symptoms pointing to organic disease should be sought on questioning. These include fever, persistent diarrhoea, especially at night, dysphagia, faecal blood loss, excessive fatigue, tenesmus, weight-loss, and severe constipation. Symptoms of this kind may indicate either treatable organic disease or malignancy and require further investigation. However, once the risk of serious disease has been reduced the context of the presenting complaint should be explored carefully, including the pattern of pain, its relationship to stress, and provoking and relieving factors. This approach may achieve more than simply gathering relevant medical information, because thorough questioning means that the patient will understand that the complaint is being taken seriously and can form the basis of meaningful explanation and the avoidance of further, unnecessary medical investigation and intervention.

Examination

Observation of the abdomen may reveal asymmetry, a mass or abdominal distension. Surgical scars may provide further clues and auscultation may identify abnormal bowel signs or vascular abnormalities. Physical examination in any abdominal complaint should include a digital rectal examination, because pathology is often located in the colorectum. In addition, pelvic examination in female patients with chronic abdominal complaints is required to exclude ovarian tumours and other gynaecological conditions possibly related to the presenting symptoms. However, examination of the abdomen often adds little specific differential diagnostic information about the cause of the disease that gives rise to these symptoms. Tumours will seldom be found; tenderness of the sigmoid colon may indicate colonic disease or IBS but can also indicate a degree of constipation, and is therefore a rather non-specific finding.

Diagnosing irritable bowel syndrome

IBS is generally regarded as a functional disorder and many physicians only consider this diagnosis after a number of investigations have proven negative. The syndrome, which is thought to be due to a combination of intestinal dysmotility and altered visceral perception, modified by psycho-social and probably post-infectious factors, is, however, a distinct entity for which a positive diagnosis is desirable in the primary care setting.[4] In 1978, Manning et al. proposed criteria for the diagnosis of IBS,[5] and in this definition abdominal pain was to be accompanied by at least two of the six so-called Manning criteria (Box 1).

A more recent attempt to permit a positive diagnosis of IBS was the elaboration of the first Rome criteria, later to be updated to the Rome II criteria[1] which are shown in Box 2. The Rome criteria can also be used to categorize patients into the IBS sub-types of predominant diarrhoea, predominant constipation, and alternating diarrhoea and constipation.

Young patients fulfilling the Rome criteria for IBS, and having no other symptoms suggestive of serious disease, do not need to undergo further investigation, and it is possible for the diagnosis to be made with a good degree of confidence in primary care. Elderly patients with symptoms of recent onset should be investigated in order not to overlook malignancy. However, there is some evidence that the Rome criteria are too complicated for routine use in primary care practice although it has been shown that general practitioners in the United Kingdom, at least, are capable of making the diagnosis of IBS with a reasonable degree of accuracy without using formal diagnostic criteria. The Rome criteria are, however, important in selecting patients for therapeutic trials and it is likely that future treatment recommendations will be based on data from patients studied in this way. It seems important, therefore, to attempt to incorporate the use of the Rome criteria into clinical practice in primary care, as far as possible.

Functional (non-ulcer) dyspepsia

Functional dyspepsia (also termed non-ulcer dyspepsia) refers to patients who have upper abdominal complaints and normal endoscopic findings.[6] Patients with endoscopy negative reflux disease (ENRD) may be part of this patient group. Non-ulcer dyspepsia accounts for the majority of patients complaining of upper GI symptoms in primary care. It is a complex diagnosis, for which no clear pathophysiologic mechanism is found. Symptoms may be various, but upper abdominal pain, nausea, flatulence, and bloating are predominant. Symptoms may be attributed to acid reflux, to delayed GI motility, to visceral hypersensitivity, or perhaps even to inflammation. A considerable proportion of patients with functional dyspepsia also suffer from functional lower digestive tract disease, mainly constipation or IBS. The prognosis of functional dyspepsia in primary care is in general good; after 1 year the majority (70 per cent) are symptom free.

In gastroscopy series, either in hospital GI clinics or in open access facilities in primary care, the proportion of normal results (which is equivalent to the proportion of patients with functional dyspepsia) varies between 40 and 60 per cent. Additional diagnostic investigations such as motility studies have no additional diagnostic value in functional dyspepsia.

From a primary care point of view, functional dyspepsia is a pragmatic diagnosis; as only 10–20 per cent of dyspeptic patients in primary care actually undergo endoscopy a 'true' diagnosis of functional dyspepsia is only established in a minority of patients. In a true sense, most patients with functional dyspepsia in primary care have uninvestigated dyspepsia.

Investigation

Investigations will be chosen on the basis of provisional diagnoses. A number of simple, office-based tests are useful in differentiating between possible causes of abdominal pain. Abnormal urinalysis should point to further investigation of the urogenital tract. Positive faecal occult blood testing, performed on 3 consecutive days with avoidance of red meat or brushing the teeth, may demonstrate occult blood loss caused by a neoplasm in the lower digestive tract, although given the low sensitivity of this test a negative faecal occult blood test is not particularly helpful in ruling out such blood loss. Routine haematological investigations are rarely helpful, although a high ESR might indicate an inflammatory process or even malignancy, and should point to further colonic investigation, whilst an elevated white blood count should similarly raise the possibility of an inflammatory or infective cause for the pain.

Upper or lower GI endoscopy is a relatively expensive investigation, but a very efficient diagnostic procedure, not least because biopsies and simple therapeutic interventions may be carried out during the course of the investigation. Many primary care physicians, however, still tend to prefer radiology for the investigation of the stomach and colon, not only because of its availability, but also because of its presumed patient-friendliness. However, elderly patients may find the contortions of contrast radiology more challenging than an endoscopy conducted under light benzodiazepine sedation. From a diagnostic point of view, radiological investigations are generally regarded as the second best option for investigating the GI tract, although the choice is likely to be limited in certain health care settings. Other intra-abdominal organs that cannot be investigated by endoscopy can be visualized with ultrasound, computer tomography, or magnetic resonance imaging.

Diverticulosis and diverticulitis

Diverticulosis is often considered a normal condition of the large bowel because it is found on radiological investigation of the colon in at least one-quarter of elderly people.[7] Its occurrence may be associated with a low-fibre diet, and it generally gives rise to no complaints. However, a small proportion, probably about 10 per cent, of people with diverticular disease occasionally develop episodes of diverticulitis, which may cause more serious disease including haemorrhage, peritonitis, intestinal perforation, and septicaemia. When a patient is suspected of diverticulitis, on the basis of abdominal pain, fever, colonic tenderness, and possibly rectal bleeding, immediate radiological investigation should be avoided because of the danger of perforation. The diagnosis is likely to be made either on the basis of previous investigations or on the physical examination combined with evidence of infection on routine haematological testing. Most patients with diverticulitis improve on a regime of rest and oral fluids, sometimes with broad spectrum antibiotics. Evidence is, however, accumulating to support early surgical management of these patients, of whom a substantial proportion go on to develop complications (see Chapter 4.5).

Specialist referral

Around 25 per cent of patients presenting in primary care with chronic abdominal complaints are eventually referred to specialists, reflecting the low prevalence of serious organic disease in this group. Specialist referral should be considered when alarm symptoms suggestive of neoplastic or infection causes of chronic abdominal pain are present, where there is diagnostic uncertainty, where appropriate investigations are not available to the general practitioner, when there is significant patient pressure, or when other psychosocial factors create pressure to obtain a further opinion.

Inflammatory bowel disease

There are two major types of IBD—ulcerative colitis and Crohn's disease.[8] In primary care practice in Western Europe, the incidence of these conditions is around two new cases per general practitioner per year.[9] The incidence is lower in Southern European countries, in Africa and in Australia, and these conditions are very rare in Asia and South America. There appears to be a genetic predisposition for IBD, recently confirmed by the discovery of genetic polymorphisms associated with Crohn's disease.[10] Environmental factors which impact on the development of IBD include smoking, which is interestingly associated with a lower risk of developing ulcerative colitis, but seems, together with the use of oral contraceptives, to increase the risk of developing Crohn's disease.

Patients with IBD usually present with gradually developing diarrhoea and abdominal pain, although about 15 per cent of patients present in primary care with advanced disease. The diagnosis can be difficult to make, and the mean time from presentation to diagnosis in patients with Crohn's disease is in the region of 18 months. IBD is also associated with a number of non-colonic conditions, including inflammatory conditions of the eye, such as uveitis, a variety of joint problems, including peripheral arthritis, sacroiliitis and spondylitis, and, in Crohn's disease, aphthous ulcerations of the oral and genital mucosa. Abnormalities of liver function, including pericholangitis, and anal and pudendal fistulae may also occur.

Ulcerative colitis typically presents with bloody diarrhoea, abdominal pain, fever, and weight loss, whilst Crohn's disease tends to present with more general malaise, abdominal pain, and diarrhoea without urgency or bleeding and, more frequently, extracolonic manifestations.

The diagnosis of both conditions can only be made on histological examination of biopsies taken at colonoscopy, although the extent of the inflammation may require further radiological investigation. Patients with chronic IBD, particularly ulcerative colitis, are at significantly increased risk of developing malignancy, so that colonoscopic surveillance, with consideration of total colectomy in patients with pancolitis of more than 10 years duration, should be planned and patients referred appropriately for specialist advice.

Rare causes of chronic abdominal pain

Refractory or atypical chronic abdominal complaints may also be due to rare conditions, including mesenteric ischaemia (abdominal angina) which occurs during periods of intestinal hypoxaemia, when arterial blood flow to the intestine is insufficient, causing post-prandial pain; arterosclerosis is usually the cause, but other vascular abnormalities may cause similar symptoms. Chronic pancreatitis is another rare cause of chronic abdominal pain which may only be diagnosed after thorough investigation.

Gallstones

The occurence of gallstones varies widely worldwide.[11] In the Western world, they are found in between 10–15 per cent of adults, amongst the population in Chile their prevalence is twice as high, while gallstones do not occur at all among the Masai in Kenya. This is related to a number of pathophysiological factors: the chance of developing gallstones depends upon the composition of the bile, its tendency to crystallize, and the motility of the gallbladder. Gallstones are found twice as often amongst women. The incidence rises with age, starting from the fourth decade.

Stones in the gallbladder are often a coincidental finding, and less than half of patients have symptoms from their gallstones. In follow-up studies, gallstones became symptomatic in 10 per cent of patients over 10 years. Non-acute symptoms that are often related to gallstones include nausea, upper abdominal pain, and dyspeptic symptoms. In a meta-analysis from 21 trials, it was shown that patients with gallstones have a slightly higher chance of upper abdominal pain (OR 2.0) and nausea (OR 1.4).[12] Stones in the cystic or bile duct do have a higher chance of producing symptoms, but these are usually acute, including gallstone colic and jaundice.

Ultrasound is the most effective way of diagnosing gallstones, and abnormal liver function tests, characterized by a high alkaline phosphatase, elevated bilirubin and moderately raised transaminases, will support the diagnosis of bile duct obstruction due to stones. Endoscopic retrograde cholangio-pancreatography (ERCP) is the most effective treatment.

As the relation between gallstones and non-acute complaints is weak, the removal of the gallbladder will usually not relieve the patient from chronic abdominal complaints. Cholecystectomy for non-symptomatic stones is only recommended in relatively young patients (under 60 years) because of the cumulative risk of complications (cholecystitis, acute colic, and a slightly higher chance of gallbladder carcinoma in patients with long-standing non-symptomatic gallstones).[13]

Chronic abdominal pain in children

Abdominal pain is extremely common in children, but fortunately organic causes are rare.[14] A number of abdominal conditions may present with chronic pain: constipation, urinary tract infections, and also rare conditions such as peptic ulcers in children, gallbladder, and even pancreatic, disease. In most of these cases, additional symptoms will alert the physician: excessive vomiting, changes in stool frequency, fever, and weight loss. Sometimes simple blood and urine tests can help in differentiating chronic non-organic bellyache from abdominal pathology. In children with a high suspicion of abdominal pathology, referral to a paediatrician is indicated.

However, the majority of children with chronic pain do not have an abdominal disease; in many cases, the pain is a reflection of social or emotional stress or changes. Children with chronic abdominal pain often come from families where members suffer from physical complaints or have emotional problems. A complicating factor in the approach to children with chronic abdominal pain is parental anxiety, which can be difficult to deal with. It may be helpful to keep a diary of the complaints, specifying the type and character of complaints, the childrens' life events related to it and demonstrating a possible pattern in the week. Discussing the results of this diary with the parents may alleviate their concerns about the condition of the child.

Principles of management

One of the major challenges facing the primary care physician in the diagnosis and management of chronic abdominal pain is striking the correct balance between appropriate referral for diagnostic procedures and specialist opinions and the protection of patients from unnecessary and potentially hazardous and expensive interventions.

General

The treatment of any patient with chronic abdominal pain begins with taking a thorough clinical history which will act as a firm foundation for subsequent explanation, reassurance and management decisions. Alarm symptoms should lead to early investigation and specialist referral as appropriate, whilst a number of conditions are amenable to early and effective treatment in primary care. Recurrent urinary tract infections, peptic ulcer disease, non-ulcer dyspepsia, and GI infections, as well as IBS and the functional disorders, can safely be treated in primary care. Most differential diagnostic investigations that need to be carried out in search for the cause of the pain can also be requested and interpreted in primary care. As long as no specific organic disease mandates referral, management or treatment of the patient with chronic abdominal pain in primary care offers the best opportunity for a multidisciplinary approach to a condition which is likely to have multiple aetiologies.

When GI infection is found to be the cause of chronic abdominal pain (*Amoebiasis, Giardiasis, Salmonellosis*), specific treatment may be required. Diarrhoea is usually the predominant symptom and specific antibiotic treatment for the underlying infection should be prescribed (see Table 2 in Chapter 4.10). Treatment of urinary tract infection is usually straightforward, although antibiotics need to be prescribed with an awareness of local and specific patterns of antibiotic resistance. The investigation and management of patients with dyspepsia is discussed in Chapter 4.1, but when peptic ulcer disease is either confirmed or strongly suspected, *Helicobacter pylori* eradication therapy, using a proton pump inhibitor (PPI)-triple therapy regime, can be given by the primary care physician.

In IBS, drug therapy remains unsatisfactory. The evidence for the efficacy of antispasmodic agents is conflicting, although at least one large meta-analysis supports the use of mebeverine as a symptomatic treatment for these patients.[15] However, appropriate dietary manipulation and, in constipation-predominant patients, the addition of extra fibre to the diet is often efficacious. Antispasmodics such as mebeverine are widely used in clinical practice, in addition to which a number of non-drug therapies have been developed, including hypnotherapy and cognitive–behavioural therapy. It is likely that a number of more specific agents, such as $5HT_3$-receptor antagonists and $5HT_4$ receptor agonists will be developed to deal with diarrhoea-predominant and constipation-dominant IBS, respectively, although at present none have proven both safe and efficacious.

The results of pharmacotherapy in *functional dyspepsia* are largely determined by the placebo effect, which may be as high as 60 per cent in patients with functional complaints.[6] The additional effect of specific drug treatment is often disappointing: acid suppression with H-2 receptor antagonists or PPIs may add another 10–20 per cent to the therapeutic efficacy, as do prokinetic or even antidepressant drugs at both low and standard dosages.

The role of *H. pylori* infection in functional dyspepsia is a matter of considerable debate. *H. pylori* infection and the related gastritis appears to be present in 30–60 per cent of patients with functional dyspepsia, although this is equal to the infection rate in the background population of non-dyspeptic patients. In most trials on therapeutic efficacy in functional dyspepsia, dyspeptic symptoms and quality of life improve, and in about 20 per cent of the patients symptoms resolve completely. Results on the benefit of *H. pylori* eradication are contradictory: some trials report a small benefit, others do not.[16] Even pooled results in different meta-analysis give conflicting results. Depending on the regional prevalence of *H. pylori* infection and PUD, *H. pylori* treatment may benefit a small proportion of patients with functional dyspepsia.[17]

IBD is a condition whose management is likely to be shared with secondary care. The early decisions about treatment and follow up will be made by specialists, but the primary care physician has an important role in providing support for these patients with chronic disease. IBD is usually treated with sulfasalazine and other 5-ASA agents, which are available in several pharmaceutical forms with different release patterns.[8] Local suppository and steroid foam enemas and preparations are used to treat proctitis. Glucocorticoids are generally reserved for exacerbations, when they can be given orally, intravenously, or in enema form. Antibiotics are ineffective in ulcerative colitis, but metronidazole and ciprofloxacin are often used in Crohn's disease. Azathioprine, 6-mercaptopurine, and methotrexate all have anti-inflammatory effects, and are second line drugs in patients with serious and refractory disease. Other experimental pharmacological options are available, but most of these are at present beyond the scope of primary care practice.

Many patients with IBD will be investigated with endoscopy on a regular basis to monitor the progression of disease and, in the case of ulcerative colitis, to provide surveillance in the light of the increased risk of the development of colon cancer. In the long run, almost half of IBD patients will come to some form of surgical treatment, because of failure of conservative therapy or disease progression. Prophylactic colectomy, discussed earlier, may occasionally be undertaken.

Implications of the problem

Chronic and intermittent abdominal pain represents one of the most frequent reasons for patients to consult a primary care physician. Although empirical therapy may be appropriate for many of these patients, those with persistent complaints will require further investigation and often specialist referral. Conversely, over-treatment and over-investigation should be avoided and more research is needed into the natural history of these conditions and of the effects of drug and non-drug therapies in their management.

Key points

- Chronic or intermittent non-acute abdominal pain is one of the most frequent reasons for consulting primary care physicians.
- At least half of patients with abdominal pain suffer from a functional disorder.
- History-taking is very important in abdominal pain, not only for the physician but also to reassure the patient.
- Most diagnostic work-up can safely be organized in primary care.
- Radiology is a second-best option after endoscopy in investigating most cases of abdominal pain.

References

1. Thompson, W.G., Longstreth, G.F., Drossman, D.A., Heaton, K.W., Irvine, E.J., and Muller-Lissner, S.A. (1999). Rome II: a multinational consensus document on functional gastrointestinal disorders. *Gut* **45** (Suppl. 2), II43–7.

2. Jones, R. and Lydeard, S. (1992). Irritable bowel syndrome in the general population. *British Medical Journal* **304**, 87–90.

3. Drossman, D.A. et al. (1993). US householder survey for functional gastrointestinal disorders: prevalence, sociodemography and health impact. *Digestive Diseases and Sciences* **38**, 1569–80.

4. Van der Horst, H.E., van Eijk, J.T., and Schellevis, F.G. (1992). New insights into irritable bowel syndrome. A literature study. *Family Practice* **9**, 405–15.

5. Manning, A.P. et al. (1978). Toward positive diagnosis of the irritable bowel. *British Medical Journal* **2**, 654.

6. Fisher, R.S. and Parkman, H.P. (1998). Management of non-ulcer dyspepsia. *New England Journal of Medicine* **339** (19), 1376–81.

7. Isselbacher, K.J. and Epstein, A. (2001). Diverticular, vascular, and other disorders of the intestine and peritoneum. In *Harrison's Online* Part 11, Chapter 289 (ed. E. Braunwald, A.S. Fauci, K.J. Isselbacher et al.). McGraw-Hill.

8. Friedman, S. and Blumberg, R.S. (2001). Inflammatory bowel disease. In *Harrison's Online* Part 11, Chapter 287 (ed. E. Braunwald, A.S. Fauci, K.J. Isselbacher et al.). McGraw-Hill.

9. Rubin, G.P., Hungin, A.P., Kelly, P.J., and Ling, J. (2000). Inflammatory bowel disease: epidemiology and management in an English general practice population. *Alimentary Pharmacology & Therapeutics* **14** (12), 1553–9.

10. Van Heel, D.A., McGovern, D.P., and Jewell, D.P. (2001). Crohn's disease: genetic susceptibility, bacteria and innate immunity. *Lancet* **357**, 1902–4.

11. Greenberger, N.J. and Paumgartner, G. (2001). Diseases of the gallbladder and bile ducts. In *Harrison's Online* Part 11, Chapter 302 (ed. E. Braunwald, A.S. Fauci, K.J. Isselbacher et al.). McGraw-Hill.

12. Kraag, N., Thijs, C., and Knipschild, P. (1995). Dyspepsia; how noisy are gallstones? *Scandinavian Journal of Gastroenterology* **30**, 411–21.

13. Sheth, S. et al. (2000). Primary gallbladder cancer: recognition of risk factors and the role of profylactic cholecystectomy. *American Journal of Gastroenterology* **95**, 1402–10.

14. Scharff, L. (1997). Recurrent abdominal pain in children; a review of psychological factors and treatment. *Clinical Psychology Review* **17**, 145–66.

15. Jailwala, J., Imperiale, T.F., and Kroenke, K. (2000). Pharmacologic treatment of the irritable bowel syndrome: a systematic review of randomized, controlled trials. *Annals of Internal Medicine* **133**, 136–47.

16. **Friedman, L.S.** (1998). *Helicobacter pylori* and non-ulcer dyspepsia. *New England Journal of Medicine* **339** (26), 1928–30.

17. **Moayyedi, P., Soo, S., Deeks, J.** et al. (2003). Eradication of helicobacter pylori for non-ulcer dyspepsia. *Cochrane Database for Systematic Reviews* (1), CD002096.

4.5 Abdominal mass

Hein G. Gooszen

Introduction

The intra-abdominal mass is not a disease, or a syndrome, but a finding on physical examination. Such findings are, by definition, of a subjective nature, with all the drawbacks of inter- and intraobserver variation.

The intra-abdominal mass represents a very heterogeneous group of diseases and it is impossible to give overall data on epidemiology since, for example, both colonic cancer and empyema of the gallbladder will lead to the detection of an intra-abdominal mass. However, data on incidence and prevalence of colonic cancer and gallstone disease cannot substitute for this. A variety of other diseases can also give rise to a palpable mass, so no attempt will be made to give overall epidemiological information.

In each patient who seeks the help of his/her primary care physician because of abdominal symptoms, there is likely to be an awareness on the part of the physician not to overlook an abdominal mass, and careful examination and judicious use of investigations is required to ensure that abnormal physical findings are correctly interpreted.

Consultation rates for an intra-abdominal mass are not available, since the patient is often unaware that his/her symptoms are due to a mass in the abdomen and, even in the most complete registration systems, the intra-abdominal mass is unlikely to be included as the reason for consulting the general practitioner.

Causes of an intra-abdominal mass

Intra-abdominal masses can be sub-divided into inflammatory, cystic (primary or secondary to inflammation, as in the case of pancreatitis), and neoplastic (benign, malignant, or vascular). Soft tissue tumours, such as sarcomas and mesenteric lesions are not discussed in detail in this chapter. Diseases of the appendix, the gallbladder, the pancreas, and diverticular disease of the colon can all, after the acute phase of the disease, give rise to the development of an intra-abdominal mass. Cystic lesions of the pancreas and the liver (including hydatid disease of the liver) and the mesentery can present with a mass on physical examination. Tumours of the pancreas and colon are the most common causes of tumours giving rise to a mass as the primary presenting symptom. An aneurysm of the abdominal aorta is the only clinically relevant example of a vascular cause of an intra-abdominal mass.

Diagnosis of an intra-abdominal mass

Clinical history

An abdominal mass is a clinical diagnosis and the result of a careful physical examination. The patient is unlikely to tell the general practitioner that he has an abdominal mass although some patients do worry about a prominent xiphisternum or have discovered a hernia. Almost always the accompanying symptoms are non-specific: a dull, vague intra-abdominal pain or a sensation of fullness. Additional symptoms such as fever, weight loss, loss of appetite, dyspepsia, or changes in bowel habit may supply further information. Because of the potential causes of an intra-abdominal mass, a full history including detailed information on eating, drinking, appetite, defaecation, the menstrual cycle, and previous infectious diseases, is crucial to inform further diagnostic steps.

Physical examination

On physical examination, the general impression (weight loss, anaemia, fever) is the first step in deciding whether there is an inflammatory process, a benign cyst or tumour, or a malignant disease as the cause of the abdominal symptoms. Inspection does not usually have diagnostic value in the case of a mass. At auscultation of the abdomen, signs of obstruction can signal the presence of a tumour compressing the bowel, leading initially to small bowel obstruction, or growing into the lumen. Percussion is dull over tumours, cysts, and inflammatory masses. An inflammatory mass is difficult to exactly delineate on palpation, whereas tumours of the gastrointestinal tract, pancreas, or liver are more circumscribed. If they can be felt on palpation, this is usually a sign of advanced disease, leaving little room for a favourable prognosis. Cystic lesions are usually not fixed and move with the adjacent organ on respiration. An aneurysm of the abdominal aorta exhibits expansile pulsations. A tumour overlying the aorta can mimic these pulsations, but without being expansile. An aortic aneurysm is usually asymptomatic and if found, this must not be held responsible for the patient's symptoms too easily.

Initial diagnostic approach

Having taken a detailed clinical history and performed a physical examination, it is usually feasible to differentiate between an inflammatory mass, a cystic lesion, a tumour, and a vascular mass. Though it is common practice to start with laboratory tests like WBC and ESR, these tests are not sensitive and specific enough to differentiate between the different causes. Clinical history and physical examination are as important to initially discriminate between inflammation or neoplasia. Too often the acceptance of negative laboratory or ultrasound tests in a patient with alarm symptoms causes unnecessary delay. Instead, the addition of more sensitive and specific investigations, such as CT scanning, can prevent further delay.

Specific diagnosis

Inflammatory mass

If an inflammatory mass is suspected, this usually originates from the gallbladder, the appendix, the sigmoid colon, or the pancreas. The mass develops in a late (after 72 h or more) phase of the acute inflammation, when it has been sealed off by adjacent organs and the greater omentum. This forms an infiltrate with dull percussion and a palpable mass which is difficult to exactly delineate. If, with the knowledge of the clinical history and physical examination, the diagnosis of an abdominal infiltrate can be established, with or without the help of laboratory tests, there is no need for further investigation at this stage. None of the above-mentioned diagnoses necessitates any specific treatment, now that the disease has reached the infiltrative stage. The ideal moment for appendicectomy, cholecystectomy, or removal of the sigmoid colon has been missed. As for acute pancreatitis, there is a growing consensus that surgery should be postponed as far as possible.

If there is doubt about the diagnosis, additional investigations such as ultrasonography (to diagnose gallstones), CT scanning (to differentiate appendicitis from a caecal tumour or diverticular disease from a tumour of the sigmoid colon) is mandatory, not because of the immediate clinical consequences but to make further plans and to inform the patient. The diagnosis of 'acute cholecystitis' is a clinical one; the right upper abdominal mass may also be caused by a hydrops or empyema of the gallbladder. Ultrasonography is only helpful to demonstrate the stones, not to establish the diagnosis of an inflamed gallbladder.

Neoplastic mass

If a neoplastic lesion is suspected, there is no need for an urgent diagnosis from a prognostic viewpoint, although the patient may be very worried, requesting urgent testing. Laboratory tests are not very useful to direct the diagnostic process. If physical examination has revealed an intra-abdominal mass, and an inflammatory cause is considered unlikely, it may be a neoplasm originating from colon, pancreas, liver, stomach, or small bowel. Usually, a tumour presenting as a mass is no longer amenable to curative resection, but palliative surgical treatment may be useful in cancer of the stomach and the small or large bowel. Further diagnostic steps will reveal whether the process is amenable to surgical treatment. The first step is often endoscopy with histology. Once the diagnosis of a malignant tumour is established, CT scanning is the investigation of choice to decide whether surgery is indicated to prevent bleeding and obstruction.

If the palpable mass is localized in the *right upper quadrant* and moves on respiration, it is growing from the liver. In that case, CT scanning can differentiate between a cyst, a tumour (primary or secondary), or hydatid disease (with the typical intracystic septa).

If the palpable mass is localized in the *middle upper abdomen* and a pancreatic tumour is suspected, by far the highest diagnostic yield can be expected from a contrast-enhanced CT scan (taken with small slices in the area of the pancreas). Thus, signs of irresectability (such as invasion of adjacent vital structures) or incurability (e.g. metastatic disease in lymph nodes or liver) can be adequately demonstrated.

Cystic lesions

Cystic lesions are a rare cause of a palpable mass, usually originating from the pancreas, the liver, and the kidney. In general have, only large cysts can be palpated on physical examination.

Pancreatic cysts are usually pseudocysts which have developed in the course of acute or chronic pancreatitis. Often they are asymptomatic and apparently harmless. If diagnosed, however, treatment needs to be considered because complications such as rupture, bleeding, and infection can occur without preceding symptoms. Until about 5 years ago, surgical treatment was the standard, but endoscopic internal drainage is becoming more popular with results which, in terms of effectiveness and recurrence rates, compare with those of surgery.

Hepatic cysts may be unilocular and only require treatment when they become symptomatic, usually as a result of bleeding. A unilocular cyst can be caused by hydatid disease or by amoebiasis. Serology, ultrasound, and CT scanning help to differentiate these infections from the harmless unilocular cyst. Multiple cysts can develop in the course of adult polycystic liver disease. Like Swiss cheese there are multiple cysts with only remnants of liver in between them. Pancreatic and renal cysts also occur in this type of polycystic disease.

Renal cysts are frequently observed as an incidental finding on CT scanning. Single cysts are asymptomatic, cannot be palpated on physical examination, and have no implication for treatment. If the kidney is affected by polycystic disease, renal failure is often the first sign of disease. Pain can occur because of bleeding into one of the cysts. A mass with a tendency to move downwards on deep respiration can be palpated.

Other causes of abdominal mass

A *palpable spleen* usually indicates severe disease such as myelofibrotic syndrome, or severe portal hypertension with secondary enlargement of the spleen. A moderately enlarged spleen, as seen in sepsis, severe infectious disease and splenic vein thrombosis, is not normally palpable on physical examination.

An *enlarged uterus* usually indicates pregnancy. Only very large myomas can be diagnosed on physical examination. In the Western world, malignant tumours of the ovaries, endometrium, or cervix are usually diagnosed long before they give rise to the formation of an intra-abdominal mass, but late presentations often occur in the developing world.

An *enlarged bladder* means that the patient desperately needs catheterization!

A *palpable aorta* can erroneously lead to referral because an aortic aneurysm is suspected. Only if the pulsations of the aorta are expansile is the suspicion justified. The size of the aneurysm can easily be assessed by ultrasonography and if the diameter exceeds 6 cm, there is an increased risk of rupture and a good argument for surgical treatment if the patient represents an acceptable anaesthetic risk.

Principles of management

General principles

If the mass is caused by intra-abdominal inflammation and the period for surgical intervention has been exceeded, surgery can no longer be safely performed because anatomical dissection is hazardous due to oedema, bleeding, and the risk of causing damage to adjacent organs. General supportive measures have to be taken to allow the inflammation to subside. There is ongoing controversy about these general supportive measures and the concept of (complete) bowel rest is challenged. It is becoming clearer that early enteral feeding is superior to the 'old' approach involving intravenous nutrition. This implies that once an infiltrate has developed from appendicitis, cholecystitis or diverticulitis (and in some patients with acute pancreatitis) the patient can be safely treated by the general practitioner, provided that there is no abscess or secondary perforation. The patient needs close, daily observation. Consultation with a surgeon is required in case of complications. Localized abdominal pain becoming generalized or continuous fever becoming spiking are the signs of clinical deterioration, suggesting the development of an abcess or secondary perforation. Routine laboratory tests like WBC and ESR are not helpful in discriminating localized disease from generalized peritonitis or sepsis.

The treatment should consist of oral fluids only, for several days, followed by gradual return to a normal diet when there is improvement. Whether this should be combined with the administration of antibiotics remains controversial. Appendicitis, cholecystitis, and diverticulitis are not primarily infectious diseases. Only when perforation occurs—sealed or free—bacteria will enter into the peritoneal cavity causing peritonitis or an abscess. At this stage, there is a role for antibiotics to prevent bacteriaemia and sepsis.

Patients with *acute pancreatitis* are usually severely ill and referral will be the rule. There is, however, a sub-group of pancreatitis patients who will not be severely ill, even though they have a palpable mass in the upper abdomen. In that case, the disease will have lasted at least 1–2 weeks. Laboratory tests such as serum amylase or lipase determination are not particularly useful, as the serum levels of these enzymes are only elevated in the first 2–5 days. The main parameter guiding further action in these patients is their clinical condition. Intrajejunal feeding by a nasogastric tube is emerging as the favoured treatment. Trials are in progress to evaluate intragastric feeding but this can only be done in the inpatient setting. If the mass is due to a cystic lesion, a neoplasm, or is of vascular origin, management focuses on a rapid diagnosis, adequate treatment, and an explanation of this diagnosis to the patient.

Specific treatment

Inflammatory mass

For appendicitis and cholecystitis, operative treatment in the acute phase (<72 h) is the therapy of first choice. Whether acute resection of the sigmoid colon is the best therapy for patients with an acute attack of diverticular disease is doubtful. For acute pancreatitis, it is increasingly accepted that surgical intervention should be delayed if possible, leaving bleeding as the only indication for immediate surgery.

Once an infiltrate has developed, conservative management entails awaiting resolution of the inflammatory mass. This usually takes 8–12 weeks. In appendicular, gallbladder, and diverticular disease, this can be frustrated by the development of an abscess or generalized peritonitis. Once this occurs, the complication has to be treated surgically or by interventional radiology.

The removal of the diseased organ is harmful and is usually delayed to a later stage.

Appendicectomy '*a froid*' has essentially been abandoned. A gallbladder with stones that has caused complications (hydrops, empyema, gallstone pancreatitis, or an inflammatory mass in the course of acute cholecystitis) has to be removed to prevent further symptoms or complications. The optimal strategy for diverticulitis of the sigmoid colon is under debate.[1] Some studies lend support to an aggressive surgical approach after an acute attack. Others tend to be more conservative, only proposing sigmoid resection after several attacks. Whether diverticulitis with an intra-abdominal mass, indicating local perforation, should be treated differently from an episode without a mass, is unknown. The strategy has to be individualized and all risk factors have to be considered.

Cystic lesions

A cystic lesion usually reflects a benign disease. Treatment is only required if the risks of complications, with the ensuing morbidity and mortality, are higher than the risk of intervention, albeit radiologically or surgically (laparoscopy or open surgery).

Cystic lesions of the *pancreas* are more common than those of the liver. In case of pseudocysts developing in the course of acute pancreatitis, spontaneous resolution can be expected. Bleeding, perforation, and infection, reported in 25 per cent of the patients, are the main complications of pseudocysts. A persisting pseudocyst with a diameter of 6 cm or more needs treatment. Surgery was the 'gold standard' until about 10 years ago,[2] but more and more alternative treatments (external or internal drainage via endoscopy) are now used.[3] These modalities are far less invasive than surgery but the recurrence rate after radiological drainage is higher and the endoscopic procedure needs expert hands. If there is no history of pancreatitis, the cystic lesion may conceal a malignancy and the therapeutic approach must be more aggressive. Percutaneous diagnostic biopsy has, because of the high false negative results and complications, no place in the diagnostic work-up of these patients. The cyst should be removed.

Cysts in the *liver* are congenital—unilocular or multilocular in the course of polycystic liver disease—or can develop as a manifestation of hydatid disease.[4] Unilocular cysts, if symptomatic, can easily be 'unroofed' by a laparoscopic approach, a type of treatment that is usually successful. Polycystic disease only needs treatment if it is causing severe mechanical symptoms. A hydatid cyst that causes symptoms is usually larger than 10 cm and needs surgical treatment because of the risk of perforation.

Tumours

If the mass is caused by a tumour of the gastrointestinal tract, the chances of cure are minimal. Surgery is justified to prevent complications such as bleeding or obstruction or to perform bulk reduction before chemotherapy or radiotherapy.

Psycho-social impact

An intra-abdominal mass, once diagnosed, is a finding with major impact on the patient and his/her relatives because of the immediate association with malignant disease. With a careful history and examination, a provisional discrimination between a benign inflammatory and a malignant mass can usually be made in an early stage, helping to put the patient at ease. However, a further diagnostic work-up is usually necessary. The patient is often correct when malignant disease is suspected! If the story does not fit, do not hesitate to take a further diagnostic step instead of waiting for weeks or months to repeat another inaccurate diagnostic procedure. A locally perforated sigmoid carcinoma can mimic acute diverticular disease, gallbladder carcinoma can mimic acute cholecystitis and pancreatic carcinoma can mimic acute or chronic pancreatitis.

Long-term care and follow-up

If the inflammatory mass has subsided and the patient has undergone cholecystectomy or sigmoid resection no further long-term care is necessary.

If diverticulitis was treated conservatively, the patient needs to be instructed regarding the prevention of constipation and informed of the possible complications of diverticular disease: stenosis, perforation, and fistula (to the bladder, small bowel, large bowel, or vagina) and recurrent attacks. In the case of acute pancreatitis without gallstones, the patient should be instructed to refrain from alcohol and might need specific guidance in this. If a tumour has been resected, local protocols on specific follow-up will show how to take care of these patients. Follow-up of patients with gastrointestinal tumours is a subject of continuing debate and details will not be discussed in this chapter.

Key points in diagnosis and treatment of an intra-abdominal mass

- An intra-abdominal mass is a subjective finding, not a disease.

- Detailed transfer of subjective clinical information is increasingly important with changing patterns in health care: working pattern, legislation, and medico-legal liability.

- An uncomplicated inflammatory mass, unless caused by acute pancreatitis, can usually be treated in the home situation.

- Evidence is accumulating to support early surgical intervention in patients with an episode of acute diverticulitis because of the subsequent development of complications.

- A (pseudo)cystic lesion of the pancreas should be considered potentially malignant if there is no history of pancreatitis.

References

1. **Young-Fadok, T.M., Roberts, P.L., Spencer, M.P., and Wolff, B.G.** (2000). Colonic diverticular disease. *Current Problems in Surgery* **37**, 457–514.

2. **Cooperman, A.M.** (2001). Surgical treatment of pancreatic pseudocysts. *Surgical Clinics of North America* **81**, 411–19.

3. **Vidyarthi, G. and Steinberg, E.** (2001). Endoscopic management of pancreatic pseudocysts. *Surgical Clinics of North America* **81**, 405–10.

4. **Hansman, M.F., Ryan, J.A., and Holmes, J.H.** (2001). Management of hepatic cysts. *American Journal of Surgery* **181**, 404–10.

4.6 Nausea, vomiting, and loss of appetite

Juan Mendive

Nausea and vomiting

Nausea—a feeling of sickness with an inclination to vomit—and vomiting—the forced expulsion of gastric or intestinal contents through the mouth—are extremely common symptoms. In primary care, they are among the commonest reasons for patients to consult general practitioners. They are most frequently the symptoms of a self-limiting and often non-specific illness, but may also be the early manifestations of serious disease. Accurate diagnosis, symptom control, and management of the underlying disease are priorities in management in primary care.

Table 1 Nausea and vomiting; differential diagnosis

Infections
Viral gastroenteritis and food poisoning
Acute gastritis and peptic ulcer disease
Acute pancreatitis
Appendicitis, cholecystitis, cholangitis, hepatitis, and pyelonephritis
Otitis media
Urinary tract infection

Mechanical causes
Gastric carcinoma
Peptic ulcer disease
Pyloric stenosis
Intestinal obstruction
Paralytic ileus
Diabetic gastropathy

Metabolic causes
Diabetic ketoacidosis
Renal failure, uraemia
Hyperparathyroidism
Pregnancy
Addison's disease

Cardiac
Myocardial infarction
Heart failure

Neurologic
Vagal response
Migraine
Vestibular disturbances, travel sickness
Midline cerebellar haemorrhage and raised intracranial pressure
Post-traumatic—cerebral contusion

Drugs and intoxication
Alcohol and drug abuse
Digoxin, non-steroidal anti-inflammatories, opiates, antibiotics, chemotherapeutic agents, oral contraceptives, alcohol, salicylates

Psychogenic causes
Stress, anxiety
Anorexia nervosa, bulimia nervosa

The vomiting centre in the medullary reticular formation receives stimuli from vagal and sympathetic afferent nerves in the pharynx, gastrointestinal (GI) tract, peritoneum, mesentery and heart, and from the chemoreceptor trigger zone, which lies in the floor of the fourth ventricle, in response to chemical, metabolic, and vestibular stimuli. Nausea and vomiting can, therefore, be caused by a very wide range of disorders, the most important of which are summarized in Table 1.

Clinical presentations

The time-course and pattern of vomiting, together with its association with abdominal pain and other digestive symptoms, can provide valuable clues to its likely cause. The patient's history usually facilitates the discrimination between the benign, self-limiting causes of vomiting (GI infections, drug or alcohol related, stress induced, pregnancy) and a presentation that suggests a more serious background. For example, projectile vomiting is typically associated in infants with pyloric stenosis and in adults with raised intracranial pressure. Early morning nausea and vomiting is typical of metabolic abnormalities, including early pregnancy, diabetic ketoacidosis, and uraemia. Vomiting shortly after meals may be due both to upper GI disorders, such as peptic ulcer disease and gastritis, and also to psychogenic causes. Acute vomiting, often accompanied by abdominal pain or diarrhoea, is typical of viral gastroenteritis, frequently due to food poisoning, but with progressive abdominal pain and other symptoms, raises the possibility of more serious abdominal problems, such as intestinal obstruction, pancreatitis, appendicitis, cholecystitis, and pyelonephritis. Nausea may be physiological in circumstances of extreme exercise or physical or mental exhaustion.

Acute vomiting may also occur in a range of neurological conditions, including migraine and, more seriously, with midline cerebellar haemorrhage and space-occupying lesions associated with raised intracranial pressure. Metabolic and drug-related vomiting usually begins with anorexia, followed by nausea and vomiting. Digoxin toxicity is typically associated with visual disturbances, including yellow-tinged vision and coloured halos. Non-steriodal anti-inflammatory drugs may produce nausea and vomiting accompanied by dyspepsia. Vomiting is a surprisingly common symptom of myocardial infarction and is sometimes the only symptom of childhood infections, such as otitis media. Opiate abuse and withdrawal, as well chronic alcoholism and binge drinking, are often accompanied by nausea and vomiting. Chronic nausea and vomiting without weight loss makes an organic reason very unlikely. Psychogenic factors, such as stress or anxiety, may also induce nausea and vomiting, which may also be part of psychiatric syndromes such as depression and bulimia, and anorexia nervosa, conditions which predominantly affect young women, in whom a distorted body image is a key feature. Bulimia is more frequent than anorexia nervosa, affecting up to 15 per cent of young women in the Western world. Anorexia nervosa is characterized by extreme weight loss in a patient who persists in considering herself overweight. This irrational self-image may be accompanied by other psychiatric features, such as depression, agitation, or anxiety. Physical consequences are common and include amenorrhoea, wasting, hypotension, and bradycardia. In bulimia, patients try to control their body weight by self-induced vomiting after (often excessive) food intake. Body weight may vary, but is normal in half of bulimic patients.

Physical examination

The physical examination begins with a check for evidence of dehydration and hypovolaemia; signs include orthostatic hypotension, reduced skin turgor, and reduced muscle tone. Attention should also be paid to the heart and respiratory rates, and the presence of jaundice and hyperpigmentation. The abdominal examination should include a search for distention, visible peristalsis, abnormal bowel sounds, peritoneal signs, tenderness, organomegaly, and abnormal masses. A thorough neurological examination is essential when a neurological cause is suspected. A full ear, nose, and throat examination should be carried out in children and infants. All patients should be asked about prescribed and over-the-counter medication and the ingestion of alcohol and recreational drugs.

Investigations

Laboratory and other investigations are unnecessary in many patients presenting with nausea and vomiting in primary care, such as patients with a confirmed, early pregnancy, those with adverse effects from non-steroidal anti-inflammatory agents, and children with tonsillitis or otitis media. However, when the cause of persistent nausea and vomiting is unclear, a number of laboratory and imaging tests may be considered. Useful blood tests include sodium, potassium, urea, and creatinine electrolyte estimations, to rule out renal failure and electrolyte disturbances, liver function tests to aid the diagnosis of hepatitis, a random blood sugar, serum amylase, and liver function tests. A pregnancy test may also be helpful and urinalysis may help to rule out a urinary tract infection.

Other useful investigations include plain abdominal radiology, particularly if intestinal obstruction is suspected, electrocardiography in patients who may have ischaemic heart disease, abdominal ultrasonography, when gallbladder pathology is suspected, and referral for upper GI endoscopy or neurological imaging in appropriate cases.

Management

The primary care approach to nausea and vomiting begins with the discrimination between the benign, well-explained episodes, in which spontaneous recovery can be expected, and those with a recurrent, chronic presentation. Management consists, whenever possible, of the management of the underlying condition, and many of the disorders described here are discussed in more detail elsewhere in this textbook. Patients with clinical signs pointing towards a serious acute abdominal problem, such as bowel obstruction, hepatitis or appendicitis, or to a serious central nervous system cause for their vomiting should be referred for specialist care, and their management is not considered further in this chapter. In cases of persistent vomiting, referral to a medical specialist may be required for further analysis of an organic background. In those patients in whom a psychogenic background is suspected appropriate attention to contributing factors is indicated. In case of a true psychiatric disorder referral for psychotherapy or specialist treatment is often best. For anorexia nervosa, a multidisciplinary approach, often requiring hospitalization, is required, including psychotherapy and a supervised feeding programme. Though the prognosis of bulimia is somewhat better, a multidisciplinary coordinated approach to treatment is also required in severe cases.

In most cases of nausea and vomiting, symptomatic relief, irrespective of the cause, is important; antiemetic agents act on the medullary vomiting centre, the chemoreceptor trigger zone, and on peripheral receptors. Phenothiazines are the most useful drugs for suppressing vomiting, although their use is not recommended in children under the age of 6 years. Prochlorperazine (Stemetil, Compazine) can be given in doses of 5–10 mg every 6 h orally, rectally, or systemically. When a vestibular cause is suspected, antihistamines, such as promethazine (Phenergan), dimenhydrinate (Dramanine), meclozine or cyclizine can be used. The antidopaminergic agents metoclopramide (Maxolon) and domperidone (Motilium), which can also be given orally and systemically, are also useful. 5-HT3 receptor antagonists, such as ondansetron, granisetron, and tropisetron are particularly useful for chemotherapy and radiotherapy-induced emesis.

In case of long-standing or abundant vomiting, fluid and electrolyte imbalance, if suspected or detected, should be treated appropriately, using oral rehydration therapy in the ambulatory care setting, although more severely dehydrated or metabolically deranged patients will require intravenous fluid therapy.

Loss of appetite

Loss of appetite (anorexia) can, like nausea and vomiting, be caused by a range of conditions, and self-evidently shares a number of aetiologies. In addition to the causes mentioned in Table 1, loss of appetite may occur before nausea in patients with abdominal disorders, in the early stages of heart failure, with oral cavity problems, and with the use of amphetamines. People may lose their appetite in cases of stress or anxiety, and anorexia may also be a presenting sign of self-neglect. The causes of anorexia are likely to be different in infants, adults, and elderly people, and in Table 2 the most common organic and non-organic causes of anorexia are summarized.

Evaluation

The clinical history is important, and the psychosocial background, as well as the physical symptoms, should be explored. The time-course and duration of the loss of appetite, associated weight loss, eating pattern, alcohol consumption, smoking, and drug use must also be discussed. Bearing in mind that anorexia may be the earliest presentation of the causes of nausea and vomiting described earlier, a careful history, including an exploration of gastrointestinal, urinary and other symptoms, is needed. Recent life events, personal, professional, and family stresses, and current mental state should also be assessed at interview.

A full physical examination is, once again, important, including serial weighing on accurate scales to establish whether body weight is falling. Laboratory investigations should be used in the same way as described previously. In general, routine laboratory testing does not contribute to the evaluation of the nutritional status. Testing should be guided by the results of history and physical examination. Nutritional assessment may be helpful in assessing a dietary cause, while anthropometric measurement of muscle- or skin-fold thickness may be useful in the follow-up of the patient with anorexia to evaluate fat and protein balance.

Management

Once again, the treatment of loss of appetite is the treatment of the underlying condition, and when an organic cause has been identified, the approach to treatment will follow that described for nausea and vomiting. However, an identifiable cause for loss of appetite may not be apparent in many patients in primary care. Early discrimination between organic and psychogenic causes is essential, because management of each follows a completely different route. If required, additional diagnostic tests or referral to a medical specialist for confirmation of diagnosis should be used to achieve this. In infants, a full exploration of family circumstances and tensions is likely to be important, and the contribution of health visitors, public health nurses, and other primary care team professionals is often invaluable.

When anorexia persists in adults, in the absence of an organic explanation, a more detailed exploration of the psychological and psychiatric background, including the use of alcohol and illicit drugs, becomes more important. Patients with depression may present with loss of appetite; adolescents in whom anorexia nervosa or bulimia nervosa is suspected should be referred for specialist assessment and management (see Chapter 9.6 for a more detailed discussion).

In terminally ill patients, the loss of appetite and subsequent weight loss is a consequence of the underlying disease. Once this is incurable, nutritional support may be considered, varying from dietary advice to enteral feeding support or even total parenteral nutrition. This needs to be discussed thoroughly, as in most terminally ill patients this will not influence the life expectancy nor the quality of life.

In the elderly, it is wise to reserve a physiological explanation for anorexia until an underlying physical or psychological cause has been ruled out with certainty. Although reduced appetite, possibly related to reduced physical activity, is an expected physiological change in the elderly, other causes must be considered. Old people living in poverty may face particular problems in purchasing food which is sufficiently appetizing to provide a full range of nutrients.

Table 2 Causes of anorexia

	Infants	Adults	Elderly
Organic cause	Viral and bacterial infections Digestive intolerance Gastro-oesophageal reflux	Gastrointestinal disease Endocrine disorders Malignancy Drug side-effects	Malignancy Drug side-effects
Non-organic cause	Parental anxiety Feeding habits	Depression, anxiety, alcoholism, illicit drug use	Physiological causes Immobility Self-neglect Depression

Further reading

Marranzini, M. and Paesetto, A.G. (1995). Anorexic and pseudoanorexic child. *La Pediatria Medica e Chirurgica* 17, 545–58.

Morley, J.E. (1996). Anorexia in older persons: epidemiology and optimal treatment. *Drugs & Aging* 8, 134–55.

Spiller, R.C. (2001). Anorexia, nausea, vomiting, and pain. *British Medical Journal* 323, 1354–7.

Talley, N.J., Phung, N., and Kalantar, J.S. (2001). ABC of the upper gastrointestinal tract: indigestion: when is it functional? *British Medical Journal* 323 (7324), 1294–7.

Ross, D.D. and Alexander, C.S. (2001). Management of common symptoms in terminally ill patients: Part I. Fatigue, anorexia, cachexia, nausea and vomiting. *American Family Physician* 64 (5), 807–14.

Allan, S.G. (1992). Antiemetics. *Gastroenterology Clinics of North America* **21**, 597–611.

Chapman, K.M. and Nelson, R.A. (1994). Loss of appetite: managing unwanted weight loss in the older patient. *Geriatrics* **49**, 54–9.

4.7 Haematemesis and melaena

Pali Hungin

Haematemesis and melaena signify acute bleeding from the upper gastrointestinal tract, the oesophagus, stomach, or duodenum. This is an important condition because it can be a life-threatening emergency requiring urgent specialist intervention. Upper gastrointestinal bleeding is especially threatening in the elderly in whom there is a substantially increased risk of complications and mortality. This is due to frailty and to the increased presence of concurrent health problems contributing to serious complications. Bleeding due to peptic ulcers linked with *Helicobacter pylori* infection has declined in the developed countries because of reducing rates of infection. The major cause of bleeding is from ulcers linked to non-steroidal anti-inflammatory drug (NSAID) therapy in the elderly, and aspirin-linked problems are also becoming more common. The overall morbidity and mortality from peptic ulcers has thus not declined despite the management of ulcers linked with *H. pylori* infection. The prevention of haematemesis remains to a large extent within the domain of primary care.

Epidemiology, incidence, and prevalence

The annual incidence of acute upper gastrointestinal haemorrhage in the United Kingdom is 103 per 100 000, rising from 23 per 100 000 in those under the age of 30 years to 458 per 100 000 in those over 75 years. In Western Europe and North America, the pattern of disease has altered significantly in the last 25 years as the populations have aged. There has been a rising incidence in the elderly and 25 per cent of patients admitted to hospital in the United Kingdom with haematemesis and melaena are aged over 80 years. In UK primary care, the consultation rate for gastrointestinal bleeding is 12 per 10 000 people (7 per 10 000 for haematemesis and 3 per 10 000 for melaena)[1] and a general practitioner with an average of 2000 patients can expect to encounter two or three cases per year. The incidence of first bleeding in those who have oesophageal varices is 4.4 per 100 per year.

Presentation

The presenting symptoms depend on the source of the bleeding and the volume of blood lost. The majority of younger patients present with small amounts of fresh-looking blood on retching or vomiting, often described as 'streaks'. This is often associated with excessive alcohol intake. In others, variable amounts of blood in vomitus, mixed or fresh, indicates recent or current haemorrhage. 'Coffee ground' vomitus, traditionally indicative of recent blood loss, is the result of gastric acid action on the deposited blood. Abdominal pain is not a consistent feature and many patients have no previous or current history of pain or discomfort; the bleeding may be painless and discovered incidentally as black stool hours or days after the initial bleeding episode.

Black stool indicates the presence of denatured blood after upper gastrointestinal loss and passage through the intestine. The blood content is homogenous with stool. In contrast, lower gastrointestinal bleeding presents as fresh looking blood loss or as blood mixed with stool rather than uniformly black. However, black stool can also be caused by the intake of oral iron- or bismuth-containing compounds. Occasionally, melaena can present as fresh blood loss if intestinal transit has been rapid. This leads to confusion with colonic causes of bleeding. In cases of doubt it is safer to manage the patient as an emergency.

Haematemesis or melaena may be associated with signs of acute shock depending on the amount of blood loss. Patients who are anaemic from previous chronic blood loss are particularly vulnerable to a further acute loss. Some patients, in the absence of haematemesis, may even present only with signs of hypovolaemia if melaena has not yet developed. This should be considered in patients who present with shock without any obvious cause. The absence of abdominal tenderness is not a reliable sign for the exclusion of a cause of upper gastrointestinal bleeding and the site of abdominal pain itself is a poor predictor of the exact cause. In 50 per cent of patients with a bleeding peptic ulcer, there is no preceding history of ulcer pain, particularly in the elderly taking NSAIDs or aspirin. Patients known to have liver cirrhosis or indicators of hepatic failure or portal hypertension are at increased risk of haemorrhage from varices and from impaired blood coagulation.

Causes of haematemesis and melaena and outcomes

Non-variceal bleeding

The commonest cause of haematemesis and melaena is non-variceal blood loss. In 50 per cent, it is due to peptic ulcers and in the rest to oesophagitis or oesophageal ulcer, Mallory–Weiss tears, gastric or duodenal erosions and vascular malformations (Table 1). Duodenal ulcers are slightly more common than gastric ulcers as a cause of bleeding and oesophagitis accounts for 10 per cent of all bleeding. Mallory–Weiss syndrome is due to a mucosal tear at the gastro-oesophageal junction. Classically, this follows recurrent vomiting after a bout of high alcohol intake but it can occur without recurrent vomiting as melaena alone. The cause of gastric erosions is unknown although they can be associated with drugs or alcohol. Tumours are a relatively uncommon cause of acute haemorrhage. Leiomyoma, a benign tumour, is more likely to bleed than other tumours. Rarer causes include aortic and splenic artery aneurysms, arterial malformations, pancreatic and biliary tree cancer, and haemostatic disorders.

About 80 per cent of those with non-variceal bleeding will not have further problems necessitating any specific measures; the remaining 20 per cent are likely to have severe bleeding due to the erosion of an artery. These patients are most at risk of death, particularly the elderly, because of concomitant medical problems compromising their survival. The overall mortality rate from acute gastrointestinal bleeding in the United Kingdom is 11 per cent.

For non-variceal acute bleeding, the Rockall scoring system (Table 2) has been devised as a means of identifying those most at risk.[3,4] This assessment is based on findings at the time of admission to hospital and background factors. In addition to increasing age, especially over 80 years, hypotension, a raised pulse, and co-morbidity, particularly heart failure and ischaemic heart disease, are indicators of increased risk of complications and mortality.

The presence of a Mallory–Weiss tear or the absence of any visible lesion on endoscopy are predictors of a relatively good outcome, whilst the detection of an upper gastrointestinal malignancy is associated with a poorer immediate outcome. The absence of visible blood or the presence of a simple dark spot at endoscopy also indicates a good prognosis as opposed to the presence of blood, adherent clot, or a visible spurting vessel.

Table 1 Relative frequency of causes of acute upper gastrointestinal bleeding (%)[2]

	Country, year						
	Multinational, 1986	England, 1990	Scotland, 1986	Wales, 1986	Denmark, 1986	United States, 1981	Australia, 1985
Number of patients	4431	430	326	330	539	100	201
Percentage bleeding from:							
Oesophagitis/oesophageal ulcer	4	12	15	7	13	0 }	17
Mallory–Weiss syndrome	3	4	2	5	3	16 }	
Varices	13	4	2	3	11	20	8
Peptic ulcer	37	50	52	48	53	40	43
Duodenal		25	36	29		22	
Gastric		25	16	19		18	
Gastritis/duodenitis/erosions	7	22	6	14	12	6	12
Tumour	3	1	1	3	2	2	4
Others/multiple pathology/no lesions	34	7	23	20	5	16	17

Table 2 The Rockall scoring system for risk of re-bleeding and death after admission to hospital for acute gastrointestinal bleeding[3,4]

Variable	Score			
	0	1	2	3
Age	<60 years	60–79 years	<80 years	
Shock	No shock Systolic BP >100	Tachycardia Systolic BP >100	Hypotension Systolic BP <100	
Pulse	<100	>100		
Co-morbidity	Nil major		Cardiac failure, ischaemic heart disease, any major co-morbidity	Renal failure, liver failure, disseminated malignancy
Diagnosis	Mallory–Weiss tear, no lesion and no SRH[a]	All other	Malignancy of upper GI tract	
Major SRH	None, or dark spot		Blood in upper GI tract, adherent clot, visible or spurting vessel	

[a] SRH: stigmata of recent haemorrhage.

Re-bleeding is associated with increased mortality. Deaths following admission to hospital for acute gastrointestinal bleeding are less likely to be the result of the blood loss itself, even if copious, but to complications following surgery and the deterioration of the patient's condition due to concomitant conditions. Re-bleeding occurs in 25 per cent of patients with a chronic peptic ulcer and is associated with a mortality of 30 per cent compared with less than 10 per cent in those who do not re-bleed.

Unexplained acute haemorrhage, that is, where no cause can be identified on investigation, occurs in up to 10 per cent. Some of these patients may have bled from lesions that have healed by the time of investigation. If re-bleeding occurs it is likely that an ulcer was missed or that the bleeding occurred from some other source such as the biliary tree or pancreas, or that the patient had a haemostatic disorder.

Variceal bleeding

Gastro-oesophageal varices are the result of portal hypertension. This is usually a complication of liver cirrhosis; 30–60 per cent of cirrhotic patients are likely to have varices,[5] which tend to enlarge over time. Their size is associated with the severity of liver disease and with ongoing alcohol intake. The mortality from the first bleeding episode of varices is high at 25–50 per cent. Factors which indicate increased risk are the severity of liver dysfunction, the size of the varices, the presence of an enhanced reddened appearance of the mucosa on endoscopy, as well as the haemodynamic state of the patient as evaluated by vital signs and investigations. An episode of bleeding is clinically significant if a transfusion of two or more units of blood is required in the first 24 h or if postural hypotension is present. The subsequent outcome is influenced negatively by the degree of liver dysfunction, the presence of encephalopathy, the extent of ascites, reductions in albumin level and the extent of derangement of INR readings.

Diagnosis and management

The diagnosis of haematemesis and melaena is largely dependent upon the patient's own account or that of witnesses. When there is doubt, vomitus or faecal material, if available, should be inspected. Testing for blood in vomitus can be done using urine testing strips such as Labstix. However, the confirmation of true melaena as opposed to discolouration from confounding causes such as oral iron or bismuth compounds can be a challenge in the patient who appears otherwise well. The presence of abdominal pain, especially in a patient with a pre-existing history of upper gastrointestinal problems, such as a peptic ulcer, should arouse suspicion. Similarly, patients known to have gastro-oesophageal varices, or considered at risk of developing them because of a history of liver disease, should be considered to have the possibility of gastrointestinal bleeding. Because of the potential consequences of a misdiagnosis, patients should be considered to have had a gastrointestinal bleed if doubt exists.

The immediate task of the clinician is to assess the patient in relation to the blood loss. Whilst an estimate of the amount of blood lost might be attempted its usefulness is compromised by not knowing the extent of loss contained within the gut. Symptoms of hypovolaemia include light-headedness, weakness, breathlessness, and feeling cold and shivery. Signs of heamodynamic problems include pallor, a raised pulse, reduced blood pressure, and other signs of shock including reduced peripheral circulation. Postural hypotension is indicative of a significant loss of circulating volume.

Once acute upper gastrointestinal haemorrhage has been diagnosed or considered, the management of the patient is essentially out of the remit of primary care, although this may be necessary in remote locations, and expeditious transfer to an appropriate facility is required. The plan of action is likely to be dependent on the clinician's assessment of the patient and the prevailing situation but a decision to avoid transfer to a unit where blood loss can be compensated and support measures can be provided is fraught with risks. A few streaks of fresh blood in an otherwise well young patient following violent retching or vomiting might be considered to be a minor problem with an acceptable risk but the true extent of blood loss is difficult to ascertain. All patients require careful assessment and observation in the event of any further loss or complications. Many such patients will present several hours or days after the event in which case emergency admission to hospital is not automatically warranted. However, those at increased risk, that is, older patients, those with a previous history of ulcers, NSAID users (especially those taking multiple preparations), those on oral anticoagulants, and those with a potential for varices or a previous episode of bleeding should be transferred to appropriate secondary care even if the loss does not appear to be current because of the possibility of latent loss or a re-bleed. Variceal bleeding and that from ulcers with an exposed artery can be particularly profuse, with rapid consequences.

In some countries, primary care is provided in a setting where attached emergency services are available; it is important in these settings that facilities for endoscopic assessment and further management are available, together with emergency provision for abdominal surgery. If circumstances dictate and facilities allow, the insertion an intravenous line with an infusion of a volume expanding solution will assist further management. This is increasingly undertaken by the paramedical staff attending such emergencies and the patient is normally transferred to hospital without the general practitioner having to attend. In many instances, patients directly attend a hospital accident and emergency department. The management of patients with acute upper gastrointestinal haemorrhage is likely to be best undertaken in units which have specialized experience with the use agreed protocols and combined endoscopic and surgical opinions. This has the advantage of a combined medical and surgical approach.

NSAIDs, aspirin, and upper gastrointestinal bleeding

Despite their value as analgesics and anti-inflammatories, NSAIDs have a substantial effect in terms of upper gastrointestinal problems, especially haemorrhage. There is a three- to fourfold relative risk of upper gastro-intestinal haemorrhage or perforation in patients taking NSAIDs. Yearly, as many as 2000 deaths in the United Kingdom, 7600 deaths and 76 000 hospitalizations in the United States, and 365 deaths and 3900 hospitalizations in Canada are attributed to NSAIDs. These data need to be interpreted within the context of the widespread use of NSAIDs: 25 million prescriptions for NSAIDs in the United Kingdom and 70 million in the United States are issued annually.[6] Upper gastrointestinal side-effects occur in up to 30 per cent of those treated for more than 4 weeks and 1–3 per cent develop gastrointestinal bleeding. Bleeding is due to the development of gastric erosions, gastric and duodenal ulcers, and perforations. The mechanism of damage is related to the local solute effect of NSAIDs as well as a systemic effect influencing local cell migration and prostaglandin synthesis

in the gastroduodenal mucosa. NSAIDs cause ulcers independently of *H. pylori* infection.

A clear pattern of the role of NSAIDs in upper gastro-intestinal bleeding is demonstrated from the United Kingdom where *H. pylori* related ulcer disease has steadily declined and has been overtaken by NSAID-linked ulcers, predominantly in those over the age of 60 years.

Aspirin has effects similar to NSAIDs with regard to upper gastrointestinal bleeding and is also linked with haematemesis and melaena.[7] The ingestion of aspirin 300 mg daily for 14 days causes gastric and duodenal petechiae, erosions, and endoscopically identifiable ulcers. As many as 60 per cent of patients develop endoscopically identifiable ulcers at 4 weeks. Aspirin at a dose of 75 mg (the dose commonly used for the secondary prevention of cardiovascular and cerebrovascular problems) can cause gastric mucosal bleeding and its long-term use is associated with the development of ulcers: after 10 weeks, 10 per cent of users will have endoscopic gastric ulcers.[8] Clinically evident gastrointestinal bleeding occurs in 3 per cent of patients over the age of 70 years taking aspirin 100 mg for more than 12 months. The risk of bleeding with aspirin is not influenced by the type of aspirin used—plain, enteric-coated, and buffered aspirin have similar levels of side-effects.

NSAIDs and aspirin can be responsible for chronic blood loss but their role in acute haemorrhage is well established; such patients are likely to have had a bleeding lesion for varying periods before the clinically noted 'acute' haemorrhage and may therefore have had a degree of anaemia.

Principles of secondary care management of acute upper gastrointestinal haemorrhage

Modern treatment is reliant on endoscopic techniques, with surgery in those in whom this fails. Better outcomes have been demonstrated from units which use agreed protocols following the patient's admission and immediate resuscitation, with the endoscopy and surgical teams working together on a management plan. Specialized units have a lower mortality than those reliant on generalists.

The priority following initial resuscitation measures is to stem the bleeding. Around 80 per cent of patients with haematemesis and melaena have relatively minor bleeding and those who do not have endoscopic evidence of current bleeding are unlikely to require more than supportive therapy, intravenous fluids, and the care of concomitant problems. Those who present with clinical shock and have an actively bleeding ulcer carry a substantial risk of re-bleeding after initial treatment. A visible bleeding vessel in the stomach or duodenum on endoscopy represents an artery, sometimes covered with a clot. These carry a greater risk of ongoing bleeding or a recurrence after initial measures.

Drug therapy in non-variceal haemorrhage is based on agents which stop active bleeding and prevent a recurrence. Acid suppression with proton pump inhibitors is an effective medical contribution to the prevention of re-bleeding. Stabilization of adherent clot, a sign that the bleeding has stopped, with tranexamic acid and reduction local blood flow with somatostatin and octreotide is sometimes tried but is best achieved with the pH raising effect of proton pump inhibitors.

Endoscopic methods to stop ulcer bleeding and to reduce the risk of further bleeding are reliant on locally applied heater probes, electrocoagulation, and argon-plasma coagulation. Of these, thermal methods appear superior and have fewer complications. Direct injection therapy during endoscopy has been used for many years, essentially using adrenalin, which facilitate the cessation of the bleeding. Local injection with fibrin glue and thrombin is also used but is considered less effective. Overall, the most effective endoscopic management relies on thermal probes in conjunction with systemic proton pump inhibitors and local injections.

For variceal bleeding, endoscopic treatment with sclerotherapy is the management of choice, together with variceal ligation. Vasoactive drugs such as somatostatin are also increasingly used. For the prevention of re-bleeding, beta-blockers, which are aimed at reducing portal pressure, have been used in conjunction with variceal ligation and surgical shunting procedures.[9]

Prevention of upper gastrointestinal haemorrhage

Preventative measures for avoiding initial haemorrhage or preventing re-bleeding are within the domain of primary care. Patients who are at risk of haemorrhage should be evaluated carefully from the point of view of potential therapies and for hospital referral.

Non-variceal bleeding

In patients with a bleeding duodenal ulcer treated without surgical intervention, the risk of re-bleeding over the following 10 years is 20 per cent compared with 5 per cent who have surgical intervention. Around 20 per cent of those with bleeding due to gastric ulcers develop further bleeding over the next 8 years. The effective management of these ulcers reduces the risks. Patients who have bled and have *H. pylori* associated ulcers should have eradication therapy, with confirmation of eradication, and long-term acid suppression therapy with proton pump inhibitors.

Patients who have had NSAID-linked bleeding ulcers should cease these drugs and be treated with acid suppression drugs to promote ulcer healing and should be considered for long-term acid suppression therapy. If NSAIDs cannot be stopped, acid suppression can be used concurrently although ulcer healing is slower. The eradication of *H. pylori* alone is insufficient in these patients, as NSAID use is an independent cause of ulcers. The Maastricht 2000 consensus statement on the management of *H. pylori* advises eradication in patients who are to commence NSAIDs on the basis that this might reduce the risk of infection-related ulcers. However, this is not entirely pragmatic in the primary care setting and needs to be applied on an individual basis following as assessment of the prevalent risks.

Concomitant treatment with acid suppression drugs or misoprostil is sometimes utilized to reduce the risk of bleeding. Prophylactic treatment might be necessary for those with a history of bleeding or those who are at increased risk. Concurrent H2 receptor blockers are not particularly effective in reducing the risk of bleeding. Misoprostil provides more consistent protection, with a reduction of ulcer risk by up to 70 per cent and bleeding by 40 per cent, but its use is limited by its side-effects, particularly diarrhoea. Proton pump inhibitors provide protection against NSAID-associated ulcers of up to 75 per cent.

COX-2 specific inhibitors, which theoretically retain the therapeutic advantages of NSAIDs whilst having a better side-effect profile, are increasingly used in primary care and maybe cheaper than combination therapy. There is evidence that bleeding from the gastrointestinal tract is reduced with their use compared with NSAIDs although dyspepsia still occurs. Whilst it is rational that all potentially ulcerogenic drugs should be avoided in those at risk, COX-2 inhibitors may offer an advantage. The large scale VIGOR[10] and CLASS[11] trials confirmed that rofecoxib and celecoxib selective COX-2 inhibitors were associated with significantly fewer upper gastrointestinal events than naproxen, a non-selective inhibitor, particularly in patients not also taking aspirin. A population based observational study also confirmed a lower short term risk of upper gastrointestinal haemorrhage for selective COX-2 inhibitors compared with non-selective NSAIDs. However, unresolved issues remain about non-gastrointestinal side effects and costs of these agents.[12] Shorter-acting NSAIDs, such as ibuprofen and diclofenac are less likely to lead to ulcer complications especially during long term treatment. As the likelihood of bleeding is also associated with increased doses, the lowest effective dose should be used. The combination of NSAIDs or with aspirin escalates the risks of bleeding.

Variceal bleeding

The prevention of variceal bleeding is essentially a secondary care problem and patients should be referred to a gastroenterologist with appropriate experience, although abstinence from alcohol may require input from the patient's primary care physicians. The prevention of variceal bleeding requires a careful initial assessment of the possible risks, based on liver function tests and the endoscopic appearances of the varices. For primary prevention (i.e. in patients who have not had a bleed), the patient should have an endoscopic assessment and medical therapy with a beta-blocker or a nitrate.[13] These work by reducing the portal venous pressure. Sclerotherapy is not appropriate because of the risk of complications. In patients with a history of bleeding (secondary prevention), medical therapy as above, sclerotherapy and band ligation is used as well as portocaval shunting procedures.

Key points

1. Haematemesis and melaena can be life-threatening and should be regarded as an emergency requiring specialized intervention.
2. The commonest causes are peptic ulcer, oesophageal inflammations and ulcers, Mallory–Weiss tears, and oesophageal varices.
3. Most haematemesis and melaena in developed countries is due to NSAID- and aspirin-linked lesions in the elderly, in whom complications and mortality are high.
4. Good management is based on a combined endoscopic and surgical approach with established protocols of care.
5. Strategies for preventing initial bleeding and re-bleeding should be used in all patients who are at increased risk.

References

1. **RCGP and OPCS**. *Morbidity Statistics in General Practice*. Fourth National Study. London: HMSO, 1995.
2. **Dronfield, M.W.** (1994). Upper gastrointestinal bleeding. In *Diseases of the Gut and Pancreas* (ed. J.J. Misiewicz, R. Pounder, and C.W. Venables), pp. 376–80. Oxford: Blackwell Science.
3. **Rockall, T.A.** et al. (1996). Risk assessment after acute upper gastrointestinal haemorrhage. *Gut* **38**, 316–21.
4. **Church, N. and Palmer, K.** (1999). Acute non-variceal gastrointestinal haemorrhage: treatment. In *Evidence Based Gastroenterology and Hepatology* (ed. J. McDonald, A. Burroughs, and B. Feagan), pp. 118–39. London: BMJ.
5. **Burroughs, A.K.** (1994). Variceal haemorrhage. In *Diseases of the Gut and Pancreas* (ed. J.J. Misiewicz, R. Pounder and C.W. Venables), pp. 381–96. Oxford: Blackwell.
6. **Hungin, A.P.S. and Kean, W.** (2001). Non-steroidal anti-inflammatory drugs: overused or underused in osteoarthritis? *American Journal of Medicine* **110** (1A), 8S–13S.
7. **Rostom, A., Maetzel, A., Tugwell, P., and Wells, G.** (1999). Ulcer disease and NSAIDs: etiology and treatment. In *Evidence Based Gastroenterology and Hepatology* (ed. J. McDonald, A. Burroughs, and B. Feagan), pp. 91–117. London: BMJ.
8. **Lanas, A.I.** (2001). Current approaches to reducing gastrointestinal toxicity of low dose aspirin. *American Journal of Medicine* **110** (1A), 70S–3S.
9. **Jalan, R. and Hayes, P.C.** (2000). UK guidelines on the management of variceal haemorrhage in cirrhotic patients. British Society of Gastroenterology. *Gut* **46** (Suppl. III), iii-1–15.
10. **Bombardier, C., Laine, L., Reicin, A., Shapiro, D., Burgos-Varga, R., Davis, B.** et al. (2000). Comparison of upper gastrointestinal toxicity of rofecoxib and naproxen in patients with rheumatoid arthritis. VIGOR study Group. *New England Journal of Medicine* **343**, 1520–8.
11. **Silverstein, F.E., Faich, G., Goldstein, J.L., Simon, L.S., Pincus, T., Whelton, A.** et al. (2000). Gastrointestinal toxicity with celecoxib versus non-steroidal anti-inflammatory drugs for osteoarthritis and rheumatoid arthritis: the CLASS study–a randomised controlled trial. *Journal of the American Medical Association* **284** (10), 1247–55.
12. **Mamdani, M., Rochon, P.A., Juurlink, D.N., Kopp, A., Anderson, M.** et al. (2002). Observational study of upper gastrointestinal haemorrhage in

elderly patients given selective COX-2 inhibitors or conventional non-steroidal anti-inflammatory drugs. *British Medical Journal* **325**, 624–30.

13. **Goulis, J. and Burroughs, A.K.** (1999). Portal hypertensive bleeding. In *Evidence Based Gastroenterology and Hepatology* (ed. J. McDonald, A. Burroughs, and B. Feagan), pp. 389–426. London: BMJ.

Further reading

Hawkey, C.J., ed. (2001). Non-steroidal anti-inflammatory drugs and the gastrointestinal tract: consensus and controversy. *American Journal of Medicine* **110** (1A), 8–11.

Irvine, E.J. and Hunt, R.H. *Evidence Based Gastroenterology*. Hamilton: Decker, 2001.

4.8 Rectal bleeding

Gerda Fijten

Introduction

Rectal bleeding is defined as the visible passage of blood from the rectum, which may or may not be mixed with the stool. Occult blood loss is discussed elsewhere, in relation to the investigation of iron-deficiency anaemia (Chapter 1.12) and to screening for colorectal cancer (Vol. 1, Chapter 11.3), and melaena (black or tarry stools, usually the result of a bleeding peptic ulcer) is discussed in Chapter 4.7.

Rectal blood loss may originate from the anus, rectum, or colon. Bright red blood is most likely to come from the distal (left) colon, and dark red blood from a more proximal site. However, if intestinal transit is rapid during brisk bleeding in the upper intestine, bright red blood may be passed unchanged in the stool. The significance of rectal bleeding varies widely, from harmless to dangerous, from self limiting conditions, such as haemorrhoids, to malignant disease.

Epidemiology

Rectal bleeding is a common symptom. In the Western adult population, between 7 and 16 per cent report rectal bleeding in the past 6 months, and some 2 per cent in the previous 2 weeks.[1] The blood is mixed with stool in about 30 per cent of cases, and seen only on the toilet paper in 70 per cent. People aged under 50 years report rectal bleeding more frequently (27 per cent) than those over 50 (12 per cent).[2,3]

A minority of people with rectal bleeding consult a doctor. In one British study, 41 per cent had sought medical advice for their bleeding.[3] Common reasons for consultation include worry about serious disease (53 per cent), pain or discomfort (20 per cent), and pressure from relatives (10 per cent). Most of the non-consulters (70 per cent) believe that their symptoms are unlikely to be serious, although they are often aware of a link between rectal bleeding and cancer. Exactly how patients estimate risk, in relation to their decision to consult a doctor, is unknown. Heightened awareness and anxiety may be induced by public health education programmes, aimed at early diagnosis of cancer, or by recent experiences of relatives or others with colon cancer.

Presentation in primary care

Representative data from the Netherlands indicate that the mean annual consultation rate in general practice for rectal bleeding is seven per 1000 persons per year, with a wide interpractice variation of between two and 18 per 1000.[4] While it is clear that a selected proportion of patients present with rectal bleeding in primary care, it is unclear how appropriate this self-selection of patients is in relation to timely diagnosis of serious disease.

Perceptions of the seriousness of rectal blood loss also differ between patients and doctors. General practitioners may regard rectal bleeding differently because of the characteristics of the population they serve, their previous experiences of colon cancer, especially if this diagnosis has been delayed, and their epidemiological knowledge. There are also differences in the perceptions of the seriousness of rectal bleeding between specialists and generalists. The predictive value of rectal bleeding for a final diagnosis of colon cancer in the specialist setting is relatively high, at around 30 per cent, compared with only 3 per cent in primary care. In the community, the predictive value is less than 0.3 per cent.[1]

Causes of rectal bleeding

In a prospective study of 290 patients aged between 18 and 75 years in the Netherlands, presenting to general practitioners with rectal blood loss, 90 per cent of cases were found to have minor or self-limiting disorders, as shown in Table 1.[4]

Haemorrhoids

Haemorrhoids represent a normal anatomical state, because varicosities arising from the haemorrhoidal veins in the perianal area occur in 50 per cent or more of the population of Western countries. Symptoms only occur if these veins become enlarged or rupture. Bright red bleeding is the rule, unmixed with stool, often seen as streaks on the stool or the toilet tissue or as larger amounts of blood in the toilet after defecation. Typical symptoms include feelings of protrusion or prolapse, anal discomfort, itch or pain, mucous discharge from the rectum, and faecal soiling. Severe pain occurs with thrombosis of external haemorrhoids.

First-degree haemorrhoids are painless, and bleed at the time of defaecation. There is no prolapse, and proctoscopy reveals enlarged haemorrhoids in the rectal lumen. Secondary haemorrhoids are characterized by protrusion through the anal canal on gentle straining, but spontaneously reduce. Third-degree haemorrhoids protrude and often require manual reduction. In fourth-degree haemorrhoids prolapse is fixed. As a result of permanently prolapsed haemorrhoids, mucous discharge, soiling, irritated perianal skin, discomfort, and pain are characteristic symptoms.

External and prolapsed internal haemorrhoids may be seen on examination. If they are not visible, straining may produce prolapse. Proctoscopy is required to visualize first-degree internal haemorrhoids. Digital rectal examination is not helpful in the detection of haemorrhoids, which are usually soft, but can reveal other problems which may be associated with haemorrhoids, including rectal tumours. The most common cause

Table 1 Final diagnoses related to rectal bleeding in general practice: $n = 290$; female, 56%; male, 44%; older than 50 years, 30%

Outcome	%
Cancer	3
Polyps	2
Colitis	5
Minor ailments:	30
Haemorrhoids	16
Fissure	7
Proctitis	4
Infections	2
Diverticular disease	0.6
Unknown cause, but healthy after 1 year	60

of haemorrhoids is straining at stool, and other causes include chronic constipation, pregnancy, obesity, and portal hypertension, in which case bleeding can be profuse (see Chapter 12).

Anal fissures

A fissure, which is a crack in the mucocutaneous line, is painful, particularly on defecation. It is frequently associated with blood seen on the surface of the stool and on toilet tissue after defecation. Painful spasm of the anal sphincter may occur. Constipation results, because of fear of pain on defecation.

On examination, a sentinel pile may be observed. Gently spreading the buttocks may reveal fissures, and the inferior portion of an ulcer may also be seen. Digital examination without a local anaesthetic is not possible, and is usually unnecessary.

Common causes of fissures include irritant diarrhoea, trauma, and tightening of the anal canal secondary to nervous tension. Fissures are the commonest cause of rectal bleeding in small infants, when they are usually due to constipation.

Other less common causes of anal fissure and ulceration must be considered, particularly if the lesions do not lie in the midline; these include syphilis, Crohn's disease, and malignancy.

Colorectal cancer

Colorectal cancer presents with rectal bleeding associated with a change in bowel habit in about one-third of cases, and in a further 10 per cent as rectal bleeding with or without anal symptoms. In its early stage, which may take years, signs of bowel obstruction are often lacking and rectal bleeding may be the first and only symptom. Advanced cancer in the left colon causes signs of obstruction earlier than right-sided lesions.

The population incidence of colorectal cancer is approximately five per 10 000 each year. The incidence increases with age to 50 per 10 000 of the population in the eighth and ninth decades.

The incidence of colon cancer is significantly lower in Finland, Japan, and in the developing world.

Colonic polyps

These occur in three neoplastic forms—adenomatous, villous, and mixed adenomatous–villous—and as hyperplastic polyps, which are very small and are thought not to possess malignant potential. Adenomatous polyps are present in about 30 per cent of people over the age of 40 years. Bleeding is usually related to polyps more than 1 cm in diameter in the rectum and sigmoid colon.

Gastrointestinal infection

A range of gastrointestinal infections, with organisms such as *Salmonella, Shigella, Campylobacter jejuni, Escherichia coli, Legionella, Clostridium difficile, Cytomegalovirus*, and amoebiasis and other parasites can all produce rectal bleeding, though usually this will present as diarrhoea mixed with blood.

Inflammatory bowel disease

Rectal bleeding, accompanied by diarrhoea, is a common presentation of ulcerative colitis. Crohn's disease usually presents with abdominal pain, diarrhoea, weight loss, and fever, but bloody diarrhoea may also be a feature. Both conditions occur more commonly in white than black races, and the population incidence is reported as at between one and five cases per 10 000 per year, with a peak onset in young adults aged between 15 and 30 years.

Colitis and proctitis due to other conditions, such as adverse reactions to antibiotics, ischaemic colitis, and radiation injury can all cause rectal bleeding, which is usually associated with diarrhoea or mucous discharge.

Diverticular disease

Uncomplicated diverticular disease usually does not cause any symptoms. The incidence increases with age; the condition affects 50 per cent of the population older than 60 in the Western world. Bleeding occur in about 10–30 per cent of the patients with diverticular disease. It is usually self-limiting, but may be profuse in exceptional cases.

Angiodysplasia

This is a vascular malformation in the bowel, usually affecting people over the age of 60 years, and is otherwise asymptomatic. Bleeding is typically intermittent and rarely massive. The clinical presentations of angiodysplasia vary from acute rectal bleeding or melaena to chronic iron-deficiency anaemia secondary to blood loss.

Meckel's diverticulum

Although rare, this is the most common cause of significant bleeding in childhood. The typical presentation which resembles that of intussusception (Chapter 4.3), includes intestinal obstruction and pain, with the passage of red-currant jelly stool.

Solitary rectal ulcer

This condition is characterized by anal discharge of mucous and pus, accompanied by pain, constipation, and bleeding. It is most commonly caused by chronic constipation, but may also be related to some sexually transmitted diseases.

Endometriosis

This is a rare cause of rectal bleeding, but should be suspected when abdominal pain and bleeding coincide with the menstrual cycle.

Diagnosis

The diagnostic approach to rectal bleeding should be based on risk assessment, and the allocation of patients to high and low risk of serious disease. Those with a high probability of colon cancer or inflammatory bowel disease require early investigation, whilst those with a low probability of a serious cause can safely be managed expectantly in primary care.

Risk assessment is based on age, medical history, and features of the present episode of rectal bleeding and physical examination. Risk factors for colon cancer include a first-degree family member with colorectal cancer, particularly if diagnosed before the age of 50 years, a previous personal history of a colorectal neoplasm, a genetic predisposition (including familial adenomatous polyposis and hereditary non-polyposis colon cancer),[5] ulcerative colitis affecting the whole colon for more than 10 years and exposure to radiation.

History-taking

It is important to confirm that the bleeding came from the rectum, and to clarify the pattern and amount of bleeding, whether it was mixed with the stool or present on the toilet paper or seen in the toilet water.

It is then necessary to enquire about associated symptoms such as anal or abdominal pain, mucoid rectal discharge, a sensation of incomplete evacuation, a recent change in bowel habit, other gastrointestinal symptoms and systemic symptoms, such as weight loss and fatigue. The medical history should be reviewed to exclude relevant, co-existing disease and drug therapy, and a careful family history should be taken, with particular reference to the incidence of colorectal cancer in relatives.

Three variables have been shown to contribute significantly and independently to a patient's risk of colorectal cancer, and these are age over 50 years, a recent change in bowel habit, and blood mixed with the stool. A combination of these signs can be considered as a diagnostic test for colorectal cancer with a high discriminatory power, and application of this test has been shown to be a safe way of reducing the number of patients referred for unnecessary further evaluation.[6]

Physical examination

Whilst the history should point strongly towards the likely cause for the rectal bleeding, a careful physical examination may yield further clues. The general examination should look for evidence of systemic illness, including weight loss, anaemia, and jaundice, and the abdominal examination should concentrate on seeking evidence of an abdominal mass, tenderness, or of free abdominal fluid.

The perianal region should be inspected carefully, and a digital rectal examination must be performed on all patients suffering from rectal blood loss, unless an anal fissure makes the procedure painful and unnecessary. Many anorectal tumours are within the reach of the examining finger. The digital examination has high positive predictive value for the presence of low bowel tumours. However, a negative rectal examination does not exclude a colorectal tumour, as more than 60 per cent are out of the reach of the palpating finger. The examination glove should be inspected for the presence of blood. Proctoscopy may be useful in detecting obvious, local causes of bleeding and may also be needed to obtain stool samples for microbiological culture.

Laboratory tests

Measures of haemoglobin, white blood count, and erythrocyte sedimentation rate (ESR) are all useful in the search for a serious organic disease, but possess low positive predictive values. Although the negative predictive values for colorectal cancer are high, they are not sufficient to exclude a malignant cause. Faecal occult blood testing is unlikely to be contributory. Stool samples should be taken when an infectious cause is suspected.

Endoscopy and radiology

Although rigid sigmoidoscopy is useful in diagnosing inflammatory and neoplastic conditions, for which it has a sensitivity of 69 per cent and specificity of 95 per cent,[7] flexible sigmoidoscopy is preferred because of its greater range and acceptability. If this investigation is negative, a double contrast barium enema (DCBE) or colonoscopy should be considered. The DCBE provides 52 per cent sensitivity and 98 per cent specificity for the presence of neoplastic lesions, so there is still a risk of missing serious disease. Complication and morbidity rates are low, but the procedure may be difficult for older immobile patients. The combination of DCBE and flexible sigmoidoscopy is often used to increase diagnostic accuracy. Together this combination provides a sensitivity of 96 per cent and specificity of 76 per cent for the detection of serious disease.[7] Colonoscopy is capable of visualising the entire colon, although the examination is highly operator dependent, can be uncomfortable, and carries a small but significant mortality.

When these investigations are unproductive, and the site of persistent rectal bleeding remains obscure, angiography and technetium scintigraphy are the next steps.

Principles of management

The management of rectal bleeding consists of both the management of the underlying condition and risk management. A full discussion of the management of minor perianal conditions is provided in Chapter 4.12 and of inflammatory bowel disease in Chapter 4.4. While the definitive management of colorectal cancer lies within the domain of the surgical and oncological specialities, the important role of the primary care team in palliative care of patients with cancer is discussed in detail in Section 17.

The cause of bleeding often remains unknown, even after taking a careful history and performing appropriate investigation. If the probability of a serious cause is considered to be low a 'watch and wait' strategy is preferable, together with reassurance and information about risks. If the probability is reasonably high (this may be even in the presence of haemorrhoids), or with persistent or recurrent symptoms, further investigation or referral is indicated to diagnose or exclude cancer or inflammatory bowel disease.

Information is essential in the communication to the patient and to the specialist.

Delay in diagnosis and treatment of colorectal cancer makes it harder to cope with the disease, especially if it is incurable. Most available evidence suggest that if any benefit exists from early symptomatic diagnosis, it is likely to be small (it does not improve the prognosis), but delay may exacerbate patients' emotional suffering.

In the decision-making process attention must be paid to the availability of the diagnostic tests employed (e.g. waiting lists for endoscopy), the possible fear of the patient, and the clinical and economic costs and benefits of different management strategies.

Key points

- A precise diagnosis of the first episode of rectal bleeding may be difficult to make in primary care.

- The prognosis of patients presenting with rectal bleeding is good and the prior probability of cancer is less than 5 per cent.

- Risk stratification of patients into those at high and low risk of serious disease—cancer and IBD—is important.

- In the absence of alarm symptoms, time may safely be used as a diagnostic tool.

- Persistent, unexplained rectal bleeding requires further investigation.

References

1. **Fijten, G.H., Blijham, G.H., and Knottnerus, H.A.** (1994). Occurrence and clinical significance of overt blood loss per rectum in the general population and in medical practice. *British Journal of General Practice* **44**, 320–5.

2. **Jones, R. and Lydeard, S.** (1992). Irritable bowel in the general population. *British Medical Journal* **304**, 87–90.

3. **Crosland, A. and Jones, R.** (1995). Rectal bleeding: prevalence and consultation behaviour. *British Medical Journal* **311**, 486–8.

4. **Fijten, G.H. et al.** (1993). The incidence and outcome of rectal bleeding in general practice. *Family Practice* **10**, 283–7.

5. **Vasen, H.F.A.** (1997). Inherited forms of colorectal cancer: guidelines for management. In *Procedures in Hepatogastroenterology* (ed. G.N.J. Tytgat and C.J.J. Mulder), Chapter 28, pp. 331–7. Dordrecht: Kluwer Academic.

6. **Fijten, G.H. et al.** (1995). Predictive value of signs and symptoms for colorectal cancer in patients with rectal bleeding in general practice. *Family Practice* **12**, 279–86.

7. **Hefland, M. et al.** (1997). History of visable rectal bleeding in a primary care population. *Journal of the American Medical Association* **277**, 44–8.

Further reading

Way, L.W., ed. *Current Surgical Diagnosis and Treatment. A Lange Medical Book*, 10th edn. Norwalk: Appleton & Lange, 1994.

Sackett, D., Haynes, R., and Tugwell, P. *Clinical Epidemiology*. Boston MA: Little Brown and Company, 1985.

4.9 Jaundice

Christos Lionis

Definition

Jaundice is a clinical sign, which appears as a yellowish discoloration of the skin, sclerae, and mucous membranes. It becomes apparent when the serum bilirubin level is in excess of 2.0–2.5 mg/100 ml (34.2–42.7 mmol/l), although it may not be clinically recognizable until levels of approximately 3 mg/100 ml (51.3 mmol/l) are reached. Jaundice in itself is not a disease, but several diseases or disorders contribute to its aetiology.

Epidemiology and consultation in primary care

Patients with jaundice usually seek medical attention on an ambulatory basis. The yellow hue is not only visible in the eye sclera, but in all areas protected from the sun, including those of the mouth, the palms of the hands, and the soles of the feet. Physicians may sometimes have to distinguish between the skin's yellow hue of jaundice and that which has been produced through consumption of large quantities of food containing carotene or drugs such as rifampin or quinacrine, which mimic jaundice. The yellow hue is not present in the eye sclera in carotenemia. In some cases, jaundiced patients present a greenish tinge, which is derived from the oxidation of bilirubin to biliverdin.

Patients may also notice pale stools and dark urine, both of which may be the first signs, before the actual appearance of jaundice. At the time of consultation, patients may complain of weight loss, pruritus, nausea, vomiting, distaste for tobacco, and other general or specific symptoms, which depend on the underlying disease and type of hyperbilirubinemia.

The incidence of jaundice in primary care differs across the world, with the variablitiy in underlying disease. In developing countries, infections are the major cause, while in developed countries biliary obstruction and drug-induced jaundice are of major importance. Incidence and prevalence of viral hepatitis in the Western world is estimated at 0.1 and 0.5, respectively, per 1000 patients annually. Though comparable data from developing countries are missing, incidence is supposed to be much higher. Hepatitis markers are closely associated with age and practically all subjects older than 44 years were anti-HAV positive and more of the 22 per cent of those subjects who visited primary care physicians in a Mediterranean island have evidence of prior infection by hepatitis B.[1]

What are the possible causes?

Common causes of jaundice

Different mechanisms are responsible for the accumulation of bilirubin in the body tissues. Jaundice may be predominantly caused by increased unconjugated (indirect), or conjugated (direct) bilirubin in the serum. The mechanisms responsible for unconjugated bilirubin include increased bilirubin production, impaired hepatic uptake, and impaired conjugation by glucoronyl transferase. Those responsible for conjugated hyperbilirubinaemia can be classified as intrahepatic, including hepatocellular diseases and intrahepatic cholestasis, and extrahepatic, which includes various types and levels of obstruction. Causes of conjugated and unconjugated hyperbilirubinaemia are illustrated in Table 1.

The most common causes of obvious jaundice are malignancy, sepsis/shock, cirrhosis, gallstones, drugs, autoimmune hepatitis, and viral hepatitis.[2] Hepatitis and infections are the predominant diagnoses in younger patients, though biliary obstruction and intrahepatic cholestasis

Table 1 Causes of hyperbilirubinaemia

Conjugated	Unconjugated
Intrahepatic causes	
Hepatocellular disease	*Excess bilirubin production*
Hepatitis	Haemolytic anaemias
Cirrhosis	Haematoma
	Infarction
Intrahepatic cholestasis occurs	
at different levels	*Impaired hepatic uptake and*
Viral hepatitis	*conjugation of bilirubin*
Drugs	Gilbert's syndrome,
Sepsis	Crigler–Najjar syndrome
Primary biliary cirrhosis	Drug reactions (probenecid,
Primary sclerosing cholangitis	rifampicin, aspirin, contrast dye,
Cholangiocarcinoma	sulfonamides)
Post-operative jaundice	
	Miscellaneous
Other disorder causing hepatocellular	Fasting
damage or intrahepatic cholestasis	Hypothyroidism
or both	Thyrotoxicosis
Infectious mononucleosis	
Spirochetal infections (leptospirosis)	
Cholangitis	
Sarcoidosis	
Lymphomas	
Alcoholic liver disease	
Congenital disorders	
Rotor syndrome	
Dubin–Johnson syndromes	
Choledochoceles	
Familial disorders	
Benign recurrent intrahepatic cholestasis	
Cholestasis of pregnancy	
Extrahepatic causes (mainly biliary obstruction)	
Gallstones	
Tumours which block the flow of bile within	
the extrahepatic biliary tree	
Pancreatitis	
Parasites	
Pancreatic pseydocyst	
Cholangiocarcinoma	
Choledochal cyst	

should not be ignored. Stones and tumours are more common at advanced ages. Physicians should be aware that some drugs can cause jaundice in all age groups, by acute or chronic hepatotoxicity or by cholestasis. Acetaminophen, aspirin, chloramphenicol, chlorpromazine, chlorpropamide, chlororthiazide, chlorotetracycline, erythromycin estolate, isoniazid, nitrofurantoin, phenylbutazone, streptomycin, and sulfadiazine have all been reported as causing jaundice.

Differential diagnosis

In making an accurate diagnosis the primary care doctor should consider three diagnostic steps.

1. *Direct or indirect hyperbilirubinaemia?* Before considering the different causes, the physician should determine the predominant type of hyperbilirubinaemia. In the first case the physician has to distinguish between conjugated (direct) and unconjugated (indirect) hyperbilirubinaemia. In the majority of cases this diagnostic dilemma can be resolved at the doctor's surgery, based only on clinical assessment. The physician should ask about symptoms such as pruritus, abdominal pain and seek clinical signs of dark urine and pale stools, which suggest direct hyperbilirubinaemia, while normal-coloured urine and stools indicate indirect hyperbilirubinaemia.

Table 2 Other causes of jaundice common in developing countries

Hepatitis A, B, C, D, E, and F are uncommon in Western countries, but may have an important contribution to jaundice in some tropical areas. The majority of patients with acute hepatitis C are asymptomatic and do not develop jaundice

Leptospirosis. Usually develops 2 weeks after direct or indirect exposure to the urine of infected animals. A severe immunological response including jaundice, renal failure, disseminated intravascular coagulation, and even death can accompany this disease. The number of infected subjects in Southern Europe and the United States has increased over the last few years

Hepatic fascioliasis is caused by obstruction of the bile duct by *Fasciola hepatica*, a sheep liver fluke

Hydatid cyst. Obstruction of the biliary tree by a liver hydatid cyst may be asymptomatic, but cases have been reported in tropical and semi-tropical areas with symptoms, including abdominal pain, jaundice, or cholangitis

Schistosomiasis. Portal hypertension with jaundice, ascites and hepatic coma are included among the complications of the trematode infection

Malaria. Acute hepatopathy with centrilobular necrosis and marked jaundice may be seen as a severe complication of *P. falciparum* infection

Table 3 Uncommon causes of jaundice

Hereditary syndromes causing jaundice
Gilbert's syndrome: the most common of the hereditary syndromes in which unconjugated hyperbilirubinaemia produces a benign, asymptomatic, mild but recurrent jaundice, which is due to mild glucuronyl transferase deficiency. Jaundice usually develops after fasting, stress, fatigue, alcohol and cigarette consumption, or during a concomitant illness. No treatment is required
Crigler–Najjar syndrome: a severe, nonhaemolytic jaundice of neonates, which is characterized by a moderate deficiency or absence of glucuronyl transferase
Dubin–Johnson syndrome: a conjugated hyperbilirubinaemia which is attributed to the impaired excretion of bilirubin from the liver
Rotor syndrome: a similar disorder to the Dubin–Johnson syndrome

Intrahepatic cholestasis of pregnancy
Intrahepatic cholestasis of pregnancy is a disease which affects pregnant women, usually in the third trimester of pregnancy. It is primarily characterized by pruritus and less frequently by jaundice

Benign recurrent intrahepatic cholestasis
Benign recurrent intrahepatic cholestasis is a rare autosomal recessive disorder which is characterized by repeated episodes of pruritus and jaundice

Post-operative jaundice
This type of jaundice, which may follow any surgical operation and develops either within the first 48 h or between 7 and 10 days and has a multifactorial cause

Rare infectious and tropical diseases
These include: amoebiasis, biliary ascariasis, hepatic fascioliasis, hepatic echinococcosis, clonorhis sinensis liver infections, brucellosis, leishmaniasis, yellow fever, malaria, viral hepatitis, louse-borne relapsing fever, leptospirosis, tuberculosis, typhoid fever, rickettsial infections, Rift Valley fever, Crimean-Congo hemorrhagic fever, and other viral haemorrhagic fevers

2. *Intra- or extrahepatic jaundice?* The second step for the primary care physician is to determine whether the hyperbilirubinaemia is intra- or extrahepatic. Intrahepatic hyperbilirubinaemia is caused by hepatocellular damage or intrahepatic cholestasis, while extrahepatic is caused by biliary obstruction. The distinction should be based on the medical history, physical examination, and laboratory investigation.

3. *Considering the most common illnesses and setting diagnostic probabilities.* The next step for the primary care physician, after the above questions have been clarified, is to consider the most prevailing illnesses in the practice area. Primary care physicians who work in developing countries could consider several other causes of jaundice, which are shown in Table 2.

Uncommon causes of jaundice

The diseases and syndromes which are listed in Table 3 are uncommon causes of jaundice, and it will be unusual for the primary care physicians to meet them in the community setting. Though bilirubin is raised in the first days of life in many children, true neonatal jaundice is a rare cause of jaundice in the Western world.

How to make a diagnosis

History

History-taking plays a key role in an accurate diagnosis of the underlying disease or health problem leading to jaundice. Patients should be asked to report in detail their symptoms and complaints. They should also be asked particular questions about the presence of abdominal pain, possibly indicating obstruction, about dark urine and pale stools, which are indications of direct hyperbilirubinaemia. Malaise, anorexia, nausea, flu-like symptoms, and discomfort or pain at the right-upper quadrant may suggest a hepatocellular disease. Abdominal pain accompanied by general symptoms such as marked weight loss may be caused by cancer of the head of the pancreas or a tumour blocking the common bile duct. Rigor and pruritus are signs of biliary obstruction complicated by cholangitis.

Physicians should then ask patients about personal lifestyles and habits that might give a clue to intrahepatic disease:

- alcohol abuse;
- sexual practices, which could inform the physicians of the risks of acquiring viral hepatitis;
- blood transfusion in the past;
- drug use, including use of over-the-counter and alternative remedies.

Patients should be asked about their recent travel destinations and, if they had been in tropical climates, about prophylactic measures undertaken. A family history of episodic jaundice, which is crucial in some cases, particularly for Gilbert's disease and the history of anaemia and gallstones should also be sought. In endemic areas, recent signs of malaria should be checked.

Physical examination

Physical examination can assist the physician in detecting clinical indications of chronic liver disease. The general health status should always be assessed. Physicians should determine the presence of enlarged lymph nodes especially those of the posterior cervical chain. If present, this could support the diagnosis of infectious mononucleosis, especially when fever and a sore throat are observed. Enlarged liver and hepatic tenderness are common findings in the many causes of hepatocellular diseases suggestive of early or mild hepatocellular disease (acute viral hepatitis), but also of extrahepatic diseases and metastatic cancer. The liver is usually small in advanced hepatocellular disease, but at this time physicians may be able to detect signs of portal hypertension, such as ascites and splenomegaly, asterixis, peripheral oedema, spider naevi, and palmar erythema. Spleen enlargement may suggest an infectious cause (infectious mononucleosis) or primary biliary cirrhosis. The gallbladder is often palpable in extrahepatic obstruction, especially when the obstruction occurs gradually. A palpable gallbladder with fever may suggest a septic complication, such as cholangitis or necrotizing cholecystitis.

Laboratory tests

Physicians can initially confirm the presence of hyperbilirubinaemia by testing the patient's urine for the presence of bilirubin by a simple test, usually available at the surgery.

After confirmation a number of blood tests may be used to differentiate between different causes of jaundice.

◆ *Serum levels of direct and indirect bilirubin.* Diagnostic value of the serum bilirubin may be augmented by using the direct-to-total bilirubin ratio: a ratio of less than 20 per cent suggests haemolysis, or Gilbert's disease. Ratios between 20 and 40 per cent point to hepatocellular rather than extrahepatic disease. Ratios between 40 and 60 per cent are found in either hepatocellular or extrahepatic disease. A ratio greater than 50 per cent favours biliary obstruction.

◆ *Aminotransferases (aspartate aminotransferases/AST, alanine aminotransferase/ALT).* ALT is more specific for the liver than AST, but a much higher level of AST compared to ALT indicates a liver affected by alcohol. Both transaminases may reach very high levels in different diseases with the exception of hepatitis C and alcoholic hepatitis where they are usually only slightly elevated.

◆ *Alkaline phosphatase (ALP).* This is the most sensitive indicator of biliary obstruction. An elevated level of ALP is observed in both the intrahepatic and extrahepatic causes of conjugated hyperbilirubinemia. It is more indicative of cholestasis or malignancy.

◆ *Gamma-glutamyltransferase (GGT)* increases in parallel with the alkaline phosphatase in biliary obstruction, but GGT is normal in bone disease. Therefore it is helpful in confirming the hepatic origin of ALP. A GGT to ALP ratio greater than 5 suggests alcoholic liver disease.

In case of high suspicion of viral hepatitis, serological tests can be used to detect the type and stage of infection. Persisting antibody titres in hepatitis B have prognostic value for chronic infection.

Additonally, a number of tests may be helpful in chronic liver disease.

◆ *Prothrombin time (PT).* PT may be prolonged in jaundice caused by intrahepatic cholestasis and extrahepatic obstruction, in which case PT is at least partly reversible when vitamin K is administered parenterally.

◆ *5-nucleotidase* is elevated in parallel with the alkaline phosphatase and suggests a hepatic rather than a bone origin of the latter.

◆ *Total blood count.* Anaemia is often found in chronic hepatitis C, but may be a finding in any chronic illness. Granulocytopaenia which is followed by a lymphocytic leukocytosis accompanies infectious mononucleosis.

◆ *Serum albumin.* Protein synthesis may be reduced in advanced liver disease.

Additional tests

To complete the patient's investigation and to serve the purpose of differential diagnosis, physicians, on some occasions, may order imaging investigations. These imaging techniques can provide answers to the following questions:

◆ Is jaundice intra- or extrahepatic?

◆ Is any obstruction in the biliary tree involved?

◆ If yes, at what level and which is the specific cause of the obstruction?

◆ Is the identified cause of obstruction removable by surgery?

Several imaging techniques are available, and they differ in their validity and reliability, accessibility, and cost. Ultrasound (US) provides a good tool for detecting gallstones and bile duct dilation, examines the hepatic parenchyma and may disclose liver metastases and infiltration of the liver by tumour.[3] Its sensitivity to detect a biliary obstruction has a range of 55–95 per cent, while its specificity is higher (82–95 per cent). Primary care physicians, after training, are capable of using US for diagnostic purposes. Physicians, while investigating their patient with ultrasound investigation should answer the question whether cholelithiasis or bile duct dilatation is present.

Computed tomography (CT) is a further non-invasive technique, but is not available in many health care systems and is more expensive. CT has almost the same specificity and sensitivity as US, but it has the advantage of being capable of detecting small hepatic lesions (<5 mm).

There are some conditions in which US is not capable of revealing whether a ductal dilatation is present and the patient should be referred to a specialist for a further imaging investigation with endoscopic retrograde cholangiopancreatography (ERCP) or percutaneous transhepatic cholangiography (PTC). Both ERCP and PTC are different modalities of direct cholangiography. ERCP is an endoscopic method of direct visualization of the biliary tree and pancreatic ducts, while PTC requires a needle to pass through the skin, the hepatic parenchyma and finally to a bile duct. The sensitivity and specificity of both imaging procedures to reveal an extrahepatic obstruction are high (88–98 per cent sensitivity and 89–100 per cent specificity). ERCP has the major advantage that it allows obstruction to be treated, either by stone removal or stent implantation.

Magnetic resonance cholangiopancreatography (MRCP) is a new imaging modality which can help to define the level of extrahepatic obstruction.

Liver biopsy

This very helpful invasive diagnostic method, can clarify the type of hepatic dysfunction, although in the case of jaundice and the possibility of an extrahepatic obstruction, its use is limited because of serious complications, including bile peritonitis. Primary care physicians should consider admitting patients to hospital for a biopsy when there is clear evidence of liver damage, signs of portal hypertension, encephalopathy, or when jaundice persists for a period of 3 months and no other diagnostic methods offer a diagnosis.

Principles of management

◆ *Which patients can be safely managed at home?* Home care of jaundiced patients should be restricted to those where conservative management is appropriate after a diagnosis of a benign cause has been established. This includes most of the infectious causes of jaundice, including infectious mononucleosis or acute viral hepatitis A or B in which there is no evidence of hepatic decompensation.

◆ *When should admission and specialist referral be considered?* Suspicion of advanced hepatocellular disease, such as portal hypertension, chronic hepatitis B and C, or primary liver cancer needs a consultation with a gastroenterologist. Traditionally, patients with acute cholecystitis or extrahepatic obstruction are referred to a surgeon. However, with ERCP techniques gastroenterologists can perform endoscopic stone release in many patients. When liver metastasis or extrahepatic malignancy are considered, especially in debilitated patients, admission to hospital for additional investigation, definitive diagnosis and treatment should be considered. When US does not confirm the presence of gallstones or stones in the biliary duct, and there are no clinical signs of cholangitis, the primary care physicians should consider malignancy; in cases of duct dilatation the most common cause of obstruction is pancreatic cancer.

◆ *When should operative management be suggested?* Primary care physicians are often questioned about the necessity for operative management when ultrasound investigation has shown a ductal obstruction or gallstones. When cholangitis is suspected, the primary care physician can administer the appropriate antibiotic treatment, but adequate biliary drainage is mandatory. ERCP, transhepatic drainage, or surgery are in the hands of the hospital specialist and may be required in the management of these patients. In cases of persisting or recurrent obstruction due to gallstones, cholecystectomy is indicated, preferably by laparoscopy.

Long-term and continuing care

Long-term and continuing care of people with jaundice

This is relevant for patients affected by hepatitis B and C. It is well known that the risk of developing cirrhosis and hepatocellular carcinoma increases in patients with chronic infection. More than 80 per cent of patients with hepatitis C remain chronically infected. Cirrhosis may develop in 30 per cent of chronic hepatitis C and 50 per cent of chronic hepatitis B infections, over a period of 20–30 years. All hepatitis B and C infected patients who develop cirrhosis should be monitored and screened for hepatocellular carcinoma, which develops in 7–10 per cent, even after viral clearance.

Primary care physicians should be aware of the recent development in hepatitis management with interferon alpha-2b. Treatment with interferon and ribavirin is recommended for patients with confirmed HCV infection who are expected to benefit from antiviral therapy after a complete clinical and laboratory assessment and consideration of the main contradictions.[4]

Prevention and health promotion issues

In the case of hepatitis B, a universal vaccination strategy has been established and almost all countries have introduced a three-dose innoculation programme. Vaccination against hepatitis A is recommended for some specific groups, but universal vaccination is still under debate.

Hepatitis C has been recognized as a serious public health problem and a comprehensive strategy to prevent and control hepatitis C includes:[5]

◆ Primary preventive action: screening and testing for blood, plasma, organ, tissue, and semen donors and virus inactivation of plasma derived products.

◆ Secondary preventive action: identification, counselling, and testing of persons at risk.

◆ Professional and public education.

Public education and public health issues

Public education seems to be quite effective in societies with poor socio-economic and hygiene conditions with the aim of restricting and diminishing the incidence of hepatitis A, but this can best be achieved through the establishment of a national innoculation programme. Persons having multiple sexual partners are at risk for sexually transmitted diseases, including hepatitis B, and potentially hepatitis C, although there is a lack of consistency in data supporting the hypothesis that sexual activities contribute to transmission of hepatitis C. Primary care physicians should be involved in counselling and educating people, especially adolescents, with the aim of preventing or diminishing the risk of acquiring hepatitis through intravenously injected drug or high-risk sexual practices.

Key points

◆ Always confirm jaundice by measuring serum bilirubin.

◆ A history of drug consumption, personal habits, and travel to tropical climates may have a prognostic value in the diagnosis of jaundice.

◆ The confirmation of pale stools and dark urine can distinguish between conjugated and unconjugated hyperbilirubinaemia.

◆ Abdominal pain or right upper quadrant pain which is accompanied by general symptoms, including marked weight loss, suggest cancer of the head of pancreas, or a metastatic disease.

◆ Physicians are advised to examine the liver for enlargement, tenderness, masses, or other abnormalities on the liver surface.

◆ Ultrasound provides a good and easily accessible tool for detecting gallstones and bile duct dilatation in the primary care setting.

References

1. **Lionis, C., Koulentaki, M., Biziagos, E., and Kouroumalis, E.** (1997). Current prevalence of hepatitis A, B and C in a well-defined area in rural Crete, Greece. *Journal of Viral Hepatitis* **4**, 55–61.

2. **Whitehead, M.W., Hainsworth, I., and Kingham, J.G.** (2001). The causes of obvious jaundice in South West Wales: perceptions versus reality. *Gut* **48**, 409–13.

3. **Johnson, D.** Clinical evaluation of the jaundice patient. In *Virtual Medical Library Home*, http://www.ccspublishing.com.

4. **Gutfreund, K.S. and Bain, V.G.** (2000). Chronic viral hepatitis C: management update. *Canadian Medical Association Journal* **162**, 827–33.

5. **CDC.** *Recommendations for Prevention and Control of Hepatitis C Virus (HCV) Infection and HCV Related Chronic Disease.* WMWR 47 (RR19), 1998, pp. 1–39.

Further reading

Wallash, J. *Interpretation of Diagnostic Tests* 6th edn. Boston MA: Little, Brown and Company, 1996.

Alpers, D.H., Owyang, C., Powell, D.W., Fred, E., and Silverstein, F.E. (1996). *Textbook of Gastroenterology.* Tadakata Yamada, 2nd edn. New York: Lippincot-Raven Publishers.

Johnson, D. Clinical evaluation of the jaundice patient. In *Virtual Medical Library Home,* http://www.ccspublishing.com.

4.10 Diarrhoea

Greg Rubin

Epidemiology

Acute diarrhoea

In the developing countries of the world diarrhoea is a major health problem. Three million people die from it each year. Of these, 92 per cent are aged less than 5 years, in which age group it is the second commonest cause of death, after pneumonia. It is estimated that 90 per cent of these deaths are preventable with correct treatment.

In Western populations, however, acute diarrhoea is a common though usually mild self-limiting illness, which affects 19 per cent of the population in a 12-month period. Nevertheless, it accounts annually for 220 000 hospital admissions in the United States among children aged less than 5 years (9 per cent of all hospitalizations in this age group) and for 300 deaths. In the United Kingdom, 100 cases of food poisoning were notified to public health authorities per 100 000 population in 2000, a figure that increased fourfold in 20 years.

Chronic diarrhoea

The prevalence of chronic diarrhoea varies with definition and with population differences. Defined as loose watery stools and/or a stool frequency more than three times per day for more than 25 per cent of the time, it affects 14 per cent of adults aged over 65 years in the United States.

Traveller's diarrhoea

Travellers' diarrhoea occurs in up to 30–60 per cent of overseas travellers, notably in those who visit tropical or sub-tropical countries. It has assumed increasing importance with the growth in foreign travel, with over 500 million international journeys being made each year.

Primary care

In the United Kingdom, one in six of those experiencing a diarrhoeal illness consult their general practitioner (GP). This results in 1.5 million GP consultations annually, and accounts for 5 per cent of all British GP consultations in children under 5.

What is diarrhoea?

Diarrhoea is often defined as a stool weight exceeding 200 g/day. This definition has several drawbacks. It may be impracticable to weigh the stools of patients in primary care. The definition is also based on experience of populations in developed countries, whereas in some African countries with high intakes of dietary fibre, normal daily stool weights can be much higher.

A more practical approach is to define diarrhoea as an increase in stool frequency or a looser consistency than normal. Thus, the passage of loose or watery stools, usually at least three times in a 24-h period, is a definition proposed by the World Health Organization (WHO) in 1993. A careful history can help to identify bowel disturbances that might be erroneously termed diarrhoea by the patient, such as faecal incontinence and tenesmus. Dysentery is infective diarrhoea accompanied by blood in the stool.

There is reasonable agreement that duration of symptoms beyond 4 weeks represents chronic diarrhoea of possible non-infective aetiology and meriting further investigation. Travellers' diarrhoea is predominantly a disorder of Western populations incurred during or immediately after overseas travel, usually to countries of the developing world.

Causes of diarrhoea

Diarrhoea is, in the simplest terms, the malabsorption of water by the gut. Between 7 and 8 litres of liquid enter the duodenum daily, made up of upper gastrointestinal secretions together with 1.5 l of food and drink. Three-quarters of this is reabsorbed in the small intestine, and most of the remainder in the large bowel, leaving 1–200 ml to escape in the stool.

Physiological disturbances in motility, permeability, mucosal secretion, active absorption, or osmosis are responsible for the development of diarrhoea. In most cases, a combination of mechanisms operates. For example, in Asiatic cholera not only does the intestinal mucosa actively secretes large volumes of fluid but small intestinal motility is also markedly increased. Intestinal absorption is impaired by damage to the microvillous membrane, as with enteropathogenic *Escherichia coli*, or by enterocyte cell death, as seen in rotavirus infection.

Dysentery is characterized by the passage of blood and mucus, fever and pain, in addition to diarrhoea. The pathological process is one of invasion of the colonic mucosa resulting in cytolysis and cell death. Mucosal congestion and diffuse colitis with superficial ulceration are visible on sigmoidoscopy.

Infective causes

The commonest cause of acute diarrhoea is enteric infection, usually from contaminated water or food. In a UK population study, the commonest infecting agents were rotavirus and small round structured virus, Campylobacter spp. and *E. coli*. Other studies have additionally identified Giardia as an important agent. Worldwide, rotavirus is the commonest single infective cause in infants and young children, and accounts for 50 per cent of deaths from diarrhoea in this age group. Cholera and Shigella are

also major concerns, being responsible for continuing pandemics in Africa and Asia. The number of cholera cases reported, and the countries affected, increased dramatically in the late 1990s, with fatality rates averaging 1 per cent but ranging up to 5 per cent. Several organisms may cause dysentery, of which the most important is Shigella.

Food poisoning may be caused by ingestion of bacterial enterotoxins, for example, from *E. coli* or *Staphylococcus aureus*, or the food may be contaminated with live organisms such as Salmonella or Campylobacter.

Enteric infection may also result in chronic diarrhoea, notably with giardiasis and amoebiasis, and the presence of immunodeficiency increases this possibility. In HIV associated immunodeficiency, for example, over 80 per cent of patients with chronic diarrhoea have a potential enteric pathogen.

Travellers' diarrhoea is most commonly caused by enterotoxinogenic *E. coli* (ETEC). Other potential causes include Shigella, Salmonella, and Campylobacter, amoebiasis, giardiasis, and cryptosporidiosis. Most patients recover within 5 days and mortality is rare.

Broad-spectrum antibiotic therapy can permit the proliferation of *Clostridium difficile* in susceptible individuals, resulting in pseudomembranous colitis, a severe systemic illness with watery diarrhoea. Such antibiotics more commonly cause simple diarrhoea through the disturbance of normal gut flora.

Non-infective causes

These more commonly result in intermittent or chronic diarrhoea. They include:

- irritable bowel syndrome (see below),
- secondary disaccharidase deficiency (see below),
- inflammatory bowel disease,
- coeliac disease,
- colorectal cancer,
- diverticulosis,
- systemic disease—thyroid disease, diabetes mellitus, adrenal disease,
- previous surgery—extensive ileal or colonic resection reducing absorptive surface area, upper GI bypass procedures that allow bacterial overgrowth, cholecystectomy,
- drugs—non-steroidal anti-inflammatory drugs, drugs with anticholinergic actions, preparations that contain magnesium salts or sorbitol,
- lactose intolerance—notably in North European populations,
- alcohol abuse,
- malabsorption, for example, due to pancreatic dysfunction,
- factitious diarrhoea caused by concealed laxative ingestion,
- toddler's diarrhoea.

Functional bowel disease

Irritable bowel syndrome (IBS) is the most common cause of chronic diarrhoea. IBS affects 15 per cent of the adult population, with diarrhoea the predominant bowel disturbance in a third of individuals and further third experiencing alternating constipation and diarrhoea. An episode of infective gastroenteritis is well recognized as an important precipitating cause of IBS, particularly in Mediterranean countries.

Secondary disaccharidase deficiency

This is the most important cause of persistent diarrhoea, and results from a loss of the disaccharidase-producing brush border of the gut epithelial cells. Ingested saccharides then remain undigested and increase osmotic pressure in the gut. Persistent diarrhoea accounts for 10% of all cases but the high death rate is because it is associated with protein malnutrition immunodeficiency, and post-infective states (esp. salmonella and shigella).

Diagnosis

Acute diarrhoea

The first steps in making a diagnosis are to establish that the patient does indeed have diarrhoea and to distinguish acute from chronic or intermittent diarrhoea. A careful history, with a description or even inspection of the stool is essential. Rectal examination is appropriate in intermittent or chronic diarrhoea. Thereafter, the line of inquiry in acute diarrhoea primarily seeks to identify a causative agent, together with predisposing and risk factors. For example, food poisoning due to *Staph. aureus* enterotoxin results in diarrhoea within 1–5 h, whereas symptom onset following ingestion of food contaminated by Salmonella occurs at 1–3 days. The nature of food ingested may give clues as the likely pathogen. Contact with a child with diarrhoea makes a viral cause likely, while the patient's age and the season of the year can narrow down the possible agent (see Table 3). Blood in the stool, systemic upset, and fever make a bacterial or parasitic cause more likely. A recent history of foreign travel can signify giardiasis, shigella, or salmonellosis, though persistent diarrhoea is more likely to be due to post-infective irritable bowel syndrome.

The management of diarrhoeal illness is largely determined by the prognosis. In developed countries, acute diarrhoea is a self-limiting illness usually lasting 2–3 days and rarely persisting beyond 14 days. Traveller's diarrhoea lasts for an average of 4 days, but persists for up to a month in a small minority of patients. In developing countries, however, acute diarrhoea and dysentery are serious illnesses with, for example, a 20 per cent mortality from Shigella dysentery. For patients with persistent diarrhoea, malnutrition is the most important predictor of mortality. Risk factors for poor outcome include:

- age over 60 years,
- immunosuppressive or systemic steroid therapy,
- malnutrition,
- acid suppressant or antacid therapy,
- immunodeficiency,
- valvular heart disease,
- diabetes mellitus,
- chronic renal disease,
- inflammatory bowel disease.

Assessment of dehydration

It is essential to assess the level of dehydration in children and those with severe symptoms (Table 1).

Investigations are of limited value in acute diarrhoea. Stool culture is indicated for bloody diarrhoea or when symptoms are persistent. In primary care, however, negative results predominate but do not exclude infection. A history of recent antibiotic use or hospitalization should prompt testing for *C. difficile* toxin. Specific stool tests, for example, for ova, cysts, and parasites, or antigens (giardiasis, cryptosporidiosis) may be also indicated by recent foreign travel or other features of the patient's history.

Chronic diarrhoea

Here, the first concern is to identify those with a serious cause, particularly since many, at least in Western populations, will have irritable bowel syndrome. Associated alarm symptoms that indicate a need for prompt specialist investigation include:

- rectal bleeding,
- weight loss,
- anaemia,
- fat intolerance or steatorrhoea.

When investigating chronic diarrhoea, the goals of the primary care physician are to exclude infective causes and to initiate screening tests for organic disease. Three separate stool samples should be cultured for ova, cysts, and parasites. Screening tests should include a full blood count, ferritin, B12, folate, calcium, endomysial antibody test, and IgA. Subsequent investigations are normally carried out by a specialist gastroenterology service and may include screening for laxative abuse, endoscopic imaging, colonic and small bowel biopsy, and investigations of malabsorption. IBS is characterized by the presence of abdominal pain associated with altered bowel habit in the absence of an identifiable structural or biochemical disorder. There are three key symptoms: pain, constipation or diarrhoea, and bloating. Diagnostic criteria are useful for clinical trials but a significant number of patients with IBS in primary care will not fulfil them. The most recent are the Rome II criteria, which define IBS as abdominal discomfort or pain for 12 consecutive weeks in the preceding 12 months that has two of the three following features: relief with defaecation, onset associated with change in stool frequency, and onset associated with a change in form (appearance of stool). The following cumulatively support the diagnosis of IBS: abnormal stool frequency, abnormal stool form, abnormal stool passage, passage of mucus, bloating or feeling of abdominal distension.

Management

Acute diarrhoea

The principles of treatment of acute diarrhoea are to manage dehydration, to relieve symptoms and to give specific antibiotic therapy where appropriate.[1] Some general principles include the importance of oral rehydration therapy (ORT) for correcting mild to moderate dehydration, the benefit of restarting normal feeding as soon as possible once dehydration has been corrected, the lack of benefit from lactose-free milk or dilution of milk,[2] and the importance of continued feeding in breastfeeding infants.

Table 1 Assessment of dehydration in acute diarrhoea

Condition	Well, alert	Restless, irritable	Lethargic or unconscious, floppy
Eyes	Normal	Sunken	Sunken
Thirst	Drinks normally, not thirsty	Thirsty, drinks eagerly	Drinks poorly or not able to drink
Skin pinch (longitudinal pinch midway between umbilicus and side)	Goes back quickly	Goes back slowly (<2 s)	Goes back very slowly (>2 s)
Conclusion	The patient has no signs of dehydration	If the patient has two or more signs, there is some dehydration	If the patient has two or more signs, there is severe dehydration
Assessment of fluid deficit	<5%, <50 ml/kg	5–10%, 50–100 ml/kg	>10%, >100 ml/kg

When there is *no dehydration*, most patients can simply be advised to maintain age-appropriate feeding and to increase their fluid intake. Starving the patient is wrong. Unsweetened fruit juices, which contain glucose and potassium, and unsalted soups are particularly suitable. However, cola and other carbonated drinks are unsuitable; they are hypertonic due to their high carbohydrate content and are also extremely low in sodium, potassium, and chloride. The routine use of lactose-free milk or dilution of milk is not necessary. ORT is an appropriate measure for infants (at a rate of 10 ml/kg after every loose stool) and for adults at increased risk, in order to prevent dehydration.

Mild dehydration in children should be corrected by giving 50 ml/kg ORT over 4 h together with replacement of continuing losses as above. The patient should be reassessed after 3–4 h. Feeding can then resume together with unrestricted fluids, which can be alternate normal fluids and ORT. Adults should receive 2 l of ORT over 24 h, followed by unrestricted normal fluids together with 200 ml ORT per loose stool. As a rule, mild dehydration can be managed at home, provided the social circumstances permit.

Moderate dehydration (up to 10 per cent) is corrected by giving 100 ml/kg ORT plus replacement of continuing losses requires more rapid restoration of the circulating volume and frequent supervision. Admission to hospital is likely to be necessary.

Severe dehydration is a medical emergency requiring bolus intravenous therapy and close specialist supervision.

Oral rehydration therapy

Oral rehydration solutions (ORS) utilize the sodium–glucose co-transport mechanism of the gut to promote absorption of water and electrolytes. Their effectiveness in treating acute diarrhoea is well proven. They are less expensive, more convenient, and safer than intravenous therapy whilst being as effective in most circumstances.[3]

The WHO formulation has been used extensively worldwide for over 20 years. A number of commercial formulations are now available which differ in composition, having lower sodium content and reduced osmolarity. In comparison to WHO ORS, these offer better symptomatic response.[4] Prepared sachets of ORS are now widely available and should be used to ensure the correct composition is maintained. A further modification

to ORS formulation, the replacement of glucose by rice powder, does not have beneficial effects on stool output, apart from in patients with cholera.[5]

Drug therapies for diarrhoea

Symptomatic therapies include drugs to reduce intestinal motility and adsorbents. Loperamide, morphine, codeine phosphate, and diphenoxylate are opiate receptor agonists, which slow gastrointestinal transit by reducing smooth muscle contraction. Loperamide and diphenoxylate do not cross the blood brain barrier and are free of CNS side-effects such as drowsiness. These drugs are widely used, especially where prompt symptom suppression is important (e.g. examinations, travel) and are the first line treatment for traveller's diarrhoea. They should not be given to young children because of possible CNS side-effects or ileus. Neither should they be used for dysentery, because of the risk of ileus and toxic megacolon. Kaolin and charcoal are adsorbents. Their disadvantages, which include adsorption of nutrients and enzymes, coupled with no good evidence of efficacy, means that they have no place in the treatment of diarrhoea.

Antimicrobial therapy is rarely indicated in acute diarrhoea and should be reserved for those with positive stool cultures who are systemically unwell or whose symptoms are severe or persistent (Table 2). It may be used empirically in those presenting with dysentery, taking regard of local epidemiology. Bacterial infection is often the cause of dysentery but, in some countries, up to 40 per cent of cases are due to amoebiasis. The cornerstone of management in epidemic cholera is ORS and not antibiotics.

Though antibiotics can reduce disease duration in some instances, they have a number of disadvantages, which include antibiotic-related diarrhoea, pseudomembranous colitis, induction of drug resistance, and induction of chronic infection (with Salmonella). Quinolones are widely used but are contraindicated in pregnancy and during breastfeeding. They can cause tendon damage and induce convulsions in epileptics. Antibiotics should not be used routinely in children.

Chronic diarrhoea

The treatment of chronic diarrhoea is primarily the treatment of the underlying disease. Nevertheless, symptomatic therapies are helpful and drugs to reduce intestinal motility (see above) are commonly used. In addition,

Table 2 Antibiotic treatment of enteric infections

Pathogen	Antibiotic	Dose (adult)	Comments
Cholera	Doxycycline	300 mg stat	Give first dose as soon as vomiting stops
	Erythromycin	250 mg four times a day for 3 days	ORT, not an antibiotic, is the principal treatment of epidemic cholera
Shigella	Ciprofloxacin	500 mg twice daily for 3 days	Shortens clinical illness and duration of pathogen excretion. Alternatives are nalidixic acid (in children) and trimethoprim (in pregnant women)
Salmonella	Ciprofloxacin	500 mg twice daily for 5 days	Reserve for enteric fever. No evidence of clinical benefit in otherwise healthy children or adults but can increase adverse effects of illness and prolong Salmonella excretion
Yersinia	Ciprofloxacin	500 mg twice daily for 5 days	For septicaemia, usually in high-risk patients
Entamoeba histolytica	Metronidazole	400–800 mg three times a day for 5–10 days	Shorter, high-dose therapy for severe, extra-intestinal disease. Follow with diloxanide furoate
Clostridium difficile	Metronidazole	400 mg three times a day for 5–10 days	
Campylobacter jejuni	Erythromycin	250 mg four times a day for 3 days	Early treatment with erythromycin is most effective
	Ciprofloxacin	500 mg twice daily for 3 days	Increasing risk of resistance to ciprofloxacin
Giardia lamblia	Metronidazole	2 g daily for 3 days	Avoid alcohol
Enterohaemorrhagic *Escherichia coli*	Ciprofloxacin	500 mg twice daily for 5 days	No clear evidence of benefit, treatment in children is associated with haemolytic uraemic syndrome

patients should be advised to maintain good nutrition and adequate fluid intake, and to avoid caffeine and alcohol.

Disaccharide intolerance is treated primarily by reducing milk in the diet, whilst correcting malnutrition through increased caloric intake. Micronutrient deficiencies are common in malnutrition and will be exacerbated by chronic diarrhoea. Supplements, especially of zinc, are an important part of treatment.

Traveller's diarrhoea

In traveller's diarrhoea, although the mainstay of treatment remains ORT, antibiotic treatment is associated with a shorter duration of diarrhoea but a higher incidence of side-effects, and a greater number of patients are cured of diarrhoea by 72 h compared with placebo [odds ratio 5.9 (CI 4.06–8.57)].[6] Their empirical use is therefore arguable, and they should be reserved for patients at high risk, those whose itinerary can least tolerate an illness, and those in whom the illness is severe. Treatment with a single dose of ciprofloxacin 500 mg is effective empirical therapy. Prophylactic therapy with co-trimoxazole, doxycycline, or ciprofloxacin has been demonstrated to significantly reduce attack rates, but is not commonly advocated because of the risks already described. Cost–benefit studies also find a weak case for prophylaxis, except in selected high-risk cases, while limited empirical self-treatment seems justified.

Vaccines

Vaccination against rotavirus infection has 69–91 per cent efficacy in preventing severe disease. In 1998, the US Food and Drug Administration licensed an oral live tetravalent rhesus-based rotavirus vaccine for use in infants. Following reports of a 1 : 10 000 risk of intussusception, the vaccine was later withdrawn in the United States by its manufacturers.

Oral vaccination against cholera gives good short-term protection. Single dose intramuscular vaccination with typhoid Vi polysaccharide preparation gives good protection for 3 years.

Preventive measures

Long-term strategies to control diarrhoeal diseases include training in case management, health education, and availability of appropriate health facilities. These are particularly important in developing countries where diarrhoeal diseases are more prevalent. Interventions that have proved effective for the process of care in these settings include the use of trained health workers, quality assurance of health care facilities and in-service training in case management for general practitioners. The promotion of breastfeeding can have important benefits. In Latin America, 40–70 per cent of infant deaths from diarrhoea would be prevented by exclusive breastfeeding in the first 3 months of life

Water supply and sanitation interventions are highly cost-effective strategies for the control of diarrhoeal disease in children under 5.[7] Relatively inexpensive measures include social marketing of good hygiene practices, regulation of drinking water and monitoring of water quality. Zinc supplements are added in some countries; a combination of zinc and vitamin A supplements has been shown to reduce the persistence of acute diarrhoea in Bangladeshi children. Finally, measles vaccination can substantially reduce the incidence and severity of diarrhoeal disease.

Table 3 Characteristics of infectious causes of diarrhoea

Organism	Transmission (in addition to faecal–oral route)	Incubation	Duration (days)	Features	Comments (exclusion until 24 h after last loose stool unless otherwise stated)
Staphylococcus aureus	Cooked meats	1–5 h	1	Vomiting, cramps	
Bacillus cereus	Rice dishes	1–16 h	0.2–0.5	Vomiting, cramps	
Clostridium perfringens	Beef, turkey, chicken	8–22 h	0.3–3		
Salmonella	Eggs, meat, poultry	12–72 h	0.5–14	Fever, nausea, abdominal pain	Negative stool tests in children and food handlers
Campylobacter jejuni	Raw meat, milk, water, pets	2–10 days	1–11	Fever, abdominal pain, bloody diarrhoea	
Shigella sonnei	Mainly faecal–oral, common in nurseries	1–7 days	0.5–14	Mild illness, may be asymptomatic	Commonest form in UK. One negative stool if aged under 5 years
Shigella boydii, flexneri, dysenteriae	Milk, salads	1–7 days	0.5–14	Fever, bloody diarrhoea	Originate outside UK
Escherichia coli					
Enteropathogenic	Food, water	0.1–2 days	1–7		Mainly seen in children
Enterohaemorrhagic (0157)	Beef, milk	1–7 days	1–7	Pain, bloody diarrhoea, haemolytic uraemic syndrome	Two negative stools required
Enterotoxic	Food, water	2–7 days	1–7	Watery diarrhoea	Traveller's diarrhoea
Giardia lamblia	Water, animals	5–20 days	14	Abdominal pain, flatulence	
Rotavirus	Epidemics, winter peaks, possible respiratory droplet spread	2–4 days	5–6	Vomiting, fever, dehydration	Peak incidence at age 3–15 months
Enteric adenovirus		8–10 days	4–9		Children under 2 years
Astroviruses	Epidemics in institutions	6 days	2–3	Mild illness	Children under 2 years
Calciviruses	Epidemics, food, water	1–3 days	2–3	Mild illness	Children over 6 months
Norwalk virus	Epidemics, food, water, airborne	0.2–3 days	1–2	Vomiting, fever, myalgia, prostration	Children. Exclusion for 3 days from onset

Implications

Exclusion from nursery, school and work

Patients with diarrhoea due to an infectious cause present a communicable hazard.[8] Most of the infective agents are spread by faecal–oral transmission, but food and water are also important vectors (Table 3). In general, patients can be regarded as no longer being infectious 24 h after the diarrhoea stops. This period may need to be extended in children under 5 and those with poor personal hygiene, and special measures are indicated in Table 3. Individual countries may have statutory reporting requirements for certain causes of diarrhoea, for public health purposes.

Persons whose work requires them to handle food may be subject to specific occupational health regulations. In the United Kingdom, they should not return to work until 48 h after the last diarrhoea stool. If Salmonella is the causative organism, then three negative stool samples are necessary.

Health economics

Whilst the 1 : 10 000 risk of intussusception with rotavirus vaccination outweighs its benefits in a Western population, the balance is very different in developing countries, where risk of death from rotavirus infection is 1 : 200. Judgements about the safety, and therefore continued production, of vaccines that are dominated by a traditional, Western perspective have important implications for child mortality from this infection.

Key points

- Diarrhoea is a common problem affecting 19 per cent of Western populations in a 12-month period. In developing countries, it is a major health problem and a common cause of death in children.

- Acute diarrhoea is defined as the passage of at least three loose stools in a 24-h period.

- The commonest cause of acute diarrhoea is enteric infection, usually from contaminated food or water, or by person-to-person faecal–oral transmission.

- The assessment of dehydration is an essential step in the management of acute diarrhoeal illness.

- The correction of dehydration using oral rehydration solution and the early resumption of normal feeding are the most important principles of treatment.

- Traveller's diarrhoea is more commonly due to bacterial infection and empirical antibiotic therapy is justified in selected cases.

- In most instances, the exclusion period for infectious causes of acute diarrhoea is until 24 h after the last diarrhoeal stool (48 h if the patient is employed as a food handler).

References

1. **Banks, M. and Farthing, M.** (2000). Management of acute diarrhoea in primary care. *Prescriber* 97–104, 19 February. (Non-systematic overview of causes and treatment of acute diarrhoea.)

2. **Brown, K.H., Peerson, J.M., and Fontaine, O.** (1994). Use of non-human milks in the dietary management of young children with acute diarrhoea: a meta-analysis of clinical trials. *Paediatrics* **93** (1), 17–27. (Meta-analysis of 29 studies concluded that routine use of lactose-free milk or dilution of milk is not necessary, especially when ORT and early feeding form the basic approach to management of diarrhoea.)

3. **Gavin, N., Merrick, N., and Davidson, B.** (1996). Efficacy of glucose based oral rehydration therapy. *Pediatrics* **98** (1), 45–51. (Meta-analysis of RCTs comparing the efficacy of ORT with IV rehydration. Over-the-counter ORS

available in the United States are appropriate and effective for the treatment of well-nourished children.)

4. **Kim, Y., Hahn, S., and Garner, P.** (2001). Reduced osmolarity oral rehydration solutions for treating dehydration caused by acute diarrhoea in children (Cochrane Review). In *The Cochrane Library* Issue 3. Oxford: Update Software. (Systematic review with meta-analysis of nine trials. Reduced osmolarity ORS compared with WHO ORS was associated with fewer unscheduled intravenous infusions, smaller stool volume, and less vomiting, without increased risk of hyponatraemia.)

5. **Fontane, O., Gore, S.M., and Pierce, N.F.** (2001). Rice based ORS for treating diarrhoea (Cochrane Review). In *The Cochrane Library* Issue 3. Oxford: Update Software. (Systematic review of 22 studies. Compared with ORS containing glucose (20 g/l), ORS containing 50–80 g/l of rice powder reduced stool output in patients with cholera, but not in infants or children with non-cholera diarrhoea.)

6. **De Bruyn, G., Hahn, S., and Borwick, A.** (2001). Antibiotic treatment for travellers diarrhoea (Cochrane Review). In *The Cochrane Library* Issue 3. Oxford: Update Software. (Systematic review, meta-analysis not feasible. All trials reported a significant reduction in duration of diarrhoea with antbiotics compared to placebo.)

7. **Varley, R.C.G., Tarvid, J., and Chao, D.N.W.** (1998). A reassessment of the cost effectiveness of water and sanitation interventions in programmes for controlling childhood diarrhoea. *Bulletin of the WHO* **76** (6), 617–31. (Cost effectiveness, cost utility analysis, hypothetical population of children aged below 5 years in primary and community care.)

8. **Public Health Laboratory Service,** www.phls.co.uk/advice/index.htm. Accessed 18 August 2001.

Further reading

(1996). Practice parameter: the management of acute gastroenteritis in young children. *Pediatrics* **97** (3), 424–35.

WHO. *The Treatment of Diarrhoea. A Manual for Physicians and Other Senior Health Workers.* WHO/CDR/95.3 10/95.

Farthing, M.J.G. et al. (1996). The management of infective gastroenteritis in adults. A consensus statement by an expert panel convened by the British Society for the Study of Infection. *Journal of Infection* **33**, 143–52.

Banks, M. and Farthing, M. (2001). Current management of acute diarrhoea. *Prescriber* 83–93, 19 June.

Murphy, M.S. (1998). Guidelines for managing acute gastroenteritis based on a systematic review of published research. *Archives of Disease in Childhood* **79**, 279–84.

Prodigy guidelines. www.prodigy.org.uk.

4.11 Constipation

Villy Meineche-Schmidt and Niek J. de Wit

Introduction

The term 'constipation' (derived from the Latin *con-stipare*, meaning 'stagnation') refers to infrequent or difficult evacuation of the faeces.[1]

It is merely a statement that relates a personal condition to what the subject believes is normal, and is not a strict scientific definition. As a consequence, self-reported constipation could refer to a very broad spectrum of clinical conditions.

In a population-based study from the United Kingdom[2] it has been demonstrated that healthy people report bowel movement varying from three times daily to three times per week, leaving a 10-fold variation of bowel frequencies as 'normal'. Furthermore, for the general public the term constipation can refer to many different conditions other than low stool frequency, such as hard stool consistency, straining on passing faeces, or inability to pass faeces at will, a sensation of incomplete evacuation or even 'spending too much time at the toilet'.[3] So, faced with a patient complaining of 'constipation' it is of prime importance to understand what he or she really means. Although constipation has a personal context, from a clinical perspective it is necessary to use an accepted standard definition of constipation in the approach to the person, who by consulting the general practitioner turns himself into a patient. Primary care physicians tend to consider *stool frequency* as the most important symptom suggestive of constipation. From a practical clinical point of view, constipation is considered to be present if the patient passes stools less than three times a week for a period of at least 6 weeks.[4,5]

Specialists use a more strict and detailed definition, based on the presence of certain symptoms for a defined period of time as well as stool frequency.[6] At least two of the following symptoms must have been present in at least 25 per cent of defecations during at least 3 months within the last year: (a) straining; (b) hard stools; (c) incomplete evacuation; (d) sensation of obstruction; (e) manual manoeuvres to pass stools; and (f) less than three defecations per week. There is no consensus as to whether patients with less than three evacuations per week and no other symptoms should be regarded as constipated, indicating that constipation can only be defined if passing faeces with low frequencies is accompanied with unpleasant symptoms.

Epidemiological data

Problems with defaecation should be seen in their cultural and psychological context. Many of the international differences in the incidence of constipation can be explained by dietary habits and social aspects of the process of passing stools, including taboos and cultural norms. Constipation is rare in many developing countries, and relatively common in the Western world. Due to the difficulties in defining the condition, data on the epidemiology of constipation are not very comparable. The prevalence in the general population varies between 2 and 28 per cent.[7] In elderly people, the incidence of constipation may reach up to 25 per cent, while 2 per cent of children under 4 years suffer from constipation. Constipation is related to a number of *risk factors*. In most studies self reported constipation is more common among women compared to men. The prevalence of constipation increases with age partly because ageing leads to decrease in the total number of neurons in the myenteric plexus. Inactivity, low caloric intake, medication, low social status, and depression have been shown to be related to constipation. In a meta-analysis of case-control studies, the risk for development of colon cancer was shown to be slightly raised in patients with constipation;[8] the pooled odds ratio being 1.48 (95 per cent CI = 1.32–1.66).

Consultation for constipation

It has been estimated that constipation accounts for 1.2 per cent of consultations in primary care in the United States.[9] Less than 5 per cent of these patients are referred to specialists, and the majority will be managed in general practice. In primary care in the Western world, constipation is mainly a problem of the elderly: morbidity data from general practice in Holland indicate that 48 per cent of the consulters for constipation were older than 65 years old, while 10 per cent were children under 4 years.[10] Constipation ranks within the top five of gastrointestinal reasons for consultation in primary care. The estimated annual incidence in general practice is 5–9 per 1000 patients per year, while the prevalence of constipation is estimated between 25 and 30 per 1000 patients per year.[11]

Only 25 per cent of the people suffering from constipation consult a physician.[12,13] Complaints with which patients present their constipation vary: slow or infrequent defaecation (60 per cent), request for medication (10 per cent), or abdominal pain (15 per cent). Apart from these symptoms, other factors determine the decision to consult: anxiety, worry about cancer risk, depression, and major life events.[13]

Background and differential diagnosis

Two major *pathophysiological* mechanisms have been identified in patients with constipation: slow-transit constipation and pelvic floor dysfunction. Slow-transit constipation indicates that the transit time of the bowel contents is longer, due to either colonic inertia with decreased numbers of contractions throughout the colon or to uncoordinated motor activity leading to functional obstruction.[14] In pelvic floor dysfunction, on the other hand, the transit time of the bowel contents is normal or only slightly prolonged, but expulsion of the faeces is the problem, leading to retention in the rectum. The physiology of this condition is poorly understood, but dysfunction or dyscoordination between contraction of the pelvic muscles and relaxation of the anal sphincter is a focus of research. Although some patients present with a mixture of these conditions, from a clinical point of view it is important to distinguish between constipation due to slow transit and constipation due to outlet problems, because the therapeutic approaches differ.

Several further causes of constipation can be discriminated (Table 1). Constipation can be a side-effect of many drugs, the most important ones being opiates (long-term opiate treatment will almost always produce constipation), antidepressants, calcium channel blockers, diuretics, antipsychotics and anticholinergic agents, non-steroidal anti-inflammatory agents, iron supplements, and antacid agents. Lifestyle and dietary factors can contribute to the genesis of constipation: insufficient fibre and fluid intake, immobility of any cause, and insufficient response to the normal defaecation reflex. Metabolic conditions such as diabetes mellitus, hypothyroidism, uremia or hypercalcemia, and mechanical obstruction due to diverticulitis or colon cancer may be the cause of constipation. In the majority of patients in primary care, no clear cause can be identified, and patients are considered to suffer from 'functional' constipation. This may be part of other functional abdominal syndromes, such as irritable bowel syndrome (IBS) or pelvic floor spasm.

Constipation in *young children* is relatively common, and may present with various symptoms: abdominal pain, recurrent urinary tract infections, incontinence, soiling, feeding or behavioural problems or 'true' constipation.[16] A congenital background (malrotation or Hirschprung's disease with megacolon) is rare, but there is often a hereditary factor. Usually there is a cyclical process of abdominal pain leading to suppression of defaecation, aggravating the constipation with even more abdominal pain. The therapeutic approach should be focused on breaking this cycle, by using a combined intervention of the effective use of laxatives and training the child to respond to the reflex.

The *elderly* are more prone to constipation, due to decreased gastrointestinal motility and lack of physical exercise, changes in dietary pattern, insufficient fluid intake, and poly-medication.[17] The problem may escalate to faecal impaction in the rectum, requiring digital removal. Most elderly people have found a way of ensuring a regular stool, usually through small changes in bowel or dietary habits or over-the-counter (OTC) laxatives. However, in some cases the overuse of laxatives may cause constipation again.

How to make a diagnosis

It is of prime importance to understand the patient's complaints and start with an adaequate problem analysis. Is the consistency or the frequency of defaecation the core problem? Is it a sensation of incomplete evacuation or is the patient unable to defecate at will?

A proper history in patients presenting with constipation should answer the following six questions:

1. What is the *normal defaecation pattern* and faecal consistency, what has changed in this pattern, and when did these changes start?

Table 1 Causes of constipation[15]

Dietiary causes
Low fibre intake
Low fluid intake

Lifestyle causes
Inadequate response to defaecation reflex
Insufficient physical excercise

Metabolic disorders
Diabetes
Hypothyroidism
Hypercalcaemia

Neuropsychiatric disorders
General
   Parkinsonism
   Spinal cord disorders
   Depression
Local
   Hirschsprung's disease
   Abdominal neuropathy
   Laxative abuse

Obstructive constipation
Colorectal cancer
Constrictive diverticulitis

Drug-induced causes
General
   Antacids
   Iron supplements
   Anticholinergics
Psychotropic drugs
   Antidepressants
   Antiepileptics
   Anti-Parkinsonian drugs
   Neuroleptics
Cardiovascular drugs
   Diuretics
   Calcium channel antagonists
Analgesics
   Opiates
   Non-steroidal anti-inflammatory drugs

Functional syndromes
Irritable bowel syndrome
Spastic pelvic floor

Table 2 Fibre content of common food and fibre supplements

Low content (2 g/cup)
Apple, grapefruit, melon, orange, peach, pear, pineapple, broccoli, carrots, oatmeal, pasta from whole-wheat flour, popcorn, pumpkin

Medium content (5 g/cup)
Beans, bran flakes 40%, raisin bran

High content (8–10 g/cup)
All Bran, Fibre One, bran flakes 100%, wheat bran

Mode of action: Increases the stool bulk and the gastrointestinal motility, producing a decrease in colonic transit time

Side-effects: Bloating and flatulence. Possibly iron and calcium malabsorption

emerging defaecation reflex instantly. Systematic suppression of this reflex may cause constipation, especially when combined with an over-consumption of low-fibre 'junk food'. Working circumstances such as long meetings, factory work, or low physical activity may contribute.

Having answered these questions it should be possible to determine whether the complaints are related to constipation per se or if they represent the constipation sub-type of IBS. If IBS can be excluded, attention should be paid to whether the constipation is secondary to some other disease or condition or to concomitant medication (as mentioned above). If no cause can be identified (which will be the case in most primary care patients with constipation) it is important to identify the mechanism of constipation. The type of constipation can be assessed by asking the patient if he or she uses external (abdominal wall or perineum) or internal (vaginal) pressure to help passing stools or if digital evacuation has been used. If so, this suggests an outlet type of constipation caused by pelvic floor dysfunction. In patients with constipation due to delayed colon transit time the frequency of defaecation reflexes is decreased, causing abdominal pain and distention.

The need for a full *physical examination* in every constipated patient may be questioned. It is required in patients at a higher risk of organic disease, such as those suspected of obstruction or perianal problems. One should realize, however, that the negative predictive value of a physical examination for, for example, colon cancer is very poor. Many will agree that every chronically constipated patient should have a full examination at least once, including rectal examination. If performed, physical examination should include a number of steps. Inspection of the anal region for faecal soiling, haemorrhoids, and perianal abcesses or tears. The patient should be asked to simulate defaecation, allowing to observe pelvic floor and perineum muscular activity and rule out anorectal mucosal prolapse. The anal sphincter tone should be tested by digital examination while noticing any localized pain. In case of suspicion of neurological disease, the anal reflex should be tested by a pinprick. In women, a gynaecological examination may need to be performed to rule out gynaecological conditions that might cause constipation, such as uterine prolapse and large fibroids.

2. Are there any *alarm symptoms*, suggestive of an obstructive cause? Rapidly developing constipation in the elderly, with considerable weight loss or fatigue may be highly suspicious of colonic cancer, especially when accompanied by rectal bleeding or a positive family history of colon cancer. The same applies to persistent constipation from birth, which might be caused by a congenital megacolon.

3. Are there any *accompanying symptoms* that might give a clue to the background of the constipation, such as abdominal pain or bloating (IBS), perianal pain (anal fissure), or vaginal complaints (rectocele)?

4. Is there any *co-morbidity or pharmacotherapy* that might explain the constipation? (Table 1.)

5. Are there any *dietary factors* that might explain the constipation; is there sufficient fibre and fluid intake in the daily diet? (Table 2.) The gut transit time and faecal volume are directly related to the fibre content of the patient's diet. A daily intake of 25–30 g of fibre is considered a minimum to ensure a regular stool. This should be accompanied by at least six glasses of fluid every day, to prevent dehydration and constipation.

6. And finally, are there any *lifestyle factors* that explain the problem? In the Western 'rush culture' there is often hardly any time to deal with the

Principles of management

Constipation in primary care is in general a benign problem, which responds well to treatment. Based on the patient's background, the results of history-taking and physical examination, a risk profile can be drawn up, indicating the patient's risk of a serious cause. The most important prognostic factors in constipation are age, duration, and onset of complaints, alarming symptoms, diet and lifestyle factors, and medication use. In practice, laboratory tests may be helpful in detecting metabolic causes for constipation. Additional diagnostic tests or referral should be reserved for those patients in whom a serious cause is suspected. Serious causes are rare; the incidence of Hirschsprung's disease is one in every 5000 neonates, that of colon carcinoma is 40 per 100 000 in the Western world, with 90 per cent of the patients older than 50 years. However, in the presence of alarm symptoms or when there is a high suspicion of malignancy, the patient should be referred for urgent sigmoidoscopy or colonoscopy. When constipation persists in newborns, paediatric referral is indicated.

In cases of constipation due to drug therapy, the drug most likely to be involved should be stopped or replaced.

In many patients, explanation about the benign background of the problem may take away worry and anxiety. Proper education about the need for regular defaecation habits, the importance of physical exercise, and 'taking time' for the digestive system might be a reason for lifestyle changes. The importance of sufficient fibre in the diet and fluid intake should be addressed, either by the physician or a dietician.

Having ruled out secondary constipation, the evidence for the superiority of specific pharmacological intervention is not very strong. More than 700 therapeutic trials have been evaluated, but only 36 randomized controlled trials could be included in a meta-analysis[18] showing that both fibre and laxatives modestly improved bowel movement frequency in adults with chronic constipation. No difference between fibres and laxatives or between different laxatives on the frequency of bowel movements could be demonstrated. The therapeutic approach therefore must be based on empiric knowledge and cost effectiveness. What has been tried and what has worked?

Faced with (predominantly or partly) slow-transit constipation the first line treatment should be a gradual increased intake of fibre, either by changing the diet (Table 2) or given as supplement (Table 3) combined with extra fluids. It is recommended to start with one dose daily, weekly increasing until effect or persistent side-effects (bloating and flatulence) appear. As the effect will become apparent gradually, therapy should be continued for at least one month.

If treatment success is not obtained with fibres, a saline agent such as magnesia should be instituted in doses of 15–30 ml once or twice a day. Hyperosmolar agents as lactulose or polyethylene glycol 15–60 ml daily are alternatives, but they have not proven beneficial over other laxatives, although well conducted randomized trials are scarce.[19]

If this does not relieve the problems, the third step is to administer stimulating agents such as bisacodyl used either orally or as suppositories three times weekly. Finally, enemas may be required in the acute treatment of constipation.

Table 3 Medications commonly used for constipation

Drug	Daily dose	Side-effects
Chronic treatment		
Bulking agents		Flatulence, meteorism
Fibre	Up to 20 g	
Sterculia	20 g	
Psyllium	30 g	
Macrogol		
Osmotic laxatives		
Magnesia	15–30 ml × 2–4	Magnesium intoxication, dehydration
Lactulose	15–30 ml × 2–4	Flatulence, sweet taste
Sorbitol	15–30 ml × 2–4	Flatulence, sweet taste
Contact laxatives		
Bisacodyl	10 mg	Rectal burning, abdominal pain
Sodium picosulphate	0.5–1.0 ml	Abdominal pain
Senna	2–4 tablets × 2	Malabsorption, abdominal pain
Mineral oil	15–45 ml	Malabsorption, dehydration
Phenolphthalein	50–250 mg	Allergic reaction
Emollients		
Paraffine oil		
Sodium laurylsulfoacetate		
Acute treatment		
Enemas, soap	500 ml	Soiling, mechanical trauma, damage to rectal mucosa
Enemas, oil	100 ml	Mechanical trauma
Enemas, Sodium phosphate	133 ml	
Bisacodyl	Suppositories	

Constipation due to pelvic floor dysfunction will not be alleviated by these treatment approaches. No treatment consensus has been reached for this dysfunction. Biofeedback has in some studies shown effect but the motivation from both the patient and the physician may play an important role.[7]

In patients who do not respond to treatment, referral for a diagnostic work up in a specialist centre may be considered, in order to identify the pathophysiologic disturbance behind the constipation. Large bowel transit time can be measured using radiopaque markers. The transit time can be measured after recording the distribution of these markers in the colon on consecutive days. A defaecogram, a radiological record of the defaecation process using barium, may reveal anatomic abnormalities around the rectum which may explain the condition. Disturbances in colonic contractions can be identified using manometric probes. Endoscopic biopsies from the bowel wall may reveal a neurological or muscular cause. Though the prime cause may be identified in this extensive diagnostic process, it does not usually provide any additional therapeutic options, apart from surgery. In severe, refractory constipated patients with slow-transit constipation, surgery can be performed and total colectomy has been shown to produce the best results,[20] although the results from surgical interventions for constipation may be disappointing, and depend on proper patient selection. Referral should be reserved for those patients whose constipation proves refractory to primary care therapy and where quality of life is severely disrupted by the condition.

Long-term care and social implications of the problem

Though constipation is a very frequent problem in the community, most people will solve it using either lifestyle or diet modification or by using a simple OTC laxative. The impact of constipation on primary care reflects the high incidence of constipation in very young children and in the elderly. Most of these patients can be treated in primary care, but a long-term treatment may be required. No research data on the impact of constipation on quality of life are known, but the psycho-social aspects of the problem need the attention of the physician, especially in risk groups. Elderly people can get very focused on their stool habits, taking the problem to a disproportional level. Explanation about the background and possible reasons for a physiological delay in older age may be very helpful to bring it back to the right proportions. In children, psychosocial elements also need to be considered, as in this age group constipation often has a behavourial background, and is either due to, or causes, problems in family relations.

Key points

- Due to the wide variation in definitions and understandings of constipation, the primary care consultation should aim to identify the patient's main presenting problem.

- Only a minority of patients have secondary constipation, and this is usually drug related.

- Serious causes of constipation are rare and are usually apparent from the clinical history.

- Primary or functional constipation should be divided into constipation-predominant irritable bowel syndrome, slow transit, or pelvic floor dysfunction.

- Primary care constipation management focuses on ruling out alarm symptoms and secondary causes of constipation, and on empirical treatment.

- Laxatives and fibre are equally effective for slow-transit constipation.

- Treatment for pelvic floor dysfunction constipation is difficult and requires specialist care.

References

1. *Dorlands Illustrated Medical Dictionary*. Philadelphia PA: Saunders, 1988, p. 375.

2. **Connell, A.M.** et al. (1965). Variation of bowel habit in two population samples. *British Medical Journal* **2**, 1095–9.

3. **Sandler, R.S. and Drossman, D.A.** (1987). Bowel habits in young adults not seeking health care. *Digestive Diseases and Sciences* **32**, 841–5.

4. **Herz, M.J.** et al. (1996). Constipation: a different entity for patients and doctors. *Family Practice* **13**, 156–9.

5. **Donatelle, E.P.** (1990). Constipation: pathophysiology and treatment. *American Family Physician* **42**, 1335–42.

6. **Drossman, D.A.**, senior ed. *The Functional Gastrointestinal Disorders*, 2nd edn. Degnon Associates, 2000.

7. **Locke, G.R. III, Pemberton, J.H., and Philips, S.F.** (2000). AGA technical review on constipation. American Gastroenterology Association. *Gastroenterology* **119**, 1766–78.

8. **Sonnenberg, A. and Muller, A.D.** (1993). Constipation and cathartics as risk factors of colorectal cancer: a metaanalysis. *Pharmacology* **47**, 224–33.

9. **Sonnenberg, A. and Koch, T.R.** (1989). Physician visits in the United States for constipation: 1958–1986. *Digestive Diseases and Sciences* **34**, 606–11.

10. **Okkes, I.M., Oskam, S.K., and Lamberts, H.** From complaint to diagnosis; primary care morbidity data in the Netherlands. Bussum, Coutinho, 1998.

11. **NIVEL and Dutch Digestive Disease Foundation.** *Gastroenterological Diseases in the Dutch Community and in Primary Care*. Utrecht: NIVEL, 1992.

12. **Talley, N., O'Keefe, E.A., Zinmeister, A.R., and Melton, L.J.** (1992). Prevalence of gastro-intestinal symptoms in the elderly; a population based study. *Gastroenterology* **102**, 895–901.

13. **Jones, R. and Lydeard, S.** (1992). Irritable bowel syndrome in the general population. *British Medical Journal* **304**, 87–90.

14. **Snape, W.J.** (1997). Role of colonic motility in guiding therapy in patients with constipation. *Digestive Diseases* **15**, 104–11.

15. **Kamm, M.E. and Lennard Jones, J.E.**, ed. *Constipation*. Hampshire UK: Wrightson Biomedical Publishing, 1994.

16. **Loening-Baucke, V.** (1994). Management of chronic constipation in infants and toddlers. *American Family Physician* **49**, 397–406.

17. **Schaefer, D.C. and Cheskin, L.J.** (1998). Constipation in the elderly. *American Family Physician* **58**, 907–14.

18. **Tramonte, S.M.** et al. (1997). Treatment of chronic constipation: a systemic review. *Journal of General Internal Medicine* **12**, 15–24.

19. **Petticrew, M., Watt, I., and Brend, M.** (1999). What's the 'best buy' for treatment of constipation? Result of a systematic review of the efficacy and comparative efficacy of laxatives in the elderly. *British Journal of General Practice* **49**, 387–93.

20. **Pemberton, J.H., Rath, D.M., and Ilstrup, D.M.** (1991). Evaluation and surgical treatment of severe chronic constipation. *Annals of Surgery American Family* **214**, 403–13.

4.12 Perianal disease

Simon Travis

Introduction

Perianal disease presents in one of four ways: an itchy bottom, perianal pain, bleeding, or a palpable lump. To the layperson (and some doctors!), diagnosis is simple: everything is attributed to 'piles'. The truth is somewhat different. Accurate diagnosis and management are essential if the discomfort of recurrent symptoms is to be avoided and the functional complexity of the anal sphincter preserved.

Anal disease is a consequence of defaecation. Treatments for fissure and haemorrhoids are included in the Ayurvedic tradition and the medieval monk John of Arderne wrote a treatise on fistula in ano. Anal humour featured in Elizabethan comedy, being central to the plot of Shakespeare's All's Well That Ends Well, in which the incurable disease (a fistula in ano) of the king of France is healed by Helena, daughter of a famous physician. The prevalence of perianal disease may account for the plethora of treatments, but the current lack of consensus on the most appropriate approach for common anorectal conditions such as an anal fissure reflects a shift away from surgical intervention. Perianal disease should largely be the province of the family physician. Unfortunately research has been driven by the selected practice of colorectal specialists, rather than by population-based studies in primary care.

The diversity of perianal disease is best considered by individual diagnosis. The epidemiology, differential diagnosis, principles of management in primary care, and implications can be considered for each condition, but aspects of history-taking and rectal examination are common to all conditions.

History-taking for perianal conditions

Patients present with itchiness, pain, bleeding, or a combination of these features. The duration, speed of onset, and associated symptoms are readily established. The correct diagnosis is then commonly apparent after simple rectal examination.

Care should be taken when there are a combination of features, if there are associated symptoms, or if the problem recurs. Pain is never a feature of uncomplicated piles and bleeding with a change in bowel habit should indicate the need for further investigation even if haemorrhoids are present. Diarrhoea and an abscess or fistula should raise the possibility of Crohn's disease. The same applies for recurrent abscesses or fistulae. Recurrent pruritus often has a dermatological origin and premalignant conditions such as Bowen's disease should be considered.

Taking a family history is necessary not only for minor conditions (pruritus caused by threadworm, for instance), but also to be on the alert for rare, major conditions such as Crohn's disease and anal cancer. Questions about topical treatments, often bought over the counter, may identify a cause for pruritus ani.

More sensitive questioning is needed to establish sexual proclivity and activity, but this is essential if sexually transmitted disease is to be recognized. Sensitivity is also needed when enquiring about faecal continence. Patients frequently fail to mention 'loss of control' or 'accidents' unless asked and may disguise the description as one of 'diarrhoea', since this is more socially acceptable. Lack of continence is the symptom most strongly associated with poor quality of life. Constipation is also debilitating and if there is no painful perianal condition to account for constipation, questions about initiating defaecation are appropriate. Delay in initiating defaecation, or digital manoeuvres to aid evacuation, suggest an evacuation disorder rather than commonplace diet-related constipation.

Rectal examination

The aphorism 'If you don't put your finger in it, you'll put your foot in it' remains valid. There is, however, more to rectal examination than lubricating the anal canal.

Look first. Perianal erythema or excoriation indicate a dermatosis, while 'funny looking' (oedematous, violaceous) skin tags may be due to Crohn's disease. Large 'warts' may be a lymphoma. Consider asking the patient to strain if poor continence is suspected. Mucosal prolapse, perineal descent, or seepage may be observed.

Palpation should be gentle. Any pain in the anal canal suggests a fissure and examination should not proceed unless the anal canal is anaesthetized with 2 per cent lignocaine gel. Assess anal sphincter tone in those with poor continence. Finally, feel in four places: anteriorly, posteriorly, bilaterally, and at the tip. A rectal neoplasm at the fingertip is easily missed by a cursory examination technique.

Additional investigations such as procotoscopy are easy to perform in primary care, and may—in trained hands—be very helpful in detecting the background of perianal problems.

Itchy bottom

Individuals vary in their capacity to feel itching and the threshold varies within an individual, depending on their state of boredom or distraction. When itching is confined to the perianal area, it is termed pruritus ani.

Pruritus ani

Pruritus ani (Fig. 1) is a common and socially embarassing condition that is often poorly managed. It is usually dermatological, caused by moisture, excoriation, and infection in varying degrees (a cross between nappy rash, athlete's foot, and self-inflicted injury) (Box 1). In the absence of systemic disease (such as diabetes or primary biliary cirrhosis), or local skin conditions, a psychogenic cause is often implied. This is not substantiated by psychological assessment.

Management

If no rash is visible and no cause identified, explain the process of itching and give advice on anal hygiene. A bidet or wet cotton wool to cleanse the bottom is better than excessive bottom polishing with paper. Very dry skin may be helped by moisturising cream and excessively moist skin by a pad in the natal cleft. Otherwise avoid topical applications of creams or powders.

For those with perianal erythema or excoriation, the first step is to control infection. A cream containing 1 per cent hydrocortisone and an antifungal (such as 2 per cent miconazole) may be used for about 2 weeks. The next step is to stop all topical applications.

Refer only those patients with persistent pruritus and a visible lesion. A dermatologist is more appropriate than a colorectal surgeon. The exceptions are patients with moisture due to seepage from a weak sphincter or a perianal lesion causing difficulty in cleaning the perianal skin.

Perianal pain

Perianal pain is characterized by an association with defaecation. It is commonly caused by constipation, which then further complicates treatment, but perianal pain may also cause constipation. It must be distinguished from pelvic pain and sacrococcygeal causes. Pelvic pain is associated with dyspareunia, the menstrual cycle, or urinary symptoms. Sacrococcygeal pain is often continuous and exacerbated by local pressure on the sacrum or coccyx.

Proctalgia fugax

Proctalgia fugax is an intense, self-limiting pain experienced in the perineum. Most sufferers do not seek medical advice. The cause is unclear, but manometric studies have implicated paroxysmal contractions in the internal anal sphincter. Symptoms are often nocturnal, affecting young people and may be relieved by defaecation. When symptoms occur for the first time in the elderly, a rare presentation of rectal cancer should be considered.

Management

For those who present, an empathetic history and rectal examination, followed by explanation and reassurance is usually all that is necessary. General advice on a high-fibre diet with adequate fluid intake to avoid constipation may help.

Refer only those with frequent, persistent, and debilitating symptoms, to a gastroenterologist rather than a colorectal surgeon. Topical glyceryl trinitrate 0.2 per cent has been used for symptomatic relief, but commonly causes headache.

Anal fissure

Anal fissure (Box 2) is a tear in the lining of the anal canal. It is common, usually transient, but may persist and cause considerable morbidity in otherwise healthy young people. The usual age of onset is 30–50 years, although fissures may occur at any age, including children.

Pain in the anal canal during straining to pass a hard stool is typical. A small amount of bright red blood frequently passes during defaecation. Persistent pain develops due to spasm of the internal anal sphincter. Examination of the anus by gently parting the anal verge will reveal a tear, usually in the posterior midline and associated with a 'sentinel pile'. This is not a pile, but a small skin tag at the distal apex of the fissure that may obscure the fissure itself.

Beware splits in a position other than the posterior midline, those that have indurated or ill-defined edges, and those that are visible without parting the anal verge. In these circumstances, Crohn's disease, HIV infection, syphilis, or cancer should be suspected.

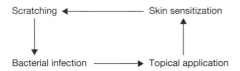

Fig. 1 The pruritus ani cycle.

Management

Treatment is designed to relax the internal anal sphincter, thereby improving local blood flow and improving healing. Forty per cent heal spontaneously, and the advent of pharmacological treatment ('chemical sphincterotomy') has led to complete reappraisal of treatment, otherwise unchanged for much of the twentieth century. Permanent incontinence occurs in a minority of surgically treated patients and the traditional 'anal stretch' should be avoided. Treatment of chronic fissures is now possible in primary care in the majority of cases. If referral is necessary, select a specialist colorectal surgeon. Lateral sphincterotomy (dividing the internal sphincter muscle by surgical incision) still has a 5 per cent risk of faecal incontinence and is best performed only after investigating anorectal physiology.

Anorectal abscess and fistula

An abscess forms following obstruction of an anal gland with resulting retrograde infection. A fistula represents the chronic phase of a perianal abscess. Recurrence is common (around 40 per cent).

Pain is the presenting symptom, sometimes associated with malaise or fever. Purulent discharge followed by rapid symptomatic relief suggests spontaneous drainage. Continuing discharge indicates a fistula. The urine should be checked for glucose and if the patient has a history of diarrhoea or other abdominal symptoms, a full blood count is appropriate: Crohn's disease will often cause anaemia or thrombocytosis.

Examination reveals a localized, tender swelling with erythema and induration. Rectal examination is extremely painful and should be avoided. The external, perianal opening of a fistula may be visible.

Management

Treatment of an abscess is immediate, adequate drainage. Antibiotics (such as metronidazole 400 mg three times daily) are often given in conjunction, but are rarely effective alone. Patients may be referred as a surgical emergency, but drainage of smaller perianal abcesses is feasible in primary care in experienced hands. The clinical distinction between perianal and ischiorectal abscess is more theoretical than practical. Uncommon intersphincteric, supralevator, or horseshoe abscesses are important to primary care only by way of recognizing that they usually indicate systemic disease such as Crohn's. Treatment is then the province of specialist colorectal surgeons.

An anorectal fistula is also treated surgically, but the variety of available procedures (eight or more) is a measure of the difficulty. Patients should be referred to a colorectal surgeon. The reason for advising specialist colorectal referral is that some of the traditional procedures (such as 'laying open the fistula') are associated with a risk of minor, but permanent, incontinence. The best chance to get treatment right is at the outset.

Bleeding

Bright red bleeding that spatters the toilet bowl or appears on the paper is the hallmark of anal canal bleeding. However, this pattern of bleeding does not preclude more serious colonic disease and if associated with frequent stools, urgency, or tenesmus, referral for further investigation is appropriate. Blood smeared on the surface of stool in the pan is unlikely to be coming from piles, since freshly shed blood disperses in water. The passage of clotted blood demands an explanation other than piles.

Haemorrhoids

Misconceptions about haemorrhoids are so widespread that any symptom attributed by a patient to 'my haemorrhoids' should be suspect until proven otherwise. The anatomy of the anal canal needs to be understood to permit rational treatment.

The anal canal is a 4-cm long tube with a highly vascular wall. Unlike anatomical drawings, the vascular anal lining *in vivo* bulges into the lumen as three (occasionally four) pads in a more or less linear array, the anal

cushions. These vascular anal cushions are protected against the shearing stress of defaecation by unique submucosal muscle and elastic tissue. The anal cushions contribute to anal closure, forming a water and air tight seal.

When the supporting structure of anal cushions is disrupted, then downward displacement occurs with consequent engorgement of the submucosal venous plexus: piles. The terms 'internal' and 'external' contribute little to management. Even the numerical classification (first degree, bleeding only; second degree, spontaneously reducing prolapse; third degree, prolapse requiring manual replacement; fourth degree, permanent prolapse) is of limited value, because the degree varies with time.

Symptoms other than bleeding and palpable prolapse are rarely attributable to uncomplicated piles. Pain with an irreducible swelling indicates thrombosis. In the absence of swelling, pain may be due to a concomitant fissure, or proctalgia. Itching is more likely to be attributable to skin sensitization from ointment used to treat often non-existent piles.

Examination can be confined to the anorectum when a careful history suggests piles and proctoscopy confirms their presence. Uncomplicated piles are impalpable. Enthusiasts advise flexible sigmoidoscopy over the age of 40, but this should be reserved for atypical bleeding patterns.

Management

Treatment of piles is most often conservative and occasionally interventional.

Referral to a colorectal surgeon for interventional treatment is appropriate if there is doubt about the diagnosis, if bleeding remains frequent in spite of conservative measures, or if prolapse is causing appreciable discomfort.

The aim is to reduce the volume of the disrupted anal cushion. Banding is generally preferrable to sclerotherapy, because it is more controllable. The general practitioner can help by starting stool softeners the day before the procedure (lactulose 20 ml twice daily, or isphagula husk) and continuing these for a week after. Advice to take regular analgesics also helps. Alternative approaches such as cryotherapy, photocoagulation, or laser therapy carry no particular advantage over simpler, more widely available techniques. Haemorrhoidectomy retains a place for piles that are too large or immobile for banding. The very painful thrombosed haemorrhoid should be treated by surgical incision and removal of the thrombus. This procedure can be performed under local anaesthesia in primary care.

Lumps and bumps

Patients sometimes present with a palpable perianal lump. In the absence of associated pain (which suggests an abscess, perianal haematoma, or infarcted pile) or bleeding (which suggests prolapsed piles), the cause is usually a skin tag or warts. Vigilance is needed to recognize the rare anal cancer.

Anogenital warts

Anogenital warts (condylomata acuminata) are caused by human papillomavirus (HPV 6 and 11). They usually represent sexually transmitted disease and one of the few cohort studies of perianal disease show that the

---

Conservative treatment of piles

- ◆ Soften the stool
- ◆ Increase dietary fibre and fluid intake
- ◆ Lactulose if stool remains hard
- ◆ Avoid prolonged straining
- ◆ Stop reading on the loo

incidence is around two per 1000 person years. It is 16-fold greater in HIV-positive individuals. Sensitive enquiry about sexual activity and practice is appropriate, with counselling and HIV testing as necessary.

The advent of topical imiquimod (5 per cent) cream, an immune modifier that promotes natural viricidal mechanisms, has transformed treatment. Ablative therapy is now rarely appropriate and self-administered imiquimod is more cost-effective than traditional podophyllin.

Anal cancer

Anal cancer is rare, being 20–30 times less common than colorectal cancer. Its importance is that it can masquerade as one of the common perianal conditions, since it presents with itchiness, pain, bleeding, or a change in bowel habit in the presence of a palpable lesion. The lesion may look like a polyp, or ulcerate like a fissure.

The message for primary care and colorectal clinics is that when there is a combination of perianal symptoms, be on your guard for uncommon causes.

The prognosis of the most common type (epidermoid cancer of the anal margin) as well as less common varieties (Bowen's and Paget's disease of the anus) is good (>80 per cent 5-year survival).

Conclusions

The initial role of the primary care physician is to explore patient expectations and misconceptions about perianal symptoms. Accurate diagnosis is possible from a careful history, rectal examination, and (sometimes) proctoscopy. The advent of non-interventional treatment for haemorrhoids, fissures, and warts means that most perianal disease can be managed effectively in primary care. This represents a substantial shift within the past decade, where surgical intervention was formerly the norm and iatrogenic incontinence after anal stretches or other procedures passed unremarked.

When advising referral, the patient's advocate is the general practitioner. Perianal conditions may be common and frequently minor, but the consequences of misdirected treatment or unrecognized disease are major. Referral to a dermatologist, colorectal surgeon, or gastroenterologist is often more appropriate than a general surgeon. Despite the prevalence of perianal disease, the paucity of population-based research into these conditions in primary care presents substantial opportunities.

Key points

- Most perianal disease can be managed effectively in primary care.
- Explore expectations and misconceptions.
- Non-interventional treatment is replacing surgery for many conditions.
- Beware combinations of perianal symptoms.
- When referring, start with specialists: simple problems become complex often through iatrogenic intervention.

Further reading

Jonas, M. and Scholefield, J.H. (2001). Anal fissure. *Gastroenterology Clinics of North America* **30**, 167–81. (Review of current treatment, illustrating the shift away from surgical intervention.)

MacRae, H.M and McLeod, R.S. (1995). Comparison of hemorrhoid treatment modalities. A meta-analysis. *Diseases of the Colon and Rectum* **38**, 687–94. (Summarizes the many trials. Different treatment are not mutually exclusive.)

Nelson, R. (2001). Operative procedures for fissure in ano (Cochrane Review). *Cochrane Database Systematic Review 3*: CD002199. (Systematic review, but already dated because the therapeutic trend is away from surgery.)

Potter, M.A. and Bartolo, D.C. (2001). Proctalgia fugax. *European Journal of Gastroenterology & Hepatology* **13**, 1289–90. (Leading article.)

Wald, A. (2001). Functional anorectal and pelvic pain. *Gastroenterology Clinics of North America* **30**, 243–51. (Review of a challenging area, often associated with frequent presentation and persistent symptoms.)

Dasan, S. et al. (1999). Treatment of persistent pruritus ani in a combined colorectal and dermatological clinic. *British Journal of Surgery* **86**, 1337–40. (Illustrates the dermatological origin of this condition.)

Conley, L.J. et al. (2002). HIV-1 infection and risk of vulvovaginal and perianal condylomata acuminata and intraepithelial neoplasia: a prospective cohort study. *Lancet* **359**, 108–13. (Recent well-controlled study of a common perianal disorder.)

Sailer, M. et al. (1998). Quality of life in patients with benign anorectal disorders. *British Journal of Surgery* **85**, 1716–19. (Analysis of 325 patients with common perianal conditions, but limited by use of historical controls.)

5

Metabolic problems

5 Metabolic problems

5.1 Obesity

Rena R. Wing and Amy A. Gorin

Obesity and overweight produce a variety of negative health consequences including increased risk of premature death. Criteria defining overweight and obesity are based on body mass index (BMI; weight divided by height; kg/m^2).[1,2] Individuals with a BMI of 18.5–24.9 are defined as normal weight, those with a BMI of 25–29.9 as overweight; and those with a BMI more than 30 as obese. The distribution of body fat affects health; abdominal fat is of greater health consequence than peripheral fat.[1]

Prevalence of obesity

The prevalence of adult obesity is increasing in both developed and developing countries across all gender, age, race, and ethnicity groups. Obesity is still relatively uncommon in Africa and Asia, but has been shown to co-exist with undernutrition (BMI < 18.5) in many developing countries. Table 1 shows the prevalence of obesity (BMI ≥ 30) in selected countries.[2]

The prevalence of overweight in children also has increased markedly over the past 40 years in both industrialized and developing countries.

Table 1 Obesity prevalence (BMI ≥30) in selected countries worldwide[a]

Country	Year	Age (years)	Prevalence (%)	
			Men	Women
Samoa (urban)	1991	25–69	58.4	76.8
Samoa (rural)	1991	25–69	41.5	59.2
US	1988–94	20–74	19.9	24.9
Saudi Arabia	1990–3	15+	16.0	24.0
Germany[b]	1990	25–69	17.0	19.0
England	1995	16–64	15.0	16.5
Canada	1986–90	18–74	15.0	15.0
Brazil	1989	25–64	5.9	13.3
Australia	1989	25–64	11.5	13.2
Finland	1991–3	20–75	14.0	11.0
Iran	1993–4	20–74	2.5	7.7
Japan	1993	20+	1.7	2.7
China	1992	20–45	1.20	1.64

[a] Data adapted from Report of a WHO Consultation titled 'Obesity: Preventing and Managing the Global Epidemic' published in Geneva, 2000.

[b] Former Federal Republic of Germany.

Although overweight children are at risk of becoming overweight adults, the most common form of obesity remains adult-onset obesity. Individuals in developed countries typically experience a gradual rise in body weight and fat over the lifespan, at least until the age of 60–65.

Causes of obesity

In simplest terms, obesity is the result of an imbalance between calories consumed and expended. Small errors in energy balance can lead to gradual weight gain. The mechanisms responsible for energy balance are not fully understood, and appear to involve the gut, adipose tissue, and brain. The discovery of leptin which is secreted by adipocytes and binds with receptors in the hypothalamus has led to increased recognition of the complexity of weight regulation.

There is a strong genetic component to obesity probably related to a variety of genes influencing energy intake and expenditure. Adoption studies and twin studies show that obesity runs in families, with a 25–40 per cent heritability.[3] Genetics also influence fat distribution, accounting for approximately 50 per cent of the individual variation. However, the dramatic increase in prevalence of obesity over the past decade clearly relates to changes in the environment, not genes. Although it is not known exactly which environmental changes are responsible, both the increasingly sedentary lifestyle, and availability of low-cost, high-fat (and high-calorie) food probably contribute.

Consequences of obesity

Overweight and obesity increase the risk of a variety of medical problems, including Type 2 diabetes, hypertension, hyperlipidaemia, coronary heart disease, stroke, osteoarthritis, sleep apnoea, gout, gallbladder disease, and cancer of the breast, prostate, and colon.[1,4] Obesity also complicates pregnancy by increasing the risk of reproductive hormone abnormalities, polycystic ovary disease, low fertility, and foetal death.

Cardiovascular disease mortality and all-cause mortality are increased in those who are overweight. In some studies, the relationship is U- or J-shaped with greater mortality in both the thinnest and heaviest individuals, whereas in other studies there is linear relationship between BMI and mortality.[4] The lowest risk of mortality appears to be in individuals with a BMI of 21–25. Health consequences relate not only to the degree of obesity, but also to fat distribution and weight gain during adulthood. Individuals who are overweight but physically active or physically fit have lower risk of mortality than those of comparable weight who are sedentary.

There are marked social consequences to overweight and obesity. Such individuals often experience discrimination; in one study, overweight adolescents were less likely to be accepted in college, to be offered employment, or to get married than their normal weight peers. Prejudice against the obese, a problem in all aspects of society, is also evidenced by health care providers. Obese individuals are less likely to receive preventive procedures such as cervical smears, due to reluctance of both patients and providers.

In addition, associated economic costs are staggering. Based on data from Australia, France, the Netherlands, and the United States, 2–7 per cent of total health care expenditure is directly attributed to overweight and obesity.[2]

Diagnosis

As noted above, the diagnosis of overweight and obesity is based primarily on BMI (kg/m^2). Independent of BMI, abdominal fat has been shown to increase the risk of Type 2 diabetes, cardiovascular disease, and mortality. In men, a waist circumference of more than 40 in (>102 cm) places the individual at high-risk of obesity-related co-morbidities, whereas in women, a waist circumference of more than 35 in (>88 cm) is of concern.[1] Pre-treatment evaluation should include family history of obesity, patterns of weight change over time, use of medications that can cause weight gain (antidepressants, antipsychotics, insulin, sulfonylureas), and other causes of obesity such as hypothyroidism.

Management of obesity in adults

The primary care physician should encourage individuals who are gaining weight and those with a family history of obesity to modify their diet and exercise habits before obesity and related co-morbidities develop. However, in one study only 6 per cent of patients with a BMI greater than 25–27 and no medical co-morbidities indicated that their physician had encouraged weight loss.

Weight loss is recommended in those with a BMI more than 30 or a BMI more than 25 plus co-morbidities.[1] An initial goal is a 10 per cent reduction in body weight, since weight loss of this magnitude improves cardiovascular risk factors and reduces the risk of developing diabetes.[5] The initial approach should combine diet, exercise, and behaviour modification.

Diet

The diet recommended for weight loss typically involves a caloric reduction of 500–1000 kcal/day from usual intake, to produce a weight loss of 1–2 lb per week.[1] Often in behavioural weight control programmes, participants who weigh less than 200 lb are encouraged to consume 1200 kcal/day, whereas those who weigh over 200 lb are encouraged to consume 1500 kcal/day. Since fat has more calories per gram (9 kcal/g) than carbohydrates or proteins (4 kcal/g), participants are often encouraged to limit their fat intake to 20–30 per cent of total calories. Low-carbohydrate/high-fat diets can produce weight loss when they lead to calorie restriction but such regimens are not recommended because of health concerns and questions regarding their long-term sustainability.

Very low calorie diets (VLCDs) (<800 kcal/day), often consumed as liquid formula, increase initial weight loss. However, even when combined with behaviour modification and ongoing contact, weight regain following VLCDs is common.[6] Use of liquid formula for one to two meals per day combined with a dinner of normal food appears to produce better long-term results.[7] Other structured diet approaches, including providing meal plans or actual food to patients, also seem to improve weight loss.

Exercise

Physical activity alone produces very minimal weight loss, but the combination of physical activity and dietary modifications appears most effective for long-term success.[8] In fact, increased physical activity is the single best predictor of long-term maintenance of weight loss, and might improve health independent of body weight.

Patients should gradually increase their calorie expenditure from physical activity, until they achieve a goal of at least 1000 kcal/week. This level can be achieved by walking 2 miles, 5 days per week. Several studies have shown that weight loss and improvements in physical fitness are comparable regardless of whether participants exercise in one long 40-min bout or in separate 10-min bouts.[9] The latter may promote better adherence.

Home-based exercise is more effective for long-term adherence and weight loss than supervised group physical activity programmes.

Behaviour modification

Behaviour modification strategies are very helpful in achieving long-term changes in diet and exercise behaviours.[10] Perhaps the most effective behaviour modification strategy is self-monitoring. Typically, patients are asked to record the number of calories and fat grams they consume and the calories they expend in physical activity or the minutes of physical activity they complete. Self-monitoring can help participants recognize small changes occurring in their diet or physical activity.

To change the cues or antecedents of overeating, behaviour therapists teach patients to remove high-calorie foods from their home, purchase low-calorie alternatives, and to look for behaviour chains by which a specific behaviour or emotion triggers maladaptive behaviour choices. Consequences or reinforcers are changed by teaching patients to praise themselves for small positive steps and to elicit support from family and friends.

Programmes combining diet, exercise, and behaviour modification

Physicians should seek programmes that combine diet, exercise, and behaviour modification, provide ongoing contact, and promote modest rates of weight loss (1–2 lb/week) with a goal of reducing weight by 10 per cent. Such programmes achieve an average 10-kg loss (10 per cent of initial weight) at 6 months and maintain a loss of 5.6 kg (60 per cent of initial loss) at 1-year follow-up.[10]

Medication

For patients with a BMI more than 30 or a BMI over 27 plus co-morbidities, weight-loss medications may be recommended in combination with diet, exercise, and behaviour therapy. In the United States, orlistat and sibutramine are the only drugs currently approved for long-term treatment of obesity;[1] mazindol, diethylpropion, phentermine, benzphetamine, and phendimetrazine are approved for only short-term use. Orlistat inhibits pancreatic lipase and thereby blocks fat absorption; approximately one-third of the fat intake is excreted through the stools. Sibutramine is a norepinephrine and serotonin reuptake inhibitor that decreases hunger and increases feelings of satiety. Both drugs have modest effects on body weight (weight losses of 4–22 lb) with most loss in the first 6 months.[1] Clinical trials have suggested that both medications also might be useful after a period of weight loss to help prevent weight regain. With orlistat, the main side-effects are oily stools and decreased absorption of fat-soluble vitamins; therefore, a multivitamin supplement is recommended. Adverse effects of sibutramine include increases in blood pressure and pulse; thus, regular monitoring of blood pressure is required. Weight loss medications must be used on a long-term basis; if these medications are stopped, patients typically regain their weight.

Weight-loss surgery

For patients with severe obesity (BMI more than 40 or over 35 plus co-morbidites) surgery might be an option. In most patients, banded gastroplasty and the Roux-en-Y gastric bypass both produce weight loss for greater than 5 years and marked improvements in obesity-related co-morbidities. The benefits of these procedures must be weighed against the risks. Bariatric surgery should be undertaken only by an experienced surgeon with support of a multidisciplinary comprehensive management programme.

Long-term management of obesity

Obesity is a chronic disease, requiring continued ongoing therapy. Longer, more intensive programmes produce better weight-loss results. Thus, it is important for patients to continue therapy through face-to-face meetings, phone calls, and/or e-mail.

Increased understanding about weight-loss maintenance has been obtained through the National Weight Control Registry, a registry of over 3000 individuals who have lost an average of 66 lb and kept it off for over 6 years.[11] Over 90 per cent of registry members maintain their weight loss through continued adherence to a low-calorie, low-fat diet, and high levels of physical activity. Seventy-five per cent report that they weigh themselves at least one time per week, with the majority weighing themselves daily.

Managing the overweight child and his/her family

Whereas in adults the goal is weight loss, in children the goal is prevention of further weight gain. Since most overweight children also have overweight parents, it is most effective to treat the child in the context of a family-based intervention. Again, the recommended approach is a combination of diet, exercise, and behaviour modification. Targeting decreased television and other sedentary activities as well as encouraging an increase in physical activity appears most effective. Epstein et al., working with children aged 8–12, have shown that an initial 8–12-week weight-control programme with monthly maintenance sessions for 12 months can effectively reduce the percentage overweight through 10 years of follow-up.[12] Thus, treating overweight children, with the goal of preventing overweight and obesity in adults, appears more effective than treating obese adults.

Key points

1. Body mass index (kg/m^2) is used to define obesity. A BMI of 18.5–24.9 is normal weight, 25–29.9 is overweight, and more than or equal to 30 is obese.

2. A waist circumference of more than 40 in in men and more than 35 in in women is associated with obesity-related co-morbidities.

3. A 10% reduction in body weight improves cardiovascular risk factors and reduces the risk for developing Type 2 diabetes.

4. Overweight individuals should be encouraged to lose weight through a combination of diet, exercise changes, and behaviour modification.

5. Medication and surgery are treatment options for obese individuals and when used, should be as an adjunct to diet, exercise, and behaviour therapy.

6. Long-term successful weight losers report continued consumption of a low-calorie, low-fat diet, high levels of physical activity, and regular body weight monitoring.

References

1. National Institutes of Health. *Clinical Guidelines on the Identification, Evaluation, and Treatment of Overweight and Obesity in Adults: The Evidence Report*. NIH Publication no. 98-4083, 1998.

2. World Health Organization. *Obesity: Preventing and Managing the Global Epidemic*. World Health Organization Report Series #894. Geneva: WHO, 2000.

3. Bouchard, C.P., Rice, T., and Rao, D.C. (1998). The genetics of obesity. In *Handbook of Obesity* (ed. G.A. Bray and W.P. James), pp. 157–90. New York: Marcel Dekker.

4. National Task Force on the Prevention and Treatment of Obesity (2000). Overweight, obesity, and health risks. *Archives of Internal Medicine* **160**, 898–904.

5. Wing, R.R., Koeske, R., Epstein, L.H., Nowalk, M.P., Gooding, W., and Becker, D. (1987). Long-term effects of modest weight loss in type 2 diabetic patients. *Archives of Internal Medicine* **147**, 1749–53.

6. National Task Force on the Prevention and Treatment of Obesity (1993). Very low-calorie diets. *Journal of the American Medical Association* **270** (8) 967–74.

7. Ditschuneit, H.H., Llechtner-Mors, M., Johnson, T.D., and Alder, G. (1999). Metabolic and weight loss effects of a long-term dietary intervention in obese patients. *American Journal of Clinical Nutrition* **69**, 198–204.

8. Wing, R.R. (1999). Physical activity in the treatment of the adulthood overweight and obesity: current evidence and research issues. *Medicine and Science in Sports and Exercise* **31**, S547–52.

9. Jakicic, J., Wing, R.R., and Wingers, C. (1999). Effects of intermittent exercise and use of home exercise equipment on adherence, weight loss, and fitness in overweight women. *Journal of the American Medical Association* **282**, 1554–60.

10. Wing, R.R. (1993). Behavioral approaches to the treatment of obesity. In *Handbook of Obesity* (ed. G. Bray, C. Bouchard, and P. James), pp. 855–73. New York: Marcel Dekker.

11. Wing, R.R. and Hill, J.O. (2001). Successful weight loss maintenance. *Annual Review of Nutrition* **21**, 323–41.

12. Epstein, L.H., Valoski, A., Wing, R.R., and McCurley, J. (1990). Ten-year follow-up of behavioral, family-based treatment for obese children. *Journal of the American Medical Association* **264**, 2519–23.

Further reading

Bray, G.A., Bouchard, C., and James, W.P.T., ed. *Handbook of Obesity*. New York: Marcel Dekker.

National Institutes of Health. *Clinical Guidelines on the Identification, Evaluation, and Treatment of Overweight and Obesity in Adults: The Evidence Report*. NIH Publication no. 98-4083, 1998.

National Task Force on the Prevention and Treatment of Obesity (2000). Overweight, obesity, and health risk. *Archives of Internal Medicine* **160**, 898–904.

World Health Organization. *Obesity: Preventing and Managing the Global Epidemic*. WHO Technical Report Series. Geneva: WHO, 2000.

Wing, R.R. and Hill, J.O. (2001). Successful weight loss maintenance. *Annual Review of Nutrition* **21**, 323–41.

5.2 Diabetes—Type 1 and Type 2

Ann Louise Kinmonth and Sean Dinneen

Introduction

Diabetes mellitus refers to a heterogeneous group of diseases characterized by raised blood glucose. Most diagnoses of diabetes are made, most routine surveillance undertaken, and most care delivered to individuals with diabetes across the world, in primary care.

The significance of hyperglycaemia lies both in the acute symptoms that trouble the sufferer, and its frequently devastating longer term consequences. These include blindness, renal failure, amputation, impotence and cardiovascular morbidity, and premature death. Diabetes is an economic scourge round the world in both developed and developing nations.

Despite microvascular complications being almost pathognomonic of the diabetic state, the majority of mortality and morbidity in diabetes is attributed to macrovascular disease. Deaths from cardiovascular disease in those with diabetes continue to rise, in contrast to overall deaths due to coronary heart disease (CHD) and stroke which have been falling steadily in developed countries.[1]

Classification

Prior to the late 1990s, the classification system for diabetes mellitus was based largely on the pharmacological therapy of the disease. Insulin-dependent diabetes mellitus (IDDM) and non-insulin-dependent diabetes mellitus (NIDDM) were the two major forms of diabetes identified. 'IDDM' patients were typically lean at presentation, prone to ketosis, and required insulin for survival. 'NIDDM' patients were typically obese at presentation, not prone to ketosis and did not require insulin for survival. This approach was problematic. Many patients with NIDDM required insulin at some point in the course of their disease and were misclassified as IDDM or had the rather confusing term 'insulin treated' NIDDM applied to them. In addition, a classification based on therapy was not always consistent with new insights into the pathogenesis of the various forms of diabetes. This led to a review of classification.[2] The main thrust was to move away from a classification based on therapy and towards one based on pathogenesis with four major categories:

1. Type 1 diabetes
    (i)   immune mediated (including latent autoimmune diabetes of adulthood—LADA),
    (ii)   idiopathic;
2. Type 2 diabetes;
3. Other specific types
    (i)   genetic defects of beta-cell function,
    (ii)   genetic defects of insulin action,
    (iii) diseases of the exocrine pancreas,
    (iv)   endocrinopathies,
    (v)   drug or chemical induced,
    (vi)   infections,
    (vii) uncommon forms of immune-mediated diabetes,
    (viii) other genetic syndromes associated with diabetes;
4. Gestational diabetes.

Type 1 diabetes

Type 1 diabetes is characterized by complete insulin deficiency. When fully developed it results, if untreated, in ketoacidosis, coma and death. The cumulative incidence is about 0.3 per cent per year and occurs throughout life with at least 50 per cent of cases presenting after childhood and adolescence.[3]

Some 90–95 per cent of children with Type 1 diabetes have HLA genotypes conferring susceptibility, but only around 5 per cent of all children with the highest risk combination will develop diabetes in childhood. Islet autoantibodies typically appear early in life, and a response involving antibodies to multiple islet antigens is highly predictive of eventual progression to diabetes.[1]

Type 2 diabetes

Type 2 diabetes is not insulin dependent but increasingly treated with insulin. Although most common after the age of 40 years, it can also present at young ages. Eighty per cent of cases of diabetes in developed countries are Type 2. It results from a combination of defects in insulin secretion and action, which vary between individuals and over time in association with progressive B-cell failure.

Other specific types

Some diabetes sub-types are now labelled according to molecular mechanism or disease associations. There is considerable interest in defining sub-types of diabetes with genetic aetiologies such as maturity onset diabetes of the young (MODY). MODY is associated with defective insulin secretion and may account for around 2 per cent of cases of Type 2 diabetes. General practitioners may occasionally encounter diabetes secondary to cystic fibrosis, or haemochromatosis. They should remember that cases of glucose intolerance can be secondary to excesses of the counter regulatory hormones, cortisol, growth hormone, glucagon, and catecholamines. Other forms of diabetes are very rare.

Gestational diabetes is defined by its onset or first recognition in pregnancy, and is associated if untreated, with macrosomia and hypoglycaemia in the neonate, and subsequent Type 2 diabetes in the mother.

The current approach to classification of hyperglycaemia is based on the epidemiologically observed risks of developing the microvascular complications of diabetes—retinopathy, neuropathy, and nephropathy.[4] This risk rises abruptly above fasting plasma glucose concentrations of 6 mmol/l. However, the relationship between hyperglycaemia and macrovascular disease is different. There is no obvious threshold of glycaemia for increased risk of CHD, with risk increasing progressively with increasing levels of blood glucose from 4 mmol/l.[5]

Current criteria

The most recently revised diagnostic criteria rely strongly on the fasting plasma glucose value, and reduce need for formal oral glucose tolerance testing (OGTT; Table 1[2]). The diagnostic fasting plasma glucose value is 7 mmol/l and the 2-h post-glucose load level is 11.1 mmol/l. It is important to have at least two 'abnormal' tests (on different occasions) before labelling asymptomatic individuals as 'diabetic'.

Practitioners should be aware of the imprecision of results including those of formal glucose tolerance testing and the many factors that can affect interpretation. These include previous diet, time of day, glucose load, and ill health. Furthermore, there remains significant individual variability in response to glucose loading on repeat testing.

Intermediate states of glucose intolerance

With the move to earlier diagnosis and surveillance of at risk groups, family doctors must also be able to interpret and advise on intermediate states of glucose intolerance. The definition of impaired glucose tolerance demands measurement of both fasting and 2-h OGTT blood glucose concentration (see Table 1). Impaired fasting glucose (IFG) is present when the fasting plasma glucose concentration is less than 7 mmol/l but greater than 6.1 mmol/l, mapping closely to the threshold for rising risk of retinopathy. These states are risk factors for both progression to diabetes and for cardiovascular disease.

Epidemiology

The prevalence of diabetes across the world is projected to double in the next decade from 100 to 215 million, largely due to Type 2 diabetes.[6] The rise in prevalence of Type 2 diabetes overall is strongly associated with obesity and global trends towards sedentary living and relative excesses in dietary energy.

Within countries, there are wide variations in prevalence of diabetes between ethnic groups. In the United Kingdom those of Asian origin have a three to six fold excess of diabetes, and African-Caribbeans a two to three fold excess compared to Anglo-Saxons.

The prevalence of diabetes rises steadily with age, reaching around 5 per cent at 65 years in the United Kingdom and up to 20 per cent in those over 85 years. The prevalence of known diabetes in residential and nursing homes can be around 10 per cent in developed countries like the United Kingdom.

Table 1 Diagnostic criteria for diabetes mellitus and other categories of hyperglycaemia

	Glucose concentration (mmol/l) (mg/dl)	
	Whole blood; capillary	Plasma; venous
Diabetes mellitus		
Fasting	≥6.1 (≥110)	≥7.0 (≥126)
or		
2-h post-glucose load or both	≥11.1 (≥200)	≥11.1 (≥200)
Impaired glucose tolerance (IGT)		
Fasting concentration (if measured) and	<6.1 (<110)	<7.0 (<126)
2-h post-glucose load	≥7.8 (≥140) and <11.1 (<200)	≥7.8 (≥140) and <11.1 (<200)
Impaired fasting glucose (IFG)		
Fasting	≥5.6 (≥100) and <6.1 (<110)	≥6.1 (≥100) and <7.0 (<126)
2-h (if measured)	<7.8 (<140)	<7.8 (<140)

Adapted from: WHO. Definition, Diagnosis and Classification of Diabetes Mellitus and its Complications: Report of a World Health Organization Collaboration. Geneva: WHO, 1999. Reference to this report should be made for whole blood venous or plasma capillary values. We show here values for the most common near-testing techniques (whole blood capillary) and laboratory assays (plasma venous).

Diabetes and its adverse consequence are linked to deprivation. The most deprived quintile in the UK population is 1.5 times more likely to have diabetes than the least deprived at any age. For those with diabetes, associated morbidity is at least three times more common in occupational class V than I.

In contradistinction to adults, the relatively low incidence of Type 1 diabetes in young children and adolescents (the average general practitioner will diagnose no more than two or three in a lifetime) can lead to missed diagnosis and poor services associated with deaths from ketoacidosis and hypoglycaemia. Type 2 diabetes although rare in childhood is being increasingly reported at younger ages mirroring the trends in physical inactivity and obesity in youth.

Health service use and disability burden

People with diabetes, especially those suffering from the macrovascular and microvascular complications, are high users of health and social services. In the United Kingdom, 9 per cent of secondary care revenue and at least 5 per cent of total health care expenditure is allocated to diabetes care across all sectors.[7] People with diabetes are admitted to hospital more frequently and remain there longer than people without diabetes; those with complications are more likely to need a carer, and to incur higher social service costs and personal expenditure than those who are complication free.

Implications

Diabetes thus presents a singular management challenge to patients, practitioners, and health services. New insights about the disorder and its optimal treatment (summarized in Table 2) have major implications for policy and practice which are reviewed below.

Table 2 New concepts in management of Type 2 diabetes and their implications for practice

Concepts		Practice
Traditional	**New**	
Diabetes is a categorical disease state due to high blood glucose	Diabetes is a syndrome or collection of diseases	All those with symptoms of diabetes should have early diagnostic testing
Acutely it causes polyuria, polydipsia, and weight loss	Hyperglycaemia represents a continuum of risk for cardiovascular disease in general as well as diabetes specific complications	All those with hyperglycaemia should be evaluated for cardiovascular risk
Long term it is associated with a range of diabetes specific complications		
Type 2 diabetes is a 'mild' disorder mainly of the elderly and often requires only symptomatic treatment	Type 2 diabetes is a serious disorder which can occur at all ages, and deteriorates over time	Diabetes should be treated intensively to minimize hyperglycaemia
	The burden of morbidity can be ameliorated by intensive treatment	It should be managed in the context of attention to all cardiovascular risk factors including smoking, hypertension, and hyperlipidaemia
Diabetes starts 'out of the blue' and cannot be prevented	Risks of diabetes can be substantially reduced by changes in health related behaviours, particularly increasing physical activity, and reducing consumption of energy rich foods, to avoid weight gain	Practitioners should challenge unhelpful traditional beliefs about diabetes in their patients and themselves
		They should model and support community based action to facilitate physical activity and healthy food choice in the population
Poor compliance with diabetes treatment is common and mainly due to ignorance or lack of will power that can be managed by information and persuasion	The burden of treatment of diabetes can outweigh the burden of the disorder in its early stages	Practitioners should learn how to move from predominantly telling patients about diabetes and the treatment they must take, to eliciting and taking account of patient ideas, concerns, and expectations regarding the treatment as well as the disease
	Apparent poor compliance may have complex explanations including structural and material barriers, socio-economic factors and beliefs about the values and consequences of treatment	Care should be organized with a view to minimizing inequities in access and structural and material barriers

Adapted with permission from: Kinmonth, A.L., Greenhalgh, P., submission to the Clarke report.

Mechanisms of hyperglycaemia

Plasma glucose concentration is determined by the rate at which glucose enters and leaves the circulation. In non-diabetic individuals, following an overnight fast, the liver is the main source of glucose production and the central nervous system is mainly responsible for glucose utilization. Rates of appearance and disappearance of glucose are precisely balanced to maintain a steady-state plasma glucose concentration of approximately 5 mmol/l. Following carbohydrate ingestion, glucose enters the circulation directly from the gut; in response to this the liver suppresses its production of glucose and insulin-sensitive tissues (mainly muscle and adipose tissue) dispose of the extra glucose through storage or metabolism. The fasting hyperglycaemia seen in patients with diabetes is a function of elevated rates of hepatic glucose production due mainly to elevated rates of gluconeogenesis. Post-prandial hyperglycaemia results from a combination of failure to adequately suppress hepatic glucose production and failure to adequately stimulate glucose uptake into insulin-sensitive tissues. Insulin is the main regulator of these metabolic processes. Defects in insulin secretion, insulin action, or both are responsible for altered metabolism.

Type 1 diabetes

Presentation

The classical presentation of Type 1 diabetes is florid with polydipsia, polyuria, and weight loss due to profound hyperglycaemia and glycosuria. The finding of ketosis or ketonuria in the presence of raised glucose is a hallmark of Type 1 diabetes and is important to look for in any newly diagnosed patient, particularly those who are lean or younger at presentation. Moderate or heavy ketonuria should alert the clinician to the probable need for early insulin therapy. Less common presentations of Type 1 diabetes include fatigue, abdominal pain, failure to thrive, and tachypnoea due to Kussmaul breathing which can be misdiagnosed as pneumonia especially in the very young.

The autoimmune predisposition can lead to other autoimmune disorders [thyroid disease, gluten-sensitive enteropathy (Coeliac disease), and Addison's disease] occurring either before or after diagnosis of diabetes. While routine screening for these disorders is not justified, a high index of suspicion should be maintained when patients with Type 1 diabetes present with unexplained symptoms.

Management

Current management of Type 1 diabetes requires daily attention to diet, exercise, self-monitoring of blood glucose, and multiple daily subcutaneous injections of insulin. The majority of patients with Type 1 diabetes use either a twice-daily mixed insulin programme or a basal/bolus programme. The former combines fast and intermediate-acting insulin either pre-mixed (using pen devices) or self-mixed (using vials and syringes). The latter combines fast-acting insulin with meals and an intermediate or long-acting insulin at night. The basal/bolus programme provides more flexibility in terms of timing and content of meals and is generally favoured in young adult patients. Patients should have a blood glucose goal range agreed with their diabetes team and should have strategies for dose adjusting their insulin to achieve this goal. The main approaches used for adjusting insulin dose are pattern recognition of self-monitoring data, and carbohydrate counting.

The Diabetes Control and Complications Trial[8] demonstrated the long-term benefits of achieving and maintaining near normal plasma glucose concentrations in terms of reducing the risk of microvascular complications. It also demonstrated the hazards of a policy of tight control, which led to a three-fold increased risk of severe hypoglycaemia. The key to getting the balance of risk versus benefit right in the individual patient is intensive education in self-management of the disease. The traditional model of the expert doctor providing advice to the non-expert patient is being replaced by a model based on the educated patient being the 'expert' in their disease and the multidisciplinary health care team providing support to the patient. Therapeutic patient education programmes[9] have demonstrated improved glycaemic control without any increase in hypoglycaemia or deterioration in quality of life. Key components of this type of programme include intensive education of patients in small groups over several days, and focusing on adaptation of the insulin programme to the individual's lifestyle rather than fitting the patient's lifestyle into their insulin programme.

Understanding Type 2 diabetes

Both insulin resistance and beta cell dysfunction are important parts of the syndrome of Type 2 diabetes, with the primary defect remaining controversial. A widely held view is that insulin resistance predominates prior to diagnosis of overt diabetes and is responsible for the transition from a state of normal to impaired glucose tolerance and eventually to overt diabetes. The UKPDS demonstrated that after diagnosis progressive loss of beta cell function occurs leading to an inexorable deterioration in glycaemic control.[10]

The conditions associated with Type 2 diabetes—obesity, dyslipidaemia, and hypertension—lead to a significantly increased risk of adverse cardiovascular outcomes. The obesity, typically abdominal, is seen in up to 80 per cent of patients at diagnosis. The dyslipidaemia is characterized by elevated triglycerides, and low levels of high-density lipoprotein (HDL) cholesterol. Type 2 diabetes has been described as a state of premature atherosclerosis with concomitant hyperglycaemia. This non-glucocentric view of the condition is very important when planning therapy since the majority of patients die from macrovascular rather than microvascular complications. While hyperglycaemia may be the key to the pathogenesis of microvascular complications, it is only one of several factors involved in the pathogenesis of macrovascular complications.

Managing Type 2 diabetes

Presentation

Unlike patients with Type 1 diabetes, those with Type 2 may have few or no symptoms at diagnosis (see Fig. 1).

The importance of lifestyle

In the majority of patients with newly diagnosed Type 2 diabetes, appropriate first-line therapy involves lifestyle modification alone. Once the patient

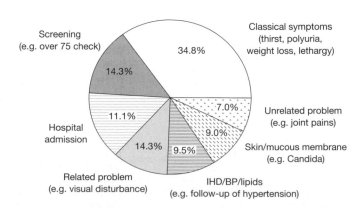

Fig. 1 Mode of presentation of Type 2 diabetes among 443 patients presenting with diabetes among 41 Hampshire practices participating in the diabetes care from diagnosis study.[11] (Published with permission from S. Griffin DM thesis, 1999.)

has an understanding of the nature of the disease and the benefits of improving metabolic control, and approaches to achieving this, the primary care team should help the patient set and achieve realistic goals for lifestyle modification. This can be assisted by review of the individual's patterns of eating, alcohol use, physical activity, and smoking. Advice is best tailored to the individual based not only on their age, cultural background, and co-morbid conditions, but also their personal motivation, social context, and ability to engage.[12] Targets set in recent trials include 150 min of additional physical activity per week (e.g. walking) five fruits and vegetables per day, and 30 per cent of calories from fat.[13] Average weight loss of 5 kg was achieved among patients in the first 3 months of the UKPDS, and while this was slowly regained over the next decade, it provided an important contribution to management.

Managing cardiovascular risk

Given that patients with Type 2 diabetes have a significant risk of cardiovascular disease,[14] many experts have argued that a policy of 'secondary prevention' is justified for all Type 2 patients. There is now strong clinical trial evidence to support widespread use of blood pressure lowering agents, lipid-lowering agents, hypoglycaemic agents, angiotensin-converting enzyme inhibitor therapy (separate from their blood pressure lowering effects), and aspirin for vascular protection in these patients.[15] Furthermore, the target levels in national guidelines for blood pressure, lipids, and glucose are becoming more rigorous (e.g. blood pressures of 130/80 mmHg, LDL cholesterol of 2.6 mmol/l, and blood glucose levels 'as close to normal as possible'[15]). This means that multiple drug therapy is usually required and it is not unusual to see patients on up to 10 different medications aimed at lowering their vascular risk (see relevant chapters on cardiovascular risk reduction.)

Managing blood glucose

Blood glucose monitoring

While the efficacy of self-monitoring of blood glucose (SMBG) in Type 2 diabetes has not been proven, many patients find it a useful adjunct to a self-management programme. The glycosylated haemoglobin or HbA1c level should be measured at intervals to guide medical management. An HbA1c level within one percentage point of the upper limit of the non-diabetic reference range can be considered to reflect reasonable glycaemic control. Values persistently greater than two percentage points above the upper limit of the reference range call for additional therapeutic action.

Use of oral agents

If after a period of 3–6 months, the blood glucose levels remain high, despite all efforts by patient and practitioner, oral hypoglycaemic therapy should be commenced. Metformin has become the first choice for monotherapy, based on results from UKPDS showing improved survival among obese patients randomized to this drug. Metformin is contraindicated in patients with renal impairment (creatinine above approximately 130 μmol/l) and in states of low tissue perfusion (such as cardiac failure) where the risk of drug-induced lactic acidosis is increased. While gastrointestinal side-effects are common on starting the drug, they can often be reduced by slow dose titration. Alternatives to metformin include members of the sulfonylurea class of insulin secretagogues and the closely related fast-acting insulin secretagogues (repaglinide and nateglinide), the thiazolidinediones (rosiglitazone and pioglitazone) and the alpha-glucosidase inhibitors, for example, acarbose. The main characteristics of these agents are outlined in Table 3. While there are many short-term studies reporting on the glucose-lowering properties of these agents few have looked at their long-term cardiovascular effects.

Progression of diabetes and introduction of insulin

As beta-cell function deteriorates over time, maintaining optimal glycaemic control requires use of multiple agents and frequently the introduction of insulin therapy. Many patients and health care providers view the need for insulin therapy in Type 2 diabetes as a negative event. Fear of self-injecting, fear of hypoglycaemia, and the stigma associated with 'severe' diabetes frequently lead to long delays before insulin therapy is commenced.

With appropriate education and follow-up patients can manage very well with the transition from tablets to insulin. Unlike Type 1 diabetes, the need for sophisticated programmes combining different types of long and short-acting insulin does not usually apply to patients with Type 2 diabetes. Instead, the amount of insulin is usually more important than the manner in which it is delivered. Patients must to be encouraged to increase their insulin dose until agreed blood glucose goals are achieved.

Weight gain is a common occurrence after initiation of insulin therapy. This phenomenon is not well understood but is partly related to the lowering of plasma glucose levels below the renal threshold with resultant conservation of calories previously lost in urine. Yki-Jarvinen et al. have looked at different ways of initiating insulin in patients with Type 2 diabetes and found that a combination of insulin and metformin was associated with better glycaemic control and less weight gain.[16] The approach termed 'bedtime insulin daytime sulphonylurea' or BIDS is popular in the United States although its efficacy compared to twice-daily insulin has not been well established.

A review of diet and exercise is very important at the time of commencement of insulin. While patients are often referred to specialist centres for initiation of insulin, there is an increasing tendency for this to happen in primary care. This can be safely done in association with training and clear protocols.

Diabetic retinopathy

Annual retinal screening is recommended from diagnosis in patients with Type 2 diabetes and from 5 years after diagnosis in patients with Type 1 diabetes. The method of screening varies widely between countries with screening undertaken mainly by ophthalmologists in the United States and by primary and secondary care physicians in the United Kingdom. The National Screening Committee in the United Kingdom has recently recommended a move towards digital retinal photography as the preferred method. A critical part of any screening programme is a robust call–recall system. The clinical stages of diabetic retinopathy are: (i) background (microaneurysms and haemmorhages); (ii) pre-proliferative (soft exudates, intraretinal microvascular anomalies, and venous beading); (iii) proliferative (neovascularization); and (iv) maculopathy (macular oedema). The extent of disease and the proximity of changes to the area of central vision should determine when patients are referred for consideration for laser photocoagulation. Marked improvement in glycaemic control reduces the progression of retinopathy over the long-term; however, for reasons that are not well understood it can be associated with an early worsening of retinopathy particularly during pregnancy. Retinal screening is therefore important ahead of any period of anticipated rapid improvement in glycaemic control.

Diabetic nephropathy

Microalbuminuria is defined as an albumin excretion rate (AER) of 20–200 μg/min (equivalent to 30–300 mg per 24 h) and represents the earliest clinical sign of diabetic nephropathy. Patients with microalbuminuria are negative to testing of urine for protein with dipsticks, and are diagnosed by measurement of albumin on a timed urine collection or a measure of the urinary albumin-to-creatinine ratio on a single sample. The presence of microalbuminuria is a risk factor for future progression to overt nephropathy (clinical grade proteinuria) and end-stage renal failure. However, more importantly, it represents a major risk indicator for future cardiovascular events, particularly in patients with Type 2 diabetes. There is increasing evidence that the ACE-inhibitor class of drugs has beneficial effects both in terms of renoprotection and also in terms of reduction in cardiovascular events in this high risk population over and above any effect on raised blood pressure alone.

Table 3 Main oral agents for the treatment of Type 2 diabetes mellitus

Class generic name	Approved daily dosage (mg)	Duration of action [(h)ours or (w)eeks]	Site of action	Mechanism of action	Effect on glucose [mmol/l (mg/dl)]	HbA1c reduction (%)	Effect on weight	Adverse effects
Sulfonylureas								
Tolbutamide	500–3000 (2500)	6–12 h	β-cell	↑Insulin secretion	↓ FPG [3.3–3.9 (60–70)] and 24-h mean glucose	1–2	↑	Hypoglycaemia, headache, dizziness, disulfiram-like reactions, hyponatraemia
Chlorpropamide	100–500	>48 h						
Tolazamide	100–1000	12–24 h						
Glipizide	2.5–40 / 5–20	12–18 h / 24 h						
Glyburide[a]	1.25–20 / 1.25–20 / 0.75–12	12–24 h / 12–24 h / 12–24 h						
Glimepiride	1–8	24 h						
Biguanides								
Metformin	500–2550	6–12 h	Liver, muscle	↓Hepatic glucose production; ↑Muscle insulin sensitivity	↓ FPG [3.3–3.9(60–70)]	1–2	↓, ↔	GI disturbances 20–30% (diarrhoea, nausea, metallic taste), lactic acidosis
Alpha-glucosidase inhibitors								
Acarbose	25–300	<4 h	Small intestine	↓ GI absorption	↓ Post-prandial increase; ↓ FPG [1.4–2 (25–36)]	0.7–1.8 (monotherapy)/ 0.2–1.4 (combination)		GI disturbances 30% (bloating, flatulence, diarrhoea)
Miglitol	150–300							
Thiazolidinediones								
Rosiglitazone	2–8	0.3–4 w	Muscle, fat, liver	↓Hepatic glucose production; ↑Muscle insulin sensitivity	↓ FPG [1.9–2.2 (35–40)] and post-prandial glucose	0.9–1.5	↑	Haemodilution oedema, required LFT monitoring
Pioglitazone	15–45	0.3–4 w						
Meglitinide analogues								
Repaglinide	1–16	2–6 h	B-cell	↑Insulin secretion	↓ FPG [3.3–3.9 (60–70)] and post-prandial glucose	1.5–1.7	↑	Hypoglycaemia, headache
Nateglinide	60–360	2–6 h						

[a] Glyburide is known as glibenclamide in Europe; other sulphonylurea agents used in Europe include gliclazide and gliquidone.

↔, no change; ↑, increase; ↓, decrease; FPG, fasting plasma glucose; Tg, triglycerides; GI, gastrointestinal.

Diabetic neuropathy

Diabetic neuropathy is most commonly seen as an asymptomatic peripheral sensorimotor neuropathy. Foot care is an essential component of primary care of diabetes. The absence of protective sensation is best demonstrated using a monofilament and is associated with an increased risk of lower extremity amputation. Appropriate education in foot care is an effective preventative and early referral of the ulcerated foot can prevent progression. Painful neuropathy can be difficult to manage. Amitriptyline and gabapentin are the most widely used agents. Other clinical manifestations include diabetic amyotrophy (which is a painful femoral neuropathy) which can be present at diagnosis of Type 2 diabetes, radiculopathy which can lead to trunk pain and be confused with cholecystitis or even myocardial infarction, and mononeuritis which most commonly leads to self-resolving diplopia. Nerve entrapment including carpal tunnel syndrome is more common in patients with diabetes than non-diabetic individuals. Autonomic neuropathy can be difficult to recognize and extremely difficult to manage. As well as postural hypotension and gastropareisis other manifestations include diabetic diarrhoea, erectile dysfunction, bladder dysfunction, and gustatory sweating. Specialist investigation and management is usually required to optimize outcomes.

Cardiovascular disease

The mechanisms for the link between chronic hyperglycaemia and accelerated atherosclerosis are not as well established as those between hyperglycaemia and microvascular complications. Many of the steps involved in atheroma formation are accelerated in patients with diabetes. Atherosclerosis is more widespread in those with than without diabetes and involves more distal parts of the vasculature. Angina and even myocardial infarction can be painless or 'silent' if associated with autonomic dysfunction. Finally, survival following vascular events is poorer for patients with diabetes than non-diabetic individuals. Beta-blockers, aspirin, ACE-inhibitors, and statins all have important roles in management of coronary artery disease in patients with diabetes and should be used unless there are clear contraindications.

Special groups and emergencies

Childhood

Type 1 diabetes in childhood is managed against the backdrop of normal growth and development. Management can be extremely demanding especially in the toddler years and requires careful monitoring of height and weight velocity to inform decisions on insulin and dietary adjustments. The primary care team is often called upon for management of intercurrent illness (see below) and psychological difficulties but overall supervision should be in a children's specialist diabetes clinic.

Adolescence

The physical, psychological, and emotional changes that occur as part of normal adolescence frequently lead to problems with diabetes management. Insulin omission and non-attendance at practice or hospital clinics are common. Eating disorders are more prevalent among young women with diabetes than non-diabetic women. Strategies for dealing with these problems include an emphasis on a non-paternalistic approach, close links with clinical psychologists (who should be seen as part of the diabetes team), and an emphasis on promoting *interdependency with* the patient's family rather than *independence from* the family.

Pregnancy

Women with Type 1 diabetes are encouraged to plan their pregnancies and to strive for near normal plasma glucose levels before conception. Supplementary folic acid beginning at least 3 months before conception is recommended to reduce the risk of neural tube defects. Antenatal care is best coordinated through a multidisciplinary team involving obstetricians, diabetologists, specialist nurses, and midwives. Increasingly, women with onset of Type 2 diabetes in the reproductive years are contemplating pregnancy. Conversion from tablets to insulin should ideally occur before conception. Tight glycaemic goals are important to reduce the risk of congenital malformations (early) and macrosomia or neonatal hypoglycaemia (later).

Elderly

The renal threshold for glucose is higher in the elderly which means that significant hyperglycaemia can occur without the typical symptoms. This, combined with multiple co-morbidities and polypharmacy makes optimal diabetes management challenging. While management targets (for glucose, BP, lipids) are frequently modified in this setting it is important not to resort to therapeutic nihilism and abandon the principles of good diabetes care.

Hyperglycaemic crises

The best treatment for diabetic ketoacidosis (DKA) is undoubtedly prevention. Patients with Type 1 diabetes must be aware of the importance of managing 'sick days' with closer monitoring of blood sugar and urine ketones, attention to adequate fluid intake, and to giving *enough* insulin to prevent metabolic de-compensation. A frequent error is omitting insulin because the patient is not eating. The primary care team can support patients in sick day management by reviewing these principles but must also know when and how to call for hospital intervention. Recurrent episodes of DKA should lead to a review of the individual's psychosocial situation.

Hypoglycaemia

The body has elaborate (counter-regulatory) mechanisms in place to respond to a fall in plasma glucose levels. Normally adrenergic responses (and symptoms) precede neuroglycopaenia. Patients and their diabetes team need to be aware of how to appropriately treat symptomatic episodes of hypoglycaemia. Fear of hypoglycaemic episodes among patients and carers, can lead to failure to achieve goal range blood sugars. A hierarchy of therapeutic options exists, from ingestion of simple carbohydrate to delivery of rapidly absorbed forms of dextrose (e.g. Hypostop) to parenteral administration of dextrose or glucagon. Frequent episodes of hypoglycaemia can lead to loss of awareness of symptoms which in turn can lead to severe hypoglycaemic episodes. Complete avoidance of hypoglycaemic episodes for several weeks or months has been shown to improve symptom awareness in these individuals.

Prevention of Type 2 diabetes, early detection and screening

Primary prevention

Given the insidious nature of Type 2 diabetes, and its long-term morbidity despite treatment, prevention is an attractive option. Strategies to increase healthy eating and physical activity decreased the incidence of Type 2 diabetes by almost 60 per cent over 3 years among high risk-volunteers with impaired glucose tolerance in the USA Diabetes Prevention Program.[13] Modelling studies suggest that such strategies also may be cost effective at a population level.

Primary care team members can contribute to population strategies through involvement in personal modeling of healthy behaviours, community action, and practice activities such as brief advice given at new patient checks. The frameworks set up for primary prevention of coronary heart disease in many countries offer another opportunity for prevention of Type 2 diabetes because of the clustering of glucose intolerance with other cardiovascular risk factors.

Early detection and screening

There is interest in screening for hyperglycaemia and intensive intervention in the progress of diabetes at an early stage. Although many of the criteria for screening are now met in relation to Type 2 diabetes, there is currently no clear justification for universal screening for diabetes. Moreover the introduction of widespread screening could swamp current resources. Currently, neither primary prevention strategies, nor good clinical management of clinically diagnosed cases are fully in place. Until primary care can optimize the treatment of blood pressure and glucose in people with known diabetes and ensure universal screening for eye disease and prompt treatment of other complications, it is unlikely that extended screening for diabetes could significantly improve outcomes.[17]

Organization of care

Most patients receive routine diabetes care in general practice, and are more likely to attend well-organized primary care clinics than hospital out patients. Worldwide, there are many examples of care integrated between primary and secondary care to meet patients' needs. However, overall care of Type 2 diabetes remains patchy and a large proportion of patients remain at greater risk than they would if their diabetes and cardiovascular status were better managed. Recent systematic reviews have established a range of organizational features at the level of the service, the practitioners and the patients, which can narrow the gap between what is known to be effective in diabetes care and what is currently provided. These features are summarized in Table 4.

At the population or district health services level, many organizations and countries have defined standards of care and mandated audit of providers against these standards. These approaches have demonstrated wide geographical variation in resource availability and service performance. In terms of organization, randomized trials have demonstrated the effectiveness of recall systems in general practice in achieving regular review of patients with Type 2 diabetes and standards of primary care as good or better than hospital outcomes on the short-term.[18] There is also good evidence to support the effectiveness of focused education of practitioners and patients in improving the provision and uptake of diabetes care, but effects on patient outcomes have not yet been reliably assessed.

The beneficial effect of a wide range of educational interventions for people with diabetes has been demonstrated in individual studies, both in hospital and primary care, and by meta-analysis. Despite considerable methodological shortcomings all forms of education produced small to moderate effects on short-term outcomes including knowledge, self-report of dietary change, and glycaemic control. Effects were smaller for didactic teaching and larger for behavioural, and experiential approaches enhancing motivation and skills in self-management.[19]

Table 4 Factors associated with better diabetes care

Health service	Agreed protocols, audit processes and IT support of district wide structured care to support effective communications and decision making Easy access to secondary care and support services, e.g. dietician, chiropody, ophthalmology, smoking cessation clinics
General practice	Up to date registers and recall for regular review with agreed criteria Inclusion of uncomplicated patients, clear referral criteria for others, e.g. with at risk foot
Practitioners	Continuing education Lead practitioner—especially trained nurse
Patients	Continuing education to support motivation and good self-management habits based on cognitive, emotional, and behavioural principles and skills acquisition

The most successful approaches to enhancing delivery of care for patients with diabetes have been complex and focused on all levels of care. For example, a centrally organized computerized database to make arrangements for follow-up, to track patient appointments, and generate reminders in combination with practitioner education is associated with better monitoring of diabetes status. The addition of a nurse to support management is associated further with improvements in metabolic control.[20]

WHO has recommended an organizational approach to diabetes care, which recognizes that what can be delivered universally to the population at primary and secondary care level will vary according to resource. It is increasingly recognized that the organization of diabetes care is as important as the technical competence of service providers in assuring proper access of care to all, and that participation of those with diabetes in the development of services offers significant opportunities for more effective patient-centred care delivery.

Key points in practice

Type 1 diabetes

- Type 1 diabetes is an autoimmune disorder associated with an absolute lack of insulin. It can present symptomatically at all ages.

- The average GP will diagnose one to three children and few adults with the condition in a lifetime, such that vigilance is required to test the urine of all those presenting with:
  - frequency of passing urine;
  - thirst (drinking at night);
  - weight loss;
  - unexplained fatigue; or
  - abdominal pain, nausea, or fast breathing (differential diagnosis of pneumonia in infants).

- Urgent referral for insulin initiation is required and emergency referral in children to avoid dehydration, ketoacidosis, coma, and death.

- Individuals and their families should be supported in self-management by an integrated specialist and generalist health care team.

- Integrated primary care supports management of intercurrent illness, comorbidity, timely referral (e.g. of the at risk foot) social support and equitable service access, including psychological support of patient and family.

- Management incorporates:
  - balancing of food choice and physical activity/inactivity with insulin type, dose, and frequency;
  - self-monitoring of blood glucose against achievable goals;
  - monitoring of glycosylated haemoglobin (HbAlc) to assess disease progression (care should be taken to avoid managing the HbAlc and not the whole patient);
  - monitoring of diabetes complications (eyes, feet, blood pressure, renal function) and other cardiovascular risk factors; and
  - early intervention to treat complications.

Type 2 diabetes

- Type 2 diabetes is a heterogeneous group of conditions associated with hyperglycaemia due to a relative lack of insulin and/or impaired insulin action.

♦ The presentation of Type 2 diabetes can be insidious and a diagnostic blood test should be considered in those presenting with: lethargy, thirst, polyuria, weight loss, blurred vision, persistent or recurrent infections, or with any evidence of complications of diabetes especially if in a high-risk group.

♦ In asymptomatic individuals, at least two diagnostic tests are required before labelling. The fasting plasma glucose diagnostic cut-off point is currently 7 mmol/l.

♦ The burden of treatment can initially well exceed the apparent burden of the disorder, and time and expertise are needed to explore the patient's ideas, concerns, and expectations about diabetes and its treatment, and to challenge them where they diverge from the known natural history, to establish informed choice.

♦ Self-management is critical and centred on:

  ▪ weight loss or avoidance of weight gain through reduction in sedentary activity and high-energy diets;

  ▪ the use of medication and insulin; and

  ▪ the overall reduction of cardiovascular risk including avoidance of smoking.

♦ Treatment is centred on tight control of blood glucose and cardiovascular risk. Hypoglycaemic therapy should be intensified to achieve blood glucose control, and insulin added as soon as necessary. Metformin is the first-line treatment for obese patients.

♦ Surveillance is centred on regular recall for

  ▪ review of glycaemia and cardiovascular risk profile; and

  ▪ early detection and treatment of microvascular and macrovascular complications.

References

1. Williams, R., Wareham, N., Kinmonth, A.L., and Herman, W. *The Evidence Base of Diabetes Care.* New York: Wiley, 2002.

2. World Health Organization. *Definition, Diagnosis and Classification of Diabetes Mellitus and its Complications.* Report of a World Health Organization Collaboration. Geneva: WHO, 1999.

3. Onkamo, P., Vaananen, S., Karvonen, M., and Tuomilehto, J. (1999). Worldwide increase in incidence of Type 1 diabetes—the analysis of the data on published incidence trends. *Diabetologia* **42**, 1395–403.

4. McCance, D.R., Hanson, R.L., Charles, M.A., Jacobsson, L.T.H., Pettitt, D.J., Bennett, P.H., and Knowler, W.C. (1994). Comparison of tests for glycated haemoglobin and fasting and two hour plasma glucose concentrations as diagnostic methods for diabetes. *British Medical Journal* **308**, 1323–8.

5. Coutinho, M., Wang, Y., Gerstein, H.C., and Yusuf, S. (1999). The relationship between glucose and incident cardiovascular events. *Diabetes Care* **22** (2), 233–40.

6. Amos, A.F., McCarty, D.J., and Zimmet, P. (1997). The rising global burden of diabetes and its complications, estimates and projections to the year 2010. *Diabetic Medicine* **14** (5), 1–85.

7. Currie, C.J. et al. (1997). NHS acute sector expenditure of diabetes: the present, the future and excess inpatient cost of care. *Diabetic Medicine* **14**, 686–92.

8. The DCCT Research Group (1993). The effect of intensive diabetes treatment on the development and progression of long-term complications in insulin-dependent diabetes mellitus. The Diabetes Control and Complications Trial. *New England Journal of Medicine* **329**, 977–86.

9. Therapeutic Patient Education. Report of a WHO study group. Geneva: World Health Organization, 1998.

10. UKPDS (33) (1998). Intensive blood-glucose control with sulphonylureas or insulin compared with conventional treatment and risk of complications in patients with Type 2 diabetes. *Lancet* **352**, 837–53.

11. Kinmonth, A.L., Woodcock, A., Griffin, S., Spiegal, N., and Campbell, M.J. (1998). Randomised controlled trial of patient centred care of diabetes in general practice: impact on current well-being and future disease risk. The Diabetes Care from Diagnosis Research Team. *British Medical Journal* **317**, 1202–8.

12. Rollnick, S., Mason, P., and Butler, C. *Health Behaviour Change.* London: Churchill Livingston, 1999.

13. Diabetes Prevention Program Research Group (2002). Reduction in the incidence of Type 2 diabetes with lifestyle intervention or metformin. *New England Journal of Medicine* **346** (6), 393–402.

14. Stamler, J., Vaccaro, O., Neaton, J.D., and Wentworth, D. (1993). Diabetes, other risk factors, and 12-year cardiovascular mortality for men screened in the multiple risk factor intervention trial. *Diabetes Care* **16**, 434–44.

15. American Diabetes Association (2002). Clinical practice recommendations. *Diabetes Care* **25** (Suppl. 1), S1–147.

16. Yki-Jarvinen, H., Ryysy, L., Nikkila, K., Tulokas, T., and Heikkila, M. (1999). Comparison of bedtime insulin regimens in patients with Type 2 diabetes mellitus. A randomised, controlled trial. *Annals of Internal Medicine* **130**, 389–96.

17. Wareham, N.J. and Griffin, S.J. (2001). Should we screen for Type 2 diabetes? Evaluation against the National Screening Committee criteria. *British Medical Journal* **322**, 968.

18. Griffin, S. and Kinmonth, A.L. (2002). Systems for routine surveillance for people with diabetes; from the Cochrane Library Issue 4. Oxford: Update Software Ltd.

19. Griffin, S.J., Kinmonth, A.L., Skinner, C., and Kelly, J. *Educational and Psychosocial Interventions for Adults with Diabetes.* London: British Diabetic Association, 1999.

20. Renders, C.M., Valk, G.D., Griffin, S.J., Wagner, E.H., Eijk, J.V., and Assendelft, W.J.J. (2002). Interventions to improve the management of diabetes mellitus in primary care, outpatient and community settings; from the Cochrane Library, Issue 4. Oxford: Update Software Ltd.

5.3 Insulin resistance/ syndrome X

Gerald M. Reaven

Introduction

This chapter summarizes the abnormalities associated with insulin resistance, differentiates the effects of insulin resistance from those due to compensatory hyperinsulinaemia, and describes an approach to the diagnosis and treatment of syndrome X.

Consequences of insulin resistance

Insulin-mediated glucose disposal varies widely in apparently healthy humans. When insulin-resistant individuals cannot secrete enough insulin to maintain glucose regulation, Type 2 diabetes supervenes. However, the ability of hyperinsulinaemia to prevent decompensation of glucose tolerance is a mixed blessing. Individuals that are insulin resistant and hyperinsulinaemic are more likely to be hypertensive and have a dyslipidaemia characterized by a high plasma triglyceride (TG) and low high-density lipoprotein (HDL) cholesterol concentration. These changes increase risk of coronary heart disease (CHD), and in 1988[1] these relationships were explicitly addressed and designated as comprising a syndrome (X). Since then, several other abnormalities have been shown to be related to insulin resistance and/or compensatory hyperinsulinaemia and CHD (Table 1). For example, the dyslipidaemia associated with syndrome X also includes the appearance of smaller, denser low-density lipoprotein (LDL) particles and enhanced post-prandial lipaemia; both have been identified as increasing risk of CHD.[2,3] The well-known association between uric acid concentration and CHD is linked via insulin resistance/compensatory hyperinsulinaemia.[4] Insulin resistance/compensatory hyperinsulinaemia are also associated with a procoagulant state, characterized by increased plasminogen activator inhibitor-1 and fibrinogen.[5] Sympathetic nervous system activity appears to be increased in insulin-resistant, hyperinsulinaemic individuals[6] and this might help explain why approximately 50 per cent of patients with essential hypertension are insulin resistant/hyperinsulinaemic.[7] The ability of insulin to decrease urinary sodium excretion almost certainly contributes to the risk of hypertension in insulin-resistant/hyperinsulinaemic individuals, and explains why these subjects tend to be salt-sensitive.[8] Finally, polycystic ovary syndrome (PCOS), the most common endocrine abnormality in premenopausal women, appears to be secondary to insulin resistance and compensatory hyperinsulinaemia.[9] Although there is evidence that variations in insulin action are under genetic regulation, probably as much as 50 per cent of the variability in insulin-mediated glucose disposal within a population of normal volunteers is secondary to difference in lifestyle.[10] In this context, obesity and decreased physical activity play particularly crucial roles, each contributing approximately equally to the variability in insulin-mediated glucose disposal. Finally, powerful ethnic differences exist, with essentially every other ethnic group being more insulin resistant than individuals of European ancestry.

Insulin resistance versus compensatory hyperinsulinaemia

Insulin resistance, per se, is necessary for the components of syndrome X to develop, but many of its manifestations are the result of the compensatory hyperinsulinaemia acting on normally insulin-sensitive tissues. For example, the compensatory hyperinsulinaemia associated with muscle insulin resistance acts on a normally insulin sensitive kidney to increase sodium re-absorption and decrease uric acid clearance; contributing to the hypertension and increase in plasma uric acid concentration seen in patients with syndrome X. Another example, is polycystic ovary syndrome, in which the compensatory hyperinsulinaemia, associated with muscle insulin resistance, acts on an ovary, that may even be hypersensitive to insulin stimulation, to secrete increased amounts of testosterone. The most important example of this combination of insulin resistance and insulin sensitive tissues in the same individual involves the dyslipidaemia of syndrome X. Muscle and adipose tissue insulin resistance lead to day-long circulating elevations of free fatty acid (FFA) and insulin concentrations, and these changes stimulate hepatic TG synthesis and very low density lipoprotein—TG secretion, leading to hypertriglyceridaemia.[11] Once the plasma TG concentration increases, there will be enhanced post-prandial lipemia, smaller and denser LDL particles, and a decrease in HDL cholesterol concentration.[12] Thus, the development of many of the manifestations of syndrome X are dependent upon the interaction between insulin resistant muscle and adipose tissue, compensatory hyperinsulinaemia, and action of the elevated insulin levels on insulin-sensitive tissues.

Diagnosis and treatment of syndrome X

Diagnosis

Although hyperinsulinaemia/compensatory hyperinsulinaemia are the basic abnormalities leading to the manifestations of syndrome X, their measurement is not the simplest approach to the diagnosis. Direct estimates of insulin resistance are not practical, and there is no standard for classifying an individual as being hyperinsulinaemic, or relating a given insulin concentration to a clinical outcome. It is simpler to see whether or not the manifestations of syndrome X are present. For this purpose, measurement of: (i) plasma glucose concentrations (fasting and 120 min after a 75 g glucose challenge); (ii) lipoprotein concentrations; and (iii) blood pressure provide an effective and economical way to search for syndrome X. If all of these values are normal, it is highly unlikely that the individual is either insulin resistant or hyperinsulinaemic. On the other hand, Table 2 presents values that make it quite likely that insulin resistance and compensatory hyperinsulinaemia exist.

Treatment

The only specific treatment of insulin resistance currently available in patients with syndrome X is to change lifestyle. More specifically, changes in both diet and level of physical activity can substantially improve the manifestations of syndrome X. In this section, the principles of therapeutic approaches to both of these issues will be briefly summarized, but a more detailed description, and one appropriate for patient use, is provided at the end of the reference list.

If an overweight person is insulin resistant, weight loss of 10–15 lb will be associated with improved insulin sensitivity, lower day-long insulin

Table 1 Manifestations of syndrome X

Dysglycaemia
±Oral glucose tolerance
Impaired glucose tolerance

Dyslipidaemia
↑ Plasma triglyceride
↓ HDL cholesterol
↑ Post-prandial lipaemia
↓ LDL-particle diameter

Uric acid metabolism
↑ Plasma, uric acid
↓ Renal uric acid clearance

Haemodynamic
↑ Sympathetic nervous system activity
↑ Renal sodium retention
↑ Blood pressure

Procoagulant
↑ Plasminogen activator-1
↑ Fibrinogen

Reproductive
Polycystic ovary syndrome

Table 2 Laboratory values indicative of insulin resistance

Variable	Value
Fasting glucose concentration	>110 <126 mmol/l[a]
Post-challenge glucose concentration	>160 <200 mmol/l[b]
Fasting triglyceride concentration	>175 mmol/l
Fasting HDL cholesterol concentration	<40 mmol/l

[a] A value >126 mmol/l is diagnostic of diabetes.

[b] A value >200 mmol/l is diagnostic of diabetes.

concentrations, and attenuation of other manifestations of syndrome X.[13] Aerobic exercise for ~30 min, three to four times per week, will also enhance insulin sensitivity. Although the benefits of these two approaches to improving insulin sensitivity have not been directly compared, they appear to be reasonably similar in terms of efficacy. However, they differ in one important aspect. The metabolic benefits of weight loss will persist for as long as weight is maintained. In contrast, the ability of aerobic exercise to enhance insulin sensitivity is relatively evanescent, and will dissipate quickly if the exercise programme is not continued. Not all insulin-resistant individuals are willing and/or able to exercise to the degree necessary to improve insulin sensitivity, and the dangers of inappropriate exercise programmes must be appreciated. Finally, although more moderate increases in level of physical activity might not significantly enhance insulin-mediated glucose disposal, such efforts are quite useful in weight loss programmes, as well as in helping to maintain normal body weight.

Despite popular claims to the contrary, variations in macronutrient content of the diet will neither affect the ability to lose weight, nor insulin sensitivity. On the other hand, changes in the macronutrient content of the diet are very important in the treatment of syndrome X.[14] Replacement of saturated fat (SF) with carbohydrate (CHO) will lower LDL cholesterol concentrations, but the more CHO in an isocaloric diet, the more insulin secretion will be stimulated. Thus, low-SF–high-CHO diets will accentuate hyperinsulinaemia in patients with syndrome X, increasing plasma TG concentrations and day long accumulation of remnant lipoproteins. In addition, HDL cholesterol concentrations will decrease further as will LDL particle diameter. If SF is replaced with monounsaturated (MUF) and polyunsaturated fat (PUF), LDL cholesterol concentration will decrease as much as with low-SF–high-CHO diets, without untoward effects on manifestations of syndrome X. Thus, weight maintenance diets containing (as per cent of total calories) 15 per cent protein, 40 per cent fat (<10 per cent SF, ~20 per cent MUF, and the rest as PUF), and 45 per cent CHO will be safe and beneficial for individuals with a high LDL cholesterol, or syndrome X, or both.

There are no drugs currently approved for treating insulin resistance in non-diabetics. Although thiazolidinedione compounds appear to work by enhancing insulin sensitivity, they are only approved for the treatment of Type 2 diabetes. Furthermore, there is little evidence that they would reduce CHD risk in patients with syndrome X. In the absence of specific pharmacological treatment of insulin resistance, drug treatment should focus on the manifestations of syndrome X. For example, high TG and low HDL cholesterol concentrations are characteristic of syndrome X, and there is evidence that the use of fibric acid derivatives can reduce CHD in individuals with these findings.[15] Approximately 50 per cent of patients with hypertension have one or more of the components of syndrome X, and attention should be given to avoid the use of antihypertensive agents that will accentuate insulin resistance and/or its manifestations. However, it should be noted that low-dose thiazide diuretics (12.5 mg of hydrochlorthiazide) are effective in lowering blood pressure, without untoward side-effects on glucose or lipid metabolism, and that use of B-receptor antagonists is certainly indicated in patients with a history of prior myocardial infarction. Finally, a high LDL cholesterol concentration is not part of syndrome X, but patients can have combined dyslipidaemia (a high TG and low HDL concentration *plus* a high LDL cholesterol concentration). Such individuals are most at risk for CHD, and the use of HMG CoA reductase inhibitors considered if diet alone does not control LDL cholesterol concentrations in patients with syndrome X.

Conclusions

Insulin-stimulated glucose uptake varies widely from person to person. In an effort to maintain ambient plasma glucose concentration between ~80 and 140 mmol/l, the pancreatic β-cell will attempt to secrete the amount of insulin required to accomplish this goal. The more insulin resistant an individual, the greater must be the degree of compensatory hyperinsulinaemia. If the β-cell cannot sustain this philanthropic effort, Type 2 diabetes ensues. Although compensatory hyperinsulinaemia may prevent Type 2 diabetes in insulin-resistant individuals, the combination of insulin resistance and compensatory hyperinsulinaemia greatly increases the risk of developing one or more of the cluster of abnormalities that make up syndrome X. All of the various facets of syndrome X are involved to a substantial degree in the cause and clinical course of CHD. Consequently, it seems reasonable to suggest that resistance to insulin-mediated glucose disposal, and the response to this defect, play major roles in the pathogenesis and clinical course of what are often referred to as diseases of Western civilization.

Key points

1. Insulin-mediated glucose disposal varies ~10-fold in apparently healthy individuals.

2. Approximately 50% of the variability in insulin action is related to differences in lifestyle.

3. Insulin resistance, compensatory hyperinsulinaemia, and associated abnormalities are major coronary heart disease risk factors.

4. Weight loss in insulin-resistant, overweight individuals will improve the manifestations of syndrome X.

5. Low-fat–high-carbohydrate accentuate the manifestations of syndrome X.

References

1. **Reaven, G.M.** (1998). Role of insulin resistance in human disease. *Diabetes* **37**, 1595–607.

2. **Reaven, G.M., Chen, Y.-D.I., Jeppesen, J., Maheux, P., and Krauss, R.M.** (1993). Insulin resistance and hyperinsulinemia in individuals with small, dense, low density lipoprotein particles. *Journal of Clinical Investigations* **92**, 141–6.

3. **Abbasi, F., McLaughlin, T., Lamendola, C., Yeni-Komshian, H., Tanaka, A., Wang, T., Nakjima, K., and Reaven, G.M.** (1999). Fasting remnant lipoprotein cholesterol and triglyceride concentrations are elevated in nondiabetic, insulin-resistant, female volunteers. *Journal of Clinical Endocrinology and Metabolism* **84**, 3903–6.

4. **Facchini, F., Chen, Y.-D.I., Hollenbeck, C., and Reaven, G.M.** (1991). Relationship between resistance to insulin-mediated glucose uptake, urinary uric acid clearance, and plasma uric acid concentration. *Journal of the American Medical Association* **266**, 3008–11.

5. **Meigs, J.B., Mittleman, M.A., Nathan, D.M., Tofler, G.H., Singer, D.E., Murphy-Sheehy, P.M., Lipinska, I., D'Angostino, R.B., and Wilson, P.W.F.** (2000). Hyperinsulinemia, hyperglycemia and impaired hemostasis. The Framingham Offspring Study. *Journal of the American Medical Association* **283**, 221–8.

6. **Facchini, F.S., Riccardo, A., Stoohs, A., and Reaven, G.M.** (1996). Enhanced sympathetic nervous system activity—the lynchpin between insulin resistance, hyperinsulinemia, and heart rate. *American Journal of Hypertension* **9**, 1013–17.

7. **Zavaroni, I., Mazza, S., Dall'Aglio, E., Gasparini, P., Passeri, M., and Reaven, G.M.** (1992). Prevalence of hyperinsulinaemia in patients with high blood pressure. *Journal of Internal Medicine* **231**, 235–40.

8. **Facchini, F.S., DoNascimento, C., Reaven, G.M., Yip, J.W., Ni, P.X., and Humphreys, M.H.** (1999). Blood pressure, sodium intake, insulin resistance, and urinary nitrate excretion. *Hypertension* **33**, 1008–12.

9. **Dunaif, A.** (1997). Insulin resistance and the polycystic ovary syndrome: mechanism and implication for pathogenesis. *Endocrine Review* **18**, 774–800.

10. Bogardus, C., Lillioja, S., Mott, D.M., Hollenbeck, C., and Reaven, G.M. (1985). Relationship between degree of obesity and *in vivo* insulin action in man. *American Journal of Physiology* **248**, E286–91.

11. Reaven, G.M. and Greenfield, M.S. (1981). Diabetic hypertriglyceridemia: evidence for three clinical syndromes. *Diabetes* **30** (Suppl. 2), 66–75.

12. Reaven, G.M. (2001). Insulin resistance, compensatory hyperinsulinemia, and coronary heart disease: syndrome X revisited. In *Handbook of Physiology* Section 7, The Endocrine System, Vol. II, The Endocrine Pancreas and Regulation of Metabolism (ed. L.S. Jefferson and A.D. Cherrington), pp. 1169–97. Oxford: Oxford University Press.

13. McLaughlin, T., Abbasi, F., Kim, H.-S., Lamendola, C., Schaaf, P., and Reaven, G.M. (2001). Relationship between insulin resistance, weight loss, and coronary heart disease risk in healthy, obese women. *Metabolism* **50**, 795–800.

14. Reaven, G.M. (1997). Do high carbohydrate diets prevent the development or attenuate the manifestations (or both) of syndrome X? A viewpoint strongly against. *Current Opinion in Lipidology* **8**, 23–7.

15. Faergeman, O. (2000). Hypertriglyceridemia and the fibrate trials. *Current Opinion in Lipidology* **11**, 609–14.

Further reading

Reaven, G.M. (1998). Role of insulin resistance in human disease. *Diabetes* **37**, 1595–607.

Bogardus, C., Lillioja, S., Mott, D.M., Hollenbeck, C., and Reaven, G.M. (1985). Relationship between degree of obesity and *in vivo* insulin action in man. *American Journal of Physiology* **248** (Endocrinol. Metab. 11), E286–91.

Reaven, G.M. (2001). Insulin resistance, compensatory hyperinsulinemia, and coronary heart disease: syndrome X revisited. In *Handbook of Physiology* Section 7, The Endocrine System, Vol. II, The Endocrine Pancreas and Regulation of Metabolism (ed. L.S. Jefferson and A.D. Cherrington), pp. 1169–97. Oxford: Oxford University Press.

Reaven, G.M. (1997). Do high carbohydrate diets prevent the development or attenuate the manifestations (or both) of syndrome X? A viewpoint strongly against. *Current Opinion in Lipidology* **8**, 23–7.

Reaven, G., Strom, T.K., and Fox, B. *Syndrome X, the Silent Killer: The New Heart Disease Risk.* New York: A Firestone Book, Published by Simon and Schuster, 2000.

5.4 Hyperuricaemia

Martin Underwood

Epidemiology

Urate is the final breakdown product of purine metabolism. The balance between purine intake/synthesis and urate excretion determines serum urate (Fig. 1). Most idiopathic hyperuricaemia (70–90 per cent) is caused by a polygenetically determined reduced renal urate excretion.[1]

Hyperuricaemia is associated with obesity, diabetes, cardiovascular problems, dyslipidaemia, and hypertension, but is probably not an independent cardiovascular risk factor. These are all features of syndrome X/ insulin resistance (Chapter 5.3).[1,2]

Environmental and genetic factors affect population serum urate:[2–4]

♦ in the United Kingdom, gout is commoner in relatively prosperous areas;

♦ in black South Africans, gout is commoner in urban compared to rural areas; and

♦ gout is nearly twice as common in black American doctors as their white colleagues.

Serum urate is considered abnormal when it is more than two standard deviations above the population mean. Typically, in the United Kingdom and United States, this is a serum urate of 0.42 mmol/l for men and 0.36 mmol/l for women. Children and pre-menopausal women have lower urate levels than adult men and post-menopausal women. Symptoms are rare when the serum urate is less than 0.42 mmol/l. In men with a urate of 0.42–0.47 mmol/l the annual incidence of gout is 0.41 per cent, this rises to 4.31 per cent when serum urate is 0.45–0.59 mmol/l.[1,3]

Primary care workload

Hyperuricaemia's main presentations are gout and urolithiasis (see Chapter 13.7).

Nearly 1 per cent of the English population have been diagnosed as having gout, 85 per cent of these are male. Five per cent of men and 1 per cent of women aged over 65 have been affected.[5] A 'typical' UK general practitioner with 1700 patients conducts 12 consultations for gout annually.[6] Population factors including age, prevalence of obesity, alcohol intake, and relative prosperity affect prevalence and consultation rates.

Several rare inborn errors of purine metabolism, for example, Lesch–Nyhan syndrome, present with multiple problems in addition to hyperuricaemia.[3]

Diagnosis

Gout typically presents as an acute monoarthritis of rapid onset, most commonly the first metatarsal phalangeal joint. Demonstrating urate crystals in joint fluid is sometimes helpful in confirming gout. Large crystal deposits (tophi) may develop asymmetrically, around hands, feet, elbows and ears. These can be confused with osteoarthritis of the distal interphalangeal joints.[7]

A raised serum urate is diagnostic of hyperuricaemia but not of gout:

♦ Serum urate often falls during an attack of gout; it is normal in 40 per cent of acute cases.[8]

♦ There is no evidence to support routine screening in symptom free individuals.

♦ Assess patients with hyperuricaemia for possible causes and associated conditions (Fig. 1 and Table 1).

Management

Prevention

♦ Routine prevention is not usually indicated.

♦ Patients treated for myelo/lymphoproliferative disorders usually receive prophylactic allopurinol.

Asymptomatic hyperuricaemia

♦ Few people with asymptomatic hyperuricaemia require treatment.[1]

♦ Manage secondary hyperuricaemia, or associated conditions, as appropriate.

♦ If serum urate is more than 0.8 mmol/l *and* urinary uric acid excretion is very high (>7.2 mmol/24 h) consider using allopurinol to prevent renal stone disease.[1,3]

♦ Advise on obesity and alcohol intake.

Acute gout

♦ Resting affected joint(s) and cold applications are of some benefit.[8]

♦ Drug treatment should be started as soon as possible.[1,8]

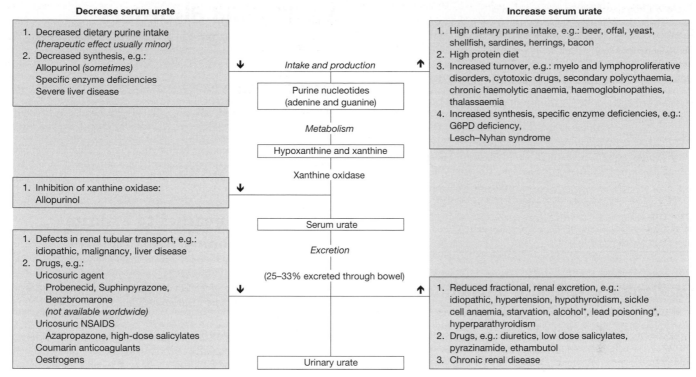

Fig. 1 Summary of urate metabolism.

Table 1 Suggested assessment of patients with hyperuricaemia

Clinical
Obesity
Blood pressure
Alcohol intake
Medication:
    Cytotoxics, diuretics, ethambutol, pyrazinamide,
    low-dose salicylates
Myelo/lymphoproliferative disorders

Laboratory
Renal function
Liver enzymes
Blood sugar
Full blood count
Erythrocyte sedimentation rate/plasma viscosity
Fasting lipids
Thyroid function[a]
Urinary urate excretion (consider if urate >8 mmol/l)[b]

[a] Up to 15–20% of patients with gout may be hypothyroid.[1]

[b] Some authorities advocate measuring before using uricosurics.[7]

♦ Both oral colchicine and non-steroidal anti-inflammatory drugs (NSAIDs), are effective. Physician preferences vary internationally.[8]

♦ Intravenous colchicine has a high incidence of serious, sometimes fatal, side-effects and should not be used.[7]

♦ Indomethacin is commonly recommended[8] but other NSAIDs are effective.[7] COX-2 inhibitors have not been assessed.[8]

♦ Intra-articular steroids are effective if one or two large joints are affected.[1]

♦ Parenteral ACTH and triamcinolone are effective, there are no data on the effectiveness of oral steroids.[1,7,8]

Symptomatic hyperuricaemia

Prophylactic treatment is not always needed. For patients with two or more attacks of gout annually, prophylaxis appears cost-effective.[1,7] In the United Kingdom, half of those with gout take regular medication.[5] A low purine diet may reduce serum urate by 0.6 mmol/l but compliance is poor.

Urate-lowering drugs may reduce incidence of acute gout by two-thirds.[8] Consider prescribing if:

♦ following review of medication serum urate levels remain high, or initial serum urate levels are very high, or the patient wants prophylactic treatment;

♦ bone or cartilage damage, gouty tophi, significant renal disease or urate stones are present.

Urate-lowering drugs

Both allopurinol and uricosurics reduce serum urate (Table 2). Allopurinol is widely used and has fewer side-effects than uricosurics. Uricosurics are contra-indicated in presence of uric acid stones or renal impairment.[1,7] The dose should be titrated according to response. Regular NSAIDs or prophylactic doses of colchicine can be used as alternatives to prevent attacks of gout.[7] Some studies suggest that benzbromarone, a uricosuric, is more effective than allopurinol at reducing serum urate. Allopurinol may be more effective than uricosurics at reducing frequency of attacks of gout.[8]

♦ Treatment with allopurinol precipitates gout in a quarter of patients.[1] Usual doses of an NSAID or prophylactic doses of colchicine (0.5 mg twice daily) for 2–3 months reduce this.

♦ A serum urate less than 0.36 mmol/l reduces crystal formation and acute attacks of gout.[8]

Table 2 Drug treatment of hyperuricaemia

Drugs	Dose
Xanthine oxidase inhibitor	
Allopurinol	100–900 mg/day
	Usual starting dose 300 mg/day
	If renal insufficiency or in older patients start on 100 mg/day
Uricosuric drugs	
A good fluid intake is required Benzbromarone	50–200 mg/day
Not available worldwide	
Sulphinpyrazone	Initial dose 100–200 mg/day. Over 2–3 weeks increase to 600 mg. Maintenance dose often 200 mg/day
Uricosuric NSAIDs	
Azopropazone or high-dose aspirin reduce serum urate	
Side-effects are common	

Continuing care/health promotion

- Monitor renal function, serum urate and blood pressure annually.
- Assess cardiovascular risk.

Key points

1. Hyperuricaemia is due to combination of genetic and environmental factors.

2. Hyperuricaemia is associated with an increased risk of cardiovascular disease.

3. Main clinical presentations are gout and urate renal stone disease.

4. Asymptomatic hyperuricaemia does not usually require treatment.

5. Treatment for acute gout is more effective if started early in the attack.

6. Allopurinol and uricosurics may precipitate acute gout. Co-prescribe an NSAID or colchicine.

References

1. **McGill, N.W.** (2000). Gout and other crystal-associated arthropathies. *Ballière's Clinical Rheumatology* **14**, 445–60. (Overview of gout and its differential diagnoses.)

2. **Wise, C.M. and Agudelo, C.A.** (1996). Gouty arthritis and uric acid metabolism. *Current Opinion in Rheumatology* **8**, 248–54.

3. **Nuki, G.** (1996). Disorders of purine and pyrimidine metabolism. In *Oxford Textbook of Medicine* 3rd edn. (ed. D.J. Weatherall, J.G.G. Ledingham, and D.A. Warrell), pp.1376–88. Oxford: Oxford University Press.

4. **Stewart, O.J. and Silman, A.J.** (1990). Review of UK data on the rheumatic diseases: 4. Gout. *British Journal of Rheumatology* **29**, 485–8.

5. **Harris, C.M., Lloyd, C.E., and Lewis, J.** (1995). The prevalence and prophylaxis of gout in England. *Journal of Clinical Epidemiology* **48**, 1153–8.

6. **McCormick, A., Fleming, D., and Charlton, J.** *Morbidity Statistics from General Practice. Fourth National Study 1991–1992.* MB5. London: HMSO, 1995.

7. **Emmerson, B.T.** (1996). The management of gout. *New England Journal of Medicine* **334**, 445–51. (Authoritative review of treatment.)

8. **Schlesinger, N., Baker, D.G., and Schumacher, H.R.** (1999). How well have diagnostic tests and therapies for gout been evaluated? *Current Opinion in Rheumatology* **11**, 441–5. (Structured review of diagnosis and treatment of gout.)

5.5 Thyroid disorders

Victor J. Pop

Introduction

Although thyroid disorders are very common and have enormous impact on quality of life, the diagnosis of thyroid disease is frequently missed. However, with modern, inexpensive highly sensitive and specific diagnostic tests it is simple to diagnose and treat thyroid disease. This chapter reviews normal thyroid function, thyroid diagnostic tests available to the GP, disorders of *function*, and disorders of *size* of the thyroid.

Diagnostic approaches to evaluate thyroid functioning

Clinical history

The signs and symptoms of thyroid dysfunction are rather non-specific—see the hyper- and hypothyroid sections below.

Physical examination

Inspection/palpation of the neck may reveal an enlarged thyroid or goitre. This may or may not be as visible when the neck is in the normal position, and the swelling moves upwards when the patient swallows. A single nodule, or multiple nodules can be palpable. Tenderness, usually due to inflammation, during palpation might contribute to the differential diagnosis.

Eye symptoms varying from eyelid symptoms to distinct exophthalmos are typical of Graves' disease. Hyperthyroidism is suggested by a tremor, warm and moist skin, tachycardia, or atrial fibrillation. Hypothyroidism is suggested by dry skin, hoarseness, myxoedema, and bradycardia.

Laboratory assessments

Biochemical tests include thyroid stimulating hormone (TSH) and free T4 (f T4) rather than total T4, the latter being influenced by the amount of circulating binding proteins (altered by oral contraceptives and other drugs) and immunological tests (thyroid antibodies) especially thyroid peroxidase antibody (TPO-Ab).

Advanced diagnostic tests

Ultrasound imaging (USI) is a non-invasive, highly sensitive method for the differential diagnosis of the causes of hyperthyroidism. Besides the morphology of the thyroid (diffuse enlarged, uni- or multinodular or cystic), the echogenicity (hypo-, normo-, or hyperechogenic) might contribute to the diagnosis. Thyroid radionuclide imaging (RNI) or scintigraphy helps to differentiate between several causes of hyperthyroidism and the functional aspects of an adenoma ('hot' versus 'cold' nodule). Fine needle biopsy is a crucial—and in experienced hands highly sensitive—test to discriminate benign from malignant nodules.

Thyroid function disorders

The definition of thyroid function disorders is based on simple biochemical criteria. The four main categories are clinical hyper- and hypothyroidism and sub-clinical hyper- and hypothyroidism (Table 1).

The terms hyper- or hypothyroidism refer to the finding of too much or little TSH in serum in combination with too little or too much thyroid hormone (f T4), respectively and do not convey anything about the causes of thyroid dysfunction. Sub-clinical hyperthyroidism is suppressed TSH with

Table 1 Biochemical definitions of thyroid dysfunction, based on assessment of TSH and free T4 (fT4) in serum, irrespective of the cause of dysfunction

TSH increased, fT4 decreased	Clinical hypothyroidism
TSH increased, fT4 normal	Sub-clinical hypothyroidism
TSH decreased, fT4 increased	Clinical hyperthyroidism
TSH decreased, fT4 normal	Sub-clinical hyperthyroidism
TSH normal, fT4 normal	Euthyroidism

No reference ranges are shown because these depend on the diagnostic kit used in the specific laboratory.

Table 2 Causes of clinical hyperthyroidism (in iodine-replete areas) relevant to general practice (estimated percentages)

Cause	% of all cases
Endogenous	90–95
Hyperthyroidism due to hyperfunction	80–90
Graves' disease	60–75
Toxic multinodular adenoma	10–15
Toxic adenoma	1–3
Hyperthyroidism due to destruction	1–5
Silent thyroiditis (autoimmune)	
Related to pregnancy: postpartum thyroiditis	2–4
Unrelated to pregnancy	0.1–0.5
Sub-acute thyroiditis (postviral)	1–3
Exogenous	1–3
Excessive intake of thyroid hormone (tablets or food)	
Drug intake (amiodarone, iodine and iodine containing drugs, radiographic contrast agents)	

an fT4 (and fT3) within the normal range, and sub-clinical hypothyroidism is increased TSH with an fT4 and fT3 within the normal range.

Clinical hyperthyroidism

Epidemiology of clinical hyperthyroidism

In iodine-replete areas, the *prevalence* rate of clinical hyperthyroidism (undiagnosed and previously treated hyperthyroidism together) is 2–3 per cent in the female and 0.2 per cent in the male population. Age-specific rates vary considerably throughout different countries partly depending on the cause (Graves' disease occurring at younger age compared to toxic nodular goitre) but mostly unexplained. Differences between races are hardly documented: only one population study in South Africa revealed a 10-fold lower prevalence rate in blacks compared to whites. There is an unexplained 10-fold excess in women compared with men. Only few (although excellent) *prospective* studies of the epidemiology of hyper-thyroidism have been carried out, mostly in the United Kingdom. The mean incidence in women in the 20-year follow-up Whickham cohort was 0.8 per 1000, the probability of the development of hyperthyroidism between the age of 35 and 60 years was 1.4 per 1000 and remained stable.[1]

In mild to moderate iodine-depleted areas, the thyroid tries to compensate for its iodine need by increasing its activity, often resulting in goitre and autonomously functioning nodule(s), and a higher proportion of hyper-thyroidism compared to hypothyroidism, even with increasing age. The *prevalence* of hyperthyroidism in one Scandinavian study was 2 per cent while the overall annual *incidence* was 0.39 per 1000, 0.63 per 1000 in women, and 0.13 per 1000 in men. Severe iodine deficiency is associated with hypothyroidism.

How common is hyperthyroidism in general practice?

Assuming an average general practice of 2000 patients with a male/female ratio of 1 : 1, the epidemiological data in the previous section imply that such a GP practice should have 20–30 women and two men with hyperthyroidism (prevalence). Over 25 years, a GP should diagnose 20–25 new cases among women, almost one per year; and two to three men over 25 years (incidence).

Causes of hyperthyroidism

These are endogenous or exogenous.[2,3] *Endogenous causes* are due to an increased *production* of thyroid hormone by the thyroid, or due to increased levels of serum thyroid hormone due to inflammatory *destruction* of thyroid tissue (thyroiditis). Thyroiditis causes a (temporary) massive release of stored thyroid hormone from the colloid into the peripheral circulation, often followed by a total depletion of thyroid hormone, leading to hypothyroidism. *Exogenous* causes of hyperthyroidism are usually related to the use of medications (Table 2).

Graves' disease is an autoimmune thyroid syndrome, as reflected by the presence of TSH receptor-stimulating antibodies in almost 100 per cent of patients and antibodies against TPO (TPO-Ab) and thyroglobulin (TG, TG-Ab). The male/female ratio ranges from 1 : 7 to 1 : 10. There is considerable genetic susceptibility to Graves' disease; some reports suggest major life events can be a trigger for Graves' disease.[3]

Ophthalmopathy discriminates between Graves' disease and other causes of hyperthyroidism. Ten to 25 per cent of Graves' patients have clinically evident ophthalmopathy, 30–45 per cent have eyelid signs, and up to 90 per cent have orbital abnormalities detectable with computerized tomography. Less than 5 per cent have severe ophthalmopathy, with a greater proportion in men. Smoking seems to be a risk factor.

In toxic multinodular adenoma (toxic multinodular goitre or struma) there are islands within the thyroid of autonomous functioning cells that escape from regulation mechanisms. Classically, when there is iodine deficiency, the normal thyroid initially enlarges to compensate for the needs of thyroid hormone production. The evolution from a diffuse goitre to a non-toxic multinodular goitre and finally to a toxic multinodular goitre is gradual (over many years) and depends highly on daily iodine intake. This explains the variation from 5 per cent in iodine-sufficient areas to almost 50 per cent in relatively iodine-deficient areas of toxic multinodular adenoma as a cause of hyperthyroidism. Moreover, it explains why this cause of hyperthyroidism preferentially occurs in older subjects (>50 years). Besides iodine, genetics and exposure to goitrogens may be important in the pathogenesis of hyperthyroidism.

Solitary toxic adenoma results in hyperthyroidism by the same mechanisms, though less frequently. Up to 80 per cent of patients with a solitary hyperfunctioning adenoma are euthyroid at diagnosis, especially when adenomas are small (<2.5 cm). The rate of developing hyperthyroidism is estimated to be 4 per cent per year, higher in older patients, those with an adenoma of 3 cm or larger at diagnosis, and those living in iodine-deficient areas.

Silent (painless) thyroiditis is rather common after pregnancy and rare otherwise. Women with elevated titres of TPO-Ab before pregnancy (5–10 per cent of fertile women) are at particular risk. Due to an immunological downregulation during normal pregnancy followed by a rebound postpartum there is lymphocytic infiltration of the thyroid cells leading to massive destruction. As a result, the thyroid stores of thyroid hormone are released into the circulation leading to hyperthyroidism, usually unrecognized. After the stores are depleted a hypothyroid phase usually occurs.

Sub-acute thyroiditis (de Quervain) is thought to be of viral origin: there is fever, general malaise, and a raised ESR. Viral antibodies can be demonstrated while titres against thyroid antibodies are low. A painful goitre is pathognomonic. It is a transient disease, rarely if ever resulting in permanent hypothyroidism.

Table 3 Differential diagnosis of causes of hyperthyroidism based on palpitation of the thyroid

	Possible diagnosis
Diffuse goitre	
Painless, regularly enlarged	Graves' disease, thyroiditis (postpartum)
Painful	Sub-acute thyroiditis
Single nodule	Solitary toxic adenoma, carcinoma (rare)
Multiple nodules	Toxic multinodular adenoma

Diagnosis of hyperthyroidism[4–6]

Differential diagnosis of hyperthyroidism is important since the cause influences choice of treatment.

Clinical signs and symptoms of florid hyperthyroidism are easy to recognize: fatigue, sweating, warm, moist skin, heat intolerance, heart palpitations (tachycardia, atrial fibrillation), weight loss, tremor, nervousness, and eyelid symptoms are classical. These signs have appropriate specificity but low sensitivity and positive predictive value. Table 3 summarizes the physical findings associated with causes of hyperthyroidism.

Laboratory tests used include TSH, fT4, and, in selected cases, thyroid antibodies. Elevated titres of TPO-Ab suggests Graves' disease or postpartum thyroiditis. An ultrasound discriminates well between Graves' disease, toxic adenoma, and toxic multinodular goitre. A thyroid scan differentiates between hyperthyroidism caused by an overproduction of thyroid hormone (increased radioactive uptake over the whole thyroid as in Graves' disease, increased uptake restricted to a solitary nodule as in toxic adenoma or in multiple nodules as in toxic multinodular goitre) and hyperthyroidism due to massive release of thyroid hormone because of thyroid damage (no uptake).

Treatment of hyperthyroidism[5–7]

Whether or not the GP treats hyperthyroidism himself, he should be aware of different treatment strategies to inform and counsel the patient about treatment options.[5,6] Drug treatment is the only therapy directly available to GPs for treatment of Graves' hyperthyroidism. Two different drugs can be used: methimazole (MMI) or carbimazole (which is rapidly converted in serum to methimazole and hence is considered as identical to MMI), and propylthiouracil (PTU). The choice of antithyroid drug is an individual matter, often based on the physician's preference. MMI and PTU are used in the United States and South America, MMI in Europe and Japan, and carbimazole in the United Kingdom. The drugs have antithyroid effects through interfering with thyroid peroxidase-mediated iodide oxidation and organification of iodine and iodothyronine coupling as well as immunosuppressive activity.

The advantages of MMI include higher compliance with a single daily dose; treated patients become euthyroid sooner; and low doses may be safer than PTU as far as agranulocytosis is concerned. The usual starting dose of MMI has been 20–30 mg daily in divided doses or once daily. For PTU, the usual starting dose is 100 mg three times daily. The arguments for combination therapy (antithyroid drug and thyroxine replacement) are unconvincing.

If thyroid function does not improve within 4–6 weeks, a dose increase is required. Thyroid function should be checked after 4–6 weeks. As thyroid function improves during the first several months after antithyroid therapy is initiated, the dose of drugs should be decreased or hypothyroidism may supervene.

Most of the side-effects of hypothyroid drugs are allergic reactions in the first few weeks or months and are more common in patients treated with higher doses. In case of minor side-effects these may subside in several days despite continuation of therapy. If these persist, the other antithyroid drug can be used with reasonable probability that the side-effect will disappear. The rare, though serious, side-effect of agranulocytosis warrants discontinuation of the drug and referral to a specialist. The GP should carefully inform the patient that its symptoms (fever and evidence of infection, most commonly oropharynx) must be reported immediately.

The primary goal of antithyroid drug therapy is euthyroidism and to anticipate a remission of Graves' disease continuing after discontinuation of therapy, which is usually given for 12–24 months. About 50 per cent of the patients will show complete remission. Most relapses of hyperthyroidism occur within 3–6 months after discontinuation of therapy.

Initially, beta adrenergic antagonist drugs can accompany antithyroid drug therapy when there are severe hyperthyroid symptoms. Propanolol 80 mg/day or atenolol or metoprolol 50 mg/day are frequently used.

Radioactive iodine therapy is the most widely used treatment of Graves' disease in the United States and is increasingly popular in Europe. Initially, radioiodine causes cellular necrosis (sometimes leading to mild thyroid tenderness) and atrophy of the thyroid. Ultimately this causes hypothyroidism: up to 90 per cent within the first year after therapy, 3–4 per cent per year thereafter. In general, 50–75 per cent of patients become euthyroid 6–8 weeks after therapy. Overall, 80–90 per cent only need one dose of radioiodine. There is no evidence that radioiodine is associated with increased risk of thyroid and other tumours. Pregnancy however, is absolutely contraindicated, at least until 3 months after treatment. No adverse effects have been documented in the offspring of patients treated with radioiodine. There is now evidence that eye disease occurs more frequently after radioiodine (especially in smokers) than after antithyroid drug or surgical therapy.

Sub-total thyroidectomy removes most of the thyroid gland, leaving a few grams of the posterior side of each lobe. Mortality is close to zero and the major complications of recurrent laryngeal nerve damage and hypoparathyroidism are infrequent (1–2 per cent). The skill of the surgeon is of major importance in predicting complications. Hypothyroidism occurs in 12–80 per cent of the patients the first year after surgery with a further onset of hypothyroidism in an additional 1–3 per cent per year, possibly reflecting the natural course of Graves' disease.

Treatment of other causes of hyperthyroidism

For toxic adenoma and multinodular goitre, antithyroid drugs are never the treatment of choice. A toxic adenoma is best treated with radioiodine although toxic multinodular goitre patients may require large and often multiple doses of radioiodine. Surgery may be the best option in patients with a large goitre because, in contrast to Graves' disease, there might be little effect of radioiodine on thyroid size.

Postpartum thyroiditis seldom requires treatment. Beta-adrenergic blockers may help women overcome the hyperthyroid phase. Subacute thyroiditis is a self-limiting viral infection seldom leading to hypothyroidism. Symptomatic treatment (paracetamol to relieve pain and fever) may be indicated.

Clinical hypothyroidism

Epidemiology of clinical hypothyroidism

In iodine-replete areas of the United Kingdom, the *prevalence* of clinical hypothyroidism is 1.5–2.2 per cent for women and 0.1 per cent for men. In contrast to hyperthyroidism, there is a substantial increase of new cases of hypothyroidism in women with increasing age. In the 20-year follow-up study in Whickham (UK), the overall mean annual *incidence* of clinical hypothyroidism in women was 4 per 1000 (all cases) comparing to 0.6 per 1000 in men.[1] Mean annual incidence was 10 times more frequent in women who originally had elevated TSH and TPO-Ab concentrations, seven times more frequent in those originally with only elevated TSH concentrations, and five times in those originally with only elevated TPO-Ab concentrations. Severe iodine deficiency is the major cause of hypothyroidism; the thyroid is no longer able to compensate for the iodine need by increasing function, resulting in goitre.

How common is hypothyroidism in general practice?

Assuming an average general practice of 2000 patients with a male/female ratio of 1 : 1, epidemiological data imply that a GP's practice would include 20–25 women and one man with hypothyroidism. Assuming clinical work for 25 years, a GP should newly diagnose 100 women (almost four per year) and 15 men over the 25 years.

Causes of hypothyroidism (Table 4)

Endogenous causes

In iodine-replete areas chronic (Hashimoto) autoimmune thyroiditis is the most common cause (up to 95 per cent) of hypothyroidism.[8] It is an autoimmune thyroid disease, reflected by the presence of elevated titres of antibodies, most commonly TPO-Ab. Classically, the process of total lymphocytic infiltration takes years, as reflected by an initially euthyroid state with only elevated titres of TPO-Ab, through a sub-clinical state with increasing TSH leading to clinical (overt) hypothyroidism with decreased fT4.

Postpartum thyroiditis can be regarded as a variant of Hashimoto thyroiditis. It occurs in 3–6 per cent of postpartum women, especially in those with elevated titres of TPO-Ab before pregnancy, as occurs in up to 10 per cent of fertile women. The relative risk of developing postpartum thyroiditis in women with elevated TPO-Ab titres is about 35–40 compared to TPO-Ab negative women. Although it is a self-limiting disease (women recover within the first postpartum year), up to 50 per cent of those with postpartum thyroiditis will have definite clinical hypothyroidism within 10 years. As such, it is believed that pregnancy precipitates clinical hypothyroidism in women who were already immunologically compromised.

Iodine deficiency is by far the most important cause of hypothyroidism in the world.[7] More than one billion people live in iodine-depleted areas with, according to the severity of deficiency, high figures of hypothyroidism. It is beyond the scope of this chapter to discuss it in detail but the interested reader is referred to a recent review.[8] GPs should know if they practice in an iodine deficient area. There are still large areas in which the iodine intake is inadequate in the United States, Germany, Italy, Spain, and most of the Eastern European countries. Even in areas with adequate iodine intake for the general population, intake might not be sufficient for pregnant women. Iodine deficiency during pregnancy has been associated with increased rates of abortions, stillbirths, and perinatal and infant mortality. Impaired mental development of the offspring has clearly been demonstrated to be associated with lower iodine intake during pregnancy.

Exogenous causes

Of the *exogenous* causes of hypothyroidism, the destructive therapies for hyperthyroidism are the most common. Almost all patients who undergo radioactive therapy for hyperthyroidism will become hypothyroid, as is the case (but to a lesser degree) with most of those treated by surgery. Radiation of the neck (for non-thyroid malignancy such as Hodgkin lymphomas) is another important exogenous cause. Of the drugs that interfere with

Table 4 Causes of hypothyroidism, relevant to general practice

Endogenous
Destruction of thyroid tissue
Chronic (Hashimoto) autoimmune thyroiditis
Postpartum thyroiditis
Defective thyroid hormone synthesis: iodine deficiency
Exogenous
Destruction of thyroid tissue
Radioactive iodine therapy for hyperthyroidism
Radiotherapy of the neck for non-thyroid malignant disease
Sub-total thyroidectomy
Defective thyroid hormone synthesis: drugs with antithyroid actions

thyroid hormone synthesis, amiodarone and lithium are most common. Amiodarone, an antiarrhythmic, contains iodine and interferes with thyroid hormone synthesis, leading to hypothyroidism in up to 20 per cent of users, patients with TPO-Ab being at particular risk. The overall prevalence of hypothyroidism in patients treated with lithium carbonate is 3.4 per cent, those with TPO-Ab also being at particular risk.

Diagnosis of hypothyroidism

Clinical signs and symptoms of overt hypothyroidism are fatigue, lethargy, constipation, hoarseness, weight gain, cold intolerance, or dry skin. In iodine-replete areas, in most cases hypothyroidism is a chronic process that takes years to develop. The onset of symptoms is similarly insidious.

Laboratory testing includes assessment of TSH, fT4, and in some cases thyroid antibodies. Elevated titres of TPO-Ab are highly suggestive of autoimmune hypothyroidism. When hypothyroidism is detected transiently during the postpartum period, the presence of these antibodies is highly predictive of definite hypothyroidism within a decade. There is no need for further diagnostic investigation before treatment is started.

Management and treatment of hypothyroidism

The precaution concerning possible harm when initiating thyroxine in ischaemic cardiac patients is mainly based on case reports and has hardly ever been confirmed by studies of large groups of patients. Exogenous causes of hypothyroidism should be looked for and whenever possible prevented.

Treatment of hypothyroidism[4,8]

At initiation of therapy, *healthy patients under the age of 60 years* without co-morbidity should receive full replacement dose of T4: 1.6–1.8 μg/kg ideal body weight per day, which is usually 75–125 μg in women and 125–200 μg in men. *Patients over 60 years* require 20–30 per cent less T4 per kg. Usually, in otherwise healthy elderly patients the initial dose is 50 μg/day. The requirement for T4 can be altered by several conditions (pregnancy) and medications (amiodarone, antiepileptic drugs).

To monitor thyroxine therapy:

- assess TSH after 8 weeks and adjust thyroxine in 25 μg increments;
- reassess after 8 weeks;
- once the dose is stable, re-assess TSH in 4–6 months;
- annually revaluate TSH; and
- reconsider the dose in the seventh or eighth decade when it might need to be decreased.

Usually, the fT4 shows the earliest normalization (within several weeks) while TSH may need up to 8 weeks. Although signs and symptoms ameliorate within weeks, most do not resolve for several months. A substantial portion of patients will present with a variety of persistent complaints even after normalization of both TSH and fT4 (muscle and joint tenderness, sleep and mood disorders). These should be taken seriously although an explanation is still lacking. Whether these patients need a small dose of T3 (12.5 μg) as well as T4 is unresolved.

Sub-clinical thyroid dysfunction

Sub-clinical hyperthyroidism (suppressed TSH with an fT4 (and fT3) within reference range) mostly has an exogenous origin: excessive substitution in hypothyroid or inadequate suppression in hyperthyroid patients. Because it has been associated with a decreased bone mineral density (in post-menopausal women) and a three-fold increased risk of atrial fibrillation, drug treatment should be adequately monitored.

Subjects with sub-clinical hypothyroidism (increased TSH with an fT4 and fT3 within the reference range) may present with vague symptoms and have an increased risk of cardiac disease. The prevalence increases with age, from 8 to 18 per cent in women (3–8 per cent in men); its progression to clinical (overt) hypothyroidism is highly dependent on the presence of TPO-Ab, the causes being similar to those of clinical hypothyroidism. Assuming an average population of 2000 patients per GP with an equal male : female distribution, there would be up to 200 women and 100 men with sub-clinical hypothyroidism. If a patient with sub-clinical hypothyroidism has signs and symptoms, a trial of low-dose (25 µg) thyroxine for several months can be used. Care must be taken to avoid sub-clinical hyperthyroidism. When a patient with sub-clinical hypothyroidism has no symptoms, an annual check of thyroid function is warranted.

A full discussion of the sub-clinical forms of hyper- and hypothyroidism is beyond the scope of this chapter and the interested reader is referred to a review elsewhere.[8]

Disturbances of thyroid size

These include a single nodule, multiple nodules, or a diffuse thyroid enlargement.

A single nodule within the thyroid

The prevalence of thyroid nodules increases with age: close to zero at 15 years to 50 per cent or higher in people over 60, but only about 10 per cent of these nodules are palpable. All patients with a single nodule of the thyroid without evidence of (sub)clinical hyperthyroidism should be evaluated or referred for evaluation. Although by far the majority of single nodules are benign tumours, thyroid cancer has to be ruled out.

Multiple nodules

The finding of multiple nodules in the thyroid also requires evaluation. In the absence of thyroid dysfunction further examination is warranted to exclude cancer. Multiple nodules with (sub)clinical hyperthyroidism favours the diagnosis of toxic multinodular goitre.

Diffuse thyroid enlargement: goitre

When a diffuse thyroid enlargement is found in the absence of thyroid dysfunction, the most likely cause is iodine deficiency and there is no need for referral. When the thyroid is enlarged together with (sub)clinical hypothyroidism, the most likely diagnosis is chronic autoimmune thyroiditis and the GP should start with thyroxine replacement. When there is thyroid goitre and (sub)clinical hyperthyroidism (and elevated titres of TPO-Ab), Graves' disease is the most likely diagnosis. Depending on the case, the GP might start drug therapy or seek further evaluation.

Key points

- For GPs, the main issue regarding thyroid function disorders is not how to diagnose or how to treat but when to think of their possible existence.
- Check thyroid function in:
  - women who present with vague complaints;
  - the elderly;
  - patients receiving drugs that interfere with thyroid function.
- Hypothyroidism can easily be treated by the GP with few further diagnostic procedures.
- Pregnant women with thyroid disorders (currently or in the past) should be referred not simply to a gynaecologist but to a doctor who specializes in the effects of pregnancy on maternal and foetal thyroid function.
- Iodine deficiency is still a major concern, not only in the developing countries but also in many parts of the Western world, including many parts of United States and Europe.

References

1. Vanderpump, M.P. et al. (1995). The incidence of thyroid disorders in the community: a twenty-year follow-up of the Whickham Survey. *Clinical Endocrinology (Oxford)* 43 (1), 55–68. (One of the best longitudinal epidemiological studies on thyroid function disorders.)
2. Singer, P.A., Cooper, D.S., Levy, E.G., Ladenson, P.W., Braverman, L.E., Daniels, G., Greenspan, F.S., McDougall, I.R., and Nikolai, T.F. (1995). Treatment guidelines for patients with hyperthyroidism and hypothyroidism. Standards of Care Committee, American Thyroid Association. *Journal of the American Medical Association* 273 (10), 808–12. (State of the art guidelines from the United States.)
3. Vanderpump, M.P., Ahlquist, J.A., Franklyn, J.A., and Clayton, R.N. (1996). Consensus statement for good practice and audit measures in the management of hypothyroidism and hyperthyroidism. The Research Unit of the Royal College of Physicians of London, the Endocrinology and Diabetes Committee of the Royal College of Physicians of London, and the Society for Endocrinology. *British Medical Journal* 313 (7056), 539–44. [State of the art guidelines from the United Kingdom (reflecting Europe).]
4. Weetman, A.P. (1997). Hypothyroidism: screening and subclinical disease. *British Medical Journal* 314 (7088), 1175–8. (Review on aetiology of hypothyroidism and arguments pro and contra screening of the general population.)
5. Lazarus, J.H. (1997). Hyperthyroidism. *Lancet* 349 (9048), 339–43. (Excellent review of all causes of hyperthyroidism.)
6. Weetman, A.P. (2000). Graves' disease. *New England Journal of Medicine* 343 (17), 1236–48. (Excellent review.)
7. Woeber, K.A. (2000). Update on the management of hyperthyroidism and hypothyroidism. *Archives of Family Medicine* 9 (8), 743–7. [An update of the previous mentioned guidelines (refs 4 and 5).]
8. Delange, F., de Benoist, B., Pretell, E., and Dunn, J.T. (2001). Iodine deficiency in the world: where do we stand at the turn of the century? *Thyroid* 11 (5), 437–47. (Very recent critical review and comments on the steps behind the battle against iodine deficiency.)

5.6 Endocrine problems (pituitary and sex hormones)

Peter Sonksen

Pituitary

Anatomy and physiology

The pituitary develops as a fusion of outgrowths from the foregut and the brain. This results in the two anatomically distinct parts (anterior, foregut; posterior, neural) and a complex system whereby hormone secretion by the anterior pituitary is regulated by neurosecretory products ('releasing hormones') manufactured and secreted by hypothalamic neurones and carried to the anterior pituitary by a portal blood supply. The posterior pituitary, however, is actually neural tissue with cell bodies in the hypothalamus and nerve endings forming the posterior pituitary. These nerve cells secrete their products, oxytocin and vasopressin, directly into the systemic circulation.

The pituitary itself is under predominantly negative feedback control, as is the hypothalamus, and investigation of pituitary disorders involves an understanding of how these mechanisms work. Prolactin secretion differs from the other hormones in that its secretion is regulated by an inhibitory factor. In the case of traumatic pituitary stalk section from a head injury prolactin levels are high when all other levels are low.

These two 'case studies' illustrate some of these points:

Case 1: An otherwise healthy woman of 43 complains of menstrual irregularity, she thinks it might be the menopause and would like your advice.

Normally, in a pre-menopausal woman, oestradiol (E2) production from the ovary feeds back and inhibits follicle stimulating hormone (FSH) secretion by the pituitary and the respective values of E2 and FSH vary slightly throughout the menstrual cycle but within their normal ranges. After ovarian failure has occurred the feedback loop is 'opened' and FSH levels rise dramatically. A single blood sample sent to the laboratory for measurement of oestradiol and FSH will often provide a clear answer. If the oestradiol (40 pmol/l) is low and FSH high (40 U/l), then the patient is clearly right, she is entering the menopause. The oestradiol measurement is not strictly needed, as a high FSH alone is diagnostic in this case but it does add confirmatory evidence.

Case 2: A man of 53 has had a pituitary tumour removed and this has been followed by a course of radiotherapy to reduce risk of recurrence. He has been taking hydrocortisone since the operation. The hospital consultant endocrinologist has advised him to have an 'insulin stress test'—he is now asking your advice about the need for this test.

The demonstration of an intact feedback loop is part of many endocrine investigations. Thus the ability of the classical insulin-induced hypoglycaemia test to evaluate pituitary function is based on the potency (and safety) of hypoglycaemia to stimulate the release of adrenocorticotropic hormone (ACTH) and growth hormone (GH). Measurement of cortisol and GH before and after dropping the blood glucose transiently below 2.2 mmol/l with 0.15 U/kg insulin intravenously is still the best 'gold standard' test of pituitary function. If he can mount a normal response then he can discontinue the cortisol. If his GH response is inadequate, then recombinant growth hormone (rhGH) replacement should be considered.

Pathophysiology

Endocrine diseases of the pituitary can originate in either the hypothalamus or the pituitary and with the power of the modern endocrine laboratory, it has often become possible to pinpoint the exact functional lesion and this can have important therapeutic implications. Although magnetic resonance imaging (MRI) has revolutionized our ability to investigate pituitary disorders, many but not all functional lesions are visible.

Endocrine conditions are intrinsically very simple; they involve either over- or underproduction of a hormone. Although these disturbances can occur in any of the endocrine systems some are much more common than others. For example, tumours secreting GH, prolactin (PRL), and ACTH are much more common that tumours producing thyroid stimulating hormone (TSH), luteinizing hormone (LH), or FSH.

Overproduction of a hormone is usually due to a benign proliferation of a clone of cells producing a single hormone. Rarely, this clone can produce two hormones—some cases of acromegaly also have very high prolactin levels and histological examination shows that the two hormones actually arise from the same cells. These cells lack the normal regulatory processes governing secretion and we use this property to establish a diagnosis.

Underproduction of a hormone, especially when onset is in childhood, is usually due to a developmental failure of the cells needed for production of the releasing hormone in the hypothalamus. When there is a 'secondary' failure in hormone production (it once was normal but now is subnormal), the cause may be degenerative or due to destruction by a pituitary or parapituitary tumour.

Investigation of the endocrine problem usually consists of two components:

1. screening and assessment of current endocrine status; and

2. detailed investigation to confirm or refute provisional diagnosis.

The first part of this is now easily carried out in general practice settings with access to good modern endocrine laboratories. The second component usually requires referral to specialist endocrine services; a telephone conversation with the consultant about what should be done before referral is always welcome and often significantly shortens the time to diagnosis and effective treatment.

Growth hormone

Until 1989 it was thought that GH was really only needed in childhood and was redundant in adults. We now know that GH is probably the most potent anabolic agent known and is the hormone mainly responsible not only for developing a 'normal body' but maintaining it throughout life.

GH secretion is pulsatile with the major peaks occurring in the first few hours of sleep. Random blood samples are therefore of limited value in investigation (see more below under acromegaly) and dynamic pituitary function tests are usually required. Normally, as much as 70 per cent of 24-h GH secretion occurs at night and disturbances of sleep disrupt normal GH secretion. Exercise is another potent stimulus of GH secretion and thus plenty of exercise and a good night's sleep are, as our mothers told us, essential components not only of 'growing up' but also staying fit and healthy!

Daily GH secretion increases throughout childhood, reaches a maximum around puberty (where it causes the pubertal growth spurt) and then declines throughout life. Beyond the age of 50–60, daily GH production rates are very low and of the same order of magnitude as is seen in young people with severe GH deficiency. This fall in GH with ageing is known as the somatopause and is probably the main reason for the loss of lean body mass (muscle, soft tissues, and bone) and increase in body fat (particularly intra-abdominal) with increasing age and the eventual development of frailty.

GH receptors exist on virtually all cells in the body and influence many processes of great importance. Amongst its many actions it stimulates the formation of insulin-like growth factors (IGF-I and -II). The local (autocrine and paracrine) production of IGF-I in tissues (under the control of GH) regulates local growth and development.

Acromegaly is the clinical syndrome associated with excess GH production, most commonly from a benign adenoma of the pituitary. It is usually diagnosed incidentally when a patient is being seen for some other reason, although it may present through one of its complications such as diabetes mellitus. It can be diagnosed by demonstrating a raised GH and IGF-I in a single random blood sample in a person who has the well-known clinical features of the disease. A positive test should always be confirmed and the patient should be referred to the local endocrinologist.

In acromegaly, the adenoma can usually be demonstrated on MRI scanning. Transphenoidal removal is the treatment of choice, followed by post-operative monitoring of GH and IGF-I levels, and an insulin stress test to demonstrate normal cortisol and GH responses. If GH and IGF-I levels do not return to normal post-operatively, a course of deep X-ray therapy (DXT) is usually indicated to destroy residual adenoma and prevent recurrence. The effects of DXT are gradual and may take many years to complete the cure. Pituitary function needs evaluating once treatment is complete as it is not unusual to find hypopituitarism requiring hormone replacement developing as long as 20 years post-DXT.

The typical facial changes in a man developing acromegaly over many years are illustrated in a textbook of endocrinology published in 1916.[1] Note that the patient was one of Harvey Cushing—the Boston neurosurgeon who pioneered pituitary surgery.

GH deficiency may present in childhood as a growth delay, although it may occasionally present through a complication such as hypoglycaemia. In adults, the syndrome of growth hormone deficiency in adults (GHDA) was only discovered in 1992 as a result of a double-blind, placebo-controlled trial of rhGH.[2] The syndrome is characterized by:

◆ low mood and poor quality of life;

◆ lack of energy, stamina, and strength;

◆ abnormal body composition (reduced lean body mass and increased fat, particularly intra-abdominal fat);

◆ reduced life expectancy due to excess cardiovascular and cerebrovascular disease; and

◆ abnormal lipoprotein metabolism (high LDL and low HDL cholesterol).

The diagnosis is confirmed by demonstrating a complete lack of GH response to insulin-induced hypoglycaemia.

These patients are often severely incapacitated and describe their lives as 'existing rather than living'. All these symptoms have been demonstrated to be completely eliminated by physiological rhGH replacement under double-blind and placebo-controlled conditions. Even in those with severely low mood and poor quality of life, things were completely restored to normal by rhGH in physiological replacement doses.

GH replacement should be given by nightly subcutaneous injections starting at 125 µg nocte and increasing the dose slowly on the basis of measured IGF-I levels not more often than every 2–4 weeks. Sensitivity varies considerably between individuals and women are more GH resistant than men. The average maintenance dose is around 500 µg/day. Side-effects are very unusual with this schedule and if they do develop are usually short-lived and self-limited and may well reflect reactivation of muscle and cartilage growth as many patients liken them to 'growing pains' of adolescence.

Assessing GH status: In someone with a history of a pituitary disorder and symptoms and signs in keeping with GHDA, a random GH and IGF-I level should be measured and if the GH is undetectable and the IGF-I below the age-related reference range of the laboratory, the patient most likely has GHDA and should be referred to hospital for a specialist opinion and most likely, an insulin stress test.

If the IGF-I level is within the lower half of the normal range this is still quite compatible with GHDA and in the presence of an appropriate history the patient should also be referred for further investigation. The presence of symptoms and signs of GHDA in a person without pituitary pathology should alert one to the possibility of an occult tumour.

In a patient with suspected acromegaly where random GH values are undetectable, the diagnosis can be excluded. If the GH and/or IGF-I values are ambiguous, then measuring GH during an oral glucose tolerance test will resolve any uncertainty. A normal response is to suppress GH levels to below 1 mU/l at some stage.

Prolactin

Prolactin is normally only concerned with milk production in the post-partum period. It is not known to have any physiological role in men (although men do get galactorrhoea with prolactinomas). Prolactin deficiency is not associated with any known abnormality apart from the inability to lactate postpartum. This occurs in Sheehan's syndrome (postpartum pituitary necrosis) but often does not get diagnosed until many years later when the full-blown condition of panhypopituitarism develops. Unlike other pituitary hormones, prolactin secretion is regulated by an inhibitory factor—dopamine. Thus, dopamine agonists inhibit prolactin secretion while dopamine blockers cause hyperprolactinaemia. Transection of the pituitary stalk leads to low levels of all pituitary hormones except prolactin, which rises.

Prolactinoma

Benign pituitary adenomas secreting prolactin are quite common. They usually present clinically at an earlier stage in women than in men. The presenting features are amenorrhoea and galactorrhoea due to disruption of the gonadotrophin/ovarian axis by prolactin. In men, although prolactin lowers LH, FSH, and testosterone levels, it is unusual for men to present with impotence and although this symptom may be present for years, it is usually ignored. Most commonly it is only when the adenoma begins to impair vision through encroachment on the visual pathway that the patient seeks help and the diagnosis is made.

Surgery is now rarely needed for treatment of prolactinomas and the majority respond (lower prolactin levels and a shrinking of the tumour) to dopamine agonist treatment with a drug such as bromocriptine that has revolutionized management.

ACTH

ACTH regulates cortisol production through direct stimulation of cortisol synthesis in the adrenal. It normally exhibits a diurnal rhythm with lowest values around midnight and levels rising in the early hours before waking. This rhythm takes about 2 weeks to fully adjust when moving from one time zone to another and is the main endocrine cause of jet lag. Taking small doses of melatonin on retiring may speed the adjustment to a new time zone. ACTH also responds to stress and the induced cortisol response, together with GH are responsible for recovery from hypoglycaemia (GH is probably more important than cortisol in this respect).

Cushing's syndrome

Cushing's syndrome is due to excess cortisol production or administration. Cushing's disease is the combination of a (usually) very small pituitary adenoma with bilateral adrenal hyperplasia. Even with high-resolution MRI scanning, it is not possible to visualize the micro-adenoma in the majority of cases. This makes establishing the correct diagnosis one of the most challenging of endocrine tasks. The role of the GP in this complex condition is to screen possible cases and refer those who test positive. The classical features are well known, but less often recognized is the frequency with which the condition presents via psychiatric conditions (classically a severe psychotic depression) and osteoporosis with pathological fractures. The central obesity with wasted limbs (so called 'lemon on match-sticks') is highly characteristic and due to cortisol blocking protein synthesis and stimulating lipid deposits, particularly centrally.

The ability to suppress ACTH (and thus cortisol) levels with a dose of the potent synthetic steroid dexamethasone forms the basis of diagnosing Cushing's syndrome. The 'overnight dexamethasone suppression test' has been established as a very reliable simple screening test for Cushing's syndrome. If 1 mg of dexamethasone is taken between 11 p.m. and midnight it suppresses the normal rise in ACTH that occurs in the morning and as a result plasma cortisol at 9 a.m. falls below 70 nmol/l in normal people. Failure to suppress cortisol indicates a failure of the feedback process and the likely diagnosis of Cushing's syndrome, and indicates that the patient should be referred to hospital for further investigation. The measurement of ACTH helps to distinguish an adrenal adenoma (where the values are indistinguishable from zero) from a pituitary adenoma. Unfortunately, ectopic ACTH production from a carcinoid tumour can be extremely difficult to diagnose correctly.

Both diagnosis of the cause of Cushing's syndrome and treatment are challenging. It is not uncommon that hypophysectomy fails to remove all the tumour and only cures around 50 per cent cases, even in the best hands. Subsequent radiotherapy and/or adrenalectomy are often needed and it is not uncommon to render a patient panhypopituitary but not cure the Cushing's syndrome. The treatment of adrenal adenomas is much more straightforward. It is usual in these cases however, to require cortisol replacement for as long as a year post-operatively before the ACTH secretion (that was inhibited by the autonomous adrenal cortisol response) recovers and the cortisol replacement can be safely stopped.

ACTH deficiency

ACTH deficiency is an exceedingly rare condition when it occurs alone but is a frequent feature of hypopituitarism and should be suspected in anyone with a pituitary or parapituitary condition or someone who has had treatment for such conditions. Contrary to popular views, it is quite possible for a patient to lead what they think is a normal life with a pituitary tumour and hypopituitarism with zero cortisol values. The classical Addisonian crisis does not occur with ACTH deficiency alone—it requires loss of aldosterone as well as cortisol and most of its features are actually due to salt depletion.

Deficiency of cortisol with normal aldosterone, as happens with ACTH deficiency, is often discovered only after the results of an insulin stress test come back—the patient having survived the test without any untoward effects occurring. It is associated with prolonged insulin-induced hypoglycaemia and spontaneous hypoglycaemia in the presence of a long fast. Patients do feel much better on cortisol replacement!

Glucocorticoid replacement therapy is most commonly given with hydrocortisone (identical to cortisol). Existing replacement regimes are probably too generous and may have negative effects on body composition (reduced lean body mass and increased fat). Targets should probably be less than 20 mg hydrocortisone a day. It is best given in divided doses such as: 10 mg on waking, 5 mg at lunch, and 5 mg at dinner. Fludrocortisone is only needed in people with Addison's disease. 'Steroid cover' for surgery and other illnesses need only provide a maximum of 150 mg in any 24-h period. For intercurrent illness a doubling of the usual replacement dose for 1 or 2 days with return to usual dose thereafter is usually sufficient.

Gonadotrophins

Gonadotrophin releasing hormone (GnRH) stimulates secretion of both LH and FSH, the exact amounts of each being determined by existing sex hormone status. LH regulates testosterone production in men and (mainly) progesterone production by the corpus luteum in women. FSH stimulates gametogenesis in men and ovulation in women.

Gonadotrophin levels rise at the onset of puberty and thereafter remain fairly constant in the male with a gentle background pulsatile pattern of secretion. There is a reduction in both LH and testosterone in older men and some may benefit from testosterone replacement. In women, LH and FSH vary throughout the menstrual cycle until the menopause when both rise to very high levels and when FSH rises higher than LH. Testosterone and oestradiol normally feedback and inhibit GnRH, LH, and FSH secretion. Primary testicular (e.g. after mumps orchitis or orchiectomy) or primary ovarian failure (e.g. Turner's syndrome or premature menopause) is associated with very high LH and FSH levels.

Hypogonadotrophic hypogonadism usually results in delayed puberty but can develop later in life. Classically, it occurs in weight-related amenorrhoea in women but it is also very common in male and female elite endurance athletes and ballet dancers. It occurs in the rare but interesting Kalman's syndrome where a diagnosis can be made without any blood tests simply by enquiring about the patient's sense of smell. In Kalman's syndrome, anosmia is associated with agenesis of the olfactory bulb and the hypothalamic centre for GnRH production. GnRH offers a logical form of treatment in most cases of hypogonadotrophic hypogonadism and was introduced in the 1980s but went out of fashion when *in vitro* fertilization developed but is now reappearing and can be very effective. GnRH has to be given in 90-min pulses via a subcutaneous needle and a special pump. Its major advantage is that it is 'natural' and takes advantage of the normal feedback processes.

Hormone replacement therapy with sex steroids is now best given using non-oral routes since the liver conjugates both oestrogens and androgens after absorption from the gut. Now that patches are readily available, they are the preferred method of steroid delivery as they avoid this 'first pass' effect and this significantly alters their therapeutic profile. Patches have the additional advantage that they deliver oestradiol and testosterone in their natural form that can be readily measured in the endocrine laboratory. This means that doses can be monitored and adjusted on an individual basis simply by checking the serum testosterone or oestradiol level. In men, the patch has advantages over depot injections since the levels produced can not only be more easily tailored to individual metabolism, but also the levels remain relatively constant.

Pituitary tumours

Non-functioning adenomas and other tumours such as craniopharyngiomas and optic nerve gliomas, usually present with visual field disturbances and here the first priority is saving vision. Headaches may be a feature but raised intracranial pressure from pituitary tumours is very rare. Hormone secreting adenomas present with their classical syndromes. Tumours of the posterior pituitary are extremely rare.

Diagnosis can readily be made with modern radiological techniques, particularly MRI scanning. Visual field testing, particularly with a red hatpin is clinically simple and very useful. Every GP should have a red and white hatpin for checking visual field in the surgery. Early field defects are more easily picked up with the red pin.

Hypopituitarism

Pituitary tumours and their treatment are the commonest cause of hypopituitarism in adults. Sheehan's syndrome (pituitary infarction) can present many years after the relevant pregnancy. Radiotherapy may not induce hypopituitarism for 10 or 20 years, so anyone who has had head or neck radiotherapy should have their endocrine status evaluated from time to time and if the index of suspicion is raised.

Although any combination of hormones can be lost in hypopituitarism, growth hormone deficiency is commonest. Next most common is gonadotrophin deficiency that usually presents as oligomenorrhoea or secondary amenorrhoea in women and much less commonly as impotence in men (who do not usually seek advice for something that they usually attribute to growing older). Loss of ACTH is not uncommonly part of panhypopituitarism but rarely occurs on its own.

The clinical features of hypopituitarism are usually insidious and by their nature tend not to bring the patient to seek advice until something as dramatic as visual loss or amenorrhoea occurs. Patients tend not to complain, particularly when they have, for example, had their vision saved by brain surgery. They think that feeling awful is the down side of successful surgery and that they should just get on with life and not complain. As depression is so common in these patients, it is important to ask patients specific questions about their mood (including queries about 'black thoughts' and 'how do you see the future'), energy level, and quality of life.

Posterior pituitary

Diabetes insipidus (DI) is the main condition associated with pathology of the posterior pituitary. It can occur with any pituitary or peripituitary tumour or transiently (or permanently) immediately after pituitary surgery (most commonly transcranial surgery). Post-operative DI may recover spontaneously within a few days or become permanent. Not uncommonly post operatively it progresses to the syndrome of inappropriate antidiuretic hormone secretion (SIADH), which again usually lasts only a few days and is self-limiting but needs to be managed carefully with water restriction if water intoxication is to be avoided. Patients who have had transcranial surgery often lose their normal thirst sensations as part of the damage from the tumour or its treatment and need to have their water balance watched extremely carefully for them. Permanent DI is usually quite easy to manage but it always remains a serious disorder and appropriate treatment and careful management of water balance at times of other surgery and illnesses in essential.

Mild water intoxication is surprisingly common in people with DI and regular checks on serum sodium often reveal asymptomatic hyponatraemia. This is most commonly due to over dosage with DDAVP (desmopressin), which, generally should not be given more often than once a day.

The presence of gross thirst and polyuria in someone with a pituitary tumour or someone who has had pituitary surgery should raise suspicion. The diagnosis of DI can be confirmed by a random urine (negative for glucose) and plasma electrolytes and osmolality. If the plasma osmolality and sodium are high and the urine osmolality very low, the diagnosis is confirmed.

DDAVP (desmopressin) is the drug of choice for treating DI. In mild cases tablet treatment may be sufficient and is very safe. In more severe cases, nasal solution and spray are effective and injections are rarely needed. Correct education in delivery is essential and should be reviewed if problems appear.

The finding of incidental hyponatraemia in someone on DDAVP should lead to paired serum and urine samples being sent to the laboratory for osmolality measurements. If the urine osmolality exceeds serum osmolality the DDAVP regime should be reviewed and reduced. Once a day DDAVP at bedtime lasts 20 h in most people and the 4 h of diuresis is a valuable 'safety valve' that protects against DDAVP over dosage. Any use of DDAVP more often than once a day should be reviewed regularly and in the presence of hyponatraemia, the dosage of DDAVP should be reduced even in the face of protests from the patient.

Key points

- Growth hormone deficiency is the commonest hormonal abnormality associated with pituitary disease.

- The low mood commonly associated with GH deficiency in adults responds better to rhGH replacement than antidepressants.

- Cushing's syndrome commonly presents via its complications—diabetes, depression, hypertension, and osteoporosis.

- Checking LH/FSH together with testosterone (men) and oestradiol (women) in a random blood sample is an effective way of assessing sex hormone status.

- Examining status of feedback system is the basis of most pituitary function tests.

References

1. Schafer, Sir Edward. In *The Endocrine Organs*. London: Longmans, Green, & Co, 1916.
2. Cuneo, R., Salomon, F., McGauley, G., and Sonksen, P.H. (1992). The growth hormone deficiency syndrome in adults. *Clinical Endocrinology* 37, 387–97.

5.7 Endocrine problems (calcium, water, and adrenal)

Robert D. Murray

Hypercalcaemia

The diagnosis of hypercalcaemia has increasingly been made since the routine use of multichannel biochemical analysers. Once the metabolic anomaly has been confirmed, the underlying diagnosis needs to be established.

Presentation

The majority of patients with hypercalcaemia are asymptomatic. The presence of symptoms relates to both the rate of rise, and absolute calcium level. Calcium levels above 2.9–3.0 mmol/l result in neuropsychiatric (fatigue, depression, confusion, proximal muscle weakness, coma), gastro-intestinal (anorexia, nausea, vomiting, constipation, non-specific abdominal pains, pancreatitis, peptic ulcer disease), renal (polyuria, dehydration, nephrocalcinosis, nephrolithiasis), skeletal (bone resorption, chondrocalcinosis, pseudogout), and cardiac symptoms (shortened QT interval, arrhythmias, cardiac arrest).

Causes

Hypercalcaemia is due to either primary hyperparathyroidism or malignancy in more than 90 per cent of cases. Hyperparathyroidism results from a solitary adenoma in 80 per cent, four gland hyperplasia in 15 per cent, and multiple adenoma or rarely carcinoma in the remaining cases. Hyperparathyroidism secondary to four gland hyperplasia is frequently associated with hereditary syndromes including multiple endocrine neoplasia (MEN) type 1 and 2A. Excessive secretion of parathyroid hormone (PTH) increases serum calcium and reduces serum phosphate. Fifty to 80 per cent of patients are asymptomatic, and many patients with mild hypercalcaemia run a benign course for many years, even life. In addition to the symptoms of hypercalcaemia, the direct action of PTH leads to local (osteitis fibrosa cystica, resorption of phalangeal tufts, 'salt and pepper' skull), and generalized bone resorption (preferentially cortical bone). Peak incidence of hyperparathyroidism is between the third and fifth decades, but may occur at any age. The prevalence in undiscovered asymptomatic patients is estimated to be as high as 1 per cent.

Malignancy-related hypercalcaemia is due to either local invasion and destruction of bone (haematological malignancies, small cell and adenocarcinoma of the lung, breast and prostate cancer), humoral factors (squamous cell carcinomas, renal and urogenital tract malignancies), or a combination of both. Humoral hypercalcaemia results from PTH-related peptide (PTHrp) which binds to and activates the PTH receptor in a manner indistinguishable to PTH. Less common causes of hypercalcaemia include:

- vitamin D and vitamin A intoxication,
- familial hypocalciuric hypercalcaemia (FHH),
- sarcoidosis,
- idiopathic hypercalcaemia of infancy (William's syndrome),
- hyperthyroidism,
- Addison's disease,
- immobilization,
- milk-alkali syndrome (Burnett's syndrome),
- tertiary hyperparathyroidism,
- medications (thiazide diuretics, lithium therapy).

Diagnosis

It is important in all cases to take a detailed history and examination with particular attention to any family history of endocrine disease, drugs, and vitamins. The underlying diagnosis in asymptomatic hypercalcaemia is hyperparathyroidism in over 90 per cent of patients. Chronic hypercalcaemia of greater than 12 months rarely relates to occult malignancy, and is usually due to hyperparathyroidism.

A raised PTH value is characteristic of primary and tertiary hyperparathyroidism, but may also be mild to moderately elevated with lithium therapy and FHH. PTH is suppressed in all other causes of hypercalcaemia. 1,25-dihydroxyvitamin D is elevated in hyperparathyroidism, vitamin D intoxication, and sarcoidosis. Additional investigations in the diagnosis of hypercalcaemia include 24 h urinary calcium (increased in hyperparathyroidism, reduced in FHH), PTHrp, thyroid function tests, serum protein electrophoresis, serum angiotensin converting enzyme, bone isotope scan, and chest X-ray. A hydrocortisone suppression test will result in a lowering of the serum calcium in cases of vitamin D intoxication, sarcoidosis, and malignancy.

Acute referral should be made for patients with severe hypercalcaemia and significant symptomatology. Routine referral for assessment should be made when the cause of the hypercalcaemia is not clear, and when chronic treatment and monitoring is required (i.e. malignancy, sarcoidosis).

Management

Immediate therapy is not required in mild to moderate hypercalcaemia (<2.8 mmol/l) when there are no significant symptoms. Calcium and vitamin supplements should be discontinued if safe to do so. Investigations to establish the underlying cause and to determine any complications of hypercalcaemia should be initiated under primary care or outpatient specialist care.

Severe hypercalcaemia requires hospital admission, especially if profound neuropsychiatric symptoms are present. The most important step in the immediate management of severe hypercalcaemia is rehydration, which corrects the associated dehydration and reduces the serum calcium. The addition of loop diuretics further decreases urinary calcium resorption. Bisphosphonates are pyrophosphate analogues that are stable in bone and inhibit bone resorption by osteoclasts. These drugs can be given intravenously for acute onset of action and are the primary therapy in reducing and maintaining serum calcium levels.

Specific therapies for hypercalcaemia include parathyroid surgery for hyperparathyroidism. Surgery should be considered where the patient's age is less than 50 years, serum calcium is over 2.9 mmol/l, creatinine clearance is reduced, or complications present (nephrolithiasis/calcinosis, severe osteopaenia, etc.). Glucocorticoids increase urinary calcium excretion and reduce intestinal calcium absorption thereby lowering serum calcium in the hypercalcaemia of malignancy, sarcoidosis, and vitaminosis D. Glucocorticoids produce no effect on serum calcium in normal subjects or patients with hyperparathyroidism. When renal function is compromised, dialysis may be required to enable calcium loss from the body. Now rarely used therapies for hypercalcaemia include calcitonin, plicamycin, and gallium nitrate.

Continuing care

Long-term management and surveillance is dependent on the underlying aetiology. Post-operatively, in hyperparathyroidism the patient should be monitored daily for 4–5 days for hypocalcaemia. The hypocalcaemia is usually mild and transient, and results from suppression of function of the normal glands during the period of hypercalcaemia and remineralization of the skeleton. No intervention is usually required. Occasionally hypocalcaemia may be more severe (<2.0 mmol/l) requiring calcium and vitamin D supplementation. Therapy will periodically need to be withdrawn during the first 3 months, to establish whether the remaining parathyroid glands have recovered or have been damaged during surgery.

Mild to moderate hypercalcaemia due to hyperparathyroidism requires long-term follow-up for any change in serum calcium levels, and the development of complications. Malignancy-related hypercalcaemia requires specialist follow-up and treatment of the underlying tumour. Management will thus be directed at the tumour, but calcium levels should be monitored regularly. Where drugs or vitamin supplements have been withdrawn as the probable cause the serum calcium should be monitored periodically to confirm normocalcaemia, as it is possible the patient may also have mild hyperparathyroidism. Hypercalcaemic sarcoidosis requires regular monitoring of serum calcium levels and slow withdrawal of the corticosteroid therapy over 12–24 months once normocalcaemia is achieved. Idiopathic hypercalcaemia of infancy generally resolves spontaneously after the first year of life. Patients with milk-alkali syndrome should minimize calcium containing foods in their diet and avoid calcium containing antacids.

Key points

- ◆ Most patients with hypercalcaemia are asymptomatic. Symptoms when present may be neuropsychiatric, gastrointestinal, renal, skeletal, or cardiac.

- ◆ Hypercalcaemia is due to hyperparathyroidism or malignancy in over 90% of cases.

- ◆ Definitive management is of the primary cause.

- ◆ Serum calcium can be lowered by rehydration, loop diuretics, and bisphosphonate therapy where necessary.

Hypocalcaemia

Chronic hypocalcaemia is less common than hypercalcaemia. Transient acute hypocalcaemia however is not uncommon, usually mild, and rarely requires intervention.

Presentation

Transient acute hypocalcaemia is usually asymptomatic and normalizes spontaneously following resolution of the underlying cause. Chronic hypocalcaemia is usually symptomatic. Symptoms may be neuromuscular (muscle spasms, carpopedal spasm, facial grimacing, intestinal cramps, chronic malabsorption), neurological (irritability, depression, psychosis, convulsions, raised intracranial pressure with papilloedema), or cardiac (prolonged QT interval, arrhythmias). Chvostek's and Trousseau's signs are usually positive.

Causes

Transient acute hypocalcaemia is observed during critical illness, acute pancreatitis, transfusion of citrated blood, and with use of heparin and glucagon. Chronic hypocalcaemia results from hypoparathyroidism, chronic renal failure (CRF), vitamin D deficiency, defective metabolism or resistance to vitamin D, pseudohypoparathyroidism (PHP), or acute severe hyperphosphataemia. Hypoparathyroidism may be hereditary or acquired. Hereditary hypoparathyroidism is associated with developmental defects (PHP, DiGeorge syndrome) and failure of additional endocrine glands, alopecia, candidiasis, basal ganglia calcification, extrapyramidal manifestations, raised intracranial pressure, and papilloedema. Hereditary hypoparathyroidism generally manifests in the first decade of life and may be autosomal dominant, recessive, or X-linked. PHP is typically associated with skeletal and developmental defects. The classical skeletal defect in PHP is Albright's hereditary osteodystrophy (AHO) comprising short stature, round facies, brachydactyly, and extraosseous calcification. The syndrome is an autosomal dominant trait resulting in deficient end-organ response to PTH. Pseudopseudohypoparathyroid patients have signs of AHO, but no hypocalcaemia. Acquired hypoparathyroidism is usually the result of parathyroid or thyroid surgery, though may be autoimmune in nature. Severe magnesium deficiency (<0.4 mmol/l) leads to impaired PTH release and reduced peripheral response to PTH. Loss of renal parenchyma and tubular damage in CRF leads to phosphate retention and failure of 1-hydroxylation of vitamin D, leading to hypocalcaemia, secondary hyperparathyroidism, and renal osteodystrophy. Vitamin D deficiency is present in up to 25 per cent of the elderly in Western Europe as a consequence of inadequate intake of dairy products and reduced sunlight exposure. Vitamin D deficiency also occurs with deficient metabolism (vitamin D dependent rickets type 1, anticonvulsant therapy), and end-organ resistance to vitamin D (vitamin D dependent rickets type 2).

Diagnosis

A thorough history and examination may reveal chronic malabsorption, impaired renal function, poor diet, previous neck surgery, excessive alcohol intake (magnesium deficiency), family history, skeletal abnormalities, or developmental defects. Preliminary investigations include serum calcium, phosphate, magnesium, and PTH. PTH is inappropriately low in hypoparathyroidism and magnesium deficiency, and elevated in PHP, vitamin D deficiency/resistance, and chronic renal failure. High serum phosphate levels are observed in hypoparathyroidism and PHP. Patients with secondary hyperparathyroidism have low or low normal serum phosphate (vitamin D deficiency and resistance). Vitamin D levels are of low specificity in the diagnosis of hypocalcaemia.

Management

Acute transient hypocalcaemia is generally mild and requires no intervention. Treatment is aimed at the cause of the hypocalcaemia. Occasionally, the hypocalcaemia is more severe and may require therapy similar to that for chronic hypocalcaemia on a temporary basis.

In chronic hypocalcaemia, the underlying cause is generally irreversible and therapeutic interventions are aimed at restoration of calcium levels. General principles of management include ensuring the diet has sufficient calcium, and if not, instituting supplemental calcium of 1000–1200 mg/day. The mainstay of treatment is vitamin D and its analogues. In severe hypocalcaemia, vitamin D should be replaced using 1α-calcidol or calcitriol and serum calcium monitored on a daily basis.

In simple vitamin D deficiency due to inadequate intake, replacement will be in the region of 1000–2000 U/day. In hypoparathyroidism and PHP, therapy is usually initiated with 1α-calcidol or calcitriol at a dose of 0.25 μg/day and increased slowly until symptoms have resolved and the serum calcium is normalized. In the absence of PTH action, and therefore failure of renal resorption of calcium, it is preferable to keep the serum calcium in the lower part of the normal range to prevent excess renal calcium excretion and consequent nephrocalcinosis. In CRF, vitamin D therapy needs to be with an analogue of vitamin D that is 1α-hydroxylated (1α-calcidol, calcitriol); and phosphate-binding antacids reduce hyperphosphataemia-associated extraosseous calcium deposition. Vitamin D dependent rickets type 1 and 2 are similarly treated with vitamin D, but they require larger doses. Hypomagnesaemia may be corrected by attention to the underlying cause and magnesium supplements.

Continuing care

Most patients with transient hypocalcaemia require no further management once the acute precipitant has been resolved. Patients with chronic hypocalcaemia require continued monitoring of their serum calcium. Up to 4 weeks are required for vitamin D analogues to achieve their peak effect on serum calcium. Hence once normal calcium levels have been restored serum calcium levels require monitoring on a monthly basis until completely stable to avoid precipitating hypercalcaemia. Thereafter, it is sensible to monitor the serum calcium every 3–4 months.

Key points

- Transient hypocalcaemia frequently occurs in association with illness, is generally mild and requires no treatment.
- Chronic hypocalcaemia is rare and results directly or indirectly from deficiency or resistance to PTH and/or vitamin D.
- Chronic hypocalcaemia is usually symptomatic presenting with neuromuscular, neurological, or cardiac features.
- The cause of chronic hypocalcaemia is rarely reversible and treatment entails the use of calcium supplements and vitamin D analogues to restore serum calcium.

Diabetes insipidus (DI)

DI is a state of excessive water intake and hypotonic polyuria due to a failure of arginine vasopressin (AVP) release (neurogenic) or action (nephrogenic). DI most frequently presents in childhood to early adult life, and is more common in males than females.

Presentation

The onset is characteristically sudden with the individual complaining of polyuria (3–24 l/day), excessive thirst, and polydipsia. Symptoms are present throughout the day and night. Dehydration occurs only where thirst does not compensate for the fluid loss.

Causes

The majority of cases of neurogenic DI are idiopathic or result from neoplastic or infiltrative disease of the hypothalamus, head injury, post-hypophyseal surgery, or lymphohypophysitis. Idiopathic DI is usually isolated, but may be part of the syndrome of DIDMOAD (DI, diabetes mellitus, optic atrophy, deafness). Neoplasia may be primary or secondary. Infiltrations are usually granulomatous diseases, of which sarcoidosis and histiocytosis X are the commonest. Post-surgical DI is frequently transient, but if persistent is usually associated with panhypopituitarism. Psychogenic polydipsia is a condition of compulsive water drinking and consequent polyuria. Water turnover is variable, but if extreme may result in dilutional hyponatraemia.

Nephrogenic DI is a consequence of failure of the kidney to respond to AVP. The causes entail renal disease (post-obstructive uropathy, unilateral renal artery stenosis, etc.), hypokalaemia, hypercalcaemia, drugs (i.e. demeclocycline, lithium), and systemic disease (multiple myeloma, amyloidosis, sickle cell disease, etc.).

Diagnosis

The history and examination should rule out more common causes of polyuria including diuretic therapy, diabetes mellitus, and chronic renal disease. The history should distinguish between frequent passing of small volumes of urine (urinary tract infection) and the passing of large volumes of urine. In psychogenic polydipsia both urine and plasma osmolality are low. Urinary volume can be confirmed by 24-h urine collection. Morning plasma and urine osmolality generally shows a dilute urine and high plasma osmolality. Serum biochemistry shows raised sodium and urea. In neurogenic DI, the posterior pituitary hyperintense signal on T1-weighted MRI images is lost. Urgent referral to an endocrinologist is warranted if hypernatraemia, dehydration, or symptoms are present, or daily urine output is over 5 l. Referral is less urgent when the patient is asymptomatic, has normal biochemistry, and is passing less than 5 l of urine per day.

The diagnostic test of choice for DI is the water deprivation test during which the patient's response to dehydration and AVP are examined. This test allows the diagnosis of DI to be confirmed, and distinguishes between neurogenic and nephrogenic forms.

Management

Nephrogenic DI is managed by correction of electrolyte disturbances and treatment of the underlying cause. Neurogenic DI is treated with desmopressin which has a prolonged antidiuretic action and no significant pressor effects. Desmopressin may be administered subcutaneously (1–4 μg), intranasally (10–20 μg), or orally (100–200 mg) once to thrice daily. Patients on desmopressin must be educated to avoid excess water intake to prevent water intoxication and dilutional hyponatraemia. Patients with psychogenic polydipsia should be treated with fluid restriction, and in some cases may need psychological help.

Continuing care

Most patients with neurogenic DI remain well on maintenance desmopressin and require only infrequent measurement of serum electrolytes and osmolality. Absorption of intranasal desmopressin may be reduced by respiratory tract infections and allergic rhinitis requiring temporary use of oral or parentral formulations. Patients with nephrogenic DI will require appropriate long-term care directed at the underlying pathological process.

Key points

- Diabetes insipidus results from deficiency (neurogenic) or resistance (nephrogenic) to AVP.
- Symptoms are polyuria (3–24 l/day) and excessive thirst which occur throughout the day and night.
- Investigations show a dilute urine and elevated serum osmolality, sodium, and urea. The water deprivation test is used to establish the diagnosis.
- Neurogenic DI is treated with AVP replacement using desmopressin. Nephrogenic DI is managed by treatment of the underlying cause.

Syndrome of inappropriate ADH secretion (SIADH)

SIADH occurs commonly within the elderly and in patients where it is associated with a number of disease processes, and medications. The AVP secretion is considered inappropriate as it is associated with a low plasma osmolality and concentrated urine.

Presentation

Symptoms of SIADH are dependent on the rate of fall and absolute serum sodium concentration. The majority of cases are mild and asymptomatic, being diagnosed on routine biochemistry. In general serum sodium levels down to 130 mmol/l may be associated with anorexia, and nausea. With sodium levels below 130 mmol/l, weight gain and vomiting occur, and the likelihood of symptoms of cerebral oedema increases (irritability, restlessness, confusion, convulsions, coma). Oedema and hypertension are classically absent.

Causes

SIADH may result from drug-induced release or potentiation of the action of AVP (i.e. chlorpropamide, carbamezepine, tricyclic antidepressants); disease-induced release of AVP (i.e. head trauma, subarachnoid haemorrhage, cerebral thrombosis, brain tumour, acute encephalitis); and ectopic AVP release from neoplastic tissue (i.e. small cell carcinoma of the lung, pancreatic carcinoma, lymphoma) or inflammatory lung disease (i.e. tuberculosis, pneumonia, lung abscess).

Diagnosis

The diagnosis should be suspected in the presence of hyponatraemia and concentrated urine (>300 mosm/l) with no concurrent oedema, dehydration, or orthostatic hypotension. Plasma osmolality, urea, and uric acid are low secondary to dilution. The diagnosis can only be made if appropriate causes of AVP secretion are excluded, in particular oedematous and hypovolaemic states. Pseudohyponatraemia due to vastly elevated triglycerides or glucose should be excluded. The underlying aetiology should be looked for. Patients who are symptomatic or with serum sodium levels below 130 mmol/l should be referred urgently for specialist assessment and acute management.

Management

As the hyponatraemia is dilutional, the mainstay of treatment is fluid restriction to 800–1000 ml/day. In nearly all patients, this results in a negative fluid balance and correction of the hyponatraemia. Addition of demeclocycline (900–1200 mg/day), a potent inhibitor of AVP action, may be necessary in resistant cases. In the acute setting, the patient should be weighed and plasma osmolality and sodium monitored daily. In severe cases with cerebral oedema management is supportive. Small volumes of 3 or 5 per cent NaCl infused over several hours have been used with effect. Larger volumes may precipitate cardiac failure or correct the hyponatraemia too quickly with resultant pontine myelinosis.

Continuing care

Long-term management seeks to define the underlying cause of the SIADH, and when identified treatment should then be directed towards the cause. In many cases, the cause either remains undefined or is not curable. In these patients, fluid restriction and demeclocycline may be continued long-term. The serum sodium and osmolality should be monitored regularly.

Key points

- SIADH is common in the elderly and in inpatients.
- Symptoms depend on the rate of fall and absolute sodium level. As the sodium level falls anorexia, nausea, and symptoms of cerebral oedema develop.
- The main causes are drugs, neoplasia, intracranial pathology, and chronic inflammatory lung diseases.
- Treatment is of the underlying cause, however, serum sodium levels can be controlled by fluid restriction and antagonism of AVP (demeclocycline).

Cushing's syndrome

Cushing's syndrome is the clinical syndrome resulting from chronic excessive glucocorticoid exposure. This section will concentrate on Cushing's syndrome of primary adrenal origin.

Presentation

Cushing's syndrome presents with weight gain, truncal obesity, plethoric 'moon' face, 'buffalo hump', fatigue, proximal myopathy, purple abdominal striae, insulin resistance and diabetes mellitus, hypertension, osteoporosis, amenorrhoea, hirsutism, acne, peripheral oedema, and personality changes. Symptoms are usually of insidious onset and may be mild or florid at the time of presentation.

Causes

After exclusion of iatrogenic Cushing's syndrome, over 90 per cent of cases of Cushing's syndrome are due to an ACTH secreting pituitary adenoma. The majority of the remaining 10 per cent are due to adrenal neoplasms. Fifty per cent of adrenal neoplasms producing hypercortisolism are malignant. Rarely, Cushing's syndrome results from ectopic secretion of either ACTH or CRH, or from nodular hyperplasia of the adrenal. Pseudo-Cushing's relates to a Cushingoid appearance classically occurring in patients with obesity, depression, or chronic alcoholism.

Diagnosis

When the diagnosis of Cushing's is suspected excessive secretion of cortisol is confirmed by measurement of urinary free cortisol. Loss of cortisol diurnal rhythm can be demonstrated by measuring cortisol levels at 09:00 h and midnight. An overnight dexamethasone suppression test (1 mg dexamethasone at midnight, with measurement of cortisol at 09:00 h the next morning) can be used to demonstrate failure of physiological suppression of the cortisol axis. Measurement of ACTH at 09:00 h, in contrast to pituitary driven Cushing's disease, will show low or undetectable levels. If investigations favour an adrenal origin the adrenal should be imaged with a fine cut CT scan.

Management

All patients with non-iatrogenic Cushing's syndrome should be referred for specialist management. Cortisol-secreting adrenal neoplasms should be removed surgically via laparotomy or laparoscope. Atrophy of the contralateral adrenal gland may take weeks to months to recover normal function. Hydrocortisone cover should therefore be given pre-operatively and continued until adrenal function is re-assessed in the early post-operative period. Adrenal carcinomas are usually larger, have an irregular edge, and metastasise to the liver and lung. If it is not possible to remove a malignant tumour in its entirety, mitotane (maximum dose 8–10 g/day) is selectively cytotoxic to cortisol-secreting cells and may be used to control the tumour and cortisol production. Whilst awaiting surgery, or where surgery is contra-indicated, cortisol production can be controlled with ketoconazole (600–1200 mg/day) or metyrapone (2–4 g/day). Liver enzymes must be monitored when using ketoconazole. All three drugs mentioned above may potentially produce cortisol insufficiency.

Continuing care

Patients with Cushing's syndrome should remain under the care of a specialist unit whilst the disease is active. If cured by unilateral adrenalectomy many specialist units continue follow-up for at least 2 years post-operatively. Attention should be paid to monitoring and treatment of the associated hypertension, diabetes mellitus, and osteopaenia if these do not improve spontaneously post-operatively.

Key points

- ◆ Cushing's syndrome is the clinical consequence of chronic excessive glucocorticoid exposure. A primary adrenal cause is present in around 10% of cases.
- ◆ Symptoms and signs are of a classical appearance associated with muscle weakness, hypertension, and diabetes mellitus.
- ◆ Investigations reveal excess glucocorticoid secretion, loss of regulatory feedback, and the normal cortisol diurnal rhythm.
- ◆ Treatment is surgical removal of the adrenal neoplasm.

Primary hyperaldosteronism (Conn's syndrome)

Conn's syndrome is the result of excessive and inappropriate aldosterone production. Peak age of occurrence is 30–50 years, and it is twice as common in females as males. It is present in 1 per cent of unselected hypertensive adults.

Presentation

Hyperaldosteronism produces hypokalaemia and hypertension. Hypokalaemia may cause muscle weakness, fatigue, polyuria and cardiac arrhythmias, particularly premature beats. Prominent 'U' waves are observed on the ECG. The hypertension is typically diastolic.

Causes

Conn's syndrome is the consequence of a unilateral adrenal adenoma in the majority of cases, but may also be the result of bilateral adenomas or idiopathic bilateral nodular hyperplasia. Glucocorticoid remediable hyperaldosteronism (GRH) is an autosomal dominant condition with a similar biochemical and clinical picture to primary hyperaldosteronism. GRH is due to duplication of the gene for aldosterone synthase so that it is expressed in the zona fasciculata where its activity is stimulated by ACTH. Some forms of congenital adrenal hyperplasia (CAH) result in overproduction of steroid precursors with mineralocorticoid activity.

Diagnosis

Biochemical profile reveals hypokalaemia, and a metabolic alkalosis. Diuretic therapy and chronic liquorice ingestion must be ruled out. The aldosterone level is raised in association with an undetectable renin level. Imaging of the adrenal by fine cut CT scan should be followed by selective adrenal vein sampling if no obvious adenoma is visualized. In contrast to patients with solitary adenomas, patients with nodular hyperplasia reveal a fall in the aldosterone level with posture. GRH responds to replacement doses of cortisol which suppress ACTH.

Management

Management of an isolated adenoma is surgical resection via laparotomy or laparoscopy. Where surgery is inappropriate or in nodular hyperplasia the hypokalaemia and hypertension may be managed medically by sodium restriction and spironolactone, an aldosterone antagonist, or other potassium sparing diuretics. Side-effects of spironolactone include gynaecomastia and reduced libido.

Continuing care

If surgical cure is achieved, no regular follow-up is required other than routine blood pressure checks. In patients managed medically, blood pressure and serum potassium should be checked every 3–6 months.

Key points

- ◆ Conn's syndrome results from autonomous production of aldosterone from the adrenal gland.
- ◆ Presentation is with hypertension and hypokalaemia.
- ◆ Management entails surgical removal of an isolated adenoma, or dietary salt restriction and spironolactone in bilateral nodular hyperplasia.

Secondary hyperaldosteronism

This condition describes an elevated aldosterone level secondary to a raised renin. This condition is usually the result of renal disease (renal artery stenosis, hypertensive glomerulosclerosis), renin producing tumours, Barter's syndrome (juxtaglomerular hyperplasia), or oedematous conditions (cirrhosis, cardiac failure, nephrotic syndrome).

Congenital adrenal hyperplasia (CAH)

CAH is the most common adrenal defect of infancy and childhood. The defect is inherited as an autosomal recessive trait.

Presentation

Presentation usually occurs before adult life. 21-Hydroxylase deficiency usually presents in the neonatal period with acute adrenal insufficiency, salt wasting, and virilization. Partial forms can be expressed after adolescence with hirsutism and oligomenorrhoea. Other enzyme defects present with acute adrenal insufficiency combined with excessive or deficient mineralocorticoids and/or androgens. Virilization in the female at birth produces ambiguous genitalia (pseudohermaphroditism). Post-natal androgen excess produces sexual precocity, virilization, and excessive early growth but reduced final height due to early fusion of the long bones.

Causes

CAH is the consequence of an enzyme defect in the steroid synthetic pathway. The most common defect is 21-hydroxylase deficiency. 17α-hydroxylase, 11β-hydroxylase, and 3β-hydroxysteroid dehydrogenase account for a minority of patients.

Diagnosis

Adrenal insufficiency presenting in the neonatal period, infancy, childhood, or adolescence should raise the possibility of CAH. Symptoms of mineralocorticoid and androgen deficiency or excess should be actively looked for. Acute adrenal insufficiency can be confirmed by a short synacthen test. Measurement of androgens and metabolites such as 17-hydroxy progesterone can help in establishing the diagnosis.

Management

CAH requires specialist care to provide patient education, continued monitoring, psychological support, and reconstructive surgery if necessary. Glucocorticoid replacement prevents adrenal crisis and suppresses the excess androgen/ mineralocorticoid production. Mineralocorticoids should be replaced as necessary with fludrocortisone. Partial syndromes may not require intervention, however, glucocorticoid sufficiency should be fully assessed.

Continuing care

Monitoring of the adequacy of glucocorticoid and mineralocorticoid replacement should be performed intermittently. Over-replacement of glucocorticoid should be avoided to prevent growth inhibition. It is important that the excess androgens are suppressed to prevent early fusion of the epiphysis.

Key points

- ◆ CAH is an autosomal recessive condition leading to defects in the steroid synthetic pathway.
- ◆ The clinical picture reflects hypocortisolaemia combined with deficiency or excess of mineralocorticoids and/or adrenal androgens.
- ◆ Management requires careful replacement with hydrocortisone to reduce excess steroid metabolites and avoid glucocorticoid side-effects.

Other adrenal masses

Adrenocortical adenoma are present in 10–20 per cent of autopsy specimens. The majority of these 'incidentalomas' are not functional. Improved imaging techniques have resulted in frequent identification of these masses. Initially investigations should determine whether an incidental adrenal mass is functional. Blood pressure should be measured and 24-h urine collected for analysis of urinary free cortisol and catecholamines. Serum biochemistry, androgens, and lying and standing renin and aldosterone should be measured. Adrenal masses are usually benign adenomas but may be adrenal carcinoma or metastasis. Large tumours greater than 4 cm and an irregular margin are suggestive of carcinoma.

Androgen secreting tumours may be 'pure' or co-secrete glucocorticoids. Androgen secretion from adrenal tumours usually presents acutely and in females produces hirsutism, oligomenorrhoea, acne, and virilization. Treatment of secretory adrenal tumours is surgery. Non-functioning adrenal tumours of greater than 4 cm should also be removed due to the risk of carcinoma. Growth of smaller non-functioning tumours should be reassessed after 6 months by repeat CT scan.

Primary adrenal insufficiency (Addison's disease)

Addison's disease is rare. Destruction of over 90 per cent of the adrenal cortex is needed to precipitate glucocorticoid, mineralocorticoid, and adrenal androgen insufficiency. The incidence is equal in males and females.

Presentation

Patients present with insidious onset of weakness, fatigue, anorexia, nausea, vomiting, diarrhoea, weight loss, diffuse abdominal pain, postural hypotension, and cutaneous and mucosal pigmentation. Cutaneous pigmentation is greatest at the elbows and skin creases and is a diffuse brown coloration, whilst mucosal pigmentation is blue-black. Hypoglycaemia is a frequent feature of neonatal hypocortisolaemia. Females may notice reduced axillary and pubic hair. Presentation is often precipitated by a stressful event (infection, surgery) resulting in acute on chronic adrenal insufficiency. Patients show hypovolaemia, circulatory collapse, hypoglycaemia, and somnolence. Acute presentation may also be seen with abrupt withdrawal of chronic corticosteroid therapy, surgical removal of the adrenal glands, and Waterhouse–Friderichsen syndrome.

Causes

Primary adrenal failure is usually the result of autoimmune disease. At presentation, 50 per cent have adrenal antibodies. Autoimmune adrenal failure may be associated with other autoimmune diseases (pernicious anaemia, vitiligo, myaesthenia gravis), or endocrine failure (premature gonadal failure, diabetes mellitus, hyper/hypothyroidism, hypoparathyroidism). These associations are frequently part of the autosomal recessive polyglandular autoimmune syndromes.

Rarely, other causes of adrenal failure are encountered, such as infection (tuberculosis, coccidiomycosis, cytomegalovirus), metastasis, sarcoidosis, CAH, surgical removal, bilateral haemorrhage, adrenoleukodystrophy, and drugs (ketoconazole, metyrapone).

Diagnosis

Biochemical profile typically shows hyponatraemia, hyperkalaemia, elevated urea, and a hypochloric acidosis. Serum calcium is elevated in 10–20 per cent of patients. Aldosterone levels are reduced in association with an elevated renin. ACTH levels are elevated. The diagnosis can be confirmed with a short synacthen test. A peak cortisol of greater than 500 nmol/l at 30 min is observed in normal subjects. Patients with Addison's disease should be referred for specialist assessment, education, and optimization of replacement therapy. Acute or acute on chronic presentations require urgent hospital admission.

Management

Life-long glucocorticoid and mineralocorticoid replacement is required. Glucocorticoids are replaced with hydrocortisone, 10 mg on waking, 5 mg around midday, and 5 mg in the late afternoon to reflect normal diurnal rhythm. Mineralocorticoid replacement is with fludrocortisone 50–100 μg/day as a single daily dose. Acute presentations are treated with aggressive rehydration, intravenous hydrocortisone 100 mg qds, and dextrose.

Continuing care

Patients with Addison's disease require long-term observation and education. It is important that they understand that their hydrocortisone dose needs to be doubled during intercurrent illness. It is also essential that patients have hydrocortisone for parenteral administration, and are taught to administer this when vomiting is associated with illness. Patients should understand that their hydrocortisone dose needs to be increased before surgery and dental work. Cortisol profiles and renin levels help to optimize replacement regimens, and reduce side-effects, of hydrocortisone and fludrocortisone, respectively. Patients should wear a pendant or bracelet identifying their condition and medications.

Key points

- ◆ Adrenal insufficiency is primarily due to autoimmune disease, but in the Third World is most likely to be the consequence of infection.
- ◆ The disease process is usually insidious but acute presentation may be precipitated by stressful events.
- ◆ Symptoms are fatigue, gastrointestinal, weight loss, pigmentation, and postural hypotension.
- ◆ Management of adrenal insufficiency is replacement hydrocortisone and fludrocortisone.

Phaeochromocytoma

Phaeochromocytoma is reported to be present in around 0.1 per cent of hypertensives. There is a slight female preponderance, and the peak age of incidence is the third to fifth decade.

Presentation

The usual presentation is hypertensive crisis or paroxysmal attacks suggestive of anxiety. Rare presentations include shock during surgery or trauma, or end-stage cardiomyopathy. Hypertension is sustained but labile in 60 per cent, and present only during attacks in 40 per cent. Paroxysms occur in over 50 per cent of patients, becoming more frequent and of greater severity with time. They are of sudden onset and may last minutes to hours. Symptoms during these paroxysmal attacks include headache, palpitations, arrhythmias, pallor, sweating, apprehension, nausea, vomiting, and abdominal pain. Chronically, weight loss and carbohydrate intolerance is observed. Postural hypotension may result from depleted plasma volume and blunted sympathetic reflexes. Angina and myocardial infarction may occur in the absence of coronary artery disease due to the high myocardial oxygen demand and coronary spasm.

Causes

Phaeochromocytoma is a tumour of the sympathetic nervous system. This highly vascular tumour occur predominantly in the adrenal medulla. However, 10 per cent are extraadrenal, 10 per cent are bilateral, and less than 10 per cent are malignant. Malignant tumours metastasise to the lung and bones. Around 5 per cent of cases are familial and associated with autosomal dominant syndromes including MEN2A and 2B, neurofibromatosis, and Von Hippel Lindau. Bilateral tumours should raise the possibility of these syndromes. Extra-adrenal tumours are predominantly abdominal with 1 per cent present in each of the thorax, neck, and bladder.

Diagnosis

The diagnosis is confirmed by measurement of 24-h urinary catecholamine excretion. Ideally, urine should be collected when the patient is symptomatic and off all medications, though this may not be logistically possible. ^{131}I-metaiodobenzylguanidine (MIBG) is concentrated in the sympathetic nervous system and is useful in confirming the presence and locality of a suspected phaeochromocytoma. CT and MRI scans help localize adrenal and extra-adrenal tumours. In difficult cases, abdominal aortography and selective venous sampling may aid tumour localization.

Management

All patients with high suspicion of a phaeochromocytoma should be under specialist care for investigation and management. Once a diagnosis of a phaeochromocytoma has been established, α-blockade is established with phenoxybenzamine, a long-acting non-competitive antagonist. Phenoxybenzamine is commenced at 10 mg bd and increased by 10–20 mg/day until the blood pressure and paroxysms are controlled. The usual maintenance dose is 40–80 mg/day. Acute α-blockade can be established with intravenous phentolamine if necessary. Once α-blockade is established, β-blockade (propranolol 10 mg qds) can be instituted to control the tachycardia. Definitive treatment is surgical removal of the tumour which must be performed in centres experienced in the associated anaesthetic complications. When it is not possible to fully resect malignant tumours long-term treatment with metyrosine may be established to inhibit tyrosine hydroxylase and thus catecholamine production. Malignant phaeochromocytomas are

resistant to radiotherapy and chemotherapy. High-dose ^{131}I-MIBG has been used with limited success.

Continuing care

After surgery 5-year survival is 95 per cent and recurrence is less than 10 per cent. If malignant, 5-year survival is around 50 per cent. Urinary catecholamines should be reassessed yearly or earlier if symptoms recur. Hypertension resolves in 75 per cent of patients, and responds to antihypertensives in the remaining patients.

Key points

- Phaeochromocytomas are rare tumours usually localized in the adrenal medulla.
- Presentation is with hypertension and paroxysmal attacks involving headaches, palpitations, pallor, and sweating.
- Diagnosis is by confirmation of excess catecholamine secretion.
- The mainstay of management is surgical removal of the tumour.

Further reading

Baylis, P.H. (1998). Diabetes insipidus. *Journal of the Royal College of Physicians of London* **32**, 108–11. (Review of the management of diabetes insipidus.)

Bilezikian, J.P. (1993). Management of hypercalcemia. *Journal of Clinical Endocrinology and Metabolism* **77**, 1445–9. (Review of the current management of hypercalcemia.)

Grinspoon, S.K. and Biller, B.M. (1994). Laboratory assessment of adrenal insufficiency. *Journal of Clinical Endocrinology and Metabolism* **79**, 923–31. (Review of the assessment of adrenal insufficiency.)

Grossman, A. *Clinical Endocrinology*. London: Blackwell Science, 1998. (In-depth endocrinology reference text covering the above metabolic anomalies.)

Guise, T.A. and Mundy, G.R. (1995). Evaluation of hypocalcemia in children and adults. *Journal of Clinical Endocrinology and Metabolism* **80**, 1473–8. (Review of current management of hypocalcemia.)

Newell-Price, J., Trainer, P., Besser, M., and Grossman, A. (1998). The diagnosis and differential diagnosis of Cushing's syndrome and pseudo-Cushing's states. *Endocrine Review* **19**, 647–72. (In-depth review of Cushing's syndrome.)

Robertson, G.L. (2001). Antidiuretic hormone. Normal and disordered function. *Endocrinology and Metabolism Clinics of North America* **30**, 671–94, vii. (Review of management of DI and SIADH.)

Weatherall, D.J., Ledingham, J.G.G., and Warrell, D.A. *Oxford Textbook of Medicine* 3rd edn. Oxford: Oxford University Press, 1996. (General medical reference text for endocrine problems.)

Werbel, S.S. and Ober, K.P. (1995). Pheochromocytoma. Update on diagnosis, localization, and management. *Medical Clinics of North America* **79**, 131–53. (Review of the management of pheochromocytoma.)

6

Genito-urinary problems

6 Genito-urinary problems

6.1 Urinary tract infections

Tjerk Wiersma

Introduction

Most urinary tract infections are limited to the bladder and cause only a superficial inflammation of the bladder mucosa. The most common presenting symptoms are urinary frequency and burning, and this type of infection is commonly called cystitis or an uncomplicated urinary tract infection. Other types of urinary tract infections known as complicated urinary tract infections can involve either the upper (pyelonephritis) or lower urinary tract and are characterized by inflammation that is more invasive. Frequent symptoms include fever (body temperature 38.5°C or above), and possibly also chills, nausea, or colicky pain suggesting the possible presence of urinary tract stones. Invasive infections of the upper and lower urinary tracts cannot be distinguished from each other simply on the basis of the clinical picture, with the exception of acute prostatitis which is usually accompanied by pain in the perineum and a painful, swollen prostate upon rectal examination.

Urinary tract infections are common. Among sexually active women, an incidence of 0.5–0.7 per person year has been reported. Because some of these infections are self-limiting, many are not seen by general practitioners. In general practice, the incidence of urinary tract infections is 30–40 per 1000 patients per year. In 80–90 per cent of the cases the patient is female and the frequency of infection increases markedly with age.

Causes and backgrounds

The probable reason that urinary tract infections are far more common in women than in men is that women have a shorter urethra, which means bacteria have to travel a shorter distance to reach the bladder. In 80–90 per cent of cases the pathogen is *Escherichia coli*. Less frequently, urinary tract infections are caused by enterococci, *Staphylococcus saprophyticus*, *Proteus mirabilis*, and *Klebsiella* species. Urethritis caused by *Chlamydia trachomatis* sometimes causes symptoms similar to those of a urinary tract infection.

The gold standard for diagnosis of a urinary tract infection is a concentration of at least 10^5 colony forming bacteria per millilitre of urine, as established by culture. In women with typical complaints of acute onset of painful and frequent urination, the chance of detecting at least 10^5 bacteria/ml in freshly voided urine is approximately 60 per cent.

If a urine specimen contains 10^5 colony forming bacteria per millilitre of urine, the term 'significant bacteriuria' is often used. However, this term should be handled with caution, because episodes of asymptomatic bacteriuria are quite common in the population, especially in the elderly. In non-pregnant patients, this is a harmless condition which does not need treatment.[1,2]

While isolated urinary tract infections in women are generally of little significance, *recurrent urinary tract infections* are more often due to an underlying condition:

- In *children*, congenital abnormalities such as vesico-urethral reflux and the risk of permanent renal damage should be considered.[3] The younger the child, the greater the risk of renal damage. The risk of new renal damage decreases markedly by the third year of life.[4]

- In *elderly men*, important causes are obstruction and incomplete emptying of the bladder due to prostatic hyperplasia.

- In *women*, post-menopausal atrophy of the urogenital tract mucosa and submucosa, as well as incomplete emptying as a result of a prolapsed uterus or a cystocele, are possible underlying causes.

- In *both sexes*, other causes of urinary tract infections include neurological disorders of the bladder, bladder or kidney stones, indwelling catheters, and impaired resistance to infection due to diabetes mellitus, radiation, or other causes.

How to make a diagnosis

History

Most patients with a urinary tract infection report symptoms of frequent, painful, or burning urination, sometimes accompanied by painful cramping in the lower abdomen, or by haematuria. In young children, elderly patients, and patients with an indwelling catheter, there may be no obvious complaints related to urination and a urinary tract infection may only be expressed in the form of general malaise.

If a patient complains of acute symptoms of frequent or painful and burning urination, the general practitioner should obtain the following information:

- duration of symptoms;

- presence of fever;

- location of pain, if present;

- occurrence of previous urinary tract infections or kidney disease.

If the patient is female, the general practitioner should also ask whether she has any gynaecological symptoms such as vaginal itching or discharge, and if an older man, the practitioner should enquire about signs which may indicate difficult urination.

Physical examination

Physical examination of the female patient is not necessary unless she has lumbar pain, a fever, or a history of kidney disease or frequently recurring urinary tract infections. The examination should consist of an abdominal and a pelvic examination, with particular attention to the presence of a distended bladder and the possible presence of a prolapsed uterus, a cystocele, or mucous membrane atrophy. In men and children presenting with signs of a urinary tract infection, a physical examination should always be carried out.

In older men, a rectal examination should be carried out to investigate the possible presence of prostatic hyperplasia.

Urinalysis, dipslide, and urine culture

In patients with acute symtoms of frequent or painful and burning urination or in children or the elderly with unexplained symptoms of general malaise and fever, the prior probability of a urinary tract infection of 60 per cent can be raised considerably by a dipstick analysis of the urine for nitrites. The *nitrite test* is based on the fact that some bacteria produce nitrite in urine. The number of false-positive results is so small that the diagnosis of urinary tract infection may be made on the basis of a positive nitrite test result. However, the number of false-negative results is considerable. If the result is negative and the clinical situation demands a definitive diagnosis, the options are either a semi-quantitative urine culture using a dipslide or a microscopic examination of the sediment to establish the presence of bacteria.

The *dipslide analysis* is a highly reliable semi-quantitative culture. *Microscopic examination of the sediment* is only sufficiently reliable if it is carried out by someone who is properly trained in the technique and who has access to a well-maintained and regularly cleaned microscope. If these conditions cannot be fulfilled, diagnosis by means of dipslides is preferable. At least 20 bacteria per high-power field ($400\times$) of the centrifuged sediment are required for a positive result. The presence of epithelial cells indicates contamination. The sediment analysis cannot be used to determine the site of the infection, even if it contains cylinders or leucocyte clumps, for example.

Urine culture with antibiotic sensitivity testing is only indicated if there is a complicated urinary tract infection or if two blindly initiated treatments for an uncomplicated infection were ineffective (see treatment).

Microscopic examination of the sediment to detect the presence of leucocytes, as well as the leucocyte esterase dipstick test, is less reliable. Although the absence of leucocytes makes a urinary tract infection less likely the risk of obtaining a false positive test result is considerable because the presence of leucocytes in urine may also occur as the result of contamination, urethritis, or, in children, due to other fever-inducing diseases.

Other dipstick tests (such as haemoglobin, pH, protein, etc.) are not advised because their test characteristics are worse than those of the nitrite test and the leucocyte esterase test, so their results are of no consequence to the subsequent course of action.

Analysis and culture of urine stored at room temperature is only reliable if the urine is tested within 2 h of collection. Mid-stream urine should be used for analysis wherever possible. It has been demonstrated that the number of bacteria detected in midstream urine is comparable with that found in urine obtained by means of catheterization or puncture.[5] To avoid contamination, women should be instructed to spread the labia when collecting the urine and men should retract the foreskin. For children who cannot yet urinate on request, urine is collected in a urine pouch which is taped to the child after the genitalia have been washed with clean water. The pouch is checked every 10 min to see if the bladder has been emptied. Contamination is likely with this method.

Evaluation

- In patients complaining of frequent and painful urination and with a positive nitrite test, at least 10^5 colony forming units per millilitre urine on the dipslide, or at least 20 bacteria per high-power field, one should diagnose a urinary tract infection.

- If the symptoms suggest a urinary tract infection, despite a negative urinalysis, the urinalysis described above should be repeated using a fresh urine sample.

- In the case of acutely painful urination but no demonstrable urinary tract infection upon repeat analysis of urine, it is likely that the patient has urethritis.

- Blind antibiotic treatment, commenced before the results of culture and sensitivity tests are known but after the urine sample has been collected, is generally appropriate in primary care settings.

Treatment

Non-pharmacological therapy

It is generally assumed that the risk of a urinary tract infection can be reduced by promoting a large volume of urine by drinking large amounts of liquids, by regularly emptying the bladder and not delaying urination when there is an urge to urinate, and completely emptying the bladder at each urination. In addition, prompt emptying of the bladder after sexual intercourse can be beneficial in women.[6] The regular intake of cranberry juice seems to diminish the risk of recurrence as well.[7]

Drug therapy

Most studies comparing the efficacy of various antibacterials in urinary tract infections have been small and have not been placebo-controlled. Regardless of the drugs used, cure rates have been almost always been in the order of 80 per cent.

Of far more importance are data concerning the susceptibility of the causative microorganisms, in particular *E. coli*, especially if these data are derived from populations representive of those found in general practice. One has to bear in mind that susceptibility data may be subject to regional variation, and only data from one's own setting are really reliable. With these limitations in mind, generally speaking, the resistance to older and widely used antibiotics such as sulfonamides and amoxicillin can be as high as 30–40 per cent. The resistance to trimethoprim is still relatively low, but has been growing in recent years, while resistance to nitrofurantoin, in spite of its widespread use, has not increased significantly recently.[8,9]

The susceptibility of uropathogens to cephalosporins or quinolones such as norfloxacin and ofloxacin is high, but these drugs are generally considered to be 'reserve' drugs which should only be prescribed on the basis of the results of culture and sensitivity testing.

The choice of drugs partly depends on whether the patient has an uncomplicated or a complicated urinary tract infection. In an uncomplicated urinary tract infection, blind treatment with the traditional drugs such as nitrofurantoin or trimethoprim may be sufficient initially.

For complicated urinary tract infections, initiation of treatment should be preceded by collection of a urine sample for culture and sensitivity testing. Treatment should preferably be with drugs with good tissue penetration and should be prolonged. For urinary tract infections in children and pregnant women, different regimens apply.

- For an *uncomplicated urinary tract infection in a patient aged 12 years or older*, nitrofurantoin (50 mg four times daily) and trimethoprim (300 mg once daily) are the first-choice drugs, unless the patient is pregnant. Breastfeeding is not a contra-indication. In uncomplicated cases, the duration of treatment is 3 days for women and 7 days for men. Follow-up is not necessary if the symptoms subside. If they do not, the urinalysis should be repeated and if it is positive the other drug of choice should be given. If symptoms still persist then a urine culture and sensitivity test should be carried out and treatment should be based on the results. For a *complicated urinary tract infection in a patient of 12 years or older* as well as for *acute prostatitis*, treatment with an antibiotic which penetrates tissues is desirable, which makes nitrofurantoin less suitable. The preferred agents are amoxicillin/clavulanic acid 500/125 mg three times daily for 10 days, in case of hypersensitivity to amoxicillin to be replaced by co-trimoxazole 960 mg twice daily for 10 days.

- The subsequent course of action is determined by the response to the initial treatment and the results of the culture and sensitivity testing. If the symptoms subside, further check-ups are not necessary.

- For a urinary tract infection in a *child below 12 years of age*, the policy is largely the same as for a complicated urinary tract infection. After urine has been collected for culture and sensitivity testing, the urinary tract infection should be treated with amoxicillin/clavulanic acid for 1 week in doses adjusted to body weight. In children aged 6 months or older with hypersensitivity to amoxicillin, co-trimoxazole is a suitable alternative.

In very young children parenteral treatment may be indicated. The subsequent course of action is determined by the response to the initial treatment and the results of the culture and sensitivity testing. In contrast to complicated urinary tract infections in elderly patients, the urine from children of up to and including 6 years should be checked once per month using a dipslide, to enable prompt treatment if there is evidence of a relapse. In older children, a single check-up is sufficient after the course of treatment has been completed.

◆ After collection of urine for culture and sensitivity testing, treatment for a *pregnant woman* with a urinary tract infection should consist of a 1-week course of nitrofurantoin unless there are contractions, because of the risk to induce haemolytic anaemia in the newborn infant due to its immature enzyme system. In that case nitrofurantoin can be replaced by amoxicillin. After the course has been completed, the urine should be checked using a dipslide. Checks for asymptomatic bacteriuria during the remainder of the pregnancy are not necessary.

Long-term care

Prophylactic treatment

◆ *Prophylaxis* should be considered when the urinary tract infections recur frequently. It has been demonstrated that prophylactic treatment with antibiotics significantly reduces the number of relapses, even in the period after prophylaxis.[10] In sexually active women, prophylaxis immediately after intercourse is often found to be sufficient.[11] There is insufficient evidence to support the use of a drug other than nitrofurantoin or trimethoprim for prophylactic treatment. Prophylaxis should consist of a dose of 50–100 mg nitrofurantoin or 100 mg trimethoprim every evening or post-coitus, for at least 3 months. Prophylaxis should be terminated after a maximum of 12 months.

◆ An alternative to regular prophylaxis consists of *self-administration of a single dose* as soon as the first signs of infection arise.[12]

◆ Whether the use of oestrogens in post-menopausal women contributes to the prevention of recurrences is not clear, because the available studies contradict each other. The efficacy of such treatment appears to be lower than that of antibiotics and might be based primarily on reducing urethral complaints resulting from mucous membrane atrophy.

Referrals

Further investigations and referral are dependent on the patient's age and gender. In particular, in young children and in boys who are not yet sexually mature there is a high probability of underlying abnormalities. Routine investigation of women with recurrent uncomplicated urinary tract infections, on the other hand, is unlikely to be beneficial. It is advisable to refer the following patients:

◆ children upto 1 year of age;

◆ boys upto 12 years of age;

◆ girls aged 1–12 years with one relapse or more;

◆ male patients from 12 years of age onwards with more than one urinary tract infection within a relatively short period of time;

◆ patients with signs of underlying abnormalities such as urine retention in the bladder, kidney or bladder stones, prostatic hyperplasia, prolapsed uterus, and bladder or pelvic tumours;

◆ women with frequently recurring urinary tract infections that do not respond satisfactorily to prophylactic treatment.

Matters of dispute

Research carried out in the 1980s showed that even at 10^2–10^3 bacteria/ml, women could experience symptoms of a urinary tract infection which could not be differentiated from those seen at higher bacteria concentrations and which responded comparably to antibiotic treatment. If the threshold for diagnosis is lowered to 10^2 bacteria/ml, the probability of a urinary tract infection in women with typical symptoms would be 80 per cent. This lower threshold until now has not been generally accepted and the test characteristics of several methods of urinalysis with this gold standard remain unclear.[13]

Screening for the presence of asymptomatic bacteriuria in pregnant women has been recommended in America in particular, but its value is still under debate. Those in favour of screening believe that treatment of asymptomatic bacteriuria not only leads to fewer symptomatic urinary tract infections, but also to fewer premature births and children with low birth weight.

The conviction that detection and treatment of asymptomatic bacteria in pregnant women is valuable because it results in fewer children with a low birth weight and fewer premature births is primarily based on a meta-analysis.[14] However, its reliability is questionable, as it may be distorted by a publication bias in favour of the studies with positive results. Only four of the eight individual trials showed a significant effect of antibiotic treatment. Monthly screening of pregnant women with asymptomatic bacteriuria with the aim of preventing symptomatic urinary tract infections, and particularly pyelonephritis, cannot be recommended, as the benefits are unclear. The amount of infections that can be prevented by such a regimen is not known.

In developed countries, there is a long-standing debate about the question of whether routine circumcision of newborn boys should be recommended. In the United States and Canada, circumcision is common, largely because of cultural habits. Several cohort studies suggest that circumcision can diminish the chance of getting a urinary tract infection by a factor of 5–10. Recent guidelines, however, state that the procedure is not essential to the child's current well-being and that routine circumcision of newborns should not be routinely performed.[15]

It is still unclear whether vesico-urethral reflux in young children needs surgical correction to prevent renal scarring. Medicinal prophylaxis might be equally effective.[16]

Key points

- Urinary tract infections are far more common in women than in men and the incidence increases markedly with age.

- The diagnosis rests on a typical history together with urinalysis which consists of a nitrite test, in negative cases to be followed by a dipslide culture or a microscopic examination of the sediment.

- In uncomplicated cases nitrofurantoin and trimethoprim are the drugs of first choice.

- Investigation of underlying abnormalities responsible for urinary tract infections are generally not necessary.

References

1. Nicolle, L.E. (1997). Asymptomatic bacteriuria in the elderly. *Infectious Disease Clinics of North America* **11**, 647–62.
2. Kemper, K.J. and Avner, E.D. (1992). The case against screening urinalyses for asymptomatic bacteriuria in children. *American Journal of Disease in Children* **146**, 343–6.
3. Dick, P.T. and Feldman, W. (1996). Routine diagnostic imaging for childhood urinary tract infections: a systematic overview. *Journal of Pediatrics* **128**, 15–22.
4. Vernon, S.J., Coulthard, M.G., Lambert, H.J., Keir, M.J., and Matthews, J.N.S. (1997). New renal scarring in children who at age 3 and 4 years had normal scans with dimercaptosuccinic acid: follow up study. *British Medical Journal* **315**, 905–8.

5. Stamm, W.E., Counts, G., Running, K.R., Fihn, S., Turck, M., and Holmes, K.K. (1982). Diagnosis of coliform infection in acutely dysuric women. *New England Journal of Medicine* **307**, 463–8.

6. Hooton, T.M. et al. (1996). A prospective study of risk factors for symptomatic urinary tract infection in young women. *New England Journal of Medicine* **335**, 468–74.

7. Kontiokari, T., Sundqvist, K., Nuutinen, M., Pokka, T., Koskela, M., and Uhari, M. (2001). Randomised trial of cranberry-lingonberry juice and Lactobacillus GG drink for the prevention of urinary tract infections in women. *British Medical Journal* **322**, 1571–3.

8. Trienekens, T., Stobberingh, E., Beckers, F., and Knottnerus, A. (1994). The antibiotic susceptibility patterns of uropathogens isolated from general practice patients in southern Netherlands. *Journal of Antimicrobial Chemotherapy* **33**, 1064–6.

9. Beunders, A.J. (1994). Development of antibacterial resistance: the Dutch experience. *Journal of Antimicrobial Chemotherapy* **33** (Suppl. A), 17–22.

10. Brumfitt, W. and Hamilton-Miller, J.M. (1995). A comparative trial of low dose cefaclor and macrocrystalline nitrofurantoin in the prevention of recurrent urinary tract infection. *Infection* **23**, 98–102.

11. Melekos, M.D., Asbach, H.W., Gerharz, E., Zarakovitis, I.E., Weingaertner, K., and Naber, K.G. (1997). Post-intercourse versus daily ciprofloxacin prophylaxis for recurrent urinary tract infections in premenopausal women. *Journal of Urology* **157**, 935–9.

12. Wong, E.S., McKevitt, M., Running, K., Counts, G.W., Turck, M., and Stamm, W.E. (1985). Management of recurrent urinary tract infections with patient-administered single-dose therapy. *Annals of Internal Medicine* **102**, 302–7.

13. Stamm, W.E. et al. (1980). Causes of the acute urethral syndrome in women. *New England Journal of Medicine* **303**, 409–15.

14. Romero, R., Oyarzun, E., Mazor, M., Sirtori, M., Hobbins, J.C., and Bracken, M. (1989). Meta-analysis of the relationship between asymptomatic bacteriuria and preterm delivery/low birth weight. *Obstetrics and Gynecology* **73**, 576–82.

15. Task Force on Circumcision (1999). Circumcision policy statement. American Academy of Pediatrics. *Pediatrics* **103**, 686–93.

16. Olbing, H. et al. on behalf of the International Reflux Study in Children (1992). Renal scars and parenchymal thinning in children with vesico-ureteral reflux: a 5-year report of the international reflux study in children (European branch). *Journal of Urology* **148**, 1653–6.

Further reading

Practice Guideline on Urinary Tract Infections. Dutch College of General Practitioners, English edition (http://www.artsennet.nl/nhg). A lot of background information and references are presented.

Kunin, C.M. (1987). *Detection, Prevention and Management of Urinary Tract Infections*. An influential monography on urinary tract infections. Philadelphia: Lea & Febiger.

Clinical Evidence. *A Compendium of the Best Available Evidence for Effective Health Care*. London: BMJ Publishing Group, 2000. This book provides up-to-date information about treatment of pyelonephritis in non-pregnant women, recurrent cystitis in non-pregnant women, and urinary tract infections in children.

6.2 Haematuria and proteinuria

Bert Aertgeerts, Frank Buntinx, and Kanwaljit Sandhu

Diseases affecting the kidneys, ureters, and bladder often do not present until they are quite advanced and the discovery of haematuria and/or proteinuria on dipstick testing should prompt further investigation leading to an earlier diagnosis.

Haematuria

Blood in the urine is either readily visible, when it is termed *macroscopic haematuria*, or detected only on dipstick testing, when it is termed *microscopic haematuria*. The dipstick test relies on the reaction between haemoglobin released from lysed erythrocytes and *o*-toluidine, producing a colour change. It will detect as few as 1 erythrocyte per cubic millimetre of unspun urine. The test cannot distinguish between haematuria and haemoglobinuria, so that microscopy of urine is required to enable the distinction to be made. False negative dipstick haematuria occurs in patients taking ascorbic acid and rifampicin. Though macroscopic haematuria is relatively rare, microscopic haematuria is not an uncommon finding, with prevalence estimated to lie between 0.18 and 16.1 per cent.[1] Table 1 lists the major causes of haematuria.

Macroscopic haematuria

Initial haematuria

Blood seen only at the beginning of micturition suggests a lesion at the level of the urethra. There may be a history of trauma; if not a mid-stream urine (MSU) specimen is needed to look for the presence of infection. A referral to a urologist is required for those whom neither cause is found and for all men who have no history of trauma: urethroscopy and further investigation are necessary in looking for other causes such as strictures, tumours, and stones of the urethra.

Terminal haematuria

Blood present at the end of micturition points towards a bleeding point in the prostate or bladder. Symptoms of bladder neck irritation and bladder outflow obstruction should be sought, including increased urinary frequency, hesitancy, urgency, poor stream, and post-micturition dribbling. Infection is the most likely cause and should be confirmed with an MSU. Other causes include bladder tumours and calculi, and prostatic enlargement, either malignant or benign. All females not having a simple urinary tract

Table 1 Causes of haematuria

Kidney	Bladder
Glomerulonephritis	Cystitis
Tubulo-interstitial nephritis	Papilloma
Polycystic kidney disease	Transitional cell carcinoma
Calculi	Calculi
Renal cell carcinoma	Schistosomiasis
Transitional cell carcinoma	
Tuberculosis	*Prostate*
Papillary necrosis	Benign prostatic hypertrophy
Trauma	Carcinoma
Ureter	*Urethra*
Calculi	Trauma
Transitional cell carcinoma	Infection
	Tumour

infection and all men should be referred for further urological assessment, which will initially include cystourethroscopy.

Pan-micturition haematuria

Blood present for the entire duration of micturition suggests bleeding from any point in the urinary tract, from the bladder upwards. Occasionally, the urine can look dark brown if it has been present in the bladder for a prolonged period of time before voiding.

Determination of the bleeding point is helped by the presence of localizing symptoms.

Symptoms of bladder neck irritation and bladder outflow obstruction are often present when the *bladder* is the source of bleeding. *Ureteric bleeding* occurs secondary to stones or transitional cell carcinoma. Stones typically present with renal colic, that is, pain in the distribution from the loin to the groin which is severe, unremitting and lasting for several hours. A tumour may rarely cause mild colic but is otherwise silent. If the patient is unwell with fever, infection secondary to obstruction proximal to the lesion must be considered. Such patients need analgesia and urgent urological assessment with plain abdominal radiography and usually an intravenous urogram (IVU). Calculi less than 5 mm in diameter tend to pass spontaneously whereas larger stones need urological intervention. In those situations where a secondary infection is suspected, not only is it important to institute empirical antibiotic therapy immediately, but there is a much greater urgency to remove the stone(s). Lesions suspicious of malignancy need to be assessed histologically following endoscopic biopsy.

There are a number of *renal* causes of haematuria. The presence of fever and loin pain suggests pyelonephritis and an MSU is necessary to confirm this. Quite often, these patients need parenteral antibiotics and admission to hospital. All males and most females will need further urological assessment, initially with ultrasound imaging of the renal tract, looking for stones or anatomical abnormalities predisposing to infection. Patients from regions of the world where tuberculosis is endemic will need treatment as above initially but a high suspicion for renal tuberculosis is required.

Loin pain and haematuria in the absence of infection may be a manifestation of a cystic kidney disorder and a renal tract ultrasound is the investigation of choice. Autosomal dominant polycystic kidney disease will be associated with a positive family history unless the patient is one of the minority subject to a spontaneous genetic mutation. Assessment of renal function and blood pressure is necessary, as well as referral to a renal physician. More than half will develop renal failure requiring dialysis. It is therefore important to recognize hypertension early, not only to reduce the adverse cardiovascular risk profile but also to delay any decline in renal function. A small number have 'loin-pain haematuria syndrome'. These patients are normotensive and have normal investigations but are troubled so much by their loin pain that they occasionally manage to persuade a urologist to perform an ipsilateral nephrectomy for pain relief.

Macroscopic haematuria occurring at the same time as an upper respiratory tract infection is very suggestive of IgA nephropathy (Berger's disease). This is the most common glomerulopathy worldwide. Defined histologically by the presence of mesangial IgA deposits within the glomerulus, it is interesting in that it has several different clinical phenotypes. It can present with intermittent macroscopic haematuria, persistent microscopic haematuria, slowly deteriorating renal function associated with microscopic haematuria and proteinuria and very rarely as either the nephrotic syndrome or as acute renal failure. As up to 50 per cent of these patients can develop renal failure requiring dialysis, it is important that they are regularly followed up by a nephrologist. Tight control of blood pressure is the mainstay of treatment, especially with ACE inhibition and diuretics if there is significant proteinuria. There are emerging but still controversial data showing that treatment with fish oils[2] and steroids[3] may retard the decline in renal function seen in those with proteinuria.

If the haematuria occurs 2–3 weeks after an upper respiratory tract infection, then the patient most likely has a post-infectious glomerulonephritis. This is now less common in the Western world and is most often associated with group A *Streptococcus* though it can occur following other bacterial infections such as *Staphylococci* and *Shigella*. Proteinuria is nearly always present. The majority will have some reduction of renal function and so it is important to assess blood pressure and renal function; if either is abnormal then an urgent referral to a renal physician is appropriate. All patients should be given a 10-day course of a penicillin, cephalosporin, or erythromycin to eradicate residual infection though there will be no effect on the renal lesion. This condition is often self-limiting resolving within 1–2 weeks. Very occasionally, nephrotic syndrome is seen and very rarely the patient may have acute renal failure requiring dialysis.

Rapidly progressive glomerulonephritis and nephrotic syndrome (i.e. haematuria, hypertension, and impaired renal function) may present with dark urine, hypertension, and features of fluid retention. This very rare scenario can be secondary to Goodpasture's disease, anti-neutrophil cytoplasmic antibodies (ANCA)-associated small vessel vasculitis such as Wegener's granulomatosis, or glomerular immune complex deposition associate with infective endocarditis. These patients need urgent nephrological assessment as to the underlying cause, nearly always dialysis and in the case of the former two aggressive immunosuppression with steroids, cyclophosphamide and sometimes plasma exchange (especially for Goodpasture's disease). These life-threatening illnesses are now associated with a lower mortality but greater morbidity especially from septic complications arising from the use of immunosuppression.

No localizing symptoms

A significant number of patients with haematuria have no localizing symptoms. In these it is initially important to send an MSU to check for infection. In the absence of infection, the process of subsequent investigation must be driven primarily either towards the kidney or lower urinary tract. Urine microscopy, to the skilled observer, may yield red cell casts or dysmorphic red cells or acanthocytes. Acanthocytes are specific for glomerulonephritis and the former two findings are consistent with either glomerulonephritis or tubulo-interstitial nephritis. Where urine microscopy is unreliable or unhelpful, initial investigation should be a renal tract ultrasound with patients under the age of 40 years referred for nephrological assessment and those older for a urological opinion. The age of 40 is generally accepted as a reasonable cut-off above which there is a significant chance of finding malignancy in a patient with haematuria who is otherwise asymptomatic.[4] In a meta-analysis assessing the diagnostic value of macroscopic haematuria for urological cancer, the sensitivity for bladder cancer was 83 per cent, for ureteral cancer 66 per cent, and for renal cancer 48 per cent. In referred patients, the positive predictive value of macroscopic haematuria for urological cancer was 22 per cent for all ages and 41 per cent in patients aged over 40 years.[5]

Many of these young patients with normal renal function and blood pressure will have a minor glomerular disorder such as thin basement membrane disease, which is usually associated with an excellent long-term prognosis.

The presence of hypertension and haematuria should always alert the physician to the possibility of underlying renal pathology necessitating the measurement of creatinine and possible referral to a nephrologist. An ultrasound scan will detect autosomal polycystic kidney disease. In those with a normal scan auto-immune disorders should be sought by direct questioning and testing for anti-nuclear antibodies (ANA) and ANCA.

Anticoagulation

Haematuria in patients who are anticoagulated may be severe enough for them to require hospital admission for resuscitation. Haematuria is very rarely spontaneous: one study found that anticoagulation with warfarin was not associated with an increase in the incidence of haematuria.[6] These patients will require further assessment as would someone with normal clotting.

With a prevalence of 51 per cent (1995) among 11 primary schools (2500 children) in Tanzania, *urinary schistosomiasis* is a common cause of macroscopic and microscopic haematuria in Africa. Nevertheless, one single dose of 40 mg/kg Praziquantel, at the beginning of the school year, decreased the incidence to 23 per cent in 1999. According to the Cochrane review in 1997,

Praziquantel (single dose) appears to be more effective than other drugs, but the reinfection rate remains high.

Special circumstances

Patients with sickle cell disease may have haematuria from papillary necrosis. In those returning from Africa, schistosomiasis and malaria should be considered.

Other causes of red urine

A number of foods and drugs can discolour the urine including beetroot and rifampicin.

Microscopic haematuria

Patients do not complain of microscopic haematuria that is detected fortuitously, as part of a screening examination, or when looked for specifically in certain situations. It is surprisingly common with a prevalence of 38.7 per cent in a cohort of 1000 men aged 18–33 tested yearly over a 15-year period.[7]

If found as part of a screening examination, for example, on registration with a new general practitioner, then the approach should be for macroscopic haematuria as outlined above.

Mild to moderate chronic renal failure (i.e. GFR 90–30 ml/min) is usually asymptomatic and may be detected only after finding microscopic haematuria on screening, often in conjunction with proteinuria. Use of the serum creatinine in the Cockroft–Gault equation[8] (see Table 2) allows an estimate of the glomerular filtration rate to be made and any impairment of renal function confirmed. An ultrasound scan of the kidneys will reveal them to be small, consistent with a chronic scarring process. If renal function is stable then it is paramount that blood pressure be tightly controlled. Unless renal function has been stable for a number of years referral to a nephrologist is advisable.

The other occasions on which microscopic haematuria is sought include severe hypertension (discussed below) or when an auto-immune condition is suspected. In the case of the latter, the patient may present with any one or a combination of symptoms over a period of weeks or months. Symptoms include lethargy, malaise, weight loss, arthralgia, skin rashes, alopecia, mouth ulcers, and uveitis/scleritis. The presence of haematuria confirms the multiorgan nature typical of many auto-immune conditions and should prompt assessment of blood pressure and renal function and measurement of ANA and ANCA, following which an urgent renal opinion should be sought.

Proteinuria

A healthy adult will excrete up to 150 mg protein in the urine during a 24-h period. The majority of this is Tamm–Horsfall protein, though there will be a small amount of albumin and a trace of globulin. Tamm–Horsfall protein is a 200-kDa glycoprotein secreted by the thick ascending limb of the loop of Henle and the distal convoluted tubule into the tubular fluid. Excess proteinuria can occur as a result of damage to the glomerulus (*glomerular* proteinuria), damage to the proximal tubule (*tubular* proteinuria) or when levels of plasma proteins are so high that the tubular reabsorption of these proteins in the filtrate is exceeded (*overflow* proteinuria). Very occasionally a patient will present with frothy urine indicating severe proteinuria (>3 g/day) associated with a glomerulopathy, but the majority of patients do not present with proteinuria, which is detected as part of screening or looked for specifically in certain situations. The dipstick contains acid–base indicators and the pH at which they change colour is lowered by increasing

Table 2 Cockroft–Gault equation

GFR (women) = 1.04 × [140 − creatinie (μM)] × weight (kg)/age (years)
GFR (men) = 1.23 × [140 − creatinine (μM)] × weight (kg)/age (years)

amounts of urinary protein; the detector becomes progressively greener with increasing proteinuria. This test is most sensitive for albumin and is insensitive for low molecular weight proteins, for example, Bence Jones protein. The dipstick urinalysis will detect urinary protein concentrations as low as 150 mg/l as a trace positive. The main causes of proteinuria are given in Table 3.

Screening

The majority of proteinuria is detected as part of an initial consultation with a new general practitioner and may be found in as many as 17 per cent of selected populations.[9] Though it can indicate serious renal disease, proteinuria is also a reflection of the glomerular filter's high sensitivity to 'extra-renal factors'. Hence, vigorous exercise, fever, smoking, heart failure, and changes in posture can all increase the normal physiological proteinuria to levels detectable by dipstick urinalysis. In the healthy normotensive patient the test for proteinuria should be repeated two or three times, looking for persistent proteinuria. Similarly, if the patient had a coincidental infection then the test should be repeated a few weeks later.

Even in the absence of symptoms, in persistent proteinuria a MSU for microscopy and culture is required to exclude urinary tract infection.

A significant number of healthy individuals have 'orthostatic proteinuria', that is, an increase in proteinuria upon standing that is reversed with recumbency. This can be confirmed by detecting proteinuria in a daytime urine but not in an early morning specimen. Orthostatic proteinuria warrants no further assessment.

In cases of persistent proteinuria it is necessary to not only quantify the 24-h urinary protein excretion but also to evaluate blood pressure and renal function and assess renal tract anatomy with an ultrasound scan.

Haematuria and proteinuria

If haematuria is detected at the same time as proteinuria on dipstick urinalysis then the diagnostic approach is similar to that for haematuria.

Nephrotic syndrome

This is a triad of proteinuria (usually >3 g/day), hypoalbuminaemia, and peripheral oedema. The clinical presentation consists of leg swelling with or without frothy urine. Trivial proteinuria (<1 g/day) with leg oedema is consistent with heart failure and clinical features in the history and examination should confirm this. Having established that the patient has nephrotic syndrome it is important to measure the renal function and blood pressure and to refer urgently to a renal physician. Most children with nephrotic syndrome have minimal change nephropathy, which is sensitive to steroid therapy and are started on a trial of steroids, with renal biopsy performed in the 10 per cent or so who do not respond. In adults the common causes are membranous nephropathy, minimal change nephropathy and focal segmental glomerulosclerosis (FSGS). For the nephrologist, the initial

Table 3 Causes of proteinuria

Factors increasing proteinuria
  Exercise
  Fever
  Cigarette smoking
  Heart failure
Urinary tract infection
Orthostatic proteinuria
Nephrotic syndrome
  Diabetes mellitus
  Minimal change nephropathy
  Membranous nephropathy
  Focal segmental glomerulosclerosis
Haematuria associated conditions
Chronic renal impairment

investigation is renal biopsy to determine diagnosis and thence treatment as minimal change nephropathy is often sensitive to steroids whereas there is controversy over their role in FSGS. In those cases where it is not possible to treat the underlying glomerulopathy, medical management rests on tight blood pressure control primarily through ACE inhibition and diuretics, control of hypercholesterolaemia using a statin and anticoagulation if the serum albumin is less than 20 g/l. It is also important to look for conditions which are associated with such glomerulopathies and patients may be assessed for systemic lupus erythematosus, myeloma and hepatitis B or C.

Hypertension and/or impaired renal function

Most patients who appear well with impaired renal function and proteinuria without haematuria will not have acute renal failure secondary to a glomerulonephritis. Instead, they will probably have chronic renal impairment which may be stable or gradually deteriorating over time. The degree of proteinuria as determined by a 24-h urine collection will positively correlate with the rate of decline in GFR. This group of patients benefit from ACE inhibition even if normotensive, and the benefit is greater in those with higher degrees of proteinuria.

The assessment of the hypertensive patient always includes looking for secondary causes of hypertension and the presence of end-organ damage. The intimate role of kidney function in blood pressure control necessitates dipstick urinalysis of all newly diagnosed or increasingly difficult to control hypertensive patients. If proteinuria is present then not only is it important to quantitate the proteinuria but also to evaluate renal function critically through the use of the Cockroft–Gault equation, which will provide an estimation of the GFR.

The serum creatinine can often lie in the normal range despite a significant loss of renal function, especially in the older patient. If the GFR is less than 90 ml/min mild renal impairment is present and there a high risk of further loss of renal function in the presence of both proteinuria and hypertension. The rate of decline of renal function worsens with increasing proteinuria and hypertension. This group of patients needs tight control of blood pressure initially with ACE inhibition and diuretics. ACE inhibitors have been shown to significantly reduce the rate of decline of renal function with the effects more pronounced in those with significant proteinuria (i.e. >3 g/day).[10] It is not uncommon to use at least 3–4 antihypertensive agents. Renal function needs to be monitored frequently and regularly. A low threshold for a nephrological opinion is necessary.

Diabetes mellitus

Patients with either Type 1 or 2 diabetes mellitus are at risk of developing nephropathy, ultimately leading to renal failure requiring dialysis. The initial manifestation of diabetic nephropathy, microalbuminuria, typically occurs 6–15 years after the diagnosis of Type 1 diabetes mellitus. It is defined as a urinary albumin excretion of 30–300 mg/day. It is worth noting that this is below the range detectable with the normal urinary dipstick. For a firm diagnosis of microalbuminuria to be made this level of urinary albumin excretion must be present in two out of three consecutive samples over a 6-month period when the patient is well, without fever, and free of urinary tract infection. The renal function at this stage is normal. This will progress to a stage of increasing proteinuria (overt nephropathy), sometimes leading to nephrotic syndrome, which will be associated with rising blood pressure and a relentless decline in GFR and to renal failure requiring dialysis. A significant proportion of newly diagnosed Type 2 diabetes will already have evidence of nephropathy. (See Chapter on diabetes.)

References

1. Cohen, R.A. and Brown, R.S. (2003). Microscopic haematuria. *New England Journal of Medicine* **348**, 2330–8.
2. Donadio, J.V. et al. (1994). A controlled trial of fish oil in IgA nephropathy. *New England Journal of Medicine* **331**, 1194–9.
3. Pozzi, C. et al. (1999). Corticosteroids in IgA nephropathy. *Lancet* **353**, 883–7.
4. Grossfeld, G.D. et al. (2001). Evaluation of asymptomatic microscopic haematuria in adults: the American Urological Association best practice policy. II. Patient evaluation, cytology, voided markers, imaging, cystoscopy, nephrology evaluation, and follow-up. *Urology* **57**, 604–10.
5. Buntinx, F. and Wauters, H. (1997). The diagnostic value of macroscopic haematuria in diagnosing urological cancers: a meta-analysis. *Family Practice* **14**, 63–8.
6. Culclasure, T.F., Bray, V.J., and Hasbargen, J.A. (1994). The significance of hematuria in the anticoagulated patient. *Archives of Internal Medicine* **154**, 649–52.
7. Froom, P., Froom, J., and Ribak, J. (1997). Asymptomatic microscopic haematuria: is investigation necessary? *Journal of Clinical Epidemiology* **50**, 1197–200.
8. Cockroft, D. and Gault, M.K. (1976). Prediction of creatinine clearance from serum creatinine. *Nephron* **16**, 31–41.
9. Wingo, C.S. and Clapp, W.I. (2000). Proteinuria: potential causes and approach to evaluation. *American Journal of Medical Sciences* **320**, 188–94.
10. The GISEN Group (Gruppo Italiano di Studi Epidemiologici in Nefrologia) (1997). Randomised placebo-controlled trial of effect of ramipril on decline in glomerular filtration rate and risk of terminal renal failure in proteinuric, non-diabetic nephropathy. *Lancet* **349**, 1857–63.

Further reading

Grossfeld, G.D. et al. (2001). Asymptomatic microscopic haematuria in adults: summary of the AUA best practice policy recommendations. *American Family Physician* **63**, 1145–54.

Carroll, M.F. and Temte, J.L. (2000). Proteinuria in adults: a diagnostic approach. *American Family Physician* **62**, 1333–40.

6.3 Acute urinary retention in adults

Joseph L. Chin

Acute urinary retention refers to the unexpected sudden inability to void despite the need and urge to do so. The problem is relatively uncommon in men under 60 years of age but 10 and 30 per cent of men, respectively, in their 70s and 80s will encounter the problem within 5 years.

Aetiology

The causes of urinary retention are: (i) increased outflow resistance from either mechanical or functional/dynamic bladder outlet obstruction; (ii) sudden overstretching of the bladder detrusor muscles; or (iii) interference of the sensory or motor innervation to the bladder. The most common cause of mechanical outflow resistance is benign prostatic hyperplasia (BPH), often with other exacerbating factors. Less common causes are locally advanced prostate cancer, acute prostatitis, prostatic abscess, urethral strictures, and meatal stenosis.

Examples of functional obstruction include increased sphincter tone due to medications (alpha adrenergic agents, antihistamines) and increased anal sphincter tone from pain. Acute overdistention of the bladder leading to weakened detrusor contractions most commonly occurs post-anaesthesia, and postpartum (possibly regional anaesthesia use). It is also associated with excessive alcohol intake and medications such as tricyclics, anticholinergics, and antineoplastic agents (Vinca alkaloids). Neurological problems such as spinal cord compression or injury, cerebral vascular accidents and multiple sclerosis can interfere with bladder sensory or motor innervation at various levels including the cortex, brain stem, spinal cord as well as neuroreceptors in detrusor and bladder outlet areas.

History

Most patients with urinary retention present with significant suprapubic discomfort. One should elicit a history of antecedent symptoms of prostate disorders, provocative events such as recent regional or general anaesthetic, significant alcohol intake, history of recent urinary tract infections, drug intake (especially sympathomimetics, anticholinergics, and antihistamines), recent perineal or anal infection, childbirth, perineal surgery, as well as constipation.

Neurological symptoms such as paresthesia and other sensory or motor deficits should be elicited. In young males, a history of urethral stricture disease as well as sexual habits (especially anal intercourse) should be sought. In young females, gynaecologic trauma, especially rape, incest, as well as difficult childbirth may be a factor. Some patients may give only a history of a slow stream or involuntary dribbling and present with overflow incontinence.

Physical examination

A distended bladder should present as a palpable suprapubic mass. Signs of uraemia should be sought. One should check for inflammation and other abnormalities of the urethral meatus and penis. Careful digital rectal examination is performed to assess prostatic size, contour, consistency, symmetry, and the presence or absence of nodules. Anal sphincter tone and perianal sensation should be noted. Neurological examination, especially motor and sensory function in the lower extremities, should be conducted carefully. In females, pelvic examination is essential, noting uterine and adnexal as well as vaginal abnormalities, including the presence of foreign bodies.

Investigations

Laboratory investigations include urinalysis and urine culture. Serum electrolytes and creatinine should also be measured to assess renal function. Risk of prostate cancer in men can be assessed by measuring prostate specific antigen (PSA) levels—see Chapters 6.10 and 6.11 for more information about this test. A complete blood count showing anaemia might suggest chronicity of the problem. Imaging studies should include renal ultrasonography to assess for hydronephrosis as well as the status of the renal parenchyma, which would be prognostic for renal function recovery. Pelvic ultrasound examination provides information on the bladder as well as any obstructive mass. In patients where a neurological deficit is either likely or evident, neurological consultation is sought. Urgent magnetic resonance imaging of the spinal cord, if available, is most helpful in such situations. Urodynamic studies are also indicated.

Initial management

Time-honoured simple manoeuvres such as turning on a tap and getting in a bathtub of warm water may be tried first although the success rate is usually suboptimal. Urethral catheterization using a 16F or 18F catheter with retention balloon is the first step, regardless of suspected aetiology. Adequate lubrication, preferably with topical anaesthesia, and sustained gentle pressure facilitate the catheter insertion. If resistance is encountered at the bladder neck, a 'coude' catheter can be tried. If meatal stenosis or urethral stricture are the cause of the retention, definitive intervention such as urethral meatotomy or urethral dilatation is necessary. In inexperienced hands, urethral sounds may cause serious damage and should be left to the urologist who may also employ 'filiforms and followers' or may elect to perform flexible cystoscopy, cannulate the urethral lumen and then employ special coaxial urethral dilators. In extenuating circumstances, for patients without prior lower abdominal surgery, an experienced primary care physician may perform suprapubic bladder aspiration (preferably with 14F or 16F plastic 'angiocath' cannulae) and provide temporary relief.

If a pharmacological agent is implicated, the offending agent should be discontinued. One has to decide whether to leave an indwelling catheter with a balloon for a period of time or to use an in-and-out catheterization to decompress the bladder and allow the patient to have a trial of voiding.

Predictors of subsequent voiding function

Over 50 per cent of patients will have recurrent retention within 1 week and close to 70 per cent will have recurrent retention in a year. Several factors help to predict the likelihood of successful resumption of voiding. One key factor is the presence of a clear, provocative event leading to retention, the most common of which is a recent anaesthetic or childbirth. Overt postpartum retention occurs in approximately 5 per cent of vaginal deliveries and is influenced by the duration of the first and second stages of labour and by the use of epidural anaesthesia. The majority of postpartum patients promptly resume spontaneous voiding.

Other favourable prognostic factors include the volume of urine drained being less than 500 ml, and with a trial of voiding, the patient being able to have a flow rate of greater than 5 ml/s and being able to void more than 150 ml. Conversely, the patient will most likely have recurrent retention if there is no provocative event and if greater than 500 ml is drained initially. The patient most likely will require definitive surgical correction if: (i) over 1500 ml is drained; (ii) there is absence of unstable bladder contraction; and (iii) urodynamic studies show an atonic bladder.

If the patient is likely to have recurrent retention, an indwelling catheter should be left in for a few days instead of an in-and-out catheterization only. A longer duration of drainage usually results in a higher likelihood of successful resumption of voiding.

Alternative bladder drainage methods

Alternatives to an indwelling Foley catheter include percutaneous suprapubic cystostomy and intermittent urethral catheterization. Percutaneous insertion of a suprapubic catheter, usually by a urologist, allows uroflowmetry studies and also facilitates a trial of voiding. There is usually less discomfort and less likelihood of infection. A contraindication for percutaneous suprapubic cystostomy is previous lower intra-abdominal surgery because of possible bowel injury. Intermittent catheterization is more labour-intensive and requires specialized care. It has a lower rate of bacteriuria and permits trials of voiding.

Subsequent management

The use of alpha-blockers such as terazosin or tamsolusin improves the chance of successful resumption of voiding. If BPH is the offending condition and the patient has failed a trial of voiding, definitive surgery such as transurethral prostatectomy may be necessary. With successful resumption of voiding following the acute episode, management is directed at prevention of future retention problems. For men with BPH, long-term pharmacological therapy with alpha-blockers and 5-alpha reductase inhibitors (e.g. finasteride) may improve the urine stream, lower post-void residual volumes and may obviate the need for surgery. For those who require urgent surgery because of recurrent or persistent urinary retention, there is a higher risk of peri- and post-operative complications compared to patients who undergo elective transurethral prostatectomy.

Acute urinary retention in children
Definition

The definition is acute retention of a volume of urine greater than the expected bladder capacity for the child [(age in years + 2) × 30 ml]. One should recognize that some children without organic neurologic deficits could withhold urine for up to 18 h.

Aetiology

The most likely causes of acute urinary retention in children are neuro-muscular dysfunction including spina bifida, urinary tract infections such as cystitis, constipation, and drugs such as antihistamines, pseudoephedrine, and neuroleptics. A condition whereby chronic overdistention has resulted in a large 'lazy' bladder is the so-called 'non-neurogenic neurogenic bladder'. Structural causes of retention include posterior urethral valves, bladder diverticuli, urethral polyps, and ureteric orifice stones. Rare aetiologic conditions include tumours such as rhabdomyosarcomas, neurofibromatosis, neuroblastoma, and ependymomas.

The age of presentation is a useful clue for diagnosis. In a newborn, hypermagnesaemia may result if the mother had been given magnesium sulfate for treatment of toxaemia during pregnancy. The babies are usually born with poor muscle tone including poor respiratory effort, flaccid limbs, and urinary retention. In an infant, posterior urethral valves in the male and other congenital conditions such as an ectopic ureterocele in the female are more likely. In the older child, urinary tract infection and spinal dysraphism are more common. There is also a gender difference in the various possible aetiologies for acute retention, with benign bladder outlet obstruction being more prevalent in males and urinary tract infection and constipation being more common in females.

History

The appropriate birth history needs to be elicited along with possible precipitating events, voiding symptoms, bowel problems, and constitutional signs and symptoms. Neurological symptoms including gait abnormalities should be elicited. Although non-organic causes are less common in young children than adults, any history of possible psychological and social trauma should be sought. There may have been prior unpleasant or painful experience from sexual abuse or medical treatment involving the genital area.

Physical examination

Careful examination of the external genitalia should be conducted in both sexes. Attention should be paid to the back and sacral area for evidence of spina bifida occulta such as sacral dimpling and a hairy nevus. The gait should be observed. Digital rectal examination is essential for the anal sphincter tone and possible prostatic and rectal mass. Sensory function at the sacral level needs to be assessed. A distended bladder presenting as a palpable abdominal mass and presence of excessive amounts of stool indicating constipation or obstipation should be noted.

Management

An attempt to induce voiding such as a warm bath and appropriate analgesics may be indicated. Unlike in some adults, 'in-and-out' catheterization will not suffice, as the child most likely will fail to resume voiding. An indwelling urethral catheter and possibly intermittent catheterization are preferable as the initial step. Investigations include urinalysis and culture for bacterial growth. Serum electrolytes including magnesium should be taken. If an adverse drug effect is suspected, the implicated agent is discontinued or substituted and a trial of voiding instituted a few days later. Constipation warrants the use of an enema and improved bowel habits and preventative measures such as stool softeners. The bladder can be retrained with timed-voiding by reminding and encouraging the child to empty his/her bladder every few hours regardless of bladder sensation. The infrequent voider requires similar bladder retraining and behavioural modification. Suspicion of a neurological problem warrants urgent spinal cord imaging and neurological consultation. If an acute urinary tract infection is the cause, intermittent catheterization or an indwelling catheter should be followed by empiric antibiotic therapy. Renal and bladder ultrasonography as well as voiding cystourethrogram may help rule out vesico-ureteral reflux. Cystoscopy is helpful in the diagnosis of obstructive anatomic lesions. If there is a suspicion of malignancy, imaging with computerized tomography or preferably, magnetic resonance of the pelvic area, followed by the appropriate surgical or oncologic consultation, if available, should be sought.

Chronic retention

Signs and symptoms

Patients with chronic retention may be asymptomatic and their condition is brought to light either by some exacerbative factors precipitating acute retention or by presenting with a sequela of chronic retention. Patients may have symptoms of voiding dysfunction including frequency, hesitancy, infrequent voiding, or overflow incontinence.

Underlying conditions may include diabetic neuropathy or other neurologic lesions. Sequelae of chronic retention include impaired renal function, hydroureteronephrosis, vesico-ureteral reflux, recurrent urinary tract infection, bladder stones, and diverticulae. In addition to a distended bladder and high post-void residual volume, one should check for signs of uraemia and for neurological deficits.

Management

Initial management includes for bladder decompression with an indwelling urethral catheter or percutaneous suprapubic catheter. Gradual drainage of the bladder (e.g. only 300 ml every 30 min) is important, in order to avoid sudden decompression which often results in gross haematuria due to disruption of bladder mucosal vessels.

Post-obstructive diuresis

With sudden relief of bilateral chronic renal obstruction, post-obstructive diuresis is a distinct possibility. Excessive loss of fluids and electrolytes may be a serious problem unless adequate hydration is ensured. Aetiologic factors include osmotic diuresis from excess retained solutes, release of excessive fluid, and compromised renal concentrating ability. Vigilant monitoring of blood pressure for postural hypotension with hourly urine output volume and adequate fluid replacement are crucial in the initial resuscitation.

Investigations

Laboratory investigations should include serum creatinine, blood urea nitrogen and in men, PSA levels. For those with elevated serum creatinine, creatinine clearance determination from 24-h urine collections may be useful for more accurate assessment of renal function. Renal ultrasonography will assess for hydroureteronephrosis and renal parenchymal thickness.

Definitive management

Definitive therapy include correction of underlying conditions such as transurethral resection of the prostate for BPH and correction of other obstructive lesions. Rarely, in some patients with a severely hypotonic bladder from chronic overdistention, more drastic surgical measures such as reduction cystoplasty or supravesical urinary diversion may be indicated to improve urine drainage. For those who either do not have a surgically correctible defect or are a poor anaesthetic risk for major urinary tract surgery, options include long-term suprapubic cystostomy drainage and teaching the patient to perform clean (not sterile) intermittent self-catheterization.

Key points

1. Acute urinary retention in adults often involves an underlying condition (e.g. BPH) and a precipitating event/factor (e.g. drugs, pain).

2. Detailed history is important in diagnosing the underlying aetiology and formulating treatment.

Continued

Further reading

Baldew, I.M. and Van Gelderen, H.H. (1983). Urinary retention without organic causes in children. *British Journal of Urology* **55**, 200–2.

Emberton, M. and Anson, K. (1999). Acute urinary retention in men: an age old problem. *British Medical Journal* **318**, 921–5.

Gatti, J.M. et al. (2001). Acute urinary retention in children. *Journal of Urology* **165**, 918–21.

Klarskov, P. et al. (1987). Symptoms and signs predictive of the voiding pattern after acute urinary retention in men. *Scandinavian Journal of Urology and Nephrology* **21**, 23–8.

Peter, J.R. and Steinhardt, G.F. (1993). Acute urinary retention in children. *Pediatric Emergency Care* **9**, 205–7.

Pickard, R., Emberton, M., and Neal, D.E. (1998). The management of men with acute urinary retention. *British Journal of Urology* **81**, 712–20.

Yip, S.K., Brieger, G., Hin, L.Y., and Chung, T. (1997). Urinary retention in the post-partum period. The relationship between obstetric factors and the post-partum post-void residual bladder volume. *Acta Obstetricia et Gynecologica Scandinavica* **76**, 667–72.

6.4 Testicular and scrotal problems

Joseph L. Chin

Overview

Excluding dermatological conditions, testicular and scrotal lesions include hydrocele, hernia, spermatocele, varicocele, tumours, haematocele, and two painful conditions, epididymitis/orchitis and torsion of the spermatic cord ('testicular torsion'). These problems are commonly encountered by primary care physicians. For instance, acute epididymitis is one of the leading causes of disability of men in the military, and had been one of the leading urological diagnoses requiring hospitalization. Testicular torsion affects one in 4000 males under 25 years of age. Varicoceles are rare before puberty, but affect 15 per cent of the adult population. Testicular tumours have variable incidences in different races, but typically afflict young men in the productive years of life.

History and physical

The initial management of scrotal and testicular problems relies heavily on the history and physical examination since the correct diagnosis can often be arrived at without extensive invasive investigations. The patient may have been asymptomatic and the abnormality noted on routine self-examination. Dysuria, microhaematuria, or urethral discharge may suggest epididymo-orchitis. Sudden onset of severe pain would suggest testicular torsion. Any history of trauma and constitutional signs and symptoms should be elicited. 'Referred pain' to the scrotal area from other sites should be kept in mind.

Scrotal and inguinal examination should be conducted in a warm room, both with the patient standing and supine. Attention should be paid to the size of any mass, its location, and its relationship to the normal anatomical structures. Note should be made of the size, shape, consistency, and orientation of *both* testes. The cremasteric reflex should be elicited in cases of painful scrotal masses, since if the reflex is present, testicular torsion unlikely (vide infra). Transillumination of the scrotum should be performed (to assess the presence and nature of fluid collections) with a flashlight placed under the scrotum in a darkened room. Clear fluid collections, as in hydroceles and spermatoceles, should transilluminate as a 'glow' whereas blood and solid lesions will not (vide infra).

Cryptorchidism

An undescended or ectopic testis may have arrested or strayed from the normal descent route. The most common ectopic location is the prepubic area, superficial to the external oblique aponeurosis. Cryptorchid testes, often dysgenetic, are clinically important because of a much higher incidence of malignancy than a normally descended testis, and may also compromise fertility potential. There may be pain with spontaneous torsion in their abnormal location. If a cryptorchid testis is discovered under the age of 5, hormone therapy (human chorionic gonadotrophin) to induce descent is first instituted and if unsuccessful, orchiopexy should be performed. Although the risk of malignancy is not lessened by orchidopexy, the testis in the intrascrotal location would be more amenable to monitoring for malignancy.

Varicocele

A varicocele is the dilation of the pampiniform plexus of spermatic veins, usually occurring on the left side due to difference in gonadal venous drainage between the two sides. This occurs in up to 15 per cent of men and is usually asymptomatic. Some patients complain of a dragging sensation. The typical appearance is that of a bag of worms within the superior aspect of the scrotum. The testis may be atrophic. Although large varicoceles are evident in the supine position, the subtle cases may only be elicited with the patient performing a Valsalva manoeuvre while standing. Presence of a right varicocele should increase the suspicion of possible venous obstruction from retroperitoneal lymphadenopathy (e.g. from lymphoma or testicular cancer) or tumour thrombus within the vena cava, most commonly from renal cell carcinoma.

Varicoceles may be associated with oligospermia and infertility. Possible explanations include venous congestion and unfavourably high temperature for spermatogenesis. Some fertile patients may have large varicoceles, whereas a sub-fertile male does not necessarily have one. Atrophy of the ipsilateral testis is suggestive of an infertility problem. If the varicocele is discovered during infertility work-up, surgical correction to decrease venous back-flow may result in improvement in semen analysis in approximately 60 per cent of cases, with subsequent improved fertility potential. Occasionally, varicocele surgery is performed for severe discomfort from testicular congestion.

Haematocele

A haematocele is a collection of blood between the tunica vaginalis and tunica albuginea. There often is a history of blunt trauma from sports injuries or other physical contact. There usually is significant discomfort with an expanding scrotal mass and possibly bleeding from scrotal skin violation. Haematoceles do not transilluminate. Testicular rupture from high-energy impact should be ruled out by careful examination of the testis, but since the testis is often obscured by haematoma formation, scrotal ultrasound examination (if available) is recommended. Suspected testicular rupture expanding haematoma or penetrating trauma to the scrotum warrant surgical exploration.

Hydrocele

A hydrocele is a fluid collection between the visceral and parietal layers of the tunica vaginalis. The etiology is often idiopathic. However, rapid enlargement would suggest an underlying infectious or malignant process. A hydrocele usually covers the anterior testicular surface and may extend into the spermatic cord area. However, the examining fingers should be able to reach above the swelling as opposed to a hernia where the swelling continues up along the spermatic cord. Careful palpation of the testis and epididymis is important. Hydroceles should transilluminate. If the tense swelling precludes adequate testicular examination, scrotal ultrasound examination, if available, should be performed. Aspiration of the fluid for diagnostic purposes risks bleeding, infection, and possible tumour spillage and is not recommended unless ultrasonography is not available. An asymptomatic 'idiopathic' hydrocele may be treated conservatively with observation. Definitive treatment, if necessary, should be by open surgery to avoid reaccumulation of fluid, which would occur with transcutaneous needle aspiration.

In an infant or child, hydroceles usually indicate patency of the processus vaginalis with communication between the scrotal sac and peritoneal cavity, associated with an indirect inguinal hernia. Typically, these hydroceles fluctuate in size. The parents may notice a sudden increase in the scrotal swelling when the child cries. If the communication has not closed by 1 year of age, surgical repair is recommended.

Spermatocele

A spermatocele is a usually painless spherical cystic mass distinct from the testis, typically arising near the junction of the 'testis proper' and the head of the epididymis. Occasionally, a large spermatocele may mimic a hydrocele or hernia. The whitish fluid of a spermatocele should be transilluminable. Surgical excision can be undertaken if the lesion has become large and causes limitation to physical activities.

Epididymo-orchitis and epididymitis

The main challenge is to distinguish this painful lesion from testicular torsion. Epididymo-orchitis usually occurs in sexually active young men and older men with urinary difficulties. Torsion more commonly occurs in adolescents although there is overlap between the two age distributions. Epididymitis usually presents with gradual onset of pain, often without clear precipitating events. Associated urinary tract symptoms may include dysuria, frequency, and urethral discharge. The epididymis is tender and may be very swollen while the testis is non-tender. In contrast, testicular torsion has a rock-hard consistency and has a horizontal lie. Although relief of pain with scrotal elevation has been described as a sign suggestive of epididymitis and conversely aggravation of pain as suggestive of torsion, this ('Prehn's') sign is considered unreliable. Urinalysis and smear of urethral discharge are useful diagnostically. If one cannot clinically differentiate with reasonable certainty between the two, Doppler scrotal ultrasound (if available) is helpful. In torsion, there should be no flow in the affected testis whereas there is high flow from inflammation in epididymo-orchitis. Nuclear scintigraphy (scrotal scan) is a more labour-intensive alternative in assessing blood flow. Testicular torsion is a urological emergency (see below). With epididymitis, the recommended treatment includes antibiotics (see Chapter 6.6) and avoidance of strenuous physical activities. In some countries, tuberculosis infections may involve the epididymis and testis, often presenting as draining sinuses or scrotal abscesses.

Testicular torsion

Testicular torsion is associated with abrupt onset of pain typically affecting pre-pubescent or adolescent boys although adults may also be afflicted. There may have been previous episodes which settled spontaneously. The testis lies horizontally, instead of vertically, due to a developmental anatomic deficiency in anchoring to the inferior scrotum. The defect is often bilateral. The 'freely hanging' testis is prone to rotate on its axis, either spontaneously or with provocation, 'twisting' the cord and becoming elevated. Venous flow is obstructed first with ongoing arterial inflow, engorging the testis. Eventually arterial flow ceases. Testicular infarction results if blood flow is not re-established within 6–8 h. The presence of the cremasteric reflex indicates that there is *no* torsion. The diagnostic challenge of a painful non-traumatic scrotal mass is to distinguish between testicular torsion and epididymitis (vide supra). If testicular torsion is suspected, urgent exploration is imperative. If confirmatory imaging studies are not available in equivocal cases, surgical exploration is indicated.

One may attempt manual de-torsion prior to surgical exploration. With the examiner standing on the supine patient's right side facing him cephalad, the left testis is manually turned clockwise and the right testis counter-clockwise. Even with successful de-torsion, subsequent formal bilateral orchidopexy to prevent future recurrences is indicated.

Torsion of testicular appendages

A vestigial remnant of the Wolffian or Mullerian duct may suddenly infarct with torsion, usually in a child. This pea-sized lesion presents as a discrete tender spot near the epididymal head or tail. In fair-skinned children, a blue dot indicating haemorrhagic engorgement of the lesion may be evident. This condition can be treated conservatively. However, in the absence of definite clinical signs and when the diagnosis is uncertain, surgical exploration is indicated to rule out testicular torsion.

Testicular tumours in adolescents and adults

Testicular cancer, most commonly germ cell tumour (GCT), comprises only 1 per cent of all malignancies in males, with a peak incidence at between 20–35 years of age. It is, apart from lymphoma, the most common malignancy at that age group in Caucasians. Overall incidence in Europe and North America is approximately five per 100 000 males. The condition is uncommon in Asians and rare in African races.

The most commonly accepted predisposing factor is cryptorchidism. GCTs are classified as seminomas and non-seminomas (embryonal cell carcinoma, yolk cell tumour, teratomas, and choriocarcinoma).

Clinical presentation

The most common presentation is an asymptomatic painless hard testicular mass. It may also be associated with a hydrocele. Patients occasionally present with systemic symptoms from metastatic disease. The first site of lymph node involvement is in the renal hilar area (presenting as an abdominal mass), subsequently spreading to iliac, mediastinal, and cervical nodes. The cancer also disseminates haematogenously to lungs and less commonly, liver and brain. Thus, patients may present first with pulmonary symptoms or a chest X-ray showing lung nodules and pleural effusions.

Physical examination

Neck, chest, abdomen, and both testes should be examined carefully keeping in mind potential ectopic testicular locations. If a hydrocele precludes adequate testicular examination, scrotal ultrasound examination (if available) should be performed rather than needle aspiration.

Investigations

Initial investigations should include baseline blood serum markers [alpha feto-protein (*a*FP) and beta human chorionic gonadotrophins (*b*HCG)] and chest X-ray. Elevated markers strongly suggest a diagnosis of germ cell tumour (seminoma or non-seminomas). However, normal markers do not preclude the possibility of a GCT. Seminomas do not have elevated *a*FP and rarely may have abnormal *b*HCG. Serum markers are invaluable for monitoring disease progress and response to treatment. Other useful markers include lactate dehydrogenase (LDH) and placenta-like alkaline phosphatase.

Management

Any suspicious testicular masses should be explored through an inguinal incision (not scrotal) with early control of the spermatic cord, to minimize possible tumour dissemination. Radical orchidectomy involves dividing the spermatic cord high at the internal inguinal ring area. Subsequent management is determined by: (i) tumour cell type; and (ii) stages of disease. Staging studies include computerized tomography of the abdomen and chest (if available). Seminomas are more radiosensitive than non-seminomas and both are chemosensitive. Management includes treatment of possible retroperitoneal lymph node involvement (even with a normal CT scan and serum tumour markers) and treatment of metastatic disease. Options include close surveillance, radiotherapy, retroperitoneal lymph node dissection, chemotherapy, or combinations thereof, depending on cell type and stage. The prognosis is favourable with expected 5 year survival of 99 per cent for tumours confined to the testis, 95 per cent for tumours with limited metastatic retroperitoneal disease, and 75–80 per cent for widespread distant metastatic disease. The main challenge is to minimize the treatment-related morbidity without compromising the therapeutic effect.

Testicular tumours in children

The majority of childhood testicular tumours occur under 2 years of age and comprise only 1 per cent of childhood neoplasms, 75 per cent of which are malignant. Most are GCTs, but a smaller percentage are stromal tumours, gonadoblastoma, leukaemia, and lymphoma infiltrates. GCTs, mostly yolk sac tumours, account for about 60–70 per cent. Leydig cell tumours are relatively common with typical presentation of precocious puberty and gynaecomastia. Yolk sac tumours have a more favourable prognosis if diagnosed and treated at less than 1 year of age. In many instances, radical orchidectomy with follow-up suffices. In more advanced cases, chemotherapy, radiation, and retroperitoneal lymph node dissection are also performed.

Paratesticular tumours

A solid non-tender mass in the epididymis suggests a neoplastic process when epididymitis has been ruled out. Adenomatoid tumours are the most common, benign paratesticular tumours being most prevalent in ages 30–40 and are solid, spheroid masses, which are usually asymptomatic. Confirmation of the epididymal location can be made on ultrasound examination. Treatment is by local excision (epididymectomy).

Other common paratesticular neoplasms include sarcomas, most commonly rhabdomyosarcoma. Often, there is a delay in seeking medical attention, with the lesions being mistaken for hernias and hydroceles. One has to be suspicious of gradually enlarging painless scrotal swellings, especially if the presentation is atypical for a benign entity. Rhabdomyosarcomas disseminate lymphatogenously and haematogenously, involving lymph nodes, lungs, and liver.

Key points

- Detailed history and physical examination is crucial.
- Surgical exploration is mandatory for suspected torsion.
- Tumours are often asymptomatic hard masses.

Further reading

Berger, R.E., Kessler, D., and Holmes, K.K. (1987). The etiology and manifestations of epididymitis in young men: correlation with sexual orientation. *Journal of Infectious Diseases* 155, 1341–4.

Berger, R.E. (1998). Sexually transmitted diseases: the classic diseases. In *Campbell's Urology* 7th edn. (ed. P. Walsh, A. Retik, E.D. Vaughan, and A. Wein), pp. 663–79. Philadelphia PA: WB Saunders.

Bomalaski, D.M., Garver, K., and Bloom, D.A. (1995). Assessment of testicular torsion. In *Topics in Clinical Urology: New Diagnostic Tests* (ed. M. Resnick). New York: Igaku-Shoin Medical Publishers.

Caesar, R.E. and Caplan, G.W. (1994). Incidence of the valve clapper deformity in an autopsy series. *Urology* 44, 114–16.

Chin, J. (2000). Recent developments in the management of testicular germ cell tumors. *Canadian Journal of Urology* 7(4), 1060–5.

Dresner, M. (1973). Torsed appendage: blue dot sign. *Urology* 1, 63–4.

Mostafi, F.K. (1973). Testicular tumours: epidemiologic, etiologic and pathologic features. *Cancer* 32, 1186–90.

6.5 Genital ulcers and warts
David Portnoy

Genital ulcers are frequent manifestations of sexually transmitted diseases and the annual worldwide incidence of genital ulcer disease probably exceeds 20 million cases. In North America and in most developed nations, the most frequent cause is herpes followed by syphilis and to a much lesser extent chancroid, which, in the United States, is frequently associated with prostitution and crack cocaine abuse. In other parts of the world such as Southeast Asia, India, Africa, and South America, chancroid, lymphogranuloma venereum, and granuloma inguinale are common occurences. Genital ulcers may be associated with other illnesses such as Crohn's disease, Behcet's syndrome, malignancy, or simply induced by trauma. Individuals with genital ulcers have an increased risk of acquiring or transmitting HIV infection. A diagnosis based on the appearance of the lesion or clinical history is often erroneous, and consequently all patients with genital ulcers should undergo testing for syphilis, herpes, and if warrented, chancroid.

Chancroid

Chancroid is caused by a gram negative bacillus, *Haemophilus ducreyi*. The incubation period is usually 3–7 days but may be up to several weeks. The initial lesion, an inflammatory papule or pustule with surrounding erythema, erodes to form a deep non-indurated painful ulcer with ragged undermined margins and a friable base covered with a purulent exudate. Males usually have single lesions while women often have multiple lesions via autoinoculation often with opposing ulcerations (kissing lesions). Female carriers may be asymptomatic with no detectable lesions. Within 1 week, a unilateral tender inguinal adenopathy develops in 50 per cent of patients which if left untreated may suppurate (bubo formation) and rupture spontaneously. It is estimated that 10 per cent of individuals with chancroid may be co-infected with herpes or syphilis.

Diagnosis

A definitive diagnosis of chancroid requires isolation of the organism using selectively enriched chocolate-based agar or a polymerase chain reaction assay which are not always available. A presumptive diagnosis is usually based on the exclusion of both syphilis and herpes in conjunction with a painful ulcer and tender inguinal adenopathy.

Treatment

Azithromycin 1 g orally in a single dose; ceftriaxone 250 mg IM in a single dose; ciprofloxacin 500 mg orally twice a day for 3 days; or erythromycin base 500 mg orally four times daily for 1 week.

Several isolates with intermediate resistance to either ciprofloxacin or erythromycin have been reported worldwide.

Patients with a fluctuant node not resolving with antibiotic therapy may require needle aspiration or incision and drainage of the bubo.

All recent sexual contacts of patients with chancroid, even those who are asymptomatic, should be notified and treated as well.

Lymphogranuloma venereum

Lymphogranuloma venereum (LGV) is a sexually transmitted disease caused by *Chlamydia trachomatis* serovars L1, L2, and L3, which are different strains from those causing chlamydial urethritis. Although LGV occurs worldwide, it is endemic in Africa, India, Southeast Asia, South America, and parts of the Caribbean but rare and sporadic elsewhere. In parts of India and Africa, it can account for 2–10 per cent of genital ulcers.

The primary lesion follows an incubation period of 3–40 days and consists of a painless papule or vesicular lesion which may ulcerate, but heals within a few days without scarring. This primary lesion goes unnoticed in the majority of patients. With penile or vulvar lesions, the bacteria spread via the regional lymphatics to the inguinal and femoral nodes, to the hypogastric and deep iliac nodes following rectal infection and to the obturator and iliac nodes with cervical lesions. This secondary or inguinal stage occurs 1–4 weeks after the primary lesion and results in a painful lymphadenopathy along with systemic symptoms such as fever, chills, headache, myalgia, and arthralgia. Other infrequent complications include meningitis, arthritis, and hepatitis. The painful nodes may suppurate and rupture, resulting in fistulas which may continue to drain for months. Inguinal involvent is the most frequent finding and 10–20 per cent of patients manifest the 'groove sign' consisting of enlarged inguinal nodes above and femoral nodes below Poupart's ligament. This is suggestive but not specific for LGV. Individuals who engage in receptive anal intercourse may develop proctitis, proctocolitis, fistulas, and rectal strictures. Progressive tissue destruction and extensive scarring may result in genital elephantiasis in both sexes.

Diagnosis

Growth of the organism in cell culture is diagnostic but recovery rates are 50 per cent at best. The diagnosis is usually based on clinical findings, excluding other causes of inguinal adenopathy, along with a complement fixation titre of greater than 1:64. Cross-reactions occur with other chlamydial infections but titres are usually less than 1:16.

Treatment

Doxycycline 100 mg orally twice daily for 21 days; or erythromycin base 500 mg orally four times daily for 21 days. Recent sexual contacts should be examined and treated as well.

Granuloma inguinale (donovanosis)

Granuloma inguinale is a chronic, progressively destructive, sexually transmitted disease caused by *Calymmatibacterium granulomatis*, a pleomorphic intracellular gram negative bacterium. The disease is endemic in India, southern Africa, parts of South America, the Caribbean, Papua New Guinea, and amongst aborigines in central Australia.

The incubation period is usually 1–4 weeks but may be several months or more. Single or multiple subcutaneous nodules or papules appear. These enlarge and erode through the skin resulting in painless ulcers with a friable 'beefy red' granulomatous, non-purulent base, and raised rolled margins. The lesions enlarge by direct extension or may spread by autoinoculation on opposing skin surfaces (kissing lesions). Less common variants of the disease include hypertrophic wart like lesions, a necrotic variant, with a foul smelling exudate that is rapidly destructive, and sclerotic or cicatricial ulcerated lesions with bandlike scarring and associated lymphoedema. Non-sexual, extragenital transmission can also occur via fingers, or by direct contact with infected lesions or infected secretions. Haematogenous dissemination to bone and viscera can also occur.

Diagnosis

The diagnosis is essentially clinical but may be confirmed by punch biopsy, scrapings or a crush preparation of the lesion stained with Giemsa, Leishman's, or Wright's stain to demonstrate the presence of Donovan bodies. These are pleomorphic organisms, often encapsulated with bipolar (safety pin) staining within large mononuclear cells.

Treatment

Trimethoprim-sulfamethoxazole one double strength tablet orally twice daily; doxycycline 100 mg orally twice daily; ciprofloxacin 750 mg orally twice daily; or erythromycin base 500 mg orally four times daily. All the above antibiotics are administered for a minimum of 3 weeks or until all the lesions have healed. If there is no response after several days of treatment, combination therapy with an aminoglycoside should be considered. Relapses within 6–18 months may occur after effective treatment. Contacts should be examined and treated only if lesions are present.

Syphilis

Syphilis is a chronic, systemic sexually transmitted disease caused by the spirochete *Treponema pallidum*. According to WHO global estimates, in 1995 12.2 million cases of syphilis were reported worldwide. The highest incidence was in South and Southeast Asia (5.79 million), Sub-Saharan Africa (3.53 million), followed by Latin America and the Carribean (1.26 million). In the United States, 7500 cases of primary and secondary syphilis were reported to the Centers for Disease Control (CDC) in 1998 where the use of crack cocaine along with prostitution have been major contributing factors. Syphilis should be considered in patients with genital ulcers especially those who have had sexual contacts in highly endemic areas (e.g. Southeast Asia, Russian Federation, Eastern Europe, etc.).

Treponema pallidum may penetrate intact mucous membranes and through minor epithelial abrasions. Most cases of syphilis are transmitted through sexual and occasionally non-sexual contact with infected mucocutaneous lesions associated with the primary and secondary stages of the disease.

The primary chancre, a non-tender ulcer, occurs at the inoculation site about 3 weeks after exposure (range 10–90 days) and is associated with regional non-suppurative, non-tender lymphadenopathy. Without treatment, the chancre heals within 3–6 weeks, but the lymphadenopathy can persist for several months. Secondary syphilis (generalized dissemination) occurs 3–6 weeks after the onset of the chancre, but the two stages may overlap. Constitutional symptoms may include fever, sore throat, malaise, anorexia, weight loss, headache, arthralgia, and generalized lymphadenopathy. Dermatologic manifestations include macular, papular and pustular rashes, condyloma lata, ulcers, mucous patches, and alopecia aerata. Other findings include aseptic meningitis, anterior uveitis, iritis, glomerulonephritis, gastritis, and periostitis. These manifestations resolve spontaneously but may recur in 25 per cent of patients with latent syphilis usually during the first year, although occasionally during the first 5 years. The USCDC defines latent syphilis acquired during the the first year of infection as early latent syphilis and all other cases as late latent syphilis. This latent (asymptomatic) phase may last indefinitely. Without treatment, one-third of patients develop tertiary syphilis which includes neurosyphilis, cardio-vascular syphilis, and gummatous syphilis. The discussion of syphilis in this chapter is limited to the diagnosis and management of the primary stage.

Diagnosis

The diagnosis of primary and secondary syphilis can be made by dark-field microscopy or direct fluorescent antibody testing of serum obtained from the lesions. The serologic tests for syphilis consist of the non-treponemal antibody tests which measure IgG and IgM antibodies to lipoidal material from damaged host cells or from the *T. pallidum* as well as specific treponemal tests. Examples of non-treponemal antibody tests include: venereal disease research laboratory (VDRL), rapid plasma reagin (RPR), automated reagin screen test (ART), and toludine red unheated serum test (TRUST). Specific treponemal antibody tests include; fluorescent treponemal antibody absorbed (FTA-ABS), microhaemagglutination assay for antibody to *T. pallidum* (MHA-TP), and the haemagglutination treponemal tests for syphilis (HATTS). False positive non-treponemal tests can occur with other spirichete diseases, pregnancy, old age, connective tissue disorders, intravenous drug use, chronic liver disease, and various other infections but the titres usually are low (less than 1 : 8). False negative results can be seen in the primary, latent and tertiary disease, and consequently a negative or positive non-treponemal antibody test requires confirmation with a specific treponemal antibody test. All patients with syphilis require follow-up non-treponemal serology testing post-treatment (e.g. 3, 6, 12, and 24 months after treatment) until an adequate response is achieved (steady decrease in titre to negative or stabilization at a low level).

Lumbar puncture and CSF examination is not recommended for early syphilis except when neurologic or opthalmic involvement is suspected.

Treatment

Patients who have acquired syphilis during the preceeding year (primary, early latent) are treated with benzathine penicillin G 2.4 million units IM in a single dose (1.2 million units in each buttock). Non-pregnant patients with a penicillin allergy should receive doxycycline 100 mg twice daily or tetracycline 500 mg four times daily for 2 weeks. Most experts suggest that HIV-infected patients with early syphilis should receive benzathine penicillin G 2.4 million units weekly for 3 weeks.

Pregnant women should receive penicillin treatment appropriate for their stage of disease and those with a penicillin allergy should be desensitized. If skin testing and desensitization is not possible and erythromycin is used, the newborn infant should be treated for presumed congenital syphilis.

Herpes simplex

Herpes simplex virus (HSV-1, HSV-2) are large enveloped DNA viruses that are usually associated with oral and genital lesions. Oral lesions are almost always due to HSV-1 and up to 90 per cent of adults have antibodies to HSV-1. Genital ulcers are usually caused by HSV-2 but up to a third of genital infections are due to HSV-1. Genital infection with HSV-1 usually occurs in seronegative individuals and is unusual in individuals previously infected with HSV-2. The seroprevalence of HSV-2 in the general population in the United States is about 20 per cent, but in selected groups such as inner city residents, gay men, prostitutes, cocaine abusers, those with multiple sexual partners, and HIV-positive individuals, the seroprevalence rates are much higher. Similarly, in developing countries such as Haiti, Peru, Zaire, and Senegal the seroprevalence in selected populations often exceeds 80 per cent.

Genital infections may be symptomatic or asymptomatic and are classified as:

♦ primary infection (no antibodies to HSV-1 or HSV-2);

♦ non-primary first episode (pre-existing antibodies to the other serotype);

♦ recurrent (pre-existing antibodies to the same serotype).

The severity of the infection is usually diminished by the presence of pre-existing antibodies, so that non-primary or recurrent infections tend to be milder than the primary infection. In a study of heterosexual couples, transmission was more likely to occur with the male (16.9 per cent) rather than the female (3.8 per cent) as the source partner. In 70 per cent of the patients, transmission occurred during periods of asymptomatic viral shedding. Asymptomatic shedding is more common during the first 6 months following primary infection, immediately prior to and following a symptomatic recurrence but can occur anytime. Recurrences and asymptomatic shedding in genital herpes are more frequent with HSV-2 than HSV-1.

Primary infection with HSV usually follows an incubation period of 2–21 days and is often accompanied by systemic symptoms such as fever, malaise, headache, myalgias, and tender inguinal adenopathy. Complications include aseptic meningitis and autonomic nervous dysfunction with urinary retention (occurs more frequently with HSV proctitis). The lesions may be macular, vesicular, pustular, or painful ulcers which form crusts and gradually heal within 1–2 weeks. The genital lesions occur on the penis and perianal region in men and in women may involve the labia, vulva, cervix, perineum, and perianal regions but can occur elsewhere. Recurrent episodes tend to be milder, resolve more rapidly and may be preceeded by a prodrome of itching, burning, or tingling sensations that can last from several hours to 1–2 days before the lesions appear. Initiation of antiviral treatment at the onset of the prodrome may abort the attack.

Diagnosis

Culture remains the preferred method because of its sensitivity, specificity and because it allows for strain typing (e.g. DFA). Antigen detection methods (EIA, DFA, IFA) have lower a sensitivity (50–90 per cent) and specificity (65–90 per cent) when compared to standard culture (sensitivity and specificity approaching 100 per cent). Strain typing may have prognostic importance regarding recurrences and for counselling purposes regarding partner susceptibility.

Treatment

Treatment should be initiated as early as possible following the onset of signs and symptoms.

First episode

Acyclovir 400 mg orally three times daily for 5–10 days; valcyclovir 500–1000 mg orally twice daily for 5–10 days; or famciclovir 250 mg orally three times daily for 5–10 days.

Recurrent episodes

Acyclovir 400 mg orally three times daily for 5 days; valcyclovir 500 mg orally twice daily for 5 days; or famciclovir 125 mg orally twice daily for 5 days.

Suppressive therapy

Chronic suppressive therapy should be considered in individuals with six or more recurrences per year. Suppressive therapy reduces the frequency of recurrences (>75 per cent) and reduces but does not eliminate asymptomatic viral shedding. Interruption of therapy at yearly intervals should be discussed with the patient to reassess the frequency of episodes since they may decrease over time in many patients.

Chronic suppressive regimes include acyclovir 400 mg orally twice daily; famciclovir 250 mg orally twice daily; or valcyclovir 500 mg orally once daily or 250 mg orally twice daily.

Pregnancy

Although the safety of acyclovir use during pregnancy has not been established, Glaxo-Wellcome registry findings have not shown an increased risk for major birth defects when inadvertent acyclovir use during pregnancy was compared with the general population. While the routine use of acyclovir during pregnancy is not recommended, most experts would recommend the use of acyclovir in primary genital herpes or serious maternal infection such as HSV encephalitis, pneumonitis, hepatitis or disseminated disease. Some investigators have also reported on the use of suppressive antepartum acyclovir therapy in women with frequently recurring genital herpes in preventing symptomatic recurrences and the need for caesarean section.

Genital warts

Of the more than 80 human papillomavirus (HPV) genotypes identified about 20 are spread through sexual contact. Up to 20–40 per cent of sexually active adults are infected although most have sub-clinical infection. About 90 per cent of genital warts are caused by HPV 6 and 11. They are usually visible and occur on the penis, scrotum, vulva, perineum, perianal, and pubic region but also involve the cervix, vagina, and urethra. These HPV types are considered 'low risk' because they are rarely associated with cancer. Other types especially HPV 16 and 18 are considered 'high risk' because of their association with cervical dysplasia and anogenital cancer.

The incubation period for external genital warts is usually 3–4 months but ranges between 4–6 weeks and 2 years. Genital warts can appear as condylomata acuminata (cauliflower shaped) or as papular (dome shaped), keratotic (thick, horny) and flat (macular). Condyloma acuminata usually involve moist surfaces, keratotic and papular appear on keratinized epithelium, while flat warts often involve both.

Genital warts are contagious and are spread during oral, vaginal, and anal intercourse. Approximately two-thirds of individuals who have sexual contact with an infected partner will develop this disease. Non-sexual transmission of HPV can occasionally occur. HPV 1–4 , commonly found on the hands, have been associated with anogenital warts in young children. The child (or the parent) via a finger wart may inadvertently infect the oral or anogenital region. Transmission among children may also occur during sexual play. HPV DNA has also been detected on the fingers of some individuals with genital warts. Although transmission of genital HPV may occasionally occur via fingers, most infections involve direct genital to genital contact. Perinatal transmission of HPV occurs infrequently and can result in respiratory papillomatosis and anogenital warts in the infant or young child. Since the incubation period of genital HPV is usually several months, genital warts especially in a child more than 2 years old may suggest sexual abuse and warrants further investigation.

Diagnosis

Exophytic anogenital warts are usually diagnosed by direct visual examination. Bright light and a hand lens with or without the use of aceto-whitening may facilitate in the diagnosis of smaller lesions especially flat warts. The use of 3–5 per cent acetic acid soaks, however, are not specific for HPV and this procedure has a high false positive rate especially in low-risk populations. HPV DNA testing and typing (PCR, hybrid capture assay) is not useful for external genital warts nor is it recommended as a means of screening for subclinical cervical infection. Cervical cytology cellular changes (ASCUS. LSIL) attributed to HPV frequently regress spontaneously but the usefullness of HPV typing in triaging these women is currently unknown.

Treatment

HPV is frequently present in clinically and histologically normal cutaneous epithelium adjacent to warts as well as other sites. Left untreated, these warts may resolve spontaneously, remain unchanged or proliferate. The removal of visible warts does not always prevent infectivity or subsequent recurrences, consequently no therapy can guarantee a cure of HPV infection. Most sexual partners of infected patients probably have sub-clinical infection but may benefit from examination to exclude the presence of visible warts, other sexually transmitted diseases and possibly counselling.

Most treatments have comparable efficacy and treatment of external warts can be administered by either the patient or provider.

Patient-applied treatment

Podifilox 0.5 per cent solution or gel applied twice daily for 3 days, then 4 days without treatment for four cycles.

Imiquimod 5 per cent cream applied three times a week and removed with soap and water 6–10 h after application for up to 16 weeks.

The use of imiquimod, podifilox, and podophyllin are contra-indicated in pregnancy.

Provider-applied treatment

Cryotherapy with liquid nitrogen or cryoprobe applied weekly.

Podophyllin 10–25 per cent in compound tincture of benzoin applied once a week for up to 6 weeks and washed off after 1–4 h for up to 6 weeks.

Trichloroacetic acid (TCA) 80–90 per cent applied weekly if necessary and excess acid neutralized with talc or sodium bicarbonate (baking soda).

Other treatments include: carbon dioxide laser therapy, electroexcision and fulgaration, surgery, subcutaneous or intralesional interferon, topical or intralesional 5-fluorouracil, and topical cidofovir.

Key points

- In most developed nations, the most frequent cause of genital ulcers is herpes followed by syphilis and to a lesser extent, chancroid. In other parts of the world, chancroid, lymphogranuloma venereum, and granuloma inguinale are common.

- A diagnosis based on the appearance of the lesion or clinical history is often erroneous, and consequently patients with genital ulcers should undergo testing for syphilis, herpes, and if warrented, chancroid.

- Up to a third of genital herpes infection is caused by HSV-1 and is unusual in individuals previously infected with HSV-2.

- In 70% of patients transmission of HSV occurs during periods of asymptomatic viral shedding.

- About 90% of genital warts are caused by HPV 6 and 11. They are considered low risk and are rarely associated with cancer.

- The incubation period for external genital warts varies between 3–4 weeks and 2 years, but is usually 3–4 months.

References

1. Mertz, G.J. et al. (1992). Risk factors for the sexual transmission of genital herpes. *Annals of Internal Medicine* **116**, 197–202.

2. Centers for Disease Control and Prevention—St Louis, M.E. and Workowski, K.I. (1999). 1998 Guidelines for the treatment of sexually transmitted diseases. *Clinical Infectious Diseases* **28** (Suppl. 1), S1–89.

3. Centers for Disease Control and Prevention. *1998 Guidelines for Treatment of Sexually Transmitted Diseases*. MMWR 1998 47(No. RR-1), 1998.

4. Hook, E.W. and Marra, C.M. (1992). Acquired syphilis in adults. *New England Journal of Medicine* **326** (16), 1060–7.

5. Beutner, K.R. et al. (1998). External genital warts: Report of the American Medical Association Consensus Conference. *Clinical Infectious Diseases* **27**, 796–806.

6. Tyring, S. et al. (1997). Perspectives on human papillomavirus infection. *American Journal of Medicine* **102** (Suppl. 5A), 1–43.

7. Mandell, G.L., Bennett, J.E., and Dolin, R., ed. *Principles and Practice of Infectious Diseases* 5th edn. New York: Churchill Livingston, 2000.

6.6 Gonorrhoea and chlamydial infections

David Portnoy

Gonorrhoea

Neisseria gonorrhoeae is a non-motile Gram negative diplococcus that primarily infects columnar and cuboidal epithelial cells. Over 600 000 new cases of *N. gonorrhoeae* are reported annually in the United States and an estimated 62 million cases worldwide, with about half occuring in Southeast Asia and a third in Sub-Saharan Africa. The incubation period for gonorrhoea is usually 2–5 days but may vary between 1 and 14 days. It is estimated that a male, following a single episode of vaginal intercourse with an infected female, will become infected 20–25 per cent of the time and that the infection rate increases to 60–80 per cent after multiple exposures. The risk of transmission from an infected male to a female after a single encounter is estimated at 80–90 per cent. Once infected, 80 per cent of women and 10 per cent of men may remain asymptomatic and serve as the major reservoir for further spread of this disease. Anorectal gonococcal infection occurs frequently in homosexual men and in up to 44 per cent of women with positive cervical cultures. Anorectal infection in women is acquired either by penile–anal contact or via infected vaginal secretions. Pharyngeal infection occur in 10–20 per cent of women, in 7 per cent heterosexual males, and in 25 per cent of homosexual men. It is acquired more efficiently by fellatio than by cunnilingus and may remain asymptomatic 98 per cent of the time but occasionally it can result in a sore throat or exudative pharyngitis. In approximately half of the patients with pharyngeal gonorrhoea, the throat is the only positive culture site. Gonococcal conjunctivitis in adults usually is the result of autoinoculation from an infected genital site.

Signs and symptoms

Urogenital infections in men

Acute urethritis is the most common manifestation. There is usually a purulent urethral discharge, dysuria, and a burning or itching sensation along the urethra. Acute epididymitis occurs in less than 10 per cent of infections and presents with unilateral scrotal pain and swelling.

Urogenital infections in women

Most women are asymptomatic. Cervicitis and a purulent endocervical discharge may be seen on pelvic examination and there may be vaginal discharge, dysuria, and intermenstrual bleeding. Infection of Bartholin's gland will result in unilateral labial swelling and pain. Upward spread of the infection from the cervix occurs in 10–20 per cent of untreated women usually at the end of or in the the first few days after menstruation and can result in endometritis, salpyngitis, tubo-ovarian abscess, or pelvic peritonitis. Extension of the infection along the paravertebral gutters or by lymphatic or haematogenous dissemination, can result in gonococcal perihepatitis which presents clinically as severe right upper abdominal pain, liver tenderness on examination and occasionally with a hepatic friction rub (Fitz–Hugh–Curtis syndrome). Pelvic inflammatory disease (PID) is manifested by lower abdominal pain, cervical motion tenderness, and adnexal discomfort on palpation. Other findings may include cervical discharge, bleeding, fever, leukocytosis, or right upper quadrant pain if perihepatitis is present. However, the sensitivity and specificity of the clinical signs are low and the presence or absence of *N. gonorrhoeae* from cervical cultures does not necessarily establish *N. gonorrhoeae* as a cause of PID or exclude the presence of other organisms such as *Chlamydia trachomatis*.

Infection in pregnancy

Gonorrhoea in pregnancy may have any of the above manifestations and is associated with spontaneous abortion, early rupture of foetal membranes, premature labour, and perinatal infant mortality.

Ocular infection

Gonococcal infection in the newborn (opthalmia neonatorum) results in a purulent conjunctivitis usually within 4 days after birth and if left untreated can rapidly progress to corneal ulceration with subsequent corneal scarring and blindness. Prior to the introduction of silver nitrate prophylaxis, this infection occurred in 10 per cent of infants born in the United States. In the adult, it can cause a purulent conjunctivitis that can result in corneal ulceration.

Pharyngeal and anorectal infection

Pharyngeal and anorectal gonococcal infections occur in both men and women and are usually asymptomatic. They can result in a pharyngitis with cervical adenitis or a proctitis with tenesmus, anal pruritis, purulent discharge, or rectal bleeding.

Disseminated gonococcal infection

Disseminated gonococcal infection (DGI) occurs in 0.5–3 per cent of infected individuals with a female to male predominance of 4 : 1. The majority of women with DGI develop symptoms during pregnancy or within 7 days of the onset of menstruation. Patients usually present with a dermatitis–arthritis syndrome or a monoarticular septic arthritis involving mostly the knees, ankles, or wrists. The dermatitis–arthritis syndrome is characterized by fever, skin lesions (papular, pustular, petechial, or necrotic), tenosynovitis, polyarthralgias, and arthritis and should not be confused with Reiter's syndrome. Other rare complications of haematogenous dissemination include Fitz–Hugh–Curtis syndrome, endocarditis, and meningitis.

Diagnosis

The laboratory diagnosis is based on the identification of *N. gonorrhoeae* at the infected site by culture or non-culture tests. Culture is the ideal method since it allows for sensitivity testing but non-culture methods may be preferred when delays in transportation or a lack of laboratory facilities may be an issue. When performed by trained personnel, the Gram stain is considered positive if Gram negative diplococci are observed within the cytoplasm of polymorphonuclear leucocytes. In urethral specimens from symptomatic men, the sensitivity and specificity can approximate 95–100 per cent but the sensitivity decreases to 40–60 per cent from endocervical specimens.

The Gram smear may be utilized for blood, skin lesions, or joint fluid in suspected systemic infections but should not be performed on rectal, conjunctival, or pharyngeal samples since this may result in confusion with other organisms. Non-culture tests include enzyme immunoassay, direct fluorescence microscopy, non-amplified DNA probe tests, and DNA amplification tests by polymerase chain reaction (PCR) or ligase chain reaction (LCR). Both the LCR and PCR tests have been shown to be very sensitive with urine specimens as well. For medico-legal purposes, a positive result obtained by an amplified nucleic acid test should be confirmed with a different set of primers or by culture. PCR and LCR can detect both *N. gonorrhoeae* and *C. trichomatis* from a single specimen. Non-amplified nucleic acid tests are not recommended for medico-legal purposes since they may yield false positive results in low-prevalence groups (populations with less than 5 per cent infected).

Treatment

The treatment of gonorrhoea has changed significantly since the introduction of sulfonamides in 1937. Sulfonamide resistance rapidly emerged and penicillin resistance has steadily increased since its introduction in the early 1940s. This resistance to penicillin is both plasmid and chromosomal mediated. In 1975, gonococcal strains completely resistant to penicillin were isolated. They were found to contain plasmids that coded for the production of beta lactamase (penicillinase producing *N. gonorrhoeae*—PPNG). In 1985, tetracycline-resistant strains of *N. gonorrhoeae* (TRNG) were isolated and in the late 1980s, strains with reduced susceptibility to the fluoroquinolones were isolated as well. Although most gonococci in the United States are susceptible to doxycycline and the quinolones, TRNG and QRNG levels are significant and increasing in other parts of the world such as the Asian and Western Pacific countries. Consequently, these drugs should not be used where resistance may be most prevalent.

Treatment guidelines for Neisseria gonorrhoeae

Treatment recommendations may vary from country to country depending on patterns of resistance.

Uncomplicated infections of the cervix, urethra, and rectum

Cefixime 400 mg orally in a single dose; ciprofloxacin 500 mg orally in a single dose; or ofloxacin 400 mg orally in a single dose; (azithromycin 2 g orally in a single dose is not recommended since it may cause gastrointestinal upset); or ceftriaxone 125 mg IM in a single dose or doxycycline 100 mg orally twice daily for 1 week.

Uncomplicated infections of the pharynx

Ciprofloxacin 500 mg orally in a single dose; ofloxacin 400 mg orally in a single dose; or ceftriaxone 125 mg IM in a single dose or doxycycline 100 mg orally twice daily for 1 week.

Conjunctivitis

Ceftriaxone 1 g IM in a single dose.

Disseminated gonococcal infection

Ceftriaxone 1 g IV every 24 h; cefotaxime 1 g IV every 8 h; or ceftizoxime 1 g IV every 8 h; ciprofloxacin 500 mg IV every 12 h; or ofloxacin 400 mg IV every 12 h; followed by oral therapy with cefixime 400 mg orally twice daily; ciprofloxacin 500 mg orally twice daily; or ofloxacin 400 mg orally twice daily or if the organism is susceptible, doxycycline 100 mg orally twice daily to complete 1 week of treatment.

Patients treated for *N. gonorrhoeae* may be co-infected with *C. trachomatis*. This has resulted in the recommendation that all patients treated for gonorrhoea should also receive empiric treatment for uncomplicated genital chlamydial infection especially where chlamydia tests are not routinely available or where patient follow-up is in doubt.

Pelvic inflammatory disease

Since the cause of PID is often polymicrobial and the specific pathogen usually unknown, treatment recommendations are discussed below under chlamydia.

Chlamydia

The genus *Chlamydia* contains three species that infect humans: *C. psittaci*, *C. pneumoniae*, and *C. trachomatis*. *Chlamydia trachomatis* infections are the most common cause of sexually transmitted disease (STD) in the United States. According to WHO annual estimates, there were approximately 89 million adult chlamydial infections worldwide of which 40 million occured in South and Southeast Asia, 15 million in Sub-Saharan Africa, and 4 million in North America. *Chlamydia trachomatis* is the most common STD in the United States and occurs most frequently in women between the ages of 15 and 24 years and in men less than 25 years old. Unlike gonorrhoea, more than 50 per cent of men and 70 per cent of women may be asymptomatic and are diagnosed as a result of routine STD screening or because a partner was symptomatic. The incubation period for symptomatic chlamydial urethritis is usually between 7 and 14 days but may be as long as 4–6 weeks, in contrast to gonococcal urethritis which usually is several days. Co-infection with gonorrhoeae may occur in up to 20–40 per cent of patients and chlamydia is the cause of 25–50 per cent of men with non-specific urethritis (NSU). Other possible causes of NSU include *Ureaplasma urealyticum*, *Mycoplasma genitalium*, *Trichomonas vaginalis*,

Herpes simplex virus and possibly on occasion, other organisms such as *Moraxella catarrhalis*, *Haemophilus influenzae*, *N. meningitidis*, or *Gardnerella vaginalis*.

Clinical manifestations

Urogenital infections in men

Chlamydia urethritis accounts for between 25 and 50 per cent of cases of NSU and is manifested by dysuria and usually a clear or whitish discharge. Chlamydia is the major cause of epididymitis in sexually active heterosexual men younger than 35 years of age and accounts for 50 per cent of the estimated 500 000 cases occuring annually in the United States. Patients often present with unilateral scrotal pain and swelling, epididymal tenderness, and fever. Coliforms are the major pathogens in the older age group and is usually associated with urinary tract infection, instrumentation, or by rectal intercourse. The role of chlamydia in prostatitis remains speculative.

Urogenital infection in women

The majority of women with chlamydial endocervical infection usually are asymptomatic. Occasionally, there is a mucopurulent cervicitis with a vaginal discharge or bleeding as well as an acute urethral syndrome with dysuria and frequency. Chlamydia may also cause bartholinitis. Ascending infection to the endometrium and fallopian tubes can result in endometritis, salpingitis, and pelvic peritonitis. *Chlamydia trachomatis* has been identified in the fallopian tubes of up to 50 per cent of patients with PID. The spectrum of disease may range from 'silent salpingitis' to overt infection with cervical motion tenderness, adnexal tenderness and lower abdominal pain and occasionally perihepatitis (Fitzhugh–Curtis syndrome). Major sequelae include chronic pelvic pain, infertility, and ectopic pregnancy.

Other manifestations in adults include proctitis, conjunctivitis as well as Reiter's syndrome.

Perinatal infections include inclusion conjunctivitis which usually occurs within 2 weeks of birth and pneumonia between the fourth and 11th weeks following delivery.

Diagnosis

Chlamydiae are obligate intracellular organisms that cannot grow on artificial media but require a susceptible tissue culture cell line for growth. Although it is more specific than non-culture methods, cultures have largely been replaced by tests which do not require viable organisms, allowing for easy transportation and faster results. These tests include antigen detection testing by direct fluorescent antibody assay (DFA) and antigen testing by enzyme-linked immunoabsorbent assay (ELISA). The sensitivity of these tests is greater than 70 per cent and the specificity is in the range of 97–99 per cent. False positive results can be a problem in low-prevalence groups (populations with less than 5 per cent infected). Nucleic acid hybridization tests have sensitivity and specificity rates similar to the above tests but are less sensitive than amplified nucleic acid tests such as PCR and LCR tests which are more sensitive and have a specificity of 98–100 per cent compared to culture. These results are adequate for medico-legal purposes when confirmed using a different set of primers. Both *C. trachomatis* and *N. gonorrhoeae* can be detected with a single swab or urine specimen. Because asymptomatic infection is frequent, sexually active adolescents and young adults less than 25 years should have annual testing. Individuals with new or multiple sexual partners especially those who inconsistently use barrier contraceptives should be tested as well.

Treatment

Uncomplicated infections of the urethra or cervix

Azithromycin 1 g orally in a single dose; doxycycline 100 mg orally twice daily for 1 week; erythromycin base 500 mg orally four times daily for 1 week; or ofloxacin 300 mg orally twice daily for 1 week.

Pregnancy

Doxycycline and ofloxacin are contra-indicated: erythromycin base (not erythromycin estolate) 500 mg orally four times daily for 7 days; amoxicillin 500 mg orally three times daily for 1 week; or azithromycin 1 g orally in a single dose.

Partners

Treating only the index case results in a high rate of re-infection, therefore, partners need to be informed and treated as well.

Pelvic inflammatory disease

Because a negative endocervical culture does not exclude an upper reproductive tract infection and since PID often is polymicrobial, treatment regimens should always provide coverage for both *N. gonorrhoeae* and *C. trachomatis* as well as anaerobes and other organisms such as *Escherichia coli* and streptococci.

Inpatient treatment

Parenteral regimens include cefoxitin 2 g IV every 6 h or cefotetan 2 g IV every 12 h plus doxycycline 100 mg IV or orally every 12 h; clindamycin 900 mg IV every 8 h plus gentamycin 1.5 mg/kg every 8 h (treatment should be continued for at least 48 h after substantial clinical improvement has occurred) followed by doxycycline 100 mg orally twice daily to complete 14 days of treatment.

Alternative parenteral regimens include: ofloxacin 400 mg IV every 12 h plus metronidazole 500 mg IV every 8 h; ampicillin-sulbactam 3 g IV every 6 h plus doxycycline 100 mg IV or orally every 12 h; ciprofloxacin 200 mg IV every 12 h plus doxycycline 100 mg IV or orally plus metronidazole 500 mg IV every 8 h.

Outpatient treatment

Ofloxacin 400 mg orally twice daily for 14 days plus metronidazole 500 mg orally twice daily for 14 days; cefoxitin 2 g IM plus probenecid 1 g PO in a single dose or ceftriaxone 250 mg IM or other third-generation parenteral cephalosporin (cefotaxime, ceftizoxime) plus doxycycline 100 mg orally twice daily for 14 days.

Epididymitis

Epididymitis most likely due to C. trichomatis or N. gonorrhoeae
Ceftriaxone 250 mg IM or cefixime 800 mg orally once plus doxycycline 100 mg orally twice daily for 10 days.

Epididymitis most likely due to enteric organisms
Ofloxacin 300 mg orally twice daily for 10 days.

Sexual partners of patients with PID and epididymitis should receive appropriate treatment and to avoid sexual intercourse until all parties are cured.

Key points

- Once infected, 80% of women and 10% of men with gonorrhoeae may remain asymptomatic.
- Pharyngeal and anorectal gonococcal infections occur in both men and women and are usually asymptomatic.
- The incubation period for symptomatic chlamydial urethritis is usually between 7 and 14 days but may be as long as 4–6 weeks, in contrast to gonococcal urethritis which usually is several days.
- All recent sex partners (within 2 months) should be referred for evaluation and treatment.
- Since PID is often polymicrobial, treatment regimens should provide coverage for both gonorrhoeae and chlamydia as well as anaerobes and other organisms.

Further reading

Centers for Disease Control and Prevention. *1998 Guidelines for Treatment of Sexually Transmitted Diseases.* MMWR 1998, 47 (No. RR-1), 1998.

Burstein, G.R. and Zenilman, J.M. (1999). Nongonococcal urethritis—a new paradigm. 1998 Guidelines for the treatment of sexually transmitted diseases. *Clinical Infectious Diseases* 28 (Suppl. 1), S66–73.

Mandell, G.L., Bennett, J.E., and Dolin, R., ed. *Principles and Practice of Infectious Diseases* 5th edn. New York: Churchill Livingston, 2000.

Holmes, K.K. et al., ed. *Sexually Transmitted Diseases* 3rd edn. New York: McGraw Hill, 1999.

Gerbase, A.C., Rowley, J.T., and Mertens, T.E. (1998). Global epidemiology of sexually transmitted diseases. *Lancet* 351 (Suppl. 3), 2–4.

6.7 HIV/AIDS

Michael Richard Kidd and Ronald McCoy

Epidemiology, prevalence, incidence, and natural history

Acquired immune deficiency syndrome (AIDS) is caused by a virus, human immunodeficiency virus (HIV), which was first isolated in 1983. The origins of AIDS remain obscure, but it is known that HIV occurred in the 1950s in isolated individuals. Widespread infection rates began in the mid-to late 1970s but, because of the long incubation period, the virus did not cause widespread disease until the 1980s. By the 1990s, AIDS had reached epidemic proportions in many countries.

The World Health Organization (WHO) has estimated that by the end of 1999, 34.3 million people were living with HIV worldwide, with 24.5 million living in Sub-Saharan Africa, the hardest hit region. It is estimated that during 1999, 5.4 million people (including 620 000 children below 15 years of age) became infected. AIDS has now become the main cause of death in parts of Africa and is responsible for the majority of adult hospital admissions in some cities. Death rates from the HIV epidemic are now starting to reverse recent gains in infant mortality in many developing countries. Many AIDS patients are never diagnosed, and their deaths may be attributed to other causes.

However, most people with HIV infection in developed countries are well. In the industrialized countries of North America, Western Europe, and the Pacific Region, the availability of effective antiretroviral therapy since 1996 has continued to reduce progression to AIDS, deaths and mother-to-child transmission of HIV. In most countries in these regions, however, the number of new HIV infections has remained relatively constant since 1996.

An understanding of the natural history of HIV infection is the key to diagnosis and treatment. The characteristic effect of unchecked HIV replication is a progressive decline in CD4 lymphocyte numbers. Together, CD4 count and viral replication are the two strongest predictors of possible clinical manifestations of HIV infection (Table 1).

HIV replication is measured by viral load assay and is the best predictor of disease progression and response to antiretroviral therapy. The routine monitoring of viral load involves measuring the level of HIV-RNA copies in the plasma using polymerase chain reaction technology. After an initial burst of uncontrolled viral replication at the time of infection with HIV, when viral load levels can be very high (>100 000 cells/μl), the plasma viral load drops to a generally steady level for many years. This is called the 'set

Table 1 Natural history and clinical stages of HIV infection in adults

Clinical stages	Common clinical features	Viral load	CD4 count
Seroconversion illness (self-limiting up to 1–3 weeks duration)	Fever, headache (may have aseptic meningitis), sore throat, maculopapular rash, lymphadenopathy, splenomegaly, atypical lymphocytes on FBE	Initial uncontrolled viral replication (>100 000 cells/µl not uncommon) followed by drop to generally steady level ('set point')	Transient decrease, commonly followed by a return to almost normal levels
Asymptomatic	Persistent generalized lymphadenopathy		Gradual decrease of 50–80 cells/µl each year
Symptomatic Early	Oral and vaginal candidiasis, oral hairy leukoplakia, seborrhoeic dermatitis, psoriasis, multidermatomal or recurrent varicella–zoster infection, cervical dysplasia, unexplained fever, sweats, weight loss, diarrhoea tuberculosis		Usually 150–500 cells/µl NB: tuberculosis can appear towards the upper end of this CD4 count range
Late	*Pneumocystis carinii* pneumonia, Kaposi's sarcoma, oesophageal candidiasis, cerebral toxoplasmosis, lymphoma, HIV-associated dementia complex, cryptococcal meningitis		Usually <150 cells/µl
Advanced	Cytomegalovirus (CMV) retinitis, cerebral lymphoma, *Mycobacterium avium* complex (MAC) infection		Usually <50 cells/µl

Table 2 Examples of AIDS-defining conditions

Candidiasis (oesophagus)

Cryptococcus (extrapulmonary)

Cervical carcinoma (invasive)

Cryptosporidiosis with diarrhoea >1 month

Cytomegalovirus of retina, brain, spinal cord, GI tract

Herpes simplex chronic ulceration >1 month

HIV-related encephalopathy

HIV-associated wasting syndrome

Isosporiasis chronic intestinal with diarrhoea >1 month

Kaposi's sarcoma

Lymphoma, primary of brain or non-Hodgkin's (B-cell or immunoblastic)

Mycobacterium avium complex or *M. kansasii* (disseminated)

Mycobacterium tuberculosis disseminated or pulmonary

Pneumocystis carinii pneumonia

Pneumonia (recurrent bacterial)

Progressive multifocal leukoencephalopathy

Salmonella septicaemia (recurrent)

Toxoplasmosis (brain)

Source: Centers for Disease Control. 1993 Revised classification system for HIV infection and expanded surveillance case definition for AIDS among adolescents and adults. MMWR 1992, 41 (No. RR-17). *See also:* Centers for Disease Control. 1994 Revised classification system for human immunodeficiency virus infection in children less than 13 years of age. MMWR 1994, 43 (No. RR-12).

point'. This level varies between people and may reflect the degree of immune system control of viral replication.

A fall in viral load levels after initiation of antiretroviral treatments is associated with improved survival. A rise in viral load is associated with disease progression and antiretroviral resistance in patients on these treatments. Increases in viral load can predict disease progression prior to any decline in CD4 counts. The progressive depletion of plasma CD4 lymphocyte numbers due to ongoing viral replication increases the risk of developing opportunistic infections (Table 2).

Most HIV-infected adults with a CD4 count of 500 cells/µl or above are asymptomatic, while a CD4 count below 200 cells/µl indicates severe immunodeficiency with a high risk of developing serious, life-threatening opportunistic infections, that is, AIDS. Between these two levels, less serious conditions are common, although they can still have a dramatic impact on an individual's quality of life. The major exception to this is the development of tuberculosis which can occur around 450 CD4 cells per microlitre.

The mean rate of CD4 decline is around 50–80 cells/µl per year in untreated patients with approximately 50 per cent of untreated patients progressing to AIDS in 10 years. This rate may be faster in people in some countries due to additional burdens of opportunistic infections and malnutrition. As a decline in CD4 counts represents immune system damage, viral load monitoring, and early antiretroviral treatment, where available, aim to prevent this decline and subsequent complications of HIV disease.

Most opportunistic infections are reactivations of dormant co-infections resulting in a pattern of opportunistic infections reflecting local prevalence of endemic infections. Tuberculosis is a common first presentation of HIV infection-related immune decline in endemic areas. However, it is rare in countries where tuberculosis is uncommon. Clinicians need to familiarize themselves with unique patterns of opportunistic infections in their region.

How common is HIV infection in primary care?

HIV infection causes multisystem disease lasting for several years. Most people with HIV infection at any one time are well, living productive lives for most of the course of the infection and able to receive most of their treatment in an ambulatory care setting. These features make primary care the ideal site for HIV disease management with appropriate referral for specialist services or hospital admission when complications arise.

The model of primary care management depends largely on the availability of investigations and treatment resources, in particular, antiretroviral drugs. The introduction of new antiretroviral treatments at the end of the twentieth century dramatically improved the survival and quality of life for many people with HIV infection, as well as producing a reduction in the risk of vertical transmission from mother to child.

The availability of increasingly effective treatments has resulted in a primary care model of early intervention which includes regular monitoring, early diagnosis, disease prophylaxis, and treatment of intercurrent illness.

Where antiretroviral access has been limited, mainly due to cost, but also for political and social reasons, treatment has been largely symptomatic, treating each complication of HIV infection as it arises. However, even when antiretroviral medications are unavailable, there are often cheap, simple, and effective measures that can improve the survival and quality of life of people with HIV. These simple health promotion interventions not only benefit the person with HIV, but also often have important public health implications for the community, such as the prevention of spread of tuberculosis.

Some primary care clinicians may not see many patients with HIV, but clinicians still need to be familiar with the range of possible presentations, as they would for any other serious condition, to enable early diagnosis and appropriate treatment. Even in parts of the world where HIV infection is less common, clinicians need to aim to detect high-risk practices among their patient populations and to intervene to help reduce the risk of HIV transmission, including the prevention of vertical transmission as a routine part of antenatal care.

In high-prevalence regions and sub-populations, some primary care clinicians have become highly experienced in the management of HIV infection and run primary care treatment services accepting referrals from other primary care clinicians. General practitioners in these clinics may offer a full range of HIV treatment services including the prescription of antiretroviral medications and offering a convenient alternative to hospital outpatient visits, which can be time-consuming and difficult to attend for patients who are working and leading active healthy lifestyles.

As in many chronic conditions, even a small number of HIV cases can require significant time, material and human resources compared to other primary care conditions. Clinicians caring for many HIV-infected patients need to ensure that their own health and stress levels are monitored.

Risk factors for HIV infection

The manifestations of HIV disease are protean, although most cases of HIV infection seen in primary care at any one time are asymptomatic. A history of high-risk behaviours or other potential exposures and the presence of characteristic clinical manifestations alert the clinician to the potential presence of HIV infection. Some patients, however, may not disclose past high-risk behaviours, often for fear of discrimination. Others may present for testing with no apparent risks. Others will present requesting post-exposure prophylaxis with antiretroviral medications after an exposure to HIV. Health care workers in high HIV prevalence areas may also be at risk.

Screening and testing of asymptomatic populations, especially pregnant women, becomes increasingly important in areas with high HIV prevalence.

Diagnosis

The diagnosis of HIV infection is different from many primary care conditions because of the potential for discrimination related to fear of infection and because of the association of HIV infection with stigmatized behaviours.

Patients need to have a risk assessment history for the detection of past possible exposures to HIV infection and to be examined for possible clinical manifestations.

Investigations

HIV infection is usually diagnosed by the detection of HIV antibodies in the plasma. These usually appear within 2–3 weeks after exposure, but may take up to 2 months. Current recommendations indicate that if HIV antibodies are not detected within 3 months after exposure, then HIV infection is unlikely to develop.

Plasma is first screened for HIV antibodies using an ELISA assay, and infection is then confirmed by Western blot.

Patients presenting with suspected acute primary HIV infection, or sero-conversion illness (Table 1), may not have developed antibodies at the time of presentation and diagnosis may require testing for HIV viral antigens including the p24 viral antigen. These patients then require repeat HIV

antibody testing over the next 3 months to confirm the presence or absence of HIV antibodies.

AIDS is diagnosed by the presence of an AIDS-defining illness (Table 2). The diagnosis of AIDS is usually more important for statistical purposes than for clinician management. Governments, insurance companies, and other funding bodies may have different funding arrangements for those with AIDS as opposed to HIV infection. Patients are treated for the AIDS-defining illness and immunodeficiency, and not for AIDS.

Pre-test HIV antibody counselling

Informed consent is necessary prior to testing for HIV antibodies to minimize the psychosocial impact of testing. Clinicians need to ensure that patients are adequately informed of the risks and benefits of HIV antibody testing so that they have sufficient information to make an informed decision about being tested. Patients need to be informed about the local HIV reporting requirements and the degree of confidentiality and privacy that they are entitled to receive. They also need to be aware of the potential risk of discrimination from family, friends, employment, housing, and other sources. Pre-test counselling is also an opportunity to further educate the patient to reduce the risk of future HIV transmission.

Post-test HIV antibody counselling

The initial reaction of patients receiving a diagnosis of HIV infection is usually shock and disbelief, and they may hear little of any information given to them by the clinician. Patients often retain little information from the consultation where the HIV diagnosis was given, and information from this session should be reviewed at the next consultation.

Specialist referral

The primary care management of HIV varies between countries. There are international differences about which medical specialties provide care for people with HIV. People with HIV in many developing countries may not have access to any specialist HIV treatment services.

Principles of management

The medical management of HIV is complex, although it follows many of the general principles of primary care. Prevention and education are essential to reduce the risk of transmission. Counselling is required both pre- and post-test and psychological support is required throughout the course of the illness. Early diagnosis is important to stage the disease and to guide the clinician and patient towards appropriate treatment options. Initial assessment and monitoring of immune function, and prevention and early detection of opportunistic infections, form the mainstay of continuing care. An ability to diagnosis the cause of medical emergencies in HIV infection is essential as prompt treatment of conditions such as acute *Pneumocystis carinii* pneumonia can be life-saving. Skills at palliative care for patients at the end of life are also essential.

The management of HIV infection is changing rapidly and clinicians need to keep up to date. Many education programmes available on the Internet and some are listed in the 'Further reading' section at the end of this chapter. The introduction of protease inhibitors in 1996 has led to a dramatic reduction in deaths from HIV infection in many developed countries. These benefits are yet to be seen in many of the developing nations of the world.

Initial assessment of people with HIV requires a full general assessment of their medical history, including their sexual history and drug and alcohol history. Full psychosocial assessment is required. Physical examination needs to include weight, oral and dental health, assessment of skin and general systems, as well as sexual health review with pelvic and/or anogenital review.

Baseline screening for infections is important. This includes a Mantoux test for tuberculosis, and serology for toxoplasma, cytomegalovirus, syphilis, and hepatitis A, B, and C. Vaccination history is required and vaccination should be provided for hepatitis A and B. Live vaccines are contra-indicated in HIV infection. The role of immunization for influenza and pneumococcal disease in people with HIV is currently controversial.

Baseline blood tests for CD4 count and HIV viral load, full blood count, renal and liver function, fasting glucose, cholesterol, and triglyceride are required. Cervical cytology is required for women at risk of cervical dysplasia.

Long-term and continuing care

People with HIV require regular clinical review. This includes a regular targeted review of possible symptoms, general physical monitoring and blood tests, as well as assessment of psychosocial function and the opportunity for patient education and health promotion. Additional monitoring is required for people taking antiretroviral medications and will be targeted towards the prevention and/or early detection of side-effects related to the specific regimen. Adherence monitoring and support is also required by people taking antiretrovirals. Compliance with antiretrovirals is critical for treatment success to prevent the emergence of viral resistance to treatments.

People with HIV are also at risk of the common conditions that affect all people in their community and require regular assessment, for example, of cardiovascular risk factors as well as appropriate screening for serious diseases, such as breast cancer and diabetes.

People with HIV are at risk of depression and HIV-related dementia and should be screened regularly for these conditions. Regular dental checks are advisable. Ophthalmological assessment is essential in all people with a CD4 count less than 100 due to the risk of cytomegalovirus (CMV) retinitis. Good nutrition has important long-term implications for survival, but is now also important due to some of the possible adverse effects of antiretroviral treatments such as chronic diarrhoea and lipodystrophy syndrome.

Prophylaxis is required by individuals depending on their immune status (e.g. the use of co-trimoxazole to prevent *P. carinii* pneumonia in people with a CD4 count <200).

There are many common conditions which can affect people with HIV and many of these are well managed in primary care. Examples include oral candidiasis, bacterial pneumonia, diarrhoea, skin infections, and sexually transmitted diseases.

Knowledge of the individual's current immune status (CD4 count and viral load) is essential in aiding diagnosis when people present with worrying symptoms. Clinicians need to be aware of the possible presenting features of a wide range of opportunistic infections and malignancies affecting people with advanced HIV infection. Patients with more severe immunodeficiency are more likely to require urgent review when they develop worrying symptoms and signs. These include increasing shortness of breath (possible *P. carinii* pneumonia), chronic cough and haemoptysis (tuberculosis or bacterial pneumonia), neurological symptoms such as paraesthesia (cerebral toxoplasmosis), eye problems such as blurred vision or visual field deficits (CMV retinitis), and loss of weight and night sweats (*Mycobacteria avium* infection or lymphoma).

Knowledge is also required of the potential side-effects of the antiretroviral medications being taken by each individual, some of which can also be life-threatening (e.g. pancreatitis with didanosine, hypersensitivity reaction with abacavir, and severe hepatitis or Stevens–Johnson syndrome with nevirapine).

Palliative care in primary care includes knowledge of the management of pain, as well as treatment of common symptoms such as diarrhoea, nausea and vomiting, peripheral neuropathy, headaches, skin problems, and insomnia.

Even in developing countries without access to antiretroviral medications or expensive investigations, basic advice can be provided to help boost the immune system or to allow early detection and treatment of clinical problems. This includes advice about a healthy diet, dental care, personal hygiene, and food preparation. Vaccinations against serious infections and screening for tuberculosis and cervical dysplasia may be available. Education to reduce the risk of transmission can be provided. Treatment for worm infestations, candidiasis, *P. carinii* pneumonia, toxoplasmosis, and turberculosis may be available.

Some of the antiretroviral medications used in adults cannot be used in children with HIV due to serious side-effects. A lack of clinical trials in children compounds this problem. In developed countries, many children with HIV are treated by paediatricians, although there may be shared care with primary care doctors. In developed nations, much of the care of children with HIV is provided solely by primary care clinicians.

Implications of the problem

A diagnosis of HIV can have a profound impact on the individual, their family, and their community. Many people with HIV are young adults and subsequent ill-health may remove them from being able to make a productive contribution to their community. Discrimination can occur in local communities and in the workplace, and can also affect health care workers with HIV infection.

Yet most people infected with HIV are well and can continue to work while on treatment or until they develop problems of chronic debilitating illness. Conditions such as intractable chronic diarrhoea, widespread Kaposi's sarcoma, CMV retinitis leading to visual loss, and HIV-related dementia can lead to a major impairment in quality of life. People also need assistance to cope with the psychological aspects of living with a chronic illness. Issues of stigmatization, low self-esteem, and isolation from family and friends can lead to depression and the risk of suicide. Poverty is common among people with HIV in all parts of the world.

There are profound implications for communities with large numbers of people infected with HIV. Often, all the members of a family may be infected with HIV. Children may be orphaned and need to be raised by elderly family members or state welfare organizations. If HIV affects the members of the family of working age then severe poverty and malnutrition may compound an already dire situation.

In some developing nations, the population of working age people is being seriously affected by HIV and in some countries past gains in infant mortality rates are now reversing. However, even in the absence of antiretroviral medication, prevention and treatment of opportunistic infections can add years of life.

Prevention of HIV, through safe sex education and needle and syringe exchanges, and the screening and treatment of pregnant women infected with HIV have all been shown to be cost effective. The major current controversy is the lack of worldwide access to antiretroviral medications, which is limited for many reasons including political and economic barriers.

Key points

1. Early diagnosis of HIV aims to minimize long-term mortality and morbidity.

2. Every patient contact is an opportunity for HIV prevention.

3. A routine sexual history and drug use history as part of the medical history helps target high-risk practices for prevention and early diagnosis of HIV infection.

4. Antiretroviral treatments significantly reduce vertical transmission (from mother to child).

5. Primary care is ideally suited for the management of people with HIV/AIDS.

Further reading

Websites

www.ashm.org.au (Australasian Society for HIV Medicine with free education resources for clinicians including a copy of the 2001 publication HIV/viral hepatitis: a guide for primary care.)

www.hopkins-aids.edu (Johns Hopkins AIDS Service provides clinicians with the latest information on antiretroviral treatments.)

www.aegis.com (Latest HIV/AIDS information, updated hourly.)

www.unaids.org (United Nations HIV/AIDS site.)

www.cdc.gov (US Centers for Disease Control and Prevention update on HIV/AIDS developments.)

References to the evidence

World Health Organization Global Programme on HIV/AIDS (global statistics and treatment and prevention programs). http://www.who.int/health-topics/hiv.htm.

US Department of Health and Human Services Panel on Clinical Practices for Treatment of HIV Infection. Guidelines for the use of antiretroviral agents in HIV-infected adults and adolescents, 2001. http://www.aidsinfo.nih.gov

USPHS/IDS (1999). Guidelines for the prevention of opportunistic infections in persons infected with human immunodeficiency virus. MMWR 1999, 48, 1–67. http://www.cdc.gov/mmwr/preview/mmwrhtml/rr4810a1.htm.

Carr, A. and Cooper, D.A. (2000). Adverse effects of antiretroviral therapy. *Lancet* **356**, 1423–30. (Update on the adverse effects of antiretroviral therapy.)

CDC (1993). Revised classification system for HIV infection and expanded surveillance case definition for AIDS among adolescents and adults. MMWR 1992, 41 (No. RR-17). http://www.cdc.gov/mmwr/preview/mmwrhtml/00018871.htm.

CDC (1994). Revised classification system for human immunodeficiency virus infection in children less than 13 years of age. MMWR 1994, 43 (No. RR-12). http://www.cdc.gov/mmwr/preview/mmwrhtml/00032890.htm.

6.8 Sexual dysfunction in men

John M. Tomlinson

What is acceptable sexual behaviour varies greatly within and among cultures. There has, for example, been widespread religious antagonism to masturbation from Biblical times. Jews and Christians regarded it as sinful, an unnatural act, as it did not lead to pregnancy and many Muslims and Hindus still believe that masturbation weakens their health.

Physicians medicalized it and in the nineteenth and early twentieth century believed and propounded (although they themselves had almost certainly masturbated in adolescence) that it caused insanity, melancholia, blindness, weakness, acne, and even early death. Nowadays, masturbation is a common, widely practised, normal behaviour even by men with a regular sexual partner, and seems compatible with a normal sexual adjustment, although it still causes guilt and embarrassment, especially in the young.[1] The mean frequency among married men is once a week, in the unmarried one to three times a week and adolescents frequently more than double or even treble that.[2]

Frequency of intercourse for couples in a regular relationship averages two to three times a week in their 20s and 30s, and falls to once a week or twice a month over 50. Many couples continue to enjoy regular intercourse into their 80s.[2]

Sexual dysfunction of any form, usually failure to obtain an erection and subsequently to have an orgasm and ejaculate, is regarded by the great majority of men in all cultures as being a catastrophe. It denotes a loss of masculinity and power and the associated distress and shame make it difficult, and in many Eastern cultures almost impossible, for an affected man to admit that there is a problem.

Sexual dysfunction

This can be divided into

1. ejaculation problems;

2. erectile problems;

3. loss of drive due to hormonal problems;

4. loss of drive due to psychological problems.

1. Ejaculation problems

Premature or accelerated ejaculation (PE)

In the younger man

The most acceptable definition of PE is qualitative: *reaching a climax and ejaculating before one or other partner is ready*. It can cause great distress to a couple, especially to the woman who is frequently left sexually aroused without release, much to her discomfort and dismay. It is very common, and possibly affects 40–50 per cent of adolescents, but declines rapidly with age. In a study of men with premature ejaculation,[3] 80 per cent ejaculated within 30 seconds of penetration, 10 per cent between 30 and 60 seconds, and only 10 per cent after 60 seconds. Most men do not complain about it, unless they ejaculate before penetration or unless their partners complain.

Treatment

1. Antidepressants such as a selective serotonin reuptake inhibitor (SSRI) slow down excitation, and paroxetine 20 mg or sertraline 50 mg at night works well. Intermittent use can be as effective as regular use, and reduces undesirable side-effects such as diminished desire.[3]

2. Behavioural methods such as Masters' and Johnson's squeeze technique[4] to reduce anxiety and improve ejaculatory control are helpful but the benefit does not seem to last beyond a year.

3. Masturbating first to lengthen the refractory period before the next orgasm helps some men but is much disliked.

4. Other methods such as using a condom or anaesthetic cream to reduce sensitivity generally do not work.

In the older man

An older man often says he has premature ejaculation when what he means is that his erection has started to go down after penetration and he has to hurry to ejaculate before it collapses. This should be treated as an erectile dysfunction (see below).

Retarded ejaculation or anorgasmia

Difficulty in reaching a climax can be due to drugs such as antidepressants or antihistamines, but is frequently psychogenic, often related to a relationship problem or fear of pregnancy. It is common in gay men, possibly due to fears of HIV infection. Treatment is difficult, but for antidepressant-induced anorgasmia, cyproheptadine 2–16 mg prn. before intercourse helps, although as it is a serotonin antagonist, relapse of the depression can occur.

Retrograde ejaculation

Also known as a 'dry come', it usually occurs after surgery around the bladder neck or prostate, or with spinal cord damage. The orgasmic sensation is unaccompanied by ejaculation, the ejaculate usually going back into the bladder and being passed later on micturition. This is a common presentation in infertility units and is managed by centrifuging the urine to collect the sperm.

2. Erectile problems

Impotence, more precisely called (but not by the patient) erectile dysfunction (ED) is defined as *the inability to get or maintain an erection firm enough for sexual activity.* Typically, the failure of erection is partial, too weak for vaginal or anal insertion. Some can penetrate but then start to lose their tumescence before orgasm.

Incidence

Although ED occurs in one man in 14 below the age of 40, it rises rapidly in the 50s and 60s, and for men between the ages of 70 and 79, the incidence is 57 per cent.[5] This is not necessarily due to age but to the physical problems and their treatment that age brings. Overall, one man in 10 is believed to have a problem.

Causes

ED can be due to psychological causes, physical causes, or a combination of the two.

Psychogenic causes

A man may occasionally have an episode of impotence due to tiredness, tension, a new partner, or too much alcohol. This is not true sexual dysfunction and most take the occasional failure in their stride. For some men, however, such a failure causes them so much anxiety that subsequent failures become inevitable (performance anxiety).

Nocturnal or early morning erections and the ability to masturbate usually remain. To avoid repeated humiliation, men who suffer from this may withdraw from their partners who may in turn blame themselves for no longer being sexually attractive or who may wrongly suspect that their partners are having an affair.

Numerous life stresses such as major physical or psychological trauma, bereavement, worrying about spouse or children, threatened job loss, or actual redundancy involving loss of personal self-esteem can all cause ED.

Sexual boredom and loss of attraction for a partner, or doubts about her fidelity can cause ED and major relationship problems. The failure can be situational, with a good erection with one partner and feeble with another.

Organic causes

ED should not be considered as an entity solely in its own right. It can be a marker for major underlying physical problems, particularly diabetes, hyperlipidaemia, and arteriopathy, as well as hormonal problems such as hypotestosteronaemia and hyperprolactinaemia.

The most common organic conditions associated with erectile dysfunction are:

- Vascular
  - hypertension
  - coronary or peripheral artery disease
  - diabetes (up to 50 per cent of diabetics suffer from ED eventually)
- Neurological
  - stroke
  - spinal cord damage
  - multiple sclerosis
  - diabetes
- Hormonal
  - hypogonadism, this may be primary (Kleinfelter's syndrome), or secondary (Kallmann's syndrome, testicular damage or mumps orchitis)
  - hypo- and hyperthyroidism

- hyperprolactinaemia; uncommon but a cause of profound loss of sexual desire in a younger man, caused by a hypophyseal prolactinoma
  - diabetes
- Pelvic trauma (iatrogenic, pathological, and accidental)
  - prostate, bladder, and rectum, surgeons now use nerve sparing procedures if they possibly can
  - pelvic fractures—frequently caused by motor cycle or car accidents
  - radiotherapy—for pelvic carcinomas
- Social drugs
  - alcohol—blood levels need to be more than 40 mg/l before any dysfunction shows ('the brewers' droop'); long-term alcoholics have testicular atrophy as well
  - smoking—can have dramatic immediate and long-term detrimental effects on erections, it is odd that this fact is not used more often to stop men smoking[6]
  - cannabis—used in India to destroy sexual appetite; there is no aphrodisiac effect although it can be a tension reliever
  - heroin—loss of sexual drive in 60 per cent of addicts
  - cocaine—drop in desire
  - amphetamines—euphoric but not sexually dampening
  - amyl nitrates—used by gay men to relax the anal sphincter; delays ejaculation, loosens inhibitions; only lasts 2 min and side-effects are flushing and headache
  - ecstasy (an amphetamine-like substance) and LSD; change perception of external stimuli. There is no sexual change for the worse.

Prescribed drugs

This is the greatest single cause of erectile dysfunction, implicated in 25 per cent of all cases. Even though the patient or his physician realize that a prescribed drug may have caused his impotence, changing it often does not allow immediate restoration of normal function, which may cause some problems with management. At least half the drugs causing the main difficulties are antihypertensives (β-blockers—propranolol, etc., timolol for glaucoma), followed by antidepressants (except nefazadone and mirtazapine), H_2 antagonists, lipid lowering agents (mainly the fibrates), nonsteroidal antiinflammatories (many are available without prescription), and antihistamines (many cold remedies include diphenhydramine).

Mechanical difficulties

It should not be forgotten that ED can arise as a result of immobility in either partner as in osteoarthritis of the hips or knees, pain, reduced effort tolerance, pain and genital abnormalities such as phimosis and Peyronie's disorder.

History-taking and examination

A careful history should be taken with sensitivity and tact. Some techniques to enable this are described elsewhere.[7]

In listening to the patient, it should be remembered that cultural issues affect the way a man may come to terms with his sexual problem. In many countries, especially in the Far East, ED is considered to be caused by too much masturbation (this is still thought to be true by some in the West, too), that sexual activity depletes the life force, and it is not good for older people or those with disabilities. Most are unaware that causes can be multifactorial and may be due to underlying disease.

Doctors can be as embarrassed and uncomfortable as their patients, causing a block to fruitful discussion. Training on sexual matters that medical students receive is still generally vestigial in the United Kingdom, yet patients assume that doctors know all about it, whereas they often know little more than their patients and are affected by the same cultural and social mores.

A social history is essential and the patient's (and particularly his partner's) view of the problem can be very enlightening, as the quality of their relationship may have a major impact on his sexual functioning.

A medical history must take into account not only past illnesses but current medication (including those bought by the patient himself, particularly antihistamines), as well as social drugs—alcohol, tobacco, cannabis, or the opiates.

Examination

A check of the blood pressure and urine for sugar is mandatory. Abnormalities of the genitalia, the abdomen, pulses, reflexes, and the prostate should be excluded. Other useful tests are a full blood count and an androgen profile.

Treatment

Treatment should not concentrate only on the penis but on the whole person and his relationship.

Reassurance after physical examination, and correcting myths and misinformation is very valuable. Psychosexual counselling or therapy, to cope with marital discord or negative emotions, needs to be encouraged in appropriate cases.

First, discuss lifestyle management, such as weight loss, cigarette use, and alcohol intake. Then treat any underlying disorder. The patient and his partner should then be involved in the choice of management.

Oral treatment is usually the preferred first method over more invasive techniques.

The first oral treatment to be introduced, sildenafil, is a phosphodiesterase inhibitor (PDE_5) potentiating the effect of nitric oxide (NO) which enhances the erectile response, but it only works with concomitant sexual and physical arousal. A drawback is that it cannot be taken by anyone using nitrates for angina or hypertension. It also takes from 30 to 45 min to work, but there is then a 4–5 hour window of opportunity for sex. It has gained worldwide acceptance and popularity, and apart from its reaction with nitrates, seems to be a very safe drug with only minor side-effects (headache, flushing, dyspepsia, and nasal congestion). Newer PDE_5 inhibitors (vardenafil and tadalafil) are also available which act more quickly and have a longer window of opportunity for sex (in tadalafil, up to 36 hours).

Apomorphine, a dopamine-agonist which enhances erectile signals to the penis by activating dopamine receptors acting on the hypothalamus, has been reformulated for ED as a sublingual pellet, in 2 and 3 mg form (compared with 6–12 mg used in the past as an emetic). It has acceptable minor side-effects (headache 7 per cent, nausea 7 per cent, yawning 4 per cent, dizziness 4 per cent), its great advantage being that it can be used concurrently with most drugs, including nitrates, and if it works, does so within 10–15 min. None of the drugs is an aphrodisiac.

Intracavernosal injection of alprostadil was historically the first breakthrough in treating ED effectively. Despite a 90 per cent success rate, most men prefer to use a non-invasive treatment, although it can be a useful adjunct in men who have failed to respond to other treatments.

Intraurethral insertion of alprostadil pellets is not so effective as the injections, but they have a place in the management of some men.

The vacuum pump has been available for many years and is very effective, although many men find it cumbersome and off-putting. It has the disadvantage of using venous blood, producing an erection which can be blue and cold, and to many is not acceptable but in combination with an oral treatment, can be very effective.

Prostheses are expensive and are only used as a last resort, because insertion destroys the erectile tissue. The only solution to a failed operation is a replacement prosthesis. There is a 2–10 per cent risk of infection, the penis will be colder and the glans will not be filled.

3. Loss of drive due to hormonal problems

A low serum testosterone is seemingly commoner than previously realized but many men are not affected by it. It is known that physical or psychological

trauma, bereavement and depression can be causes of a temporary fall. If the fall persists, characteristic symptoms may arise, some of which seem so nebulous that they may be confused with the ageing process, or with depression. These include a general loss of drive, both physical and sexual, hot flushes and sweats during the day, profuse nocturnal sweating with pillows or nightwear having to be changed, stiff cracking ankle and knee joints on getting out of bed, loss of sexual desire or sexual thoughts and fantasies, unusual and excessive tiredness, irritability, and muscle weakness.

There is an ongoing debate about treating those who are discovered to have a low testosterone, whether or not they have ED. Treatment should not be started until the hypogonadism has been investigated. Androgens should not be used to treat ED unless there is a testosterone deficiency. Erections are note solely dependent on normal levels of serum testosterone. It is well documented that severely hypogonadal men can achieve rigid erections. However, those who also have ED may benefit from a PDE_5 inhibitor as well as replacement therapy. There is a suggestion they may have a synergistic effect. Testosterone treatment can be oral, but although this is popular, it is not recommended by the British National Formulary because of possible hepato-toxicity. It suggests intramuscular depot preparations, either a deep gluteal injection of testosterone enantate 250 mg/ml every 2–3 weeks, or implants 600–1200 mg, deep into the gluteal area every 5–6 months. Patches are also available for skin and scrotum attachment. These can cause skin irritation. Two testosterone gels are now available which are more acceptable to the majority of men, especially as the hormonal blood level peaks and troughs are levelled.

4. Loss of drive due to psychological problems

Paradoxically, there are men who retain the ability to get an erection but get no joy or satisfaction from sex. They don't want to initiate it and tend to avoid it, much to the distress of their partner. Management of these men is difficult. Once a full history and examination have ruled out an organic cause, help from a psychotherapist with training in sexual and relationship problems is probably the best line of management.

Key points

- ◆ ED can be a marker for serious underlying disease.
- ◆ Always ask the patient what *he* thinks the cause is.
- ◆ His partner should also be involved, especially in management.
- ◆ Do not treat the penis alone; psychogenic as well as organic causes should be sought.
- ◆ It is mandatory to check the urine, BP, and genitalia.
- ◆ Testosterone replacement should only be used if the serum level is low.

References

1. **Bancroft, J.** *Human Sexuality and its Problems.* Edinburgh: Churchill Livingstone, 1989. (Although this book is now a little old and in need of revision, it remains one of the best comprehensive textbooks in the subject.)

2. **Gebhard, P.H. and Johnson, A.B.** *The Kinsey Data.* Philadelphia PA: Saunders, 1979. (A useful interpretation of Kinsey's vast mass of data on human sexual behaviour.)

3. **Waldinger, M.D.** et al. (1998). The effect of SSRI antidepressants on ejaculation: a double blind, randomised, placebo-controlled study with fluoxetine, fluvoxamine, paroxetine and sertraline. *Journal of Clinical Psychopharmacology* **18** (4), 274–81. (Confirmatory evidence of the value of antidepressants in treating premature ejaculation.)

4. **Masters, W.H., Johnson, V.E., and Kolodny, R.C.** *Human Sexuality* 5th edn. New York: Harper Collins, 1995. (An eminently readable, well written, and illustrated textbook for everyone, with a huge bibliography.)

5. **Whitehead, E.D.** et al. (1990). Diagnostic evaluation of impotence. *Postgraduate Medicine* **88** (2), 123–36.
6. **Hirshkowitz, M.** et al. (1992). Nocturnal penile tumescence in cigarette smokers with dysfunction. *Urology* **39**, 101–7.
7. **Tomlinson, J.M.**, ed. *ABC of Sexual Health*. London: BMJ Books, pp. 12–15, 1999. (This book contains comprehensive, up-to-date information, and a practical analysis of sexual health. An ideal reference book for doctors, nurses, students of all interests, and all those not normally involved in this area of sexual health.)

Further reading

Eardley, I., Sethia, K., and Dean, J. *Erectile Dysfunction: A Guide to Management in Primary Care*. London: Mosby-Wolfe Medical Communications, 1999. (This is a well-illustrated clearly laid out overview of ED from the primary care perspective, with a valuable bibliography. Available from Pfizer Ltd.)

6.9 Female sexual dysfunction

Alan Riley

Female sexual dysfunction occurs frequently in the general population with a reported overall prevalence among women aged 18–59 years of 43 per cent.[1] The prevalence is increased in many clinical conditions such as diabetes mellitus, renal failure, and some neurological diseases.

Although some women present directly with their sexual problems, many more present with a variety of complaints such as request to change their oral contraceptive, recurrent uro-genital symptoms for which no organic cause is found, depression, anxiety, and functional gastrointestinal disorders (e.g. irritable bowel syndrome). Another important indicator of possible sexual dysfunction, especially vaginismus, is the woman who continually finds excuses (e.g. menstruating, no time, 'I'll come back when I've bathed') for not permitting vaginal or pelvic examination.

The extent to which the primary care physician will be involved in the management of female sexual dysfunction varies greatly. At one extreme, some doctors may wish to provide comprehensive management while others may not wish to be involved at all. In the latter situation, the doctor should consider early referral to minimize the detrimental effects sexual problems can have on the patient's self-esteem and her relationship with her sexual partner.

Aetiology

The aetiology of female sexual dysfunction is multifactorial with possible organic, psychological, and behavioural elements being involved. There is increasing evidence that organic factors involved in the aetiology of male sexual dysfunction may also impair female sexual response. Hence vascular, neurologic, and endocrine abnormalities should be considered as possible aetiologic factors in female sexual dysfunction.

History

Obtaining a comprehensive history of sexual dysfunction is not always easy. For example, a woman who says she is unable to become sexually aroused may mean she fails to experience the physiological changes normally associated with sexual arousal (e.g. increased genital lubrication), or she may, on questioning, confirm that she does lubricate but fails to experience any pleasure or excitement from sexual stimulation. So, often the outcome of treatment is poor entirely because the nature of the patient's symptoms has not been precisely defined. It is also essential to ascertain the impact the symptoms have on the woman herself, on her sexual partner and on their sexual and non-sexual relationship. Whenever possible, it is helpful to interview the patient's sexual partner.

Examination

Clinical examination in cases of sexual dysfunction has four main objectives: (i) to discover pathology; (ii) to assess the patient's response and attitude to physical examination; (iii) to look for unreported bruising that might suggest an abusive relationship; and (iv) reassurance for the patient. The extent of examination will be determined by the presenting symptom and concomitant symptoms. It is essential to explain to the patient (and her partner if he/she attends the clinic) how the examination might help them and what it entails. It is also necessary to have a chaperone present even if the doctor is the same sex as the patient. Care should be taken in undertaking vaginal examination; difficulty in inserting a speculum could be misinterpreted by the patient as meaning she is too small or tight.

Investigation

The extent of investigations will likewise be determined by the presenting symptom and concomitant symptoms. Organic conditions should always be considered and appropriate investigations undertaken.

Treatment

Treatment will to a large extent be determined by the presenting and concomitant symptoms but some approaches are common to all forms of female sexual dysfunction, such as 'sensate focus'. Details of this and other therapeutic approaches may be found elsewhere (see Further reading).

Whenever possible, therapeutic approaches should include both the patient and her partner. When significant relationship conflict is apparent, treatment specifically directed at the sexual symptom should be delayed until the conflict is improved by couples therapy.

Absent or low sexual desire

Loss of sexual desire is the most frequent sexual symptom in the population at large and among women attending sex therapy clinics.

Spontaneous sexual desire is not always the first step in the sexual response. Perhaps as many as 30 per cent of women never experience spontaneous feelings of sexual desire, their desire being triggered by sexual activity. However, this is not widely known among women who consider lack of spontaneous sexual desire to be abnormal and may present for treatment, often as a result of pressure from their partners who would like the woman to be sexually proactive.

Loss of sexual desire and reduced ability to fantasize and experience sexual daydreams may point to an organic cause. Sexual desire is androgen dependent. Androgen deficiency should be considered when loss of sexual desire follows bilateral oophorectomy or chemotherapy; desire in such patients may be improved by testosterone treatment. Hypothyroidism and hyperprolactinaemia should also be considered in the assessment of loss of sexual desire. Any debilitating condition or chronic pain is also likely to reduce sexual desire. Loss of sexual desire is a frequent symptom of depression.

Loss of desire for sexual activity with a partner in a woman who continues to experience sexual daydreams or can generate sexual fantasies is

Table 1 Effective sexual stimulation

Positive (sexually enhancing) stimuli
Central
  Sexual drive—fantasies etc.
  Positive feedback arising from enjoying sexual experience
Peripheral
  Sexually arousing input from special senses, for example, visual, olfactory, auditory
  Touch—especially erogenous zones, clitoris, vagina, breasts, etc.

Negative (sexually inhibiting) stimuli
Historical
  Sexual abuse or trauma
  Restrictive upbringing
  Insecurity in psychosexual role
  Lack of sexual education (factual and practical)
Current
  Unmet (unrealistic) sexual expectations
  Relationship conflict
  Restricted foreplay
  Poor communication (unable to tell partner her sexual needs and
    preferences)
  Impaired self-image
  Depression
  Performance anxiety
  Fear of intimacy
  Guilt
  Interruption/distraction (e.g. baby crying, telephone ringing)
  Pain (especially genital)
  Hyperprolactinaemia
  Drugs known to impair sexual response (e.g. antidepressants,
    antihypertensive agents, antipsychotics, dopamine
    antagonists, etc.)

behavioural or psychological in aetiology. Loss of attraction, sexual boredom, or general relationship conflict should be considered. All the negative stimuli in Table 1 should also be considered as possible aetiological factors in loss of sexual desire. An important reinforcing factor for sexual desire is sexual satisfaction. Gaining satisfaction from an activity makes us want to do it again; not gaining satisfaction does not have this reinforcing effect. As many people have unrealistic expectation of sex, they are rarely satisfied and hence lose desire. It is always important to assess the patient's personal criteria for sexual satisfaction; when they are judged to be unrealistic, explanation and education to lower her expectation often enhances sexual desire.

Treatment of loss of sexual desire depends on the cause. Most treatment will involve cognitive–behavioural therapy and psychodynamic approaches with couples therapy being required when relationship issues are considered significant. Empirical use of antidepressants, especially trazedone, is sometimes helpful. Androgen treatment is not without risk but is sometimes effective as the last resort or when androgen deficiency is present.

Sexual arousal disorder

Some women may complain directly of inability to become sexually aroused but more frequently women present with dyspareunia due to failure of lubrication and genital vasocongestion. One approach to identifying the likely cause of arousal disorder is to consider what is required for sexual arousal [adequate blood supply to genitalia; intact nerve supply (both autonomic and sensory); appropriate hormonal milieu (especially oestrogen and maybe androgen); functional end organ (clitoris, vagina, erectile tissue); intact sexual drive; effective sexual stimulation]. Hence, any impairment in any of these factors, by disease, surgery, radiotherapy, or pharmacotherapy may result in failure of arousal. One factor, 'effective sexual stimulation' requires clarification. This can be regarded as the balance between positive (sexually enhancing) stimuli and negative (sexually inhibiting) stimuli (Table 1).[2]

The management of arousal dysfunction involves identifying and treating organic causes and discovering, from reviewing the patient's history, what inhibiting factors may be operating and resolving such factors by cognitive–behavioural therapy or other psychological approaches.

Female orgasm disorder

This is the persistent or recurrent delay in or absence of orgasm (anorgasmia) following normal sexual arousal. It can be global in that the woman is totally unable to attain orgasm or, more commonly, situational. This is where the woman can achieve orgasm in some situations (e.g. masturbation) but not in others. While anorgasmia can have an organic aetiology, such as neuropathy, it is usually psychological or behavioural in origin. Psychologically, women may inhibit subconsciously their attainment of orgasm for fear of losing control. Behaviourally, they may not have learnt the most appropriate stimulation techniques to trigger orgasm. Pressure from the partner for the woman to experience orgasm is also a common factor. The more frequent the woman fails to attain orgasm the harder she tries and this effort inhibits arousal. Anorgasmia also occurs when effective sexual stimulation is inadequate and hence an assessment of sexually enhancing and sexually inhibiting stimuli is required (Table 1).

The management of anorgasmia involves sex education and especially self-exploration. The woman is encouraged to explore different modes of stimulation, varying pressure and speed of manual stimulation of the clitoris, and other erogenous areas. Vibrators may be helpful in this respect. At the same time, cognitive–behavioural therapy is useful to resolve unconscious fears of orgasm and to enhance sexual arousal. Once the woman has succeeded in attaining orgasm, she can 'teach' her partner how to stimulate her.

Sexual pain disorders

Sexual pain disorders comprise conditions in which genital pain is triggered by sexual activity. Most commonly, the pain is related to vaginal penetration and may occur before, during or after this event. The pain may be felt deep in the pelvis (deep dyspareunia), often associated with penile thrusting, or superficially around the vaginal introitus. More rarely, the trigger for the pain is localized in the clitoris or labia and can occur during manual stimulation. Pain is a powerful sexual turn off and repeated sexual pain will result in impaired arousal (which, by virtue of reduced lubrication can aggravate the condition), inhibited orgasm, and loss of sexual desire.

In all patients presenting with sexual pain, assessment must include thorough examination to exclude organic causes. Patients with vulval pain or superficial dyspareunia sould be assessed for lack of lubrication, oestrogen deficiency and vulvar vaginal and urethral disorders (including use of potential irritants such as spermicides, deodorants, and latex products). Those with deep dyspareunia should be checked for conditions such as pelvic inflammatory disease, fibroids, ovarian cyst, post-operative adhesions, cystits, urethritis, inflammatory bowel disease, and constipation. Pathological conditions are not always evident on routine vulval and pelvic examination and where there is doubt about the diagnosis referral for gynaecological or dermatological opinion is recommended before labelling the cause 'psychogenic'.

While the successful treatment of detected organic disorders resolves the problem of sexual dysfunction in most women, a minority of patients will continue to experience sexual pain. In these women, the pain is probably anticipatory in nature; the cycle of pain—inhibited arousal—reduced lubrication—painful penetration persisting. Patients should be advised to use copious amounts of a water-soluble artificial lubricant prior to penetration, and encouraged to 'take charge of' sexual activity with her partner and especially of penile–vaginal penetration, perhaps by adopting the female superior squatting coital position so that she can control the rate and depth of penetration and coital thrusting. Occasionally, the patient's self-use of vaginal trainers (previously known as dilators) may help her experience pain-free penetration and hence allow her to gain confidence. In those women whose persistent pain is localized around the introitus and occurs on penetration, the use of a local anaesthetic (e.g. 1 per cent lignocaine gel) may help. One group of patients who are particularly difficult to treat are those whose sexual pain started after sexual assault or abuse. Often these patients require more intensive psychotherapy. It must also be appreciated that some women will use sexual pain as an excuse to avoid sexual intercourse. Assessment to discover the underlying psychological or behavioural problems in these cases is essential.

Vaginismus

Vaginismus is the recurrent or persistent involuntary contraction of the pelvic floor muscles when vaginal penetration is anticipated or attempted. Adduction of the thighs and arching of the back can also occur in severe cases. The condition can be primary when it has been present throughout the woman's life or secondary when it has occurred after a period, however short, of pain-free vaginal penetration. Secondary vaginismus frequently follows a genitally painful experience such as gynaecological surgery, painful gynaecological examination, forced vaginal penetration, sexual abuse or assault or childbirth. It is thus seen as a conditioned response to prevent pain by making penetration impossible. Vaginismus can also be associated with fear of pregnancy or of sexually transmitted disease.

Although vaginismus may cause the woman to withdraw from all sexual activities, other women with this complaint can participate in and enjoy all types of sexual activity except penetrative sexual intercourse. They may even be orgasmic in these non-penetrative activities. Many couples in which the woman has vaginismus are content not to have penetrative sex and present for treatment only when they want to start a family. In this situation, some couples will preferentially accept being taught how to artificially inseminate the woman rather than have treatment to overcome the vaginismus.

The vaginismic response can be global in that it occurs irrespective of the nature of the object that attempts to penetrate the vagina or selective where it occurs only in some situations. Hence a woman may have a vaginismic response to attempted penile penetration but can comfortably use tampons; or it could occur during attempted penetration of vagina by her partner's finger or penis but not during vaginal examination by the doctor. These different circumstances can lead to failure to establish the diagnosis. A differential diagnosis of sexual aversion disorder should always be considered (see below).

Some women who experience vaginismus have the ideas that their vaginae are too small to allow penetration or that their hymen is too rigid to rupture but these are rarely the case. There is no justification for examination under anaesthesia or hymenectomy in the management of vaginismus, except where an unrelated gynaecological pathology is suspected and early examination is advised.

Treatment of vaginismus usually is by cognitive–behavioural therapy. The woman learns to control her pelvic floor muscle spasm while gently introducing 'trainers' of gradually increasing size into her vagina. Specially designed trainers are available for this purpose but many therapists prefer to use less clinical objects such as tampons of increasing size and/or fingers. Once the patient can accommodate such objects without a vaginismic response, the same objects are inserted into her vagina by her sexual partner. It is preferable for the patient whilst lying on her back (or squatting) to move herself on to the object held at the vaginal introitus rather than to actively insert the object in to the vagina. Intercourse can then be attempted in the female superior squatting position so that the woman can control rate and depth of penetration.

A more detailed discussion of the approach to sexual pain disorders is given in Chapter 7.9.

Sexual aversion

In this condition, the woman has an aversion to and active avoidance of sexual contact with her partner. The aversion may be restricted to a particular element of sex or sexual contact (e.g. genital secretions, oro-genital activities) or a more generalized revulsion of anything sexual or activities that might lead to sexual activities (e.g. intimate touching, kissing). The intensity of the aversion ranges from extreme phobic anxiety reaction (panic attack) to lack of pleasure associated with mild anxiety. The treatment of sexual aversion generally requires specialist psychotherapeutic experience. Selective serotonin re-uptake inhibitors are sometimes effective, but this treatment is not evidence based.

Key points

- Female sexual dysfunction has detrimental effects on relationships which in turn aggravate the sexual dysfunction.

- Only a minority of women who experience sexual dysfunction present for treatment.

- The major treatment modality of female sexual dysfunction is psychological.

- When doctors feel unable to provide active management themselves for women presenting with sexual problems, early specialist referral is indicated.

References

1. Laumann, E.O., Paik, A., and Rosen, R.C. (1999). Sexual dysfunction in the United States. Prevalence and predictors. *Journal of the American Medical Association* **281**, 537–44.
2. Riley, A. (1997). Problems of the sexual response cycle. *Journal of the Diplomates of the Royal College of Obstetricians and Gynaecologists* **4**, 270–5.

Further reading

Gabbard, G.O., ed. *Treatments of Psychiatric Disorders* 3rd edn. Part 2. Washington DC: American Psychiatric Publishing Inc., 2001, pp. 1845–2069.

Hawton, K. *Sex Therapy: A Practical Guide.* Oxford: Oxford University Press, 1985.

Leiblum, S.R. and Rosen, R.C., ed. *Principles and Practice of Sex Therapy: Update for the 1990s.* New York and London: The Guilford Press, 1989.

Tomlinson, J., ed. *ABC of Sexual Health.* London: British Medical Journal Books, 1999.

6.10 Benign prostate disorders

Maarten Klomp

Benign prostatic hyperplasia

Introduction and definition

Benign prostatic hyperplasia (BPH) is the most common cause of voiding problems in elderly men. A distinction should be made between the histological and the clinical diagnosis of BPH. Histologically BPH is characterized by proliferation of both epithelial and stromal elements in the periurethral and transitional zones of the prostate.

The clinical diagnosis is based on three main elements: lower urinary tract symptoms (LUTS), enlargement of the prostate, and urethral obstruction. LUTS may be caused by three different pathophysiologic mechanisms. These are: static bladder outlet obstruction due to increased prostate volume, dynamic bladder outlet obstruction related to the smooth muscle tone of the prostate, and instability of the detrusor muscle of the bladder. Detrusor instability may occur with or without urethral obstruction and is the reason why one in four men with BPH derives no benefit from transurethral prostatectomy.

Epidemiology and natural course

Symptoms related to BPH affect 10–50 per cent of all men above 60 years, but only a small number of them visit the general practitioner. Both the incidence and the prevalence of BPH increase with age.

The natural course of BPH is unpredictable and can have a variable pattern. The symptoms can occur intermittently, remain stable, be progressive, or disappear. The majority of patients improve spontaneously or have stable symptoms. BPH can be complicated by urinary tract infections, as well as acute or chronic urine retention and an overflow bladder. The latter may lead to renal function disorders but the prevalence of upper urinary tract dilatation and renal impairment in BPH is only 1–3 per cent. The occurrence of these complications is not predicted by the severity of the symptoms.

Differential diagnosis

The differential diagnosis includes urinary tract infections, urethral strictures, bladder stones, bladder cancer, and neurogenic bladder. Non-urological conditions such as diabetes or congestive heart failure and the use of medications can also be responsible for LUTS. Although many men with LUTS are anxious about prostate cancer, the symptoms have a very weak link to prostate carcinoma. Micturition problems are not considered to be early symptoms of prostate cancer, which is usually asymptomatic. This corresponds to the fact that BPH is located periurethrally, while prostate cancer arises in the peripheral zone of the prostate.

Diagnostic approach

History

Initially requires a focus on:

◆ Obstructive complaints: straining to urinate, a weak stream, difficulty in emptying the bladder, post-micturition dribbling.

◆ Irritative complaints: difficulty in suppressing the urge to urinate, and an increasing diurnal and nocturnal micturition frequency.

◆ The clinical course of the complaints (how quickly they arose or worsened).

◆ The inconvenience they cause (disturbed sleep, social limitations, incontinence).

Subsequent enquiries deal with:

◆ Relevant comorbidity (diabetes, stroke, Parkinson's disease, multiple sclerosis).

◆ Previous urological investigations or treatment, urethritis.

◆ Medication which affects micturition (antipsychotics, antidepressants, antiparkinsonian medication, parasympatholytics, diuretics).

A voiding diary can be helpful to obtain a better impression of the voiding pattern and the urinary symptoms can be quantified by a symptom score.

Physical examination

The physical examination is performed after the patient urinates, to aid in detecting a distended bladder. The prepuce is examined for phimosis. A digital rectal examination with palpation of the prostate is then performed. Attention is paid to the form, consistency, size, and tenderness of the prostate. The findings are interpreted as follows:

◆ symmetric, firm, and elastic—normal;

◆ normal and enlarged—suspected BPH;

◆ normal and tender—suspected prostatitis;

◆ irregular consistency or hard node—suspected prostate carcinoma.

Urinalysis

The urine should be examined for the presence of erythrocytes and signs of urinary tract infection, by urinary dipsticks or by microscopic examination.

Additional diagnostic tests

Additional tests are available to aid in diagnosis in selected cases of LUTS.

◆ *Prostate-specific antigen:* The routine determination of prostate-specific antigen (PSA) in general practice to detect prostate carcinoma is not recommended, because symptoms of benign prostatic hyperplasia are only very weakly linked to prostate cancer. Furthermore, elevated PSA values are not specific for prostate cancer but may also occur in cases of BPH, prostate stones, and prostatitis. The finding of an elevated value may trigger additional investigations to diagnose prostate cancer, while there is no evidence that follow-up and treatment will decrease morbidity and mortality. Especially men with a life expectancy less than 10 years should be dissuaded from this measurement (see Chapter 6.11).

◆ *Creatinine and imaging of the upper urinary tract:* It is not necessary to measure creatinine routinely, because the prevalence of abnormal renal function associated with BPH is less than 2 per cent.

Ultrasound imaging of the upper urinary tract is indicated when chronic retention of urine is suspected.

◆ *Post-micturition residual urine measurement and uroflowmetry:* There is no clear evidence that either of these investigations can predict the outcome of the therapy of BPH.

◆ Urethrocystoscopy, transrectal ultrasonography of the prostate, and pressure-flow studies are optional investigations in the evaluation by the urologist.

Evaluation and diagnosis

The general practitioner can make the diagnosis of BPH on the basis of LUTS, a normal or enlarged prostate, and normal findings in the urinalysis. Excluded from this diagnosis are patients with:

◆ suspected neurogenic bladder (case history);

◆ suspected urethral stricture (case history);

◆ possible prostatitis based on painful micturition and a tender prostate detected by digital rectal examination;

◆ haematuria (>2–3 erythrocytes per high-power field) in the absence of urinary tract infection;

◆ possible prostate cancer suggested by digital rectal examination or elevated PSA.

In these patients further investigation by a urologist may be necessary for a definitive diagnosis.

Treatment of BPH

The general practitioner should explain to the patient that his complaints are due to a very common and benign change in the prostate. The severity of the complaints and the inconvenience they cause can vary with time. Some changes in lifestyle may be beneficial, including, reduction of fluid intake at specific times, moderate alcohol consumption, not postponing urinating, taking time to urinate, and urination whilst sitting. Medications taken by the patient should be reviewed for possible influence on micturition.

Watchful waiting

Watchful waiting is a satisfactory and safe alternative to treatment. Men with mild complaints are not likely to benefit from any active treatment. Those with moderate or severe complaints have the potential to improve, but they must make this decision after being well informed about the possible benefits and risks of treatment.

Clinical evidence shows that the decision whether to treat should not be based on the outcome of technical investigations such as prostate volume, post-voiding residual urine measurement, or uroflowmetry. The degree of bother to the patient appears to be the best predictor of the success of treatment and is more important than the severity of the symptoms.

Medical therapy

On average, drug therapy has little beneficial effect on the symptoms, but some men do experience significant benefit. Medication has a much smaller effect than surgery, but should be considered in patients experiencing substantial discomfort and inconvenience but who will not or cannot undergo surgery.

Alpha-blockers

Alpha-receptor-blocking sympatholytics act on the stromal smooth muscle of the prostate and reduce the urethral outflow resistance to urine. Several alpha-blockers are approved for treating BPH: prazosin, alfuzosin, terazosin, doxazosin, and tamsulosin.

Alpha-blockers have a statistically significant effect in reducing symptoms and improving quality of life scores, and in this they excel over finasteride. They also produce an earlier response, usually within 2–4 weeks. If there is no effect in 6 weeks, the medication is stopped. The main side-effects are dizziness and orthostatic hypotension. Blood pressure must be monitored while treating with alpha-blockers. Even when symptoms have improved, the treatment should be reviewed after a certain period to determine whether continuing is worthwhile.

Finasteride

The rationale for using 5α-reductase inhibitors such as finasteride is that they reduce prostate size by blocking the conversion of testosterone to dihydrotestosterone, the major intraprostatic androgen. Finasteride has been shown to reduce prostate size and improve urine flow rates. Symptom scores also improve significantly, but the improvement is limited and only occurs in men with a prostate volume more than 40 ml. Six months or more are required to achieve the maximal effect. Possible side-effects are impotence and decreased libido (<5 per cent). Finasteride also lowers the serum PSA by approximately 50 per cent, which might affect its utility in the early detection of prostate cancer.

Surgical therapy

Absolute indications for surgical treatment are recurrent acute urinary retention, recurrent urinary tract infection associated with chronic retention, or kidney function disorders due to obstruction. Surgical treatment can also be considered if the patient finds his symptoms unacceptable.

Transurethral resection of the prostate (TURP) is still the 'gold standard'; 75 per cent of all men improve, 5 per cent become impotent, 5 per cent become incontinent, and 40 per cent have transient post-operative problems, such as haemorrhage, infection, or retention. In most patients, ejaculation is retrograde following the operation. Open prostatectomy is even more effective, but it is also more invasive and causes much greater morbidity. Transurethral incision of the prostate (TUIP) is a good alternative, especially in men with smaller prostates, and it has the lowest morbidity rate.

New techniques

Various new techniques are being introduced for treating BPH. These include laser therapy, the placement of stents, and different forms of thermal therapy. Although some preliminary results are promising, the long-term effects are not yet known.

Continuing care and periodic reassessment

Except for patients being treated with medications, periodic reassessment is not automatically advised. The preferred policy is to ask the patient to return if there is an increase in his symptoms or if alarm symptoms occur such as pain or haematuria occur.

Key points on BPH

- The natural course of BPH is unpredictable. In a minority of patients the symptoms worsen.

- In most patients, diagnostic procedures should be limited to the history, physical examination, and urinalysis.

- Men visiting the general practitioner for LUTS have little or no increased risk of prostate cancer.

- Shared decision-making between doctors and their patients is necessary before treating BPH.

- In patients with mild symptoms, 'watchful waiting' is the advisable policy.

- In general, the effect of medication for BPH is small, but some patients may obtain benefit.

- Surgery still is the gold standard in treating BPH; the degree of bother is the most important issue to consider.

Prostatitis

Acute prostatitis

Epidemiology, aetiology, and presentation

Acute prostatitis is a severe infectious disease that is relatively uncommon in general medical practice. There are no reliable data on its incidence. In elderly men with urinary tract infections the prostate is often inflamed. The infection is usually caused by Gram-negative bacteria such as *Escherichia coli*, occasionally *Staphylococci* or *Enterococci*. There is seldom a relation with sexually transmitted urethritis.

Men with acute prostatitis are usually febrile and very ill. In addition to signs of a urinary tract infection such as pain and difficulty in urinating, increased frequency of urination and occasionally passage of exudate from the urethra, they often have pain in the penis, perineum, and lower back; sometimes defaecation is painful. Occasionally, prostatitis is associated with acute urinary retention, caused by oedema of the prostate.

Diagnosis

Characteristic findings on digital rectal examination are a very pressure-sensitive, swollen, and soft prostate. Excessive manipulation of the prostate should be avoided, because of the extreme pain and the chance of causing bacteraemia.

A midstream urine sample is examined for bacteriuria by means of a dip-stick or microscopic examination. A urine culture is used to determine antibiotic sensitivity.

Management

The first choice antibiotic is a quinolone, such as ciprofloxacin, 500 mg twice daily, or ofloxacin, 200 mg twice daily. If the patient does not tolerate quinolones, cotrimoxazole, 960 mg twice daily, is the best alternative. The antibiotic therapy can be changed if the results of the culture and sensitivity testing so indicate. Very ill patients and those in which no improvement is seen within 24–48 h require parenteral therapy. A patient with acute urine retention is referred for placement of a suprapubic catheter.

Duration of antibiotic therapy is controversial. Although there is no evidence that treatment for more than 10 days is beneficial, treatment is often continued for 4 weeks to avoid chronic prostatitis. Complete recovery can be expected following adequate treatment of an acute prostatitis. Persistence of the complaints may signal the presence of a prostatic abscess, which can be demonstrated by ultrasonography. If acute prostatitis recurs, further examination is indicated to detect a possible underlying cause.

Chronic prostatitis

Epidemiology, aetiology, and presentation

Chronic prostatitis is characterized by persistent or intermittent pain or discomfort in the perineum, penis, testicles, suprapubic region, lower back, and groin, together with LUTS such as urgency, dysuria, and increased frequency of urination, and sometimes painful ejaculation. Although the complaints are usually very vague, they often cause the patient great distress. Physicians find the treatment of patients with chronic prostatitis very frustrating, due to the difficulty in arriving at an exact diagnosis and therefore a rational basis for treatment.

Data on the incidence of chronic prostatitis in general practice are meagre and unreliable. Although there has been much research on the aetiology of chronic prostatitis, it remains unclear. There are hypotheses about the influence of such factors as infection, stress, sexual activity, allergy, and autoimmunity.

The disorder has long been divided into three types: (i) chronic bacterial prostatitis when evidence of bacterial infection is found; (ii) chronic aseptic prostatitis when there is inflammation without infection; and (iii) prostatodynia when no inflammation is found. In clinical practice, this differentiation has been based on the four-glass test, in which the first void, midstream, and post-prostatic massage urine, and the expressed prostatic secretion are examined for signs of infection (bacteria) and inflammation (leucocytes).

At present, most experts believe that chronic aseptic prostatitis and prostatodynia are overlapping entities. Hence, for these categories the term chronic pelvic pain syndrome has been introduced. This term is appropriate because a clear pathophysiologic concept is lacking and also a relation with the prostate is not always certain. For the general practitioner, it is also sufficient to distinguish between chronic bacterial prostatitis (10 per cent of cases) and the chronic pelvic pain syndrome (90 per cent).

Diagnosis

A careful history of the nature, the severity, and the progress of the complaints is taken. Physical examination of the external genitalia is followed by rectal palpation. In chronic prostatitis, the prostate can be sensitive to pressure, but not necessarily. Neither the symptoms nor the physical findings serve to differentiate between the different types of prostatitis. Bacteriological examination is performed using seminal fluid or the expressed prostatic secretion, or by comparing the number of bacteria in a urine sample before and after another one minute of vigorous prostate massage. This two-glass test appears to be as reliable as the classical four-glass test. If the culture is positive or if the number of bacteria in the urine after massage is 10 times greater than that in the midstream urine, the diagnosis of chronic bacterial prostatitis is made, and if not, the diagnosis is chronic pelvic pain syndrome.

Management

It is important to give the patient a good explanation of the nature of the disorder, especially its expected course and the limited possibilities for treatment.

Chronic bacterial prostatitis is treated with antibiotics. As in acute prostatitis, preference is given to quinolones, such as ciprofloxacin, 500 mg twice daily, or ofloxacin, 200 mg twice daily. If there is intolerance to quinolones, the alternatives are cotrimoxazole in a dose of 960 mg twice daily, trimethoprim in a dose of 200 mg twice daily, or doxycycline in a dose of 100 mg twice daily. Determining antimicrobial sensitivities is necessary

to avoid the use of an ineffective antibiotic. There is no consensus about the duration of treatment. The minimum is 4 weeks. Some authors advise longer treatment to prevent recurrence, but there is no evidence to support this.

The treatment of chronic pelvic pain syndrome is less well established. Many physicians routinely prescribe antibiotics, but there is no evidence to support this treatment. Incidental success with antibiotics has been reported and may be related to the existence of occult infection. Some advise trial antibiotic treatment for 2–4 weeks, to be extended only if there is clinical improvement. Several other medications are also used on a trial-and-error basis, the most important of which are alpha blockers, non-steroidal anti-inflammatory drugs, and allopurinol. There is also no hard evidence to support any of these treatments at present. There are indications that thermal therapy and perhaps management of stress can reduce the symptoms in some cases.

Because further diagnostic studies by a urologist have little additional value and an effective specialist treatment lacks, there is no unambiguous guideline for referral.

Key points on prostatitis

- In acute prostatitis, the general practitioner prescribes empirical antibiotic treatment, modified if necessary by antibiotic sensitivity testing.
- Chronic bacterial prostatitis is diagnosed by culture of seminal fluid or expressed prostatic secretion, or by using the two-glass test.
- There is no established evidence-based therapy for the chronic pelvic pain syndrome.

Further reading

Benign prostatic hyperplasia

Dutch College of General Practitioners. *Difficult Micturition in Older Men*, 1997. (Practice guideline for General Practitioners in the Netherlands.)

National Health and Medical Research Council. *The Management of Uncomplicated Lower Urinary Tract Symptoms in Men*, 2000. (Clinical practice guideline for men, general practitioners, and urologists, Commonwealth of Australia.)

Agency for Health Care Policy and Research. *Benign Prostatic Hyperplasia: Diagnosis and Treatment. Clinical Practice Guideline*, 1994. (Report on BPH for men, general practitioners, urologists, and other specialists, United States of America.)

NHS Centre for Reviews and Dissemination. *Benign Prostatic Hyperplasia*, 1995. (Review article in the series 'Effective Health Care', United Kingdom.)

Ziada, A., Roseblum, M., and Crawford, E.D. (1999). Benign prostatic hyperplasia: an overview. *Urology* 53, 1–6.

Jepsen, J. and Bruskewitz, C. (1998). Comprehensive patient evaluation for benign prostatic hyperplasia. *Urology* 51 (Suppl. 4A), 13–18.

Nickle, J.C. (1998). Long-term implications of medical therapy on benign prostatic hyperplasia end points. *Urology* 51 (Suppl. 4A), 50–7.

Jepsen, J. and Bruskewitz, C. (1998). Recent developments in the surgical management of benign prostatic hyperplasia. *Urology* 51 (Suppl. 4A), 23–31.

Barry, M. and Roehrborn, C. (2001). Benign prostatic hyperplasia. Effects of medical treatments and effects of surgical treatments. *Clinical Evidence*, 588–98.

Prostatitis

Nickel, C. *Textbook of Prostatitis*. Oxford: Isis Medical Media, 1999.

Walker, P. and Wilson, J. (1999). National guideline for the management of prostatitis. Clinical Effectiveness Group (Association for Genitourinary Medicine and the Medical Society for the Study of Venereal Disease). *Sexually Transmitted Infections* 75 (Suppl. 1), S46–50.

McNaughton Collins, M. et al. (2000). Diagnosis and treatment of chronic abacterial prostatitis: a systematic review. *Annals of Internal Medicine* **133** (5), 367–81.

Stern, J. and Schaeffer, A. (2001). Chronic prostatitis. *Clinical Evidence*, 599 604.

Nickel, C. (2000). Prostatitis syndromes: an update for urologic practice. *Canadian Journal of Urology* **7** (5), 1091–8.

6.11 Prostate cancer

Neill Iscoe

Is cure possible in those for whom it is necessary?
Is cure necessary in those for whom it is possible?
Willet Whitmore

Introduction

Prostate cancer is now the most commonly diagnosed cancer in North American, European, and Australian men. The age-specific incidence of prostate cancer rises steeply with age (Fig. 1), and it is now estimated that a North American man has a one in nine chance of developing prostate cancer during his lifetime. However, the risk of developing prostate cancer varies with age so that for a man of a given age the risk of him developing prostate cancer over the 10-year interval is never one in nine. Though the lifetime risk of a man developing prostate cancer is similar to a woman developing breast cancer, the risks by decade of life vary. Compared to breast cancer, prostate cancer rates have a later and steeper increase.

The incidence of prostate cancer is higher in North America compared to other parts of the world. In part, this is an artefact due to increased detection because of the frequent use of the prostate-specific antigen (PSA) blood test. Fortunately, the increases in incidence in North America and elsewhere have not been accompanied by similar increases in mortality from prostate cancer (Fig. 2).

Epidemiology

While prostate cancer is the most common malignancy in North American men it is far less frequent in other countries, notably those in the Orient and in the Indian subcontinent.[2] While some of current geographic variation represents detection bias (in that less frequent investigations are performed in some countries), data from the pre-PSA era revealed the incidence rate of prostate cancer in North American black males to be 40 times higher than that recorded in Japan.[3]

The documentation of a true geographic variation leads to questions about the relative importance of genetics and environment in the causation of prostate cancer. Genetic factors are important. The disease is more common in men with affected first-degree relatives and is more common in monozygotic twins than dizygotic twins.[4] However, environmental factors are also important as Japanese men who migrate from Japan to Hawaii develop incidence rates intermediate between those of men in Japan and Caucasians in Hawaii.[3] Current work on the environmental contributors to the development of prostate cancer has raised tantalizing data related to the possible protective effects of various compounds such as selenium, lycopenes (found in high concentrations in tomatoes), and soy. However, the uncertainties related to examining these and other factors are such that no recommendations about the use or avoidance of any agents can be made at this time.

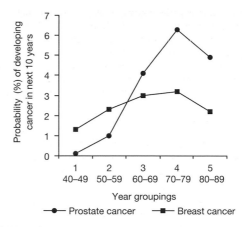

Fig. 1 Probability of developing prostate or breast cancer by age group. (Data from Canadian Cancer Statistics 2001.[1])

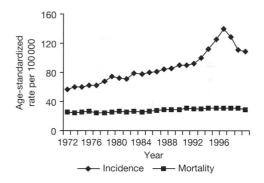

Fig. 2 Age standardized incidence and mortality—Canada 1972–1996. (Data from Canadian Cancer Statistics 2001.[1])

Prostate cancer exemplifies the difference between a diagnosis and an illness. Approximately 30 per cent of North American men above the age of 50 harbour prostate cancer if examined at autopsy. This proportion increases to more than 80 per cent for men above the age of 80. However, the number of men who are diagnosed and treated for prostate cancer is far less. This indicates there is a vast cohort or men with undiagnosed prostate cancer who never develop any clinical symptoms. Additionally, about two in three men currently diagnosed with prostate cancer die with, but not from, this illness. This is because prostate cancer generally has a long clinical course and is primarily a disease of older men who are at risk of death from other age-related illnesses.

Clinical diagnosis

Prostate cancer confined to the prostate produces few, if any symptoms. A change in urinary stream is common as men age and is rarely due to early prostate cancer. Pain is a symptom of advanced disease and usually occurs in patients with bone metastases. The diagnosis of prostate cancer is most often made in asymptomatic men by finding an abnormality of the prostate during a rectal examination, by pathologic examination of tissue removed during a procedure done for other reasons (e.g. transurethral resection of the prostate for urinary symptoms), or, as is commonly the case in North America, as a result of a PSA blood test. Rectal examinations are highly dependent on the examiner and screening for prostate cancer by rectal examination is neither sensitive nor specific. When cancers are detected by this means they are commonly more advanced and less amenable to curative therapies. In contrast, prostate cancers detected by PSA screening are more likely to be localized and, theoretically, more likely to be cured with current therapies.

Screening for prostate cancer

Will the early detection of prostate cancer with PSA screening lead to decreased mortality? Though the principles of screening were described more than 35 years ago,[5] PSA screening for prostate cancer is one of the most contentious issues in modern clinical medicine. Advocates claim that failure to promote screening will lead to needless deaths while opponents claim that promoting screening without good evidence will lead to increased morbidity from therapy and the inevitable premature deaths that occur when any therapy is applied to large populations.

Currently, two large randomized clinical trials are evaluating whether screening and treatment reduces prostate cancer mortality but results from these studies are not expected until later this decade.

PSA screening is promoted to varying degrees between countries and even within countries. The test has known sensitivity and specificity for detecting prostate cancer and, though not ideal, is comparable to mammography. As a simple blood test, PSA screening is acceptable to patients and practitioners. What is far less clear is the acceptability of the test when it is combined with the morbidity of investigations and therapies that could follow; particularly when there is uncertainty about the net clinical benefit. PSA screening appears to detect prostate cancer at an earlier stage of disease and finds tumours of lower grade more frequently than clinically detected cases.[6] However, detection of early stage disease might simply be a manifestation of lead time bias in which people are found earlier in the course of their illness but where the final outcome of the illness is not materially altered by its earlier discovery. The finding of lower grade tumours might be an example of length bias in which more slowly evolving and, therefore, more innocuous disorders are found more frequently by screening manoeuvres.

In the absence of high-quality information, the most appropriate course of action is to inform men what is known and not known about PSA screening and subsequent treatment for prostate cancer.[7] This means a practitioner needs to understand a PSA test is not entirely accurate, that all men with prostate cancer do not need treatment at diagnosis, and that therapy for prostate cancer can result in significant morbidity.

Management of prostate cancer

Though Dr Whitmore's remark at the beginning of the chapter can be interpreted as indicating therapies do not affect the course of prostate cancer, it more likely sets up the scenario whereby therapy results in one of three outcomes. Firstly, therapy is not necessary, as the disease would be better managed with an expectant approach. Secondly, therapy is necessary but is ineffective in controlling the cancer. Finally, there is likely a cohort of patients for whom therapy does lead to cure or less morbidity and should be used. The problem is we are uncertain as to how large this third cohort is *and* to what extent this cohort can be increased by a screening programme.

At the present time, the primary forms of therapy for early prostate cancer remain:

1. *Expectant management (watchful waiting).* Expectant management is generally reserved for men who have very low volume and low-grade cancers.[8] Many of these men will never require any form of treatment and will die of other disorders before their prostate cancer becomes manifest. Other men will require treatment when it becomes evident their cancer is progressing.

2. *Surgery, generally radical prostatectomy.* This therapy is used for men with organ-confined disease who are fit and wish a surgical approach to their disease.

3. *Radiation therapy.* This form of therapy may be given as external beam radiation or, for a select group of patients, as brachytherapy in which radioactive sources are inserted into the prostate gland. Currently, brachytherapy is restricted to men with low volume, low-grade prostate cancer. Radiation therapy is generally chosen because the disease is not amenable to surgery (it extends beyond the prostate gland), because the patient is not fit for surgery, or because he prefers the side-effect profile of radiation treatment to that of surgery.

4. *Hormone manipulation.* This is reserved for men with local disease who require therapy but who are not candidates for radiation or surgery. It is also used as an adjunct to these treatments and for men with metastatic disease.

Though specialists may believe surgery or radiation therapy is superior for a patient in a given clinical situation, there are no compelling data from randomized controlled trials that provide an objective assessment of their relative benefits in terms of survival. As the therapies have very different morbidities (Table 1), patients may base part of their decision on the disability associated with a particular treatment. Though radiation therapy produces more frequent bowel disturbances, prostatectomy produces more urinary and sexual dysfunction. Each man should be encouraged to discuss the risks and benefits of his treatment options with his physician before making a decision about therapy.

When prostate cancer is suspected, a PSA test should be ordered as it provides information about the likelihood of the cancer being localized. A reading of over 20 is highly suggestive of advanced disease whereas one below 10 is usually associated with localized disease. A biopsy should be done to confirm the diagnosis.

The pathologist should report on the amount of the cancer in the biopsy specimen and the histological grade of the tumour, reported as a Gleason score. Gleason scores range from 2 to 10 with a low score indicating a well-differentiated neoplasm of lower malignant potential. Predictive tables have been developed[10–12] that define the likelihood of extensive disease based on the PSA level, the Gleason score, and, where reliably assessed, the extent of the primary tumour (T stage). Investigations and therapies beyond these are based in large measure on the perceived risk of metastatic disease.

Decisions related to further investigations and therapy are generally based on consultations with specialists, primarily urologists and/or radiation oncologists. Where such individuals and the therapies they provide are not readily available the best a practitioner may be able to do is make a diagnosis based on physical examination and hopefully a PSA and biopsy. At that point, if radiation or surgery would be considered if available, but

Table 1 Percentage of men recording side-effects of radical therapy for prostate cancer—24-month survey responders[9]

	Radical prostatectomy (n = 961)	Radical radiotherapy (n = 373)
Bothered by dripping or leaking urine[a]	11.7	2.3
Bothered by frequent bowel movements, pain, or urgency	4.1	5.7
Bothered by sexual dysfunction[b]		
55–59 years of age[a]	74.9	39.9
60–74 years of age	52.8	46.6

[a] Differences statistically significant $p < 0.05$.

[b] Defined as a big or moderate problem versus small or no problem.

All values expressed as percentages and derived from logistic regression modelling after adjusting for the likelihood of treatment selection, age at diagnosis, baseline function, race/ethnicity, comorbidity, and educational attainment.

Adapted from Potosky, A.L. et al. (2000). Health outcomes after radical prostatectomy or radical radiotherapy for prostate cancer. Results from the Prostate Cancer Outcomes Study. *Journal of the National Cancer Institute* **92**, 1582–92. Reprinted with permission of the publishers.

access to these treatments is not possible it would be reasonable to treat the patient by hormone manipulation.

The goal of hormone manipulation in prostate cancer is androgen ablation. This is currently indicated not only for patients with symptomatic advanced disease but also for men who are asymptomatic but are considered at high risk for further disease. This includes men whose PSA level does not fall appropriately after radical local therapy (undetectable after surgery or less than 1 following radical radiotherapy). There are also reports that men derive benefit from adjunctive hormonal therapy when combined with radical radiation therapy for those patients with locally advanced disease.[13] Finally, men who are initially observed may be commenced on androgen ablation when a rise in PSA is observed. However, no one really knows the best threshold for commencing androgen ablation in this situation.

Methods of achieving androgen ablation include bilateral orchiectomy, the prescription of exogenous oestrogens in the form of diethylstilbestrol (DES), or the prescription of antiandrogens or luteinizing hormone-releasing hormone agonists (Table 2). All of these modalities are effective in delaying the progression of prostate cancer. However, oestrogens predispose to cardiovascular disease and many men seem unable to psychologically accept the idea of bilateral orchiectomy. For these reasons the newer, and much more expensive therapies, namely LH-RH agonists and antiandrogens, are frequently used where available. The LH-RH agonists are given parenterally in a depot formulation every 2–3 months. LH-RH agonists can be associated with a temporary flare of the disease. For patients with metastatic prostate cancer, flares can precipitate conditions like spinal cord compression. Therefore, in patients with metastatic disease non-steroidal antiandrogens are given prior to the LH-RH agonist and are often continued afterwards.

With androgen ablation all men experience, to varying degrees, loss of libido, loss of muscle mass, lassitude, and lower bone density. Currently, there is a trend to use these agents earlier in the course of the disease. If this trend continues, the long-term risks of these agents will have to be monitored and managed.

While surgery and radiation therapy hold out the promise of eradicating the cancer, hormone therapy only suppresses the cancer. The life expectancy of a patient with progressive prostate cancer following curative therapy is long compared to other cancers and depends on the stage at which recurrence is discovered. In one study of the natural history of rising PSA following radical prostatectomy a median of 8 years elapsed from the finding of a rising PSA to the development of metastases with a further 5 years from metastases to death.[14]

While many men die with but not of their cancer, it is clear that a significant number of men die from this disease and many more endure the consequences of the treatment or metastases even if they die of other causes. When cure of symptomatic disease is not possible all efforts should focus on palliation. For men with prostate cancer this can be a considerable challenge as bone metastases are an almost universal finding. Symptomatic care commonly involves a combination of analgesics and spot irradiation to painful bone lesions along with hormone therapy. While chemotherapy is used, at this time its role in palliation is secondary to these treatments.

All quality-of-life research indicates serious alterations in the physical, emotional, and sexual function of men with prostate cancer that is related to the type of therapy: surgery, radiation therapy, androgen ablation, or some combination of these. While research may lead to improvements in

one or more of these domains, there is little doubt that the prostate cancer patient's primary caregiver will continue to be a significant source of support and guidance to the patient and his partner.

Conclusions

Areas of uncertainty abound in prostate cancer. When will we have sufficient information to confidently recommend for or against preventive strategies? Is there benefit to a mass screening programme? Can we find a way to better define which patient would benefit from each of the specific management strategies available? Can we reduce the morbidity of treatments by reducing their frequency or by improving restorative therapies? Can we more effectively manage patients needing palliation? While some of these questions require highly specialized laboratory work, questions relating to screening, symptom control, and informed decision-making could benefit a great deal from a general practitioner perspective.

Key points

- Prostate cancer incidence varies widely around the world. It is high in Western societies and low in Asian societies

- Environmental contributors to the initiation and progression of prostate cancer are suspected but have not been conclusively identified to the point that recommendations about preventive action can be made

- Screening for prostate cancer is possible but it is unclear whether it produces any benefits, and if it does, whether the benefits outweigh the relatively frequent morbidity of treatment. Results from prospective randomized trials are expected towards the end of this decade. In the absence of this information, men should be counselled about the known risks (morbidity of therapy) and possible benefits of treatment before being screened

- Not all men die from their prostate cancer and for a certain group of men with very low volume and low-grade tumours, an initial policy of observation is appropriate

- The therapy of prostate cancer can significantly undermine the quality of life of the patient

References

1. **National Cancer Institute of Canada.** *Canadian Cancer Statistics 2001.* Toronto: Canada, 2001 (http://www.ncic.cancer.ca) (annual report).

2. **Muir, C.S., Nectoux, J., and Staszewski, J.** (1991). The epidemiology of prostate cancer. *Acta Oncologica* **30**, 133–40 (review).

3. **Shimizu, H., Ross, R.K., Bernstein, L., Yatani, R., Henderson, B.E., and Mack, T.M.** (1991). Cancers of the prostate and breast among Japanese and white immigrants to Los Angeles County. *British Journal of Cancer* **63**, 963–6 (primary research).

4. **Lichtenstein, P.** et al. (2000). Environmental and heritable factors in the causation of cancer. *New England Journal of Medicine* **343**, 78–85 (primary research).

5. **Wilson, J.M.G. and Junger, G.** *The Principles and Practice of Screening for Disease.* Geneva: World Health Organization, 1966 (classic monograph on screening).

6. **Madalinska, J.B., Essink-Bot, M.-L., de Koning, H.J., Kirkels, W.J., ven der Maas, P.J., and Schröder, F.H.** (2001). Health-related quality of life effects of radical prostatectomy and primary radiotherapy for screen-detected or clinically diagnosed prostate cancer. *Journal of Clinical Oncology* **19**, 1619–28 (primary research).

Table 2 Pharmacologic agents used in androgen ablation therapy

Pharmacologic class	Agents
Oestrogens	Diethylstilbesterol
Antiandrogens	
Non-steroidal antiandrogens	Bicalutamide, flutamide, nalutamide
Steroidal antiandrogens	Cyproterone acetate
LH-RH agonists	Buserelin, goserelin, leuprolide

7.   **Barry, M.J.** (2001). Prostate specific-antigen testing for early diagnosis of prostate cancer. *New England Journal of Medicine* **344**, 1373–7 (review).

8.   **Chodak, G.W.** et al. (1994). Results of conservative management of clinically localized prostate cancer. *New England Journal of Medicine* **330**, 242–8 (overview of multiple series).

9.   **Potosky, A.L., Legler, J., Albertsen, P.C., Stanford, J.L., Gilliland, F.D., Hamilton, A.S., Eley, J.W., Stephenson, R.A., and Harlan, L.C.** (2000). Health outcomes after radical prostatectomy or radical radiotherapy for prostate cancer. Results from the Prostate Cancer Outcomes Study. *Journal of the National Cancer Institute* **92**, 1582–92 (primary research).

10. **Partin, A.W., Kattan, M.W., Subong, E.N.P., Walsh, P.C., Wojno, K.J., Osterling, J.E., Scardino, P.T., and Pearson, J.D.** (1997). Combination of prostate-specific antigen, clinical stage, and Gleason score to predict pathological stage of localized prostate cancer. *Journal of the American Medical Association* **277**, 1445–51 (primary research).

11. **Gilliland, F.D., Hoffman, R.M., Hamilton, A., Albertsen, P., Eley, J.W., Harlan, L., Stanford, J.L., Hunt, W.C., and Potosky, A.** (1999). Predicting extracapsular extension of prostate cancer in men treated by radical prostatectomy: results form the population-based Prostate Cancer Outcomes Study. *Journal of Urology* **162**, 1341–5 (primary research).

12. http://box.cvl.bcm/edu/~mkattan/localized.html (summary of multiple series examining predictive indexes).

13. **Bolla, M.** et al. (1997). Improved survival in patients with locally advanced prostate cancer treated with radiotherapy and goserelin. *New England Journal of Medicine* **337**, 295–300 (primary research).

14. **Pound, C.R., Partin, A.W., Eisenberger, M.A., Chan, D.W., Pearson, J.D., and Walsh, P.C.** (1999). Natural history of progression after PSA elevation following radical prostatectomy. *Journal of the American Medical Association* **281**, 191–7 (primary research).

7

Women's health

7 Women's health

7.1 Breast pain and lumps

Helen Zorbas

How common is this presentation in primary care?

Breast symptoms are a very common presentation in general practice; on average, a general practitioner will have three consultations each week for breast symptoms. Breast lumps/lumpiness and breast pain constitute the majority of breast symptoms in general practice. In the United Kingdom, breast pain alone, or in association with lumpiness, accounts for up to half of the consultations in breast clinics. In Australia, about 65 per cent of the general practice consultations for a breast symptom are for a breast lump, about half are for breast pain, and about 20 per cent are for breast pain and breast lump. The majority of these symptoms will not be due to a breast cancer.

Epidemiology

Breast pain

Breast pain or mastalgia is a very common condition that affects most women at some point in their lives; studies have found that about 75 per cent of women admit to having recent breast pain. In the majority of women mastalgia does not affect the quality of life, but breast pain is a chronic symptom for most women who seek treatment.

The incidence of breast pain varies with the pattern of pain; cyclical mastalgia is more common in pre-menopausal women, average age 35 years, and non-cyclical mastalgia primarily affects women at least a decade later. About half of the women who have cyclical mastalgia have a change in their symptoms at some point in their life associated with a hormonal influence, for example, childbirth, breastfeeding, hysterectomy, or the use of hormone replacement therapy (HRT). Most of these cases resolve at the menopause. The Cardiff group noted that for some patients, the nature of the pain changed over time from cyclical to non-cyclical mastalgia. Follow up of patients who attended a mastalgia-specific clinic in Cardiff in Wales, United Kingdom, found that most women who presented with breast pain had been troubled by the affliction for at least 5 years. The median age of onset was 36 years, but age ranged from 12 to 63 years. The average duration of pain was 12 years and especially so if it began in the second and third decades of life. For many of these patients, the pain was chronic and relapsing.

Breast lumps

The incidence of breast lumps due to benign breast disease is high in pre-menopausal women and varies according to the aetiology; for example, fibroadenomas are more common in the second and third decades, whereas cysts are more common in the fifth decade. A lump is the most common presentation of a breast cancer; the incidence of breast cancer increases with increasing age.

The patterns of age incidence of different breast conditions assist the clinician in assessing the likelihood of a certain diagnosis and formulating the 'pre-test probability' of cancer. It should be borne in mind, however, that the increasing use of HRT has affected the incidence of breast symptoms and women taking HRT may present with conditions commonly associated with pre-menopausal years.

What are the possible causes?

Breast pain

A number of aetiologies have been suggested for breast pain, including histological differences, dietary, and hormonal factors. However, none of these has been substantiated and studies have varied in their approach and scientific rigour resulting in questionable findings. Therefore, although a hormonal relationship has been implicated and is likely, involving not only oestrogen and progesterone, but also prolactin, gonadotrophic hormones, and prostaglandins, the mechanism of pain is still not well understood.

It is important to exclude underlying chest wall pain when first assessing women with mastalgia. Musculoskeletal discomfort may commonly be experienced at the costochondral junction, along ribs, or along the mid axillary line at the lateral edge of the breast. In one breast clinic, chest wall pain accounted for up to 10 per cent of patients presenting with breast pain.

Rib cage pain can be a trap for the unwary since many women complain of breast tenderness as pressure is placed on the underlying rib. The patient may complain of a pain worse after exercise, at the end of the day, or after lying on that side. The secret is to lay the patient half on her side so that the breast tissue falls away from the ribs laterally. The fingers can be gently insinuated under the breast tissue to produce a characteristic 'catch' from the patient as the rib is pressed.

Breast pain may be localized or bilateral and cyclical or non-cyclical. Localized pain may be associated with underlying localized pathology and these are commonly benign conditions such as a tense breast cyst or area of fibrocystic change, a fibroadenoma, or an area of inflammation.

Uncommonly, breast pain may be a symptom of breast cancer. Breast pain alone is the presenting complaint in less than 7 per cent of symptomatic cancers and breast pain associated with a lump is the presenting symptom in about 14 per cent of symptomatic breast cancers.

Breast pain in a pre-menopausal woman which is cyclical and bilateral is indicative of normal physiological processes.

Most breast pain is usually mild or moderate in degree, but some women are significantly physically disabled by their pain. Those with even mild pain may be particularly concerned about underlying pathology, in particular breast cancer.

Many women who attend breast clinics with mastalgia as the presenting symptom do so because of fear of something more sinister. It is, therefore, important to consider the impact of anxiety and fear on the woman's perception of her symptoms and to address these sympathetically, once her pain has been adequately investigated.

Breast lumps

A breast lump is the most common presenting symptom of breast cancer; approximately 70 per cent of breast cancers present as a lump and 14 per cent as a lump with pain. A breast lump may be a discrete entity that stands out from the surrounding breast tissue, or it may be ill-defined and part of an area of lumpiness or nodularity.

A defined mass that is smooth and fluctuant is most likely to be a cyst. It may be soft or firm to palpation and may be painful depending on the fluid tension within the cyst. Cysts are a common breast symptom, accounting for approximately 15 per cent of all discrete breast masses. Cysts present particularly in the decade prior to menopause and the perimenopausal period, and women taking HRT may continue to experience cysts while on this therapy.

Fibroadenomas are also common symptomatic breast masses, particularly in women under 35 years, accounting for 60 per cent of masses in women aged 20 years or younger. A fibroadenoma usually presents as a defined, smooth, firm mass that is very mobile and may become more prominent and more tender pre-menstrually but may also present as a new finding in a woman taking HRT. The most important differential diagnosis in this age group is breast cancer. Breast cancer can uncommonly present as a smooth lump.

Breast lump or lumpiness in a pre-menopausal woman which occurs cyclically, is bilateral, and which may be associated with breast pain is usually due to normal physiological change. However, any asymmetrical area of nodularity that is ill-defined, particularly if it does not vary with the menstrual cycle in pre-menopausal women or is new in post-menopausal women, should be regarded with a high suspicion for cancer.

Although it is very common for women to experience breast changes such as pain or lumps, in more than 95 per cent of cases, they will not be due to breast cancer. However, even with a fully implemented mammographic screening programme, more than half of all breast cancers will be identified outside screening by a woman or her doctor as a change in her breast. Breast cancer is the most common cause of cancer death in women in Australia, with about 60 000 new cases in the world each year and is the most common cause of cancer death in women in much of the Western World. The challenge for the general practioner, therefore, is to investigate breast symptoms effectively to exclude cancer.

A number of factors bear on the probability of a particular symptom being due to a breast cancer. The factors that may increase risk for a particular woman include her age, whether she has a significant family history of breast and other cancers, whether she has had a previous breast cancer or a previous biopsy that shows atypical proliferative disease or other marker for increased risk. The history of the presenting symptom and the findings on clinical examination will additionally add to the formulation of a likely diagnosis and the risk for breast cancer.

How to make a diagnosis

There are a few important principles in the investigation of a woman who presents with a breast symptom. It is important to be attentive to the woman and her concerns, to follow a consistent step-wise approach to investigation, and to ensure that there is correlation between what the patient is describing, your clinical findings, and what any other test results indicate. Most importantly, it is vital that the investigative process results in a diagnosis that is confirmed by test results and adequately accounts for the symptom.

The 'triple test', which utilizes a systematic approach to the investigation of breast symptoms with clinical examination, imaging, and percutaneous biopsy, is accepted as the most effective way to maximize the detection of cancer and to provide an accurate diagnosis for a localized abnormality. However, not all women will require investigation with all three tests;

indeed, as the majority of symptoms are due to normal physiological changes, most women can be reassured after providing a history and having a clinical breast examination. Imaging may then support this diagnosis.

However, if any of the tests raises the suspicion of malignancy, or if the results do not correlate with one another, irrespective of any other normal test results, further evaluation and referral to a breast surgeon or specialist breast clinic is required (see Chapter 7.11).

History and clinical breast examination

A detailed history and thorough clinical breast examination provide important information on which to base further investigation, and should be accurately documented.

History

Relevant history includes details of:

- current medications or recent changes in medication, especially exogenous hormones;
- hormonal status/menstrual history;
- previous breast problems, results of previous investigations;
- risk factors, particularly strong family history of breast/ovarian cancer.
- History of presenting symptom:
  - site—constant or changing;
  - duration—when and how first noted, any changes since first noted;
  - relationship to menstrual cycle or exogenous hormones;
  - associated symptoms.

Clinical breast examination

Patient seated/standing

Inspection should take place in good light and with the patient seated or standing:

1. with arms by her side;
2. with arms raised above her head;
3. pressing on hips (tensing pectoral muscles) and leaning slightly forward.

It is important to inspect the breasts from the side as well as the front. Paying particular attention to the breast contours and the nipple region, look for any skin changes such as erythema, discoloration, dimpling or puckering, visible lumps, discoloration, inversion or ulceration of the nipple.

While the patient is still seated or standing:

1. *Palpate the supraclavicular fossae*, with the patient's shoulders relaxed.
2. *Palpate the breast*, examine the upper breast by sliding down from the clavicles with the middle three fingers, and also bimanually palpate the whole breast. Palpation with the woman seated sometimes demonstrates abnormalities otherwise difficult to detect.
3. *Palpate the axillae*, the axillary fossa is best felt with the patient's arm completely supported by the non-examining hand. A good way to get the patient to relax her arm is to ask her to 'let the shoulder drop'.

Patient lying down

Palpate the breast with the middle three fingers feeling with the distal pulp—use the flat of the fingers, not the tips. Palpate using a rotating or walking action of the finger pulps, gently then more firmly so as to palpate superficially and then more deeply. The patient's ipsilateral arm should be raised behind her head so that the breast tissue is spread out against the underlying chest wall. Examine all four quadrants, including the nipple and subareolar region and the axillary tail. The axillary region may be further examined with the patient's arm resting by her side.

Women with very large breasts may require a pillow to be placed under the ipsilateral shoulder to assist examination of the lateral breast and axilla.

In addition, it is important to lift large or very lax breasts to enable examination of the inframmary ridge region, where lesions could go undetected for some time. The non-examining hand may be used to either immobilize a large breast or fix breast tissue to assist examination.

Record details of any abnormality including exact position, size, shape, consistency, mobility, fixation, tenderness. Any area of interest that requires further investigation should be brought to the woman's attention and she should be assisted to feel the area herself if she wishes.

Investigating mastalgia

Taking a history and performing a clinical breast examination will provide much information to the clinician about the nature and likely cause of the presenting symptom. For example, the history may indicate hormonal activity due to starting the oral contraceptive pill; or clinical examination may indicate that the pain originates from the chest wall rather than the breast.

A thorough history is taken to determine the duration, location, and extent as well as the timing of the breast pain to try to distinguish cyclical from non-cyclical mastalgia. This history will also provide an indication of the impact of the pain on quality of life such as interfering with work, sport, sexual relations, or hugging children. In addition, a menstrual history, information about the use of any exogenous hormones or other drugs, and a family history of breast cancer should be taken.

For the majority of symptoms seen by primary care practitioners, these investigations will be sufficient to provide adequate reassurance; for example, for those women who present with typical cyclical mastalgia, no clinical abnormality, and no risk factors. Breast imaging may or may not be performed for this group of women and this is primarily at the discretion of the general practitioner and may be influenced by whether the patient is due for a screening mammogram or her level of anxiety. It is advisable to organize a follow-up appointment in 6–8 weeks to review the patient and her symptomatology.

Breast imaging should be performed if:

- there is any concern arising from the history or clinical examination;
- there are any risk factors for breast cancer;
- the symptom is unilateral and persistent;
- at the follow-up visit the symptom persists;
- the woman is anxious.

Ultrasound examination is recommended as the first-line imaging test for women under 35 years; if there is any suspicion of cancer on clinical examination or ultrasound, then a mammogram should be performed as well. Women aged 35 years and over should minimally have a mammogram and if there is any localized symptom, an ultrasound examination is recommended as it may provide additional information about the cause of the symptom. Any clinical or imaging abnormality should be further investigated with targeted imaging and percutaneous biopsy tests.

Investigating breast lumps

The aim of the investigation of a breast symptom is to achieve an accurate diagnosis. The triple test approach will ensure that the vast majority of diagnoses are effectively achieved without the need for open surgical biopsy.

Taking a history and performing a clinical breast examination will help to categorize the lump as benign, indeterminate, or suspicious for cancer. For example, a lump that has been slowly increasing in size over 6 months might be regarded with greater suspicion than a lump that appeared overnight. In addition, the patient's previous personal history or family history of breast cancer or her age may impact on the likelihood of a woman's lump being a breast cancer. On examination, it is important to document the lump's size, position, shape, consistency, mobility, tenderness, fixation, or associated skin changes. These features will also indicate a likely diagnosis.

Imaging tests are very important diagnostic tools in the triple test approach. Mammography is the first-line imaging test recommended for women 35 years or more and ultrasound the first-line imaging test for younger women or those women who are pregnant or lactating. It is important to include all relevant details and results when making referrals to provide the radiologist with the information to perform the most appropriate imaging tests to gain maximal information about the area of interest. Often, a combination of mammography with special views and targeted ultrasound are performed to add further information about the likely diagnosis. If there is any suspicion of cancer, bilateral mammography must be performed to identify the extent of the disease in the affected breast and any asymptomatic disease in the other breast (see Chapter 7.11).

It is important that clinical examination and imaging tests are performed prior to any tissue sampling procedures. This is because any resultant tissue distortion or haematoma following biopsy could confound the subsequent clinical and imaging findings.

Any solid lesion seen on ultrasound can be sampled either by fine needle aspiration cytology or core biopsy, preferably under ultrasound guidance to maximize the likelihood of obtaining an adequate and representative sample. The choice of sampling procedure may depend on the local expertise and resources, or factors such as the type or position of the lesion in the breast.

Any abnormality seen on mammography can be sampled by stereotactic guidance or by ultrasound if it can also be visualized with this modality.

Principles of management

The primary care physician is usually the first port of call for a woman with a breast symptom. The key role for the clinician is to ascertain which women can be reassured that their symptom is normal or due to benign breast disease and which women require specialist referral. Once adequately investigated and a diagnosis is made, benign breast disease can, in most instances, be successfully managed in the general practice setting.

Breast pain

Up to 85 per cent of women with cyclical hormonal mastalgia experience improvement in their symptoms after reassurance that their pain is not due to cancer. In addition, simple measures such as wearing a bra which provides more support, or manipulation of the type or dose of oral contraceptive pill or HRT may be all that is required. Chest wall pain can be treated with anti-inflammatory drugs or, if localized, infiltration with a local anaesthetic and steroid injection can be considered.

The primary indication for treatment is pain that interferes with everyday activities. A pain chart is helpful in consolidating a woman's perceptions of her pain and in assessing the effectiveness of any treatment.

Evening primrose oil contains gamma linoleic acid and is a rich source of essential fatty acids. Studies of its effectiveness vary; while some studies have found a response rate of up to 55 per cent for patients with cyclical mastalgia and considerably lower rates for women with non-cyclical mastalgia, other studies do not demonstrate an effectiveness greater than placebo. Evening primrose oil is a natural product, virtually free of side-effects, and is a commonly prescribed therapy for moderate pain. It can be bought over the counter in pharmacies or health food stores; a daily dose of 3000 mg is usually recommended for a period of 3–4 months as onset of improvement, if it occurs, is slow.

Hormonal therapies are reserved for intractable or more severe mastalgia. These are usually best prescribed either under the supervision of or in consultation with an endocrinologist or specialist breast surgeon. Danazol, an antigonadotrophin, is the first-line treatment here. About 70 per cent of women with cyclical mastalgia and fewer with non-cyclical mastalgia respond to Danazol. However, about 20 per cent of women may experience side-effects, some of which can be severe enough to discontinue treatment and include headache, nausea, vomiting, acne, and weight gain. Bromocriptine is a prolactin inhibitor and can be used as either first- or second-line therapy for moderate/severe mastalgia with about a 50 per cent response rate for cyclical mastalgia and 25 per cent for non-cyclical mastalgia. Adverse effects are common and can be severe, such as postural hypotension and depression.

Common breast lumps

If the lump is seen on ultrasound to correspond to a typical cyst, it may either be aspirated or left alone. This aspiration may more readily be performed under ultrasound guidance at the time of the imaging examination with prior discussion and consent of the woman. Commonly, asymptomatic cysts are also found by chance on breast ultrasound examination and these do not require treatment. If the symptomatic cyst is aspirated no further investigations are required provided that the lump does not persist and that the cystic fluid is normal in appearance (straw coloured to dark green) and is not blood stained. However, if any of these signs are present, the aspirated fluid should be sent for cytology. Any remaining lump requires independent further evaluation with imaging and biopsy. This may be performed by the radiologist at the time of aspiration with prior discussion with the referring doctor and the woman. The woman should be referred to a breast or specialist breast clinic for coordination of further evaluation of the lump.

Any solid lesion seen on imaging requires triple assessment to confirm a diagnosis and exclude cancer. This may best be achieved by referral to a breast surgeon or specialist breast clinic.

Follow-up

It is important that the investigation leads to a firm diagnosis of the cause of breast symptoms. Reviewing a woman in 3–6 months, for example, should not be used to delay making a diagnosis.

Women should be encouraged to return for review if their symptoms change or worsen or if they remain worried. Follow-up and review of women whose symptoms are found to be benign or due to normal hormonal changes in 6–8 weeks will help to identify those symptoms which persist or change in a way which may require further investigation or treatment. In addition, it is important to be prepared to reconsider and review the original diagnosis based on more recent history or symptom changes.

Key points

- The majority of breast symptoms will not be due to a breast cancer.
- All symptoms should have a diagnosis.
- The 'triple test' approach to diagnosis is the most effective means of maximizing the detection of cancer.
- Any woman with a triple test positive result, or where there is inconsistency of test results, requires further investigation and/or surgical referral *irrespective of other normal test results*.
- Reassurance that cancer is not responsible for their symptom and an explanation of the hormonal basis of their pain may be the only treatment necessary in up to 85 per cent women with cyclical mastalgia.

Further reading

Maddox, P. and Mansel, R.E. (1989). Management of breast pain and nodularity. *World Journal of Surgery* **13** (6), 699–705.

Morrow, M. *Management of Common Breast Disorders: Breast Pain. Breast Diseases*. JB Lippincott Company, 1991, pp. 63–73.

National Breast Cancer Centre. *The Investigation of a New Breast Symptom: A Guide for General Practitioners*. Woolloomooloo NSW: NHMRC National Breast Cancer Centre, 1997.

Irwig, L. and Macaskill, P. *Evidence Relevant to Guidelines for the Investigation of Breast Symptoms*. Woolloomooloo NSW: NHMRC National Breast Cancer Centre, 1997.

Pit, S., Cockburn, J., and Zorbas, H. *Investigation of a New Breast Symptom: An Audit in General Practice*. Woolloomooloo NSW: NHMRC National Breast Cancer Centre, 1999.

Dixon, J.M., ed. *ABC of Breast Diseases*. London: BMJ Publishing Group, 1999.

7.2 Nipple discharge

Rebecca B. Saenz

Introduction

The primary concern of most women presenting to their primary care physician with nipple discharge is the possibility of malignancy. Unless the discharge is serosanguinous, bloody, or associated with a palpable mass, the patient may be reassured that the cause is most likely benign. A careful history and physical examination will reveal the cause in many instances.

Definitions

Lactation is the normal physiologic function of the female breast. This subject is covered in detail in Chapter 8.9. Expressible milk may be present for up to 2 years after weaning, and may occasionally be reported as nipple discharge.

True nipple discharge is the spontaneous flow of fluid from the nipple apart from pregnancy or lactation. Fluid may be milky, clear, creamy, yellow, green, brown, black, serous, serosanguinous, or bloody. Nipple bleeding is a subset of nipple discharge, and except in late pregnancy or early lactation, is probably the most troublesome sign.

Galactorrhoea is the production of milk unrelated to pregnancy or breastfeeding. Breast pathology is rarely a cause. Primary galactorrhoea may be caused by mechanical nipple stimulation, chest wall trauma, or nerve irritation. Secondary galactorrhoea may be caused by a variety of endocrine conditions, neoplastic processes, chronic disease states, and pharamacologic agents.

Conditions that may mimic nipple discharge include discharge from Montgomery's tubercles, seen in adolescent girls, and exudate from various skin lesions of the nipple or areola.

Epidemiology

About 20 per cent of female patients will have nipple discharge with squeezing and 50–80 per cent report discharge with application of suction, as with a pump. Most of these will be physiologic in nature, secondary to a hormonal cause or a pharmacologic side-effect. It is estimated that 20–25 per cent of women will experience spontaneous galactorrhoea at some time in their lives.

About 10–15 per cent of women with benign breast disease will present to their primary care physician with the complaint of nipple discharge and 2.5–3 per cent of women with breast malignancy will present with nipple discharge as the primary complaint. Likelihood of malignancy increases with age.

Approximately 80–90 per cent of newborns of either gender will also exhibit nipple discharge within the first 2–3 weeks of life, and up to 5 per cent will continue to do so for up to a month.

Nipple discharge in men is extremely rare.

Although nipple discharge without an associated mass in women is associated with malignancy in only 10–20 per cent of cases, there is wide variability among studies of association between nipple discharge and malignancy in men.

Differential diagnosis and natural history

Physiologic discharges

Lactation

Lactogenesis begins during pregnancy. Occasionally, the pregnant patient may present with 'nipple discharge', in which case reassurance and anticipatory guidance regarding her body's preparation to breastfeed her baby is all that is required. In approximately 0.1 per cent of mothers, the secretions may be blood-stained, a condition referred to as 'rusty pipe syndrome'. Unless accompanied by a discrete mass, this is not a cause for concern. After delivery, colostrum and milk may be blood-tinged for up to 2 months due to this condition, which spontaneously resolves over time. However, if bleeding persists, or a mass becomes evident, investigation is warranted.

Primary galactorrhoea

Physiologic primary galactorrhoea may occur at the stages of life during which there is rapid hormonal change. The first of these is the neonatal period, during which newborns may produce an expressible nipple discharge known as 'witch's milk' or neonatal lactation. After delivery, the infant is no longer exposed to the high levels of maternal sex steroids as during pregnancy via the placenta, but the infant pituitary continues to secrete high prolactin levels for a few weeks after birth, producing a hormonal milieu conducive to lactation. Neonatal lactation is benign and self-limited, resolving as infant prolactin levels decline. Transient galactorrhoea may also be seen at menarche, due to rapid breast development, and at menopause, due to rapid drops in oestrogen while prolactin levels remain steady.

Primary galactorrhoea may also be seen as the result of mechanical nipple stimulation, such as by tight-fitting clothing or in sexual foreplay. Intentional mechanical stimulation by use of a breast pump can induce lactation.

Galactorrhoea has also been reported in association with chest wall trauma, burns, surgery, and after mammography. Chest wall nerve irritation due to herpes zoster may also induce galactorrhoea. More central irritation of a nerve root due to a cervical spine lesion has also been reported to cause galactorrhoea. Cessation of mechanical stimulation or treatment of the nerve or nerve root irritation usually allows cessation of milk production.

Secondary galactorrhoea

Secondary galactorrhoea may occur as the result of various hormonal disturbances in the hypothalamic–pituitary axis. The most common of these is pituitary adenoma. Others include pituitary stalk resection, emptysella syndrome, multiple sclerosis, and infiltrative conditions such as sarcoidosis, tuberculosis, and schistosomiasis.

Some systemic diseases may cause secondary galactorrhoea. Hypothyroidism results in high levels of thyrotropin-releasing hormone, which then increases the prolactin level. Chronic renal failure may result in higher circulating prolactin levels due to decreased prolactin clearance by the kidneys. The hypersecretion of cortisol due to Cushing's disease may induce a hyperprolactinaemic state, as can the increased growth hormone levels associated with acromegaly.

Several other neoplastic processes may be the cause of secondary galactorrhoea due to ectopic release of prolactin. These include craniopharyngioma, bronchogenic carcinoma, renal adenocarcinoma, lymphoma, hydatidiform mole, hypernephroma, mixed growth hormone-secreting and prolactin-secreting tumours, and null-cell adenomas. Achievement of hormonal balance by medical or surgical means usually results in cessation of secondary galactorrhoea, regardless of the underlying cause.

Pharmacologic causes of secondary galactorrhoea include hormonal preparations, dopamine antagonists, and herbal preparations. Practically speaking, these drugs include the categories of oral contraceptives, hormone replacement therapies, antioestrogens, antipsychotics, tricyclic anti-depressants, selective serotonin reuptake inhibitors, benzodiazepines, antithyroids, gastrointestinal agents, some antihypertensives, some antiepileptics, and several herbal preparations. See Table 1 for the full list. Secondary galactorrhoea due to pharmacologic causes usually ceases when the offending agent is withdrawn.

Table 1 Pharmacologic causes of galactorrhoea

Antidepressants and anxiolytics	Antipsychotics	Antihypertensives	Gastrointestinal agents	Hormonal preparations	Other drugs	Illicit drugs	Herbs
Alprazolam	Acetophenazine	Atenolol	Cimetidine	Conjugated oestrogens	Amphetamines	Amphetamines	Anise
Amitriptyline	Amisulpride	Diazoxide	Cisapride	Cyproterone	Anaesthetics	Cannabis	Blessed thistle
Amoxapine	Benperidol	Methyldopa	Clebopride	Medroxyprogesterone	Arginine	Heroin	Fennel
Buspirone	Bromperidol	Reserpine	Domperidone	Nafarelin	Clobazam		Fenugreek seed
Citalopram	Chlorpromazine	Verapamil	Famotidine	Oral contraceptive formulations	Cyclobenzaprine		Marshmallow
Clomipramine	Chlorprothixene		Metoclopramide	Combination oestrogen	Danazol		Milk thistle
Doxepin	Levosulpiride		Octreotide	and progestogen	Diethylstilbestrol		Nettle
Fluoxetine	Melperone		Prochlorperazine	Progestogen only	Dihydroergotamine		Red clover
Imipramine	Molindone		Ranitidine	Protirelin	Dinoprost		Red raspberry
Metaclazepam	Perazine			Tamoxifen	Isoniazid		
Moclobemide	Perphenazine				Opiates		
Nortriptyline	Pipamperone				Rimantidine		
Paroxetine	Pipotiazine				Sumatriptan		
Protriptyline	Remoxipride				Valproic acid		
Sertraline	Risperidone						
	Sulpiride						
	Sultopride						
	Triflupromazine						
	Trimeperazine						
	Veralipride						
	Zotepine						

Pathologic nipple discharge

Causes of pathologic breast discharge include both benign and malignant breast diseases. Non-puerperal mastitis may cause a purulent nipple discharge that resolves with appropriate antibiotic treatment. Fibrocystic breast disease, duct ectasia, and intraductal papilloma may present with serous, serosanguinous, or bloody nipple discharge. Occasionally, other breast malignancies, particularly intraductal carcinoma, will present with nipple discharge. Treatment of the underlying disorder results in remission of the nipple discharge as well.

Making the diagnosis

History and physical examination

A thorough history and physical examination can give important clues to possible causes of nipple discharge. How long has the nipple discharge been present? Is it spontaneous, or only apparent with manual manipulation? How copious is the discharge—merely noticeable, or a social embarrassment? Is the discharge unilateral or bilateral; from only one duct or from several? What colour is the discharge—milky, clear, purulent, coloured, or bloody? Is there any associated pain? Is there an associated mass?

Nipple discharges that are bilateral, from more than one duct, milky, painless, and not associated with any palpable mass are designated physiologic, and usually prove to be galactorrhoea. Pathologic discharges, those due to intrinsic breast disease, are more often spontaneous, unilateral, from only one duct, and may be any colour, including bloody or blood-tinged.

Once it is determined that the discharge is likely physiologic, further questioning may be directed toward eliciting possible primary or secondary causes. Could the patient be pregnant, or how recently has she breastfed? Has there been any mechanical stimulation, such as from tight-fitting clothing, repeated breast self-exams, or sexual activity? Has there been any chest wall irritation from herpes zoster, dermatitis, burns, or surgery? Is there any history of spinal cord problems or oesophageal reflux? A thorough review of systems may reveal other symptoms of hypothalamic–pituitary axis problems, such as amenorrhoea or irregular menses, infertility, visual field defects, or others that the patient may not realize are relevant. Symptoms of other systemic diseases or other neoplastic processes should also be sought.

A thorough medication history, including use of illicit substances, non-prescription medications, and herbal remedies should be reviewed. The list of pharamacologic causes of galactorrhoea is quite extensive. Patients may be hesitant to reveal use of illicit substances unless directly questioned.

If the discharge is determined to be pathologic, a history of any related fever, pain, or other signs of infection may indicate non-puerperal mastitis, especially if the discharge is purulent. Coloured non-purulent discharges may be caused by breast cysts or ductal ectasia. Colours range from creamy, yellow, brown, green, to black. Smoking history often correlates with darker colour of discharge.

Serous, serosanguinous, and bloody discharges are sticky and range in colour from yellow to pink to bloody. Ductal ectasia, epithelial hyperplasia, intraductal papilloma, and various malignancies are the causes, with a positive correlation between increasing age and likelihood of malignancy.

A thorough breast exam should be conducted to exclude the possibility of a palpable mass or adenopathy in addition to determining the character of the discharge itself. Any palpable masses discovered take precedence in the investigation. The physical exam should also include investigation of any symptomatology revealed in the history and review of systems. Large visual field defects can be revealed on gross confrontation testing, but may need to be confirmed by more formal visual field mapping. Other physical signs of secondary causes of nipple discharge should be sought, if the discharge is milky.

Laboratory studies

The nipple discharge may be tested for the presence of occult blood using any of the commonly available occult blood testing cards or the appropriate section of a urine dipstick. Cytology of the discharge is not particularly useful for excluding malignancy, due to a high false-negative rate. However, the high specificity for malignancy makes a positive result useful. Microscopy of nipple discharge can also be useful in confirming the presence of fat globules, indicative of galactorrhoea, or of other cell types that can give diagnostic clues. A few macrophages and lymphocytes are normally present in milk, and thus are also indicative of galactorrhoea. The presence of many large foamy macrophages and few, if any, epithelial cells is indicative of ductal ectasia. A predominance of segmented neutrophils may be more indicative of infection. Culture and sensitivity should be performed if the discharge appears purulent.

Several biochemical assays of nipple discharge have been investigated for their sensitivity and specificity in predicting or excluding the presence of carcinoma. Among these are lactose, sodium, potassium, casein, GCDFP-15 (a marker for apocrine metaplasia), Erb-2, and CEA levels. At present, biochemical assays remain investigational, as none has been demonstrated to be conclusive in this clinical scenario.

Measurement of serum levels of human chorionic gonadotrophin, thyroid-stimulating hormone, and prolactin are indicated if the discharge is milky. Blood urea nitrogen and creatinine levels may be helpful if chronic renal failure is suspected. Tests for the less frequent causes of secondary galactorrhoea may be guided by the history.

Imaging studies

In patients with galactorrhoea, a high prolactin level or irregular menses warrants a magnetic resonance image or computerized axial tomography scan of the brain, with special attention to the pituitary, to assess for pituitary adenoma. Less commonly, these tests may reveal other intracranial pathology associated with galactorrhoea, such as craniopharyngioma or empty-sella syndrome.

Patients with pathologic discharge should have breast imaging performed, particularly those older than 35 years. Which test should be done is controversial and often dependent on operator expertise.

Mammography is indicated in all patients over 35 years with a nipple discharge, but particularly if the discharge is serous, serosanguinous, or bloody. Microcalcifications along a duct may reveal an otherwise unsuspected intraductal carcinoma. Larger calcifications and prominent ducts are more typical of ductal ectasia. In general, the density of breast tissue in patients under 35 years of age lowers the sensitivity of mammography considerably.

High-resolution ultrasound may be used to amplify information obtained during physical exam or mammography. Occasionally, it detects small lesions or dilated subareolar ducts. As resolution continues to improve, ultrasound will continue to increase in usefulness.

Galactography, or cannulation of a duct and instillation of contrast material, has gained popularity in some settings. It can demonstrate abnormal ductal anatomy, ductal dilatation, intraductal papillomas, and communication between ducts and cysts. Lesions may be missed in dilated ducts, however, and blood clots may appear as papillomas, raising both false-negative and false-positive rates. Occasionally, galactography demonstrates a previously undetected lesion that can then be localized by ultrasound for a fine needle aspiration cytology procedure. Pre-operative galactography, with instillation of methylene blue, can serve to delineate ductal anatomy for the surgeon. Use of galactography may be limited by patient discomfort, and for this reason, is not used routinely.

Magnetic resonance imaging of the breast has recently shown promise as having a higher sensitivity than either mammography or ultrasound. It may be comparable to galactography, but is much less invasive and with greater patient comfort.

A newer technique of fibreoptic ductography, using a small diameter silica fibrescope, has recently been described. Initial reports indicate that direct visualization of breast ducts, and thus intraductal lesions, might be possible with this technique. Anaesthesia was not required in the original series, but the procedure has the potential to cause discomfort.

Triage and principles of management

Once it has been determined that a nipple discharge is physiologic rather than pathologic, the patient may be safely reassured that breast malignancy is not the cause. Many physiologic causes of nipple discharge can be determined by history alone. If the cause is not readily apparent, serum tests for hormone levels can differentiate between a hyperprolactinaemic state and the other hormonal causes. In many cases the more expensive imaging studies may not be necessary.

The evaluation of a pathologic discharge should be more aggressive. Any palpable mass should take precedence in the evaluation. If no mass is palpable, mammography and ultrasound imaging should be performed according to screening guidelines. Suspicious lesions identified should then be biopsied. If no suspicious lesions are revealed on mammography or ultrasound, or if screening guidelines did not indicate those investigation, galactography may be performed. Cytology should be performed as an adjunct to these studies, to ascertain the likelihood of ductal ectasia. Culture and sensitivity testing should be performed as indicated. Any infection or malignancy discovered should then be treated appropriately.

If malignancy is ruled out after thorough evaluation of pathologic discharge, further treatment may be guided by the patient's wishes. If discharge is not copious and the patient wishes to preserve her future ability to breastfeed, surveillance by serial breast examination and mammography may be an option. If the discharge is copious enough to be a social embarrassment, or if the patient's family history places her at high risk for breast cancer, terminal duct excision may be considered.

Key points

1. Classification of nipple discharge as physiologic or pathologic based on history and physical characteristics, guides the remainder of the evaluation of nipple discharge.

2. Evaluation of any associated mass takes precedence over evaluation of the nipple discharge.

3. Physiologic nipple discharge may be caused by stimulation, chest wall trauma or irritation, hormonal imbalances, or pharmacologic agents.

4. Pathologic nipple discharge may be caused by infection, intraductal papilloma, ductal ectasia, breast cysts, or various breast malignancies.

Further reading

Bassett, L.W., Jackson, V.P., Jahan, R., Fu, Y.S., and Gold, R.H. *Diagnosis of Diseases of the Breast.* Philadelphia: W.B. Saunders Company, 1997. (Comprehensive text on breast problems.)

Morrow, M. (2000). Evaluation of common breast problems. *American Family Physician* **61**, 2371–8. (Review article on breast pain, nipple discharge, and breast masses.)

Pena, K.S. and Rosenfeld, J.A. (2001). Evaluation and treatment of galactorrhea. *American Family Physician* **63**, 1763–75. (Comprehensive review article.)

Webster, D.J.T. (2000). Nipple discharge. In *Benign Disorders and Diseases of the Breast: Concepts and Clinical Management* 2nd edn. (ed. L.E. Hughes, R.E. Mansel, and D.J.T. Webster), pp. 171–86. St Louis: WB Saunders.

Freeman, J.J., Altieri, R.H., Freeman, A.H., Kuo, T., Sardinha, F., Buckingham, C.C., Sklar, J.J., Dyroff, K., and Floyd, A. (1994). Inappropriate breast secretions of possible bacterial etiology in the parous nonpuerperal female. *Journal of the National Medical Association* **86**, 203–8. (A case series.)

Kavanagh, A.M., Giles, G.G., Mitchell, H., and Cawson, J.N. (2000). The sensitivity, specificity, and positive predictive value of screening mammography and symptomatic status. *Journal of Medical Screening* **7**, 105–10. (A recent large retrospective study.)

Makiti, M. et al. (1991). Duct endoscopy and endoscopic biopsy in the evaluation of nipple discharge. *Breast Cancer Research and Treatment* **18**, 179–81.

Merlob, P., Aloni, R., Prager, H., Mor, N., and Litwin, A. (1990). Blood-stained maternal milk: prevalence, characteristics, and counselling. *European Journal of Obstetrics, Gynecology, and Reproductive Biology* **35**, 153–7. (Landmark prospective study of blood-tinged milk in puerperal period.)

Orel, S.G., Dougherty, C.S., Reynolds, C., Czerniecki, B.J., Siegelman, E.S., and Schnall, M.D. (2000). MR imaging in patients with nipple discharge: initial experience. *Radiology* **216**, 248–54. (A recent retrospective study.)

Rongione, A.J., Evans, B.D., Kling, K.M., and McFadden, D.W. (1996). Ductography is a useful technique in evaluation of abnormal nipple discharge. *The American Surgeon* **62**, 785–8. (Recent prospective study.)

Slawson, S.H. and Johnson, B.A. (2001). Ductography: how to and what if? *Radiographics* **21**, 133–50. (Instructional article on the procedure itself, with several examples of radiographs showing various lesions discovered at ductography.)

Sweetman, S., ed. *Martindale: The Complete Drug Reference.* London: Pharmaceutical Press. Electronic version. MICROMEDEX, Greenwood Village, Colorado (edition expires 6/01).

7.3 Vaginal discharge

Tim Stokes

Epidemiology

Vaginal discharge and other associated lower genital tract symptoms such as vulval itching and soreness are common in adult women. In one Swedish population-based survey, one in four women aged 19–25 years reported such symptoms within the previous 6 months.[1]

How common is this presentation in primary care?

One in 10 women presenting in UK general practice complains of vaginal symptoms. Vaginal symptoms (chiefly attributable to vulvovaginal candidiasis) account for approximately 1200 consultations per 10 000 women aged 16–44, half of whom consult more than once for the same problem.[2]

What are the possible causes?

A normal vaginal discharge is clear or white and its amount and fluidity can vary depending on the stage of the menstrual cycle. A change in terms of colour and/or amount, often associated with symptoms of itching, soreness, and a 'bad' smell, represents an abnormal vaginal discharge.

An abnormal vaginal discharge is usually caused by infection. The two commonest causes of vaginal infection in pre-menopausal women in primary care are bacterial vaginosis and vulvovaginal candidiasis.[3] Other infections include trichomoniasis, chlamydia, gonorrhoea, and genital herpes. Table 1 shows the underlying diagnosis of vaginal discharge among pre-menopausal women consulting in one Swedish general practice.[3] Women consulting with the same symptoms in the developing world will have higher prevalences of trichomoniasis, chlamydia, and gonorrhoea.[4]

Table 1 Diagnosis in 101 women aged 15–50 consulting in general practice due to vaginal discharge (The number of women who were also given the definite diagnosis as a preliminary diagnosis at presentation are given in brackets.)

Endogenous conditions	No. of patients	Sexually transmitted infections (STIs)	No. of patients	Other causes	No. of patients
Bacterial vaginosis	34 (33)	Chlamydial infection	15 (5)	Psychological factors	5
Vulvovaginal candidiasis	23 (20)	Trichomoniasis	9 (7)	Cytolysis	5
		Genital herpes	7 (7)	IUD-associated	5
		Gonorrhoea	1 (1)	Urinary tract infection	3 (3)
		Mucopurulent cervicitis	1 (1)	Other/unknown	7
Total no. of patients	56[a]		29[b]		25

[a] Of the 56 patients, nine also had an STI.

[b] Among the 29 patients with an STI, four had two sexually transmitted agents.

Source: ref. 3.

Table 2 Clinical features of infective causes of vaginal discharge in pre-menopausal women

	Vulvovaginal candidiasis	Bacterial vaginosis	Trichomoniasis	Chlamydia and gonorrhoea
Symptoms				
Key symptom	Vulval itching	Abnormal vaginal discharge Slightly increased amount Abnormal smell ('fishy')	Abnormal vaginal discharge Increased amount Yellow-green colour Abnormal smell	Symptoms listed below are non-specific and poor predictors of infection
Other symptoms	Vaginal discharge Vulval pain/burning Dysuria Superficial dyspareunia	No vulval soreness or itching	Vulvar soreness	Vaginal discharge Dysuria Postcoital or intermenstrual bleeding Low abdominal pain
Signs				
Vulval examination	Erythema Oedema Fissures	No erythema	Erythema	
Speculum examination	Vaginal erythema Thick curdy discharge	No vaginal erythema Increased vaginal discharge	Vaginal erythema Yellow-green vaginal discharge Profuse vaginal discharge Strawberry appearance of cervix	Vaginal discharge Cervical mucopus Cervical ectopy Cervix bleeds when touched

Bacterial vaginosis (BV)

BV is a clinical syndrome that results from the replacement of the normal vagina flora (*Lactobacillus*) with a mixed flora consisting of *Gardnerella vaginalis*, anaerobes, and *Mycoplasma hominis*. It is not regarded as a sexually transmitted infection (STI). The only proven consequence of untreated BV is in pregnant women where it is associated with late miscarriage, pre-term birth, premature rupture of membranes, and postpartum endometritis.[5]

Vulvovaginal candidiasis (VVC)

VVC is a clinical syndrome that results from the transformation of asymptomatic vaginal carriage of the yeast *Candida albicans* into symptomatic vaginitis. Predisposing factors include pregnancy, poorly controlled diabetes, and antibiotic usage. It is not regarded as an STI. An estimated 75 per cent of women will have at least one episode of VVC or 'thrush' during their lives. Less than 5 per cent of women experience recurrent VVC (defined as four or more episodes of VVC annually). The pathogenesis of recurrent VVC is poorly understood.

Trichomoniasis

Trichomoniasis is caused by the protozoan *Trichomonas vaginalis*. It is an STI and an important risk marker for other STIs. Untreated trichomoniasis in pregnant women is associated with pre-term birth and low birth weight.[6]

Chlamydia

Chlamydial cervicitis is caused by the bacterium *Chlamydia trachomatis* and is the commonest bacterial STI in women in the developed world. It is asymptomatic in up to 70 per cent of women. A diagnosis on the basis of symptoms is problematic as none of the reported symptoms is strongly predictive of infection (see Table 2).[7] Untreated chlamydia is a cause of significant morbidity, the three important complications being pelvic inflammatory disease (PID), tubal infertility, and ectopic pregnancy.

Gonorrhoea

Gonorrhoeal cervicitis is caused by the bacterium *Neisseria gonorrhoea* and is rarely seen in primary care in developed countries. Gonorrhoea shares many of the features of chlamydia as diagnosis on the basis of symptoms is problematic[7] and if untreated it also leads to PID, tubal infertility, and ectopic pregnancy.

Genital herpes

Genital herpes is caused by *Herpes simplex* virus. It should be considered in the differential diagnosis of a vaginal discharge in primary care although its key symptoms are pain, genital ulceration, and dysuria.[8]

Non-infective causes

These must not be overlooked and include oral contraception, local genital tract pathology (e.g. cervical polyp) or a retained foreign body such as a tampon. Vulvovaginitis may be caused by eczema or chemical irritants. In post-menopausal women, atrophic vaginitis can present with a watery vaginal discharge.

How to make a diagnosis

History

The key clinical features of the common infective causes of vaginal discharge are presented in Table 2.

A presenting complaint of vaginal discharge is suggestive of a vaginal infection (BV/trichomoniasis).[8] Clarification of the discharge should focus on recent changes in amount, smell, and colour. The presence of any associated symptoms such as vulval itching, soreness, pain/burning, ulceration, and dysuria should also be sought.

A presenting complaint of vulval itching is suggestive of VVC and that of vulvar ulceration suggestive of genital herpes.[8] A history of previous episodes should be sought as both VVC and genital herpes are often recurrent. First episode genital herpes may present with severe symptoms; subsequent recurrences are self-limiting and associated with mild symptoms.

If an STI (trichomoniasis, chlamydia, gonorrhoea) is suspected then a sexual history should be taken. It is important to determine demographic and risk factors for infection. These include age less than 25, being single, recent change in sexual partner or recent multiple partners, and no use of barrier methods of contraception. The presence of two or more of these risk factors should increase the index of suspicion for a diagnosis of an STI.

The woman's reasons for consultation are important. She may find her symptoms intolerable or she may have been prompted to consult because of her partner's sexual behaviour. Has she considered the possibility of an STI and, if so, how does she feel about being tested for one? Women with VVC may already have treated themselves with over-the-counter preparations.

The psychological and social impact of symptoms must be determined. Women may find the symptoms embarrassing and a chronic discharge, in particular, can have a devastating effect on a sexual relationship.

Examination

The vulva should be inspected for signs of oedema, erythema, and ulceration. A speculum examination should be performed to assess the consistency, location, and amount of vaginal discharge. A thick curdy vaginal discharge is predictive of VVC. The cervix should be inspected for signs of cervical mucopus (mucopurulent cervicitis), cervical ectopy, and contact bleeding. Mucopurulent cervicitis is predictive of chlamydia or gonorrhoea.[7,8] A bimanual examination allows signs suggestive of PID (adnexal tenderness, cervical motion pain) to be sought.

Investigation

Primary care physicians in different countries will have variable access to near patient tests for vaginal discharge (microscopy and tests for BV):

- Microscopy of wet mounts of vaginal discharge may reveal fungal hyphae (VVC), motile trichomonads or clue cells (BV).

- BV can be tested for by checking the pH of the vaginal discharge (>4.5 is significant) and performing the 'whiff' test (the discharge has a fishy odour either before or after the addition of 10 per cent potassium hydroxide).

Gram staining can also diagnose BV by determining the relative concentration of the bacterial morphotypes characteristic of its altered vaginal flora.

A high vaginal swab (HVS) in appropriate culture medium will detect trichomoniasis and organisms that can cause VVC (*C. albicans*) and BV

(*G. vaginalis*). VVC and BV should be diagnosed on the basis of a positive culture result *plus* suggestive clinical symptoms and signs. Asymptomatic colonization of pre menopausal women is common with both *C. albicans* (10–20 per cent of women) and *G. vaginalis* (>50 per cent of women) and is *not* an indication for treatment.

An endocervical swab is necessary if chlamydial and/or gonorrhoeal infections are suspected. Swabs for gonorrhoea should be sent for culture while swabs for chlamydia may be analysed using antigen assays, nucleic acid amplification techniques, or culture, depending on local laboratory facilities.

Confirmation of a diagnosis of genital herpes requires viral culture of swabs taken from the ulcers.

Referral

All women with an STI should be considered for referral to a specialist genito-urinary medicine (GUM) clinic. The decision should be made on a 'case-by-case' basis and in collaboration with the woman.

Referral to a GUM clinic is recommended on the following grounds:

- a full counselling service is available to provide advice on risk reduction;

- screening for other STIs can be performed;

- the provision of contact tracing to ensure that partners are treated.

If a woman does not wish to attend a GUM clinic, she should use barrier methods of contraception until she and her partner(s) have completed a course of drug treatment. She should also advise her partner(s) to seek medical advice regarding treatment for the STI.

Principles of management

There is more to managing a woman with vaginal discharge than simply treating the infection with an appropriate antimicrobial. The possibility of an STI should always be considered.

The doctor must be reasonably sure of the diagnosis before starting antibiotic therapy. Often this will necessitate an examination and appropriate investigations. It is, however, common practice in primary care to treat women with a discharge with an appropriate antimicrobial *without* conducting an examination or performing swabs. Such practice is acceptable in women who give a history strongly suggestive of either VVC or BV and in whom there is no suspicion of an STI. Such women should be advised to return for further assessment if their symptoms persist following treatment.

All members of the primary health care team who deal with women likely to present with a vaginal discharge—this includes women requiring contraceptive advice and cervical screening—should know how and when to take a sexual history, take appropriate swabs, and refer the woman for further management.

Specific conditions

The *Centers for Disease Control and Prevention Guidelines for Treatment of Sexually Transmitted Diseases* offer detailed advice on treatment, including drug regimes for pregnant women.[9]

Vulvovaginal candidiasis

Treat if symptomatic.

- Topical azole treatment (e.g. clotrimazole 500 mg vaginal tablet as a single dose); or

- Oral fluconazole 150 mg as a single dose.

VVC is not usually acquired through sexual intercourse. Partners should be treated if they are symptomatic.

Recurrent VVC

The diagnosis must be confirmed by a clinical examination and microscopy and/or culture before the patient is 'labelled' with this difficult-to-treat condition. It can easily be confused with a non-infectious cause such as eczema. Non-drug options include advice on loose-fitting clothing, avoidance of chemical irritants or allergens when bathing and the use of oral yoghurt containing *Lactobacillus* species. Drug treatment must be continued long-term as the aim is to eradicate *C. albicans*. None of the recommended drug regimes has been evaluated in randomized controlled trials. The following may be both safe and easy to comply with:

◆ fluconazole 100 mg weekly for 6 months.

Bacterial vaginosis
Treat if symptomatic.

◆ metronidazole 400–500 mg orally twice daily for 7 days; or
◆ metronidazole 2 g as a single dose.

Routine treatment of sexual partners not recommended.

Trichomoniasis

◆ metronidazole 400–500 mg orally twice daily for 7 days; or
◆ metronidazole 2 g as a single dose.

Sexual partners must be treated.

Chlamydial cervicitis

◆ doxycycline 100 mg twice daily for 7 days; or
◆ azithromycin 1 g orally as a single dose.

Sexual partners must be treated.

Gonorrhoeal cervicitis
Drug choice is determined by local resistance patterns.

◆ ciprofloxacin 500 mg orally as a single dose; or
◆ ofloxacin 400 mg orally as a single dose.

Sexual partners must be treated.

Genital herpes
First episode:

◆ acyclovir 200 mg five times daily for 7–10 days.

Recurrent episodes:

◆ acyclovir 200 mg five times daily for 5 days.

Taking a saline bath may also be beneficial. Sexual partners should be treated if symptomatic.

Long-term and continuing care: opportunities for prevention and health promotion

As vaginal discharge is often caused by STI the prevention and control of STIs is crucial. This can be achieved by:

◆ educating patients on how to reduce the risk of contracting a STI (e.g. advice on 'safe sex');
◆ being aware of the need to test for other STIs when one is suspected (e.g. test for chlamydia and gonorrhoea when trichomoniasis is suspected);
◆ emphasizing the need for the sexual partners of patients with an STI to be treated.

Implications of the problem

Vaginal discharge can have a significant adverse effect on a woman's quality of life. One study of UK women who self-treated for 'vaginal thrush' (VVC) found that their symptoms made them feel miserable, unable to work,

embarrassed, or even stigmatized.[10] About half of the women knew that they could take simple measures to prevent the symptoms of thrush, but others wanted more information. This study highlights the fact that vaginal discharge should never be viewed as a trivial complaint. Women want information about what causes their vaginal discharge and what they themselves can do to prevent it recurring—they do not just want treatment with an antibiotic.[10,11]

Key points

◆ An abnormal vaginal discharge is predictive of bacterial vaginosis or trichomoniasis.

◆ Vulval itching associated with a thick curdy vaginal discharge and burning is predictive of vulvovaginal candidiasis.

◆ Clinical symptoms are poorly predictive of chlamydial and gonorrhoeal cervicitis.

◆ Bacterial vaginosis and vulvovaginal candidiasis are clinical syndromes, not microbiological diagnoses.

◆ Women with a diagnosis of trichomoniasis, chlamydia, and gonorrhoea require testing for other STIs.

◆ Women with a diagnosis of trichomoniasis, chlamydia, or gonorrhoea should encourage their partner to seek appropriate medical advice.

References

1. Jonsson, M. et al. (1995). The silent suffering women—a population based study on the association between reported symptoms and past and present infections of the lower genital tract. *Genitourinary Medicine* **71**, 158–62.
2. Office of Population Censuses and Surveys. *Morbidity Statistics from General Practice Fourth National Study 1991–1992*. London: HMSO, 1995.
3. Wathne, B., Holst, E., Hovelius, B., and Mardh, P.A. (1994). Vaginal discharge—comparison of clinical, laboratory and microbiological findings. *Acta Obstetricia et Gynecologica Scandinavica* **73**, 802–8.
4. Gerbase, A.C., Rowley, J.T., Heymann, D.H., Berkley, S.F., and Piot, P. (1998). Global prevalence and incidence estimates of selected curable STDs. *Sexually Transmitted Infections* **74** (Suppl. 1), S12–16.
5. Flynn, C.A., Helwig, A.L., and Meurer, L.N. (1999). Bacterial vaginosis in pregnancy and the risk of prematurity: a meta-analysis. *Journal of Family Practice* **48**, 885–92.
6. Cotch, M.F. et al. (1997). *Trichomonas vaginalis* associated with low birth weight and preterm delivery. The Vaginal Infections and Prematurity Study Group. *Sexually Transmitted Diseases* **24**, 353–60.
7. Sloan, N.L., Winikoff, B., Haberland, N., Coggins, C., and Elias, C. (2000). Screening and syndromic approaches to identify gonorrhea and chlamydial infection among women. *Studies in Family Planning* **31**, 55–68.
8. Ryan, C.A. et al. (1998). Risk assessment, symptoms, and signs as predictors of vulvovaginal and cervical infections in an urban US STD clinic: implications for use of STD algorithms. *Sexually Transmitted Infections* **74** (Suppl. 1), S59–76.
9. Centers for Disease Control and Prevention (1998). Guidelines for treatment of sexually transmitted diseases. *MMWR—Morbidity & Mortality Weekly Report* **47**, 1–111. http://www.cdc.gov/nchstp/dstd/1998_STD_Guidlines/1998_guidelines_for_the_treatment.htm.
10. Chapple, A., Hassell, K., Nicolson, M., and Cantrill, J. (2000). 'You don't really feel you can function normally': women's perceptions and personal management of vaginal thrush. *Journal of Reproductive & Infant Psychology* **18**, 309–19.
11. O'Dowd, T.C., Parker, S., and Kelly, A. (1996). Women's experiences of general practitioner management of their vaginal symptoms. *British Journal of General Practice* **46**, 415–18.

Further reading

Holmes, K.K. and Stamm, W.E. (1999). Lower genital tract infection syndromes in women. In *Sexually Transmitted Diseases* 3rd edn. (ed. K.K. Holmes, P. Mardh, P.F. Sparling, S.M. Lemon, W.E. Stamm, P. Piot, and J.N. Wasserheit), pp. 761–81. New York: McGraw-Hill. (This review offers an evidence-based approach to the diagnosis and management of infective causes of vaginal discharge.)

Carr, P.L., Felsenstein, D., and Friedman, R.H. (1998). Evaluation and management of vaginitis. *Journal of General Internal Medicine* 13, 335–46. (A comprehensive review of infective and non-infective causes of vaginitis.)

Clinical Effectiveness Group (Association of Genitourinary Medicine and the Medical Society for the Study of Venereal Diseases) (1999). National guidelines for the management of sexually transmitted infections. *Sexually Transmitted Infections* 75 (Suppl. 1), S4–8 (*Chlamydia trachomatis*), S13–15 (Gonorrhoea), S16–18 (Bacterial vaginosis), S19–20 (Vulvovaginal candidiasis), S21–3 (*Trichomonas vaginalis*), S24–8 (Genital herpes). http://www.agum.org.uk/guidelines.htm. Clinical Effectiveness Guidelines. (These evidence-based UK guidelines are regularly updated.)

7.4 Amenorrhoea

Danielle Mazza

Definition

Amenorrhoea, or the absence of menstruation, can be classified into two types. Primary amenorrhoea occurs when there is failure to establish menstruation and is generally regarded as abnormal by the age of 14 years in girls without signs of secondary sexual development or by the age of 16 in the presence of normal secondary sexual characteristics.[1] These age limits, while arbitrary, allow for variability in the normal rates of sexual maturation and the increasingly lower mean age of menarche due to improved nutrition. Secondary amenorrhoea is defined as the absence of menstruation for 6 consecutive months in a woman who previously had regular periods.[2] It does not include those physiological causes of amenorrhoea, namely pregnancy, lactation, and menopause.

How common is it in the community?

In general, secondary amenorrhoea (prevalence of between 1 and 3 per cent)[3] is much more common than primary amenorrhoea (prevalence of about 0.3 per cent).[4] However, when considering certain population groups such as the infertile (between 10 and 20 per cent[5]) competitive runners training 80 miles per week (up to 50 per cent[2]) and ballet dancers (up to 44 per cent[2]), the prevalence of amenorrhoea is much higher.

It is difficult to determine how common the presentation of amenorrhoea is in primary care. This is because studies that document patient reasons for encounter and problems managed in primary care do not go into sufficient level of detail. They do, however, document that 'menstrual problems' as a general category account for 0.6 per cent of all patient reasons for encounter,[6] and is the seventh most common reason for referral to a specialist.

Possible causes

Broadly speaking, there are four major causes of amenorrhoea:

1. pregnancy;
2. hypothalamic—pituitary dysfunction;
3. ovarian dysfunction;
4. alteration of the genital outflow tract.

However, from a clinical perspective, after ruling out the possibility of pregnancy, causation of amenorrhoea is best considered by classifying the problem as either primary or secondary amenorrhoea.

Primary amenorrhoea is then classified according to the presence or absence of secondary sexual characteristics. These characteristics consist of breast development, pubic and axillary hair development, and the growth spurt. The onset of menstruation should usually occur within 2 years of the onset of these changes.[1] Table 1 lists the possible causes of primary amenorrhoea when secondary sexual characteristics are present and Table 2 shows the causes of primary amenorrhoea when secondary sexual characteristics are absent. In this latter situation, classification is assisted by consideration of height.

Secondary amenorrhoea, on the other hand, is best classified according to whether or not androgen excess exists. Table 3 shows the causes of secondary amenorrhoea when there are no features of androgen excess present and Table 4 shows the causes of secondary amenorrhoea when androgen excess is present.

Table 1 Causes of primary amenorrhoea when secondary sexual characteristics are present (adapted with permission from ref. 1)

Constitutional delay
Pregnancy

Genito-urinary malformation
    Imperforate hymen
    Transverse vaginal septum
    Absent vagina ± a functioning uterus

Androgen insensitivity
    XY female
    Testicular feminization

Resistant ovary syndrome

Table 2 Causes of primary amenorrhoea when secondary sexual characteristics are absent (adapted with permission from ref. 1)

Normal stature	Hypothalamic dysfunction
	    Chronic illness
	    Anorexia, weight loss, exercise, 'stress'
	Isolated gonadotrophin-releasing hormone deficiency
	    Kallman's syndrome
	    The olfactogenital syndrome
	Hyperprolactinaemia
	Ovarian dysgenesis/agenesis
	Premature ovarian failure
	Galactosaemia
	Gonadal dysgenesis

Short stature	Hydrocephalus Trauma Empty sella syndrome Tumours Turner's syndrome

Table 3 Causes of secondary amenorrhoea when no features of androgen excess are present (adapted with permission from ref. 2)

Physiological	Pregnancy
	Lactation
	Menopause
Uterine	Cervical stenosis
	Ashermann's syndrome (intrauterine adhesions secondary to instrumentation)
Ovarian	Premature ovarian failure
	Resistant ovary syndrome
Hypothalamic	Weight loss
	Exercise
	Psychological distress
	Chronic illness
	Idiopathic
Pituitary	Hyperprolactinaemia
	Hypopituitarism
	Sheehan's syndrome
Causes of hypothalamic/ pituitary damage	Tumours
	Cranial irradiation
	Head injuries
	Sarcoidosis
	Tuberculosis
Systemic disease	Chronic illness
	Hypo/hyperthyroidism
Iatrogenic	Post pill and Depo-Provera injection (temporary)
	Radiotherapy
	Chemotherapy

Table 4 Causes of secondary amenorrhoea when androgen excess is present (adapted with permission from ref. 2)

Polycystic ovary syndrome
Cushing's syndrome
Late onset congenital adrenal hyperplasia
Adrenal or ovarian androgen producing tumour

From a primary care perspective, common causes of primary amenorrhoea include constitutional delay, Turner's syndrome, and more rarely, an absent vagina with a non-functioning uterus.

Many young women will have constitutional delay as the cause of their primary amenorrhoea. This delay is caused by an immature pulsatile release of GnRH, which eventually matures spontaneously. There is often a family history of delayed menarche or puberty in these girls.[7]

Turner's syndrome is caused by a chromosomal abnormality whereby there is either complete absence or a partial abnormality of one of the two X chromosomes. The incidence is one in 2000 female births.[8] The features of Turner's syndrome are variable but consist of: short stature; webbed neck; lymphoedema; a shield chest with widely spaced nipples; scoliosis; a wide carrying angle; coarctation of the aorta and streak ovaries.

Rokitansky–Kuster–Hauser syndrome is the name given to a condition where there is either partial or complete absence of the vagina and a rudimentary uterus. It accounts for up to 15 per cent of primary amenorrhoea cases.[9] While ovarian development is normal, up to 40 per cent of girls

Table 5 The clinical manifestations of PCOS (adapted with permission from ref. 2)

Symptoms	Endocrinology	Possible sequelae
Obesity	↑Androgens (testosterone and androstenedione)	Diabetes mellitus
Menstrual disturbance	↑LH	Dyslipidaemia
Infertility	↑Fasting insulin	Hypertension
Hyperandrogenization	↑Prolactin	Cardiovascular disease
	↓Sex hormone binding globulin ↑Oestrodiol, oestrone	Endometrial carcinoma

with this syndrome have associated renal tract abnormalities and 12 per cent skeletal abnormalities.[10]

Where secondary amenorrhoea occurs, GPs will most commonly be faced with either polycystic ovarian syndrome (PCOS), premature ovarian failure, hyperprolactinaemia, weight/exercise-related amenorrhoea, or contraceptive-induced amenorrhoea.

PCOS is present in 30 per cent of women with amenorrhoea. Its prevalence amongst women of reproductive age is thought to be between 5 and 10 per cent.[11] It is a disorder with a spectrum of clinical manifestations which are outlined in Table 5.[2]

Ovarian failure or menopause is considered premature if it occurs before the age of 40. In 20–40 per cent of cases, it is caused by autoantibodies,[12,13] however. Other causes include mumps, surgery, radiotherapy, or chemotherapy.

Up to one-third of cases of secondary amenorrhoea are caused by a prolactin-secreting adenoma.[14] In women with amenorrhoea associated with hyperprolactinaemia, the main symptoms are usually those of oestrogen deficiency.[15] Galactorrhoea is only found in up to one third of hyperprolactinaemic patients although its appearance is not correlated either with prolactin levels or with the presence of a tumour.[16]

In order to sustain a normal menstrual cycle a woman's body mass index needs to be greater than 19 (normal = 20–25 kg/m^2).[2] Amenorrhoea is induced when a woman loses 10–15 per cent of her normal weight for height.[2] This weight loss can be due to a number of causes from illness to anorexia to exercise. Exercise-induced amenorrhoea is found in women undertaking endurance events and in those who participate in activities where appearance is important such as ballet and gymnastics.

Some women taking the combined oral contraceptive pill will suffer from 'post-pill amenorrhoea'. This reflects the period of time it takes for the hypothalamic–pituitary–ovarian axis to return to its normal functioning after being suppressed by the synthetic hormones in the combined pill. In most women, 'post-pill amenorrhoea' either does not occur or is only of 1–2 months duration. Women who experience a longer duration of amenorrhoea after discontinuing the pill will usually be uncovering some organic reason that is halting normal menstruation, usually PCOS. It is likely that taking the pill was actually disguising the problem which emerged on discontinuation.

The majority of women using the progestogen only contraceptive agent Depo-Provera or the levonorgestrel releasing intrauterine system will become amenorrhoeic after 6–9 months' use of these contraceptive agents. This is a direct result of the progestogen that thins the endometrial lining and in the case of Depo-Provera (and in some women the progestogen only pill) suppresses ovulation. Normal menstruation and fertility returns in these women after discontinuation of these agents. For Depo-Provera this takes an average of nine months after the last injection unless there is an underlying organic problem.

Making a diagnosis in cases of primary amenorrhoea

At intial presentation, the family physician needs to take a history detailing the following issues:

- Family history of:
  - delayed puberty;
  - genetic anomalies.
- Symptoms associated with possible causes of the amenorrhoea, for example:
  - cyclical lower abdominal pain possibly suggesting haematocolpos (accumulation of menstrual blood in the vagina);
  - symptoms of hypothyroidism;
  - absence of a sense of smell which may be associated with gonadotrophin deficiency.
- The presence of chronic illness such as diabetes, coeliac disease, chronic renal or heart disease.
- History of chemotherapy.
- Recent emotional upsets or change in body weight.
- Level of exercise.

During examination, height and weight should be measured in order to calculate the girl's body mass index. The presence of secondary sex characteristics (such as breast tissue and pubic and axillary hair) should be noted as should features of Turner's syndrome and signs of androgen excess, thyroid disease, and galactorrhoea. It is important not to examine the breasts prior to prolactin estimation as the level may then be falsely elevated. The external genitalia should be examined to look for clitoromegaly (indicating virilization). A pelvic examination to assess whether or not a uterus is palpable is inappropriate in young girls who are not sexually active and can be assessed later using an ultrasound if necessary. Pregnancy must be excluded.

The investigative pathways recommended[1] are shown in Figs 1 and 2, respectively, for a patient with and without secondary sexual characteristics.

Making a diagnosis in cases of secondary amenorrhoea

When taking a history in a woman with secondary amenorrhoea the following issues are important:

- previous menstrual, obstetric, and gynaecological (endometrial curettage, oophorectomy) history;
- recent contraceptive use, that is, progestogens or combined oral contraceptive pill;
- risk of pregnancy;
- associated symptoms, for example, galactorrhoea, hirsutism, hot flushes and/or dry vagina, symptoms of thyroid disease;
- history of an eating disorder, recent change in body weight or emotional upsets;
- level of exercise;
- previous abdominal, pelvic, or cranial radiotherapy or history of chemotherapy;
- family history of early menopause.

The important aspects of the examination include:

- height and weight;
- hirsutism, acne, or signs of virilization such as deep voice or clitoromegaly;
- signs of thyroid disease or galactorrhoea;
- acanthosis nigricans (hyperpigmented thickening of the skin folds of the axilla and neck which is a sign of profound insulin resistance and is associated with PCOS);
- fundoscopy and assessment of visual fields if a pituitary tumour is suspected;
- pelvic examination for enlarged polycystic ovaries.

After conducting a pregnancy test, the next step is to perform thyroid function tests and measure prolactin levels. The thyroid function tests will rule out both hyper or hypothyroidism. Prolactin levels may be moderately and transiently elevated in response to stress, a breast examination and

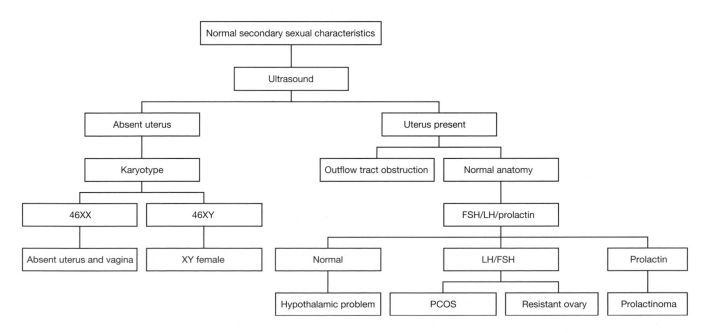

Fig. 1 Investigative pathway for a patient with normal secondary sexual characteristics (adapted with permission from ref. 1).

venepuncture, returning to normal levels (<400 miu/l) within 48 h. More permanent, elevation at levels more than 700 miu/l can result from PCOS or pronounced hypothyroidism (thyrotrophin-releasing hormone stimulates the secretion of prolactin). A prolactin level above 1000 miu/l on two occasions warrants further investigation (e.g. CT or MRI scan of pituitary fossa) and is suggestive of a microadenoma; a level greater than 5000 miu/l is usually associated with a macroadenoma.[2]

The third step is to assess the woman's oestrogen status. Serum oestradiol levels can be misleading and are not generally recommended.[17] A progestogen challenge test is a more reliable way of assessing oestrogen status and is carried out by giving the woman oral medroxyprogesterone acetate to take in a dose of 5–10 mg for 5–7 days. Women with adequate circulating oestrogen and a normal genital outflow tract will have a withdrawal bleed (positive test) usually 2 days after discontinuing the progestogen. If no withdrawal bleed occurs (negative test), oestrogen levels are likely to be low. A negative test will also result from destruction of the endometrium (Ashermann's syndrome) or an outflow obstruction. These possibilities may be indicated by the history and can be confirmed by the use of a cyclic oestrogen and progestogen challenge (i.e. giving the woman a combined oral contraceptive pill to take for 1–2 months) or hysteroscopy.

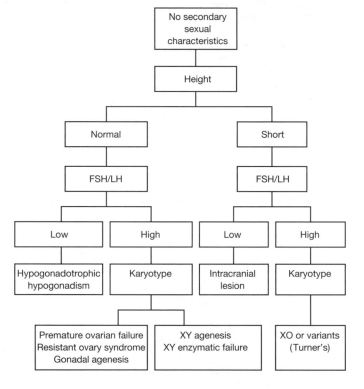

Fig. 2 Investigative pathway for a patient with no secondary sexual characteristics (adapted with permission from ref. 1).

Serum gonadotrophin levels (FSH and LH) are used to distinguish between hypothalamic or pituitary failure and gonadal (ovarian) failure. Four common pictures emerge. These are summarized in Table 6. An elevated FSH of more than 50 iu/l as an indication of ovarian failure or premature menopause. Low FSH and low LH levels in the presence of a negative progestogen challenge is an indication of amenorrhoea secondary to exercise, low weight, and/or stress. Normal or mildly raised gonadotrophin levels particularly with a raised LH : FSH ratio in the presence of a positive progestogen challenge test and mildly elevated androgens is indicative of PCOS.

Congenital adrenal hyperplasia or Cushing's syndrome should be considered if there is mild elevation of androgens (testosterone, DHEA-S and 17-hydroxy-progesterone) in an adrenal pattern. Moderate or severe hyperandrogenism may be indicative of a steroid-producing tumour.

Principles of management

The general principles of management when a young girl or woman presents with amenorrhoea are:

♦ To treat where possible any underlying causes of amenorrhoea.

♦ To take preventive action against complications arising from long-term oestrogen deficiency.

♦ To give advice about future fertility and address any psychological distress.

Treatment of underlying causes of amenorrhoea

The GP can institute many aspects of management of amenorrhoea. Firstly, it is important to educate the patient and her family (if appropriate) about her condition and how it has arisen. General lifestyle advice on smoking, alcohol consumption, exercise, weight, and diet (including calcium intake) should also be given.

The GP will most commonly deal with cases of hyperprolactinaemia, PCOS, and weight- and exercise-related amenorrhoea in their practice.

Hyperprolactinaemia is probably best dealt with in consultation with a specialist endocrinologist. Bromocriptine is very effective and reduction in tumour volume is seen within 6 weeks of commencing therapy.[2] Surgery is reserved for cases of drug resistance.

Most management of PCOS is symptom-oriented.[19] The first line of attack in the obese is to encourage weight loss. In this group, insulin-sensitizing agents (such as metformin) have been trialled and are worth considering as improvements have been demonstrated in biochemistry and symptoms, together with an increase in fertility.[20]

In women who do not want to become pregnant, use of an oral contraceptive pill will reinstitute regular withdrawal bleeds while providing protection to the endometrium. Use of an antiandrogenic agent such as Diane 35 ED will also assist with the hirsutism and acne though it may take up to 6 months to have any effect on these symptoms. Where contraception is not needed, spironolactone can be used. It will inhibit ovarian and adrenal synthesis of androgens. It can be given at a dose of 50–150 mg/day and can also be used in conjunction with an oral contraceptive pill, which in itself may improve hirsutism by increasing the level of serum hormone binding globulin.

Table 6 Laboratory findings in common causes of secondary amenorrhoea (adapted with permission from ref. 18)

	FSH	LH	Prolactin	Testosterone	Oestrogen status
Hyperprolactinaemia	Normal or low	Normal or low	High	Normal	Low
PCOS	Normal	Raised in 40%	Normal or moderate rise in 5–30%	Slightly raised	Normal
Premature menopause	Very high	High	Normal	Normal	Low
'Hypothalamic', that is associated with weight loss, exercise, or stress	Low or normal	Low or normal	Normal	Normal	Low or normal

Women who present with infertility will require full investigation for this condition and after referral to a gynaecologist are usually commenced on clomiphene citrate (Clomid). In those who fail to ovulate using this therapy metformin can assist.

Laparoscopic ovarian 'drilling' using diathermy has been used in the treatment of PCOS for over 15 years. The major concern with this form of therapy is the high rate of post-operative adhesions.[21] The other issue is that it does not seem to be directed at any of the aetiological factors involved in the development or expression of PCOS.

Weight-related amenorrhoea is very challenging to treat given the fact that in many women an underlying eating disorder may be present. Referral to a psychiatrist may be helpful in these cases, as would the assistance of a dietitian.

Several conditions may require referral to a specialist. In primary amenorrhoea, early referral is appropriate if there are symptoms and signs of androgen excess or thyroid disease; if there is galactorrhoea or growth retardation; if genital tract malformation, intracranial tumour, chromosomal anomaly, or other pathology is suspected.[18]

In secondary amenorrhoea, GPs should refer on:

♦ Patients with hyperprolactinaemia for CT or MRI imaging.

♦ Patients with mildly raised testosterone levels who do not have polycystic ovary syndrome and patients with testosterone levels in the normal *male* range.

♦ Patients with premature ovarian failure for screening for autoimmune disease, for example, Addison's disease when this is clinically indicated; chromosomal analysis may also be considered for those under 30 years.

♦ Patients with low gonadotrophin levels that cannot be explained by stress, exercise, and weight loss.[18]

Preventive action against complications arising from long-term oestrogen deficiency

The patient's oestrogen status is a major determinant of therapy.[17] In situations where the woman has a normal oestrogen status but is anovulatory, inadequate progestogen is being produced to result in endometrial stabilization and menstruation. The woman is at risk of endometrial hyperplasia (because of the unopposed oestrogen). Using progestogens for 7–10 days of every month or a combined oral contraceptive pill in these women will decrease this risk.

When the woman is hypo-oestrogenic (where amenorrhoea is due to hyperprolactinaemia, premature ovarian failure, weight loss, or exercise) a different set of problems arise, the most important being the risk of osteoporosis. Compared with women who have normal menstrual cycles, a 10–20 per cent decrease in lumbar bone density has been found in women with hypo-oestrogenic amenorrhoea, irrespective of the cause.[22,23] Oestrogen replacement should therefore be given to all women who have been amenorrhoeic for longer than 6 months. It is more appropriately and conveniently given in the form of the combined oral contraceptive pill,[24] as the optimal dose in the form of hormone replacement therapy is unknown. Calcium supplementation (1500 mg/day) is also recommended.[25]

The question of whether or not women who are amenorrhoeic secondary to the use of Depo-Provera as contraception are at risk of developing osteoporosis is controversial. One recent longitudinal study[26] suggesting that the rate of bone loss is probably non-linear, with a rapid loss in the first 5 years and a levelling off afterwards. It may be appropriate to check oestradiol levels or bone mineral density in long-term users who have other risk factors for osteoporosis, or symptoms of oestrogen deficiency.

Another concern for hypo-oestrogenic women is the risk of cardiovascular disease. However, few studies have evaluated this risk. One small study[27] looking at lipids in women with hypothalamic amenorrhoea (HA) found that, in contrast to menopausal oestrogen deficiency, young women with HA and oestrogen deficiency have increased levels of high density lipoprotein (HDL) and no increases in total cholesterol (TC), low density lipoprotein (LDL), and triglycerides. This study suggests that the negative effects of oestrogen deficiency on cardiovascular risk factors may be modified in women with HA.

Women with PCOS also have an increased risk of developing cardiovascular disease, hypertension, and diabetes. It is believed that the main underlying disorder is insulin resistance and this results in an associated dyslipidaemia (with raised triglycerides, raised LDL levels, and reduced HDL levels) and elevated plasminogen activator inhibitor-1 levels.[11]

Giving advice about future fertility and addressing psychological distress

Amenorrhoea is a sign for women that 'something' is not working properly. It can therefore be associated with considerable anxiety, altered self-image, and loss of self-esteem. The diagnosis of Turner's syndrome or some other congenital anomaly when young women present with primary amenorrhoea will be very traumatic for both the girl and her family.[28] These families may benefit from genetic counselling.

It is important to advise women with secondary amenorrhoea that if any sporadic ovulation is occurring then pregnancy is still a possibility. Contraception should therefore be used if they do not wish to conceive. For most, however, the concern is for future fertility. Reassuringly, treatment of the underlying cause of the amenorrhoea is usually all that is required to restore fertility.

Women with PCOS may respond to weight loss and can be treated with clomiphene to induce ovulation. If this is not effective, gonadotrophins can be used. Women with HA may also have their fertility restored by pulsatile gonadotrophins. Hyperprolactinaemia can be treated with bromocriptine and women with premature ovarian failure can achieve pregnancy with *in vitro* fertilization techniques using ovum donation.

Key points

♦ Pregnancy is the most common cause of amenorrhoea.

♦ Menarche usually occurs within 2 years of the development of secondary sex characteristics and prior to the age of 16.

♦ Common causes of secondary amenorrhoea include hyperprolactinaemia, polycystic ovarian syndrome, and weight- and/or exercise-related amenorrhoea.

♦ Preventive action against complications arising from long-term oestrogen deficiency should be taken.

♦ Treatment of the underlying cause of the amenorrhoea is usually all that is required to restore fertility.

References

1. **Edmonds, D.K.** (1999). Primary amenorrhea. In *Dewhurst's Textbook of Obstetrics & Gynaecology for Postgraduates* 6th edn. (ed. D.K. Edmonds), pp. 34–42. London: Blackwell Science.

2. **Balen, A.H.** (1999). Secondary amenorrhea. In *Dewhurst's Textbook of Obstetrics & Gynaecology for Postgraduates* 6th edn. (ed. D.K. Edmonds), pp. 42–61. London: Blackwell Science.

3. **Pettersson, F., Fries, H., and Nillius, S.J.** (1973). Epidemiology of secondary amenorrhea. I. Incidence and prevalence rates. *American Journal of Obstetrics & Gynecology* 117, 80–6.

4. **Singh, K.B.** (1981). Menstrual disorders in college students. *American Journal of Obstetrics & Gynecology* 140, 299–302.

5. **Franks, S.** (1987). Primary and secondary amenorrhoea. *British Medical Journal (Clinical Reserve Edition)* 294, 815–19.

6. **Britt, H., Sayer, G.P., Miller, G.C., Charles, J., Scahill, S., Horn, F., Bhasale, A., and McGeechan, K.** *General Practice Activity in Australia*

1998–99. AIHW Cat. No. GEP 2. Canberra: Australian Institute of Health and Welfare (General Practice Series No. 2), 2000.

7. **Rosenfeld, R.G.** (1987). Constitutional delay in growth and development. *Seminars in Adolescent Medicine* **3**, 267–73.

8. **Saenger, P.** (1996). Turner's syndrome. *New England Journal of Medicine* **335**, 1749–54.

9. **Pletcher, J.R. and Slap, G.B.** (1999). Menstrual disorders: amenorrhea. *Pediatric Clinics of North America* **46**, 505–18.

10. **Griffin, J.E.** et al. (1976). Congenital absence of the vagina. The Mayer–Rokitansky–Kuster–Hauser syndrome. *Annals of Internal Medicine* **85**, 224–36.

11. **Hopkinson, Z.E.** et al. (1998). Polycystic ovarian syndrome: the metabolic syndrome comes to gynaecology. *British Medical Journal* **317**, 329–32.

12. **Alper, M.M. and Garner, P.R.** (1985). Premature ovarian failure: its relationship to autoimmune disease. *Obstetrics & Gynecology* **66**, 27–30.

13. **Damewood, M.D.** et al. (1986). Circulating antiovarian antibodies in premature ovarian failure. *Obstetrics & Gynecology* **68**, 850–4.

14. **Schlechte, J.** et al. (1980). Prolactin-secreting pituitary tumors in amenorrheic women: a comprehensive study. *Endocrinology Review* **1**, 295–308.

15. **Jacobs, H.S.** (1981). Management of prolactin-secreting pituitary tumours. In *Progress in Obstetrics and Gynaecology* Vol. 1 (ed. J. Studd), pp. 263–76. Edinburgh: Churchill Livingstone.

16. **Jacobs, H.S.** et al. (1976). Clinical and endocrine features of hyperprolactinaemic amenorrhoea. *Clinical Endocrinology* **5**, 439–54.

17. **Kiningham, R.B., Apgar, B.S., and Schwenk, T.L.** (1996). Evaluation of amenorrhea. *American Family Physician* **53**, 1185–94.

18. http://www.prodigy.nhs.uk/guidance.asp?gt=amenorrhoea accessed 21 January 2003.

19. **Balen, A.** (1999). Pathogenesis of polycystic ovary syndrome—the enigma unravels? *Lancet* **354**, 966–7.

20. **Velasquez, E.M.** et al. (1994). Metformin therapy in polycystic ovaries reduces hyperinsulinaemia, insulin resistance, hyperandrogenaemia and systolic blood pressure while facilitating normal menses and pregnancy. *Metabolism* **43**, 647–54.

21. **Campo, S.** (1998). Ovulatory cycles, pregnancy outcome and complications after surgical treatment of polycystic ovary syndrome. *Obstetrics & Gynecology Survey* **53**, 297–308.

22. **Biller, B.M.** et al. (1992). Progressive trabecular osteopenia in women with hyperprolactinemic amenorrhea. *Journal of Clinical Endocrinology & Metabolism* **75**, 692–7.

23. **Drinkwater, B.L.** et al. (1984). Bone mineral content of amenorrheic and eumenorrheic athletes. *New England Journal of Medicine* **311**, 277–81.

24. **Seeman, E.** et al. (1992). Osteoporosis in anorexia nervosa: the influence of peak bone density, bone loss, oral contraceptive use, and exercise. *Journal Bone Mineral Research* **7**, 1467–74.

25. **Skolnick, A.A.** (1993). 'Female athlete triad' risk for women. *Journal of the American Medical Association* **270**, 921–3.

26. **Tang, O.S.** et al. (2000). Further evaluation on long-term depot-medroxyprogesterone acetate use and bone mineral density: a longitudinal cohort study. *Contraception* **62**, 161–4.

27. **Miller, K.K., Grinspoon, S., and Klibanski, A.** (2000). Cardiovascular risk markers in hypothalamic amenorrhoea. *Clinical Endocrinology* **53**, 359–66.

28. **Rees, M.C.P.** (1997). Menstrual problems: amenorrhoea. In *Women's Health: Oxford General Practice Series 39* 4th edn. (ed. A. McPherson and D. Waller), pp. 328–42. Oxford: Oxford University Press.

Further reading

Edmonds, D.K. (1999). Primary amenorrhoea. In *Dewhurst's Textbook of Obstetrics & Gynaecology for Postgraduates* 6th edn. (ed. D.K. Edmonds), pp. 34–42. London: Blackwell Science.

Balen, A.H. (1999). Secondary amenorrhoea. In *Dewhurst's Textbook of Obstetrics and Gynaecology for Postgraduates* 6th edn. (ed. D.K. Edmonds), pp. 42–61. London: Blackwell Science.

7.5 The menopause

Janice Rymer

The menopause is defined as the time of the last menstrual period, which means it is a retrospective definition made after 1 year of amenorrhoea. With increased ageing of populations and decreased mortality in the elderly, female life expectancy has increased dramatically. In the United Kingdom, the mean age of the menopause is 50 years and 9 months, with median onset of the perimenopause (the commencement of hypo-oestrogenic symptoms) being between 45.5 and 47.5 years. A woman can expect to spend nearly 40 per cent of her life span after the menopause, and post-menopausal women account for 20 per cent of the UK population. Over 80 per cent of women will experience typical menopausal symptoms, with over half of these finding one or more of the symptoms a problem.

The menopause is a physiological event, and its timing may be determined genetically. Although endocrine changes are permanent, (i.e. ovarian failure), menopausal symptoms such as hot flushes usually resolve with time. However, some symptoms may remain the same or worsen, for example, genital atrophy. Whether or not women suffer from acute oestrogen-deficient symptoms, they may be at risk of the long-term consequences of the cessation of ovarian function. Although cessation of menstrual periods is a universal recognition of menopause, the other oestrogen-deficient symptoms are not cognitively known or acknowledged by many women in different cultures. For example, Japanese and Navaho Indian women have no words for menopause or hot flush in their respective cultures. It is important to remember that each woman has been raised in her own culture with its belief systems, attitudes, and values about all facets of life and her stature after the menopause may be lowered or elevated. This means that in many Western cultures a woman may view the menopause more negatively, whereas, for example, the Meo of Northern Thailand have a celebratory menopause ceremony after which a woman may participate in roles once reserved only for men. This time in a woman's life may also be difficult as the menopause may coincide with other life events, which may bring their own psychological sequelae, for example, children leaving home and retirement.

Aetiology

The menopause is the result of ovarian failure and is preceded by a transition phase which may be named the perimenopause or climacteric, which is of variable duration. This latter time is characterized by increasing resistance of the ovarian follicles to stimulation by the gonadotrophins. Oestrogen output by the ovary declines, and gonadotrophin levels increase. Anovulation becomes more frequent and as a result progesterone deficiency occurs, which may lead to prolonged and/or irregular vaginal bleeding. Ovarian failure may not be a natural event, and may be caused by surgery, radiotherapy, chemotherapy, systemic illness, or autoimmune disease.

Diagnosis

History

The diagnosis is usually made on assessment of the symptoms, with the commonest being hot flushes or sweats, and urogenital symptoms. Hot flushes can be socially disabling and may interfere with daily activities, while night sweats result in interrupted sleep and progressive fatigue. The mechanism of menopausal vasomotor instability is uncertain but a hypothalamic mechanism has been suggested. Vaginal dryness is a common symptom and this is due to flattening and thinning of the epithelium which results in atrophic vaginitis. Loss of glycogen from the epithelial cells leads to disappearance of the lactic acid-forming Döderlein's bacilli and as a consequence the vagina becomes alkaline. The supporting structures of the genital tract may lose tone, and uterovaginal prolapse may result, causing women to complain of a 'lump down below', dragging discomfort in the pelvis, or urinary or bowel symptoms.

Other symptoms include mood changes, lack of concentration, and decrease in libido. It is important to assess the extent to which oestrogen-deficiency symptoms are interfering with quality of life.

Examination

Blood pressure should be taken as it is good practice to treat hypertension before commencing hormone replacement therapy (HRT). Further examinations, for example breast and pelvic, are only performed if there is a clinical indication from the history. Some countries recommend routine breast and pelvic examinations in women over the age of 50.

Investigations

Blood tests are not usually performed unless the diagnosis is in doubt, for example, premature ovarian failure. In menopausal women, an oestradiol concentration of less than 70 pmol/l and follicle stimulating hormone (FSH) greater than 15 iu/l are expected. In many countries, routine mammography screening is offered to women over the age of 50.

Hormone replacement therapy

The aim of HRT is to alleviate symptoms, and continuation of therapy may provide long-term benefits, although often, with relief of symptoms, women discontinue therapy. Relief of symptoms is the single most common reason for prescribing HRT. The diversity of current HRT preparations illustrates the fact that no one preparation will suit all women. The preparations vary in the types and amounts of oestrogen and progestogen, and their routes of administration. HRT consists of oestrogen replacement, and if women still have a uterus then they must take progestogen therapy as well. The progestogen therapy can either be given in a cyclical form, usually for 10–12 days of each calendar month, or continuously. The purpose of the progestogen is to protect the endometrium from being stimulated by the oestrogen. One of the major problems of adherence to HRT has been that post-menopausal women do not want to resume bleeding, hence the introduction of therapies that do not produce regular vaginal bleeding.

Why take HRT?

Perimenopausal and post-menopausal women want to know whether or not they should take HRT. Users of HRT tend to be healthier, better educated, more active, leaner, and drink more alcohol than non-users.[1] Adherence to HRT is generally poor and the reasons for this are complex. The primary care physician needs to understand the short and long-term benefits of HRT, be able to warn women about the side-effects, discuss possible risks, and to know which women should not receive HRT.

Short-term benefits

When ovarian function begins to decline, women may experience symptoms of oestrogen deficiency and the commonest of these are hot flushes, psychological symptoms, and urogenital symptoms. The natural history of the hot flushes and psychological symptoms is that they disappear, although this may happen over a very variable time period. Urogenital symptoms will persist or deteriorate.

Long-term benefits

At the time of ovarian failure, the female skeleton undergoes accelerated bone loss as well as age-related bone loss. Most women lose around 1 per cent of bone mass per year, but during the first 3–4 years after the menopause, bone loss declines more rapidly. HRT will prevent the post-menopausal skeleton from losing bone and cohort studies have shown that the fracture rate is reduced at clinically relevant sites, such as the spine and neck of femur, by 50 and 30 per cent, respectively.[2,3] After HRT is stopped, bone loss will resume within a year and bone turnover increases to the level of untreated women within 3–6 months. Therefore, to be effective, HRT has to be continued in women in their 60s and probably into their 70s to decrease the risk of hip fracture.

Cardiovascular disease rarely affects women before the menopause, strongly implicating oestrogen deficiency in the aetiology of the disease. Observational studies have shown that HRT decreases coronary heart disease but the exact mechanism is unclear. The Nurses Health Study showed the risk of coronary heart disease (CHD) was more than doubled in women who have had a bilateral oophorectomy before the menopause, compared with women of a similar age.[4] A review of population-based case-control, cross-sectional, and prospective studies of oestrogen therapy and CHD calculated the overall relative risk associated with oestrogen therapy to be reduced by approximately 50 per cent.[5] However, these observational studies are potentially flawed as HRT users tend to be thinner and healthier, thereby introducing bias. Two randomized controlled trials (RCTs) of primary prevention of heart disease by HRT in the United States (Women's Health Initiative—WHI) and the United Kingdom (Women's International Study of Long Duration—WISDOM) have been discontinued as the risks outweighed the benefits in the WHI study[6] and the WISDOM study felt that they should discontinue also. The present recommendation is that HRT cannot be recommended for prevention of cardiovascular disease. Both trials used prevart and medroxyprogesterone acetate. The prevart arm of the WHI study is still continuing. However, with regard to secondary prevention, there is confusion following the findings of the Heart and Estrogen/Progestin Replacement Study (HERS)[7] which was the first RCT comparing HRT to placebo in women who had established heart disease and investigating hard endpoints, namely myocardial infarction and death. Against an expectation of 50 per cent less events there was a statistically significant increase in CHD events in the first year in the group that took HRT and no difference in mortality rates at four years between HRT and placebo groups. The study has been criticized for using medroxyprogesterone acetate as the progestogen, because it is known to be lipid 'unfriendly' and also because the expected benefit may have occurred if the study had gone on longer, but the study cannot be disregarded.

The effects of HRT on stroke risk are not known. There is now accumulating evidence (from observational studies) that HRT may provide some protection against Alzheimer's disease[8] and colorectal cancer.[9]

Delivery systems available

Oral therapy

Synthetic oestrogen replacement has been superseded by the use of natural preparations. Oral HRT passes directly from the intestine to the liver via the portal circulation. It is metabolized in the liver before reaching the systemic circulation and the target organs. Extensive first pass metabolism of oestrogen occurs and relatively high dosages of the drug are ingested to achieve the same serum levels as those achieved with the parenteral routes. The principal metabolite oestron-3-glucuronide is excreted in the bowel and urine and is therefore not available for systemic action. Other consequences of the first pass through the liver are changes in the hepatic metabolism and an increase in the proteins produced by the liver. These include serum lipoproteins with the changes induced by oestrogen producing favourable effects. The lowering of antithrombin III, however, may not be favourable for the coagulation mechanism. Oral therapy produces a diurnal variation in oestrogen levels. As with all oral medication, adherence is a problem especially in women who experience nausea with oral preparations.

Oral therapy can be given in the form of unopposed oestrogen replacement therapy, cyclical oestrogen and progestogen replacement therapy, or continuous combined therapy. Unopposed oestrogen therapy is used in women who have had a hysterectomy. Cyclical hormone replacement therapy involves daily oestrogen and progestogen for 12 days of each month. In some of the oral therapies, the oestrogen and progestogen tablets are presented separately. This is not ideal, as women sometimes notice that when they are taking both tablets they experience progestogenic side-effects. They therefore may elect to ignore the progestogen tablets and end up taking unopposed oestrogen replacement therapy. Tablets that have oestrogen and progestogen in the same tablet for the last 12 days are superior as they improve adherence to the progestogen phase of therapy.

Transdermal therapy

Percutaneous oestradiol substitution is possible by using adhesive patches or gel application. With patches the medication is absorbed across a membrane directly into the systemic circulation, thereby minimizing any effects of first pass liver metabolism. The oestradiol levels are higher and oestrogen levels remain steady. There are no measurable effects on clotting factors and transdermal oestrogen may result in small, favourable changes in serum lipoprotein patterns, similar to but of a lesser magnitude than those seen with oral administration of oestradiol. There are two types of patches—reservoir and matrix. The reservoir patches have been largely superseded by the matrix patches which are associated with less skin reactions and the fact that the matrix patch dosage can be varied. As with oral oestrogen replacement therapy, transdermal oestrogen therapy must be given in conjunction with progestogen if the woman still has a uterus. The progestogen can be given either in the form of oral tablets for 12 days, or more recently, via a cyclical combined patch. The introduction of this patch should increase adherence as women only have to use one route of therapy rather than previously using both transdermal and oral therapy. Adherence to the progestogen component of treatment will also be higher. For the post-menopausal woman, continuous combined patches are now available, which should induce an atrophic endometrium, equivalent to the oral continuous combined preparations. More recently, oestradiol gel has been gaining in popularity. The gel is applied to the skin and the absorption is proportional to the area of application. Compared to the transdermal patches, efficacy in the relief of climacteric symptoms and protection of the female skeleton is equivalent but the gel is less irritant to the skin. However, in non-hysterectomized women, progestogen must be delivered by an alternative route.

Implants

Oestradiol implants are small pellets which are inserted into the subcutaneous fat where they dissolve and release oestrogen over a number of months. They produce higher serum levels of oestrogen than other forms of therapy and hypoestrogenic symptoms can recur despite high serum levels. This phenomenon of tachyphylaxis may occur in conjunction with supraphysiological oestradiol levels and the long-term consequences of these are uncertain. If the woman still has a uterus then she must take cyclical progestogens to avoid the risk of endometrial hyperplasia. As the release of oestrogen may continue for many months, progestogens must continue to be used until no further withdrawal bleeds occur. If women are receiving oestradiol implants, testosterone implants can also be inserted at the same time to improve tiredness and increase libido. Testosterone implants are now available in many doses. Although not yet available in the United Kingdom, testosterone patches and gel can also be used.

Vaginal preparations

Vaginal oestrogen preparations are generally used for the treatment of local atrophic symptoms but it has been shown that local application of oestriol, oestradiol, or conjugated oestrogens to the vagina is followed by absorption of a high percentage of hormone into the general circulation, especially as the atrophic vaginitis improves and local vascularity increases. Vaginal preparations are available as vaginal rings (silicone vaginal rings provide a continuous release of low doses of 17-β-oestradiol), vaginal suppositories, and vaginal cream. More recently, a vaginal ring has been developed that provides systemic doses of oestradiol but needs to be changed every 3 months.

Non-bleeding therapies

One of the major problems of adherence to HRT has been that post-menopausal women do not want to have regular vaginal bleeding. The following non-bleeding therapies are now available.

Continuous combined therapies

With these therapies, oestrogen is given daily in conjunction with progestogen, in the form of either oral or transdermal preparations. One of the major side-effects of these preparations is the high incidence of breakthrough bleeding (25–50 per cent in the first 6 months).

Progestogen-containing intrauterine system (IUS)

The IUS releases a small dose of progestogen locally to induce an atrophic endometrium. This enables oestrogen replacement therapy to be taken either orally, transdermally, intravaginally, or by implant. The advantage of this system is that the progestogen is administrated locally, eliminating the systemic side-effects that can occur from the progestogenic phase of HRT.

Tibolone

Tibolone is a unique molecule in that is has oestrogenic, progestogenic, and androgenic properties. When taken orally it is broken down into three metabolites, with the progestogenic metabolite predominating at the level of the endometrium, producing an atrophic endometrium. Women on tibolone do not need progestogen-induced bleeds every month. As with continuous combined therapy, they may experience some breakthrough bleeding in the first 6 months, although the incidence is less than with continuous combined therapy. Due to its androgenicity, tibolone is also licenced for improving libido.

Side-effects

The commonest side-effects experienced by women taking HRT are nausea, abdominal bloating, breast tenderness, oedema, and weight gain. These symptoms tend to appear in the first few weeks and generally resolve within 3 months, by which time all the oestrogen receptors are saturated. Breast tenderness may be particularly predominant in older women who have not been exposed to oestrogen for some years. The resumption of monthly bleeding after being amenorrhoeic is an unwanted effect which can be avoided by using the continuous combined therapies, tibolone, or oestrogen replacement therapy with a progestogen-containing IUS. Whilst the concept of 'no-bleed' HRT is attractive, clinical experience and published data suggest that unscheduled and often persistent bleeding can still be a significant problem.[10] Within the first 6 months, there is a 25–50 per cent incidence of breakthrough bleeding with continuous combined therapy and 10–20 per cent with tibolone.[11] Clinically, post-menopausal bleeding has been a major cause for concern but with the non-bleeding therapies it does not have the same significance in the first 6 months. However, vaginal bleeding after the first 6 months of therapy warrants investigation. A transvaginal scan should be performed and the endometrial thickness should be less than 5 mm. An outpatient endometrial biopsy can be taken in the primary care setting. If these initial investigations are not reassuring then the gold standard for assessing the endometrium is to perform a hysteroscopy, which can now be done in the outpatient setting under local or no anaesthesia. Hysteroscopy affords a panoramic view of the endometrial cavity, and a hysteroscopically directed biopsy can be taken.

The commonest findings in this group of women who have breakthrough bleeding on non-bleeding therapies are atrophic endometrium or endometrial polyps. If endometrial atrophy is present then continuation with therapy should resolve the problem, and if a polyp is present this can be removed surgically.

Risks

A major concern about HRT is its effect on the breast; many women perceive that breast cancer is the leading cause of death in women. Breast tissue is oestrogen-sensitive and oestrogen stimulates breast tumour cells *in vitro*. The latest meta-analysis (based on observational studies) has shown that long-term treatment (>5 years) leads to an increase in the relative risk of breast cancer by a factor of 1.023 for each year of use. In other words, if 1000 women use HRT for 10 years, starting at age 50, it is estimated that by the age of 70 there will be an additional six cases of breast cancer, raising the background incidence from 45 to 51 cases.[12] The limited data suggest that the use of progestogens has not diminished the excess risk associated with oestrogens.

Unopposed oestrogen will increase the incidence of endometrial hyperplasia and carcinoma. Progestogens substantially decrease the excess risk of endometrial cancer but must either be taken for 12–14 days of each month or continuously.

There appears to be an approximately threefold increase in the relative risk of venous thromboembolic disease (VTE) in women on HRT,[13,14] although the absolute risk is still low. The increase in risk appears to be restricted to the first year of use, with an odds ratio of 4.6 (95 per cent CI 2.5–8.4) during the first 6 months. This suggests that the HRT may be unmasking an underlying thrombophilic tendency.

Contra-indications

Many HRT data sheets and patient information leaflets are inaccurate with their list of contra-indications, of which most have been extrapolated from oral contraceptive data. This is unfortunate as the alkyloestrogens are very different from the esterized or micronized oestrogens used in HRT. Absolute contra-indications are pregnancy, active venous thromboembolism, severe active liver disease, and endometrial and breast cancer with recurrence. Relative contra-indications are abnormal vaginal bleeding, breast lump, previous endometrial and breast carcinoma, strong family history of breast cancer, and previous venous thromboembolism.

Adherence

Whether or not women continue with HRT depends on many factors, related to the patient, the doctor, the medication, and other factors such as contact with friends, relatives, and the media. Women who consult physicians about the menopause are different from those who do not. Their motivation to consult is influenced by their health beliefs and they may consider menopause a 'natural' phenomenon, and therefore that any resultant symptoms should not be treated. Previous experience of medication will also be influential as they will be worried about side-effects and long-term risks.

The doctor influences the consultation by the amount of time he/she has available for the patient, his/her knowledge of the menopause and HRT, and his/her confidence and competence in being able to negotiate and agree a management strategy with the women. This is the push (willingness to prescribe) and the pull (desire to use) effect.[15]

Adherence to medication also involves its perceived benefits, convenience, possible side-effects, long-term risks, and cost. The most crucial factor with adherence is whether women like taking HRT, as it is the woman who decides on a daily basis whether or not she will continue with it.

Pre-menopausal women

Other women may benefit from HRT. Women who are hypo-oestrogenic through excessive exercise or low body mass index need HRT to prevent bone resorption at a time which may be critical to their achieving a peak bone mass. The use of gonadotrophin-releasing hormone (GnRH) analogues is increasing in gynaecological practice, most commonly for treatment of endometriosis, and preoperative preparation for myomectomies and endometrial resections. If used for greater than 3 months, significant bone loss may occur. If longer-term use is planned then 'addback' therapy to prevent oestrogen deficient symptoms and bone loss must be initiated, with either continuous combined therapy or tibolone.[16]

Alternatives to HRT

Osteoporosis

Selective estrogen receptor modulars (SERMs)

Raloxifene is a SERM, and appears to be efficacious in reducing the incidence of vertebral fractures and to have a beneficial effect on the incidence of breast cancer. This protection appears to be confined to oestrogen receptor-positive tumours. SERMS will not relieve hot flushes and the commonest side-effects are hot flushes or leg cramps. Raloxifene does not appear to stimulate the endometrium.

Bisphosphonates

Bisphosphonates have a basic pyrophosphate structure. They bind avidly to hydroxyapatite, inhibit oestroclastic bone resorption and then are buried within the skeleton where they remain with a half life of 10–12 years or more. They have the potential to inhibit mineralization of bone in a dose-dependent manner. They are licenced for the treatment and prevention of osteoporosis. Etridronate sodium, the first-generation bisphosphonate, is given cyclically (2 weeks on, 11 weeks off) in order to reduce the possibility of inhibiting bone mineralization. Second- and third-generation bisphosphonates do not inhibit mineralization directly but are potent antiresorptive agents. The commonest side-effects of the bisphosphonates are gastrointestinal side-effects, and as all bisphosphonates have extremely poor bioavailability and bind calcium avidly, they should be given on an empty stomach with water only.

The SERMs and bisphosphonates are appropriate in women who wish to protect their skeleton and do not have other hyperoestrogenic symptoms.

Lifestyle changes

For prevention and treatment of osteoporosis, it is important to emphasize to women appropriate lifestyle changes. Their diet should be adequate in calcium and they should be encouraged to do regular weight-bearing exercise, stop smoking, and avoid excess alcohol intake.

Urogenital symptoms

Vaginal lubricants

If atrophic vaginitis is a problem then over-the-counter lubricants can be purchased to improve vaginal dryness. Water-soluble lubricants are advised.

Summary

Ovarian failure can produce hypo-oestrogenic symptoms and these are the commonest reasons for women to consult at the time of the perimenopause or the post-menopause. HRT will relieve the oestrogen-deficiency symptoms but may produce unwanted side-effects. If the therapy suits women, they will be more motivated to take it in the long-term, and this will prevent post-menopausal bone loss. There is controversy over whether HRT protects against cardiovascular disease. Women's main concern on commencing

HRT relates to the question of breast cancer, and it appears that the incidence of breast cancer is slightly increased with women who take long-term HRT. Adherence remains a significant problem, and if women dislike HRT, or they are concerned about the side-effects or the long-term risk then they will not take it.

References

1. **Clinical Synthesis Conference** (1999). Hormone replacement therapy. *Lancet* **354**, 152–5.

2. **Spector, T.D., Brennan, P., Harris, P.A., Studd, J.W., and Silman, A.J.** (1992). Do current regimes of hormone replacement therapy protect against subsequent fractures? *Osteoporosis International* **2** (5), 219–24.

3. **Lufkin, E.G., Wahner, H.W., O'Fallon, W.M., Hodgson, S.F., Kotowicz, M.A., Lane, A.W., Judd, H.L., Caplan, R.H., and Riggs, B.L.** (1992). Treatment of postmenopausal osteoporosis with transdermal estrogen. *Annals of Internal Medicine* **117** (1), 1–9.

4. **Colditz, G.A., Willett, W.C., Stampfer, M.J., Rosner, B., Speizer, F.E., and Hennekens, C.H.** (1987). Menopause and the risk of coronary heart disease in women. *New England Journal of Medicine* **316**, 1105–10.

5. **Stampfer, M.J. and Colditz, G.A.** (1991). Estrogen replacement therapy and coronary heart disease: a quantitative assessment of the epidemiologic evidence. *Preventive Medicine* **20**, 47–63.

6. **Writing Group for the Woman's Health Initiative Investigators** (2002). Risks and benefits of estrogen plus progestin in healthy postmenopausal women. *Journal of the American Medical Association* **288** (3), 321–33.

7. **Hulley, S.** et al. (1998). Randomized trial of estrogen plus progestin for secondary prevention of coronary heart disease in postmenopausal women. *Journal of the American Medical Association* **280** (7), 605–12.

8. **Birge, S.J. and Mortel, K.F.** (1997). Estrogen and the treatment of Alzheimer's disease. *American Journal of Medicine* **103** (3A), 365–455.

9. **Potter, J.D.** (1995). Hormones and colon cancer. *Journal of the National Cancer Institute* **87** (14), 1039–40.

10. **Udoff, L.** et al. (1995). Combined continuous hormone replacement therapy. A critical review. *Obstetrics and Gynecology* **86**, 306–16.

11. **Rymer, J., Fogelman, I., and Chapman, M.G.** (1994). The incidence of vaginal bleeding with tibolone treatment. *British Journal of Obstetrics and Gynaecology* **101**, 53–6.

12. **Collaborative Group on Hormonal Factors in Breast Cancer** (1997). Breast cancer and HRT: collaborative re-analysis of data from 51 epidemiological studies of 52,705 women with breast cancer and 108,411 women without breast cancer. *Lancet* **350**, 1047–59.

13. **Daly, E., Vessey, M.P., Hawkins, M.M., Carson, J.L., Gough, P., and Marsh, S.** (1996). Risk of venous thromboembolism in users of hormone replacement therapy. *Lancet* **348**, 977–80.

14. **Jick, H., Derby, L.E., Myers, M.W., Vasilakis, C., and Newton, K.M.** Risk of hospital admission for idiopathic venous thromboembolism among users of postmenopausal oestrogens.

15. **Topo, P., Hemminki, E., and Uutela, A.** (1993). Women's choice and physicians' advice on use of menopausal and postmenopausal hormone therapy. *International Journal of Health Sciences* **4** (3), 101–9.

16. **Rymer, J., Morris, E., and Fogelman, I.** (1991). GnRH analogues and addback therapy in current gynaecologic practice. (ed. J. Studd). Edinburgh: Churchill Livingstone.

7.6 Urinary incontinence

Toine Lagro-Janssen

Epidemiology

Urinary incontinence entails involuntary urine loss, regardless of the volume of urine lost. The condition primarily affects women and elderly people. About one in four women below the age of 65 suffers from urinary incontinence, 7 per cent of whom experience urine loss on a daily basis.[1] The majority of women under 65 with incontinence exhibit stress incontinence, while 16 per cent suffer from urge incontinence, and 18 per cent from mixed incontinence.[2] Among women over 65, 14 per cent experience daily urine loss.[3] Thirty to 50 per cent of the female population in nursing homes experience incontinence.[4] Certain conditions enhance a patient's chances of being affected by the disorder, such as being overweight, chronic coughing, congestive heart failure, or having had a hysterectomy.

Presentation in primary care

Patients generally find it difficult to consult their doctors about urinary incontinence. Research suggests that only 50 per cent of the people suffering from the condition actually go and see their doctor about it, and in most cases, only mention it as a secondary complaint, or when leaving the office at the end of a visit with an unrelated purpose.[1] The most important reason for patients not to seek medical advice is that they experience their complaints as a minor discomfort, as not sufficiently serious to warrant treatment. Most women do not worry about their condition and hardly see it as an impediment on their lives. Some women do not even regard it as something abnormal, but rather as an inevitable female complaint. A sense of shame may also prevent women from discussing their complaints with their GPs. When the incontinence takes serious forms, however, women do tend to worry about it and go ask for help. Women suffering from urge incontinence, and elderly people, are furthermore usually better known to their GPs.[1]

Possible causes

In most cases, involuntary loss of urine is related to disturbances in the continence mechanism of the bladder itself. This pertains to both stress incontinence, urge incontinence, and mixed incontinence. Rare forms of incontinence are reflex incontinence and overflow incontinence.

Stress incontinence is defined as the occurrence of involuntary urine loss when a rise in abdominal pressure causes the intravesicular pressure to exceed the maximum urethral pressure in the absence of detrusor activity. Weakness of the sphincter mechanism closing the bladder occurs under elevated intra-abdominal pressure; it is more vulnerable in women than in men. Women do not have proximal sphincters. Their bladders are only distally closed off by smooth and striated muscle tissue surrounding the urethra. The pelvic floor, with layers of connective tissue, ensures further closure. The pelvic floor muscles may be weak due to predisposition, pregnancy, or vaginal delivery. Prolonged second stage of labour and the use of forceps are notorious for causing damage to the neuromuscular function of the pelvic floor and the bladder sphincter. This explains why stress incontinence is a primarily female condition.

Urge incontinence describes the occurrence of involuntary urine loss as a result of spontaneous detrusor activity which cannot be consciously suppressed, and which may or may not be accompanied by an awareness of the desire to urinate. In these cases, we are dealing with an unstable bladder, usually caused by a disruption of the conditioned reflex mechanism. People with an average intake of liquid urinate seven times a day. The first urge to relieve the bladder occurs when it contains 300–400 ml of urine. In normal cases, the urge is suppressed till circumstances allow for relief. If people begin to urinate too frequently, the bladder loses its retaining function. Micturition patterns are susceptible to emotional influences. Bladder infections and urogynaecological surgery often entail frequent micturition and may provoke urge incontinence. Anxiety about incontinence then results in frequent urination and sustains the incontinence. Some research results describe psychiatric and psychopathological disorders in patients with urge incontinence, but studies carried out in general practice calls such results into question. With advancing age, neurological disorders acquire greater importance in the aetiology of urge incontinence.

A number of factors may contribute to the occurrence of incontinence. Caffeine or medication producing sympathetic or parasympathetic effects such as antidepressants or antipsychotics, may, by affecting the autonomic innervation of the bladder, affect the continence mechanism.[5] Diuretics, as well as alcohol, also lead to higher bladder content and pressure, and occasional loss of urine. Urologic and gynaecologic surgery are important causes of incontinence. Women who have undergone a hysterectomy are also likely to be afflicted by the condition. Neurological disorders, such as diabetic neuropathy, often lead to reflex or overflow incontinence. Lower oestrogen levels in post-menopausal women may result in a loss of peri-urethral support tissue, which in turn may cause a reduction in sphincter activity of both bladder and urethra.

Mixed incontinence is a combination of stress and urge incontinence and can be attributed to corresponding causes. Experience shows that women suffering from stress incontinence attempt to avoid loss of urine by going to the bathroom more often, and tend to develop urge incontinence as well.

Relflex incontinence is the result of abnormal spinal reflex activity in the absence of a normal urge to micturate, as in the case of spinal cord lesions.

Overflow incontinence describes involuntary loss of urine when the intravesicular pressure exceeds maximum urethral pressure as a result of the bladder filling in the absence of detrusor contractions.

These last two types of incontinence are rare and will not be discussed in this chapter.

Making a diagnosis

History

The purpose of the clinical history is first of all to establish what type of incontinence the patient is suffering from. The loss of small amounts of urine during activities that increase abdominal pressure such as sneezing, coughing, jumping, laughing, lifting, and exercising constitutes the typical clinical symptom of stress incontinence. The patient does not experience an urge to micturate while losing urine. As soon as the pressure decreases, the urine loss stops too. These losses may vary from a few drops to significant volumes. The overall pattern of micturition appears normal.

In the case of urge incontinence, the patient experiences such a strong desire to void that she may be unable to reach the bathroom in time. Once it has started, it is hard to interrupt the urine flow. The volume of urine lost tends to be larger than in the case of stress incontinence. Working with or hearing the sound of water may trigger off the desire to void. Women sometimes experience urine loss the very moment when relief seems at hand, that is, when turning the key in the front-door lock. Urge incontinence is often accompanied by additional complaints, for example, frequent urination and nocturia. Pain is not a feature of incontinence and may indicate an infection instead. In the case of mixed incontinence, the loss of urine occurs both during episodes of increased pressure and in association with a strong desire to void.

Other patterns of incontinence indicate the presence of pathology requiring specialist investigation. The presence of certain neurological disorders (spinal cord lesions) may indicate reflex incontinence. Continual loss of small volumes of urine indicates bladder overflow (rare in women) or a vesicovaginal or vesicorectal fistula.

It is helpful to ask about factors that might have contributed to the development of urine loss.[6] Apart from shedding light on the type of incontinence, the answer to this question provides insight in the seriousness of the condition. The latter may also be inferred from the frequency of incidents and the volume of urine loss, from whether or not the patient uses absorbent materials, and how often she has to change herself. Keeping a urinary diary for a week, in which patients record how often they wet themselves, what they were doing at the time, and how much urine they lost, also serves to clarify the type and seriousness of the incontinence. Such diary entries may additionally show the presence of special forms of incontinence that occur as a result of neurological disorders, or of continuous urine loss due to bladder overflow or a fistula. Secondary symptoms, such as a painful micturition, and genital complaints may indicate different diagnoses.

Examination, investigation

Physical examination focuses on the exclusion of conditions that may cause urinary incontinence, such as a distended bladder, evidence of infection, and pelvic masses. Most important is the gynaecological examination. A check is made to see whether there is any atrophy of the vulva and of the vaginal epithelium. The possibility of a cystocoele, a prolapse of the uterus, a uterine fibroid or a tumour of the adnexa, is also investigated. A prolapse of the uterus does not automatically indicate stress incontinence, since a prolapse is probably equally likely to occur with and without incontinence.

In anticipation of exercises to strengthen the pelvic floor muscles, women with stress incontinence can be asked to push the GPs inserted fingers together during the vaginal examination. If the anal muscles and the opening of the vulva contract simultaneously, there is usually no dysfunction of the pelvic floor activity. In this way, the GP is able to assess the patient's ability to voluntarily and adequately contract these muscles. A number of patients with urge incontinence experience pain in the lower abdomen, which increases during and after intercourse. For these patients, the vaginal examination is sensitive and painful while palpation does not indicate abnormalities.

Since urge incontinence and mixed incontinence can be the major symptoms of a urinary tract infection, bladder tumour, or bladder stones, the urine is tested for infections and haematuria. Because the results of the case history and those of urodynamic tests correspond, there is no need to carry out urodynamic tests before starting conservative therapy.

Certain categories of patients should be referred for further examination and treatment.[6] In the diagnostic stage, this pertains to patients whose condition does not fit the types of urge, stress, and mixed incontinence described above. It may, for instance, remain unclear exactly what type of incontinence the patient is suffering from, or whether there are indications of neurological disorders. When physical or additional examination points to underlying forms of pathology, patients should be referred as well. Women with a considerable prolapse should always be referred, since in these cases surgical treatment is indicated.

Management

Before starting treatment, GPs ask patients for which symptoms they wish to be treated, and what kind of improvements they would like to see. By exploring the significance of the complaint and its psychosocial implications, it will become clear why the patient is asking for help at this particular moment. Attention should be given to adequate incontinence aids, for which there are many possibilities.

Stress incontinence

The GP explains to the patient that the complaints, indicating stress incontinence, stem from a deficiency in the closing mechanism of the bladder. Emphasis is put on the role of the pelvic floor muscles in this process, so that patients understand why treatment, consisting of pelvic floor muscle exercises, is recommended.

Pelvic floor muscle exercises involve contracting the pelvic floor musculature for a count of five, and relaxing it for the same period of time. The pelvic floor muscles are those muscles that are contracted when fighting the urge to pass either water or wind. In order to make a woman conscious of the pelvic floor muscles, the GP may ask her to push the inserted fingers together during the vaginal examination. This makes it possible to instruct the correct muscles, and allows for correcting the involuntary contraction of the abdominal muscles, the buttock muscles, or the thigh muscles. The contraction of the pelvic floor muscles should be repeated at least 10 times, with a total of 50 times per day. Improvement can only be expected after at least 8 weeks of exercising. The better the patient sticks to the exercise schedule, the better the results. Motivating patients is crucial, for performing the exercises, especially at first, is difficult, and requires discipline. Patients should be given written instructions on how to perform the exercises. Pelvic floor muscle exercises are effective in 60–70 per cent of all female patients.[7] This improvement continues after 5 years.[8] If a woman does not succeed in contracting the correct muscles, she can be referred to an adequately experienced physiotherapist.

Alternative treatment of stress incontinence involves the use of a pessary. A circular polyvinyl pessary pushes the urethra–bladder connection upwards, with continence as a result. The option of a pessary is definitely preferred for women with a major prolapse, when surgical intervention is not a possibility due to various contra-indications. In cases where patients are unable to perform exercises as a result of reduced cognitive functions, a pessary is also the best form of treatment.

Ordinary vaginal tampons may have a positive effect on incontinence during short periods of exertion, such as dancing or practising a sport. The effect is probably due to the fact that tampons push up the bladder orifice.

It is not useful to treat stress incontinence with medication. Although some research suggests a positive effect of oestrogens on both stress and urge incontinence in post-menopausal women, few adequate placebo-controlled studies are available to confirm such results. Results of this kind of treatment are better with urge and mixed incontinence than with stress incontinence (see management of urge incontinence).

Urge incontinence

The exact causes of urge incontinence are as yet unknown. Poor urinating habits, exacerbated by emotional influences, may well play a role. Due to frequent micturition, the bladder has become oversensitive. It has, as it were, forgotten how to retain urine. The bladder's retaining capacity can be recovered through training.[9] Here too, the results largely depend on the patient's compliance with the exercise regime. The GP explains the nature and the origins of the patient's complaints in these terms. It should be emphasized that certain kinds of behaviour (micturition patterns) may sustain physical complaints (incontinence). Training is intended to boost the bladder's capacity.

Patients are asked to record the times of micturition and moments of incontinence in a urinary diary, and to postpone micturition for 15 min each day. Remaining seated facilitates postponement of micturition. In this way, the interval between micturition is gradually lengthened. An alternative is the so-called clocking micturition method. Here, the shortest period between two micturitions is extended by 5–15 min. Training only takes place during daytime, on the assumption that a positive development will automatically alleviate micturition during the night. The ultimate goal is a micturition frequency of seven times a day with normal intake of fluids.

Keeping a urinary diary has a supporting effect, as does giving patients written instructions. Training the bladder is easier if patients, in the early stages, avoid substances that particularly stimulate bladder activity, such as alcohol and coffee. The diary is used to evaluate patient progress. If bladder training fails to produce an improvement after 3 months, it is pointless to continue.

Drugs play a limited part in the treatment of urge incontinence.[6] The effectiveness of products such as spasmolytics, for instance, has not been adequately established, and there is a substantial risk of undesirable effects. Frequently noted side-effects include dryness of the mouth, urine retention, and unclear vision. In first-line care, oxybutinin and tolterodine

should, especially with elderly patients, be prescribed with the greatest care. Spasmolytics may also be indicated if bladder training proves to have no beneficial effects. Results of such medication are assessed after 2 weeks. In similar situations, treatment with oestrogens is a potential alternative. In post-menopausal women with atrophy of the vaginal epithelium, treatment with oestrogen may be indicated as well.

In cases of mixed incontinence, urge incontinence is usually experienced as the most distressing form of the disorder. Initial treatment therefore consists of bladder training. Depending on the results, this may be supplemented with pelvic floor muscle exercises.

Long-term care

Preventive measures primarily concern parturition. Although it is easy to aim for a timely termination of an inadequately progressing labour in order to avoid pelvic neuromuscular damage through overstretching and ischaemia, such an aim is not so easily achieved. How is one to decide when labour is taking too long? And is it possible to prevent this with episiotomy? What is clear is that the use of forceps should, if possible, be avoided. Gynaecological surgery generally and hysterectomy in particular may furthermore lead to prolapse and incontinence. What is more, a prolapse operation may itself result in incontinence. A strong indication for surgery and specialist care are therefore of crucial importance. To prevent damage to the pelvic floor, pelvic floor muscle exercises are recommended during pregnancy and labour. Several recent randomized clinical trials show that pelvic floor muscle exercises and bladder training result in significant lower numbers of women with stress incontinence after childbirth.[10] Rapid mobilization after labour may thus be highly effective in raising a woman's consciousness of the pelvic floor and its use, so that an increase in intraperitoneal pressure automatically and simultaneously provokes contraction of the pelvic floor muscles.

Following its aetiology, prevention of urge incontinence entails a disruption of, at the earliest possible moment, the vicious circle of anxiety about incontinence and frequent micturition, which, in its turn, leads to increased urge and subsequent incontinence.

Implications of the problem

Patients generally handle their complaints in different manners, and this includes women experiencing the involuntary loss of urine as well. Psychosocial implications depend on the seriousness of the problem and the type of incontinence. Urge and mixed incontinence in particular affect the quality of life: patients sleep badly, feel hampered in their social lives, feel emotionally unstable, and lack self-confidence.[11] The relation between the seriousness of the complaints and the experience of psychological problems is more complicated.[12] Generally speaking, there is a clear connection between subjectively experienced problems and the seriousness of the complaints. The more serious their symptoms, the more worried patients are about the future. At the same time, one in seven women with a mild form of incontinence experiences serious problems. The objective degree of seriousness therefore does not necessarily correspond to the subjective degree of suffering.

Appendix 1

Exercises to strengthen the pelvic floor muscles

The pelvic floor consists of various muscles. It supports the uterus, the bladder, and the intestines. At the front, the pelvic floor is attached to the pubic bone, while at the rear it is attached to the coccygeal bone.

There are three openings in the pelvic floor:

- the urethra (urinary opening);
- the vagina; and
- the anus.

Patients can exercise the muscles around these openings in order to strengthen the pelvic floor musculature, including the muscles that close off the bladder.

If you pause stop the flow of urine while urinating, you will be able to feel which muscles are involved. These are the same pelvic floor muscles you contract when you put off going to the bathroom to urinate.

While doing the exercises, you contract the pelvic floor musculature for a count of about six.

Next, allow the muscles to relax again (producing the same feeling as when starting to urinate).

See to it that the rest of your body remains relaxed and try to continue to breathe regularly.

You should perform this contracting and relaxing about 10 times.

Repeat the exercises 5–10 times per day.

Once you have identified the muscles to be contracting, you can perform this exercise whenever you wish during the day, even while you are carrying your daily activities. If you do this regularly, every day, you will start to notice results after 6–8 weeks.

Appendix 2

Bladder training

One of the most important jobs performed by the bladder is the collection and storage of urine. If you urinate too often, the bladder will become less efficient at retaining urine. As a result, it will stimulate the desire to urinate when it contains relatively little urine. For this reason, the bladder must be re-educated, as it were. It must re-learn how to hold more urine.

Exercises:

Keep a diary, entering the following information:

◆ the time when you feel the urge to urinate;

◆ the time when you go to the bathroom; and

◆ the time when you wet yourself.

The aim is to postpone the times that you go to the bathroom by 15 min. To make postponement easier, you may use a chair or a stool. Sitting down helps to prevent involuntary urine loss, so that you will not have to be afraid to wet yourself. You try to extend the period of postponement by 15 min each day. You keep a record in your diary of the times that you go to the bathroom. Bringing your diary, see your GP after 3 months to discuss progress.

References

1. Lagro-Janssen, A.L.M., Smits, A.J.A., and van Weel, C. (1990). Women with urinary incontinence: self perceived worries and general practitioners' knowledge of the problem. *British Journal of General Practice* **40**, 331–4.

2. Lagro-Janssen, A.L.M. et al. (1991). Controlled trial of pelvic floor exercises in the treatment of urinary stress incontinence in general practice. *British Journal of General Practice* **41**, 445–9.

3. Rekers, H. et al. (1992). Urinary incontinence in women from 35 to 79 years of age: prevalence and consequences. *European Journal of Gynecology and Reproductive Biology* **43**, 229–34.

4. Valk, M. Urinary incontinence in psychogeriatric nursing home patients. Prevalence and determinants—dissertation. Utrecht: Utrecht University Press, 1999.

5. Fantl, J.A. et al. *Urinary Incontinence in Adults: Acute and Chronic Management.* Clinical Practice Guideline No. 2, Update. Rockville MD: US Department of Health and Human Services. Public Health Service, Agency for Health Care Policy and Research. AHCPR Publication No. 96-0682, 1996.

6. Lagro-Janssen, A.L.M. et al. (1995). NHG-Practice guideline 'Urinary Incontinence'. *Huisarts en Wetenschap* **38**, 71–80.

7. Berghmans, L.C.M. et al. (1998). Conservative treatment of stress urinary incontinence in women: a systematic review of randomized clinical trials. *British Journal of Urology* **82**, 181–91.

8. Lagro-Janssen, A.L.M. and van Weel, C. (1998). Long-term effect of treatment of female incontinence in general practice. *British Journal of General Practice* **48**, 1735–8.

9. Berghmans, L.C.M. Conservative treatment for women with stress incontinence and bladder overactivity—dissertation. Maastricht: Maastricht University Press, 2000.

10. Mørkved, S. and Bø, K. (2000). Effect of postpartum pelvic floor muscle training in prevention and treatment of urinary incontinence: a one year follow up study. *British Journal of Obstetrics and Gynaecology* **107**, 1022–8.

11. Hunskaar, S. and Vinsnes, A. (1991). The quality of life in women with urinary incontinence as measured by the Sickness Impact Profile. *Journal of American Geriatric Society* **39**, 378–82.

12. Lagro-Janssen, T., Smits, A.J.A., and van Weel, C. (1992). Urinary incontinence in women and the effects on their lives. *Scandinavian Journal of Primary Health Care* **10**, 211–16.

7.7 Menstrual disorders: menorrhagia

Norma O'Flynn

Definitions and epidemiology

Menorrhagia is a Greek-derived label applied to heavy menstrual periods. The term comes from the Greek 'men' for month and 'rhegynai' to rush out. Menorrhagia is defined as the loss of 80 ml or more of blood per period. The cycle may be regular or irregular. This definition is based on the distribution of blood loss in a population study, and the associated incidence of anaemia. Eighty millilitres marked the 90th centile of blood loss and anaemia was significantly increased above 60 ml of blood loss; 80 ml was chosen as the upper limit of normal blood loss. Studies in more selected populations in developed and developing countries have found similar distributions of blood loss. However, the association between the amount of blood loss and iron-deficiency anaemia will depend on the nutritional status of the population.

Using objective measurement, menorrhagia is more common in women in older age groups. Objective measurement of menstrual blood loss is however rare in clinical practice. Presentation and treatment is dependent on an individual's perception of her periods.

In community studies, 30 per cent of women consider their periods to be heavy. Subjectively, heaviness is considered in terms of the use of sanitary protection, length of bleeding, presence of clots, colour of blood lost, and general feelings of tiredness. A complaint of heavy periods may mean that the period is now heavier than it was, or the individual may have always considered her period heavy. Less than 50 per cent of those who complain of heavy periods will fulfil the objective definition of menorrhagia.

The medical classification of disorders of menstruation may not reflect the experience of women. Medical diagnostic categories divide menstrual disorders into separate disorders affecting different aspects of menstruation such as blood loss, pain, timing, and mood. Research in primary and secondary care in the United Kingdom has shown that women treated for heavy periods also find other aspects of their period troublesome.

Presentation in primary care

A study in British general practice found a consultation rate of 5 per cent of women in the 30–49-year age-group for heavy menstrual bleeding. Results from a general practice database in New Zealand indicate that 2.3 per cent of consultations for women less than 50 years old were for heavy menstrual bleeding. Presentation may be precipitated by concern about the degree of blood loss, the associated effect on quality of life or consideration of underlying causes. Some women may fear that the bleeding will not stop.

Possible underlying causes

There are no studies of the causes of heavy periods in the general population. Information on causes comes from retrospective analyses of findings at investigation and surgery in secondary care. In many studies from specialist centres, menstrual blood loss is measured and the findings relate to women whose menorrhagia is defined objectively. A large proportion of women treated for menorrhagia do not have identifiable pathology. There is no evidence that many women with menorrhagia have anovulatory cycles.

- Local endometrial factors may account for up to 80 per cent of cases. Laboratory studies have found increased fibrinolytic activity and increased production of prostaglandins at endometrial level in women with menorrhagia.

- Uterine fibroids or leiomyomas occur in at least 20 per cent of women in their reproductive years. Fibroids are more common in black women, in the nulliparous, and the obese. They are commonly considered a cause of increased blood loss, but are likely to be coincidental rather than causal in the majority of women. A number of small studies show that fibroids are more common at extremes of blood loss. It has been suggested that only submucous fibroids that distort the uterine cavity cause heavy bleeding, but the current evidence is contradictory.

- Adenomyosis, endometrial polyps and endometrial hyperplasia have all been associated with menorrhagia. One selected case-series of women with objective menorrhagia found endometrial polyps in 4 per cent and endometrial hyperplasia in 2 per cent. Complex and atypical hyperplasia can progress to endometrial carcinoma, but this is rare in pre-menopausal women.

- Inherited bleeding disorders may be associated with menorrhagia. A complaint of heavy bleeding since the menarche and other complaints of bleeding are likely in the affected group.

- Intrauterine contraceptive devices are associated with an increase in menstrual blood loss.

- Irregularities of menstruation and changes in menstrual pattern may be associated with pelvic infection and sexually transmitted diseases.

Assessing the patient

The purpose of assessment of a patient with heavy periods is to evaluate the complaint, to ascertain if the patient is anaemic and to rule out any underlying cause that requires treatment.

An overview of management is presented in Fig. 1.

History

Menstrual problems are less likely than other problems to be discussed among family and friends before presentation. Therefore, women may have

difficulty in articulating their menstrual complaint. The clinician should enquire about number of days of bleeding, regularity of cycle, quantity of sanitary protection used, effect on work, social life, and sexual relationships. Details of other aspects of the periods such as pain and possible worries about underlying causes should be sought. Increased blood loss is correlated with extremes of reproductive age, increased sanitary protection use and length of time bleeding.

Erratic cycles may be associated with endometrial polyps and submucous fibroids.

A number of risk factors for endometrial hyperplasia are ascertainable from the history. In a hospital population, body weight more than or equal to 90 kg, age not less than 45 years, infertility, family history of colonic carcinoma, and nulliparity were risk factors for endometrial hyperplasia in pre-menopausal women with abnormal uterine bleeding (heavy, irregular, or intermenstrual bleeding). Irregularity of cycles or duration of menstrual bleeding were not risk factors for endometrial hyperplasia.

Examination

General examination should include the search for evidence of anaemia. Abdominal and pelvic examination will exclude obvious pelvic pathology.

Investigation

Full blood count is required to exclude anaemia. Haemoglobin falls with increasing blood loss. However, studies in developed countries have shown normal haemoglobin levels despite objective menorrhagia. Ferritin levels may be a more sensitive indicator in these populations.

Ultrasound/biopsy

Hysteroscopy, the direct inspection of the uterine cavity with directed biopsy, is now the best test for intrauterine pathology. It can be performed in outpatients without anaesthesia.

Transvaginal ultrasound is commonly used to evaluate the endometrium and has been compared to hysteroscopy. One study of women with objectively defined menorrhagia in a secondary care setting found 96 per cent sensitivity, 86 per cent specificity, 91 per cent positive predictive value, and 94 per cent negative predictive value in the diagnosis of intrauterine abnormality. In a less selected primary care population with a lower prevalence of abnormalities, the negative predictive values are likely to be higher, that is, a negative result is very likely to be a true negative. Ultrasonography is therefore suggested as a first-step procedure, with abnormal or inconclusive results requiring further investigation.

An endometrial thickness of more than or equal to 12 mm in pre-menopausal women is suggestive of endometrial hyperplasia and endometrial biopsy is required.

Referral

The procedures for referral will be dependent on local circumstances. Ultrasonography and Pipelle biopsy may be available in a primary care setting, or referral to secondary care may be required for these or other investigations.

Principles of management

General principles

The majority of women treated for menorrhagia will not have identifiable pathology. A full exploration of the woman's complaint, an explanation that sinister causes are rare and attention to other concerns such as fertility or fear of cancer will be helpful to most women.

The presence of anaemia indicates an individual is suffering an unsustainable degree of blood loss. Any anaemia should be treated, and continued treatment with iron can prevent development of anaemia.

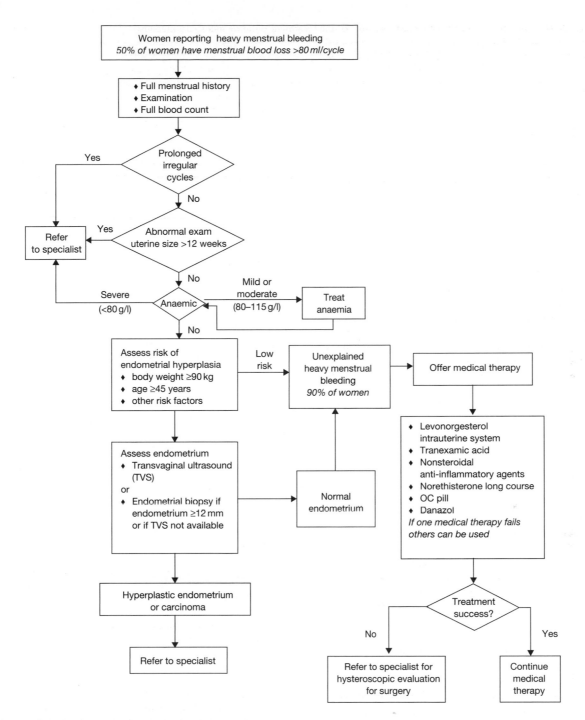

Fig. 1 Algorithm for the management of heavy menstrual bleeding. [*From:* Working Party for Guidelines for the Management of Heavy Menstrual Bleeding (1999). An evidence-based guideline for the management of heavy menstrual bleeding. *New Zealand Medical Journal* **112**, 174–7.]

The main focus of management is to reduce menstrual blood loss

Emergency treatment

Progesterone treatment will stop severe bleeding. A variety of regimes can be used; the aim is to use an adequate dose of progesterone to stop bleeding. For example, start with a high dose of norethisterone such as 30 mg bd. for 3 days, 20 mg bd. for 3 days, 10 mg bd. for 3 days, and 5 mg bd. for 10 days. Once treatment is finished, a withdrawal bleed will occur.

Ongoing treatment

A number of different medical treatments are available. The following treatments have been shown to reduce menstrual blood loss in randomized controlled trials. The efficacy of each treatment, specific benefits, and side-effects are shown in Table 1.

- Non-steroidal anti-inflammatory drugs (NSAIDs) decrease menstrual loss when taken during the menstrual cycle. This is a group effect due to their action on prostaglandin synthesis. The dosages of some of the NSAIDs used in trials are mefenamic acid 500 mg tds, ibuprofen

Table 1 Comparative table of medical therapy for the treatment of heavy menstrual bleeding

Drug	Mean reduction in blood loss (%)	Specific benefits	Adverse effects
Levonorgesterol IUS	94+	Contraception No requirement to take tablets	Menstrual cramps Expulsion of system Intermenstrual bleeding
Oral progesterone (days 5–25)	87	Cycle regularity	Bloating, mood swings Premenstrual syndrome
Tranexamic acid	47	Non-hormonal	Nausea, diarrhoea
NSAIDs	29	Relief of dysmenorrhoea and headaches	Nausea, diarrhoea
Oral contraceptive pill	43	Contraception Relief of dysmenorrhoea	Nausea Breast tenderness Headache
Danazol	50	No bleeding	Weight gain, acne
Oral progesterone (luteal phase)	4	Cycle regularity	Bloating, mood swings Premenstrual symptoms

Adapted with permission from: Working Party for Guidelines for the Management of Heavy Menstrual Bleeding (1999). An evidence-based guideline for the management of heavy menstrual bleeding. *New Zealand Medical Journal* **112**, 174–7.

400 mg tds (ibuprofen 200 mg tds also reduced blood loss but to a lesser extent), flurbiprofen 100 mg bd.

♦ Antifibrinolytic treatments, the commonest of which is tranexamic acid, also reduce blood loss when taken during menstruation (dose tranexamic acid 500 mg–1.5 g 3–4 per day).

♦ The combined oral contraceptive pill (OCP) is often used to reduce menstrual loss, in particular if contraception is also required. Although commonly used, there has been only one randomized controlled trial to test the effect of the OCP on menorrhagia. This found no significant difference between effect of OCP and NSAIDs.

♦ Oral progestogen therapy has been used in two different ways; in the luteal phase or for 21 days from day 5 to 25 of the cycle. Luteal phase progesterone is less effective than all other therapies and no longer considered as appropriate treatment. The longer course of treatment, for example, norethisterone 15 mg daily from days 5 to 25, causes a reduction in blood loss, but less than the intrauterine system (IUS). Both treatment options can increase cycle regularity which is valued by women.

♦ The levonorgesterol-releasing IUS is an intrauterine device sheathed in levonorgesterol. It reduces endometrial proliferation, and so reduces the duration and amount of menstrual loss. It is extremely effective in reduction of blood loss and at 12 months, the majority of women have amenorrhoea or only slight bleeding. The system also provides contraception and has been associated with high rates of satisfaction and continuation in studies of its use. A trial comparing the IUS with hysterectomy found no differences between treatments in health related quality of life at one year. If these findings are sustained over longer follow-up, the IUS may provide a long-term solution for many women.

If a woman's period problem also encompasses other aspects of her period, the choice of treatment may be influenced by those factors, for example, OCP or NSAIDs for dysmenorrhoea.

The available medical therapies will cause a reduction in blood loss. However, since the majority of cases of menorrhagia are subjectively defined, the preferred treatment outcome will also be subjectively defined. Some women will be content to use regular medication as long as is necessary, others will find such a regime difficult and unacceptable and may prefer a surgical solution.

Surgical treatment

Hysterectomy has been the main surgical treatment for women complaining of menorrhagia. Over the last decade, alternative techniques have become available which ablate the uterine lining and thus cause a reduction in bleeding. It has been hoped that these techniques would provide an alternative to hysterectomy. Patients have a shorter stay in hospital, with more rapid recovery and return to normal activity. However, women treated by hysterectomy experience more improvement in menstrual symptoms, higher rates of satisfaction with treatment, and superior health-related quality of life. In the United Kingdom, hysterectomy rates have remained stable despite the introduction of endometrial ablation.

Implications

Living with menorrhagia

All societies have rules regarding menstruation. Some religious and cultural groups prohibit women entering places of worship or doing daily tasks such as cooking. Even in secular societies, women learn to keep menstruation a private matter and external evidence or open discussion of menstruation is unusual. These factors can make a woman's management of her period difficult, particularly if she has to change sanitary protection frequently and is fearful of staining of clothes. Quality of life scores (using SF36) of women with menorrhagia are significantly lower than those of the general population. General energy levels, work life, social life, family life and relationships, and practical difficulties in managing menstruation have all been identified as problems by women. The financial cost of sanitary protection and treatments may be a problem for poorer women. Objective measurements of quality of life improve after all treatments.

Psychological effects

Menstrual complaints have often been attributed to psychological factors. The association is considered by some to be dismissive of women's health problems and indicative of sexual prejudice. The association has arisen partly from the discrepancy between objective and subjective menorrhagia, and the search for a reason as to why women without 'true' menorrhagia were seeking treatment. The disorders can co-exist and just as the psychological distress is improved by treatment of menorrhagia, the psychological morbidity may be caused by living with the menstrual complaint.

Future directions

The medical definition of menorrhagia is a condition based on a cut-off point of menstrual blood loss. As such it is arbitrary and removed from patient experience. Patient presentation is more likely a combination of menstrual difficulties, their functional sequlae and their effect on quality of life. Exploration of the interplay of such factors may be more productive in understanding patient complaint. A re-definition of menstrual complaints in such terms may be helpful.

Primary care practitioners are currently limited by a paucity of information as to the predictive power of menstrual symptoms for specific disorders in primary care populations. Such information may allow the primary care practitioner to reassure patients, and the effects of such reassurance and the necessity for investigations in primary care context could be evaluated.

Key points

1. Complaints of heavy menstrual bleeding are common in the community.

2. The complaint has a significant effect on quality of life.

3. Serious causes are rare.

4. Effective treatments to reduce blood loss are available.

Further reading

Hallberg, L. et al. (1966). Menstrual blood loss—a population study. *Acta Obstetricia Gynaecologica Scandinavica* **45**, 320–51. (The definition of menorrhagia emerged from this study.)

Janssen, C.A.H., Scholten, P.C., and Heintz, P.M. (1997). Menorrhagia—a search for epidemiological risk markers. *Maturitas* **28**, 19–25. (The most recent epidemiological study in the community.)

Byles, J.E., Hanrahan, P.F., and Schofield, M.J. (1997). 'It would be good to know you're not alone': the health needs of women with menstrual symptoms. *Family Practice* **14**, 249–54. (The experience of women consulting in primary care for menstrual complaints.)

O'Flynn, N. and Britten, N. (2000). Menorrhagia in general practice—disease or illness. *Social Science and Medicine* **50**, 551–61.

Warner, P., Critchley, H.O., Lumsden, M.A., Campbell-Brown, M., Dougls, A., and Murray, G. (2001). Referral for menstrual problems: cross-sectional survey of symptoms, reasons for referral and management. *British Medical Journal* **323**, 24–5.

Working Party for Guidelines for the Management of Heavy Menstrual Bleeding (1999). An evidence-based guideline for the management of heavy menstrual bleeding. *New Zealand Medical Journal* **112**, 174–7. (Guidelines aimed at general practitioners and gynaecologists.)

Vercellini, P. et al. (1997). The role of transvaginal ultrasonography and outpatient diagnostic hysteroscopy in the evaluation of patients with menorrhagia. *Human Reproduction* **12** (8), 1768–71.

Hurskainen, R. et al. (2001). Quality of life and cost-effectiveness of levonorgestrel-releasing intrauterine system versus hysterectomy for treatment of menorrhagia: a randomised trial. *Lancet* **357**, 273–7. (This paper presents the results of a randomized controlled trial comparing IUS with hysterectomy at 1 year.)

http://www.nzgg.org.nz/. (The web-page for the New Zealand guidelines group provides access to the guidelines provided for the management of heavy bleeding, how the guidelines were generated, and an extensive list of relevant references.)

Garratt, A.M., Ruta, D.A., Abdalla, M.I., Buckingham, J.K., and Russell, I.T. (1993). The SF36 health survey questionnaire: an outcome measure suitable for routine use within the NHS? *British Medical Journal* **306**, 1440–4.

Warner, P. (1998). Psychosomatic and other influences on complaints of menstrual bleeding and pain. In *Clinical Disorders of the Endometrium and Menstrual Cycle* Chapter 26 (ed. I.T. Cameron, I.S. Fraser, and S.K. Smith), pp. 331–43. Oxford: Oxford University Press. (A critique of the evidence of the psychosomatic nature of menstrual complaints.)

7.8 Menstrual disorders: dysmenorrhoea

Norma O'Flynn

Definition and epidemiology

Dysmenorrhoea is painful menstruation. It is medically classified as primary, that is, occurring in the absence of disease, or secondary to an underlying disorder. The pain is crampy and spasmodic. It is present mainly in the lower abdomen, but may be experienced suprapubically or in upper thighs.

Dysmenorrhoea is a common symptom, found in all cultural groups. Prevalence rates as high as 90 per cent are described in selected adolescent populations. The complaint is presumed to improve with age, but there is little evidence about its natural history. The only follow-up study, in a general population sample in Sweden, found a prevalence of 72 per cent at 19 years of age, and 67 per cent in the same group at 24 years. Parity was associated with a reduction in prevalence and severity of dysmenorrhoea, with no change in the nulliparous.

Risk factors for severity of dysmenorrhoea are early age at menarche, long menstrual periods, smoking, and alcohol intake.

Presentation in primary care

Although dysmenorrhoea is a common symptom, only a minority of people affected consult a doctor. Many women regard menstrual pain as a normal physiological event and self treatment with over-the-counter (OTC) medication is common. Information from a UK community study indicates that while 32 per cent of women reported a restriction in activites due to dysmenorrhoea, 12 per cent of women with dysmenorrhoea attended a GP in the previous 12 months, and 73 per cent used OTC medication.

Causes

Primary dysmenorrhoea

Myometrial hyperactivity can be demonstrated in women with dysmenorrhoea. This hyperactivity causes pain by reducing uterine blood flow, and causing uterine ischaemia. Elevated levels of vasopressin and leukotrienes are found in women with dysmenorrhoea, and increased endometrial synthesis of prostaglandins has been demonstrated. These compounds stimulate contractions of myometrium and vascular smooth muscle.

Secondary dysmenorrhoea

Secondary dysmenorrhoea is by definition associated with pelvic pathology and some of the possible causes are shown in Table 1.

Table 1 Causes of secondary dysmenorrhoea

Endometriosis
Pelvic inflammatory disease
Pelvic venous congestion (pelvic varices)
Uterine fibroids
Endometrial polyps
Intrauterine contraceptive devices
Uterine abnormalities
Previous surgery

Endometriosis

Endometriosis is the presence of endometrial glands and stroma outside the uterine cavity. There is poor correlation between endometriosis and pain symptoms. Abnormal vaginal bleeding may occur, as may bowel or bladder symptoms depending on the sites of endometrial deposits.

Pelvic inflammatory disease

Acute pelvic infection may cause secondary dysmenorrhoea. Chronic pelvic infection describes either recurrent episodes of upper genital tract infection or problems caused by damage from previous pelvic infection.

There is overlap between secondary dysmenorrhoea, chronic pelvic pain (CPP), and dyspareunia, as all three have similar underlying causes. In the community study by Zondervan et al., 46 per cent of sexually active women aged 18–49 with dysmenorrhoea had either CPP and/or dyspareunia.

CPP is defined as continuous or intermittent pain in the lower abdomen or pelvis, of at least 6 months duration, not exclusively associated with menstruation or intercourse. Although traditionally investigated by gynaecologists, it can arise from any structure related to the pelvis, including the abdominal and pelvic walls. Pain may be related to bowel, bladder, nerve, or musculoskeletal problems. There is, for example, an excess of hysterectomy in women with irritable bowel syndrome. A history of sexual abuse at any age is more common in women with CPP than other pain syndromes. Investigation is often difficult. Forty per cent of diagnostic laparoscopies find no obvious cause for pain.

Making a diagnosis

History

A diagnosis of primary dysmenorrhoea should be presumed in a nulliparous woman with a history of cyclical spasmodic lower abdominal pain and no other symptoms. In primary dysmenorrhoea the pain usually occurs over the first 1–2 days of the period. Secondary dysmenorrhoea is more likely to appear later than the menarche, or may differ from previous experiences of dysmenorrhoea. Pain may start before and continue throughout a period. Failure of response to conventional treatment or other symptoms should alert the clinician to the possibility of underlying disease.

Available evidence however would suggest that symptoms are poor predictors of underlying disease. Severe dysmenorrhoea is more likely in patients with endometriosis, but the ranges of severity in those with and without disease overlap considerably. The presence of a vaginal discharge, the past use of a coil, previous pelvic surgery, or a history of infertility all increase the possibility of intrauterine pathology.

Examination

The diagnosis of primary dysmenorrhoea is made on the history, and examination may not be required. Pelvic examination will rule out large fibroids, and in endometriosis or pelvic inflammatory disease (PID) the uterus may be immobile and there may be areas of tenderness.

Investigation

Swabs will indicate the presence of infection at the cervix, but caution is needed as infection in the lower genital tract is not necessarily proof of infection in the upper genital tract. Antibiotics can have an anti-inflammatory effect, and thus result in an improvement in symptoms even if the cause is not pelvic inflammatory disease. A pragmatic trial of antibiotic treatment is not diagnostic and further investigation should be considered if the patient returns again.

An ultrasound scan may be required for evidence of intrauterine abnormalities. The diagnosis of endometriosis, PID, and adhesions all require laparoscopy.

Principles of management

Primary dysmenorrhoea is amenable to treatment, and a high rate of success should be expected.

- Non-steroidal anti-inflammatory drugs (NSAIDs) inhibit prostaglandin synthesis. They are the drug of first choice in the treatment of dysmenorrhoea. Naproxen, ibuprofen, and mefenamic acid are all more effective than placebo, as is aspirin. The drugs should be taken at the onset of pain or period, whichever is first. The dose of ibuprofen used in trials was 400 mg four times a day.

- The oral contraceptive pill (OCP) reduces uterine contractility, produces endometrial atrophy and reduces endometrial prostaglandin concentrations.

- Failure of dysmenorrhoea to respond to NSAIDs or OCP may indicate underlying disease and further investigation should be considered.

- A variety of other treatments are available. Progestogens, for example, dydrogesterone 10 mg twice daily, or norethisterone 5 mg three times daily, from day 5 to 25, and the levonorgesterol intrauterine system (IUS) are effective at reducing dysmenorrhoea.

- More novel treatments aimed at leukotriene pathways or vasopression antagonists are not yet available. Treatments such as danazol, gonadotrophin-releasing hormone agonists, oxytocin antagonists, transcutaneous electrical nerve stimulation (TENS) and division of the uterosacral ligaments have also been suggested, but evidence to support their widespread use is lacking.

Treatment of secondary dysmenorrhoea is treatment of the cause, or the induction of amenorrhoea. Treatment is less successful than in primary dysmenorrhoea.

The management of CPP is increasingly seen to require multidisciplinary involvement. A biopsychosocial model and approach is advocated. This moves the process away from finding 'the cause' of the pain, and examines behaviour and cognitions associated with the pain. Early intervention with adequate treatment of pain is recommended to ensure that physical changes are minimized and chronic behaviour patterns do not become established.

Implications

The extent of the socio-economic implications of dysmenorrhoea are not well researched. Studies have used different definitions of dysmenorrhoea, used different ways of grading severity and the age-group of those studied has also varied. Fourteen per cent of girls in an American study of 2699 school girls missed school frequently because of dysmenorrhoea, and 10 per cent of women aged 18–49 in a UK study, reported taking time off work in the past year.

Future directions

Alternative therapeutic options, such as agents acting on leukotriene or vasopressin pathways, may provide treatment for the minority of sufferers of primary dysmenorrhoea who do not respond to NSAIDs or the OCP.

One challenge facing primary care is to identify as early as possible those whose symptoms are in keeping with chronic pelvic pain. Earlier identification may result in more appropriate treatment for the patient, and a subsequent reduction in morbidity. To achieve this, research on the predictive power of symptom complexes, and on different models of management will be required.

Key points

1. Dysmenorrhoea is extremely common.

2. Eighty to 90 per cent of women with primary dysmenorrhoea will respond to NSAIDs or the OCP.

3. Investigation should be considered if there is lack of reponse to NSAIDs or OCP.

4. There is overlap between dysmenorrhoea, chronic pelvic pain, and dyspareunia.

Further reading

Sundell, G., Milsom, I., and Andersch, B. (1990). Factors influencing the prevalence and severity of dysmenorrhoea in young women. *British Journal of Obstetrics and Gynaecology* **97**, 588–94. (This is the only follow-up study in dysmenorrhoea.)

Harlow, S.D. and Park, M. (1996). A longitudinal study of risk factors for the occurrence, duration and severity of menstrual cramps in a cohort of college women. *British Journal of Obstetrics and Gynaecology* **103**, 1134–42.

Zhang, W.Y. and Li Wan Po, A. (1998). Efficacy of minor analgesics in primary dysmenorrhoea: a systematic review. *British Journal of Obstetrics and Gynaecology* **105**, 780–9.

Mahmood, T.A. et al. (1991). Menstrual symptoms in women with pelvic endometriosis. *British Journal of Obstetrics and Gynaecology* **98**, 558–63.

Zondervan, K.T. et al. (2001). The community prevalence of chronic pelvic pain in women and associated illness behaviour. *British Journal of General Practice* **51**, 541–7.

Kennedy, T.M. and Jones, R.H. (2000). The epidemiology of hysterectomy and irritable bowel syndrome in a UK population. *International Journal of Clinical Practice* **54**, 647–50.

Moore, J. and Kennedy, S. (2000). Causes of chronic pelvic pain. *Best Practice & Research in Clinical Obstetrics and Gynaecology* **14** (3), 389–402. (An overview of causes of chronic pelvic pain.)

Grace, V.M. (2000). Pitfalls of the medical paradigm in chronic pelvic pain. *Best Practice & Research in Clinical Obstetrics and Gynaecology* **14** (3), 525–39. (Grace discusses the medical model of chronic pelvic pain, in particular the dichotomy between organic and psychogenic pain. This paper and ref. 7 above, are in an edition of *Best Practice & Research in Clinical Obstetrics and Gynaecology* dedicated to chronic pelvic pain.)

7.9 Dyspareunia

Danielle Mazza

Introduction

Despite being a source of great anxiety, it is not often that a woman presents to a general practitioner complaining of dyspareunia. Instead, the astute GP may pick up clues or use opportunities such as a routine Pap smear to inquire about sexual function and only then be told about the woman's concerns. Despite this, with a careful history and examination and over several consultations, the primary care practitioner can be of great assistance to women suffering from this difficult problem.

Definition

Dyspareunia is genital pain experienced just before, during, or after sexual intercourse.[1] It is usually classified as either being 'superficial' (occurring at the vulva when penile entry into the vagina is initiated or 'deep' (felt deep within the pelvis with penile thrusting).

The *Diagnostic and Statistical Manual of Mental Disorders*, 4th edn. (DSM-IV),[2] classifies dyspareunia as a sexual pain disorder, a sub-category of sexual dysfunction. The criteria used to define the condition under the DSM-IV are:

◆ Recurrent or persistent genital pain associated with sexual intercourse in either a male or a female.

◆ The disturbance causes marked distress or interpersonal difficulty.

◆ The disturbance is not caused exclusively by vaginismus (pain resulting from attempted insertion of the penis into the vagina due to intense involuntary contraction of the perineal muscles surrounding the outer one-third of the vagina) or lack of lubrication.

◆ The disturbance is not better accounted for by another Axis I disorder (except another sexual dysfunction) and is not due exclusively to the direct physiological effects of a substance (e.g. a drug of abuse, a medication) or a general medical condition.

Rather than considering dyspareunia a 'psychiatric' condition, increasing prominence is being given to the consideration of this condition as a 'pain syndrome' whereby an initial instigating factor is then perpetuated by confounding factors.[3]

Epidemiology

The prevalence of dyspareunia is difficult to determine given the private nature of sexual concerns. Figures vary depending on the population sampled and the specific questions asked. In the United States, a study of a national probability sample[4] found that women with dyspareunia (7 per cent) comprised a smaller group than women with decreased interest in sex, orgasmic difficulties, lack of pleasure, or arousal difficulties. Another community-based survey of women aged 35–59[5] found one-third of women had operationally defined sexual dysfunction: impaired sexual interest was identified in 17 per cent of women, vaginal dryness in 17 per cent, infrequency of orgasm in 16 per cent, and dyspareunia in 8 per cent.

In contrast to this, surveys of women in primary care settings have found much higher rates. A study of women seeking routine gynaecological care[6] in both obstetrics and gynaecology (O&G) practices as well as family practices found that a total of 98.8 per cent of the women surveyed reported one or more sexual concerns. The most frequently reported concerns were lack of interest (87.2 per cent), difficulty with orgasm (83.3 per cent), inadequate lubrication (74.7 per cent), dyspareunia (71.7 per cent), body image concerns (68.5 per cent), unmet sexual needs (67.2 per cent), and needing information about sexual issues (63.4 per cent). Another study of consecutive women attending O&G and family practices[7] found the prevalence of dyspareunia to be 46 per cent among sexually active women.

A survey looking specifically at dyspareunia[8] found that 22 (21 per cent) of 105 women who had dyspareunia reported its occurrence as 'rare', 58 (55 per cent) as 'occasional', and 25 (24 per cent) as 'frequent' or 'constant'. Although the actual frequency of intercourse was the same among all these groups, 49 (47 per cent) of the women reported that they had less frequent intercourse because of dyspareunia, and 35 (33 per cent) reported that their dyspareunia had an adverse effect on their relationship with a sexual partner.

In trying to determine whether this condition is 'psychosomatic' or 'pathological' many studies have looked at the biopsychosocial profiles of women complaining of dyspareunia. In one case control study,[9] women with dyspareunia were found to have more physical pathology on examination, and they reported more psychologic symptomatology, more negative attitudes toward sexuality, higher levels of impairment in sexual function, and lower levels of marital adjustment. Interestingly, they did not report more current or past physical or sexual abuse. Patients with dyspareunia are more likely than the general population to report pain with insertion of a tampon or digit, or during a gynaecologic examination.[9] The literature is contradictory when it comes to socio-demographic characteristics, one study[4] concluding that increasing age and college education were associated with a lower likelihood of dyspareunia, and another study[7] finding that the incidence of dyspareunia was not associated with age, parity, marital status, race, income, or educational level.

Aetiology

The aetiology of dyspareunia is varied and controversial with the debate focusing on whether the condition is psychological or organic. Causation is probably best considered according to the onset (primary versus secondary), frequency (complete versus situational), and location of the pain (superficial versus deep).

When dyspareunia has been present the whole of the woman's sexual life, it is of primary onset and is probably related to psychosocial issues. The woman may have been brought up with negative attitudes towards sex and learnt to associate sex with guilt and shame. She may have suffered from sexual abuse or be in an unwanted relationship or have had a painful first sexual experience. When the dyspareunia commences after a period of normal sexual functioning, a physical cause is more likely although psychosocial issues may come into play and exacerbate the problem.

If dyspareunia is continual despite different positions, different situations, and/or different sexual partners the aetiology could be either psychosocial or of medical origin. Equally, some women identify the fact that having sex in a certain position will bring about dyspareunia possibly due to some kind of pelvic pathology.

The location of the pain is very important when considering causation. When the pain is described as sharp, burning, or pinching occurring at the vaginal introitus at the time of penile insertion, it is likely that the pain is a learned response perhaps to a negative experience. Deep pain experienced in the lower abdomen with deep thrusting of the penis is likely to be secondary to a pelvic problem such as endometriosis or a pelvic mass. Sex occurring with the man on top or a rear entry position usually exacerbates deep pain.

GPs are most likely to encounter the commonly occurring organic conditions listed in Table 1.

How to make a diagnosis

History

Like all sexual problems, dyspareunia is difficult to diagnose accurately because doctors are hampered by both their own and the patient's reticence

Table 1 Common organic causes of dyspareunia seen in general practice

A. Lubrication inadequacy	◆ Atrophic vaginitis
	◆ Progestogen only contraceptives
	◆ Insufficient arousal
B. Scarring	◆ Episiotomy
	◆ Pelvic surgery
C. Pelvic disorders	◆ Endometriosis
	◆ Prolapse
	◆ Inflammatory bowel disease
	◆ Pelvic mass
D. Vulvovaginal conditions	◆ Vaginitis
	◆ Chemical irritation/dermatitis
	◆ Vestibulitis
E. Urologic disorders	◆ Acute or chronic cystitis/urethritis

to discuss such private matters. When discussing any sexual matters during a consultation, it is important to remain open, non-judgemental, to use simple language and to assume nothing.

Research shows the importance of doctor-initiated questioning when dealing with sexual health concerns. In a study of 887 patients only 29 (3 per cent) spontaneously cited a sexual problem. An additional 142 (16 per cent) raised sexual concerns only on direct inquiry.[10] Because patients rarely raise the fact that they are experiencing dyspareunia during a consultation (let alone present with it as their reason for attending), general practitioners should utilize their opportunities to take a full sexual history and so to uncover dyspareunia. Examples of such opportunities include when seeing a patient for the first time, when conducting a routine Pap smear or breast check, when dealing with contraceptive issues, relationship issues, menopause or other gynaecological reasons for presentation, depression, or anxiety.

In these situations, a screening history is appropriate. This consists of a minimum of four questions:[11]

1. Are you sexually active? (If no then when were you last sexually active?)

2. Do or have you had any discomfort or other problems during intercourse? (If yes do these bother you?)

3. Have you had more than one sexual partner? (If yes, how many and how long ago?)

4. Have you had any pain on passing water or unusual discharge from your genitals? (If yes, please describe it.)

Once a history of dyspareunia is elicited, the following needs to be detailed:

◆ a description of the pain;

◆ duration;

◆ intensity;

◆ location;

◆ exacerbating and ameliorating factors;

◆ partner's response to woman's dyspareunia and the impact of the problem on the individual and the relationship with her partner;

◆ whether the woman has ever had a history of successful sexual experiences;

◆ previous treatments and the degree of response to them.

A full medical, gynaecological, and obstetric history should also be taken and prescription or illicit drug use identified. Drugs that have been associated with dyspareunia are bromocriptine mesylate (Parlodel), which may cause painful clitoral tumescence, and desipramine hydrochloride (Norpramin), which may cause painful orgasm.[12]

Appropriate gynaecological questions to ask include the following:[13]

- Are there vaginal symptoms such as discharge, burning or itching suggestive of vaginitis?

- Is there a history of STDs, especially HSV or HPV?

- Is there an obstetric delivery history of lacerations, episiotomies, or other trauma?

- Is there an abdominal or genitourinary surgical or radiation history?

- Has the patient had prior gynaecologic diagnoses, including endometriosis, fibroids, or chronic pelvic pain?

- What is the patient's current contraception method and is there any history of intrauterine device use?

If the history points to primary dyspareunia or vaginismus then the woman's background should be explored with questions asked about the influence of her religion, culture, and family in forming her attitudes towards sex. Exposure to either child or adult sexual abuse should also be explored.

Examination

It is important that before conducting the physical examination, the GP explains to the woman exactly what will take place. Permission needs to be obtained to proceed and women should be given the option of delaying the examination until the next consultation should they so wish. A hand mirror can be offered to the woman so that she can watch the proceedings and understand the evaluation that is taking place.

The examination commences with inspection of the vulva and vaginal introitus. The GP should note areas of erythema, atrophy, leukoplakia, or discharge. Any traumatic, surgical, or episiotomy scars should be noted. Vulvar vestibulitis involves a constellation of findings consisting of vulvar erythema and severe pain or burning with touching of the vestibule or attempted vaginal entry.[14] The cause of vulvar vestibulitis is unknown. Focal tenderness elicited by gently touching the vestibule with a cotton-tipped applicator is indicative of this syndrome.

Insertion of a small speculum, lubricated generously with water, can then be attempted. If pain is elicited it is important to ask the woman if it is the same type of pain as she experiences with intercourse. If speculum examination is tolerated then inspection of the vagina and cervix can occur. The inspection should note any lesions, signs of infection or atrophy, presence of congenital anomalies, and evidence of trauma. If appropriate, swabs for microscopy and culture and chlamydia PCR testing and a Pap smear can be taken.

Once the speculum is removed, vaginal examination using one digit can proceed. This examination allows the GP to assess the presence of vaginismus and to do a pelvic assessment. This includes noting the presence of any adnexal masses, the size and position of the uterus, and the presence of any localized tenderness that may be associated with endometriosis or pelvic inflammatory disease.

At the conclusion of the examination, the GP should reassure the woman that all looks normal if this is in fact the case.

Investigations

Investigations are of limited value in making a diagnosis in cases of dyspareunia. If vulvar disease is suspected after examination then the patient can be referred for a colposcopy and may have a biopsy.

Interestingly though, a study of 141 consecutive adult patients with chronic vulvar symptoms referred to a dermatologist[15] showed that the commonest cause of chronic vulvar symptoms in this group of patients was dermatitis, seen in 54 per cent of patients. The other commonly seen conditions were lichen sclerosus (13 per cent), chronic vulvovaginal candidiasis (10 per cent), dysaesthetic vulvodynia (9 per cent), and psoriasis (5 per cent). In this study group, a majority (overall 72 per cent) of patients with a chronic vulvar complaint had a corticosteroid responsive dermatosis rather than a gynaecological condition. While this is not the same sample as one might suspect in general practice the prevalence of dermatitis is worth noting.

A pelvic ultrasound may be of assistance if an ovarian mass or endometriosis is suspected. The severity of cases of 'deep' dyspareunia will determine if a laparoscopy is necessary.

Principles of management

While treatment of dyspareunia should be directed at the underlying cause, all women should be offered simple reassurance and some will benefit from sexual education. For many women, the opportunity to talk openly and explicitly about their sexual life with someone who is objective and non-judgemental is very welcome. The GP can ask the woman to identify any ameliorating action she has taken or what sexual actions or positions have improved her symptoms and thus build her self-confidence and self-esteem by making her feel more 'in control'.

Discussion about and suggestions for modification of sexual technique may help reduce pain with intercourse. Increasing the amount of foreplay and delaying penetration until maximal arousal has occurred will allow increased vaginal lubrication and thus decrease pain with penile entry. The importance of explaining the normal pattern of female sexual arousal cannot be over-emphasized. Often, women may be concerned that their vagina is too small to allow entry of a penis. It can be helpful to therefore explain that in response to sexual arousal, the vagina increases in length about 35–40 per cent and expands in width at the upper end by about 6 cm.

Stressing the importance of feeling at ease in sexual situations in order to become aroused and experience pleasure may sound simple but should not be forgotten. Nor should the fact that the partner, their actions, emotions, and responses to the situation need to be explored. The woman should therefore be consulted as to whether she would like to include the partner in any further consultations so that they too can gain insight into the problem which they share.

Lubricant can be recommended as a temporary measure in cases of dyspareunia, however, many women feel that 'fussing around' with lubricant prior to intercourse takes away from the spontaneity of the sexual activity and increases their anxiety.

Vaginismus

Vaginismus, or the involuntary spasm of the introital (bulbocavernosus) muscles, has been classified by the DSM-IV as a separate entity from dyspareunia.[2] Others, however, have found that neither interview nor physical examination is useful in distinguishing the two and suggest a multi-axial description of these syndromes rather than viewing them as two separate disorders.[16]

Women with vaginismus have developed a phobia about penetration and as well as unsuccessful intercourse will also have experienced failed gynaecological examinations, an inability to use tampons and default from cervical screening.

The most effective treatment approach for vaginismus is a combination of behaviour modification and emotional counselling.[17] The aim of the treatment is to achieve a situation where the woman feels that she owns her own vagina and can share it for sexual activity should she wish.[18] Butcher suggests these steps in the treatment of vaginismus:[18]

1. sexual education;

2. control of vaginal muscles;

3. self-exploration of sexual anatomy;

4. insertion of a trainer under controlled relaxation;

5. sharing of control with partner;

6. insertion of penis, with the woman in control;

7. transfer control of insertion of penis to partner;

8. exploration of phobia.

The first step is to educate the woman regarding her reproductive anatomy and function and explain to her the pattern of female sexual responsiveness. The partner should be involved and agree to withhold from intercourse until such time as the woman is prepared to allow it to occur. The partner should be warned that this might take up to 6 months.

The behaviour modification component of the treatment involves learning how to control the vaginal musculature through relaxation and performing Kegel exercises. This can be taught by explaining to the woman that the muscles are the same ones that she uses to cut off urine flow when she is urinating. She can practice contracting and relaxing these muscles at home and should be encouraged to explore her own sexual anatomy at home using a mirror. When she feels comfortable, she can start practising insertion of a small dilator or something like a small syringe into the introitus. Initially, lubricant should be used and the woman encouraged to insert the dilator after she has contracted and relaxed the vaginal muscles three times. This should be practised three or four times a week. Gradually the size of the dilator is increased and then the partner allowed to insert it during sex play. Only after the woman feels comfortable inserting a penile-sized dilator into the vagina can intercourse be attempted. At all times the woman needs to feel in control and the partner must not thrust until the woman signals she feels ready.

Vulvodynia

The International Society for the Study of Vulvar Disease defines vulvodynia as chronic vulvar discomfort, burning, stinging, irritation, or rawness.[19] There are several sub-classifications of vulvodynia that include cyclic vulvovaginitis, vulvar vestibulitis syndrome, dysaesthetic or essential vulvodynia, papulosquamous vulvar dermatoses, vesiculobullous vulvar dermatoses, neoplastic vulvar lesions, and vestibular papillomatosis.[20] The diagnosis and management of vulvodynia is complex and patients with these conditions are probably best referred to specialist gynodermatology clinics.

Inadequate lubrication

Unfortunately, a vicious cycle between dyspareunia and lubrication develops in women. The more pain they experience, the less aroused and the less well lubricated they are during sex. If intercourse continues then the lack of lubrication worsens the pain. Although the lack of arousal and difficulty in lubrication initially stemmed from irritation or unsatisfactory sexual techniques, they then become a repetitive and expected component of coitus.[22]

Where there is inadequate arousal, patients and their partners need to be counselled in foreplay techniques. Another major reason for women to suffer from decreased lubrication is atrophic vaginitis caused by lack of oestrogenization. This occurs in several settings: during lactation, in some women using progestogen only contraception such as Depo Provera and in women who are peri- or post-menopausal.

In each of these situations, symptoms respond well to topical vaginal oestrogen. The cream is applied with an applicator initially daily for 2 weeks. After this it need only be used twice weekly.

Postpartum dyspareunia

Many women complain of dyspareunia in the puerperium. In one study,[23] 45 per cent of the patients had entry pain, a small percentage had pain at the site of vulvar repair, and the remaining 39 per cent had non-focal pain. There was only a slight difference in pain between women having a first delivery versus those having their second. In this study, over one-quarter of the women who underwent caesarean section had pain, while 41 per cent of lactating women had dyspareunia. The median time to resolution of the non-focal dyspareunia was 5.5 months, and tenderness persisted up to 1 year. Mediolateral episiotomy has been noted to cause more morbidity than the midline type.[24]

After pelvic surgery for cancer or benign conditions

Hysterectomy remains a common gynaecological procedure. To date, the concern has been that pelvic surgery, specifically hysterectomy, might be associated with sexual dysfunction and especially with dyspareunia because of the theoretical risk of vaginal shortening and decreased vaginal lubrication. However, a recent prospective trial[25] found that sexual functioning actually improved after hysterectomy, with the rate of dyspareunia decreasing from 18.6 per cent before hysterectomy to 3.6 per cent 24 months after surgery.

Pelvic surgery for cancer is, however, associated with other problems that may cause dyspareunia. Any cancer can contribute to sexual dysfunction because of the significant and varied psychological stresses placed on the individual. With pelvic surgery, the physical effects can be more problematic. Radical surgery for vulval, uterine, or cervical cancer will involve significant loss of structures and radiation and chemotherapy can cause ovarian failure and, in the case of radiation, deformation and scarring of the vagina.

Implications of the problem

If not addressed, dyspareunia can have a significant and continuing effect on a woman and her partner. In the long term, severe dyspareunia and vaginismus can also bring about problems conceiving. It is, however, a problem that is amenable to primary care practitioners who have good communication skills and an empathic manner. As with all matters concerning sexual functioning, GPs should feel comfortable dealing with this issue if they want to address it in their practice. If they do not, referral is preferable.

If, however, GPs do feel capable of dealing with this sensitive area they will be rewarded by patients who are grateful for having their problem addressed.

Key points

- Dyspareunia is genital pain experienced just before, during, or after sexual intercourse.
- It is usually classified as either being 'superficial' (occurring at the vulva when penile entry into the vagina is initiated or 'deep' (felt deep within the pelvis with penile thrusting).
- An accurate history provides the most clues to the causation of the dyspareunia.
- While treatment of dyspareunia should be directed at the underlying causes, all women should be offered simple reassurance and some will benefit from sexual education.
- It is important to address the relationship issues that will have arisen as a result of the dyspareunia in any treatment plan.

References

1. **American College of Obstetricians and Gynecologists.** *Sexual Dysfunction.* Technical bulletin no. 211. Washington DC: ACOG, 1995.
2. **American Psychiatric Association.** *Diagnostic and Statistical Manual of Mental Disorders* 4th edn. Washington DC: APA, 1994, pp. 511–18.
3. **Meana, M., Binik, Y.M., Khalife, S., and Cohen, D.** (1997). Dyspareunia: sexual dysfunction or pain syndrome? *Journal of Nervous Mental Disorders* **185**, 561–9.
4. **Laumann, E., Paik, A., and Rosen, R.C.** (1999). Sexual dysfunction in the United States: prevalence and predictors. *Journal of the American Medical*

Association **281**, 537–44 (Published erratum appears in *Journal of the American Medical Association* 1999, **281**, 1174).

5. Osborn, M., Hawton, K., and Gath, D. (1988). Sexual dysfunction among middle aged women in the community. *British Medical Journal (Clinical Reserve Edition)* **296**, 959–62.

6. Nusbaum, M.R., Gamble, G., Skinne, B., and Heiman, J. (2000). The high prevalence of sexual concerns among women seeking routine gynecological care. *Journal of Family Practice* **49**, 229–32.

7. Jamieson, D.J. and Steege, J.F. (1996). The prevalence of dysmenorrhea, dyspareunia, pelvic pain, and irritable bowel syndrome in primary care practices. *Obstetrics & Gynecology* **87**, 55–8.

8. Glatt, A.E., Zinner, S.H., and McCormack, W.M. (1990). The prevalence of dyspareunia. *Obstetrics & Gynecology* **75**, 433–6.

9. Meana, M., Binik, Y.M., Khalife, S., and Cohen, D. (1997). Biopsychosocial profile of women with dyspareunia. *Obstetrics & Gynecology* **90**, 583–9.

10. Bachmann, G.A., Leiblum S.R., and Grill, J. (1989). Brief sexual inquiry in gynecologic practice. *Obstetrics & Gynecology* **73**, 425–7.

11. Ross, M.W. and Channon-Little, L.D. *Discussing Sexuality: A Guide for Health Practitioners*. Sydney: MacLennan & Petty PTY Limited, 1991.

12. (1992). Drugs that cause sexual dysfunction: an update. *The Medical Letter on Drugs and Therapeutics* **34**, 73–8.

13. Phillips, N. (1998). The clinical evaluation of dyspareunia. *International Journal of Impotence Research* **10** (Suppl. 2), S117–20.

14. Marinoff, S.C. and Turner, M.L. (1991). Vulvar vestibulitis syndrome: an overview. *American Journal of Obstetrics & Gynecology* **165**, 1228–33.

15. Fischer, G.O. (1996). The commonest causes of symptomatic vulvar disease: a dermatologist's perspective. *Australasian Journal of Dermatology* **37**, 12–18.

16. de Kruiff, M.E., les Kuile, M.M., Weijenborg, P.T., and van Laakveld, J.J. (2000). Vaginismus and dyspareunia: is there a difference in clinical presentation? *Journal of Psychosomatic Obstetrics & Gynaecology* **21**, 149–55.

17. Canavan, T.P. and Heckman, C.D. (2000). Dyspareunia in women. Breaking the silence is the first step toward treatment. *Postgraduate Medicine* **108**, 149–52, 157–60, 164–6.

18. Butcher, J. (1999). Female sexual problems II: sexual pain and sexual fears. *British Medical Journal* **318**, 110–12.

19. International Society for the Study of Vulvar Disease Taskforce (1984). Burning vulvar syndrome: report of the ISSVD taskforce. *Journal of Reproductive Medicine* **29**, 457.

20. Metts, J.F. (1999). Vulvodynia and vulvar vestibulitis: challenges in diagnosis and management. *American Family Physician* **59**, 1547–56, 1561–2.

21. McKay, M. (1993). Dysesthetic ('essential') vulvodynia. Treatment with amitriptyline. *Journal of Reproductive Medicine* **38**, 9–13.

22. Halvorsen, J.G. and Metz, M.E. (1992). Sexual dysfunction, part I: classification, etiology, and pathogenesis. *Journal of the American Board of Family Practice* **5**, 51–61.

23. Goetsch, M.F. (1999). Postpartum dyspareunia. An unexplored problem. *Journal of Reproductive Medicine* **44**, 963–8.

24. Reamy, K.J. and White, S.E. (1987). Sexuality in the puerperium: a review. *Archives of Sexual Behaviour* **16**, 165–86.

25. Rhodes, J.C. et al. (1999). Hysterectomy and sexual functioning. *Journal of the American Medical Association* **282**, 1934–41.

Further reading

Heim, L.J. (2001). Evaluation and differential diagnosis of dyspareunia. *American Family Physician* **63** (8), 1535–44.

Canavan, T.P. and Heckman, C.D. (2000). Dyspareunia in women. Breaking the silence is the first step toward treatment. *Postgraduate Medicine* **108** (2), 149–52, 157–60, 164–6.

7.10 Abnormal cervical smear

G. Kheng Chew, Margaret E. Cruickshank, and A. Patricia Smith

Introduction

Cervical cancer is one of the leading causes of morbidity and mortality in women worldwide. Although it is now the fourth most common cancer in women in the Western world,[1] it is severely under-reported in the developing countries. There has been a decline in the incidence of cervical cancer over the last 30 years, mainly in squamous cell carcinoma. Cervical cytology screening programmes, both organized and sporadic, are thought to account for this.

The aim of cervical cytology screening is to detect abnormal squamous cells exfoliated from the cervix. Cervical cancer is thought to be a slow developing cancer because of the long natural history between pre-invasive and invasive disease. Interval sampling of the exfoliated cells detects precancer cells in the cervix so women may be directed for further investigations. Since the 1940s, the standard method of identifying abnormal cells sampled from the cervix is by the Papanicolaou (Pap) smear.

Cervical screening in the United Kingdom started in the 1960s when several local screening programmes were introduced. Ad hoc screening programmes continued to be developed over the years. In 1988, the National Health Service Cervical Screening Programme (NHSCSP) was established to coordinate a national screening programme that adopts common standards and working practices throughout the United Kingdom. A call–recall programme was set up in each health authority to identify and invite women to attend for cervical screening. Follow-up appointments were generated for further cytological examinations depending on the cytology result.

There has been a similar decrease in the incidence of squamous cell carcinoma in Scandinavia where organized cervical screening has been undertaken for some time. More recently, the success of these programmes has led to organized screening in Limerick (Ireland), Australia, New Zealand, Canada, and Italy. Since 1994, the European network for Cervical Cancer screening has been operational and the aim is to improve the quality of the national programmes for organized cervical cancer screening in the European Union. In the United States, screening still remains opportunistic. The implementation of organized screening requires a high level of infrastructure, which is often difficult to establish and maintain in a developing country. Other methods of primary screening are being researched for these countries.

Pathogenesis

The cervix is covered by both squamous and columnar epithelium. The squamous epithelium covers the ectocervix (Fig. 1) and is continuous with the vaginal squamous epithelium. The squamous epithelium is stratified, non-keratinizing, and is separated from the stroma by the basal lamina. In normal squamous epithelium, the cells differentiate as they mature; this leads to a pattern of stratification whereby the epithelium is divided into layers of progressively more mature cells. The parabasal cells are immature, with a high nuclear–cytoplasmic ratio and occasional mitotic activity. With maturation and differentiation, the intermediate cells have more abundant cytoplasm surrounding prominent nuclei. The mature squamous epithelium is flat and enucleate.

Squamous epithelium is affected by hormonal factors:

♦ Maturation of the squamous cells is influenced by oestrogen. Absence of oestrogen or counteraction by excessive progesterone leads to poor cellular maturation and differentiation. Parabasal cells are found more superficially than usual.

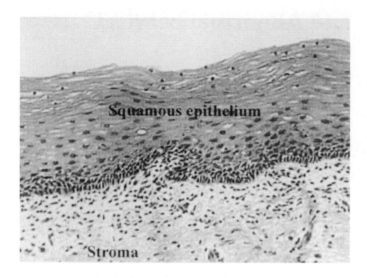

Fig. 1 Histology of normal ectocervical squamous epithelium. The squamous columnar junction is not visualized here.

◆ The menstrual cycle affects the pattern of the cells sampled. There is a higher proportion of superficial cells in the immediately post-menstrual period and an increase in intermediate cells and debris in the post-ovulation period.

Columnar epithelium of the cervix merges with squamous epithelium at one extreme and the endometrium at the other. The columnar epithelium extends into glandular crypts, which are as deep as 1 cm. Cells sampled from the columnar epithelium are endocervical cells. They tend to be present in sheets or clusters and appear not unlike the parabasal squamous cells.

The anatomical position of the squamocolumnar junction (Fig. 2) is influenced by hormonal changes. The squamocolumnar junction is originally in the endocervical canal and, as a result of hormonal changes during puberty, eversion of the cervix occurs and a new squamocolumnar junction is formed on the ectocervix. The area in between the old and new squamocolumnar junction is the transformation zone. This area often undergoes squamous metaplasia, whereby an area originally covered by columnar epithelium becomes covered by squamous epithelium, which offers a protective effect.

The presence of hostile agents such as infection or carcinogens inhibit squamous metaplasia and maturation of the squamous epithelium is arrested at varying stages (Fig. 3). If a cervical smear is taken at this time, it may well show dyskaryotic cells.

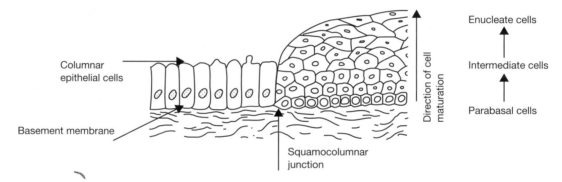

Fig. 2 The squamocolumnar junction.

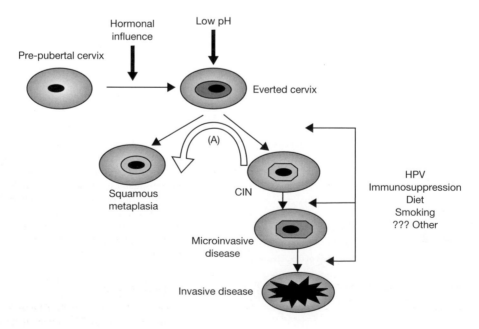

Fig. 3 Theory of pathogenesis of squamous cell carcinoma of cervix (A) CIN, particularly low-grade CIN, can spontaneously regress and revert to normal epithelium.

Natural history

In the United Kingdom, mild dyskaryosis and borderline abnormalities (low-grade abnormalities) make up the bulk of abnormal smears. Human papillomavirus (HPV) infection is associated with cervical intraepithelial neoplasia (CIN). The interval between HPV infection and change in the cervical epithelium is uncertain (Fig. 4). In most instances, the HPV infection is transient as the women's immune system effectively clears the virus. Other factors causing a low-grade cytological abnormality include inflammation and infection, such as chlamydia and bacterial vaginosis. Treating these conditions will often correct the cytological abnormalities. The smear should be repeated in 6 months to ascertain if the abnormality is still present or has regressed.

In a small proportion of women, the viral infection is chronic. The change in the epithelium can progress to a higher grade of CIN if left untreated and in some cases to malignancy. It is possible, however, that high-grade CIN develops de novo without preceding low-grade disease.

Epidemiology

In 1999–2000, about 3.9 million women in England and Wales were invited for cervical screening.[2] Approximately 3.8 million women had smears taken, 2.4 million as part of the national screening programme and 1.4 million as the result of opportunistic screening. Up to 10 per cent of tests were inadequate as they did not contain material suitable for analysis. Of the remainder, 91.8 per cent were negative, 6.5 per cent showed borderline changes or mild dyskaryosis, 0.9 per cent showed moderate dyskaryosis, and 0.7 per cent showed severe dyskaryosis or worse.

In Australia (not including Queensland or Northern Territory), 0.7 per cent of women screened (target age group of 20–69 years) in 1998 demonstrated a high-grade abnormality.[3] The incidence of high-grade abnormalities in the 20–29-year age group was 13.9 per 1000 women compared to less than two per 1000 women in the 50–69-year age group. In Canada, an estimated 8 per cent of cervical smears taken will be reported as abnormal.[4] These figures are comparable to those in the United Kingdom.

Many epidemiological studies have been carried out to study risk factors for the development of cervical cancer. The common factors are listed below.

Coitus

Squamous cell carcinoma (SCC) is not seen in women who have never had coitus. The number of sexual partners, age at first intercourse, and age of partners are also linked to SCC. These findings support the hypothesis that there is a sexually transmissible aetiological agent.

Sexually transmitted disease

Women with a high frequency of sexually transmitted disease are more susceptible to SCC. Although these infections may be a consequence of coitus, certain high-risk HPV types (HPV 16 and 18) are recognized by the World Health Organization (WHO) and International Agency for Research on Cancer (IARC) as oncogenic viruses. HPV DNA has been found in 99.7 per cent cases of SCC.[5]

Immunological factors

Women with chronic immunosuppressive disease or on immunosuppression medication are more susceptible to SCC. HPV infection is common but the infection is usually transient and any changes in the epithelium return to normal. In women who are immunosuppressed, clearance of the virus is less effective, leading to persistence of cervical disease and possible progression to malignancy.

Socio-economic factors

Women from lower socio-economic groups are more susceptible to SCC; the reasons for this are obscure.

Smoking

Cigarette smoking is associated with a higher incidence of SCC. When confounding factors such as intercourse at early age and multiple partners are removed, the association is still strong.[6]

Cervical smear results: classification

The classification of abnormal smears varies between countries and laboratories. The British Society of Cervical Cytology (BSCC)[7] uses a classification system that is based on the degree of cellular abnormality. This system is rarely used outside of the United Kingdom. The National Cancer Institute Bethesda Workshop 2001 recommends a classification based on the grade of the underlying abnormality. In this chapter, we will discuss the BSCC classification and a table is provided (Table 1) to compare the NCI Bethesda Workshop 2001 classification.[8]

Inadequate smear

A smear is reported as inadequate if it does not contain cells suitable for analysis. If, however, cells are present that are dyskaryotic or worse, it should be reported as such. Cervical smears can be reported as inadequate for the following reasons:

- If there are insufficient cells for analysis; taking into account the woman's age and hormonal status.
- If the cells are separated and superficial, suggesting that they are vaginal rather than cervical in origin.
- If the cells are obscured by inflammatory exudate, blood or other debris preventing a satisfactory reading of the smear.
- If the specimen had been air dried or poorly fixed to such a degree that assessment is not possible.
- If there are no squamous epithelial cells present on the slide, unless an endocervical cell assessment is specifically requested.

A repeat smear is recommended as soon as possible. If the cause of inflammatory exudate is due to an underlying infection, treatment of the infection is recommended before repeating the smear.

The BSCC does not regard the presence of endocervical or squamous metaplastic cells as a determinant of sampling of the entire transformation zone. It is the responsibility of the smear taker to visualize the cervical os and to adequately sample the entire transformation zone.

Negative smear

A negative smear (Fig. 5) report indicates the absence of dyskaryotic cells. A negative smear should have sufficient squamous epithelial cells taking into account the woman's age and hormonal status. The cells usually cover

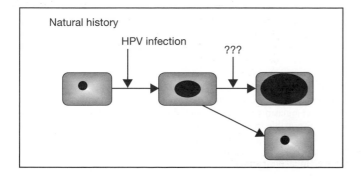

Fig. 4 Natural history of cervical cell dyskaryosis.

Table 1 Classification of cervical smear results

Bethesda classification	British classification
Negative	*Negative*
Associated infection	Associated infection
Non-neoplastic findings	Non-neoplastic findings
◆ Inflammation, radiation, IUCD	◆ Inflammation, radiation, IUCD
◆ Glandular cells post-hysterectomy	◆ Glandular cells post-hysterectomy
Epithelial cell abnormalities	
Squamous cell	
Atypical squamous cells	
◆ of undetermined significance (ASC-US)	Borderline nuclear abnormality
◆ cannot exclude HSIL (ASC-H)	
Low-grade squamous intraepithelial lesion (LSIL) (encompassing HPV/ mild dysplasia/CIN1)	Mild dyskaryosis
High-grade squamous intraepithelial lesion (HSIL) (encompassing moderate and severe dysplasia CIN2 and CIN3)	Moderate dyskaryosis Severe dyskaryosis
◆ with features suspicious for invasion	Severe/?malignant
Squamous cell carcinoma	Malignant
Glandular cell	
Atypical	
◆ Endocervical cells	Borderline nuclear abnormality
◆ Endometrial cells	
◆ Glandular cells	Glandular abnormality
Atypical	
◆ Endocervical cell, favour neoplastic	Glandular abnormality
◆ Glandular cells, favour neoplastic	Glandular abnormality
Endocervical adenocarcinoma-in-situ	Glandular abnormality/malignant
Adenocarcinoma	
◆ Endocervical	Malignant—glandular changes
◆ Endometrial	Malignant—endometrial cells
◆ Extrauterine	Malignant—extrauterine
◆ Not otherwise specified	

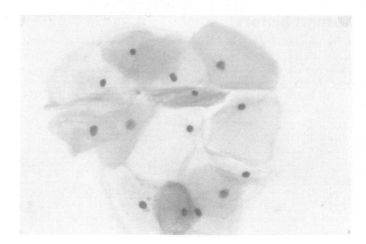

Fig. 5 Cytology showing normal squamous epithelial cells.

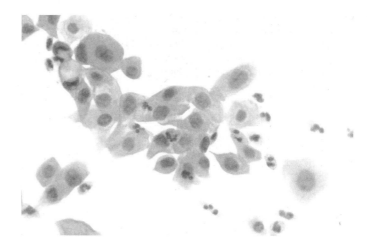

Fig. 6 Squamous epithelial cells with mild and moderate dyskaryosis.

at least one-third of the glass slide. The exception is found in smears from women with an atrophic cervix.

The presence of an infection, severe inflammation, or thick exudate does not exclude a reading of a negative smear provided the epithelial cells can be accurately assessed and dyskaryotic cells are not present. It is not uncommon to have a negative smear and infection (*Candida* spp., bacterial vaginosis or *Trichomonas* vaginalis) on the report. Women with a negative smear will be recalled for their next smear at the routine recommended interval of 3 years.

Dyskaryosis

This refers to the nuclear changes in the cells sampled from areas of CIN. The ratio of nuclear size to cytoplasm is a reflection of the degree of cytoplasmic maturation in the epithelial cells; the higher the ratio, the more severe the degree of dyskaryosis. The degree of dyskaryosis is not an absolute reflection of the degree of CIN due to possible sampling error where the most severe areas may be missed in the process. The smear must be reported according to the highest degree of dyskaryosis noted.

Mild dyskaryosis

This shows relatively normal cytoplasmic maturation to superficial cells. This abnormality is sometimes seen with squamous metaplasia and

atrophic epithelium but may be associated with CIN. This category is synonymous with the low-grade squamous intraepithelial lesion (LSIL) in the Bethesda classification. It is important to bear in mind that a significant number of women with LSIL on cervical cytology will be found to have a high grade squamous intraepithelial lesion (CIN 2 and 3) at colposcopy.[9] At the very least, the smear should be repeated in 6 months.

Moderate dyskaryosis

Moderately dyskaryotic cells do not undergo cytoplasmic maturation past the intermediate cells level. The nuclei are more prominent than in mild dyskaryosis and there is a higher nuclear–cytoplasmic ratio (Fig. 6). Women with this smear result should be referred for colposcopic assessment.

Severe dyskaryosis

In this category, there is limited cytoplasmic maturation and a high nuclear–cytoplasmic ratio. Occasionally, it can be difficult to differentiate this from possible malignant cells. All women with this smear should be referred for colposcopic assessment urgently.

Severe/?Invasive cancer

Specific features suggestive of invasive carcinoma include extensive keratinization, presence of coarse chromatin clumps and large nucleoli in dyskaryotic cells. When there is concern about coexistent invasive disease, this should be highlighted so that referral for further assessment can be expedited.

Glandular cell abnormalities

The characteristic cytologic features of cervical glandular intraepithelial neoplasia (CGIN) are nuclear crowding, pseudostratification of nuclei, 'feathering', loss of cohesion of cells at the edges of the groups, and rosette formations. The smear usually has abundant endocervical cells, focally distributed against a clean background. These changes are apparent on low-power examination. Not all the features are present all the time. The columnar cells also demonstrate dyskaryotic changes which can be divided into low and high grade. This classification into low and high grade dyskaryosis is not an indicator of the risk of malignant potential.

Invasive endocervical adenocarcinoma shows the abnormalities associated with CGIN together with 'malignant diathesis', macronuclei and 'windowing' of nuclear chromatin.

Smears characteristic of CGIN and invasive endocervical adenocarcinoma are reported as ?glandular neoplasia. If the changes are equivocal, they are reported as borderline. Women with ?glandular neoplasia are referred for colposcopic assessment, although often there are no obvious colposcopic features. An excisional biopsy is recommended for histological diagnosis. Borderline smears with glandular abnormalities must be repeated in 6 months. If the abnormalities persist, they should be referred for colposcopic assessment and excisional biopsy.

Endometrial cells

The presence of endometrial cells in the smear is normal in the first 12 days of the menstrual cycle. Without relevant clinical details of the menstrual cycle, type of contraception, hormone replacement therapy, or gynaecological complaints, a report of endometrial cells in the smear is of little clinical relevance. It is rare for women under 40 years old to have neoplastic endometrial disease. However, in women over 40 years old, the finding of abundant and/or atypical endometrial cells should be included in the report. It is the responsibility of the smear taker to pursue further investigations to exclude endometrial pathology.

Borderline changes

This classification was introduced by the BSCC for smears where there was genuine doubt as to whether the cellular changes represent a neoplastic process. Although this is possible in many situations, the three main areas of concern are:

1. Association with HPV Infection where the distinction between mild dyskaryosis and borderline nuclear change is not easily defined. In the BSCC system, this is important because of the distinction between HPV infection with or without associated CIN. The recognized spontaneous regression of changes associated with HPV infection means that women with these changes can be managed conservatively with a repeated smear in 6 months. In the Bethesda system, both are classified under LGSIL, so defining this category is less important.

2. When it is sometimes difficult to distinguish benign reactive or degenerative changes from higher degrees of dyskaryosis or even invasive cancer. Where the grade of dyskaryosis is recognized, the smear should be reported accordingly. However, where there is genuine doubt, a repeat smear is recommended in 6 months. This correlates well with the atypical squamous cells of unknown significance (ASCUS) and atypical glandular cells of unknown significance.

3. Endocervical cells which show changes but are not typical of glandular neoplastic changes associated with CGIN. As the recommended investigation for ?glandular changes is an excisional biopsy, the borderline changes are followed up with a repeat smear to see if the changes persist or regress. For those that regress, a repeat smear in

12 months is recommended. For those that persist, referral for colposcopic assessment and excisional biopsy is recommended.

Cervical smear sampling

Cervical smear sampling is carried out using a wooden spatula to collect the cells of the transformation zone of the cervix. The entire transformation zone (TZ) is sampled by rotating the spatula through 360° clockwise and anticlockwise (Fig. 7) and the sample gently spread on a clean glass slide and fixed prior to transportation to cytology laboratory. An adequately sampled smear should contain cells from the ectocervix and the endocervix. Conversely, the presence of both cell types does not confirm adequate sampling unless the cervix is properly visualized and the entire TZ sampled.

Smear-taking equipment (Fig. 8)

The Pap smear used today has not changed since its development in the 1940s. It has certain limitations such as loss of cells in the sampling device; mucus, cellular debris and/or blood obscuring the epithelial cells making it difficult to read and clumping of cells making analysis unsatisfactory. This accounts for a significant proportion of inadequate and borderline results. A meta-analysis[10] was conducted to ascertain the most effective sampling device. If a spatula was used, the extended tip spatula (Aylesbury) is superior to the classical Ayre spatula in sampling both ectocervical and, in particular endocervical cells. It is also found to be superior in the detection of dyskaryosis. The combination of the extended tip spatulas and endocervical brush produced the best sampling results.

To overcome the problem of contamination by cellular debris, a liquid-based slide preparation method has been developed. The cells are collected from the transformation zone, using a plastic (Cervex) broom and transferred into a liquid medium. The liquid is filtered to get rid of the

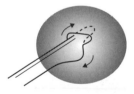

Fig. 7 Taking a cervical smear using an Aylesbury spatula. The spatula should be rotated 360° clockwise and anticlockwise.

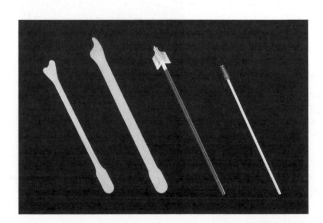

Fig. 8 Different cervical samplers (left to right) Ayres spatula, Aylesbury spatula, Cervex broom and endocervical cytobrush.

non-cellular material and the cells are deposited in a monolayer on a slide. Reports of ASC or borderline abnormality are reduced with this method. The true positive rate is also increased, at 92 per cent.[11,12] The increased detection of SIL is confirmed by histological diagnosis. The kit for liquid-based cytology is more expensive than the conventional Pap smear, but the increase in sensitivity, savings in cost of repeated smears and emotional cost to women should be considered in the cost analysis. Several pilot programmes are currently running to evaluate the replacement of the Pap smear with liquid-based cytology.

Screening programmes

Cervical screening is most effective when screening is centrally organized and high coverage of the target population is more important than the screening interval. Nevertheless, the recall interval for women with a negative result concerns system management as well as the individual woman. False negative results are an inherent problem, but given the long natural history of CIN, regular recall will diminish the risk of interval cancers. Indeed a reduction in sensitivity may be accepted against improved specificity. This reduces the number of 'false positive' results which generate not only unnecessary investigation and intervention but also considerable anxiety. It is paramount that women participating in screening are informed of its limitations in terms of false negatives and false positives and also the probability of being recalled either for a repeat smear or referral to colposcopy. This is the responsibility of the smear taker. The management of cervical cancer is fully discussed in Chapter 7.12.

Management

The cervical smear is usually obtained from asymptomatic women. When the smear is reported as showing HSIL or worse, colposcopic examination is recommended. Follow-up smears are deferred until colposcopic examination done and recommendations are made for cytological follow-up.

Colposcopy examination involves examination of the cervix under magnification. It allows the study of the vasculature of the cervix, where an abnormal vessel pattern can suggest neoplastic disease. The cervix is stained with acetic acid, 3 or 5 per cent solution, to identify areas of acetowhite epithelium (Fig. 9). The degree of acetowhite is often an indicator of the degree of dyskaryosis. Conversely, areas of dyskaryotic epithelium will not

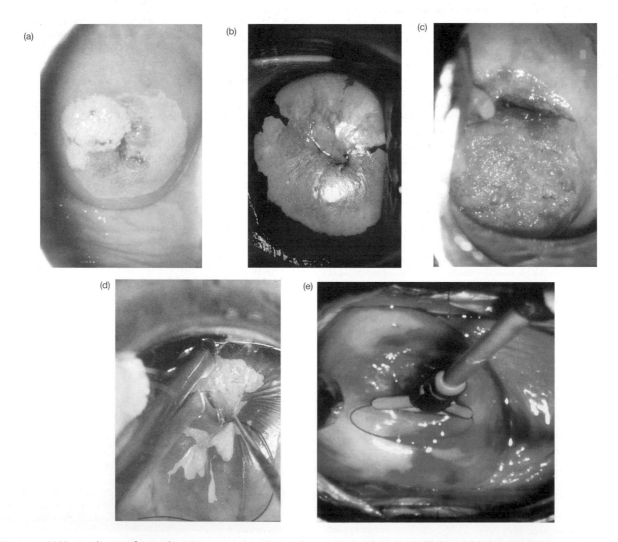

Fig. 9 Clockwise: (a) Varying degrees of acetowhite changes noted on the transformation zone of the cervix. (b) Areas of dyskaryosis that are negative to Lugol's Iodine staining. (c) Cervical cancer involving posterior lip of cervix. (d) A punch biopsy being taken for histological analysis. (e) LLETZ (LEEP) being carried out to remove the abnormal epithelium.

stain black with Lugol's iodine. Colposcopy allows directed biopsy of abnormal epithelium for histological diagnosis.

Smears reported as LSIL or atypical squamous changes of undetermined significance should be repeated in 6 months time. There are conflicting ideas on the management of low-grade cytological abnormalities. While it may appear that a low-grade smear corresponds to low-grade disease, this is not entirely true. It is possible for a high-grade lesion to be missed when the smear is taken, hence the smear under-represents the true diagnosis. The discrepancy between smear cytology and histology is supported in a large series by Flannelly et al.[13] At present, in some health authorities in the United Kingdom, women with a low-grade smear will be recommended colposcopy at the first abnormal reading. However, as most low-grade changes resolve spontaneously, secondary investigations may be too intrusive and cost-ineffective. Testing for high-risk HPV may be the discerning factor for closer follow-up for those who are HPV positive. Two multicentre studies are being carried out in the United Kingdom (TOMBOLA*) and the United States (ALTS†) to evaluate the use of HPV testing in the management of low-grade cytological abnormalities.

Treatment options

The available treatment options have changed over the years. As CIN is increasingly detected in young women, a conservative treatment approach for CIN was preferred in order to preserve reproductive function.

Initially, ablative measures were used widely. These methods include cold coagulation, diathermy, and laser ablation. As this is a destructive therapy, histological diagnosis is essential to confirm the presence of CIN and to exclude invasive disease in order to prevent under treatment. This obviously relied on stringent practice and colposcopic examination by skilled colposcopists. Follow-up and good compliance from the women were imperative in order to detect treatment failures and recurrences. A long-term follow-up study in a stable population in Aberdeen, UK[14] showed this to be an acceptable form of treatment, if diagnostic and follow-up criteria were met.

By 1993, colposcopy centres throughout the United Kingdom were leaning towards excision treatment to allow for histological analysis of the excised transformation zone. Large loop excision of transformation zone (LLETZ) or LEEP (loop electrosurgical excision procedure) as it is known in the United States was the preferred mode of treatment in the majority of centres.[15] This procedure allows excision of the abnormal area using a diathermy loop and can be carried out under local anaesthetic in the outpatient area. Short-term side-effects from this treatment include haemorrhage (both primary and secondary) and infection. Cruickshank et al.[16] showed that there was no association between single LLETZ treatment and cervical incompetence in later pregnancies.

Current practice therefore includes an LLETZ if the abnormal area can be visualized in its entirety. If the abnormality extends into the endocervical canal, a cone biopsy is still the recommended treatment. Cone biopsy is also an acceptable form of conservative treatment for microinvasive disease. Small volume invasive disease or recurrent CIN in women who have completed their family are treated with hysterectomy.

Follow-up

Follow-up following conservative treatment of CIN is important in the detection and early treatment of recurrence and/or treatment failure. Women who have received conservative treatment for CIN are at five times higher risk of developing invasive cancer than the general population. Careful follow-up with cervical cytology is recommended for the first 10 years following treatment.[17] There is no evidence of benefit of follow-up with colposcopy and cytology over cervical cytology alone.

A meta-analysis was carried out by Yabroff et al.[18] to study the factors associated with delayed or incomplete follow-up of abnormal

* TOMBOLA—Trial of Management of Borderline and Low Grade Abnormalities.
† ALTS—ASCUS/LGSIL Triage Study.

screening. These include both older (>65 years) and younger (<20 years) women, financial barriers, lower levels of education, lower levels of social support, and non-white race. Reasons for non-compliance include a fatalistic approach to the screening test results, a reluctance to find out if something is wrong, fear of diagnostic procedure or cancer and feeling that they are too old for treatment anyway.

Physicians and other providers play an important role in patient adherence to follow-up testing after an abnormal smear. Physician–physician communication (between primary care provider and specialist) is the first pathway for communication of an abnormal screening test result. Lack of communication can lead to confusion about the primary responsibility for patient notification. Once the abnormal test result is received, the primary care provider must communicate the results to the patient. Physician–patient communication can play a role in patient delay or lack of follow-up of abnormal screening results. The information must be precise and the importance of follow-up tests must be communicated to the patient, bearing in mind that most women are asymptomatic at the time of screening.

Key points

- ◆ Cervical smear screening is aimed at detecting premalignant disease (CIN) to allow early treatment.

- ◆ Organized screening programmes have successfully reduced the incidence of cervical cancer.

- ◆ Women should be appropriately counselled about the results of the smear and encouraged to attend follow-up investigations.

References

1. Vizcano, A.P., Moreno, V., Xavier-Bosch, F., Munoz, N., Barros-Dios, X.M., Borras, J., and Parkin, D.M. (2000). International trends in incidence of cervical cancer in squamous cell carcinoma. *International Journal of Cancer* **86** (3), 429–35.

2. Cervical Screening Programme, England: 1999–2000. *Bulletin 2000/30.* Published November 2000.

3. Commonwealth of Australia. *Screening for the Prevention of Cervical Cancer*, 1998.

4. Stuart, G.C.E. and Parboosingh, J. (1991). Implementation of comprehensive screening for cervical cancer in Canada: impediments and facilitators. *Journal of Canadian Medical Association* **145** (10).

5. Walboomers, J.M., Jacobs, M.V., Manos, M.M., Bosch, F.X., Kummer, J.A., Shah, K.V., Snijders, P.J., Peto, J., Meijer, C.J., and Munoz, N. (1999). Human papillomavirus is a necessary cause of invasive cervical cancer. *Journal of Pathology* **189** (1), 1–3.

6. La Vecchia, C., Franceschi, S., Decarli, A., Fasoli, M., Gentile, A., and Tognoni, G. (1986). Cigarette smoking and the risk of cervical neoplasia. *American Journal of Epidemiology* **123** (1), 22–9.

7. Johnson, J. and Patnick, P., ed. *Achieveable Standards, Benchmarks for Reporting, and Criteria for Evaluating Cervical Cytopathology.* NHSCSP publication No. 1, 2000.

8. The NCI Bethesda 2001 Workshop.

9. Jones, B.A. and Novis, D.A. (2000). Follow-up of abnormal gynecologic cytology: a college of American pathologists Q-probes study of 16 132 cases from 306 laboratories. *Archives of Pathology & Laboratory Medicine* **124**, 665–71.

10. Martin-Hirsch, P., Lilford, R., Jarvis, G., and Kitchener, H.C. (1999). Efficacy of cervical-smear collection devices: a systematic review and meta-analysis. *Lancet* **354** (9192), 1763–70. [Erratum appears in *Lancet* 2000 **355** (9201), 414.]

11. Brown, A.D. and Garber, A.M. (1999). Cost-effectiveness of 3 methods to enhance the sensitivity of Papanicolaou testing. *Journal of the American Medical Association* **281** (4), 347–53.

12. Bishop, J.W. et al. (1998). Multicenter masked evaluation of Auto-Cyte PREP thin layers with matched conventional smears. Including initial biopsy results. *Acta Cytologica* **42** (1), 189–97.

13. Flannelly, G., Anderson, D., Kitchener, H.C., Mann, E.M., Campbell, M., Fisher, P., Walker, F., and Templeton, A.A. (1994). Management of women with mild and moderate cervical dyskaryosis. *British Medical Journal* **308** (6941), 1399–403.

14. Chew, G.K., Jandial, L., Paraskevaidis, E., and Kitchener, H.C. (1999). Pattern of CIN recurrence following laser ablation therapy: long term follow up. *International Journal of Gynaecological Cancer* **9**, 487–90.

15. Kitchener, H.C., Cruickshank, M.E., and Farmery, E. (1995). The 1993 British Society for Colposcopy and Cervical Pathology/National Coordinating Network United Kingdom Colposcopy Survey. Comparison with 1988 and the response to introduction of guidelines. *British Journal of Obstetrics & Gynaecology* **102** (7), 549–52.

16. Cruickshank, M.E., Flannelly, G., Campbell, D.M., and Kitchener, H.C. (1995). Fertility and pregnancy outcome following large loop excision of the cervical transformation zone. *British Journal of Obstetrics & Gynaecology* **102** (6), 467–70.

17. Soutter, W.P., de Barros Lopes, A., Fletcher, A., Monaghan, J.M., Duncan, I.D., Paraskevaidis, E., and Kitchener, H.C. (1997). Invasive cervical cancer after conservative therapy for cervical intraepithelial neoplasia. *Lancet* **349** (9057), 978–80.

18. Yabroff, K.R., Kerner, J.F., and Mandelblatt, J.S. (2000). Effectiveness of interventions to improve follow-up after abnormal cervical cancer screening. *Preventive Medicine* **31** (4), 429–39.

Table 1 Mammographic abnormalities

Soft tissue
Mass
Parenchymal distortion
Oedema
Microcalcification

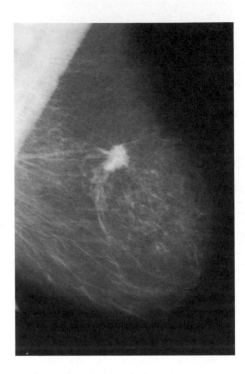

Fig. 1 Spiculate mass due to an invasive cancer.

7.11 Abnormal mammogram

Ian S. Fentiman and Michael J. Michell

Introduction

There are three main indications for mammography:

1. as part of the assessment of symptomatic women;

2. screening of women aged more than 50 or high-risk cases aged less than 50; and

3. follow-up of breast cancer patients.

Indiscriminate use of mammography may, at best, lead to uninformative images, with unnecessary radiation exposure and may also be responsible for false negative findings and delays in diagnosis.

Abnormal mammographic findings

Mammographic abnormalities appear as either soft tissue lesions or microcalcification as outlined in Table 1.

Soft tissue mass

Soft tissue mammographic masses may have a spiculate, irregular, or smooth outline. A spiculate mass, the commonest mammographic appearance of a carcinoma, comprises a central soft tissue tumour with spicules extending into the surrounding tissue (Fig. 1). Ninety-five per cent of spiculate masses are due to invasive carcinoma. Less common causes are shown in Table 2.

Table 2 Causes of a mammographic soft tissue mass

	Spiculate mass	Irregular mass	Well-defined mass
Common causes	Invasive cancer	Invasive cancer Fibroadenoma Papilloma	Cyst Fibroadenoma
Less common causes	Non-invasive cancer	Non-invasive cancer	Invasive cancer (mucinous, medullary types)
	Radial scar (complex sclerosing lesion)	Abscess	Phyllodes tumour Intracystic cancer Abscess Metastasis
	Surgical scar		Lymphoma

An irregular soft tissue mass appears as a soft tissue opacity with an irregular or lobulated outline, sometimes with a poorly defined margin between the mass and the surrounding tissue. Irregular masses may be due to carcinoma, fibroadenoma, or papilloma. Well-defined masses have smooth curved margins and are usually cysts and fibroadenomas, (Fig. 2)

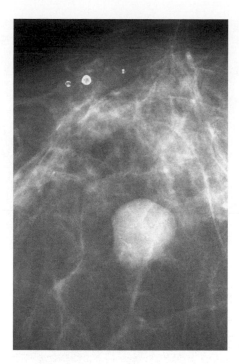

Fig. 2 Well-defined mass due to a fibroadenoma.

Table 3 Causes of microcalcification

Ductal carcinoma in situ
Invasive carcinoma
Fibrocystic change
Fibroadenoma
Papilloma
Epithelial hyperplasia

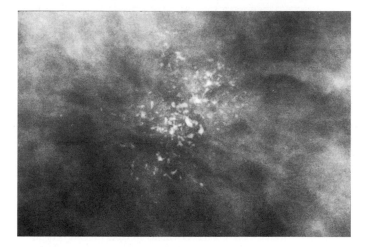

Fig. 3 Microcalcification due to ductal carcinoma in situ.

but may also be caused by cancers, particularly medullary, mucinous, intracystic and, high-grade invasive sub-types.

Parenchymal distortion

Distortion of the breast parenchyma is recognized by straightened lines radiating towards a central area devoid of a recognizable mass. The commonest cause is a surgical scar, usually confidently diagnosed with knowledge of the site of previous surgery. In the absence of previous surgery, approximately 50 per cent of such lesions are due to malignancy, usually well-differentiated or tubular carcinomas. The commonest benign cause is a radial scar (known as a complex sclerosing lesion). Some show complex histological features with both benign and malignant lesions present.

Oedema

The oedematous breast is enlarged with skin thickening and diffuse increase in parenchymal density. Unilateral breast oedema may be due to locally advanced carcinoma, lymphatic or venous obstruction, cardiac or renal failure. In malignant cases there may be diffuse, irregular microcalcification.

Microcalcification

Microcalcification is the sole mammographic abnormality in up to 25 per cent of screen-detected carcinomas. Commonly caused by benign breast disease, it has resulted in many excision biopsies of benign lesions (Table 3). Microcalcification in malignant disease occurs within necrotic debris in the lumen or within the tumour matrix of the neoplastic duct wall. Benign microcalcification may occur within the lobular spaces in microcystic change, within fibroadenomas or papillomas and also occurs within ducts showing simple epithelial hyperplasia. Malignant microcalcification may show typical features including linear and branching shapes allowing a near definitive diagnosis to be made (Fig. 3). Often, however, the appearances of benign and malignant cases are very similar and cannot be confidently diagnosed without needle biopsy.

Triple assessment

For a patient with a breast lump or very localized nodularity, a definite diagnosis is sought by triple assessment (clinical evaluation, radiological investigation, and needle biopsy).

- *Clinical evaluation*
  - History
  - Examination
- *Imaging*
  - Ultrasound
  - Mammography
- *Needle biopsy*
  - Fine needle aspiration cytology
  - Core needle biopsy

Clinical evaluation

The major points requiring attention in history-taking are summarized in Table 4. A suddenly painful lump in a pre-menopausal woman or in a woman taking HRT is likely to be a cyst. A painless lump in an older woman is likely to be a carcinoma and in a younger woman a fibroadenoma. The examination should pay particular attention to measurement of the size of any palpable abnormalities. Once the clinical evaluation has been completed and a working diagnosis made the patient undergoes appropriate imaging tests, informed by a description and diagram of the clinical findings.

Radiological investigation

The aim of further radiological assessment of breast abnormalities is to characterize the type and extent of an abnormality as accurately as possible.

Table 4 Major points in history-taking from symptomatic breast patients

Symptoms	Lump/pain/discharge/nipple inversion/lumpiness
Duration	
Prior breast history	Biopsies/breast cancer/abscess
Past medical history	Major operations/serious illness
Drugs	OC/HRT/other endocrine therapy
Reproductive history	Menarche/cycle/LMP/menopause/births/lactation
Family history	First/second degree/age at diagnosis/ovarian cancer

This information is then considered, together with the clinical findings and, where appropriate, needle biopsy to determine further management.

Special mammographic techniques: localized compression and magnification views

Localized compression views involve compressing one area of the breast to displace and spread the glandular tissue. This is particularly useful in the evaluation of soft tissue mass lesions because the margins become more easily visible. Possible areas of parenchymal distortion are also investigated using this technique to distinguish summation shadows due to overlying normal breast stroma from true distortion. Magnification mammography produces images with both magnification and increased resolution allowing detailed analysis of microcalcification. This determines whether they are benign and need no further investigation, or are suspicious for malignancy and require needle biopsy for further investigation.

Ultrasound

Modern real-time high-frequency ultrasound (10–15 MHz) provides high-quality images of the breast tissue and lesions as small as 2–3 mm can be demonstrated. It is used for initial imaging in women aged less than 35 years with a lump and for the further investigation of a mammographic mass. Simple cysts can be accurately diagnosed and are aspirated only if they are symptomatic (Fig. 4). Solid benign lesions such as fibroadenomas usually have well-defined margins and are round or oval in shape. Malignant masses characteristically have less well-defined or irregular margins (Fig. 5). Although the ultrasound features may strongly suggest whether a mass is benign or malignant, there is considerable overlap in the findings and needle biopsy is required to establish a definite diagnosis.

Image-guided needle biopsy

Needle biopsy of highly suspicious mammographic abnormalities is performed to confirm the diagnosis of malignancy so that treatment can be planned. For equivocal abnormalities where the differential diagnosis includes both benign and malignant causes, needle biopsy is performed to establish the diagnosis. Advantages of obtaining a non-operative diagnosis for mammographic abnormalities include:

- pre-operative surgical planning for women with cancer;
- fewer benign surgical excision biopsies;
- fewer operations for women with cancer;
- more effective pre-operative counselling for women with cancer.

Most soft tissue lesions detected by mammography are visible on ultrasound which is used to guide the biopsy needle so that the lesion is accurately sampled. Most microcalcification clusters and parenchymal distortions are either poorly seen or invisible on ultrasound so X-ray stereotaxis is used for needle guidance (Table 5).

Biopsy procedures are carried out under local anaesthetic and may either involve removal of material for cytological examination (FNAC—fine

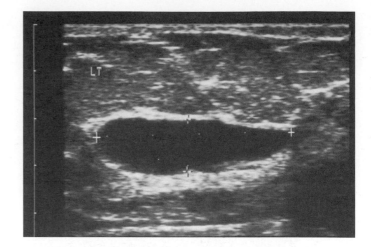

Fig. 4 Ultrasound of a simple breast cyst.

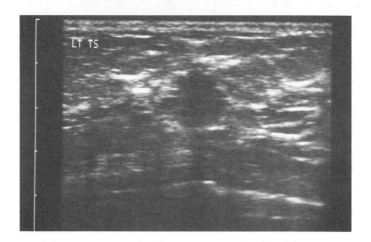

Fig. 5 Ultrasound showing an irregular hypoechoic mass due to an invasive cancer.

Table 5 Image-guided breast biopsy

Image guidance
Ultrasound—soft tissue mass
X-ray stereotaxis
Microcalcification
Parenchymal distortion
Sampling
Fine needle aspiration cytology (FNAC)
Core biopsy (CB)
Vacuum-assisted core biopsy (VACB)

needle aspiration cytology) or removal of a tissue sample for histological examination (CB—core biopsy). Vacuum-assisted core biopsy (VACB) allows more tissue to be removed for histological examination and increases the accuracy of biopsy for some types of lesion, particularly microcalcification. Use of modern image-guided breast biopsy techniques allows a definitive pre-operative diagnosis of malignancy to be made in more than 90 per cent

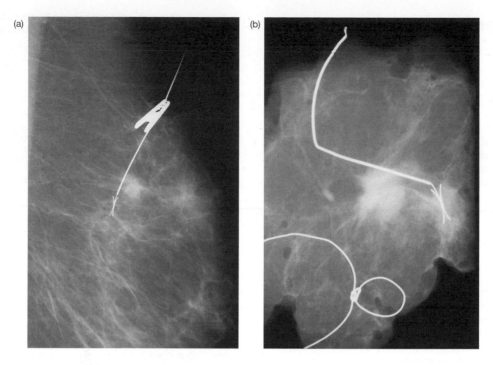

Fig. 6 Needle localization and surgical excision of a non-palpable cancer. (a) The wire has been inserted to mark the position of the cancer. (b) The specimen radiograph confirms that the cancer has been removed.

of breast cancer patients. When needle biopsy has not provided a specific diagnosis consistent with the mammographic findings, diagnostic surgical excision is required.

Needle localization breast surgery

Non-palpable lesions requiring surgical excision for either therapeutic or diagnostic purposes are marked prior to surgery to ensure that the appropriate tissue is identified and excised. This is carried out under either ultrasound guidance for soft tissue lesions or X-ray for microcalcification as for image-guided needle biopsy. A needle containing a fine wire is positioned under local anaesthetic and image guidance with its tip either through or adjacent to the lesion. The needle is then removed leaving the marker wire within the breast. After surgical excision the tissue specimen containing the wire is X-rayed to ensure the abnormality has been removed (Fig. 6). After detailed histological examination further management may be planned.

Magnetic resonance imaging (MRI) of the breast

MRI images of the breast are obtained using an MR machine with dedicated breast imaging equipment. Images are taken before and after intravenous injection of an MR contrast agent. Tumours show a higher signal than surrounding normal tissue following contrast because of the neovascularization which accompanies tumourigenesis. The technique has high sensitivity for the detection of breast cancer but has low specificity because benign lesions like fibroadenomas are also demonstrated, with imaging features not allowing them to be confidently differentiated from cancer. The current indications and possible future applications of breast MRI are shown in Table 6.

Table 6 Indications and possible applications for breast MRI

Differentiation of surgical scar from carcinoma on post-treatment mammograms
Investigation of breast implant abnormalities
Staging of breast cancer—detection of mammographically occult tumours
Monitoring local response of breast cancer to chemotherapy
Screening in young women with a high risk of developing breast cancer

Further reading

Tabar, L. and Dean, P.B. *Teaching Atlas of Mammography* 2nd edn. Stuttgart: Thieme, 1985.

Michell, M.J. (1998). The breast. In *Textbook of Radiology and Imaging* (ed. D. Sutton), pp. 1429–60. Edinburgh: Churchill Livingstone.

Madjar, H. *The Practice of Breast Ultrasound*. Stuttgart: Thieme, 2000.

Heywang-Kobrunner, S. *Contrast-Enhanced MRI of the Breast*. Basel: Karger, 1990.

Michell, M.J. (2000). FNAC and core biopsy of impalpable breast lesions. In *Breast Cancer: Diagnosis and Management* (ed. J.M. Dixon), pp. 31–41. Amsterdam: Elsevier Science.

7.12 Screening for cancer in women

Marie-Dominique Beaulieu and Isabel Rodrigues

Gynaecological cancers, along with lung and colorectal cancers, are among the most frequent to affect women in their lifetime. The goal of this chapter is to present the most recent information on prevention and screening for breast, ovarian, cervical, and endometrial cancers.

Breast cancer

Epidemiology

The lifetime incidence of breast cancer for a woman who reaches her 90s is one in eight in North America and Europe, although these rates vary by race and ethnicity. For example, the incidence of breast cancer in Caucasian Americans is 115.2 per 100 000 and drops to 78.1 per 100 000 in Asian and Pacific Islanders.[1] Incidence has increased in the last 10 years, largely due to increased detection of ductal carcinoma in situ, which represents 88 per cent of new cases.[1] The 5-year survival rate for all stages is 85 per cent, ranging from 97 per cent for localized cancers, to 77 per cent for regional cancers, and 21 per cent for tumours found with distant metastasis.[1]

Risk factors

Assessing an individual's risk

The most important risk factor for breast cancer is still age, most cancers occurring after age 50. Seventy per cent of women with breast cancer have no other identifiable risk factors. Only 5–10 per cent of breast cancer cases demonstrate a pattern of autosomal dominant inheritance. Nevertheless, assessing the risk of breast cancer may be important to guide counselling on decisions related to hormone replacement therapy, mammography screening before age 50, chemoprevention, and genetic screening.[2]

Some factors have been consistently associated with breast cancer and are currently used to assess breast cancer risk. They are:

- a family history of breast cancer in a first-degree relative [relative risk (RR), 1.4–13.6], depending on the number of relatives and age at diagnosis
- a family history with second-degree relatives (RR, 1.5–1.8)
- age at menarche: under 12 years old (RR, 1.2–1.5)
- age at menopause: over 55 years old (RR, 1.5–2.0)
- age at first live birth: over 30 years old (RR, 1.3–2.2)
- benign breast disease (any finding, RR, 1.5–1.8; atypical hyperplasia, RR, 4.0–4.4)
- hormone replacement therapy (RR, 1.0–1.5).[2]

Other risk factors have been less consistently associated with breast cancer (diet, alcohol consumption, sedentary lifestyle, lactation, and oral contraceptives) or are very rare in the general population (exposure to radiation therapy). They are not used in any of the current prediction models.[2]

Four models are currently used to assess breast cancer risk.[2] The most common is that developed by Gail et al. from the Breast Cancer Detection Demonstration Project.[3] Because of the interactions between the risk factors, individual risk is better calculated with a software which is available on the web site of the National Cancer Institute.[4] This tool enables professionals to obtain a woman's individual 5-year and lifetime risk of developing breast cancer.[2]

No risk assessment procedure has been formally evaluated for use in routine screening or case-finding. Most experts consider that there is no evidence to support its routine use by physicians. However, it may guide women and physicians concerned about increased risks to decide whether or not there is a need to pursue further discussion or to obtain referrals for expert advice.[5]

Genetic-susceptibility testing

Family physicians are in a key position to assess the risk of inherited breast cancer in an asymptomatic woman. They are often asked for advice by their patients. Hence, they must be able to identify when referral for genetic testing is indicated. Two major genes, *BRCA1* and *BRCA2*, have been linked to breast cancer susceptibility. Women with mutations on either of these genes have a lifetime risk of breast cancer of 60–85 per cent.[2] The familial characteristics which increase the likelihood of carrying a *BRCA1* or *BRCA2* mutations are:

- known *BRCA1* or *BRCA2* mutations;
- two or more family members under 50 with breast cancer;
- male breast cancer;
- breast and ovarian cancer; and
- Ashkenazi Jewish ancestry.

The presence of one of these characteristics may warrant a referral to a genetic cancer screening centre.[2]

For women from families without these risk factors, genetic testing is unlikely to provide any useful information. In high-risk families, however, genetic testing may be useful for two reasons. First, women who test negative can be reassured that their risk is comparable to that of women of their own age with comparable risk factors without genetic mutations. They can be counselled on this basis about prevention and screening. Second, in families at increased risk, testing may identify a substantial number of carriers, thus clarifying the status of this family as regard to mutations. Since the benefit to women who test positive remains controversial (see below), genetic testing should not be offered without appropriate counselling.[2] Practice guidelines have been produced in the United Kingdom to help family physicians make appropriate referrals to genetic screening facilities.[6]

Primary prevention

Some 5 years ago, there was not much to tell women about primary prevention of breast cancer, other than give sound healthy lifestyle advice based on relative risk data rather than on strong evidence of any efficacy. The question of counselling women about hormone replacement therapy in relation to the risk of breast cancer will not be addressed in this chapter (see Chapter 7.5). The relative risks associated with hormone replacement therapy are not higher in women with a family history of breast cancer. The issue is more about the addition of risks.

Some primary prevention interventions are now available to some women at high risk of breast cancer: chemoprevention and prophylactic mastectomy—two options which are not without adverse consequences.

Chemoprevention of breast cancer

The most recent clinical practice guideline on the question of chemoprevention of breast cancer has been released jointly by the Canadian Task Force on Preventive Health Care (CTFPHC) and the Canadian Breast Cancer Initiative's Steering Committee on Clinical Practice Guidelines for the Care and Treatment of Breast Cancer.[5] Both expert panels conclude that there is fair evidence to recommend against the use of tamoxifen in women at low or normal risk of breast cancer (D recommendation). For women at higher risk (Gail's Index at or above 1.66 per cent at 5 years), evidence support counselling on the potential benefits of prevention with tamoxifen and its harmful effects (B recommendation). As the 5-year risk of breast cancer increases above 5 per cent, the benefits of tamoxifen outweigh the harmful effects. In such situations, the duration of tamoxifen use is 5 years, based on trials of tamoxifen in the treatment of early breast cancer.[5] Tamoxifen is associated with an increased risk of endometrial cancer and thromboembolic events. The effectiveness of raloxifen as chemoprevention therapy is under study. This last molecule does not increase the risk of endometrial cancer.

Prophylactic bilateral mastectomy

To date, there are no practice guidelines on the indications for prophylactic mastectomy, an option which some women with genetic mutations on the *BRCA1* or *BRCA2* genes may consider. Some cohorts of women have been followed in the United States and the Netherlands.[7] Experience bears on surveillance of close to 300 women with proven mutations, about 80 having chosen prophylactic mastectomy. To date, none of these women have been reported with breast cancer; however, the cohort with the longest follow-up (16 years) is small (12 cases of prophylactic mastectomy). The decision to choose this option remains controversial for obvious reasons. Prophylactic oophorectomy is another option.[8] Chemoprevention with tamoxifen or raloxifen remains the hope for the future. Family physicians must remain alert to new knowledge in the field and establish strong links with local experts and centres specialized in cancer genetics counselling.

Screening

Three screening manoeuvres are available: mammography, clinical breast examination by a health professional, and breast self-examination (BSE).

Screening mammography

Screening mammography with or without clinical examination has been shown to be effective in women between the ages of 50 and 69 in seven randomized controlled trials (RCTs) conducted in Europe or North America.[9] Most industrialized countries have screening programmes which actively reach out to women of this age group. A 70 per cent coverage of the population is expected to lead to a 25 per cent reduction in the mortality rate due to breast cancer. Such level of effectiveness has been shown for screening intervals between 1 and 3 years.[9] These programmes also include women considered at an increased risk either because of their family history or because they have had a previous diagnosis of atypical hyperplasia of the breast. For high-risk women, particularly those between 40 and 49 years of age, screening is generally recommended on an annual basis.[9] Exposure to hormone replacement therapy has been consistently associated with a reduction in the sensitivity of screening mammography although the impact of this phenomenon on the effectiveness of screening programmes is not known.[10]

The effectiveness of screening women between the ages of 40 and 49 at an average risk of breast cancer has been a source of debate for the last 15 years. Most programmes do not reach out to women of this age, and some actually discourage them by not reimbursing the intervention. However, in the light of a meta-analysis of long-term follow-up studies including women in this younger age group upon entry, some expert panels have revised their recommendations from a 'D', which excludes screening mammography for women of this age with average risk of breast cancer, to a 'C' recommendation, which means that there is no strong evidence for or against it and that decisions must be taken 'on other grounds'.[11] This meta-analysis suggests that screening mammography in women 40–49 years old at average risk of breast cancer may bring a relative risk reduction of 18 per cent after 13 years of follow-up.[12] Estimates of the number needed-to-screen range from 500 to 1540 in the trials showing a positive benefit, as compared to 526 at age 50 and 169 at age 60. Physicians are advised to counsel women on the potential benefits and potential harms of screening mammography at ages 40–49 (increased biopsy rates; anxiety; false reassurance; and potential diagnostic delay for women with false negative results). The Gail scoring system may assist physicians in evaluating the individual's lifetime risk of breast cancer, although no cut off point at which benefits clearly outweigh drawbacks has been identified.[2]

However, a new meta-analysis produced by the Cochrane Collaboration has stirred up the debate again.[13–15] The authors of this review claim that two of the RCTs were flawed (the New York and the Edimburg trials), three were of poor quality, and two (the Canadian and the Malmo trial) were of medium quality. The overall results (including women aged between 40 and 69 years) of the two better trials does not show any benefit of screening (OR: 1.02; 95 per cent CI 0.95–1.10). Still, data from all eligible trials (excluding the two flawed ones), shows a benefit from screening in women aged between 50 and 69 years upon entry in the trials (OR: 0.75; 95 per cent CI 0.62–0.89). The fact that some editors of the Cochrane Collaboration disagreed with the authors of the review[13,15] is not helped to settle the controversy.

Clinical examination of the breast

In the year 2000, there were few data to support the worldwide recommendation to examine women's breast to screen for breast cancer starting at the age of 40.[9] Clinical examination by a professional was part of screening in only one of the six screening mammography RCTs. Still, it was deemed common sense to recommend it, based on the knowledge that some palpable tumours are missed on mammography.[9] The Canadian National Breast Screening Study-2 showed that after 13 years of follow-up, yearly clinical examination by a professional can yield results comparable to clinical examination and mammography for women between 50 and 59 years of age.[16] The authors urged caution in the interpretation of their trial which should not be regarded as a plea for abandoning screening mammography. Indeed, the observed efficacy was the result of performance of clinical examination by highly trained professionals (nurses for the most) in conditions not found in most actual care settings. However, such data can be of great interest to countries that have not developed or may not afford screening mammography programmes, or to individuals who refuse mammography after appropriate counselling.

Breast self-examination (BSE)

There have been some new data on BSE in the last 5 years, but nothing extraordinary for either women or professionals. BSE has been given grade C recommendations by most expert panels due to the lack of strong evidence in its favour, despite the belief in its effectiveness. Indeed, expressing a negative view or any doubt about the manoeuvre is seen as heretical in many circles. Many cancer organizations and women's groups recommend it strongly, sometimes starting at age 20. In 2001, the Canadian Task Force on Preventive Health Care issued a grade D recommendation—that is, it recommended excluding BSE from the screening interventions against breast cancer.[17] Needless to say, this recommendation provoked a strong negative reaction in Canada and the United States. What is the evidence on BSE?

Two large RCTs, a quasi-randomized trial, one large cohort study, and several case-controlled studies have failed to show benefit from regular performance of BSE on breast cancer mortality as compared to no BSE.[17] The CTFPHC gave weight to the negative results reported in the Shanghai and the Russian RCTs showing an increase in the number of biopsies for benign breast disease at 5 years without benefits in terms of mortality (rate of biopsy of 1.1 versus 0.5 per cent in the Shanghai trial and RR of 1.5 in the Russian trial). The CTFPHC was criticized for having given such weight to these observations, considering that the follow-up of 5 years was not long enough to show any benefits in terms of breast cancer mortality. The CTFPHC recommendation must be viewed on a population basis and not on an individual basis. There is certainly no strong evidence to support investment in population-based interventions to teach BSE as an effective intervention to reduce breast cancer mortality. Large-scale performance of BSE may increase unnecessary biopsy rates, particularly in young women.

Ovarian cancer

Epidemiology

Ovarian cancer ranks second in frequency among gynaecological cancers. It represents about 4 per cent of all cancers in women. Incidence does not vary much with race and ethnicity in industrialized countries. Its incidence is stable: between 9 and 15 per 100 000 population.[1] Ovarian cancer has the highest mortality rate of all gynaecological cancers (5-year survival between 30 and 50 per cent, all stages).

Risk factors

The single risk factor for ovarian cancer is family history. The odds ratio of developing ovarian cancer in relatives of ovarian cancer cases compared to controls is 3.6 for first-degree relatives and 2.9 for second-degree relatives. About 5–10 per cent of all ovarian cancers are hereditary. *BRCA1* and *BRCA2* genes mutations have been associated with this increased risk.[1]

Other factors consistently associated with a decreased risk of developing ovarian cancer are pregnancy and exposure to oral contraceptives. Having carried one pregnancy to term is associated with a 40 per cent decrease in relative risk and five pregnancies with a 67 per cent decrease. Any use of oral contraceptives is associated with a 34 per cent decrease in the relative risk and 6-year use or longer with a 70 per cent decrease.[1]

Prevention and screening

To date, no primary or secondary prevention measure has been shown to be effective in reducing mortality from ovarian cancer.[18] Three large RCTs combining pelvic ultrasound and CA-125 dosage are in progress.

Under the most optimistic assumptions, annual pelvic examinations of 40-year-old women would reduce the 5-year mortality rate from ovarian cancer by 0.0001 per cent.[19] A CA-125 tumour marker has a sensitivity of 29–75 per cent in Stage I tumours and 67–100 per cent in Stage II. Specificity is also limited since up to 1 per cent of healthy women have increased CA-125 levels, as do 6–40 per cent of those with benign ovarian masses. CA-125 is increased in 30 per cent of women with non-gynaecological cancers.[19] Reported sensitivity for ultrasound imaging ranges between 50 and 100 per cent for abdominal and 76–97 per cent for transvaginal techniques.[19]

There is no good evidence to support any specific course of action in women at high risk. The number of cases in relatives and/or the association with breast cancer may warrant referral to a specialized centre where the indications for tumour marker and ultrasound follow-up as well as of genetic testing will be discussed. This is particularly encouraged in regions where women can be enrolled in a trial. Options for mutations carriers are the same as discussed in the breast cancer section.[18]

Endometrial cancer

Epidemiology

Endometrial cancer is the most common cancer of the female reproductive tract. Its incidence is higher in Caucasian (22.6 per 100 000) than in Black women (15.3 per 100 000). Five-year survival rates at all stages is 84 per cent, rising to 92 per cent when detected at Stage I. Close to 90 per cent of endometrial cancers bleed early in the natural history of the disease. Consequently, up to 70 per cent of all cancers are diagnosed while the disease is still confined to the uterus.[1]

Risk factors

Unopposed exogenous oestrogen replacement therapy is the strongest risk factor (RR: 10–30 after 5 years of unopposed use). Endometrial hyperplasia is the second most important risk factor. It is estimated that 23 per cent will progress to endometrial cancer if not treated. Obesity, diabetes, and early menarche are other known risk factors.[1]

Primary prevention and screening

The only preventive measure is the addition of a progestin to oestrogen replacement therapy. To date, only continuous combined and sequential once-a-month exposure to progestins have proven effective in reducing the relative risk of endometrial cancer to 1 as compared to women without oestrogen replacement.[20] Trials are underway to evaluate the effectiveness of less frequent cyclic exposure.

No screening manoeuvre has proven to be of any benefit over prompt evaluation of uterine bleeding in peri- and post-menopausal women.[1]

Cervical cancer

Epidemiology

In developing countries, cervical cancer was the most frequent cancer in women until the early 1990s when breast cancer became the most common. In developed countries, it is still the third most frequent cancer after breast and colorectal cancer. Central and South America, Southern and Eastern Africa, and the Caribbean are the highest risk areas for this type of cancer, with incidence rates of at least 30 new cases per 100 000 women per year. The lowest incidence and mortality rates are reported in Canada.[21]

A significant reduction in the incidence of cervical squamous cell carcinoma was observed during the last few decades. However, in the last years a trend for increased incidence has been observed among white women under 50 years of age in the United States and many European countries. Franco et al.[21] suggest this trend could be explained by an increased detection of cancer with Pap smears, the use of new diagnostic techniques, or a cohort effect. It has also been reported (United States, Sweden, Australia, and Canada) that rates of adenocarcinomas and adenosquamous carcinoma, which usually account for about 10–15 per cent of all cervical cancers, have been steadily increasing in young women.[22] It is still unclear why, but it is of concern since this type of cancer has a poorer prognosis.

Risk factors

Cervical cancer is the long-term consequence of a sexually transmitted disease (STD) caused by human papillomavirus (HPV).[23] This infection is very common among young sexually active people. Furthermore, in the vast majority of women, the infection is transient and resolves spontaneously.[21,24] Harbouring high-risk types such has HPV 16, 18, 31, and 33, for a prolonged time (persistent infection) increases the risk of progression to high-grade pre-invasive dysplastic lesions. An estimated 40 per cent of untreated high-grade lesions will further progress to invasive cancer over an average of 10 years.[23] Other co-existing factors could act as promoters of the transformation into neoplasia. These include smoking, STD other than HPV infection, high parity, long-term use of oral contraceptives (>12 years), and possibly diet (reduced risk with beta carotene and vitamin C).[21] This is why periodic screening is so important in order to discover and treat pre-invasive lesions.

Screening

The Pap smear

The decrease in incidence of cervical cancer has been related to the widespread use of Pap tests which started in the late 1960s.[21,23] It is one of the most effective preventive interventions performed by clinicians. Most women with invasive cervical cancer have not had a Pap test in the 3 years before their diagnosis, even though 75 per cent were seen in a primary care outpatient clinic.[23] Nevertheless, up to 47 per cent of invasive cervical cancers occur among women under 70 years of age with a past history of regular cervical cancer screening tests.[25] This suggests that the actual screening test is still not optimal.

Problems with sensitivity of the test have been reported.[25] Its limitations come mainly from inadequate sampling, slide preparation that do not contain abnormal cells from the cervix, or slide misinterpretation, where few abnormal cells are missed among the vast majority of normal cells. Sensitivity of 40–80 per cent has been reported.[25] (See also Chapter 7.10.)

Newer methods

To address the limitations of cytology smears, several screening methods have been developed and evaluated.

Thin-layer liquid-based cytologic collection

This technique improves the quality of the sample and minimizes the reading error, since most (versus 20 per cent for the conventional Pap) of the material sampled is available for reading. The exfoliated cervical cells are transferred in a cell-preserving solution. The cell processor separates and discards the inflammatory cells and red blood cells. A sample of suspended cells are smeared onto a slide in a thin layer fashion and read by cytotechnologists. The US Food and Drug Administration approved the ThinPrep Pap Test (1996) and the AutoCyte PREP System (1999). However, increased costs and lack of large-scale data using histological verification of samples limit its widespread use.[21,26]

Computer-assisted automated cytology (AutoPap Primary Screening System)

A high-speed video camera scans about 200 Pap smears daily. According to morphometric algorithms, it detects and shows images of the abnormal cells to be screened manually. High-volume laboratories could benefit from this device although additional costs may be incurred and its approval for automated reading is still pending.[21]

HPV testing (Hybrid Capture-II)

This test detects the 13 most oncogenic HPV types in cervical samples by means of signal amplification and immunocapture of DNA and RNA hybrids. The test is also suitable for self-sampling that could improve participation rates in screening programmes.

HPV testing is more sensitive than the regular Pap smear in detecting high-grade lesions. However, there are concerns about its lesser performance among younger women. Potential patient anxiety related to additional investigation and clinical management for HPV as an adjunct to or substitute for the conventional Pap smear has not been properly evaluated in large clinical trials.[21,23]

When to start? When to end?

While data on efficacy and cost analysis are becoming available on newer methods of screening, the Pap smear remains the gold standard test suggested for screening for cervical cancer. The use of a spatula in combination with an endocervical brush appears to increase the rate of detection of disease without increasing the rate of false positive findings.[23] Recommendations are not uniform and vary according to different sources. The youngest age at which screening should begin is 18, although the Finnish Cancer Association suggests screening women only after the age of 30[23] (Table 1).

Screening is generally no longer recommended after the ages of 65–69 although all sources agree to stop screening only in women with a past history of regular screening tests with normal results. Older women with a history of previous hysterectomy for benign conditions also fall in this category[23,27,28] (Table 2).

Frequency of screening

Intervals between tests may be extended to 3 years if two or three consecutive tests are normal. Some suggest that continued annual screening should be considered in women with risk factors such as a first occurrence of sexual intercourse before the age of 18, multiple sexual partners, smoking, or low socio-economic status.[27]

Further reduction in the incidence and mortality from cervical cancer is possible if access to optimal cervical cancer screening is expanded, thus encouraging clinicians to offer screening tests to all women consulting outpatient clinics and prompting women to be screened.

Clinicians need to be continually updated on technological advances in screening techniques such as liquid-based cytologic collection and analysis, HPV testing, and self-sampling so as to more accurately identify women with precursor lesions.

Table 1 Recommendations on when to start screening

When to start screening	Source
18 years regardless of sexual activity	American Cancer Society (http://www.cancer.org) American College of Obstetricians and Gynaecologists (http://www.acog.org)
When women become sexually active	Canadian Task Force on Preventive Health Care (http://www.ctfphc.org) American Academy of Family Physicians (http://www.aafp.org) American College of Preventive Medicine (http://www.acpm.org)
18 years if history unknown or unreliable	American College of Preventive Medicine National Health Service of the United Kingdom (http://www.cancerscreening.nhs.uk/cervical/
21 years old	index.html)
30 years old	The Finnish Cancer Organization[23]

Table 2 Recommendation on when to stop screening

When to end screening	Source
65 years if previous regular screening and normal results; two satisfactory smears and has had normal results in the previous 9 years	American College of Preventive Medicine
69 years if previous regular screening and normal results	Canadian Task Force on Preventive Health Care

References

1. **American Cancer Society** (2000). *Cancer Facts and Figures*. http://www.cancer.org.
2. **Armstrong, K., Eisen, A., and Weber, B.** (2000). Primary care: risk of breast cancer. *New England Journal of Medicine* **342**, 564–71.
3. **Gail, M.H.** et al. (1989). Projecting individualized probabilities of developing breast cancer for white females who are being examined annually. *Journal of the National Cancer Institute* **81**, 1879–86.
4. **Prevention of endometrial cancer.** *CancerNet*, 2001, http://cancernet.nci. nih.gov/cgi-bi.
5. **Levine, M.** et al. (2001). Chemoprevention of breast cancer. A joint guideline from the Canadian Task Force on Preventive Health Care and the Canadian Breast Cancer Initiative's Steering Committee on Clinical Practice Guidelines for the Care and Treatment of Breast Cancer. *Canadian Medical Association Journal* **164** (12), 1681–90.
6. **Eccles, D.M.** et al. (2000). Guidelines for a genetic risk based approach to advising women with a family history of breast cancer. *Journal of Medical Genetics* **37** (3), 203–9.
7. **Eisen, A. and Weber, B.L.** (2001). Prophylactic mastectomy for women with BRCA1 and BRCA2 mutations—facts and controversy. *New England Journal of Medicine* **345** (3), 207–8.
8. **Rebbeck, T.R.** et al. (1999). Breast cancer risk after bilateral prophylactic oophorectomy in BCRA1 mutation carriers. *Journal of the National Cancer Institute* **91** (17), 1475–9.
9. **US Prevention Services Task Force** (1996). Screening for breast cancer. In *Guide to Clinical Preventive Services*. Report of the US Prevention Services Task Force, pp. 73–87. Baltimore MD: Williams & Wilkins.
10. **Banks, E.** (2000). Hormone replacement therapy and the sensitivity and specificity of breast cancer screening: a review. *Journal of Medical Screening* **8** (1), 29–34.
11. **Ringash, J., with the Canadian Task Force on Preventive Health Care.** (2001). Preventive health care, 2001 update: screening mammography among women aged 40–49 years at average risk of breast cancer. *Canadian Medical Association Journal* **164** (4), 469–76.
12. **Hendrick, R.E.** et al. (1997). Benefit of screening mammography in women aged 40–49: a new meta-analysis of randomized controlled trials. *Journal of the National Cancer Institute Monography* **22**, 87–92.

13. Olsen, O. and Gotzsche, P.C. (2001). Screening for breast cancer with mammography. In *The Cochrane Library* Issue 4. Oxford: Update Software.

14. Olsen, O. and Gotzsche, P.C. (2001). Cochrane review on screening for breast cancer with mammography. *Lancet* **358**, 1340–2.

15. Horton, R. (2001). Screening mammography—an overview revisited. *Lancet* **358**, 1284–5.

16. Miller, A.B. et al. (2000). Canadian National Breast Screening Study-2: 12-year results of a randomized trial on women aged 50–59 years. *Journal of the National Cancer Institute* **92** (18), 1490–9.

17. Baxter, N., with the Canadian Task Force on Preventive Health Care. (2001). Preventive health care, 2001 update: should women be routinely taught breast self-examination to screen for breast cancer? *Canadian Medical Association Journal* **164** (13), 1837–46.

18. Bell, R. et al. (1998). Screening for ovarian cancer: a systematic review. *Health Technology Assessment* **2** (2), i–iv, 1–84.

19. US Prevention Services Task Force (1996). Screening for ovarian cancer. In *Guide to Clinical Preventive Services*. Report of the US Prevention Services Task Force, pp. 159–66. Baltimore MD: Williams & Wilkins.

20. Lethaby, A. et al. (2001). Hormone replacement therapy in post menopausal women: endometrial hyperplasia and irregular bleeding. In *The Cochrane Library* Issue 4. Oxford: Update Software.

21. Franco, E.L., Duarte-Franco, E., and Ferenczy, A. (2001). Cervical cancer: epidemiology, prevention and the role of human papillomavirus infection. *Canadian Medical Association Journal* **164** (7), 1017–25.

22. Liu, S., Semenciw, R., and Mao, Y. (2001). Cervical cancer: the increasing incidence of adenocarcinoma and adenosquamous carcinoma in younger women. *Canadian Medical Association Journal* **164** (8), 1151–2.

23. Sawaya, G.F. et al. (2001). Current approaches to cervical-cancer screening. *New England Journal of Medicine* **344** (21), 1603–7.

24. Kuhn, L. et al. (2000). Human papillomavirus DNA testing for cervical cancer screening in low-resource settings. *Journal of the National Cancer Institute* **92**, 818–25.

25. Cuzick, J. et al. (2000). A systematic review of the role of papillomavirus (HPV) testing within a cervical screening programme: summary and conclusions. *British Journal of Cancer* **83** (5), 561–5.

26. Ferenczy, A. et al. (1996). Diagnostic performance of hybrid capture human papillomavirus deoxyribonucleic acid assay combined with liquid-based cytologic study. *American Journal of Obstetrics and Gynecology* **175**, 651–6.

27. National Guideline Clearinghouse. Washington DC, http://www.guideline.gov.

28. National Cancer Institute, http://www.cancernet.nci.nih.gov.

7.13 Violence as a women's health issue

Barbara Lent

Since the mid-1980s, a growing number of physicians and medical organizations have recognized gender-based violence as a tremendous social problem with significant consequences for the physical and mental health of women and children. Experiences of violence and abuse can affect victims' presentations to the health care system, their responses to suggestions for investigation and/or management of their health problems, and their relationships with individual caregivers. As primary care providers and gatekeepers to other health services, family physicians have a unique opportunity to assist those who have experienced abuse in their personal lives, and to collaborate in the prevention of further abuse.

Definition of violence against women

The United Nations has defined violence against women as 'any gender-based violence that results in, or is likely to result in, physical, sexual or psychological harm or suffering to women, including threats of such acts, coercion or arbitrary deprivations of liberty, whether occurring in public or private life'.[1] While this definition is extremely broad, encompassing all aspects of violence experienced by females, whether in the family, in the community, at work or at school, whether perpetrated or condoned by family members, coworkers, strangers, and/or the state, this chapter will focus largely on the health impact of the most endemic form of violence against women: abuse in intimate relationships. The terms 'violence' and 'abuse' will be used interchangeably to mean the use of physical force, sexual coercion and/or verbal threats, used to intimidate or control the behaviour of another person, with whom one has an intimate or other close family relationship.

Prevalence of abuse

Irrespective of nationality, very large numbers of adult women experience abuse by their current or former partners,[2] with numbers varying across studies, from 10 to 60 per cent, depending on the definition of abuse, the way the information was sought, the relationship between the woman and the assessor, and the prevailing societal attitudes to abuse in intimate relationships, and to its disclosure. The lifetime prevalence of sexual coercion is reported as high as 50 per cent,[3] particularly for women living in war-torn countries.[4] Population-based studies and studies from clinical settings caring for children who are pregnant and/or suffering from STDs demonstrate that, for an alarming number of both male and female children under 18, the experience of abuse by family members or intimate partners begins early in life.[5]

Natural history

Abused women themselves describe a pattern of abuse that typically escalates in frequency and severity over time, resulting in substantial injuries, mental and physical health problems, and impaired social and personal functioning, often combined with a pattern of poor self-care. Many women experience repeated violence before they disclose to friends, family members or physicians, or other potential helpers. Particularly alarming are the international data demonstrating the substantial murder and suicide rates for both victims and perpetrators of abuse in intimate relationships.[2]

Health consequences

Women with a history of abuse may present to the health care system with a wide range of acute and chronic physical and psychological health problems,[6–8] and use the health care system proportionately more than non-abused women.[9–11] (Table 1). Certain constellations of symptoms and signs should particularly alert family physicians to ask patients about the possibility that abuse in a current or previous relationship may be contributing to health problems. These include:

♦ multiple bruises, lacerations and abrasions, especially if the explanation of injury does not fit well with physical findings (e.g. bilateral injuries are more likely to have been inflicted by someone than to be the result of falls);

♦ repeated visits to emergency departments;

♦ vague, somatic complaints, that do not fit typical descriptions of organic problems;

♦ chronic pain syndromes (e.g. irritable bowel, chronic pelvic pain, chronic headache);

♦ anxiety, depression, and/or suicidal ideation;

Table 1 Potential clinical indicators of abuse[a]

Physical findings
Dental trauma
Any injury, especially to the head and neck (even with a seemingly good
    explanation), and any fatal injury

General findings
Chronic abdominal, pelvic, or chest pain
Somatic disorders
Irritable bowel syndrome
Chronic gynaecologic symptoms
Sexually transmitted diseases and exposure to human immunodeficiency virus
    through sexual coercion
Exacerbation of symptoms of a chronic disease such as diabetes, asthma, or
    coronary artery disease
Chronic joint or back pain, headaches, numbness, and tingling from injuries
Noncompliance with medical regimen

Psychological symptoms
Depression and suicidal ideation
Anxiety symptoms and panic disorder
Eating disorders
Substance abuse
Post-traumatic stress disorder

Findings during pregnancy and childbirth
Any of the above
Unwanted pregnancy
Complications such as miscarriage, low birth weight of infant, abruptio placentae,
    premature rupture of membranes, and antepartum haemorrhage
Lack of prenatal care

Incidental findings
Delay in seeking treatment or inconsistent explanation of injuries
Repeated visits to the emergency department or clinic
Evasiveness of patient or jumpiness, fearfulness, or crying
Overly attentive or verbally abusive partner
Identifiable social isolation
Abuse of child or elderly adult in a household

[a] One or more of these factors may be present.
Reproduced from Eisenstat, S. and Bancroft, L. (1999). Domestic violence. *The New England Journal of Medicine* **341**, 886–92.

- substance abuse by patient and/or partner;
- post-traumatic stress disorder.

In addition, a history of abuse may result in poor self-care, as manifested by inappropriate use of alcohol, prescription drugs and/or illicit drugs, inappropriate use of health care services, poor nutritional status, and/or limited social or recreational pursuits. Abuse in a current relationship has also been found to be associated with delayed entry into pre-natal care.[12]

In a recent report on the economic impact of violence on the health of women aged 15–44, rape and domestic violence were shown to account for 9.5 million disability-adjusted life years lost worldwide, comparable to the impact of all cancers[2] (Table 2).

Asking about abuse

The high prevalence and significant health effects of violence against women and the special nature of the often long-term relationship between family physicians and their patients makes it important that family physicians ask about the possibility of abuse. In addition to addressing any concerning symptoms or signs, family physicians can use periodic health examinations, routine pre-natal care,[13] and even well-child visits[14] to screen for abuse. Some physicians prefer to ask direct, non-judgemental questions specifically about patients' histories of abuse in their current or previous relationships or in their families of origin, while others prefer to

Table 2 Estimated global health burden of selected conditions for women aged 15–44

Condition	Disability-adjusted life years lost (millions)
Maternal conditions	29.0
Sepsis	10.0
Obstructed labour	7.8
STDs (excluding HIV)	15.8
Pelvic inflammatory disease	12.8
Tuberculosis	10.9
HIV	10.6
Cardiovascular disease	10.5
Rape and domestic violence[a]	9.5
All cancers	9.0
Breast	1.4
Cervical	1.0
Motor vehicle accidents	4.2
War	2.7
Malaria	2.3

[a] Rape and domestic violence are included here for illustrative purposes. They are risk factors for disease conditions, such as STDs, depression, and injuries, not diseases in themselves.
From: Heisi, L., Pitanguy, J., and Germain, A. *Violence Against Women: The Hidden Health Burden.* Washington DC: World Bank, 1994.

use standardized tools. The Woman Abuse Screening Tool is one such instrument with demonstrated reliability and validity in English,[15] French,[16] and Spanish;[17] it has been shown to be effective in identifying abuse in adult women patients attending their regular family physicians for pre-natal care or periodic health examinations or for assessment of particular health problems[15] (Table 3).

Detection in primary care settings

Detection rates in primary care settings remain low,[18,19] reflecting institutional and organizational factors, gaps in physicians' skills knowledge and attitudes, and patient discomfort and/or reluctance to disclose.[20]

Various interventions have been suggested to improve detection rates, such as offering focused educational programmes to physicians,[21] incorporating simple screening tools into regular history-taking,[15,22] and enhancing the office environment to demonstrate to patients the appropriateness of discussing abuse and violence during clinical encounters. However, a recent systematic review of studies of interventions demonstrated that interventions to increase health care provider screening required both an educational and a behavioural component (e.g. provision of screening questions) to be effective.[20]

What to do on disclosure

When patients disclose a history of abuse, it is crucial that family physicians respond in a way that makes these patients feel believed and supported. It is inappropriate to ask victims about how their behaviour contributed to the abusive episodes or to minimize the seriousness of the abuse. Appropriate attention to health problems should be provided, in addition to information about how to get help in dealing with the non-medical consequences of abuse. Depending on their own comfort levels and on the availability and/or expertise of local resources, family physicians can refer women for assistance in obtaining shelter, sorting out financial options, exploring legal options, and/or arranging further psychological counselling for themselves or their children.

Table 3 Woman Abuse Screening Tool

1. In general, how would you describe your relationship?
   ◆ a lot of tension
   ◆ some tension
   ◆ no tension

2. Do you and your partner work out arguments with:
   ◆ great difficulty
   ◆ some difficulty
   ◆ no difficulty

3. Do arguments ever result in you feeling down or bad about yourself?
   ◆ often
   ◆ sometimes
   ◆ never

4. Do arguments ever result in hitting, kicking, or pushing?
   ◆ often
   ◆ sometimes
   ◆ never

5. Do you ever feel frightened by what your partner says or does?
   ◆ often
   ◆ sometimes
   ◆ never

6. Has your partner ever abused you physically?
   ◆ often
   ◆ sometimes
   ◆ never

7. Has your partner ever abused you emotionally?
   ◆ often
   ◆ sometimes
   ◆ never

8. Has your partner ever abused you sexually?
   ◆ often
   ◆ sometimes
   ◆ never

From: Brown, J. et al. (2000). Application of the Woman Abuse Screening Tool (WAST) and WAST-short in the family practice setting. *Journal of Family Practice* **49**, 896–903.

If the patient disclosing abuse has an ongoing relationship with the abuser, the family physician should ensure the patient has an appropriate safety plan, in case the threatened or actual violence escalates. Many community agencies can provide women with written materials to help delineate safety plans.

Caring for other family members

Because of the strong overlap between woman abuse and child maltreatment, family physicians caring for women and their children must consider the possibility of child maltreatment whenever concerns about woman abuse arise; similarly, when considering the possibility of child maltreatment, the physician should ask about woman abuse. An extensive review of the literature found that in 32–53 per cent of families where women are abused by their partners, the children are also being victimized by the same perpetrators.[23] Abused women themselves may perpetrate the physical and/or emotional abuse of the children.[24] Even witnessing the ongoing abuse of their mothers has been shown to have an effect on children's emotional, social, cognitive, and behavioural functioning.[25] Any concerns must be reported to the appropriate child protection agencies.

In addition, family physicians are unique among health care providers in that they might find themselves caring for both the victims of abuse within an intimate or family context, and the perpetrators of the same abuse. In such situations, physicians must ensure that the needs of the abused women and the perpetrators are addressed independently, such that their

rights to autonomy, confidentiality, honesty, and quality of care are maintained.[26] Couple or marital therapy is contra-indicated unless the woman's safety can be ensured and the man has taken responsibility for his abusive behaviour.

Confidentiality and reporting issues

Women will feel more comfortable disclosing abuse if they know that their caregivers will keep the details of their disclosure confidential, except when risk to third parties is disclosed. This issue is particularly important for family physicians who also provide care to other family members.

Confidentiality issues can also arise when family physicians consider referring patients with a history of physical or sexual abuse for procedures which might be deemed intrusive or invasive procedures, such as vaginal examinations or endoscopies. In such situations, family physicians should discuss with patients whether relevant information, provided to them in confidence, can be shared with other health professionals (e.g. consultants, midwives).

Although some jurisdictions mandate health care providers to report cases of domestic violence to law enforcement authorities, many health care professionals and community advocates argue that such laws interfere with patient autonomy, and will deter women from disclosing their history of abuse or from seeking care at all for fear of retaliation by their abusive partners.[27]

Prevention

Family physicians can help to minimize the long-term complications of abuse by sensitively asking about the possibility of abuse in current or previous relationships when following up on specific symptoms or signs that raise clinical suspicions of abuse. Screening for abuse during periodic health examinations, pre-natal assessments, and well-child assessments may lead to earlier detection, and thus limit the extent of physical and psychological disability among abused women and their children. In addition, physicians can use their status in the community to promote initiatives to make violence less socially acceptable, to reduce sex-role stereotyping and to move away from social relationships of male dominance and female submission.

Key points

1. Family physicians have a unique opportunity to address and identify woman abuse, because of their long-term relationships with patients and their focus on both physical and psychological health.

2. Violence in intimate relationships has significant consequences for the mental and physical health and well-being of women and children.

3. Family physicians should ask about the possibility of abuse, both when sorting out concerning signs or symptoms, and as part of the screening done during periodic health examinations, routine pre-natal visits, or well-child examinations.

4. After violence is disclosed, the family physician must validate the woman's experience and reinforce for her that such behaviour is socially unacceptable and is not her fault, while attending to any acute or chronic clinical concerns.

5. In order to reduce the extent of woman abuse and its serious negative consequences for women, their children, their partners, and the community, physicians can use their status in their own communities and work with other community leaders to promote changes in social attitudes towards violence between men and women.

References

1. **Declaration on the elimination of violence against women**. Resolution No. A/RES/48/104. New York: United Nations, 23 February 1994.

2. **Heisi, L., Pitanguy, J., and Germain, A.** *Violence Against Women: The Hidden Health Burden.* Washington DC: World Bank, 1994.

3. **Haskell, L. and Randall, M.** *The Women's Safety Project: Summary of Key Statistical Findings.* Ottawa, Canada: Canadian Panel on Violence Against Women, 1993.

4. **Swiss, S. and Giller, J.** (1993). Rape as a crime of war: a medical perspective. *Journal of the American Medical Association* **270** (5), 612–15.

5. **World Health Organization**. Violence against women: a priority health issue, 1997, http://www.who.int/violence_injury_prevention/vaw/infopack.htm.

6. **Coker, A.** et al. (2000). Physical health consequences of physical and psychological intimate partner violence. *Archives of Family Medicine* **9**, 451–7.

7. **Koss, M. and Heslet, L.** (1992). Somatic consequences of violence against women. *Archives of Family Medicine* **1**, 53–9.

8. **Eisenstat, S. and Bancroft, L.** (1999). Domestic violence. *New England Journal of Medicine* **341**, 886–92.

9. **Wisner, C.** et al. (1999). Intimate partner violence against women: do victims cost health plans more? *Journal of Family Practice* **48** (6), 439–43.

10. **Sansone, R., Wiederman, M., and Sansone, L.** (1997). Health care utilization and history of trauma among women in a primary care setting. *Violence and Victims* **12** (2), 165–72.

11. **Finestone, H.** et al. (2000). Chronic pain and health care utilization in women with a history of childhood sexual abuse. *Child Abuse & Neglect* **24** (4), 547–56.

12. **Dietz, P.** et al. (1997). Delayed entry into prenatal care: effect of physical violence. *Obstetrics and Gynecology* **90**, 221–4.

13. **Council on Scientific Affairs, American Medical Association** (1992). Violence against women: relevance for medical practitioners. *Journal of the American Medical Association* **267**, 3184–9.

14. **Siegel, R.** et al. (1999). Screening for domestic violence in the community pediatric setting. *Pediatrics* **104**, 874–7.

15. **Brown, J.** et al. (2000). Application of the Woman Abuse Screening Tool (WAST) and WAST-short in the family practice setting. *Journal of Family Practice* **49**, 896–903.

16. **Brown, J.** et al. (2001). Depistage de la violence faite aux femmes: epreuves de validation et de fiabilite d'un instrument de mesure francais. *Canadian Family Physician* **47**, 988–95.

17. **Brown, J. and Ryan, B.** *Woman Abuse: A Ten-Year Program of Research.* Working Paper Series #01–02. London, Canada: Centre for Studies in Family Medicine and Thames Valley Family Practice Research Unit, 2001.

18. **Abbott, J.** et al. (1995). Domestic violence against women: incidence and prevalence in an emergency department population. *Journal of the American Medical Association* **273**, 1763–7.

19. **Hamberger, L., Saunders, D., and Hovey, M.** (1992). Prevalence of domestic violence in community practice and rate of physician inquiry. *Family Medicine* **24**, 283–7.

20. **Waalen, J.** et al. (2000). Screening for intimate partner violence by health care providers: barriers and interventions. *American Journal of Preventive Medicine* **19**, 230–7.

21. **McLeer, S.V.** et al. (1989). Education is not enough: a systems failure in protecting battered women. *Annals of Emergency Medicine* **18**, 651–3.

22. **Sherin, K.** et al. (1998). HITS: a short domestic violence screening tool for use in a family practice setting. *Family Medicine* **30**, 508–12.

23. **Edleson, J.** Mothers and children: understanding the links between woman battering and child abuse, 1995, http://www.mincava.umn.edu/papers/nij.htm.

24. **Trainor, C. and Mihorean, K.** *Family Violence in Canada: A Statistical Profile 2001.* Catalogue no. 85-224. Ottawa: Statistics Canada, Canadian Centre for Justice Statistics, 2001.

25. **Jaffe, P., Wolfe, D., and Wilson, S.** *Children of Battered Women.* Newbury Park CA: Sage Publications, 1990.

26. **Ferris, L.** et al. (1997). Guidelines for managing domestic abuse when male and female partners are patients of the same physician. *Journal of the American Medical Association* **278**, 851–7.

27. **Hyman, A., Schillinger, D., and Lo, B.** (1995). Laws mandating reporting of domestic violence. *Journal of the American Medical Association* **273**, 781–7.

Further reading

World Health Organization. Violence against women: a priority health issue, 1997, http://www.who.int/violence_injury_prevention/vaw/infopack.htm. (An excellent compilation of international studies on the epidemiology and health consequences of violence against women.)

Waalen, J. et al. (2000). Screening for intimate partner violence by health care providers: barriers and interventions. *American Journal of Preventive Medicine* **19**, 230–7. (A comprehensive article that reviews the potential benefits of screening for intimate partner violence as well as the barriers and difficulties in promoting such interventions.)

Council on Scientific Affairs, American Medical Association (1992). Violence against women: relevance for medical practitioners. *Journal of the American Medical Association* **267**, 3184–9. (An early report that summarizes the health consequences of violence against women and that clearly reviews the role of physicians in these issues.)

8

Conception, pregnancy, and childbirth

8 Conception, pregnancy, and childbirth

8.1 Pre-conception care

Stefan Grzybowski and Colleen Kirkham

Pre-conception care is part of a seamless continuum of care from well woman and contraceptive visits to pre-natal care. It represents a huge as yet largely unrealized opportunity to improve the health of mothers and their babies.

Introduction

Pre-conception care is ideally provided in the context of a carefully planned pregnancy in which health promotion strategies can be integrated with optimal risk reduction based on best evidence. Unfortunately, this is rarely the case as conception is difficult to predict, and patterns of care vary dramatically dependent on socio-economic status, education, and ability to access care.

This chapter presents an overview of best practices for physicians, midwives, and nurses who have the opportunity to improve the preparedness of the mother for the physiologic and psychosocial challenges of pregnancy. While there are huge differences in the social structures defining the provision of primary care between countries, the evidence base of our discipline is broadly applicable. The risks associated with pregnancy over the age of 35 are as relevant in Australia as they are in Canada and the United States. The potential benefits of a pre- and periconceptional intake of 0.4 mg/day of folic acid are as important in reducing the primary risk of neural tube defects in Calcutta as they are in the Indian population of London.

Practitioners need to better utilize opportunities to address pre-conception care issues in the course of regular visits such as those for well women check-ups and contraceptive counselling. These should include not only screening for infectious diseases and genetic risk factors, but also immunizations and advice regarding diet and exercise. These initiatives can be strengthened by educational interventions in schools, the workplace, and through the media.

Pre-conception care is ideally part of an integrated continuum of comprehensive family-centred maternity and newborn care, which addresses not only the medical but psycho-social and spiritual dimensions of care.

Lifestyle issues

Counselling to promote healthy lifestyle choices is an important component of pre-conception care. Common sense advice needs to be weighted with evidence-based information about issues such as diet, exercise, and exposure to potentially harmful agents.

Diet

For women with no special nutritional challenges, a well-balanced diet with representative servings of fruit, vegetables, meat or alternatives, grains, and milk products is appropriate. Usual caloric requirements will increase in pregnancy by 100 cal per day before 12 weeks and then by 300 cal per day until delivery and when breastfeeding. There are increased requirements for folic acid, calcium, and iron. Moderate amounts of caffeine and aspartame (artificial sweetener) appear to be safe. Because of the potential risks of such infections as toxoplasmosis and listeria, women planning a pregnancy should avoid eating raw meat, fish and eggs, unpasteurized milk and cheeses, most soft cheeses, and unwashed fruit and vegetables. Women with special nutritional needs or those whose body mass index (BMI) falls outside of a normal range (BMI approximately 20–25) should have the benefit of consultation with a nutritionist.

Folic acid supplementation

There is good evidence from randomized controlled trials to show that the ingestion of folic acid from 4 weeks pre-conceptionally to 12 weeks after conception prevents neural tube defects (NTDs). NTDs vary in manifestation from relatively mild spina bifida occulta to severe meningomyelocele with associated paraplegia and bladder and bowel incontinence or lethal anencephaly. Women at increased risk are those with a previously affected infant or a positive family history of a NTD.

The worldwide incidence varies from one to nine per 1000 births and 90–95 per cent of cases occur in families with no previous history of an affected infant.

The dose of folic acid for primary prevention is 0.4 mg per day (relative risk reduction, RRR of 40–60 per cent) and for secondary prevention is 4.0 mg per day (RRR of 50–72 per cent) starting at least 1 month before conception (Box 1). Many authors recommend that women take folic acid throughout the reproductive years, as more than 50 per cent of pregnancies are unplanned.

The average diet contains less than 0.2 mg of folic acid per day from foods such as green vegetables, fruits, and grains. Furthermore, folates are inactivated by prolonged food storage and cooking, making adequate dietary intake without supplementation difficult to achieve.

A number of studies show that few women take folic acid in the 4 weeks prior to conception. There is some evidence to suggest that improved pre-conception counselling will lead to improved rates of folate ingestion.

There are recent examples of public health programmes of enrichment of commercial food with folic acid notably in the United States with the addition of folic acid to enriched grain products and associated evidence of a 19 per cent relative decrease in the incidence of NTDs. This promises to be the most effective strategy to reach the population at risk.

Dietary supplements

There are increased requirements for both calcium and iron in pregnancy and a pre-conception visit provides an excellent opportunity to assess for women

Box 1 Folic acid supplementation

Primary prevention	0.4 mg/day
Secondary prevention	4.0 mg/day
Starting at least 1 month before conception	

at risk of inadequate stores. Teenagers and women of low socio-economic status are at particularly increased risk.

Calcium and vitamin D are important for maintenance of maternal bone as well as to support the developing foetal skeleton. Women at highest risk are those with limited intake of dairy products or minimal sun exposure due to climate or culture. Recommended daily intake of calcium during pregnancy is 1200–1500 mg per day and vitamin D is 200 IU per day (5.0 µg). One cup of milk contains approximately 300 mg of calcium.

Inadequate iron stores are a common finding amongst women both pre-pregnancy and in early pregnancy. Iron deficiency is associated with intrauterine growth retardation, premature delivery, and even foetal death. It is prudent to screen women at high risk for iron-deficiency anaemia and supplement as necessary. High-risk groups include women of low socio-economic status, high parity, women with a history of menorrhagia or multiple gestations, vegetarians, regular blood donors, and adolescents.

High doses of vitamin A are known to increase the risk of cranial–neural crest defects. Women should be cautioned against excessive use (greater than 5000 IU/day).

The safety of many herbal preparations, including some herbal teas, has not been adequately studied.

Exercise

Exercise is an important part of a healthy lifestyle. It is encouraged in uncomplicated pregnancies. A routine of 20–40 min three to five times weekly is reasonable. Inactive women planning a pregnancy may want to begin an exercise programme prior to conceiving. Women should be cautious about vigorous exercise in the first trimester because of the at least theoretical risk of maternal hyperthermia affecting the closure of the neural tube. A similar proscription applies to hot tubs and saunas.

Smoking and drug use

Tobacco use is increasingly common amongst teenage women. In the United States, 25 per cent of women between the ages of 18 and 24 smoke tobacco on a daily basis. Risks associated with smoking can be raised in the pre-conception period and a smoking cessation strategy can be undertaken. Risks include intrauterine growth retardation, prematurity, abruptio placenta, placenta previa, spontaneous abortion, and stillbirth.

Illicit drug use presents a broad range of problems often calling for specialized interventions ideally framed within a non-judgemental harm reduction strategy. Stabilization on a methadone maintenance programme of an opiate-addicted woman may be life-saving. Intravenous heroin or cocaine addiction is often associated with hepatitis B, hepatitis C, and/or HIV infection. Pre-conception screening and counselling provide an important window of opportunity for intervention in the drug-dependent woman.

Alcohol use

Excessive alcohol use during pregnancy is associated with the development of foetal alcohol syndrome (FAS), a constellation of growth retardation, facial deformities, and central nervous system dysfunction including mental retardation and behavioural abnormalities. Growth retardation or neurologic involvement in the absence of full FAS is termed foetal alcohol effect (FAE). The safe dose of alcohol consumption during pregnancy is unknown. Abstinence is ideal and to be encouraged in the woman planning imminent pregnancy.

Medication usage and exposure to potential teratogens

The 8 weeks after conception represent the greatest developmental risk to the foetus. Pre-conceptionally, a careful review of medications and potential work or home-related chemical exposures is essential. There are relatively few medications with proven teratogenic effects, but these include isotretinoin prescribed for acne, antiepileptic agents such as phenytoin, valproic acid and carbamazepine, tetracycline, warfarin, lithium, ACE-inhibitors, and non-steroidal anti-inflammatory drugs. The safety of many other medications and herbal remedies in pregnancy has not been

adequately studied and consequently avoidance where possible is the best course. Exposure to metals such as lead, copper or zinc, anaesthetic gases, organic solvents, and radiation can also be harmful. Information is emerging suggesting that widely available lawn and garden pesticides have teratogenic effects. Women considering pregnancy should avoid such exposure.

Risk assessment

History and physical examination should include a systematic identification of preconceptional risks through assessment of reproductive, medical, and family histories. This includes a detailed menstrual, sexual, contraceptive, and prior pregnancy and delivery history.

Increased maternal age

With increasing frequency, women are planning a pregnancy over the age of 35. Particularly when this is a first pregnancy, the decision is often associated with considerable anxiety.

Pre-existing maternal disease is more commonly encountered. Hypertension and diabetes mellitus need to be screened for and if present investigated and optimally controlled prior to pregnancy. Women need to know that pregnancy complications are also more common. The risk of spontaneous abortion increases significantly with age. In one study, risk was 8.9 per cent in women aged 20–24 and 74.7 per cent in those aged 45 years or more. Twin pregnancies are up to three times more likely. Placental problems of abruption and placenta previa are seen more frequently as is gestational diabetes. Interventions such as rates of caesarean section have been reported to be two to three times more frequent than in younger women. Nevertheless, with appropriate pre-conception and antenatal care, healthy maternal and newborn outcomes are the norm.

Pre-natal genetic screening assumes an increased importance as the cumulative risk of a chromosomal abnormality increases with maternal age to approximately 1 : 200 at age 35, 1 : 100 at age 38, and 1 : 20 for women aged 40–44.

Fertility drops significantly as women age. Approximate pregnancy rates after 1 year of trying to conceive are 74 per cent in women 30 years and under, compared to 54 per cent in women over 35.

Domestic violence, sexual assault, and abuse

Physical, sexual, and emotional abuse by an intimate partner is common and is recognized as a significant risk to the health of both mother and infant. Also, pregnancy, labour, and delivery can be particularly difficult for women with histories of sexual assault or childhood sexual abuse. Structured direct screening questions about experiences of physical and sexual violence should be routinely included in the same way as questions eliciting other risk factors such as diabetes and smoking.

Female genital mutilation is common in some African countries and increasingly seen in migrant populations. It is estimated that as many as 100 000 women worldwide may be affected. These women may pose a special challenge for caregivers. Female attendants may be indicated and early consultation helpful.

Infectious disease history

There are a number of important infectious disease issues that should be addressed pre-conceptionally.

Sexually transmitted diseases

During pregnancy, sexually transmitted diseases (STDs) including chlamydia, gonorrhoea, genital herpes, syphilis, human immunodeficiency virus (HIV), and hepatitis B can lead to adverse outcomes for mother and infant.

Chlamydial and gonococcal infections increase the risk of pelvic inflammatory disease, infertility, ectopic pregnancy, prematurity, low birth weight, intrauterine foetal death, postpartum endometritis, and ophthalmia neonatorum. Active maternal chlamydial infection has a vertical transmission rate of 50–60 per cent.

Syphilis infection during pregnancy may result in spontaneous abortion, stillbirth, premature delivery, or congenital syphilis. Risk of transmission to the foetus is 70–100 per cent for untreated primary syphilis. Women at high risk should be screened prior to conception and several times during pregnancy.

Genital herpes is common and appropriate management is discussed in the chapter on pregnancy care.

For many STDs (chlamydia, gonorrhoea, syphilis), treatment of the partner(s) is also required to prevent re-infection. Risk factors for STDs include age under 25, low socio-economic status, history of prior STD, and multiple sexual partners.

Counselling about safe sexual practices is important before pregnancy.

Human immunodeficiency virus

The prevalence of HIV infection amongst women of child-bearing age varies dramatically. In North America, it is currently estimated to be less than three per 1000 women. In some parts of Sub-Saharan Africa, as many as 250 per 1000 women are infected. When a woman is infected with HIV and untreated, vertical transmission of the virus occurs in approximately 15–40 per cent of cases. Treatment can be effective in significantly reducing this risk to less than 1 per cent with optimal antenatal combination antiretroviral therapy tailored to the HIV disease and with intrapartum and neonatal antiretroviral therapy. The risk of maternal–infant HIV transmission is increased by advanced stage HIV disease, low CD4 lymphocyte count, and high viral load. All women of child-bearing age should be offered counselling and testing for HIV in the pre-conception period.

Rubella

All women of child-bearing age should be screened for rubella immunity by serology or proof of vaccination. Non-immune women should be vaccinated prior to pregnancy (Box 2). An acceptable alternative for non-pregnant women is to offer vaccination against rubella without screening. Women should avoid pregnancy for 1 month following immunization.

Varicella

Chicken pox infections during pregnancy can lead to severe illness in the mother, including pneumonia, as well as congenital varicella syndrome in up to 2 per cent of cases if contracted prior to 20 weeks. Varicella infections around delivery can lead to severe neonatal varicella. Women planning a pregnancy should be asked about a past history of varicella—a highly reliable and valid way to determine if an individual is immune. There is mounting evidence that women without a history of chicken pox should be offered serologic testing and vaccination if they are not immune, prior to pregnancy. Varicella vaccine is not considered safe during pregnancy though there are no data to show that inadvertent vaccination will cause the congenital varicella syndrome.

Hepatitis B and C

Screening for active hepatitis B infection by measuring hepatitis B surface antigen (HbsAg), is currently recommended for all pregnant women at the first pre-natal visit. However, women at increased risk of infection should be screened pre-conceptionally and vaccinated if sero-negative. Risk factors include injection drug use, multiple sexual partners or sexual partner in a high-risk group, household contacts of hepatitis B infected individuals, travellers to countries where hepatitis B is endemic (Southeast Asia, China, Eastern Europe), and health care workers exposed to blood or blood products. Some jurisdictions are moving towards universal vaccination of all young adults. Hepatitis B vaccination is not contra-indicated in pregnancy.

Women at risk for blood borne pathogens or with multiple sexual partners should also be screened for hepatitis C which has a 6–10 per cent vertical transmission rate.

Toxoplasmosis

Routine serologic testing for toxoplasmosis in the pre-conception period is not currently recommended. Women should be counselled before pregnancy about avoiding raw meat and unpasteurized dairy products, washing fruits and vegetables well, and avoiding contact with cat litter or soil that may contain faeces as these are potential sources of infection.

Chronic medical illness

Women with chronic medical illnesses such as diabetes or hypertension should be assessed on a case by case basis. Pre-conception assessment includes evaluating the potential impact of the chronic illness on a woman's capability to carry a pregnancy as well as the potential effect the stress of pregnancy might have on progression of the illness. Once these risks are projected and understood, women can be counselled with respect to optimal management and timing of pregnancy.

Genetic risks

Pre-conception genetic counselling is recommended for couples with a previous foetus or child affected with a genetic disorder (e.g. cystic fibrosis, Duchenne muscular dystrophy), a positive family history of genetic disorder or birth defect, or recurrent miscarriage (increased risk of chromosomal translocation). Individuals who belong to an ethnic group with a high incidence of a recessive condition should also be offered disease specific screening. For example, one in 30 Ashkenazi Jews is a carrier of Tay Sachs disease. The carrier state for Tay Sachs can be detected by measuring serum hexosaminidase A activity in non-pregnant women and men and WBC hexosaminidase A in pregnant women.

Individuals of Mediterranean, Southeast Asian, East Indian, African, Hispanic, and Middle Eastern descent are at increased risk of carrying the genes for alpha and beta thalassaemia. The screening test for thalassaemia is a red blood cell mean cell volume (MCV) of less than 80 fl. If the screen is less than 80 then haemoglobin electrophoresis and morphology should be pursued. If a woman is found to be a carrier, her partner should be screened.

The incidence of sickle cell abnormality is high amongst individuals of African heritage. These patients should be offered testing for sickle cell (haemoglobin S) trait.

Genetic testing for cystic fibrosis should be offered to women with a positive family history.

Planning the pregnancy

Ideally, a couple will actively plan their pregnancy and a woman will present to her caregiver for pre-conception counselling. There are a number of books and tools available to support a couple in their planning and preparation. One of these tools is the Pregnancy Planning Guide developed by the authors at the Department of Family Practice at the University of British Columbia and Children's and Women's Health Centre of British Columbia. It is a rotational calendar designed to present information both pictorially and in text to guide a woman through planning a safe and satisfying pregnancy. It serves as both a guideline and a prompting agent to encourage evidence-based and timely care (see Fig. 1). The references that are the foundation for the information on the guide are available at http://www.bcricwh.bc.ca/ or www.pregnancyplanningguide.com.

Box 2 Immune status assessment

Assess immune status and vaccinate if indicated

- Rubella
- Varicella
- Hepatitis B (women at increased risk)

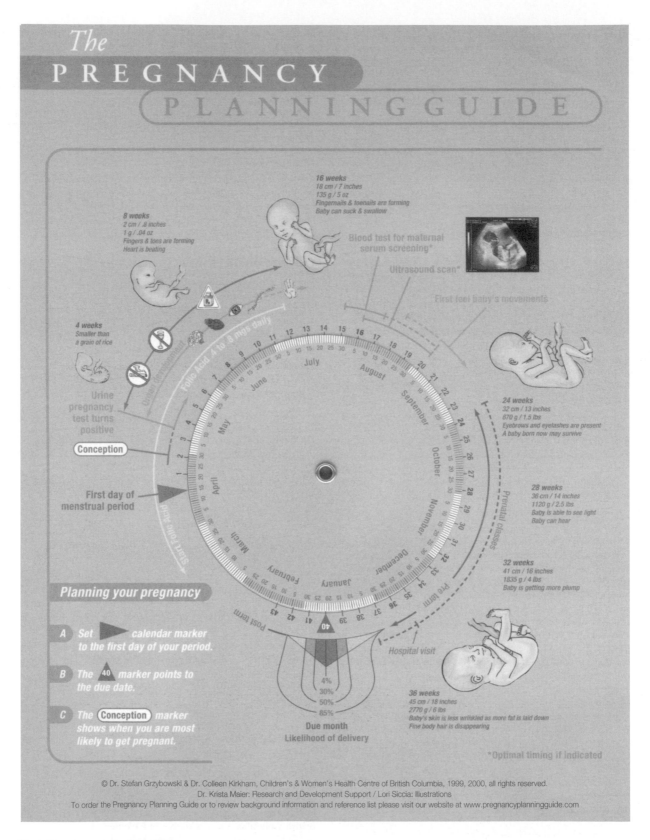

Fig. 1 The pregnancy planning guide.

Acknowledgements

We are grateful to Dr Deborah Money and Dr Sylvie Langlois for their very helpful review of sections of the chapter and suggestions for revisions.

Overview and further reading

Jack, B. and Culpepper, L. (1998). Preconception care. In *Family Medicine—Principles and Practice* 5th edn. (ed. R. Taylor), pp. 78–83. New York: Springer-Verlag. (Thoughtful and in-depth review of subject upon which we structured our chapter.)

Health Canada, Family-Centred Maternity and Newborn Care: National Guidelines. Minister of Public Works and Government Services, Ottawa, 2000. Website: http://www.hc-sc.gc.ca. (Chapter 3 review of pre-conception care, useful summary and accessible on Web.)

Canadian Task Force on the Periodic Health Exam. *The Canadian Guide to Clinical Preventive Health Care*. Ottawa, Ontario: Health Canada, 1994. Website: www.ctfphc.org.

United States Preventive Services Task Force. *Guide to Clinical Preventive Services* 2nd edn. Baltimore MD: Williams and Wilkins, 1996. Website: http://www.ahcpr.gov/clinic/uspstfix.htm. (Both the Canadian Task Force on Preventive Health Care and the US Preventive Services Task Force use a similar, standardized method to systematically review evidence for a variety of preventive health care interventions. Explicit criteria are used to judge the quality of evidence from published clinical research, and then clinical practice guidelines are developed using a rating scale from grade A to grade E to classify the evidence.)

Cochrane Library: http://www.updateusa.com/Cochrane/default.HTM. (The Cochrane database of systemic reviews contains highly structured reviews with evidence included or excluded on the basis of explicit quality criteria to minimize bias.)

Cunningham, F. et al. (2002). *Williams Obstetrics*, New York, McGraw-Hill. (A useful desk reference for the medical complications of pregnancy.)

Diet and nutrition

Health Canada. *Nutrition for a Healthy Pregnancy: National Guidelines for the Childbearing Years*. Ottawa: Minister of Public Works and Government Services, Canada, 1999. Website: http://www.hc-sc.gc.ca.

Pesicka, D., Riley, J., and Thomson, C. *Obstetrics/Gynecology Nutrition Handbook*. New York: Thomson Publishing, 1996.

Barrett, J. and Pitman, T. *Pregnancy and Birth: The Best Evidence*. Toronto: Keystone Porter Books Limited, 1999.

Kolasa, K.M. and Weismiller, D.G. (1995). Nutrition during pregnancy. *American Family Physician* 56, 205–12.

Brown, J.E. and Kahn, E.S.B. (1997). Maternal nutrition and the outcome of pregnancy. *Clinics in Perinatology* 24, 433–49.

Smith, J.L. (1999). Foodborne infections during pregnancy. *Journal of Food Protection* 62, 818–29.

Folic acid

MRC Vitamin Study Research Group (1991). Prevention of neural tube defects: results of the Medical Research Council Vitamin Study. *Lancet* 338, 131–7.

Czeizel, A.E. and Dudas, I. (1992). Prevention of the first occurrence of neural-tube defects by periconceptional vitamin supplementation. *New England Journal of Medicine* 327, 1832–5.

Werler, M.M., Shapiro, S., and Mitchel, A.A. (1993). Periconceptional folic acid exposure and risk of occurrence of neural tube defects. *Journal of the American Medical Association* 269, 1257–61.

Hall, J.G. and Solehdin, F. (1998). Genetics of neural tube defects. *Mental Retardation and Developmental Disabilities* 4, 269–81.

Honein, M.A., Paulozzi, L.J., Matthews, T.J., Erikson, J.D., and Wong, L.Y.C. (2001). Impact of folic acid fortification of the US Food Supply on the occurrence of neural tube defects. *Journal of the American Medical Association* 285 (23), 2981–6.

Exercise

Wang, T.W. and Apgar, B.S. (1998). Exercise during pregnancy. *American Family Physician* 57, 1846–52.

Lokey, E.A., Tran, Z.V., Wells, C.L., Myers, B.C., and Tran, A.C. (1991). Effects of physical exercise on pregnancy outcomes: a meta-analytic review. *Medicine and Science in Sports and Exercise* 23, 1234–9.

Stevenson, L. (1997). Exercise in pregnancy. Part 2. Recommendations for individuals. *Canadian Family Physician* 43, 107–11.

Medication usage and exposure to potential teratogens

Koren, G., Pastuszak, A., and Ito, S. (1998). Drug therapy: drugs in pregnancy. *New England Journal of Medicine* 338, 1128–37.

Maternal age

Jolly, M., Sebire, N., Harris, J., Robinson, S., and Regan, L. (2000). The risks associated with pregnancy in women aged 35 years or older. *Human Reproduction* 15, 2433–7.

Domestic violence

Fishwick, N.J. (1998). Assessment of women for partner abuse. *Journal of Obstetric, Gynecologic, and Neonatal Nursing* 27, 661–70.

Mayer, L. and Liebschutz, J. (1998). Domestic violence in the pregnant patient: obstetric and behavioral interventions. *Obstetrical and Gynecological Survey* 53, 627–35.

Petersen, R. et al. (1997). Violence and adverse pregnancy outcomes: a review of the literature and directions for future research. *American Journal of Preventive Medicine* 13, 366–73.

McFarlane, J., Parker, B., Soeken, K., and Bullock, L. (1992). Assessing for abuse during pregnancy. *Journal of the American Medical Association* 267, 3176–8.

Human immunodeficiency virus (HIV)

Tessier, D., Dion, H., Grossman, D.W., and Rachlis, A. *HIV Care: A Primer and Resource Guide for Family Physicians*. Mississauga, Canada: The College of Family Physicians of Canada, 2001.

Samson, L. and King, S. (1998). Evidence-based guidelines for universal counselling and offering of HIV testing in pregnancy in Canada. *Canadian Medical Association Journal* 158, 1449–57.

Lorenzi, P. et al. (1998). Antiretroviral therapies in pregnancy: maternal, fetal and neonatal effects. Swiss HIV Cohort Study, the Swiss Collaborative HIV and Pregnancy Study and the Swiss Neonatal HIV study. *AIDS* 12 (18), F241–7.

Money, D.M. et al. (2000). Obstetrical complications, maternal/fetal toxicities and vertical transmission in combination antiretroviral-treated pregnant women. *Infectious Diseases in Obstetrics/Gynecology* 8, 205.

Morris, A. et al. (1999). A review of protease inhibitors (PI) use in 89 pregnancies. *6th Conference on Retroviruses Opportunistic Infections*, 1999, Abstract No. 687.

Varicella zoster screening

Smith, W.J., Jackson, L.A., Watts, H.D., and Koepsell, T.D. (1998). Prevention of chickenpox in reproductive-age women: cost-effectiveness of routine prenatal screening with postpartum vaccination of susceptibles. *Obstetrics & Gynecology* 92, 535–45.

Chapman, S. (1998). Varicella in pregnancy. *Seminars in Perinatology* 22, 339–46.

Seidman, D.S., Stevenson, D.K., and Arvin, A.M. (1996). Varicella vaccine in pregnancy. *British Medical Journal* 313, 701–2.

Glantz, C.J. and Mushlin, A.I. (1998). Cost-effectiveness of routine antenatal varicella screening. *Obstetrics & Gynecology* 91, 519–28.

Genetic screening

Milunsky, A. *Genetic Disorders and the Fetus: Diagnosis, Prevention, and Treatment* 4th edn. Baltimore MD: Johns Hopkins University Press, 1998.

Canadian Guidelines for Prenatal Diagnosis—Genetic Indications for Prenatal Diagnosis (2001). *Journal SOGC* **23** (6), 525–31.

Genetic Testing for Cystic Fibrosis (1999). National Institutes of Health Consensus Development Conference Statement on Genetic Testing for Cystic Fibrosis. *Archives of Internal Medicine* **159**, 1529–39.

8.2 Sub-fertility

Jan Grace and Alison Taylor

Introduction

Sub-fertility is a common condition with important psychological, economic, and medical implications; 15 per cent of all couples in the Western world are involuntarily childless. Approximately one-half will go on to conceive either spontaneously or with simple advice or therapies, but 8 per cent of couples will have unresolved sub-fertility and require more sophisticated treatments. The likelihood of spontaneous pregnancy in sub-fertile women is strongly influenced by age, the duration of infertility, and the occurrence of a previous pregnancy. Despite the stable population prevalence of sub-fertility, the demands on the sub-fertility services have grown substantially over the last two decades during which major technological advances have developed.

Worldwide patterns of fertility are similar with a few exceptions. In India, couples tend to present late for evaluation and only 7.2 per cent of sub-fertility is related to tubal disease. African couples are more likely to have secondary sub-fertility, with a history of sexually transmitted disease or pregnancy complications. Their infertility diagnoses such as bilateral tubal occlusion or pelvic adhesions are suggestive of previous genital infection.

Definition

Sub-fertility is the inability to conceive after 1 year of intercourse with the same partner without contraception. Conception should occur in 80–90 per cent couples within 12 months of ceasing contraception and in 95 per cent by 2 years. Primary sub-fertility affects couples who have never conceived. Secondary sub-fertility applies to couples who have had a pregnancy previously although this may not necessarily have had a successful outcome. Most couples who present have relative *sub-fertility* (reduced chance of conception) rather than absolute *in*fertility. It is important to remember when discussing treatment options that many couples have a chance of conceiving spontaneously.

The impact on primary care

Approximately 50 per cent of sub-fertile women in Western societies seek advice or treatment. The investigation and management of infertility is a large public health problem and the limited resources available need to be used prudently. National, regional, and local protocols on primary care management and indications for referral of an infertile couple to a secondary or tertiary care centre should be developed.

Causes of sub-fertility

The main causes of sub-fertility can be divided into male factors, anovulation, tubal factors, endometriosis, and unexplained infertility. These categories are based on functional considerations that facilitate treatment rather than the diagnosis. The categories and their frequency in primary and secondary sub-fertility are summarized in Table 1. However, not all couples fit neatly into one category and several problems may have to be managed simultaneously. Male factors may be the main cause in 20–25 per cent of couples and will contribute to sub-fertility in a further 25 per cent. It is always important to investigate both partners, even if there is an obvious female factor present.

Male factor infertility

Between 20 and 25 per cent of cases of sub-fertility are due to male factors alone and in another 25 per cent, causes can be identified in both men and women. Sperm count, motility and morphology are the basic parameters used to estimate male fertility, and normal values for these are shown in Table 2.

In 40–60 per cent of cases of male factor sub-fertility, a cause for diminished semen quality can be determined; the remainder can be regarded as idiopathic. Lifestyle factors that affect semen quality include smoking, alcohol, recreational drugs, and high temperature. Oestrogenic environmental pollution and other industrial toxins such as lead and cadmium have also been implicated. The relationship between good nutrition and reproduction is well established. Further studies are required to establish whether there is any benefit from the use of antioxidants such as vitamins C and E, and mineral supplementation such as zinc and selenium.

Physical causes are important. There is strong evidence of a worldwide increase in the frequency of testicular cancer and of congenital abnormalities such as cryptorchidism and hypospadias. Testicular maldescent, also associated with male sub-fertility, occurs in 3–6 per cent of males at birth.

Varicocoele is present in 25–40 per cent of sub-fertile and 8–13 per cent of fertile men. Its presence is associated with decreased sperm concentration, but surgical intervention does not always lead to improvement of semen quality and pregnancy rates.

Table 1 Diagnostic categories and distribution of couples with primary and secondary infertility

	Primary (%)	Secondary (%)
Male	25	20
Anovulation	20	15
Tubal	15	40
Endometriosis	10	5
Unexplained	30	20

Table 2 Normal semen analysis parameters (World Health Organization)

Parameter	Normal	Terminology if abnormal
Volume of ejaculate	2–5 ml	Oligospermia
Sperm count	$>20 \times 10^6$/ml	Oligozoospermia; severe oligozoospermia if $<5 \times 10^6$/ml; azoospermia if no sperm in ejaculate
Motility	>50% progressive with >25% rapidly progressive	Asthenozoospermia
Morphology	>20% normal	Teratozoospermia

Genital tract obstruction most commonly follows vasectomy. Other causes such as infection or congenital absence of the vasa deferentia (CAVD) should be suspected in patents with azoospermia with normal testicular volume and clinical evidence of active spermatogenesis. CAVD is associated with a mild variant form of cystic fibrosis for which both partners should be screened. Sub-fertility can be related to coital dysfunction including ejaculatory failure or difficulties, erectile problems, loss of libido, impotence, and retrograde ejaculation. A primary psychosexual cause is rare, and most disorders can be attributed to medical or iatrogenic causes, but having a sub-fertility problem can cause difficulties in relationships resulting in secondary coital dysfunction compounding the problem.

Antisperm antibodies (ASAs) are immunoglobulins that bind to spermatozoa and in some cases affecting their motility. Significant risk factors for the development of ASAs include vasectomy, with up to 70 per cent of males post-operatively, and infections such as epididymo-orchitis.

Hypogonadotrophic hypogonadism can be congenital or acquired and low levels of gonadotrophins lead to lack of spermatogenesis and low testosterone levels. A man will present with varying degrees of secondary sexual development and small atrophic testes. Although uncommon, it is an important diagnosis to make because it is amenable to treatment with gonadotrophins.

The most common chromosomal abnormality to interfere with spermatogenesis is Kleinfelters syndrome (47, XXY); 15 per cent of azoospermic and 4 per cent of men with severe oligozoospermia have an abnormal karyotype.

Treatment with certain drugs (Table 3) or exposure to radiation or chemicals can interfere with spermatogenesis. Cytotoxic drugs used for the treatment of testicular cancer, Hodgkin's disease, non-Hodgkin's lymphoma and leukaemia, and the diseases themselves can affect fertility.

Table 3 Drugs that may affect male fertility

Drug type	Drugs	Effect
Antihypertensive	Methyldopa Thiazides Propranolol	Sexual dysfunction (ejaculatory problems, impotence, reduced libido)
	Calcium channel blockers	Sperm function affecting acrosome reaction and fertilization
Antipsychotics	Thioridazine Fluphenazine	Sexual dysfunction
Antidepressants	Tricyclics Trazodone Fluoxetine Phenelzine	Sexual dysfunction
Chemotherapy	Alkylating agents Methotrexate Vincristine	Germ cell toxicity leading to oligozoospermia or azoospermia
Androgens	Anabolic steroids	Sexual dysfunction Suppression of spermatogenesis
Gastrointestinal	Sulfasalazine Cimetidine Metoclopramide Omeprazole	Impaired spermatogenesis Sexual dysfunction
Recreational	Tobacco Alcohol Marijuana	Sperm motility and count reduced Sexual dysfunction Sexual dysfunction Reduced sperm count
	Cocaine	Reduced sperm motility
	Heroin methadone	Sexual dysfunction Reduced ejaculate volume Reduced sperm motility

Anovulation

Anovulation is a factor in one-fifth of all sub-fertile couples and may be divided into ovarian, hypothalamic, and pituitary causes. Ovarian failure can occur at any age, but is regarded as premature before the age of 40 years and is associated with high levels of gonadotrophins and low oestradiol levels. Chromosomal abnormalities such as Turners XO and Turners mosaicsm (XO XX) are found in 70 per cent of patients with primary amenorrhoea, while 2–5 per cent of women with secondary amenorrhoea caused by premature ovarian failure have chromosomal abnormalities.

Autoimmune processes underlie most causes of premature ovarian failure. Other aetiological factors include infection, previous surgery, and chemo- and radiotherapy. Familial forms of premature ovarian failure are associated with a fragile X mutation. Hypothalamic dysfunction may result in abnormal secretion of gonadotrophin-releasing hormone (GnRH) from the hypothalamus, for example, Kallman's syndrome which is characterized by anosmia and hypogonadotrophic hypogonadism. Weight loss, excessive exercise, and stress can also alter GnRH secretion. This in turn affects the release of follicle-stimulating hormone (FSH) and leutinizing hormone (LH) from the pituitary gland and is characterized by low FSH and LH levels.

Hyperprolactinaemia may result from a prolactin-secreting pituitary adenoma or disruption of the inhibitory release of dopamine on prolactin secretion, causing anovulatory amenorrhoea.

Polycystic ovary syndrome (PCOS) is defined as the detection of polycystic ovaries by ultrasound scan together with symptoms of oligomenorrhoea, obesity, and hyperandrogenism. Endocrine features include raised serum LH and testosterone levels but these are only found in 40 and 48 per cent of patients, respectively. PCOS is the commonest cause of secondary amenorrhoea and anovulation.

Tubal disease

Tubal damage accounts for 25 per cent of all cases of infertility and accounts for more than half of infertility in women. Pelvic inflammatory disease (PID) is the single most important cause of tubal damage. The two organisms most frequently related to upper genital tract infection are *Neisseria gonorrhea* and *Chlamydia trachomatis*. The incidence of Chlamydial genital infection is increasing worldwide. It is recognized to be associated with at least 50 per cent of cases of acute PID in developed countries and in 50–80 per cent of women is asymptomatic. Other organisms may play a lesser role but tuberculosis must be considered in women from high-risk areas such as African and the Indian subcontinent. Any lower abdominal surgery is also a risk factor for tubal factor infertility, due to the development of adhesions. Previous ectopic pregnancy is a further risk factor for tubal damage, and may have resulted in the loss of a fallopian tube.

Endometriosis

The association of endometriosis and infertility is unclear; it is diagnosed in 10–20 per cent of women undergoing investigation for infertility compared to 1–5 per cent of women undergoing sterilization. The pathophysiology of infertility associated with endometriosis is complex. It involves a combination of factors including defective folliculogenesis, disorders of ovulation, and distortion of pelvic anatomy by adhesions.

Unexplained infertility

The diagnosis of unexplained infertility is made when no specific cause of infertility can be identified after a full diagnostic evaluation and is applied to 10–25 per cent of infertile couples. There should be evidence of normal ovulation and tubal patency and a normal semen analysis. The chance of these couples conceiving spontaneously in the first 3 years following investigation is high at between 40–89 per cent.

The diagnosis of infertility

The diagnosis of infertility is based on taking an accurate history and performing appropriate examination and investigations on both the male and female partner. Key features of history-taking and examination are summarized in Tables 4 and 5, respectively.

Table 4 History

Male	
Infertility	Duration of infertility
	Previous pregnancies in present and past relationships
	Previous investigations and treatment
Medical	Sexually transmitted disease, epididymitis, orchitis
	Testicular maldescent
	Drug and alcohol abuse
	Chemotherapy
Surgical	Testicular injury, torsion, orchidopexy, herniorraphy
	Vasectomy and reversal
Occupational	Exposure to toxins
	Time away from home
Sexual	Onset of puberty
	Coital frequency and timing, knowledge of the fertile period
	Difficulties with coitus
Female	
Infertility	Duration of infertility
	Previous pregnancies in present and past relationships
	Previous investigations and treatment
Menstrual	Amenorrhoea, oligomenorrhoea, details of cycle
	Pain, menorrhagia, abnormal bleeding
Obstetric	All pregnancies including ectopic, terminations, miscarriage
	Any complications
Surgical	Abdominal and pelvic surgery
Medical	Thyroid disease
Family	Premature menopause
Sexual	Coital frequency and timing
	Knowledge of fertile period
	Difficulties with coitus

Table 5 Examination

Male	
General	Height, weight, body mass index, blood pressure
	Evidence of hypoandrogenism and gynaecomastia
Groin	Exclude inguinal hernia
Genitalia	Palpate testis, testicular volume, site in scrotum
	Palpate epididymes for nodularity or tenderness
	Presence and normality of vasa deferentia
	Check for presence of varicocoele
	Examine penis for structural abnormality
Female	
General	Height, weight, body mass index
	Acne, hirsuitism, balding
	Increased muscle mass and deep voice
	Signs of hyper- and hypothyroidism
Breast	Lumps and galactorrhoea
Pelvic	Assess hymen, clitoris, and labia
	Vagina for infection, septae, and nodules
	Cervix for polyps
	Endocervical swabs and smear
	Uterine size, tenderness, mobility, position
	Adnexal masses

Fertility investigations should be initiated after a year of unprotected intercourse for most couples, but may be started sooner in females over the age of 35 years, or those with an obvious risk factor for sub-fertility. It should be possible to perform the basic screening tests within 2–3 months and to provide the couple with a management plan. This may involve reassurance or simple remedies. Alternatively, they may require referral to a secondary or tertiary referral unit for more detailed investigations and treatment. Table 6 summarizes the investigations for both partners in primary and secondary care.

Ovulation is likely if the woman has a regular monthly cycle, but laboratory evidence may be obtained by measuring a serum progesterone level on day 21 of a 28-day cycle, or 7 days prior to expected menses in cycles of other lengths. A level in excess of 30 nmol/l indicates ovulation, and a level of 20–30 nmol/l usually suggests that ovulation is occurring, but also that the progesterone measurement has been mistimed, and should be repeated after checking the length of the cycle.

If a cycle is irregular or there are spells of amenorrhoea or a history of galactorrhoea, hirsutism, or obesity, then additional tests are appropriate. These include day 2–6 FSH, LH, oestradiol, TSH, testosterone, and prolactin levels. A raised FSH level is a more accurate reflection of reduced ovarian reserve of oocytes than chronological age and if the level is elevated (>10 iu/l) the patient should be referred early to specialist care. There is no evidence that the use of temperature charts and LH detection kits to time intercourse improves outcome, and their use should be discouraged.

Laparoscopy is the gold standard investigation for the evaluation of tubal disease but it is an invasive and costly procedure. It is particularly useful in detecting peritoneal adhesions and endometriosis. Hysteroscopy can be used to evaluate the uterine cavity at the same time. Therapeutic interventions such as division of adhesions and ablation of endometriosis may also be performed at the same time. Hysterosalpingography (HSG) is less invasive and is useful in screening for tubal patency and uterine cavity abnormalities in low-risk women. It involves the intrauterine instillation of radio opaque dye while X-ray images are taken (Fig. 1).

Hysterocontrastsonography (HyCoSy) uses ultrasonography with intrauterine injection of contrast. It has benefits in terms of better visualization of the uterine cavity and no radiation exposure but requires skilled ultrasonography to detect tubal patency (Fig. 2). As both tests involve uterine instrumentation they should be performed in the first half of the cycle with antibiotic prophylaxis.

Investigations such as endometrial biopsy to evaluate the luteal phase, the postcoital test, and specialized sperm function tests are no longer recommended as routine investigations.

Table 6 Investigations in sub-fertility

Sex	Setting	Investigation
Male	Primary care	Accurate semen analysis
		×2 if first abnormal
	Sub-fertility clinic	Male hormone profile if azoospermic
		Genetic counselling and screening
		Testicular biopsy if azoospermic
Female	Primary care	Baseline endocrine profile
		(day 2–6 FSH, LH, oestradiol,
		prolactin, TSH, testosterone)
		Luteal phase progesterone
		(day 21 or 7 days prior to onset of
		next menses)
		Rubella status
		Chlamydia swab
		Cervical smear
	Sub-fertility clinic	USS pelvis
		HSG/HyCoSy
		Laparoscopy and dye test

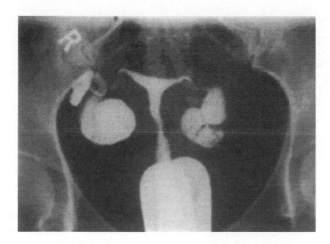

Fig. 1 Hysterosalpingogram revealing bilaterally blocked tubes with hydrosalpinges.

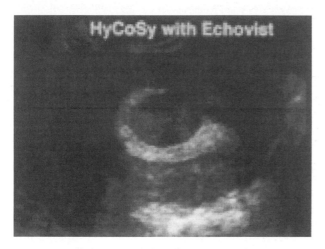

Fig. 2 Hysterocontrastsonography view of uterine cavity showing fibroid polyp.

Management

Conservative

An initial period of expectant management may be worthwhile in young couples, with less than 3 years of unexplained infertility. Conservative management of endometriosis can also be considered in mild to moderate cases before more invasive techniques are used. Medical treatment of endometriosis does not lead to increased conception rates after discontinuing therapy and, because the mechanism of action usually involves suppression of ovulation, is counterproductive. A period of conservative management may also be appropriate in young couples with mild oligozoospermia.

Danazol and bromocriptine are not effective in treating unexplained infertility. Endocrine disorders such as thyroid disease and hyperprolactinaemia should be corrected medically or surgically and male hypogonadism is amenable to medical therapy.

Surgical

Apart from microsurgical reversal of tubal sterilization and some selected cases of mild tubal damage, surgery for more serious tubal damage is generally limited in effectiveness. Even if surgery restores tubal patency, it will not improve the integrity of the damaged ciliated lining needed for tubal function and gamete/zygote transport. Laparoscopic ablation of minimal or mild endometriosis has been reported to improve fertility.

Laparoscopic drilling of polycystic ovaries by laser or diathermy is as effective as gonadotrophins in inducing ovulation resistant to clomiphene. Some cases of obstructive azoospermia may be amenable to surgical correction.

Ovulation induction

Women who are overweight with anovulation secondary to polycystic ovaries should be advised to lose weight as a first-line management option as ovulation may resume spontaneously in up to 70 per cent of cases.

The effectiveness of clomiphene citrate has been clearly demonstrated in the treatment of infertility associated with oligo-ovulation or anovulation. An initial starting dose of 50 mg on day 2–6 of the cycle is recommended. Ovulation should be confirmed by a day 21 progesterone serum level and the dose of clomiphene should be increased stepwise by 50 mg to a maximum of 150 mg. This represents a sensible first-line treatment given its low cost, ease of administration, and low incidence of side-effects. Use beyond six cycles is contra-indicated because of an increased risk of ovarian cancer with prolonged use.

An alternative to clomiphene is tamoxifen, given at a starting dose of 20 mg and increased by 20 mg to a maximum of 60 mg. In cases of prolonged amenorrhoea, it may be necessary to induce a withdrawal bleed with norethisterone.

If clomiphene is not successful or has been used for at least 6 months, ovulation can be induced with gonadotrophin (FSH) injections. These require careful ultrasound monitoring to reduce the risk of multiple pregnancy. Patients who have hypogonadotrophic hypogonadism may respond to a subcutaneous GnRH pump to stimulate FSH and LH secretion, resulting in ovulation.

Assisted conception

The term assisted conception is used to describe a number of techniques employed to treat sub-fertility. Most techniques consist of gonadotrophin stimulation of the ovaries to induce superovulation, preparation of a sperm sample, and approximation of the gametes. They should be performed in a secondary or more commonly tertiary referral unit with ongoing support from the couple's general practitioner.

The techniques include intrauterine insemination (IUI), donor insemination (DI), *in vitro* fertilization (IVF), intracytoplasmic injection (ICSI), surgical sperm retrieval (PESA or TESE), egg donation (OD), embryo and sperm cryopreservation (OS/SS), pre-implantation genetic diagnosis (PGD), and surrogacy.

Superovulation and IUI

This technique is suitable for unexplained infertility or mild sperm abnormalities. Ovulation induction of one to three follicles is achieved using gonadotrophins and semen is prepared. The rationale is to increase the density of motile sperm reaching the fallopian tube and to overcome an undiagnosed cervical factor. Pregnancy rates of 10–20 per cent can be expected after each IUI cycle with a cumulative pregnancy rate of approximately 35 per cent after three cycles. The risks of ovarian hyperstimulation and multiple pregnancy must be carefully considered.

Donor insemination

Donor insemination is an option with or without superovulation in couples with severe male factor sub-fertility or for lesbian couples or single women wishing to become pregnant.

Other assisted conception techniques are summarized in Table 7.

The outcome of treatment is determined by the age of the woman, any previous pregnancies, initial FSH levels, duration of infertility, and the number of eggs or embryos available for replacement at the end of treatment.

The complications of assisted conception can be divided into drug side-effects, ovarian hyperstimulation, and pregnancy complications such as multiple and ectopic pregnancy and miscarriage.

Table 7 Assisted conception techniques

Technique	Principle	Major indications	Outcome (live birth per cycle)
IVF	Superovulation, oocyte retrieval under ultrasound guidance, insemination of eggs with sperm to achieve fertilization, embryo culture and transcervical embryo replacement	Severe tubal disease Endometriosis Male factor infertility Unexplained infertility	20–25%
ICSI	IVF in which a single sperm is injected into the oocyte cytoplasm to allow fertilization	Severe impairment of sperm quality Previous failed fertilization at IVF	20–25%
PESA/TESE	IVF or ICSI where fresh sperm is extracted from the epididymis or testicle	Obstructive and non-obstructive azoospermia with confirmed spermatogenesis	20–25%
OD	IVF/ICSI using donated oocytes with transcervical replacement of embryos into the recipient's endometrial cavity	Absent or non-functioning ovaries/premature ovarian failure Significantly reduced ovarian reserve/poor quality oocytes in IVF	20–25%
	Cryopreservation of sperm or embryos in liquid nitrogen	Storage if surplus embryos available with IVF/ICSI or prechemotherapy for use at a later date	15–20%
PGD	Biopsy of embryos to identify unaffected embryos to be replaced	Life-threatening congenital diseases carried by parents who wish to avoid antenatal testing and termination or delivering an affected child	20–25%

Ovarian hyperstimulation syndrome (OHSS) is an iatrogenic complication of superovulation. It is characterized by enlarged ovaries and increased vascular permeability causing ascites and pleural effusions with intravascular volume depletion and haemoconcentration. If severe, it can be life-threatening causing thrombosis and multiorgan failure. It is most commonly seen with gonadotrophins but is also rarely seen with clomiphene. Risk factors include young age, low body weight, and PCOS. Management is preventative; patients with risk factors are given a lower dose of stimulation and cycles can be cancelled or embryos can be frozen and replaced when the patient has recovered.

There has been a 30 per cent increase in twin pregnancies over the last two decades. This has been attributed to assisted conception techniques and has obstetric, perinatal, and social risks. The risk of twins with IUI is 5–10 per cent and with IVF is 20–25 per cent. Decreasing the number of embryos replaced can reduce the risk of multiple pregnancy, particularly triplets. The Human Fertilisation and Embryology Authority (HFEA) guidelines are to reduce the number of embryos replaced to two in the majority of cases.

The incidence of ectopic pregnancy with IVF and ET is 2–5 per cent of pregnancies as opposed to 1 per cent in the general population. There is also an increased risk of heterotopic (combined intrauterine and ectopic pregnancy) and bilateral tubal ectopic pregnancy. The main risk factor is tubal damage. It may be possible to reduce this risk by ultrasound guided replacement of embryos. In order to minimize the morbidity and mortality of ectopic pregnancy early diagnosis with transvaginal sonography and serial measurement of serum hCG is essential. Current therapeutic options include expectant, medical, and surgical methods and the choice of treatment depends on the site and size of the ectopic pregnancy, the condition of the patient, level of expertise of the surgeon, and whether laparoscopic facilities are available.

Miscarriage is common with a rate of about 25 per cent for all spontaneous pregnancies and the rate is no different for pregnancies conceived after fertility treatment. Women are often older when going through assisted conception or have conditions such as PCOS that increase the risk of miscarriage. It is important to make an early diagnosis and to provide easy access to services to manage the miscarriage medically and emotionally.

Health promotion and patient education

Simple measures and advice can improve a couple's chance of conception and increase the chance of successful treatment. In young patients, recommendations regarding safe sexual practice to avoid genital infection can reduce the risk of damage to the fallopian tubes, epididymis, and testes. Basic advice about the correct timing of sexual intercourse during the fertile period may be helpful. If the body mass index of the female partner is greater than 30 kg/m^2 a supervised weight loss programme should be advised whether she is ovulatory or not. Although weight loss in the male will improve general health, there is little evidence that it improves fertility.

Both partners should be advised to give up smoking. Women should drink no more than 2–4 units of alcohol per week. In men, there is evidence that excessive drinking can adversely affect reproductive health.

Men with poor sperm quality should be advised to wear loose-fitting underwear and trousers and to avoid social and occupational situations that can cause testicular hyperthermia if possible.

The rubella status should be checked and if the woman is sero-negative then vaccination should be offered. Pregnancy should be avoided for 1 month after vaccination. Folic acid should be taken while trying to conceive and for the first 12 weeks of pregnancy to reduce the risk of neural tube defects. The daily dose is 0.4 mg and should be increased to 5 mg if there is a history of a previous neural tube defect or of treated epilepsy.

Quality of life issues
Psychological

In order to minimize the inevitable emotional consequences of sub-fertility, a number of important measures should be initiated. There should be easy access to services and adequate provision of accurate and comprehensive information, both verbal and written. Investigations should be carried out efficiently according to a protocol and waiting times for clinics should be kept to a minimum. An awareness among health professionals of the psychological and emotional impact of infertility is paramount. It is essential to be a good listener and to be supportive. Providing counselling can reduce distress, which may improve the outcome of treatment. Couples commonly feel frustrated that the situation appears to be outside their control. This can be alleviated by involving them with clear explanations of the implications of test results, their likelihood of conceiving with and without treatment, and the treatment options open to them, including the possibility of conservative management. Consideration should also be given to psychosexual problems, which in some couples may be pre-existing and be exacerbated by investigation and treatment.

Health economics

Health economists use the principle of sacrifice in order to gauge the need for treatment and its value in the population. In areas where state funding is not provided, couples often use up most of their savings. The average savings used per couple are around £4000 (US$ 6000)causing significant changes in lifestyle and day to day living. Infertility causes significant stress and suffering and should be regarded as a valid health need.

Key points

1. Sub-fertility is a common problem affecting one in six couples.

2. Many couples have a chance of conceiving spontaneously and conservative management may be an appropriate option after investigation.

3. Local protocols should be agreed for general practice management and referral of sub-fertile couples.

4. Advice should be given to couples to improve their general health and chances of successful reproduction.

5. Patients should be fully informed and involved with decisions regarding their treatment and have easy access to expert advice and counselling.

6. Most causes of sub-fertility are amenable to treatment either by correction of the primary problem or by using assisted conception techniques.

7. The secondary and tertiary management of infertility should take place in a dedicated fertility unit with facilities to investigate and manage couples, staffed by an appropriately trained multiprofessional team.

Further reading

Royal College of Obstetricians and Gynaecologists. *The Initial Investigation and Management of the Infertile Couple.* London: RCOG Press, 1998. (Evidence-based Guidelines No 2.)

Royal College of Obstetricians and Gynaecologists. *The Management of Infertility in Secondary Care.* London: RCOG Press, 1998. (Evidence-based Guidelines No 3.)

Rowe, P.J., Comhaire, F.H., Hargreave, T.B., and Mellows, H.J. *WHO Manual for the Standard Investigation and Diagnosis of the Infertile Couple.* Cambridge: Cambridge University Press, 1993.

Gunnell, D.J. and Ewing, P. (1994). Infertility prevalence, needs assessment and purchasing. *Journal of Public Health Medicine* 16, 29–35.

Wong, W.Y. et al. (2000). Male factor sub-fertility: possible causes and the impact of nutritional factors. *Fertility and Sterility* 73 (3), 435–42.

ESHRE (1996). Guidelines to prevalence, diagnosis, treatment and management of infertility. *Human Reproduction* 11, 1775–807.

Marcoux, S., Maheux, R., and Berube, S. (1997). Laparoscopic surgery in infertile women with minimal or mild endometriosis. *New England Journal of Medicine* 337, 217–22.

Hughes, E., Collins, J., and Vanderkerckhore, P. (1998). Clomiphene citrate versus placebo for ovulation induction in oligoamenorrheic women (Cochrane Review). In *The Cochrane Library* Issue 2. Oxford: Update Software.

Hughes, E.G. (1997). The effectiveness of ovulation induction and intrauterine insemination in the treatment of persistent infertility: a meta-analysis. *Human Reproduction* 12, 1865–72.

Clark, A.M. et al. (1995). Weight loss results in significant improvement in pregnancy and ovulation rates in anovulatory obese women. *Human Reproduction* 10, 2705–12.

Hughes, E.G. and Brennen, B.G. (1996). Does cigarette smoking impair natural or assisted fecundity? *Fertility and Sterility* 66, 679–87.

Templeton, A. The epidemiology of infertility. In *Infertility* (ed. A.A. Templeton and J.O. Drife), pp. 33–58. London: Springer-Verlag.

Van Steirteghem, A., Liebars, I., and Devroey, P. (1996). Assisted reproduction. In *Scientific Essentials of Reproductive Medicine* (ed. S.G. Hillier, H.C. Kitchener, and J.P. Neilson), pp. 230–41. New York: Saunders.

Appleton, T. (1999). The distress of infertility: impressions from 15 years of infertility counselling. In *A Textbook of In Vitro Fertilization and Assisted Reproduction* (ed. P.R. Brinsden), pp. 401–6.

Brent and Harrow Health Authority (1997). *Clinical Guidelines for the Management of Subfertility in Brent and Harrow.*

8.3 Contraception

Susan Harris and Sharon Thomson

Introduction

Contraception represents a major public health issue for this planet. UN figures report that of 185 million pregnancies each year at least 75 million are unwanted; 45 million abortions take place annually and 20 million of these are unsafe. Contraception is a relatively inexpensive way to improve the health of women and their families.

Contraceptive choice must be individualized and a number of factors need to be considered. These include: effectiveness, importance of avoiding or delaying pregnancy, cultural milieu, religious background, age, other health considerations, role of the partner, need for protection against sexually transmitted infections (STIs), accessibility, and cost. The World Health Organization has developed medical eligibility criteria for initiation and continuation of all methods of contraception. This document is referenced worldwide and provides excellent guidelines.

Fertility awareness or natural methods

Natural or fertility awareness methods are based on identification of the days of a menstrual cycle when pregnancy is likely to occur. The actual fertile time lasts for about 6 days of each cycle (sperm living up to 5 days and the egg living less than 1 day). During these days couples may abstain, or use a barrier method or withdrawal. Efficacy depends on the method used (see Table 1). Most unintended pregnancies are related to the failure to abstain or use a barrier method and misidentification of the fertile time. Advantages include absence of side-effects, minimal cost, acceptability to certain religions, and increased understanding of fertility. Fertility awareness methods are unreliable postpartum, after hormonal contraception, when breastfeeding, or in the presence of vaginal infection.

The *calendar method* is used to determine the fertile time based on previous cycle length. *Basal body temperature* (BBT) is based on the increase in temperature that occurs at ovulation; barrier or abstinence may be used through the first part of the cycle until the temperature change is observed. Identification of the clear, stretchy, slippery *cervical secretions* of

Table 1 Contraceptive effectiveness

Effectiveness group	Contraceptive method	Pregnancies per 100 women in first 12 months of use	
		As commonly used	Used correctly and consistently
Always very effective	Implants	0.1	0.1
	Vasectomy	0.2	0.1
	Combined injectables	0.3	0.3
	DMPA and NET-EN injectables	0.3	0.3
	Female sterilization	0.5	0.5
	TCu-380A IUD	0.8	0.6
	Progestogen-only oral contraceptives (during breastfeeding)	1	0.5
Effective as commonly used Very effective when used correctly and consistently	Lactational amenorrhoea method	2	0.5
	Combined oral contraceptives	6–8	0.1
	Progestogen-only oral contraceptives (not during breastfeeding)		0.5
Only somewhat effective as commonly used Effective when used correctly and consistently	Male condoms	14	3
	Withdrawal (coitus interruptus)	19	4
	Diaphragm with spermicide	20	6
	Fertility awareness-based methods	20	1–9
	Female condoms	21	5
	Spermicides	26	6
	Cap with spermicide—Nulliparous women	20	9
	Cap with spermicide—Parous women	40	26
	No method	85	85

Emergency contraceptive pills: Treatment initiated within 72 h after unprotected intercourse reduces the risk of pregnancy by at least 75%.

Adapted from Hatcher, R.A. et al. *Managing Contraception*, Millennium edition. Tiger GA: The Bridging the Gap Foundation, 1999.

Adapted from World Health Organization. *Improving Access to Quality Care in Family Planning: Medical Eligibility Criteria for Contraceptive Use* 2nd edn. Geneva: World Health Organization, 2000 (WHO/RHR/00.02).

ovulation indicates the need to abstain or use a barrier method. *Symptothermal* methods indicate fertility by cervical secretions, BBT, change in cervical position, ovulation pain, midcycle spotting, breast, and skin changes. Over the counter *home test kits* rely on the detection of luteinizing hormone (LH) at ovulation.

> *Lactational amenorrhoea:* If an infant is fed only breast milk and the mother has not had postpartum menses, breastfeeding provides more than 98% protection against pregnancy in the first 6 months after birth. Guidelines include less than 4 h between daytime feeds, less than 6 h intervals at night, and less than 5–15% of feeds supplemented.

Vaginal methods

Vaginal methods consist of physical and chemical barriers with use related to coitus. These methods are simple, non-invasive, and controlled by the woman. They may also provide protection against STIs. They require that a woman be comfortable with insertion and may require fitting by a health care provider. Efficacy varies with the method used and may be influenced by parity (see Table 1).

The *diaphragm* is a dome-shaped latex rubber cup with a flexible rim available in varying sizes and types. Correct placement of the device, retention for at least 6 h after coitus and utilization of spermicide for each episode of intercourse determine efficacy. A higher risk of urinary tract infection with diaphragm (and cervical cap) use is most likely related to *Escherichia coli* colonization secondary to the spermicide. Other risks include latex allergy, vaginal irritation, and risk of Toxic Shock Syndrome. New silicone diaphragm-like devices are currently available in some countries. The *cervical cap* is a soft deep rubber cap with a firm rim that fits around the base of the cervix. It is used with spermicide and can be left in place for 48 h. The *female condom* is a soft loose-fitting lubricated polyurethane sheath. It has a large outer rim, which remains outside the vulva and a smaller ring on the inner closed end, which encircles the cervix. The condom is used once only and can be inserted up to 8 h before intercourse. It is less likely to rupture than a male condom. It provides protection against STIs. The contraceptive *sponge* is a polyurethane device that contains spermicide. The sponge is inserted deep into the vagina and provides protection for 12 to 24 h, regardless of the number of episodes of intercourse. It should be left in place for at least 6 h after intercourse. *Spermicides* consist of active spermicidal agent(s) and a carrier or base. The mechanism of action is through immobilization or destruction of sperm. The most commonly used active agent is nonoxynol-9. The carrier may be gel, foam, cream, film, suppository, or tablet. Efficacy depends on correct placement no longer than 1 h prior to intercourse. Spermicide use may lead to increased vaginal and urinary tract infections.

Male methods

Male methods have been widely used for centuries. They provide inexpensive, easily accessible contraception with few risks but are coitally dependent. Efficacy depends on correct and consistent use.

The *male condom* consists of a thin sheath placed over the penis, which acts as a barrier to the passage of semen. It must be used throughout the act of intercourse. Condoms can be made of latex rubber, natural membrane, plastic, or polyurethane. Failure may be related to incorrect use or breakage and slippage. Disadvantages may include decreased sensitivity and spontaneity, which may lead to erection problems. Latex allergy has become an issue for some but can be avoided with the polyurethane type of condom.

> Condoms have the advantage of providing STI protection. They are portable, hygienic, and provide visible proof of protection.

Withdrawal (coitus interruptus) relies on the prevention of contact between sperm and the egg. Penile–vaginal intercourse takes place until ejaculation is imminent at which point the male partner 'withdraws' from the vagina and away from the external genitalia of the female. Sperm in the pre-ejaculate may increase pregnancy risk. The method has no cost, involves no chemicals or devices, and is free of side-effects. The risk of STIs may be decreased (probably because of decreased volume of semen entering the vagina) but it is not eliminated. Disadvantages are that it requires consistent and correct use as well as a high level of self-control. Withdrawal may decrease the pleasure of the sexual act.

Hormonal methods

Oral contraception

An oral contraceptive is a substance or combination of substances administered by mouth to prevent pregnancy. The oral contraceptives that are most commonly prescribed are those containing oestrogen and a progestogen, referred to as combined oral contraceptives (COCs). Progestogen-only pills (POPs) are often prescribed to women who are unable to tolerate oestrogen-related side-effects or are lactating. Oral contraceptives are safe, effective, and used extensively by women throughout the world.

Combined oral contraceptives

COCs disrupt ovulation and implantation. The oestrogen in the pill causes suppression of follicle stimulating hormone (FSH) and luteinizing hormone (LH). The progestogen in COCs causes the cervical mucus to thicken, disrupts ovulation, interferes with sperm penetrability, and produces a decidualized endometrial bed, which hampers implantation.

COCs are comprised of 35 μg or less of the oestrogenic compounds ethinyl estradiol or mestranol. COCs also contain first-, second-, or third-generation progestogens. COCs come in preparations that are either fixed-dose (the daily ratio of oestrogen and progestogen remains constant) or phasic (the ratio of the oestrogen and progestogen changes once or twice in a 21-day course). There has traditionally been a 7 day pill-free interval (PFI) between cycles as it takes 7 days to shut down follicular development. This regimen may contribute to an increase in unintended pregnancies, due to ovulation, if more than 7 days elapse before the next cycle is initiated.

> It is appropriate to shorten or eliminate the PFI for up to three cycles (tricycling) using a fixed-dose pill. Tricycling is also frequently used for such problems as headaches (including migraines with non-focal aura that occur during the hormone-free interval), heavy or painful withdrawal bleeds, and premenstrual syndrome.

Effectiveness is one of the primary reasons a woman or couple will choose COCs (see Table 1). COCs are also safe, reversible, and offer a reproductive lifetime option (may be used until menopause if there are no contra-indications). Non-contraceptive benefits of COCs include protective effects against endometrial cancer, ovarian cancer, ovarian cysts, benign breast disease, ectopic pregnancy, pelvic inflammatory disease (PID), and endometriosis as well as treatment for acne, hirsutism, chronic anovulation, and anaemia. The pill also provides menstrual benefits of decreased pain, PMS, and blood loss. Disadvantages include troublesome side-effects in the first 3–6 months, which may lead to discontinuation. COCs provide no protection against STIs. This option is contra-indicated with the following: age over 35 and smoking, hypertension (160/100 or higher), diabetes with neuropathy/retinopathy, vascular disease, history of or active deep vein thrombosis or pulmonary embolism, major surgery with prolonged immobilization, history of a stroke, complicated pulmonary hypertension, atrial fibrillation, history of subacute bacterial endocarditis, migraines with focal neurologic symptoms at any age, current breast cancer, or liver disease.

Physical examination and laboratory tests prior to a woman receiving COCs are unnecessary barriers to access. Written and oral instructions should always be provided with an invitation to return within 3–6 months to discuss any concerns, check the blood pressure, and reinforce correct use. COCs are currently being supplied by non-physician providers in many parts of the world where access to medical care is limited.

Progestogen-only oral contraceptives (POPs, Minipill)

POPs contain a small dose of one of the progestogens levonorgestrel, norethisterone, or ethynodiol diacetate. POPs are an excellent choice for women who are breastfeeding or who cannot take oestrogen. The progestogens in POPs act in the same manner as those in COCs with thickening of cervical mucus being the primary mechanism. POPs are generally less effective than COCs (see Table 1). Missing a pill by more than 3 h requires a back up method for at least 48 h and emergency contraception if unprotected intercourse occurred during this time. There is no PFI with POPS. All of the pills in the packet contain hormone.

Relative contraindications to POPs include severe arterial wall disease, liver disease, undiagnosed pregnancy, trophoblastic disease, and porphyria. As with other progestogen-only methods, irregular bleeding is not uncommon, but amenorrhoea may also occur after prolonged use. Breast tenderness and depression are less common.

POPS are underutilized in spite of the fact that with good counselling and more willingness to provide this method, more women would have access to a reliable and appropriate contraceptive.

Hormonal vaginal rings and patches

For women who have difficulty remembering to take a pill every day, both of these devices offer an alternative hormonal delivery system of oestrogen and progestogen. The ring is inserted in the vagina and remains in place for 3 weeks; it is removed for 1 week before reinserting. The patch is worn for 1 week at a time and is changed on the same day of the week three times a month with the fourth week being patch-free.

Subdermal implants

Implants containing a progestogen in a slow-release carrier are surgically inserted in the upper arm. Implants are highly effective for up to 5 years (see Table 1), are oestrogen free, and readily reversible. Mechanisms of action and side-effects are similar to those attributed to other progestogen-only methods.

Injectable contraception

Injectable contraception refers to the injection of hormones to prevent pregnancy. Choices include depot medroxyprogesterone (DMPA) acetate 150 mg every 12 weeks, norethisterone oenanthate 200 mg every 8 weeks, and, more recently, medroxyprogesterone 25 mg/estradiol cypprionate 5 mg every month. The mechanism is the prevention of ovulation. The method is convenient, safe, reversible, and highly effective (see Table 1). It provides long-acting contraception and is controlled by the woman. Progestogen-only injectables are also suitable for lactating women and for those in whom oestrogen is contra-indicated. They may also reduce seizure frequency in epileptics. Injectable contraception may cause menstrual irregularity (management: low-dose COC for one or more cycles, Premarin 1.25 mg daily for 21 days or moving up the timing for the next dose). Other side-effects may include weight gain, breast tenderness, depression, decrease in bone density as well changes in lipids (decrease in HDL). The hormones cannot immediately be withdrawn and infertility may sometimes persist for 18 months after discontinuing treatment. Injectable contraception is contra-indicated in pregnancy and by undiagnosed vaginal bleeding, thromboembolic disorders, and breast cancer.

> Injectable contraception requires return visits to the caregiver. Innovative means to improve access and facilitate re-injection need to be sought, such as work site or pharmacy injection or self-administration.

Emergency contraception

Emergency contraception refers to any method used after intercourse and before implantation. There are two main methods—*hormonal and intrauterine contraceptive devices*. The *Yuzpe* method refers to the use of a regimen of a COC in two doses 12 h apart commenced within 72 h of the earliest act of unprotected intercourse. A second hormonal regimen utilizes 750 μg of levonorgestrol repeated in 12 h. Both methods can be used at any time in the cycle and regardless of the number of episodes of intercourse. The mechanism of action is similar to that of other hormonal methods. Emergency contraception prevents 75–85 per cent of the pregnancies that would have occurred if emergency contraception had not been used (98 per cent efficacy rate). Efficacy improves with treatment prior to 72 h. The progestogen-only method has slightly higher efficacy and fewer side-effects than the Yuzpe. The main contra-indications are pregnancy, acute migraine, allergy to hormones, and ethical objection to its use after fertilization.

> Emergency contraception can provide a safe effective method, which is unrelated to coitus and can be controlled by the woman. It can be prescribed in advance and in some countries it can now be obtained at a pharmacy.

An *intrauterine contraceptive device* can be inserted up to 5–8 days after intercourse. The failure rate of this method is less than 0.1 per cent but it requires a surgical procedure and carries the risk of PID and pain. It is useful when there is an absolute contra-indication for oestrogen or progestin or when this is the long-term method desired.

Intrauterine contraceptive device

The intrauterine contraceptive device (IUCD) more commonly called an intrauterine device (IUD) or coil is a solid object, usually made of a plastic material that may be coated with copper or medicated with a progestogen. Most IUDs have frames, but two frameless or implantable IUDs are now available. The IUD is placed in the uterine cavity for the purpose of preventing pregnancy primarily by preventing sperm from fertilizing ova. Copper IUDs also alter tubal and uterine transport. There is no evidence to support the belief that the IUD is an abortifacient. Progestogen IUDs act hormonally as in oral contraceptives.

Effectiveness is determined by size, shape, presence of copper or progestogen, user age, and parity. IUDs are very effective (see Table 1). Some IUDs may be used for up to 12 years making them highly cost-effective. IUDs are indicated for women who cannot use hormonal methods and want long-term reversible contraception. They are contra-indicated for those with copper allergy and increased risk for STIs. IUDs offer safe contraception independent of intercourse, and do not require remembering to take a pill every day. Hormone-releasing IUDs are also being used as an effective treatment for menorrhagia. Some women experience heavier, longer menses, and dysmenorrhoea, especially during the first few months after insertion. Pelvic inflammatory disease is a complication attributed to insertion of the IUD and subsequent exposure to sexually transmitted infection. Expulsions and pregnancy complication are less common complications.

> Approximately 110 million women worldwide use IUDs; 50 million of these are in China. This method is underutilized in the rest of the world, most likely due to previous problems with older types of IUDs. Accurate education for women and providers would improve access and provision of this highly effective method.

Sterilization

Since women may be fertile up to the age of 50 or more years and males are fertile for most of their lives, more permanent contraception is often sought once childbearing has been completed. This is one of the most widely utilized methods throughout the world. Safety of both male and female sterilization has improved with better patient selection, improved general anaesthesia, the increased use of local anaesthetics, improved surgical techniques, and better-trained personnel.

Female sterilization

Sterilization involves blocking the fallopian tubes to prevent sperm from uniting with an egg. Ligation, mechanical occlusion, and electro-coagulation are the main methods used under local or general anaesthesia. Sterilization can be performed in the interval period (more than 4 weeks after delivery), postpartum, or post-abortion. Sterilization is one of the most effective contraceptive methods (see Table 1). Advantages are safety and permanence. It is also woman-controlled, unrelated to coitus, and offers privacy. Immediate complications are rare and pertain to haemorrhage, injury to organs, or respiratory problems; the use of general anaesthesia increases the risk. Long-term problems include regret (associated with younger age and life events such as loss of a child or new spouse). Non-contraceptive effects include decreased incidence of ovarian cancer, possible enhanced sexuality, and decreased PID.

Vasectomy (male sterilization)

Vasectomy refers to the blockage of the vas deferens to prevent sperm from passing into the ejaculated seminal fluid. Conventional methods include a small incision or puncture wound over the vas, following which the vas is cut and occluded. This is a safe minor surgical procedure with few complications. Effectiveness is not well researched but pregnancy rates are thought to be 0.1 per cent in the first year. Advantages are similar to those from female sterilization, aside from the fact that it is male-controlled. Concerns have arisen over long-term side-effects of development of sperm antibodies and increased risk of prostate cancer; the literature has not confirmed a significant risk of either of these.

Conclusion

Contraceptive technology offers many choices to women and their partners. However, the challenge remains to educate women and providers about these options. Patient information and education in the appropriate language and literacy level is critical in order for people to change personal behaviour and reduce health risks. Teaching should be offered in a non-judgemental manner and tailored to the readiness of the woman. Written, verbal, and pictorial information helps to reinforce learning, enhance retention, and empower women to be more successful contraceptors. Finally, the approach to education about fertility control should also include discussions about disease prevention as well as pregnancy. Providers must be diligent in sharing the concept of 'Dual Protection' as it reflects the reality of HIV, AIDS, and other STIs, which are major health concerns worldwide.

Further reading

Guillebaud, J. *Contraception: Your Questions Answered*. London: Harcourt Publishers, 1999.

Dunn, S. (2001). Emergency contraception and family physicians. An ounce of prevention when it really counts. *Canadian Family Physician* **47**, 1159–60.

Hatcher, R.A. et al. *Managing Contraception*. Tiger GA: Bridging the Gap Foundation, 1999.

Hatcher, R.A. et al. *Contraceptive Technology* 17th revised edn. New York: Ardent Media Inc, 1998.

The Society of Obstetricians and Gynaecologists of Canada. *Sex Sense: Canadian Contraception Guide.* Ottawa: Society of Obstetricians and Gynaecologists of Canada, 2000.

Acheson, L.S. and Danner, S.C. (1993). Postpartum care and breast-feeding. *Primary Care* **20**, 729–47.

World Health Organization. *Improving Access to Quality Care in Family Planning: Medical Eligibility Criteria for Contraceptive Use* 2nd edn. Geneva: World Health Organization, 1996.

Speroff, L. and Darney, P. *A Clinical Guide for Contraception.* Baltimore MD: Williams & Wilkins, 1996.

Nelson, A.S. (2000). The intrauterine contraceptive device. *Obstetrics and Gynecology Clinics of North America: Update in Contraception* **27** (4), 723–40.

Kaunitz, A. (2000). Injectable contraception: new and existing options. *Obstetrics and Gynecology Clinics of North America: Update in Contraception* **27** (4), 741–80.

Lavalleur, J. (2000). Emergency contraception. *Obstetrics and Gynecology Clinics of North America: Update in Contraception* **27** (4), 817–40.

Gilliam, M.L. and Derman, R.J. (2000). Barrier methods of contraception. *Obstetrics and Gynecology Clinics of North America: Update in Contraception* **27** (4), 841–58.

Hatcher, R.A. et al. (2001). Contraceptive patch, ring: in US by 2001. *Contraceptive Technology Update* **22** (8), 88–9.

Dickinson, J. et al. *Contraceptive Patient Handout Manual.* Atlanta GA: American Health Care Consultants, 2000.

8.4 **Normal pregnancy**

Elizabeth Shaw and David Price

Pregnancy is a normal biological process that is supported and nurtured by good pre-natal care (Chapter 8.1). Wherever possible this involves using the best available evidence to: (i) maintain excellent physical and psychological health for the woman and her unborn child in the context of her family and community; and (ii) prevent and screen for problems which may arise. As positive pregnancy outcomes are linked to caregiver relationships and consistency, the family physician is ideally suited to this task.[1] The paradigm of pregnancy as a natural, physiologic event is philosophically consistent with our discipline and we have the unique capacity to provide continuity of care for the entire family. The goal of this chapter is to assist with the provision of this essential care.

The content of pre-natal care

The optimum number of pre-natal visits has not been established. Recent trials indicate that between four and nine visits are compatible with good maternal and neonatal outcomes in low-risk women. In a recent randomized controlled trial examining a reduced number of antenatal visits in low risk women (average 8.6) in the United Kingdom, there were no differences in measures of maternal or perinatal morbidity. However these women had poorer psychosocial outcomes (worry, negative attitudes toward their babies) and reduced satisfaction with their pre-natal care.[2,3] The Society of Obstetricians and Gynecologists of Canada recommend visits every 4–6 weeks until 30 weeks, every 2–3 weeks until 36 weeks and every 1–2 weeks until delivery.[4] This is similar to 1989 recommendations from the US Expert Panel on the Content of Prenatal care.

There are many tools to assist the clinician in implementing evidence-based care. One of these is the Maternity Care Calendar and Guidelines checklist developed in British Columbia, based on the Canadian Task Force on the Periodic Health Examination and the United States Preventive Services Task Force. Further information is available in refs 5 and 6.

Antenatal psycho-social assessment

The comprehensive psycho-social assessment of the mother and her partner is now recognized as an essential component of routine prenatal care. Child and woman abuse and postpartum depression are strongly associated with lack of social support, recent life stressors, and maternal psychiatric disease. A history of previous abuse, and poor maternal self-esteem also strongly correlate with child abuse.

The Antenatal Psychosocial Health Assessment Form (ALPHA) was designed following a systematic review of the literature to assist practitioners with the psychosocial assessment of their pregnant patients.[7] Easily incorporated into one or several pre-natal visits, it assesses 15 antenatal factors which show a strong association with adverse postpartum outcomes such as child abuse, couple dysfunction, and depression. In a recent qualitative study, its use was well accepted by clinicians and patients. It allows the early identification of issues that may be amenable to intervention and increased support, as well as the enhancement of physician–patient rapport.[8]

Care during the first trimester

History and physical

The establishment of an accurate last menstrual period (LMP) and estimated date of delivery (EDD) is one of the most important goals of the first pre-natal visit. These have implications for the timing of investigations and interventions, particularly with the post-term pregnancy. Naegle's rule determines the EDD by taking the date of the last menstrual period, adding 7 days and subtracting 3 months.

At the first pre-natal visit a previous pregnancy history, history of major medical illnesses, genetic history, and family history focusing on high-risk groups (e.g. Tay Sachs, sickle cell) should be obtained. This is the most important time to discuss a woman's plans for breast-feeding, as most women decide this issue very early in pregnancy. A directed physical exam with emphasis on blood pressure, breast exam, nutritional status, and uterine size should be done. Diagnosis of breast lumps should be pursued as some types of breast cancer are accelerated by pregnancy.

Screening

Blood work

Initial blood tests should include a haemoglobin, blood type, Rh factor, an antibody screen, and rubella. If the rubella titre is non-immune, the patient should be offered vaccination postpartum. Serologic screening for syphilis is recommended even when prevalence rates are low as curative treatment is available that also prevents foetal transmission. Similarly, antiretroviral therapy for the human immunodeficiency virus (HIV) reduces foetal transmission rates by greater than 60 per cent. In North America, 70 per cent of female HIV cases had no risk factors. Counselling for HIV testing should occur with all pregnant women.

Other sexually transmitted diseases

Consider screening for chlamydia and gonorrhoea depending on the prevalence of disease in the community and the risk factors in individual patients. Neonatal conjunctivitis, acquired at the time of delivery, is the major risk to the foetus. Bacterial vaginosis is associated with preterm birth before 37 weeks. A recent double blind randomized controlled trial in 500 UK women has shown that screening and treating pregnant women with asymptomatic bacterial vaginosis was associated with a reduction in the rate of preterm birth (number needed to treat = 14). Bacterial vaginosis is also associated with late miscarriage after 13 weeks, but is not a strong factor for first trimester miscarriage.

Papanicolau smear (PAP)

The first pre-natal visit presents an opportunity to screen women who have not had a recent PAP. If the patient undertakes regular screening, and has had a normal PAP within the past 2 years, the PAP may be deferred to the postpartum period. PAP smears taken in pregnancy are less likely to contain cells from the transformation zone, and are thus less reliable for diagnosis.

Health maintenance and prevention

Common symptoms in early pregnancy

First trimester bleeding occurs in approximately 30 per cent of all pregnancies and one in seven will miscarry. Bed rest and hormone administration does not prevent pregnancy loss. The woman should contact her family physician if the bleeding is more than just mild spotting or is associated with abdominal pain.

At least half of all pregnant women experience nausea and vomiting in the first trimester. Small, frequent meals, eating upon wakening, and salty foods may control symptoms. Accupressure at the Neiguan point (on the inner aspect of the wrist proximal to the flexor crease) is also effective. More severe nausea or hyperemesis gravidarium may respond to a combination of doxylamine succinate 10 mg with pryidoxine HCl 10 mg (marketed in Canada as Diclectin). The usual dose is two tablets at bedtime. Another can be added in the morning and mid day if needed. This medication has been shown to be extremely safe in pregnancy.

Dietary recommendations/supplements

One of the most effective pre-natal manoeuvres, as discussed in the previous chapter, is the use of folic acid to prevent neural tube defects. No specific dietary supplementation has been shown to reduce the risk of pre-term birth or low birth weight. Similarly, there is nothing to support dietary restriction of any type during pregnancy. Calcium supplementation may reduce the risk of high blood pressure including pre-eclampsia during pregnancy, but there is no proven reduction in perinatal mortality. Current recommended daily intake in Canada is 12–1500 mg daily. Routine iron supplementation improves women's iron stores, but has no other effect on maternal or foetal health. If there is clear evidence of iron deficiency (Hgb <10, with microcytic indices, or low iron levels), iron supplementation is indicated.

Weight gain recommendations in pregnancy are controversial. No experimental evidence relates improved perinatal outcomes to weight manipulation. Observational studies show an association between pre-term birth and weight gain below the recommended range (11.5–16 kg) in women with a normal pre-pregnancy BMI (20–25). Similarly, weight gain above this range is associated with an increased risk of macrosomia, cesarean section, and postpartum weight retention.[9] High-risk groups who are malnourished, and adolescents may need to gain more weight. Weight gain should not fall below 6.8 kg regardless of pre-pregnant weight.

Lifestyle issues

There is no reason in a low-risk pregnancy to limit a woman's activities, assuming there are no risks of exposure to environmental toxins or excess physical stress (see pre-term birth prevention). Likewise, there is no reason to curtail sexual activity. Regular moderate exercise (defined as the ability to carry on a conversation during exercise) in a low-risk pregnancy has positive benefits for cardiorespiratory fitness with no obvious adverse maternal or foetal effects.

There is strong evidence that cigarette smoking reduces birthweight and is associated with pre-term birth and perinatal death. Behaviourally focused smoking cessation programmes have been shown to be effective. Regular alcohol use in pregnancy (2×1 oz drinks/day) also affects foetal growth and the foetal brain adversely. Although the 'safe' limit of alcohol during pregnancy has not been established, many clinicians recommend abstention. As women often consume alcohol prior to knowledge of their pregnancy, care should be taken not to instill excessive guilt, as moderate alcohol intake has not been associated with adverse foetal outcomes. A discussion of recreational drug use is beyond the scope of this chapter, but there is certainly some data to suggest adverse effects on foetal growth, and/or neuropsychological function. The reader is directed to the additional resources.

Infectious diseases

Infections such as varicella, toxoplasmosis, and parvovirus (Fifth's disease) are of concern as they have potentially severe consequences for the newborn. The issue often arises after exposure when pregnant woman questions her risk. More than 85 per cent of women with no history of varicella are immune, however if in doubt, a rapid latex agglutination test for varicella IgG can be performed. If this test is unavailable then varicella immune globulin should be given within 96 h of exposure. More common in Europe than in North America, toxoplasmosis is a parasite found in cat faeces. Screening is not recommended in low endemic areas. Primary prevention by eating well-cooked meat and pasteurized milk products, washing hands after handling raw meat or vegetables and wearing gloves while gardening, or changing the litter box is recommended. As most of the parasite resides in soil and water, risks from soil exposure are actually higher than that from cats. Parvovirus, a common viral illness in children, may cause haemolytic disease of the newborn if acquired in utero. An assay for specific IgG can confirm immunity. Although the risk of transmission is small, close ultrasound examination to detect hydrops is suggested in exposed non-immune women.

Pre-natal classes

Antenatal education classes which focus in part on coping mechanisms during labour and delivery have been shown to reduce the amount of analgesic required during labour and increase satisfaction with some aspects of childbirth.[10] If accurate and unbiased information on childbirth options is made available, the well-informed consumer may help to influence the implementation of evidence-based care.

Care during the second trimester

Screening

Routine ultrasound

Although a meta-analysis of routine early ultrasound shows a reduction in perinatal mortality, this is entirely due to elective termination of abnormal foetuses detected.[11] Induction rates for post-dated pregnancies are reduced but this does not translate into improved foetal outcomes. An 18–20-week ultrasound is recommended as it gives good assessment of foetal anatomy and still allows women options for termination. Overall, about 50 per cent of abnormalities are detected with a false positive fate of 0.2–1.0 per 1000. Women value ultrasound, which generally reduces anxiety and increases confidence in the pregnancy. There is fair evidence to include routine ultrasound in pre-natal care.[12]

Foetal growth

Measurement of the symphisis-fundal height (SFH) by a consistent observer has fair sensitivity and specificity for predicting low birth weight, and may be a useful screening test prompting ultrasound evaluation for foetal growth restriction. Maternal weight gain does seem to correlate with foetal growth at extremes and poor weight gain may be a marker for emotional, financial, or social problems in the pregnancy. Assessment of weight and SFH should be part of every second and third trimester visit.

Congenital/chromosomal abnormalities

The use of a risk score combining a woman's age with serum levels of alpha foetoprotein, unconjugated estriol and human chorionic gonadatrophin (HCG) measured between 15 and 21 weeks of gestation (triple screening), can detect up to 70 per cent of trisomy 21 (Down syndrome) and 60 per cent of trisomy 18. With a risk cut-off of 1/385, the false positive rate is about 9.5 per cent. Alpha foetoprotein also screens for neural tube defects, with a positive test result usually considered greater than 2.2 multiples of the mean. The accuracy of the test depends upon accurate dating. In North America, all women are offered triple screening, and those with positive results are offered amniocentesis as are women 35 and older at the time of delivery.

In parts of Europe, combining a 10–13-week ultrasound for nuchal fold thickness with serum HCG, pregnancy-associated placental protein (PAPP-A) levels, and maternal age has a 75–85 per cent sensitivity for Down syndrome. Studies are ongoing in North America.

Amniocentesis is usually performed between 16 and 18 weeks gestation and carries a 0.5–1.0 per cent risk of miscarriage and a 0.5 per cent risk of very low birth weight babies. Although chorionic villus sampling (CVS) provides first trimester diagnosis, the risks are higher. Transabdominal CVS is available prior to 16 weeks, but is currently experimental.

Pregnancy-induced hypertension (PIH)

PIH may occur at any time in the second half of pregnancy but rarely prior to 28 weeks. Screening involves the use of a mercury sphygmomanometer and a stethoscope with the patient sitting or in the left lateral position with the arm at the level of the heart. Both the fourth and fifth Korotkoff sound should be used to record the diastolic pressure, with the fourth being used to initiate investigation, due to its wider margin of safety. An absolute blood pressure of 140/90 or greater is considered abnormal and should signal the need for closer monitoring. The presence of 1+ protein or greater on a urine dipstick is also significant, however in the presence of persistent hypertension, a negative urine cannot be relied upon, and a 24-h urine for protein should be ordered. Oedema is common in normal pregnancy, and is not useful as a screening test for PIH. Blood pressure readings and a urine dip for protein should be a part of each visit during the second and third trimesters. As PIH is a multisystem disease, it can occasionally present without hypertension or proteinuria. Patients who present with right upper quadrant pain, central nervous system symptoms or signs of placental insufficiency (poor foetal growth) should be evaluated for this condition (see Chapter 8.6).

Health maintenance and prevention

Most of the health maintenance and prevention issues discussed in the first trimester apply to the entire pregnancy. There are a few additional issues which now become relevant.

Pre-term birth prevention

Pre-term birth is the leading cause of perinatal morbidity and mortality. Treatment of asymptomatic bacteriuria and smoking cessation have been shown to reduce pre-term birth rates. There does appear to be a 1.2–1.5 times higher risk of pre-term birth in women who stand for prolonged periods (>2 h). Although there is no clear guideline, risks/benefits should be discussed with women who have physically stressful jobs. Otherwise population-based strategies must educate women to present early for care with any signs or symptoms of pre-term birth. Pre-term birth should be discussed at every second and early third trimester visit.

Common discomforts of pregnancy

Women frequently complain of fatigue, backache, heartburn, constipation, leg cramps, and oedema. Most of these symptoms will respond to reassurance and common sense such as limiting activity and avoidance of aggravating activities. Heartburn can be controlled by eating small frequent meals, and avoiding food prior to bed. Antacids can be safely prescribed when necessary. H_2 blockers are probably safe to use in resistant cases. Constipation responds best to an increase in dietary fibre and fluids with the addition of stool softeners if necessary. Mineral oil and saline cathartics should be avoided. Leg cramps respond to massage and stretching of the affected muscles. There is no evidence of benefit from sodium or calcium supplements. Leg oedema is experienced by 80 per cent of women, and is not a sign of pre-eclampsia. Support stockings may give temporary relief, but can be very uncomfortable.

Gestational diabetes

Although screening for gestational diabetes in the second trimester is a routine part of pre-natal care in many countries, no data support this practice. Screening is normally done at 24–28 weeks gestation by measuring the blood sugar 1 h after a 50-g glucose load. At a cut-off point of 7.8 mmol/l, the sensitivity and specificity for predicting an abnormal glucose tolerance test is 79 and 83 per cent, respectively.[13] The screening test is only valid during this narrow time window however, and the gold standard 100 mg glucose tolerance test (GTT) is reproducible less than 50 per cent of the time. There is also no convincing evidence that treatment of women with an abnormal GTT reduces perinatal mortality or morbidity.[14] A large study involving two regions in the province of Ontario, Canada with opposing policies on universal screening for gestational diabetes, examined 8 years of data and over 800 000 women. Despite a significant rise in the prevalence of gestational diabetes in the universal screening region, there was no difference in rates of foetal macrosomia, caesarean delivery or other pregnancy complications.[15] Both the 50 g glucose challenge and 100 g GTT can be used for case finding (i.e. in obese women, or women with a history of previous macrosomia). Women in whom diabetes is suspected should be followed with fasting and 2 h post-prandial blood sugars during their pregnancies.

Care during the third trimester

Screening

Group B strep

Group B Streptococcus bacteria exist asymptomatically in the GI/GUI tract of many women and is transmitted to a small number of neonates during the birth process. Intrapartum prophylaxis is effective at reducing the morbidity and mortality associated with neonatal infection. Currently accepted strategies for preventing this transmission include screening at 36 weeks (lower 1/3 of the vagina and rectal swab) and giving intrapartum antibiotics to positive mothers once labour ensues. The other alternative is to treat risk factors while in labour. These include prolonged rupture of membranes (>18 h), maternal fever, pre-term labour, previous group B strep bacteriuria and prior history of an infant infected with group B strep. Treatment usually consists of intravenous penicillin. Attempts to eradicate the bacteria prior to delivery are not successful.

Health maintenance and prevention

Monitoring of SFH, weight, measurement of blood pressure, and urine dip for protein should continue with each visit. Routine vaginal exams do not offer any added information and are not recommended.

Foetal movement counting

Formal maternal monitoring of foetal movement does not improve perinatal mortality and may increase maternal anxiety. Subjective feelings of decreased foetal movement, however, should prompt assessment for foetal well-being with a non-stress test (NST) or biophysical profile (BPP). These standardized tests of doppler measurement of the foetal heart rate (NST) or ultrasound measurement of foetal rate, movement, amniotic fluid levels and foetal breathing patterns allow for reassurance of both the patient and clinician.

Breech presentation

Assessment of foetal position is important near term as breech version after 37 weeks by a skilled operator is associated with a 58 per cent reduction in the relative risk of a non-cephalic presentation and a corresponding reduction in cesarean sections. The value of this is emphasized by the results of the Term Breech trial, which indicate a higher perinatal mortality in breech presentations delivered vaginally.[18] The knee–chest position prior to labour may also reduce non-cephalic presentations, but trials were small.

Labour preparation

At or before the 36th week visit is an ideal time to review expectations/plans for delivery. Administrative details (when and whom to phone, procedure to follow once in labour) should also be discussed. The role of the partner in support and pain management should be discussed. This is an area which is often overlooked but may have a significant positive effect not only on the delivery but on the couple's postpartum relationship.

Perineal massage in the third trimester reduces the incidence of perineal trauma in primiparous but not multiparous patients. Information on the technique can be found in the additional resources.

Based on a meta-analysis of randomized controlled trials showing a reduction in perinatal mortality, women with reliable dates should be offered induction after 41 weeks gestational age.[19] Some form of foetal monitoring should occur after 41 weeks in women who elect a more conservative approach. This is further discussed in Chapter 8.7.

Concluding remarks

Family physicians who provide evidence-based family-centred birthing for their low-risk patients have excellent outcomes.[20–22] Effective maternity care recognizes the importance of balance between both the biomedical and psycho-social needs of pregnant women. It empowers women to make informed choices, and respects diversity. Women appear to value relationships, communication, involvement in decision-making, and continuity of pre-natal caregiver over continuity in intrapartum care.[1,23] This makes it reasonable and feasible for family physicians to join with like-minded colleagues in providing complete pregnancy care; allowing an acceptable lifestyle, while maintaining the capacity to develop the relationships that are essential to patient and provider satisfaction.

References

1. Hodnett, E.D. (2001). Continuity of caregivers for care during pregnancy and childbirth (Cochrane Review). In *The Cochrane Library* Issue 2. Oxford: Update Software.

2. Sikorski, J., Wilson, J., Clement, S., Das, S., and Smeeton, N. (1996). A randomised controlled trial comparing two schedule of antenatal visits: the antenatal care project. *British Medical Journal* 312, 546–53.

3. Clement, S., Sikorski, J., Wilson, J., Das, S., and Smeeton, N. (1996). Women's satisfaction with traditional and reduced antenatal visit schedules. *Midwifery* 12, 120–8.

4. Health Canada. *Family-Centered Maternity and Newborn Care: National Guidelines.* Ottawa: Minister of Public Works and Government Services, 2000.

5. Grzybowski, S., Nout, R., and Kirkham, C.M. (1999). Maternity care calendar wheel-improved obstetric wheel developed in British Columbia. *Canadian Family Physician* 45, 661–6.

6. Kirkham, C.M. and Grzybowski, S. (1999). Maternity care guidelines checklist to assist physicians in implementing clinical practice guidelines. *Canadian Family Physician* 45, 671–8.

7. Wilson, L.M., Reid, A.J., Midmer, D.K., Biringner, A., Carrol, J.C., and Stewart, D.E. (1996). Antenatal psychosocial risk factors associated with adverse postpartum family outcomes. *Canadian Medical Association Journal* 154, 785–99.

8. Reid, A.J., Biringer, A., Carroll, J.D., Midmer, D., Wilson, L.M., Chalmers, B., and Stewart, D.E. (1998). Using the ALPHA form in practice to assess antenatal psychosocial health. *Canadian Medical Association Journal* 159, 677–83.

9. Abrams, B., Altman, S.L., and Pickett, K.E. (2000). Pregnancy weight gain: still controversial. *American Journal of Clinical Nutrition* 71 (Suppl.), 1233S–41S.

10. Enkin, M.W., Keirse, M.J., Neilson, J.P., Crowther, C.A., Duley, L., Hodnett, E.D., and Hofmeyr, G.J. (2000). Antenatal education. In *A Guide to Effective Care in Pregnancy and Childbirth.* Oxford: Oxford University Press.

11. Neilson, J.P. (2001). Ultrasound for fetal assessment in early pregnancy (Cochrane Review). In *The Cochrane Library* Issue 2. Oxford: Update Software.

12. Denianczuk, N.N. et al. (1999). Guidelines for ultrasound as part of routine prenatal care. *Journal SOGC* 78, 1–6.

13. Canadian Task Force on the Periodic Health Examination (1992). Periodic health examination, 1992 update: 1. Screening for gestational diabetes. *Canadian Medical Association Journal* 147, 435–43.

14. Enkin, M.W., Keirse, M.J., Neilson, J.P., Crowther, C.A., Duley, L., Hodnett, E.D., and Hofmeyr, G.J. (2001). Gestational diabetes. In *A Guide to Effective Care in Pregnancy and Childbirth.* Oxford: Oxford University Press.

15. Wen, S.W. et al. (2000). Impact of prenatal glucose screening on the diagnosis of gestational diabetes and on pregnancy outcomes. *American Journal of Epidemiology* 152, 1009–14.

16. Hannah, M.E., Hannah, W.J., Hewson, S.A., Hodnett, E.D., Saigal, S., and Willan, A.R. (2000). Planned caesarean section versus planned vaginal birth for breech presentation at term: a randomised multicentre trial. Term Breech Trial Collaborative Group. *Lancet* 356, 1375–83.

17. Crowley, P. (2001). Interventions for preventing or improving the outcome of delivery at or beyond term (Cochrane Review). In *The Cochrane Library* Issue 2. Oxford: Update Software.

18. Klein, M. et al. (1983). A comparison of low risk women booked for delivery in two different systems of care. Part II. Labor and delivery management and neonatal outcome. *British Journal of Obstetrics and Gynaecology* 90, 123–8.

19. Krikke, E.H. and Bell, W.R. (1989). Relation of family physician or specialist care to obstetrics interventions and outcomes in patients at low risk: a western Canadian cohort study. *Canadian Medical Association Journal* 140, 637.

20. Reid, A.J., Carroll, J.C., Ruderman, J., and Murray, M.A. (1989). Differences in intrapartum obstetric care provided to women at low risk by family physicians and obstetricians. *Canadian Medical Association Journal* 140, 625–33.

21. Morgan, M., Fenwick, N., McKenzie, C., and Wolfe, C.D. (1998). Quality of midwifery led care: assessing the effects of different models of continuity for women's satisfaction. *Quality in Health Care* 7, 77–82.

Futher reading

Canadian Academy of Sports Medicine: Position Statement—Exercise in Pregnancy, July 1998. http://www.casm-acms.org/Committees/WIISM/Pspreg.htm (July 16, 2001). (Evidence-based guidelines for exercise in pregnancy.)

Information on obtaining the maternity care calendar is also available at www.bcricwh.bc.ca

Additional information on drugs/chemicals in pregnancy.

Briggs, G.G., Freeman, R.K., and Yaffe, S.J. *Drugs in Pregnancy and Lactation: A Reference Guide to Fetal and Neonatal Risk.* Baltimore MD: Williams and Wilkins, 2001.

MotheRisk on-line: http://www.motherisk.org/. (This is a searchable internet resource for evidence-based information about the safety or risk of drugs, chemicals and disease during pregnancy and lactation. The Motherisk Team is affiliated with the University of Toronto.)

Labreque, M. et al. (1999). Randomized controlled trial of prevention of perineal trauma by perineal massage during pregnancy. *American Journal of Obstetrics and Gynecology* 180, 593–600. (A description of perineal massage, and information on obtaining patient handouts.)

8.5 Teenage pregnancy

Caroline Free

The term 'teenage pregnancy' emerged in industrialized countries in the late 1960s. It gradually replaced the terms 'unwed mother' and 'illegitimate child'.[1] In many societies pregnancy during teenage years is the norm, but in industrialized countries teenage pregnancy is generally considered undesirable. The problem of teenage pregnancy has been debated within medicine, education, policy, social science, and the media. The source of the problem of 'teenage pregnancy' has been located as social, individual, moral, technical, and educational. This chapter aims to provide an approach to the primary care of pregnant teenagers and the prevention of unwanted teenage pregnancies.

Epidemiology

Internationally there are large variations in teenage conception rates, birth rates, termination of pregnancy rates, and their trends. Pregnancy rates range from 10 per 1000 women aged 15–19 in Japan to 102 per 1000 women aged 15–19 in the Russian Federation.[2] Abortion rates range from 4 per 1000 women aged 15–19 in Germany to 56 per 1000 in the Russian Federation. Variations in teenage pregnancy rates between areas in the same country are large. In the United Kingdom, the highest area teenage pregnancy rates are more than six times the lowest area rates.[3]

What causes variations in teenage pregnancy

Higher rates of teenage pregnancy are associated with socio-economic deprivation, lower levels of education, and family disruption (divorce or separation).[4] Groups at particularly high risk include: young people in or leaving social services care, school non-attendees, aboriginal status, homeless teenagers, and daughters of teenage mothers. In Northern European countries, where generally lower teenage pregnancy rates are found, there is a greater openness about sexuality, sex education, and accessible services.[5] The provision of educational programmes linked to accessible services are associated with falls in teenage pregnancy.[5]

How common is this presentation in primary care

Consultation rates vary according to the area, country, and the service's acceptability to teenagers. Consultation rates specifically for pregnant teenagers in primary care are not routinely available. In the United Kingdom, consultation rates for pregnant 16–24 year olds are 421 per 10 000 person years at risk.[6] Whilst the numbers of pregnant teenagers attending primary care practices is generally low, their health and social needs make considerable demands on primary care resources.

Presentation of teenage pregnancy

Teenagers may be unwilling or unable to tell primary care physicians that they are or may be pregnant. Teenagers may not know that they are pregnant due to non-specific signs and symptoms of early pregnancy or they may deny the possibility of pregnancy. Denial of pregnancy can be due to fear, embarrassment, a sense of invulnerability, or a way of avoiding facing up to the consequences of pregnancy. The significance of menstrual changes can easily be missed for the following reasons:

- the implantation bleed which occurs when the trophoblast implants into decidua may be mistaken for a normal period;
- teenagers with irregular periods may miss the significance of 'another' late/missed period;
- bleeding in early pregnancy may be mistaken for a period;
- pregnancy may have occurred after finishing contraception which stopped their period (such as the contraceptive injection) and before the onset of a regular period.

Diagnosis of teenage pregnancy

Primary care physicians will have a range of views regarding teenage sexuality and pregnancy—some of which may be negative. Reflective practitioners should be aware of their views and how these may impact on their interaction with patients. In order to obtain an accurate history, good communication and open discussion about confidentiality are essential. Teenagers find it easiest to talk to someone who is friendly, understanding, and non-judgemental.[7]

Late and non-presentation of pregnancy in teenagers means that clinicians should have a low threshold for considering and testing for pregnancy. The usual symptoms and signs should be sought in order to make the diagnosis of pregnancy. Conditions that mimic pregnancy should be considered. The usual confusions about pregnancy diagnosis apply to the teenager but may be compounded by the fact that many teenagers have irregular menses, especially the very young teenager.

Principles of management

Initial management and assessment

1. Diagnose pregnancy and determine the gestational age.
2. Identify and assess for pregnancy complications or concurrent medical conditions which require referral.
3. Seek the teenager's views regarding the pregnancy.
4. (a) provide counselling regarding pregnancy options or (b) provide early pregnancy advice and initial care.
5. Make referrals for termination of pregnancy, adoption agencies.
6. Refer to social or educational services if appropriate.
7. If indicated, make arrangements for further antenatal care. Antenatal care may be provided by the primary care physician themselves, community midwife, specialist teenage pregnancy team, or hospital antenatal care according to the local arrangements and services.

Teenagers views regarding pregnancy

The significance of teenage pregnancy varies according to the cultural and social expectations of teenagers in relation to motherhood, marriage, education, and career. In some societies, marriage during teenage years is common and children are expected within a year or two of marriage. In this social context, teenage pregnancy is both anticipated and welcome. In other settings, a teenager may value the social role of motherhood whether or not the pregnancy was planned. A teenager who has high expectations of education or a job may see pregnancy as a 'disaster'. The attitude to the pregnancy may be shaped by negative attitudes regarding the morality of termination of pregnancy. Key people such as parents or the sexual partner may also influence attitudes. There may be considerable parental support for an ongoing pregnancy or parental pressure to have a termination. Parents or the sexual partner may strongly disapprove of termination of pregnancy.

Counselling regarding pregnancy options

Conflicting pressures and emotions can be confusing for the teenager trying to reach a decision about a pregnancy. Referral can be made to a counsellor if they are available and access can be arranged within the time frame required.

Supporting the teenager to reach a decision about the pregnancy involves:

1. *Establishing good communication.*

2. *Establishing a time frame for decisions.* Accurate determination of gestation gives a time frame for active or passive decisions about termination of pregnancy.

3. *Providing information about options.* Factual information about the options available should be provided. Teenagers often have misconceptions about what is involved and may have concerns about the effect of termination of pregnancy on future fertility.

4. *Exploring the teenagers views about options.* The teenagers' thoughts about and expectations of pregnancy, motherhood, fertility, and termination should be explored. Steps that can be taken to do this include getting her to talk about/write down her positive and negative thoughts about the pregnancy. Asking her to think about/write down: What would it be like to have a baby/have an abortion/get the baby adopted? Why would she do or not do this? What do other important people think about the pregnancy? How does this affect her decision? How would her life or future plans change if she did any of these?

Initial and continuing care

The chapter on normal pregnancy (Chapter 8.4) provides a detailed account of the provision of routine antenatal care that teenagers should also receive. The majority of teenagers will not have planned to become pregnant and will, therefore, miss out on pre-conception care such as folic acid supplementation. The absence of pre-conception care and an unplanned pregnancy means tetarogenic medication may have been taken in early pregnancy (e.g. acne medications: isotretinoin, oxytetracycline). Teenagers usually first attend the doctor much later in pregnancy than older women. One-fifth of pregnant teenagers delay their first appointment for antenatal care until after the 20th week of pregnancy. In view of this delay, it is important for primary care clinicians to initiate antenatal care at the time of diagnosis to those teenagers presenting with an ongoing pregnancy. The consultation at the time of presentation of an ongoing pregnancy should cover: antenatal advice, a full history, examination of the blood pressure, urine and depending on gestational age foetal size, foetal heart rate, and foetal movements, and initial blood test investigations. Teenagers are more likely to smoke prior to pregnancy and more likely to continue smoking during pregnancy than older mothers. Advice regarding the effects of smoking and means of smoking cessation should be offered.

Complications

Generally, pregnancy itself is physically well tolerated, even in the under 16 year olds. Serious *biological risks* conferred by teenage pregnancy are low. Teenagers without medical complications are likely to do well in the intra-partum period. There are some complications and problems that teenagers (especially younger teens) are more prone to, including hypertension and anaemia. In a pregnant teenager aged less than 16 years, the relative risk for anaemia is 2.5 (95 per cent CI 2.19–2.92). The relative risk of gestational hypertension is 1.7 (95 per cent CI 1.28–2.4).[8] After the delivery teenagers are half as likely to breast feed than older mothers. Post-natal depression is three times as common amongst teenage parents. Rates of depression can be as high as 40 per cent.

Whilst the majority of teenage pregnancies, as among older women, result in a normal health baby, there are increased risks of low birth weight, prematurity, and a higher infant mortality rate. These poorer outcomes associated with teenage pregnancy, however, are partly the result of social deprivation and lack of social support rather than age itself. After adjusting for marriage, educational level, and antenatal care, teenagers in the 13–17-year-old age group compared to the 20–24-year-old age group have a relative risk of low birth weight of 1.7 (95 per cent CI 1.5–2.0), premature delivery of 1.9 (95 per cent CI 1.7–2.1), and small for gestational age of 1.3 (95 per cent CI 1.2–1.4). In 18–19-year-old age group compared to the 20–24-year-old age group, after adjusting for education, antenatal care, and marriage, the relative risk of low birth weight is 1.2 (95 per cent CI 1.1–1.4), prematurity 1.5 (95 per cent CI 1.4–1.6), and small for gestational age 1.1 (95 per cent CI 1.0–1.2).[9] The impact of the problems associated with teenage pregnancy are moderated by good antenatal, intra-partum, and post-natal medical care and social support. Teenagers receiving inadequate care have twice the risk of having a low birth weight baby than teenagers receiving adequate care. Teenager's attendance for ongoing care, however, may not fit a predetermined pattern, and opportunistic care may need to be provided. Of concern in the teenage population is the presentation of a pregnancy complication in a woman with a concealed pregnancy or the late presentation of complications due to poor attendance for antenatal care. Clinicians must be vigilant for the possibility of pregnancy and pregnancy complications as key differential diagnoses, so that appropriate treatment of the rare serious or life-threatening conditions is not delayed.

The experience of teenage pregnancy and social aspects of teenage pregnancy in industrialized societies

Women who planned their pregnancy in their teenage years typically cite a high value placed on the role of motherhood and few aspirations relating to school or education.[10] These teenagers typically view themselves as being ready to start a family and view themselves as being with the right partner. A minority of women who plan pregnancies anticipate that pregnancy will be a means of change and gaining independence. Unplanned teenage pregnancies are associated with denial of pregnancy and fear about parental reactions. In the UK context, however, only a small minority of pregnant teenagers experience deteriorating relationships with parents following pregnancy.

Most teenage parents see real advantages in having had a child.[10] They are proud of their children and cite the positive impacts of having a child. Whilst teenagers do not regret having children, many feel in retrospect they had been too young to be parents and acknowledge that they had not really thought through the implications, particularly in terms of the responsibilities involved. Teenage parents face a number of difficulties: they report financial pressures, that their housing is poor and is often located in areas with high levels of crime and drug-related problems.

Relationship problems are often experienced during pregnancy. The arrival of the baby may result in rising tensions within relationships. Few teenagers stay with the natural fathers, some develop new relationships whilst others are on their own. Family networks for some young mothers are very strong. Mothers of teenage mothers may be heavily relied upon for advice, emotional support, and considerable amounts of child care. Teenagers without strong family support face greater difficulties adapting to the parental role. Teenagers in the most difficult social circumstances struggle with poor housing, partners in prison, drug and alcohol problems, and the demands of a small child. Pregnant teenagers leaving social service care face particular difficulties. Despite good intentions in doing a better job than they felt their parents had done, they experience poor social support, family networks are not available to them, and when housing is provided it is mostly in socially deprived areas. Temporary housing provides limited opportunity to develop social networks and the configuration of housing in deprived areas (such as bed and breakfasts or high-rise flats) gives little opportunity to interact with others. Such teenage mothers may feel out of place in mother and toddler programmes designed where the other women are in very different circumstances and from different backgrounds. When attempting to restart education or work, teenagers experience considerable difficulties due to child care, preceding lack of education, and monetary difficulties.[10]

The experience of teenage pregnancy and motherhood highlights the importance of social issues for teenagers including housing difficulties, family support, relationship difficulties, and educational issues. Where these are available, social services or support groups for pregnant teenagers/young mothers should be contacted. In countries with compulsory education standards, educational providers will need to be informed about teenagers who are below the legal age for ending education.

Preventing teenage pregnancy

Services for teenagers need to be flexible, easily accessible outside school hours, informal, confidential, and advertised as such. Both male and female providers should be available. Access is easiest if the service can be provided on a walk in basis.[7] Teenagers who become pregnant are more likely than their peers to have previously sought contraception advice or a pregnancy test.[11,12]

Good relationships between providers and clients, offering a wide choice of methods and the encouragement of switching among methods as opposed to dropping out, have been linked to increased uptake of contraception and falls in fertility.[13]

Teenagers' views regarding different contraceptives and their own priorities should be sought. Primary care physicians should provide clear explanations and written information about contraceptives, their effects, and side-effects in order to support the teenager in reaching a decision. Written and oral instructions about how to use the contraceptive should be given. Practical skills, such as how to put a condom on, can be demonstrated and observed using plastic models. Future contraception should be discussed with the teenager who is pregnant and opting for termination of pregnancy. Women who opt for the oral contraceptive after termination of pregnancy should receive supplies of this before the termination so that it can be started immediately. Similarly, plans regarding contraception antenatally and again immediately after childbirth should be discussed. The use of condoms to protect against STDs and cervical abnormalities should be raised.

Legal issues and confidentiality

Different countries vary in the legal provision of confidential contraceptive and medical care to teenagers (Table 1). Primary care physicians should familiarize themselves with the legal framework regarding confidentiality in their own country.

Table 1 Legality of provision of services to teenagers in different countries

Provision	Countries
Legal to under 16 and confidential	Canada, New Zealand, Denmark, Spain, Portugal, Sweden, Switzerland, Germany
Provision of contraception under the age of 16 is legal: the adolescent must be capable of understanding the medical issues/consequences	Australia, Scotland
Parental permission is required for provision in under 15s	France
Federal family planning programme maintains confidentiality. Private and state funded clinics enforce different consent conditions	United States of America
Provision under 16 is legal. The visit, but not the nature of the visit, will be recorded on the health insurance documents sent to the parents	Netherlands
Provision legal and confidential: for contraception the young person should understand the moral, social, and emotional implications; cannot be persuaded to tell their parents. It must be in the young person's best interests, i.e. otherwise likely to have unprotected sex or to suffer in physical or mental health	United Kingdom

Adapted from The Department of Health. *Teenage Pregnancy.* London: The Stationary Office, 1999.

Implications of the problem

Longer term implications of teenage pregnancy include impacts on the health of the children and poor social and economic outcomes. Health impacts for the children include a twofold increase in the rates of hospital admission for gastroenteritis and childhood accidents. Children of teenagers score less well on verbal and non-verbal ability tests in pre-school developmental checks. Ultimately, there is a higher risk of the child themselves becoming a teenage parent.

Teenage pregnancy is also linked to poor socio-economic outcomes for mothers and their children. In the United Kingdom, teenage parents by the age of 33 are more likely than others to fail to complete secondary school, be in receipt of state benefits, and be divorced or separated. If working, teenage parents are more likely in their mid-20s to be in semi-skilled or unskilled manual occupations. Teenage parents and their children are more likely to live in poverty, have poor housing, and poor nutrition.[4,5]

Summary and further research

The particular health and social needs of teenagers who are pregnant means that providing good primary care may be time consuming and necessitate the involvement of other agencies and professionals. Providing good initial care remains a challenge for primary care physicians working in busy clinics. Further research is required to support primary care practice. Different models for providing coordinated care to teenagers from a range of professionals should be evaluated. Services specifically targeted at the most vulnerable teenagers should be developed and evaluated. Mechanisms for linking sex education in schools to primary contraceptive services require more robust evaluation. Factors within primary care practices that result in effective contraception use need to be identified and educational interventions developed.

Key points

1. Teenage pregnancy is associated with poorer socio-economic outcomes for mother and baby.

2. Whilst the majority of teenage pregnancies result in the birth of a healthy baby, and teens generally do well intrapartum, there are increased risks of infant mortality, prematurity, maternal depression, anaemia, and pre-eclampsia.

3. Good antenatal care and multidisciplinary support for teenagers can reduce adverse outcomes.

4. A high index of suspicion, a careful menstrual history, and easy access to immediate pregnancy tests are key to diagnosing pregnancy and initiating either good antenatal care or early referral for termination of pregnancy.

5. Primary care can play a key role in preventing teenage pregnancy through providing accessible and confidential contraceptive services; ideally, services should be linked to sex education in schools.

References

1. Arney, W. and Bergen, B. (1984). Power and visibility: the invention of teenage pregnancy. *Social Science and Medicine* **18**, 11–19. (This provides a historical background to teenage pregnancy.)

2. Singh, S. and Daroch, J. (2000). Adolescent pregnancy and childbearing levels and trends in developed countries. *Family Planning Perspectives* **32** (1), 14–23.

3. Smith, T. (1993). Influence of socio-economic factors on attaining targets for reducing teenage pregnancies. *British Medical Journal* **306**, 1232–5.

4. The Department of Health. *Teenage Pregnancy*. London: The Stationery Office, 1999. (This provides an overview of teenage pregnancy in the UK context. Comparative international data, a review of the literature, and practice from other industrialized countries are presented.)

5. NHS Centre for Reviews and Dissemination (1997). Preventing and reducing the adverse effects of unintended pregnancies. *Effective Health Care* **3**, 1–12. (This is based on a systematic review and synthesis of research and presents the evidence regarding health care and educational interventions that prevent teenage pregnancy or reduce the adverse impacts of teenage pregnancy.)

6. OPCS. *Morbidity Statistics from General Practice. Fourth National Study 1991–1992*. London: HMSO, 1995.

7. Peckham, S., Ingham, R., and Diamond, I. *Teenage Pregnancy: Prevention and Programmes*. Institute for Health Policy Studies, University of Southampton, 1996. (This provides an overview of the literature regarding effective contraceptive services and presents a framework for developing and evaluating services.)

8. Fraser, A., Brockert, J., and Ward, R. (1995). Association of young maternal age with adverse reproductive outcomes. *New England Journal of Medicine* **332**, 1113–18.

9. Konje, J., Palmer, A., Watson, A., Hay, A., and Imrie, A. (1992). Early teenage pregnancies in Hull. *British Journal of Obstetrics and Gynaecology* **99**, 969–73.

10. Hughes, K., Cragg, A., Taylor, C., Goodrich, J., and Christophers, W.J. (1999). *Reducing the Rate of Teenage Conceptions. Young People's Experiences of Relationships, Sex and Early Parenthood: Qualitative Research*. London: Health Education Authority, 1999.

11. Churchill, D., Allen, J., Pringle, M., Hippisley-Cox, J., Ebdon, D., and MacPherson, M. (2000). Consultation patterns and provision of contraception in general practice before teenage pregnancy. *British Medical Journal* **321**, 486–9.

12. Zabin, L.S., Sedivy, V., and Emerson, M.R. (1994). Subsequent risk of childbearing among adolescents with a negative pregnancy test. *Family Planning Perspectives* **26**, 212–17.

13. Jain, A. (1989). Fertility reduction and the quality of family planning services. *Studies in Family Planning* **20**, 1–15.

8.6 Vaginal bleeding in early pregnancy

Sander Flikweert and Tjerk Wiersma

Introduction and background[1]

Vaginal bleeding in early pregnancy means blood loss in the first trimester of pregnancy—the period up to 14 weeks following the first day of the last menstruation—and occurs in about 30 per cent of all pregnancies. In about half of these cases the blood loss indicates an imminent miscarriage, while in most of the remainder it stops, and the pregnancy remains intact. While the significance of the blood loss for the outcome of the pregnancy is unclear, the term 'threatened miscarriage' is used. Other causes of blood loss during the first trimester of pregnancy include ectopic pregnancy, vaginal or cervical abnormalities, such as polyps, or rarely trophoblastic disease.

Complications of the first trimester of pregnancy are common: half of conceptions miscarry before 12 weeks, most before ever becoming clinically apparent. However, about 15–20 per cent of all pregnancies end in a clinically recognizable miscarriage. About three-fourths of these occur between the 8th and 14th week of pregnancy. The general practitioner's diagnostic effort is first directed at excluding other causes of blood loss during the first trimester of pregnancy, such as an ectopic pregnancy (estimated to occur one-tenth as often) or a polyp.

It is generally not possible, on the basis of the case history and a physical examination, to predict the outcome of pregnancy with any certainty. If diagnostic signs of an ectopic pregnancy are lacking and with good explanation and instruction to the pregnant woman, a wait-and-see policy can be adopted. If the blood loss eventually results in a miscarriage, expulsion of the foetus occurs within 4 days in two-thirds of cases and within a week in 80 per cent. Medical intervention is not indicated in these cases.[2] The general practitioner will only make a referral for curettage in cases in which the blood loss is considerable, persistent, or associated with fever.

Differential diagnosis

Other causes of blood loss in the first trimester of pregnancy include:

- An ectopic pregnancy. The major symptom is pain. Women with fallopian pathology suggested by a history of pelvic inflammatory disease (PID), a previous ectopic pregnancy, or subfertility, women who became pregnant after sterilization, use of *in-vitro* fertilization (IVF) or comparable techniques, and women who became pregnant whilst using an intrauterine contraceptive device (IUD), have an increased risk of an ectopic pregnancy.

- Vaginal or cervical abnormalities such as a bleeding polyp or a bleeding ectropion. The prevalence of (pre-)malignant conditions of the cervix in women of fertile age is very low.

- A molar pregnancy (trophoblastic disease). The incidence of a molar pregnancy in Europe is low; figures vary between one in 1600 to one in 3000 pregnancies. The incidence is also low in North America, while in Asia, Africa, and South America it is higher.

Diagnosis

Blood loss in early pregnancy is likely to cause the woman much uncertainty and concern but there is usually no reason for alarm from a medical point of view. Initially, telephone advice and information is sufficient, as long as there are no known risk factors for an ectopic pregnancy and no symptoms indicative of one, if the quantity of blood lost is not alarming, and the woman is not unduly concerned. The physical examination can then take place several hours later.

History

The history covers the following points:

- When was the first day of the last menstruation and how long was the cycle? Has pregnancy been established by means of a test? When? Was the last menstruation normal?

- What number pregnancy is this? Has miscarriage(s) occurred previously?

- What has been the patient's experience of the pregnancy until now?

- When and in what quantity did the blood loss begin? If there have been blood clots or tissue fragments, when and in what quantities? Have they been saved?

- Are there other symptoms, such as labour-like pain, continuous pain, an ill feeling, or an elevated temperature?

- Are there risk factors for an ectopic pregnancy (see differential diagnosis)?

- How is the patient managing the experience emotionally?

Physical examination

The physical examination covers the following points:

- Percussion and palpation; pain, dullness, abdominal rigidity, rebound tenderness, distension?
- A foetal heartbeat may be heard with a Doppler at 9–10 weeks, and can be made more audible by elevating the uterus during the bimanual examination.
- Speculum investigation and vaginal palpation: are there blood clots in the vagina? Is blood coming through the cervix or from elsewhere? Is the cervical os open or closed? Is there tissue in the cervical os? What is the size, consistency, and position of the uterus? Are the adnexae palpable or painful? Is the intraperitoneal space sensitive?

If the patient has brought the material lost, it should be examined. Blood clots can best be examined and palpated in a tray of water with alcohol, the purpose being to assess whether there are really blood clots, or decidua tissue (usually fragments that are rough on the outside and smooth on the inside, sometimes a complete 'cast' of the uterine cavity), or an amniotic sac (a vesicle with flocculated chorionic villi). Usually, a foetus is not present or recognizable; however, a virtually empty amniotic sac is quite often found.

It can only be concluded that the miscarriage is complete if a complete gestational sac has been found. In the remaining cases, investigations of the 'clots' in the aborted material usually provide little information and, therefore, these do not need to be saved by the woman. The value of assessing this material is marginal and no special effort should be made to collect it.

The diagnostic process

A threatened miscarriage is, in part, diagnosed by excluding other disorders. On the basis of the history and the physical examination, the general practitioner ascertains whether there are reasons to suggest another diagnosis.

- In women with risk factor(s) for an ectopic pregnancy, or when ectopic pregnancy should be suspected.
- If pain is prominent. Symptoms due to an ectopic pregnancy often occur at an early stage of the pregnancy, usually before the 8th week. Often, the last 'menstruation' was shorter than usual and was in fact an abnormal blood loss from the ectopic pregnancy. The adnexae or the intraperitoneal cavity are often painful on palpation, or there are other signs of peritoneal irritation. In severe cases, the patient complains of dizziness and has an elevated pulse rate and a low blood pressure. When an ectopic pregnancy is suspected, an emergency referral is indicated.
- Vaginal or cervical abnormalities such as a bleeding polyp or a bleeding ectropion may be the cause of the blood loss. A polyp can be removed by twisting it off with forceps.
- A trophoblastic pregnancy is also a possible cause of blood loss during the first 16 weeks of pregnancy. The probability of trophoblastic disease increases with age. Blood loss occurs almost exclusively after the 14th week of pregnancy. Other indicative symptoms include extreme nausea, uterine size greater than would be expected for the stage of pregnancy concerned, and loss of a hydatidiform mole. A trophoblastic pregnancy can be demonstrated by an ultrasound scan and, when diagnosed, mandates specialist referral.

If there are no indications for one of these diagnoses, the general practitioner needs to differentiate between a miscarriage and blood loss that is of uncertain significance for the outcome of the pregnancy. Features that indicate that the blood loss will result in a miscarriage include profuse blood loss with tissue fragments, protrusion of the amniotic sac through the cervical os, and an open cervical os. Pain similar to that of labour or menstruation and a loss of pregnancy feelings are indicative of a miscarriage. The uterus is smaller and firmer than expected for the assumed stage of pregnancy.

On the basis of the case history or the results of the physical examination, an imminent miscarriage cannot be definitely excluded. If symptoms indicative of a miscarriage are lacking, there is an equal chance that the pregnancy will proceed normally or that there will be a miscarriage.

Supplementary investigations

For a pregnancy duration of more than 6 weeks, transabdominal or transvaginal ultrasound scanning can provide further clarification about the prognosis of the blood loss. If the uterus contains an intact foetus (having a beating heart), the probability that the pregnancy will remain intact is 95 per cent. The predictive value of a negative finding for a pregnancy of 8 or more weeks is also about 95 per cent, although for a shorter pregnancy the predictive value is less, as there is a reasonable chance that the foetal heart action has not been detected. For this reason if there is a blood loss at 6–8 weeks, a transvaginal ultrasound scan is the preferred option. In incomplete miscarriage, ultrasound may reveal a variety of cystic or echogenic findings. If the thickness of the uterine contents exceeds 5 mm, retained tissue is almost certain, although not all patients will require suction curettage. Complete spontaneous miscarriage results in an empty uterus with a bright 'endometrial stripe' indicating that the uterine walls have collapsed against each other. Ultrasound scans to establish the viability of the foetus at less than 6 weeks are of no value, because the foetal heart is not yet beating. The general practitioner needs to discuss with the pregnant woman the place of the scan, which, although helping to determine foetal viability, is unlikely to have an immediate effect on management. Many women, anxious about the outcome of the pregnancy, are likely to press for a scan to reassure them that all is well.

The woman's blood group should be determined at this stage, if it is not already known. Rhesus D-negative women should be considered for administration of anti-D immunoglobulin following a miscarriage. Other tests such as determining the progesterone level do not contribute to the diagnosis. Pregnancy tests following a miscarriage will only give a negative result after a number of days have elapsed, because the elevated hCG levels return slowly to normal.

Principles of management

For women experiencing a miscarriage as well as women for whom the outcome of the blood loss is still unclear, the appropriate policy is to await the outcome, as events run their natural clinical course, and to provide advice, instruction, and appropriate follow-up or referral.[3] Management also has to focus on identifying women with incomplete miscarriages, who are at risk of bleeding and infection, and who may benefit from medical or surgical intervention.

Information

If the pregnancy remains intact, the blood loss will remain limited and will soon stop. If the blood loss ends in a miscarriage, there is a high probability that the foetus was abnormal. A miscarriage can, therefore, be viewed as a natural event. There are no measures available that can facilitate the continuation of the pregnancy or an uncomplicated clinical outcome of the miscarriage. Routine medical intervention is unnecessary. In three-fourths of cases, expulsion of the uterine contents occurs within a week. Usually, the expulsion is associated with the loss of some blood clots and a moderate quantity of blood (about as much as during a heavy menstruation), and labour-like pain. A more rapid removal of the pregnancy product by means of curettage is only indicated if the bleeding is persistent or heavy or is associated with much pain or fever. In all other cases, curettage is an unnecessary medical intervention.[4]

For many if not most women, experiencing a miscarriage is a great disappointment. Feelings of rebellion, anger, guilt, despondency, and grieving about the loss of the unborn child—certainly at the start—are not uncommon and are very understandable. Time is needed to deal with these feelings. There is no need to ignore or suppress them and equally no reason to feel ashamed. If the aforementioned feelings strongly dominate everyday life it is sensible to discuss these with the partner, family and friends, or the general practitioner. It is important not to trivialize the woman's experience by suggesting that she can 'try again'. It is preferable to take cues from the woman as to her need for information.

Information for patients

If nothing unusual occurs, a follow-up appointment should take place a week after the start of the blood loss. An earlier appointment should be sought by the woman if the blood loss becomes heavy, the pain becomes more severe and is no longer intermittent but becomes continuous, and if a fever develops. At this stage, the speculum examination and vaginal palpation should be repeated. Patients may also wish to contact their general practitioner to discuss their emotional reaction to these events.

Sometimes, the increase in complaints is caused by a lump of tissue that is visible in the cervix. Removal of this manually or with a sequestrum forceps is advisable. The symptoms will then cease within several hours. If there is heavy blood loss, increased pain that cannot be attributed to powerful uterine contractions, or fever, a referral for further investigation and possible treatment should take place.

Quite often contact is made because the woman requires further information, for example, about the question as to whether or not her situation is normal, or reassurance after hearing stories from others which have made her anxious. In such cases, a conversation in which the general practitioner offers understanding and a listening ear along with a clear explanation is generally sufficient.

Check-up after a week

A check-up takes place after about a week. If it is already clear that the blood loss was due to a miscarriage, the check-up involves determining whether or not the miscarriage is complete. If the outcome is still not clear, it involves determining whether or not the pregnancy is still intact. To this end, the general practitioner first enquires about the presence, duration, and amount of blood loss and then repeats the speculum examination and the vaginal palpation.

The following possibilities are now considered:

◆ If in the previous week much blood with tissue fragments has been lost, the blood loss has stopped, the cervical os is closed, and fever or pain are absent, then it can be concluded that the miscarriage is complete. If vaginal palpation reveals a small and firm uterus, the diagnosis is confirmed. Further investigation or treatment is not indicated.

◆ Protracted and intermittent blood loss associated with a uterus that is not small and firm and an os that is not tightly closed indicate an incomplete miscarriage. Unless already performed, an ultrasound scan is requested. In the case of a pregnancy of less than 8 weeks duration, a transvaginal ultrasound scan is necessary. An impression of the quantity of blood lost can be gained by determining the haemoglobin level, the pulse rate, and the blood pressure. Especially if the ultrasound scan suggests residual foetal fragments in the uterus, the general practitioner discusses with the woman whether she will be referred for curettage or whether she will wait for a couple of days to see what happens.

◆ If the blood loss was slight and brief, the size of the uterus is in accordance with the duration of pregnancy, and the pregnancy feelings have not disappeared, the pregnancy is probably still intact. The treatment policy for this pregnancy does not differ from that of any other pregnancy. If there are still doubts about the vitality of the foetus, an ultrasound scan can clarify this.

Referral for curettage

Indications for dilatation and curettage following a miscarriage include heavy blood loss (heavier than a normal period), increasing pain, fever, and blood loss lasting for more than a week.

Antirhesus (D) immunoglobulin

Prior to the 12th week of pregnancy, rhesus (D) immunization of a rhesus (D)-negative pregnant woman by rhesus (D)-positive foetal blood is unlikely. Administration of anti-D immunoglobulin in the case of a spontaneous miscarriage without subsequent curettage is, therefore, not indicated prior to the 12th week of pregnancy. For such cases, after the 12th week of pregnancy, anti-D immunoglobulin should be administered intramuscularly within 24–48 h. This form of rhesus prophylaxis can be worthwhile for up to 2 weeks after the miscarriage.[5]

Long-term and continuing care

If a miscarriage has occurred, the general practitioner should offer a follow-up appointment several weeks later, to discuss coming to terms with the loss of the foetus. This check-up could reveal whether there is a continuing discharge or whether menstruation has occurred in the meantime. If necessary, haemoglobin can be measured.

A period of grief following a miscarriage is quite common, but not inevitable.[6] Women who have had a miscarriage are more likely to suffer from depression, especially during the first month after the miscarriage. The greatest risk for depression is among women who have been depressed previously.[7]

Criticism is regularly expressed about the counselling provided by medical practitioners with respect to the level of support and information provided. The criticism mostly concerns the attitude towards the patient, advice, organizational circumstances in the hospital, and the aftercare. Research has revealed that patients highly value attention being paid to their feelings, being involved in determining the treatment policy, empathy, and support, as much as they value clear information and a substantial investment of time by the doctor.[8]

Particularly if a woman experiences three or more consecutive miscarriages, an underlying cause requiring further medical examination or treatment can be considered. Whereas about 10 per cent of all pregnancies end in a miscarriage, the probability of recurrence is about 16 per cent after one miscarriage, about 25 per cent after two previous miscarriages, and about 45 per cent after three.[9] However, even after consecutive miscarriages, the probability that a subsequent pregnancy will result in a healthy child is estimated to be at least 60–70 per cent (as opposed to 85 per cent for women with a miscarriage in the case history).[10] Although the chances of finding a treatable underlying abnormality are slight, it is appropriate to exclude the antiphosphololipid syndrome and other thrombophilic disorders. Recurrent miscarriages are not a reason for check-ups during pregnancy by the specialist or for a hospital delivery.

From cytogenetic studies with aborted material, it is clear that in about 60 per cent of cases the miscarriage was caused by a chromosomal abnormality in the foetus. More than half of the chromosomal abnormalities are autosomal trisomnies. A numeric chromosomal abnormality in a foetus from healthy parents has no consequences, as it is a unique event and is thus in no way connected with a clearly increased probability of a recurrent miscarriage or numeric chromosomal abnormality.

After the second consecutive miscarriage, chromosomal analysis of both partners should be considered. In 2–3 per cent of cases, a structural chromosomal abnormality will be found. This prevalence is five to ten times higher than in the general population. Finding a genetic cause can help to predict the probability of a new miscarriage but even more so to predict the probability of a child with serious abnormalities being born.

Establishing that one of the partners carries a chromosome abnormality enables genetic counselling about the probability of a miscarriage and the health of the offspring. In the event of a possible pregnancy, pre-natal chromosomal investigation by means of a chorionic villi sampling or amniocentesis is indicated. Investigation of the family can be offered in order to identify and advise other carriers of the chromosomal abnormality.

The general practitioner discusses the possibility of karyotyping and the possible consequences of this with the couple and whether they are interested in this option. If karyotyping is desired, the submission of a tube of sterile heparinized blood from both the man and the woman to the regional clinical genetic centre is sufficient.

Key points

- About 30% of all pregnant women experience vaginal bleeding in early pregnancy. In about half of these cases the bleeding stops and the pregnancy remains intact.

- About 15% of all pregnancies end in miscarriage. In most cases expectant management in general practice ('wait-and-see' policy) is used. A miscarriage can be viewed as a natural event.

- If there is any diagnostic sign of an ectopic pregnancy, referral to a specialist is recommended.

- Ultrasound scan can help to determine foetal viability, but is unlikely to have an immediate effect on management.

- Administration of anti-D immunoglobulin in the case of a spontaneous miscarriage without subsequent curettage, is only indicated after the twelfth week of pregnancy.

- After the second consecutive miscarriage, chromosomal analysis of both partners should be considered. In 2–3% of cases a structural chromosomal abnormality will be found. This prevalence is 5–10 times higher than in the general population.

References

1. The Dutch College of General Practitioners (NHG) issued a practice guideline based on the expectant management of miscarriage. This guideline is on Internet in English. Dutch College of General Practitioners (NHG) Standard M3 'Miscarriage' (http://www.artsennet.nl/nhg).

2. Everett, C. (1997). Incidence and outcome of bleeding before the 20th week of pregnancy: prospective study from general practice. *British Medical Journal* 315, 32–4.

3. Ankum, W.M., Wieringa-de Waard, M., and Bindels, P.J.E. (2001). Management of spontaneous miscarriage in the first trimester: an example of putting informed shared decision making into practice. *British Medical Journal* 322, 1344–6.

4. Nielsen, S. and Hahlin, M. (1995). Expectant management of first-trimester miscarriage. *The Lancet* 345, 84–6.

5. Use of anti-D immunoglobulin for Rh prophylaxis (http://www.rcog.org.uk).

6. Janssen, H.J.E.M. A longitudinal prospective study of the psychological impact of pregnancy loss on women (thesis). Nijmegen: Catholic University Nijmegen, 1995.

7. Neugerbauer, R. et al. (1997). Major depressive disorder in the 6 months after miscarriage. *The Journal of the American Medical Association* 277, 383–8.

8. Fleuren, M. et al. (1998). Does the care given by general practitioners and midwives to patients with (imminent) miscarriage meet the wishes and expectations of the patients? *International Journal of Quality in Health Care* 10, 213–20.

9. Knudson, U.B., Hansen, V., Juul, S., and Secher, N.J. (1991). Prognosis of a new pregnancy following previous miscarriages. *European Journal of Obstetrics & Gynaecology and Reproductive Biology* 39, 31–6.

10. Cook, C.L. and Pridham, D.D. (1995). Recurrent pregnancy loss. *Current Opinion in Obstetrics and Gynecology* 7, 357–66.

8.7 Complications of pregnancy

Andrew Shennan and Tim Overton

This chapter will consider both maternal and foetal complications of pregnancy that commonly present to the primary care physician. Maternal conditions may either be pregnancy related or coincidental; therefore also included are common medical conditions which have a significant impact on pregnancy or vice versa. In primary care, a detailed knowledge of prenatal diagnosis is essential so this will be considered in addition to complications involving the foetus.

Maternal conditions

Hypertension and pre-eclampsia

Epidemiology

Hypertension occurs in more than 10 per cent of the antenatal population and is the commonest medical complication of pregnancy. Less than 5 per cent of women will get pre-eclampsia, with associated morbidity or mortality to mother or baby in less than 1 per cent. Eclampsia (seizures) are rare (about one in 2000 pregnancies in developed countries) but are associated with a 2 per cent maternal mortality rate. Although pre-eclampsia is 10 times more common in first pregnancies, it is more dangerous in a multiparous woman. As the course and onset of pre-eclampsia are unpredictable, antenatal care is largely geared towards identifying women with hypertension and proteinuria. Essential hypertension occurs in about 2 per cent of pregnant women; the risk of developing superimposed pre-eclampsia is at least doubled and it is also more likely to be early onset and more serious.

Clinical features

Essential hypertension may be masked in early pregnancy due to the normal physiological fall in blood pressure. Secondary causes of hypertension, including renal, cardiac, or endocrine origins should be sought when women present in early pregnancy with new hypertension; appropriate referral is required.

Pre-eclampsia is a syndrome characterized by hypertension (diastolic ≥90 mmHg, on two occasions >4 h apart) and proteinuria (urinalysis ≥1 + dipstick or ≥300 mg/24 h) developing in the second half of pregnancy. It is a multisystem disorder and can involve hepatic, renal, blood, and central nervous systems. The foetus may develop intrauterine growth restriction, although this is rare with late onset disease. Pre-eclampsia usually resolves within 6 weeks of delivery, but blood pressure can remain elevated up to 3 months postpartum. It is now established that the risk of ischaemic heart disease in later life is doubled in women who have had pre-eclampsia. Isolated hypertension ('pregnancy-induced-hypertension' or PIH) may be the first sign of pre-eclampsia; the gestation at onset determines the risk of developing proteinuria and perinatal risk (i.e. before 30 weeks up to 50 per cent, at term <10 per cent will). Women are usually asymptomatic, and even in severe disease the classical symptoms of headache, epigastric pain, and nausea and vomiting are often absent. However persistent epigastric pain unresponsive to antacids should alert the clinician to pre-eclampsia with liver involvement. Hypertension and proteinuria are not always the first signs of the disease.

Management

Blood pressure measurement and urinalysis must be performed regularly in all pregnant women, and particularly in women at increased risk such as those with essential hypertension, diabetes, and other vascular disease. In hypertensive women, other indications of pre-eclampsia, such as symptoms, small-for-dates foetus or epigastric tenderness should be sought. Any additional sign, including proteinuria, indicates the need for prompt referral for further assessment.

Women with chronic hypertension on treatment should remain on antihypertensive medication, although angiotensin-converting enzyme inhibitors should be avoided and an alternative used if necessary. Diuretics should also be avoided. Methyldopa is often used as it has an established safety profile, but beta-blockers and calcium channel blockers have fewer side-effects and are equally efficacious. Treatment of blood pressure does not prevent the development of pre-eclampsia, but reduces severe hypertension. It is not known whether PIH should be treated with antihypertensive agents, but severe hypertension (>170/110 mmHg) should be avoided. Postpartum blood pressure is frequently highest after the third day, and treatment may need to continue till the 6-week check.

Low-dose aspirin (75 mg) reduces the incidence of pre-eclampsia (by about 15 per cent) as well as the perinatal death rate and can be used from 12 weeks gestation in women at high risk.

Diabetes

Epidemiology

A clear distinction between pre-existing and gestational diabetes in pregnancy must be made as risk status and management are very different. Approximately 2 per cent of women will have pre-existing diabetes. Gestational diabetes occurs in less than 1 per cent of Caucasian populations, but more than 5 per cent of Asian women, and depends on the definition of glucose intolerance used.

Clinical features

Pre-existing diabetes

Diabetes should be tightly controlled from the time of conception onwards. Congenital abnormalities of the heart, bones, and neural tube are related to poor glycaemic control in early pregnancy (up to 25 per cent if HbA1c >10 per cent).

Increasing doses of insulin are required in women with pre-existing diabetes as pregnancy progresses, to approximately double by term. Diabetic retinopathy is twice as likely to progress or develop in pregnancy (secondary to improvement in glycaemic control). For the same reason hypoglycaemia is more common, but diabetic ketoacidosis is rare, possibly due to close supervision during pregnancy. Diabetic renal disease can deteriorate, but usually improves after delivery.

The risks of miscarriage, pre-eclampsia, and infection are all increased in diabetic pregnancy, and the perinatal mortality rate is more than doubled. Unexplained intrauterine death can occur, usually after 36 weeks, and is related to poor glycaemic control. Insulin is anabolic and can cause macrosomia, which increases the risk of traumatic delivery, particularly shoulder dystocia.

Gestational diabetes (GDM)

GDM is associated with an increase in perinatal morbidity and mortality, but to a lesser degree than pre-existing diabetes. There is no increase in perinatal mortality unless GDM represents the first time pre-existing diabetes is diagnosed, and in this case the risks will be the same. Women diagnosed with GDM will have a 50 per cent chance of developing non-insulin dependant diabetes in the next 10–15 years and therefore should have annual glucose checks and advice about presenting symptoms. Women at risk of GDM are offered screening by a short 50 or 75 g glucose tolerance test, usually performed at around 28 weeks. Criteria for screening vary considerably but are based on ethnicity, age, previous obstetric complication, or family history.

Management

Pre-existing diabetes

Referral to a specialist clinic with obstetrician, physician and specialist nurses, dieticians, and midwives should be made as soon as possible. The aim is to maintain normoglycaemia with fasting blood glucose less than 5 mmol/l, and less than 7.5 mmol/l post-prandial. Hyperglycaemia and particularly ketoacidosis are not well tolerated by the foetus, while hypoglycaemia is. Oral hypoglycaemics cross the placenta and should be avoided. Starvation should be avoided but a strict low sugar/fat diet encouraged with high fibre content. Increased home blood-glucose monitoring is required to obtain optimal control along with self-adjustment of insulin. However, frequent snacking is required to avoid hypoglycaemia, and women (and their partners) are taught to use intramuscular glucagon.

Prenatal diagnosis must be offered to rule out congenital abnormalities; cardiac and neural tube defects can be identified by ultrasound at 18–20 weeks. Regular scans are performed to assess growth. Elective delivery is usually offered before 40 weeks, as the increased risk of intrauterine death cannot be predicted by foetal monitoring, but this will depend on the level of glycaemic control achieved.

Gestational diabetes

Diet is the mainstay of treatment, although postprandial or fasting hyperglycaemia is an indication to start insulin. Early delivery is not usually recommended if there is good control and a normal size foetus. GDM usually recurs, and women must be advised about their future risks of diabetes.

Thromboembolic disease

Epidemiology

This is the leading cause of deaths directly attributed to the pregnancy in developed countries. A combination of increased clotting factors and venous stasis (particularly in the left leg) increase the risk of deep vein thrombosis sixfold. The risk is greatest immediately after delivery, and lasts at least 6 weeks postpartum. The risk is at least doubled again in women who have a Caesarean section; a deep venous thrombosis (DVT) occurs in 1–2 per cent of these women.

Clinical features

Most DVTs are iliofemoral (72 per cent), unlike non-pregnant cases (9 per cent) and 85 per cent occur on the left. Clinical signs, such as swelling, pain and redness are unreliable in pregnancy, and are wrong in half of cases. Pleuritic chest pain and breathlessness must always be investigated (see below). Increasing age (>35 years), weight (>80 kg) and parity (>3), immobility, pre-eclampsia, and large varicose veins are all risk factors in pregnancy. Any operative delivery increases the risk, particularly emergency Caesarean sections.

Management

Any suspicion of DVT or pulmonary embolus requires immediate referral for assessment. Definitive diagnosis is essential in all cases, and venography and chest X-rays give negligible radiation to the foetus. Doppler scanning can be used for detection of DVTs in the leg above the calf. A ventilation perfusion scan does not involve unacceptable levels of radiation. A thrombophilia screen for both inherited and acquired defects should be sought in all confirmed cases, and in women planning a pregnancy with a previous history of thromboembolism. Some functional tests such as activated protein C resistance and protein S levels maybe abnormal due to pregnancy, and need to be repeated postpartum if abnormal. Acute phase management is similar to non-pregnant cases, but prophylaxis with heparin must be continued into the puerperium. Heparin is the drug of choice for treatment and prophylaxis as it does not cross the placenta. Warfarin is teratogenic and can result in intracerebral foetal and retroplacental bleeding; it is only used in very high risk women such as those with metal prosthetic heart valves. Low molecular weight heparins are now used extensively in pregnancy.

Heparin prophylaxis is recommended in high-risk cases, that is, thromboembolic disease in the current pregnancy, identified thrombophilia, or recurrent previous thromboembolism. Low-dose aspirin is safe in lower-risk cases; heparin is added intra- and postpartum, but not earlier, to reduce the risks of heparin-induced osteoporosis.

Asthma

Asthma occurs in 3 per cent of pregnant women. It can improve, remain unchanged, or deteriorate, usually due to non-compliance with treatment. Only severe asthma has been associated with foetal growth restriction and neonatal morbidity. Treatment and management is similar to non-pregnant cases, but with an emphasis on prevention rather than acute treatment. Increasing the dose or frequency of inhaled steroids is a good first measure. Counselling regarding the safety of the drugs, including inhaled or oral steroids which are safe in pregnancy, is essential. Poor control is more dangerous to the pregnancy than the medication used. All drugs can be safely used while breast feeding.

Epilepsy

One in 200 pregnant women will have epilepsy. Eclampsia must be ruled out in any women presenting with a seizure in the second half of pregnancy. Fits may occur only in pregnancy (gestational epilepsy). A first fit in pregnancy requires immediate referral for investigation, including CT or MRI scan and EEG. In the majority of women, the frequency of fits remains unchanged, but in over 25 per cent will increase. This may be due to reduced drug compliance, or reduced blood levels of anticonvulsants due to altered pharmacokinetics in pregnancy. Problems with sleep in later pregnancy may precipitate an increase in seizure rate. Fit-free women will remain so, as long as anticonvulsant medication continues.

Single fits are generally well tolerated by the foetus (unless there is direct trauma to the abdomen), but status epilepticus is dangerous for both mother and baby. The child has an increased risk of congenital abnormalities (independent of anticonvulsant medication) and epilepsy. Most anticonvulsants cross the placenta and are teratogenic, increasing the risk of both major and minor malformations from 3 to 6–7 per cent. No one drug is less teratogenic, but risk increases with number of drugs used. Pre-conceptual (for 12 weeks) and first trimester folic acid high-dose supplementation (5 mg) is likely to reduce the risk of neural tube defects. The safety of newer anticonvulsants has not been established, but benzodiazepines are not teratogenic.

Drugs should not be changed if fits are well controlled, and in spite of altered pharmacokinetics there is no need to check drug levels unless there is a fit. Vitamin K (10 mg) should be given to all women from 36 weeks gestation. Breast-feeding is safe, and is recommended with some drugs, which could be associated with neonatal withdrawal reactions (e.g. phenobarbitone).

Prior to pregnancy, control of epilepsy should be optimized, preferable on a single or as few agents as possible. Fit-free women may consider stopping medication, although there is a risk of recurrence with implications for driving. High-dose oestrogen (50 µg) or progesterone pills are required in women taking some anticonvulsants due to induction of hepatic enzymes.

Liver disease and related disorders

Hyperemesis in pregnancy may be associated with abnormal liver (and thyroid) function, with elevated transaminases in about 50 per cent of cases associated with severe vomiting. Women with ketonuria and unable to maintain hydration should be referred for intravenous therapy. Commonly used antiemetics such as metoclopramide are not teratogenic.

Intrahepatic cholestasis of pregnancy can present in the second half of pregnancy with severe pruritis, classically on the palms and soles in association with abnormal liver function tests. There is no rash, other than excoriations from stratching. Other causes of abnormal liver function must be excluded. There is a risk of postpartum haemorrhage in the mother and therefore vitamin K (10 mg daily) is given before delivery. Rates of both intrauterine foetal death and foetal distress are increased, and women should be referred for monitoring and induction of labour. Antihistamines, cholestyramine, steroids, and ursodeoxycholic acid have all been used to alleviate symptoms in the mother, but are not known to reduce foetal risk.

Pre-eclampsia may present with epigastric pain and abnormal liver function. Severe vomiting and abdominal pain in the third trimester may indicate acute fatty liver of pregnancy. Although this is rare, it has a high maternal mortality and requires immediate referral.

Anaemia and thrombocytopaenia

A haemoglobin concentration of less than 10.5 g/dl is considered low in pregnancy, although lower levels may still be physiological due to haemo-dilution. Women already depleted in iron (e.g. from menorrhagia or a short interval from the previous pregnancy) may rapidly drop their haemoglobin with the extra demands of pregnancy. Red cell indices will help give clues to the aetiology and all are reduced in iron deficiency, particularly the mean cell volume (MCV) which is the first to fall. Ferritin levels are the best indicator of iron deficiency (<15 µg/l). Folate deficiency is the next commonest cause, and is usually due to dietary insufficiency, although it may be related to haematological disease such as thalassaemia or to anticonvulsant medication. Standard oral supplements of iron are combined with folate and can be used for prophylaxis or treatment. Routine supplementation is controversial but will increase the haemoglobin concentration.

A spuriously low MCV (compared with the haemoglobin concentration) may indicate a haemoglobinopathy and the need for haemoglobin electrophoresis. Those with sickle cell or thalassaemia trait will need counselling about prenatal diagnosis, and their partners may need testing. Sickle cell disease is associated with increased perinatal morbidity and mortality and requires specialist referral.

Thrombocytopaenia (platelet count $<100 \times 10^9$/l) is often an incidental finding in pregnancy. It is often physiological (gestational), but autoimmune thrombocytopaenia (ITP) should be considered, as well as other rare causes such as the antiphospholipid syndrome. Infection, including HIV, can cause a low platelet count, as well as drugs. Further investigation is needed in all patients with unexplained thrombocytopaenia.

Bleeding

Antepartum haemorrhage (APH) is any bleeding from the genital tract between 24 weeks and the onset of labour, and requires immediate assessment. It is associated with a sevenfold increase in perinatal mortality. Bleeding identified from the placental site occurs in 2 per cent of women. Retroplacental bleeding is known as an abruption, is often associated with pain, and requires urgent admission due to its potential to compromise the foetus. A low placenta may bleed when the lower segment forms, typically after 28 weeks gestation, and is known as placenta praevia. This may require Caesarean section if it remains below the presenting part of the foetus. Incidental causes, such as those from the cervix (e.g. carcinoma) or even rectum (e.g. haemarrhoids) must be considered. Vaginal assessment should not be performed until an ultrsound excludes placenta praevia. Placenta praevia can be managed at home if asymptomatic (diagnosed incidentally on scan) or after a single early bleed. However severe bleeding is possible and warrants urgent transfer to hospital. Women with APH who are rhesus negative require anti-D prophylaxis.

Pre-term labour

Premature delivery (between 24 and 37 weeks gestation) occurs in 6–7 per cent of women. A quarter of cases are not related to spontaneous labour, that is, are for iatrogenic reasons, the commonest of which is pre-eclampsia. Delivery before 30 weeks is associated with significant morbidity. Between 24 and 28 weeks, survivors are prone to physical disability, but up to 32 weeks more subtle problems can be found at school age, such as learning disability, hyperactivity, and attention-deficit disorders. Women with threatened pre-term labour usually do not deliver but urgent referral is required. Antenatal steroids are given up to 36 weeks to reduce respiratory distress in the baby, and referral to a unit that has appropriate neonatal facilities is required. Foetal fibronectin vaginal swabs and cervical ultrasound are better than symptoms or risk factors at predicting delivery. Cervical sutures may be considered in women with previous early delivery, but rarely improve the outcome.

Common obstetric risk factors

Previous Caesarean section

Women presenting with a previous Caesarean section are now common but have an 80 per cent chance of a vaginal delivery. The reason for delivery, for example, delay in labour, has little influence on this success rate. The risk of complications is low, particularly if labour begins spontaneously.

Breech presentation

Vaginal breech deliveries at term have a 3 per cent incidence of severe morbidity or mortality to the baby. External cephalic version can significantly and safely convert breech to cephalic presentations, particularly if undertaken after 36 weeks, and should be encouraged.

Foetal conditions

The foetus can be affected by congenital problems, either genetic or structural, or by problems acquired from the mother. A broad understanding of these issues for the primary care physician is essential for appropriate counselling and preparation for delivery. With the increasing sophistication of imaging techniques, opportunities now exist for in utero therapy to maximize the chances of foetal and neonatal well-being.

Congenital foetal abnormalities

Congenital foetal abnormalities are either genetic or structural in origin. Down syndrome, one of the commonest chromosomal abnormalities, has an overall incidence of approximately 1 per 700 livebirths, whereas the gene for cystic fibrosis is present in about 1 per 22 Caucasian individuals. Fifteen per cent of newborns have single minor congenital abnormality and 3 per cent of deliveries have a major malformation.

Genetic problems

Genetic problems either affect the number or structure of the 46 normal chromosomes (aneuploidy) or individual genes on the chromosomes. Chromosomal disorders account for 60 per cent of first trimester miscarriages and are present in 4–5 per cent of stillbirths. Antenatal screening programmes are now commonplace and identify women at particular risk of carrying an aneuploid foetus, to whom definitive testing by invasive means (such as amniocentesis) can be offered.

Antenatal screening for chromosome disorders

Screening programmes for Down syndrome have developed during the last decade. Eighty per cent of Down syndrome occur in women under 35 years old. Current screening programmes offer invasive testing to approximately 5 per cent of the pregnant population and detects about 70 per cent of foetuses with Down syndrome. Screening is by ultrasound assessment (nuchal or anomaly screening) or maternal blood tests (serum screening) taking in to account the maternal age.

Nuchal screening

This ultrasound screening test is performed between 11 and 14 weeks gestation and measures the thickness of fluid at the back of the foetus's neck (Fig. 1). The maternal age and gestational-age-related prevalence for Down syndrome is taken into account when calculating the risk. The gestational age is calculated from the crown–rump length (ref. 1).

Anomaly screening

The 'routine' 20-week scan is perceived by most as the opportunity for checking that the baby is developing normally, but it is another screening test. With increasing sophistication of ultrasound equipment the routine detection of foetal anomalies is more common. Whilst the early diagnosis of problems requiring planning for delivery, such as congenital heart disease, have obvious benefits, the identification of 'markers' that indicate that the

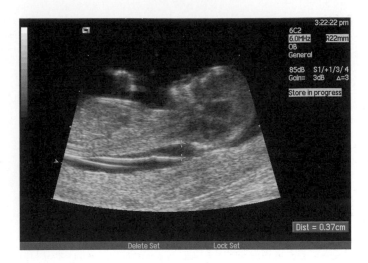

Fig. 1 Increased nuchal translucency at 13 weeks gestation.

foetus *may* be affected by an underlying chromosome or genetic problem can be upsetting. It is not at all unusual to perform such a scan on a woman who earlier in the pregnancy decided not to have screening for Down syndrome. Faced with the news that there are features (such as echogenic bowel, short femurs, renal pelviceal dilatation, etc.) that indicate a foetus is at increased risk of having Down syndrome parents may be angry and feel the scan was conducted without proper informed consent. Accurate information beforehand is very important. Conversely, it is vital that patients appreciate the limitations of ultrasound assessment. Even in the best foetal medicine centres, the detection rate for foetal anomalies is only in the region of 60–70 per cent and in the average unit detection rates are much lower.

Serum screening

Serum screening involves the measurement of various pregnancy associated substances in the mothers' blood usually around 15 weeks gestation. In the 'triple test' maternal serum levels of human chorionic gonadotrophin (hCG), oestriol (uE_3) and alpha foetoprotein (AFP) are measured between 15 and 20 weeks gestation; in pregnancies at risk of Down syndrome, the levels of AFP and uE_3 are lower and the level of hCG higher than in normal pregnancies. The results are combined in a mathematical algorithm with the maternal age and the gestation and a risk of the pregnancy being affected by Down syndrome calculated in the same way as for nuchal screening. When the risk is greater than one in 250, definitive testing by amniocentesis is usually offered. A cut-off value of this order aims to identify 5 per cent of the population who are then offered amniocentesis. Detection rates (sensitivity) may be as high as 75 per cent assuming complete uptake of the test and subsequent amniocentesis. The addition of other serum markers (e.g. inhibin A) may improve the detection rate and there is increasing interest in the use of markers sensitive earlier in pregnancy (e.g. PAPP-A) to bring forward serum screening to the end of the first trimester. The validity of the original demonstration projects have been questioned, and the optimal methods of identifying Down syndrome will continue to develop.

Future screening

The aim of screening is to provide accurate information with no risk to the pregnancy. Much interest over the past decade has been generated by the potential for isolating foetal cells or foetal DNA from the maternal blood stream enabling definitive diagnosis from a maternal blood sample. At the time of writing, this is some years off being a reality. It is likely that isolation of foetal genetic sequences from maternal blood will be used initially to refine screening programmes to reduce the false-positive rate without compromising the detection rate.

Definitive testing

Whilst a low screening risk can be very reassuring, couples with a high risk will often request a definitive test. Chorionic villus sampling (CVS) is performed between 11 and 14 weeks gestation and amniocentesis from 14 weeks. CVS is associated with a miscarriage rate of between 1 and 2 per cent, whereas amniocentesis has a loss rate of just under 1 per cent. Whilst it is technically feasible to perform amniocentesis earlier than 14 weeks, it is then associated with a higher miscarriage rate than CVS. Following the widespread introduction of CVS, there was concern that the test was associated with foetal limb deformities. However, numerous studies have now confirmed that, providing the CVS is performed after 11 weeks gestation, the risk of transverse foetal limb defects is not increased. Both tests are carried out under continuous ultrasound guidance enabling visualization of the needle at all times to minimize the chance of accidental foetal trauma (Fig. 2). With conventional cytogenetic techniques a full karyotype is usually available after about 2 weeks although newer molecular techniques (such fluorescent in situ hybridization and polymerase chain reaction) allow a preliminary chromosome count (which will effectively exclude major trisomies such as Down syndrome) within 24 h. Foetal blood provides a rich source of DNA. Rapid karyotyping after 20 weeks gestation in the past has relied on foetal blood sampling which requires considerable expertise. With recent advances in molecular techniques foetal blood sampling has been largely superseded by amniocentesis which is safer and more widely available.

Gene disorders

With the ability for early prenatal diagnosis, the importance of single gene disorders in the aetiology of congenital defects is becoming increasingly recognized. Autosomal dominant disorders are caused by the inheritance of a single gene from one parent. The consequence may be mild in conditions such as polydactyly or severe especially with conditions that manifest themselves in adulthood, for example, Huntingdon's Chorea. Counselling of potentially affected couples is complicated by the variable expression and incomplete penetrance which can significantly affect the severity of the condition. Autosomal recessive disorders require the inheritance of the faulty gene from both parents to produce an affected offspring. In cystic fibrosis, one in 22 people in the United Kingdom are carriers which means that one in 500 couples are at a one in four risk of having an affected child. Many of the genes that cause these defects have now been identified enabling prenatal diagnosis of an affected foetus by CVS at 11 weeks. With rapid advances in molecular techniques and the cloning of new genes each day it is important that each pregnancy potentially affected by a genetic disorder is assessed because it is quite possible that a prenatal diagnostic test has been developed since the last pregnancy. Websites such as the 'On-line Mendelian Inheritance in Man' (OMIM) can give valuable up-to-date information (http://www.ncbi.nlm.nih.gov/Omim/).

Structural foetal abnormalities

The incidence of major structural abnormalities is in the region of 30 per 1000 births of which the central nervous system contributes approximately 10 per 1000, cardiovascular system 8 per 1000, renal tract 4 per 1000, and skeleton 2 per 1000. Although the incidence remains quite low, this group accounts for 20–30 per cent of perinatal mortality in developed countries. Routine ultrasound examination in the mid-trimester, which is widespread in Europe, aims to identify many of these. Unfortunately, the majority of such malformations occur in low risk pregnancies and the overall detection rates remain low, although recent studies report detection rates for major anomalies in the region of 50–60 per cent.

Despite the failings in some studies to demonstrate an impact on perinatal survival, the offer of an ultrasound examination remains popular with most parents. Unfortunately, there is not always the appreciation that this is a screening test and that it can be declined. Most women who decline serum screening for example, attend for the anomaly scan and may be justifiably upset if markers for Down syndrome are detected.

Nevertheless, detection of certain anomalies in the antenatal period may have considerable benefit. There may be an underlying genetic problem or other associated abnormalities. For example, 30 per cent of foetuses with exomphalos (herniation of the foetal bowel into the umbilical cord) will have Down syndrome and 10 per cent will have an associated cardiac problem. With certain congenital abnormalities, such as major congenital heart disease, neonatal preparation for delivery may be needed with the added benefit of enabling the parents to meet the team who will be involved in the care of their baby.

Some structural abnormalities are very disfiguring (facial clefting and gastroschisis) and antenatal detection allows valuable time for parental preparation not only in terms of what to expect when their child is born but also what can be done (Figs 3 and 4).

With increasing availability of fertility treatment the multiple pregnancy rate has increased from 10.4 per 1000 maternities in 1985 to 14.4 per 1000 maternities in 1997. Perinatal mortality rates are 37, 52, and 231 per 1000 live and stillbirths for twins, triplets, and higher-order multiple births, respectively. Whilst knowing whether or not twins are identical is of great

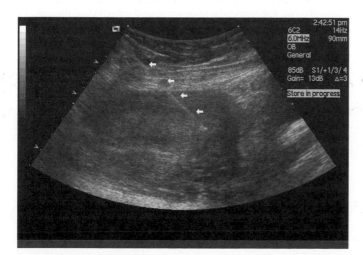

Fig. 2 Chorionic villus sampling showing needle (arrows) lying within the placenta at 12 weeks gestation.

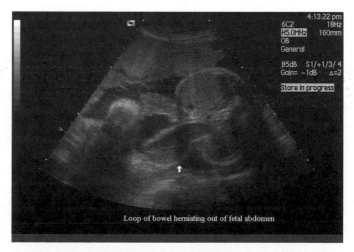

Fig. 3 Ultrasound diagnosis of gastroschisis at 24 weeks gestation with loops of bowel herniating from the anterior abdominal wall.

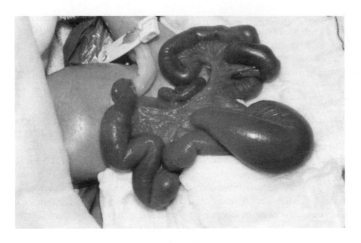

Fig. 4 Appearances of the gastroschisis immediately after birth.

interest to parents, of more concern to the obstetrician is whether twins share the same placenta (monochorionic) or have separate placentas (dichorionic). Monochorionic twins are always identical (monozygous) whereas dichorionic twins are usually non-identical (dizygous) but can be identical. It follows, therefore that the only way dizygosity can be confirmed on ultrasound examination is by demonstration of discordant genitalia. Determination of chorionicity is important because monochorionic twins have a five times higher rate of late miscarriage and perinatal mortality, an increased risk of genetic and structural abnormalities and a greater incidence of intrauterine growth restriction. With monochorionic placentation, there are vascular communications between the twins and in 15–20 per cent twin–twin transfusion syndrome occurs. This ultimately leads to overtransfusion of one twin (the recipient) causing a compensatory polyuria resulting in polyhydramnios, and oliguria in the co-twin (donor) which presents with severe oligohydramnios giving the appearance of a 'stuck twin' as it becomes shrouded in its own amniotic membrane. Untreated, this condition is usually fatal to both twins so early detection is vital to allow the opportunity for in utero therapy. Because of all these complications, most foetal medicine centres advise fortnightly scans from early in the second trimester. Chorionicity can be accurately determined by ultrasound examination at the time of the dating scan at the end of the first trimester. It becomes increasingly difficult thereafter and if there is any doubt at this stage prompt referral is vital so as not to miss the opportunity for accurate diagnosis.

Finally, some structural abnormalities require in utero intervention to maximize the chances for the baby. Isolated pleural effusions may prevent adequate lung development in utero. Pleural-amniotic shunts can be inserted via the maternal abdomen and uterus so that one end of the shunt lies within the pleural space of the foetal chest and the other allows drainage of the fluid into the amniotic cavity. At delivery, immediate clamping of the shunt is required to prevent a developing pneumothorax with the onset of spontaneous respiration.

Medical therapy

Under certain circumstances medical treatment can be offered to the pregnant woman with the aim of the drugs passing across the placenta to treat an underlying foetal problem. Occasionally, idiopathic polyhydramnios develops in the second trimester increasing the risk of pre-term labour. If severe, fluid can be aspirated from around the foetus by passing a needle through the maternal abdominal wall under ultrasound guidance into the amniotic cavity (amniodrainage) but carries a small risk of pre-term labour. An alternative is for the mother to take a prostaglandin inhibitor. This will pass into the foetus, and by a direct action on the foetal kidneys, reduce foetal urine output, decreasing the quantity of amniotic fluid.

Rarely, a foetus will develop a sustained cardiac arrhythmia. This often presents with decreased foetal movements in the second or third trimester. Ultrasound assessment may demonstrate a foetal tachycardia and secondary signs of cardiac failure (foetal hydrops). Although delivery will allow the opportunity for direct therapy, such babies delivered prematurely have a poor outcome. Maternal administration of antiarrhythmics such as digoxin or flecainide can cause cardioversion with subsequent resolution of the cardiac failure allowing the pregnancy to continue with delivery of a healthy infant nearer to term.

Certain maternally transmitted congenital infections will benefit from in utero medical therapy. If toxoplasmosis is suspected in pregnancy, the administration of spiramycin to the mother will reduce the chance of transplacental passage to the foetus. If foetal infection is confirmed either by ultrasound examination or analysis of amniotic fluid samples for toxoplasma specific genetic sequences by PCR, treatment with pyrimethamine, sulfadiazine, and folinic acid in alternating courses with spiramycin may decrease the foetal sequelae.

Surgical therapy

One of the greatest advances in foetal medicine over the last 20 years has been the ability to gain access to the foetal circulation by ultrasound-guided needling procedures. This can either be at the point of insertion of the umbilical vein into the placenta, in a free loop of umbilical cord or directly into the foetus itself, usually where the umbilical vein courses through the foetal liver. This allows a pure sample of foetal blood to be aspirated and also enables life-saving transfusions if the foetus is severely anaemic.

Rhesus alloimmunization

Red cell alloimmunization results in the passage of antibodies across the placenta to the developing foetus. If the foetus has the same blood group as the antibodies the red blood cells will be destroyed causing foetal anaemia. The commonest example of this is with the Rhesus blood group system. Women who are rhesus negative may produce antibodies against the D antigen if the foetus is Rhesus positive. This so-called sensitization usually occurs when there has been leakage of small quantities of foetal blood into the maternal circulation. This can occur in the pregnancy without any warning. Certain events will increase the risk of sensitization such as amniocentesis, antepartum haemorrhage, external trauma, for example, following a road traffic accident, and of course, delivery of the baby. Under these circumstances, the chance of sensitization occurring can be reduced by the administration of anti-D immunoglobulin to the mother within 72 h of the sensitizing event. The widespread use of prophylactic anti-D has significantly reduced the incidence of rhesus alloimmunization. Nevertheless, occult sensitization still occurs. This is usually diagnosed when routine antenatal blood tests detect the presence of antibodies. When the quantity of antibodies reaches a certain level referral to a foetal medicine centre for further assessment is necessary. The degree of risk may be quantified by performing an amniocentesis and looking for the breakdown products of foetal red blood cells in the amniotic fluid. The levels of these products can be plotted on well validated graphs against the maternal gestation (Liley's charts) and when the 'action line' is crossed foetal blood sampling performed with the facility to carry out an in utero transfusion should the foetus be anaemic. Depending on the gestation at which foetal anaemia is diagnosed multiple transfusions may be required until the foetus achieves sufficient maturity to allow safe delivery. This treatment is now commonplace and is generally safe allowing the delivery of a healthy infant which would otherwise die in utero from hydrops foetalis.

With the reduction in rhesus alloimmunization due to the widespread use of anti-D, other red cell antigens, such as Kell and anti-c, are becoming increasingly important causes of foetal anaemia.

Although serial amniocentesis remains the accepted method of monitoring such foetuses each procedure carries a small risk of miscarriage or pre-term labour and worsening sensitization. Recently, more reliance has been placed on non-invasive means. In anaemic foetuses, blood is preferentially shunted towards the foetal brain. Doppler assessment of the blood flow in the foetal middle cerebral artery can detect a decreased resistance and increased flow indicative of foetal anaemia. At this point invasive testing can be performed. Using this approach, fewer invasive tests are required minimizing the risk to the foetus.

Another important cause of severe foetal anaemia is infection with parvovirus (Fifth disease). This is particular amenable to treatment as the infection is self-limiting usually requiring only a single red blood cell transfusion. As the virus causes no long-term problems providing the transfusion is tolerated, the foetus usually makes a complete recovery.

Conclusion

Foetal and maternal medicine is a rapidly developing subject, and the primary care physician require a broad understanding of the problems and opportunities for therapeutic interventions. In particular, accurate pre-pregnancy counselling helps potential parents have realistic expectations of what to expect in pregnancy.

Key points

- ◆ Pre-eclampsia is a multisystem disease and is more than hypertension and proteinuria; women with persistent epigastric pain may have severe disease.

- ◆ Women with pre-existing diabetes are at risk of congenital abnormalities. This is reduced by tight glycaemic control before conception.

- ◆ Gestational diabetes is associated with a 50% risk of subsequent non-insulin dependant diabetes, and women should have annual glucose checks.

- ◆ Any suspicion of DVT or PE warrants immediate referral; chest X-ray and venography are safe in pregnancy and are associated with negligible radiation to the foetus.

- ◆ Drugs, including inhaled or oral steriods for asthma are safe in pregnancy and while breast-feeding.

- ◆ Most anticonvulsant drugs are equally teratogenic, and this risk increases with multiple agents. Women taking them should receive 5 mg of folic acid from 3 months pre-conceptually.

- ◆ Severe pruritus in the second half of pregnancy, particularly on the palms and soles, may indicate intrahepatic cholestasis of pregnancy. Abnormal liver function tests require urgent referral for investigation and foetal monitoring.

- ◆ Screening for Down syndrome results in invasive testing in 5% of pregnancies, and detects 70% of affected babies.

- ◆ Ultrasound scanning will detect 60–70% of foetal anomalies at best.

Further reading

CEMD: **Department of Health**. Why Mothers Die. Report on confidential enquiries into maternal deaths in the United Kingdom 1996–1999. London: Stationery Office, 2001. (This triennial publication outlines the management issues surrounding the maternal deaths that occur in the United Kingdom. Many issues concern primary care.)

Duley, L., Henderson-Smart, D., Knight, M., and King, J. (2001). Antiplatelet drugs for prevention of pre-eclampsia and its consequences: systematic review. *British Medical Journal* **322**, 329–33. (This article is a systematic review demonstrating the benefit of antiplatelet therapy in the prevention of pre-eclampsia.)

Nelson-Piercy, C. (2001). Asthma in pregnancy. *Thorax* **56** (4), 325–8 (review). (This provides a comprehensive review of the management of asthma in pregnancy.)

Nelson-Piercy, C. *Handbook of Obstetric Medicine*. Isis Medical Media, 1997. (This handbook provides easy reference, including charts, algorithms, and key points on the management of most medical problems in pregnancy.)

Shennan, A. and Bewley, S. (2001). How to manage term breech deliveries. *British Medical Journal* **323** (7307), 244–5. (This editorial outlines the evidence for avoiding breech deliveries at term, while stressing the need for external cephalic version.)

Snijders, R. (2001). First-trimester ultrasound. *Clinical Perinatology* **28**, 333–52. (This review explains the value of early ultrasound in the diagnosis of foetal problems.)

Taylor, M.J.O. and Fisk, N.M. (2000). Multiple pregnancy. In *The Obstetrician and Gynaecologist*. RCOG (2000). (This article provides a concise but comprehensive review of the problems associated with multiple pregnancies.)

8.8 Caring for women in labour

Matthew K. Cline and Phillipa M. Kyle

Introduction

Pre-natal care is instituted with the goal of establishing a relationship with the pregnant woman and detecting, treating, or minimizing risk factors to the mother and foetus throughout the pregnancy. Providing care during labour and birth continues this process. The clinician must remain vigilant to not only detect abnormalities that occur during the course of labour, but also to avoid unnecessary interventions that could interfere with it. Research into the interventions used during labour has helped clarify which interventions are beneficial, unnecessary, or potentially harmful. In many areas, the evidence is inconclusive, and in these instances it is important for the patient's preferences to guide care. The World Health Organization's, 'Care and Normal Birth: a Practical Guide', is summarized in Table 1, and was designed to be used regardless of level of care, setting, or specific training of birth attendant.

Diagnosis of labour

Labour is defined as the 'progressive dilatation of the uterine cervix with repetitive uterine contractions'. Pre-natal education can have an important role, as one randomized study showed that a 10-min educational meeting with the clinic nurse about when to come to the hospital for labour decreased outpatient hospital visits for false labour from 57 per cent of nulliparous women to 30 per cent.[1]

Patients in early or latent phase labour are often observed in an outpatient setting for several hours to monitor dilatation. To evaluate whether nursing care in early labour could reduce unnecessary hospitalizations, McNiven et al. randomized nulliparous women who were contracting and who presented to the hospital at less than 3 cm dilated to a usual care group (admitted) or a reassurance group (sent home with instructions). Those sent home, when subsequently admitted in active labour, had a decrease in Caesarean delivery from 10.6 to 7.6 per cent, lower rates of oxytocin augmentation, reduced use of pain medication or epidural, shorter labour duration, and a shorter second stage. They also had significantly higher satisfaction scores.[2]

Table 1 Effective and ineffective practices during birth (modified from the WHO Grading of Practices in Labor[26])

Practices supported by evidence
   Personal birth plan
   Offering oral fluids during labour and delivery
   Providing care as close to woman's home as feasible and safe
   Respecting right of women to privacy in birth
   Empathic support by caregivers, and respect for women's choice of
      companions, during labour and birth
   Giving women as much information and explanation as they desire
   Non-invasive, non-pharmacological methods of pain relief during labour,
      for example, massage and relaxation techniques
   Foetal surveillance by intermittent auscultation as first choice in women at
      no apparent risk
   Freedom in position and movement throughout labour
   Active management of the third stage of labour
   Early skin-to-skin contact between mother and child. Support initiation
      breastfeeding within 1 h postpartum

Practices which are clearly harmful or ineffective and should be eliminated
   Routine enema or pubic shaving
   Routine intravenous infusion in labour
   Routine use of supine position during labour
   Sustained, directed bearing down efforts (Valsalva) during the second
      stage of labour
   Use of oral tablets of ergometrine or prostaglandins in the third stage of
      labour to prevent haemorrhage
   Routine manual exploration of the uterus after delivery

Practices for which insufficient evidence exists to support a clear recommendation
   Non-pharmacological methods of pain relief during labour, e.g., herbs,
      immersion in water, and nerve stimulation
   Routine early amniotomy in the first stage of labour
   Nipple stimulation to increase uterine contractions during the third stage
      of labour

Practices which are frequently used inappropriately
   Restriction of food/fluids during labour
   Pain control by systemic agents or epidural analgesia
   Continuous electronic foetal monitoring
   Oxytocin augmentation
   Routinely moving labouring woman to different room at onset of second stage
   Encouraging woman to push when full dilatation or nearly full dilation of the
      cervix has been diagnosed, before woman feels urge to bear down more
   Rigid adherence to stipulated duration of the second stage if maternal and
      foetal conditions are good and if there is labour progress
   Operative delivery
   Liberal or routine use of episiotomy

A prolonged latent phase of labour, defined as over 20 h in nulliparas and 14 h in multiparas, often responds to therapeutic rest with sedation. Choices for sedation include morphine or other narcotics given in sufficient doses to allow the patient to sleep. The majority of these patients will awaken in active labour, while about 15 per cent will have stopped contracting and were in false labour.[3] It is important to make a correct diagnosis of labour and manage false, early, and latent phase labour well as a prolonged latent phase is associated with subsequent dystocia and an increased rate if Caesarean delivery.[4]

Progress of labour

First stage of labour

Latent phase

Friedman described the period of increased uterine contractions that precedes active labour, lasting from 1 to 20 h, as the latent phase of labour.

Active phase

As the uterine contractions become regular, more painful, and longer, the active phase of labour begins. This begins when the cervix is dilated 3–4 cm, but individual variation exists. When plotted as cervical dilatation or descent against hours in labour, it is noticeable as a distinct change in slope of the curve. Knowledge of this graphical representation of labour has led to creation of 'action lines' suggesting when intervention might be necessary. Such partographs often use a 1 cm/h rate of dilatation as the minimum acceptable without intervention, but it is important not to adopt rigid guidelines based exclusively on cervical dilatation.

Descent of the foetal head

With a singleton in vertex presentation, the foetal head can become engaged at any point before or during labour, but a ballotable head at term requires further investigation, especially in a primigravid woman.

Second stage of labour

The second stage of labour begins with complete dilatation of the cervix and ends with birth. While in the past various unsupported time limits have been suggested, it is recognized that epidural analgesia can prolong the first and second stages, and if progress is being made in descent of the foetal head, and the mother and foetus are tolerating labour well, labour should continue.

Third stage of labour

The third stage begins at birth and ends when the placenta is delivered. It is during this phase that potential complications such as postpartum uterine atony with maternal haemorrhage can occur, and this has led to the evaluation of active versus physiologic management of the third stage.

Care during labour

Position changes and ambulation during labour

Many authors have discussed the multiple benefits that occur when a labouring patient is allowed to modify her position based upon personal comfort. There is good evidence that position change is useful in achieving good progress in labour, is well tolerated, and can safely be accomplished. Position change may be more important than a 'best' position.[5]

If position change is important during the first stage, it may be even more important at minimizing dystocia in the second stage. Many labour units still utilize the dorsal lithotomy position for the birth, mainly due to caregiver convenience. However, evidence suggests significant benefit of other positions; upright delivery reduces lumbar lordosis, directs the foetal head towards the outlet of the pelvis, and increases the pressure exerted by the presenting part.[6]

Maternal support during labour

In many cultures, it is characteristic for the labouring patient to be supported by other women who are not directly providing medical care for the patient. Evidence of multiple benefits of having a doula, or labour support person, present throughout the labour has led to use of this type of assistance in many maternity settings. A Cochrane review showed that the presence of a doula was associated with a reduced need for: medication for pain relief, operative vaginal delivery, Caesarean delivery, and a reduced number of neonates with APGAR score below 7 at 5 min. Maternal satisfaction was also significantly improved.[7] Criteria for doula selection include having had a positive vaginal birthing experience, being willing to be available throughout the labour, and speaking the same language as the patient. While support by the patient's partner can also be beneficial, the value attributed to the doula in trials is in addition to family or partner support. While nursing support is of course very beneficial, the trial data demonstrates that hospital nursing staff cannot replace doulas.

Pain relief during the first stage

As pain perception during labour is variable, no single approach works for all labouring patients. However, in order to have multiple options for providing assistance to the labouring patient, the clinician should be familiar with a number of interventions. Childbirth education often stresses psychoprophylaxis, and can be practiced by the patient at home, and has been noted to provide benefit.

Transcutaneous electrical nerve stimulation and nitrous oxide are commonly used methods of pain relief, as are intracutaneous sterile water injections, massage, showers, and other forms of water therapy. Birth in water has been extensively reviewed and found, with professional guidance, to be safe.

Parenteral narcotics such as morphine or its synthetic analogues can provide some relief during labour, but can also cause nausea and sedation in the mother, and decreased variability of foetal heart tones and depressed respiration in the neonate. Diamorphine has been shown to be the most effective of this group.[8] In some settings, intravenous fentanyl has been employed, as its rapid onset and short duration of action make it an attractive alternative.

Epidural analgesia is perceived as the most effective at diminishing maternal pain, and for those who request pharmacologic pain relief, patient satisfaction is higher and pain scores during labour are lower with epidural analgesia compared to narcotics. While the most recent Cochrane meta-analysis concludes that epidural analgesia does not increase labour dystocia or Caesarean delivery rates, recent data show that there is an increased rate of assisted vaginal delivery with epidural use.[9] This remains a controversial area, with many clinicians feeling certain that outside the rarified conditions of a randomized controlled trial, epidural analgesia, especially very early employment, indeed does increase the Caesarean section rate. This effect is likely mediated, in part, by keeping women in bed attached to a monitor, thereby reducing mobility. It is likely that it is not epidural analgesia per se that increases the use of various interventions but the *routine* employment of this modality early and often as a substitute for attentive care and before less complex pain management strategies have been attempted. Moreover, well-timed use of epidural analgesia can normalize labour and reduce other interventions.[10,11] Additionally, a recent prospective trial suggests that low-dose epidural techniques compared to traditional higher dose techniques may lead to a higher normal vaginal delivery rate.[12]

Pain relief during the second stage

Several options, including epidural analgesia, exist for relief of pain during the second stage of labour. As the pain is related to distention of the vagina and perineum, somatic rather than visceral nerves are stimulated, making narcotics (intrathecal or systemic) less effective. Local infiltration of an anaesthetic such as 1 per cent lidocaine is an option for perineal analgesia, but the place of infiltration can weaken the tissues and lead to perineal tearing at that point. Women who are prepared for the sensations of crowning—the 'ring of fire' referred to by midwives—find that the pressure they exert on the perineum decreases their perception of pain. The pudendal block, utilized to block the pain impulses along the dorsal perineal nerve, can be quite effective for perineal analgesia or for assisted vaginal birth.

Evaluation of the foetus during labour

Both in North America and the United Kingdom, continuous electronic foetal monitoring has become the standard for foetal surveillance, with at least 85 per cent of labouring patients being monitored in this fashion. However, randomized trials performed after the technology had been adopted did not show significant benefit for low-risk mothers. Numerous expert groups state that the choice of technique of foetal monitoring during labour, whether continuous electronic foetal monitoring (EFM) or intermittent auscultation (IA), should be based on the risk profile of the patient and the judgement of the individual physician and patient. A Cochrane review of trials comparing the two methods (including over 50 000 patients) concluded that continuous EFM was associated with a slightly decreased risk of a 1 min APGAR score less than 4 and a decreased risk of neonatal seizures. The increase in neonatal seizures was observed in settings where oxytocin was used routinely without EFM, whereas today, use of oxytocin for induction or augmentation is a specific indication for use of EFM. The decreased risk of neonatal seizures was only noted in centres in which foetal scalp pH sampling was available when an abnormal foetal heart tracing occurred; therefore, these seizure-associated factors were likely site-specific. No significant differences were seen in rate of admissions to neonatal intensive care units or perinatal deaths. EFM was associated with an increased rate of Caesarean delivery and total operative delivery.[13] The current recommendations for method of foetal surveillance involve assessing the risk of the patient and if considered low risk proceed to IA every 15 min during the first stage of labour and every 5 min during the second stage of labour (monitoring throughout a contraction and for 1 min afterward). Previously, the use of a 15–20 min EFM 'admission test strip' upon arrival had been utilized along with a patient's known history to decide whether or not the patient was appropriate for intermittent auscultation. Recent data suggest that this increases the operative delivery and intervention rates with no demonstrable benefit on perinatal outcome.[14]

Interventions not found to be beneficial during labour

Several interventions that were previously a standard part of admission to a labour ward have been found to be either unnecessary or possibly harmful. These include perineal shaving, and routine use of enemas. There is no clinical evidence to justify these practices. Oral intake is often limited during labour, as some are concerned about the possibility of aspiration should a patient require general anaesthesia for an unexpected Caesarean delivery. Routine access to oral liquids does not seem to have significant risk to the patient and is recognized as appropriate by the American College of Obstetrics and Gynecology, and some even consider a light diet as acceptable although preferably in combination with H2 antagonists. Routine reliance on intravenous hydration may lead to potential fluid overload and decreases maternal mobility.

The birth

The traditional pushing method taught to caregivers in many settings is closed-glottis pushing with full dilatation, whether or not the patient feels the urge to bear down. A recent study has suggested that allowing the head to descend until it distends the pelvic floor may result in more effective pushing, less maternal exhaustion, and a lower risk of foetal malpresentation, especially in the setting of epidural analgesia.[15] A randomized trial of the use of oxytocin in the second stage in patients with an epidural revealed lower rates of operative vaginal delivery and Caesarean delivery with similar infant outcomes.[16] This trial suggests that oxytocin use, rather than as a routine part of the second stage, in the presence of deep epidural analgesia, is an alternative prior to instrumentation. As the head distends the perineum, many birth care providers assist with perineal stretching by use of perineal massage, either with lubricants or a topical anaesthetic. However, recent evidence suggests that the benefits are minimal.[17] In nulliparas, however, perineal massage during the weeks before labour can decrease perineal trauma during birth.[18]

The use of pressure on the foetal occiput to maintain flexion potentially results in fewer perineal lacerations. Routine episiotomy is not beneficial,[19] as its use is associated with increased rates of rectal trauma, increased postpartum pain, and dyspareunia. British and other international studies addressed only mediolateral episiotomy and birth attendance generally by midwives. The only North American study[20] evaluated median episiotomy and physician practice, demonstrating that routine median episiotomy was associated with a 20-fold increase in severe rectal trauma, even after controlling for the factors that might lead to episiotomy use. Mediolateral episiotomy marginally reduces rectal trauma over medial episiotomy but is the more painful of the two.[21] Therefore, episiotomy should be employed only for specific indications. Moreover, forceps or vacuum use is not an obligatory indication for episiotomy. In settings where episiotomy was separated from instrumentation, rectal trauma was significantly decreased.[22]

Third stage of labour management

Recent evaluation of the third stage of labour has divided it into physiologic (or expectant) management versus active management. Expectant management involves delayed cord clamping and waiting for spontaneous placental delivery with the cord intact without the use of uterotonic drugs. Active management involves administration of an oxytocic after delivery of the anterior shoulder with cord traction and massage of the uterus to hasten placental separation. Benefits of active management of the third stage are decreased postpartum haemorrhage, increased postpartum maternal haemoglobin, and reductions in need for maternal blood transfusion. Adverse effects include increased nausea and vomiting, increased pain during the third stage, and increased postpartum hypertension.[23]

After the birth

Following birth, skin-to-skin contact between the mother and newborn and support of early breastfeeding are important. The placenta should be examined for completeness. Attention should then focus on exploring the vagina and perineum for lacerations and ascertaining uterine tone. First-degree lacerations involve the mucosa, generally are superficial, and do not require repair unless significant bleeding is noted. Second-degree lacerations penetrate into subcutaneous fascia or muscle of the perineum, but do not disrupt the rectal mucosa or sphincter. Episiotomy is an induced second-degree laceration, and both are repaired with a continuous absorbable suture started above the apex of the vaginal portion of the laceration and continued out to the introitus into the subcutaneous tissue of the perineum to complete repair of the perineal body and perineal skin. Third-degree lacerations extend into the fibres of the rectal sphincter and repair involves reapproximating the rectal sphincter capsule in addition to the routine second-degree laceration repair that overlies this area. Fourth-degree lacerations extend through the rectal sphincter and into the rectal lumen. This repair requires a submucosal layer in the rectum, reinforcing of the rectovaginal fascia, and a repair of the rectal sphincter and then completion of the remaining laceration repair. A third- or fourth-degree repair should only be performed by the experienced. For significant perineal injury, anti-inflammatory drugs assist in pain relief.

Suture material

Randomized controlled trials have assessed both type of suture and the technique used. Evaluation of polyglycolic acid versus catgut or chromic suggests that polyglycolic acid (Dexon or Vicryl) causes less short-term pain and results in lower incidence of wound dehiscence. A subcuticular technique is associated with less short-term pain in the perineum than interrupted transcutaneous sutures.[24]

Conclusion

Providing pre-natal and maternity care is an ideal role for the primary care practitioner. As a continuation of the pre-natal plan of detecting, reducing, and intervening for risk factors that develop in the mother or foetus during the pregnancy, appropriate attention should be given to abnormalities that may occur at the time of admission to labour and delivery and throughout the birth. Maternal preferences remain an important part of decision-making during birth care, and are especially important in guiding the clinician when current medical evidence in inconclusive. Primary caregivers

have a responsibility to enhance the atmosphere of birth while preserving safety, to empower women in this intensely personal and spiritual event, and to remain vigilant in keeping childbirth the normal physiologic experience that it is, rather than a technology-driven event.[25]

References

1. Bonovich, L. (1990). Recognizing the onset of labor. *Journal of Obstetric, Gynecologic, and Neonatal Nursing* 19, 141–5.
2. McNiven, P.S., Williams, J.I., Hodnett, E., Kaufman, K., and Hannah, M.E. (1998). An early labor assessment program: a randomized, controlled trial. *Birth* 25, 5–10.
3. Cohen, W.R., Acker, D.B., and Friedman, E.A., ed. *Management of Labor* 2nd edn. Rockville MD: Aspen Publishers, Inc., 1989, pp. 13–14.
4. Chelmow, D., Kilpatrick, S.J., and Laros, R.K. (1993). Maternal and neonatal outcomes after prolonged latent phase. *Obstetrics and Gynecology* 81, 486–91.
5. Smith, M.I. et al. (1991). A critical review of labor and birth care. *Journal of Family Practice* 33, 281–92.
6. Fenwick, L. and Simkin, P. (1987). Maternal positioning to prevent or alleviate dystocia in labor. *Clinical Obstetrics and Gynecology* 30 (1), 83–9.
7. Hodnett, E.D. (2001). Caregiver support for women during childbirth (Cochrane Review). In *The Cochrane Library* Issue 1. Oxford: Update Software.
8. Fairlie, F.M., Marshall, L., Walker, J.J., and Elbourne, D. (1999). Intramuscular opioids for pain relief in labour: a randomised controlled trial comparing pethidine with diamorphine. *British Journal of Obstetrics and Gynaecology* 106, 1181–7.
9. Howell, C.J. et al. (2001). A randomised controlled trial of epidural compared with nonepidural analgesics in labour. *British Journal of Obstetrics and Gynaecology* 108, 27–33.
10. Janssen, P.A., Klein, M.C., and Soolsma, J.H. (2001). Differences in institutional cesarean delivery rates—the role of pain management. *Journal of Family Practice* 50, 217–23.
11. Klein, M.C., Grzybowski, S., Harris, S., Liston, R., Spence, A., Le, G., Brummendorf, D., Kim, S., and Kaczorowski, J. (2001). Epidural analgesia use as a marker for physician approach to birth; implication for maternal and newborn outcomes. *Birth* 28 (4), 243–8.
12. COMET Study Group UK (2001). Effect of low-dose mobile versus traditional epidural techniques on mode of delivery: a randomised controlled trial. *Lancet* 358, 19–23.
13. Thacker, S.B. and Stroup, D.F. (1999). Continuous electronic heart rate monitoring versus intermittent auscultation for assessment during labor (Cochrane Review). In *The Cochrane Library* Issue 2. Oxford: Update Software.
14. Mires, G., Williams, I., and Howie, P. (2001). Randomised controlled trial of cardiotocography versus Doppler auscultation of fetal heart at admission in labour in low risk obstetric population. *British Medical Journal* 322, 1457–62.
15. Fraser, W.D. (2000). Multicenter, randomized, controlled trial of delayed pushing for nulliparous women in the second stage of labor with continuous epidural analgesia. The PEOPLE (Pushing Early or Pushing Late with Epidural) Study Group. *American Journal of Obstetrics and Gynecology* 182 (5), 1165–72.
16. Saunders, N.J. et al. (1989). Oxytocin infusion during second stage of labor in primiparous women using epidural analgesia: a randomized double blind placebo controlled trial. *British Medical Journal* 299, 1423–6.
17. Stamp, G., Kruzins, G., and Crowther, C. (2001). Perineal massage in labour and prevention of perineal trauma: randomised controlled trial. *British Medical Journal* 322, 1277–80.
18. Labrecque, M., Eason, E., Marcoux, S., Lemieux, F., Pinault, J.J., Feldman, P., and Laperriere, L. (1999). Randomized controlled trial of prevention of perineal trauma by perineal massage during pregnancy. *American Journal of Obstetrics and Gynecology* 180 (3 Pt 1), 593–600.
19. Caroli, G. and Belizan, J. (2001). Episiotomy for vaginal birth (Cochrane Review). In *The Cochrane Library* Issue 3. Oxford: Update Software.

20. Klein, M., Gauthier, R., Robbins, J., Kaczorowski, J., Jorgensen, S., Franco, E., Johnson, B., Waghorn, K., Gelfand, M., Guralnick, M., Luskey, G., and Joshi, J. (1994). Relation of episiotomy to perineal trauma and morbidity, sexual dysfunction and pelvic floor relaxation. *American Journal of Obstetrics and Gynecology* **171** (3), 591–8.

21. Coats, P.M., Chan, K.K., Wilkins, M., and Beard, R.J. (1980). A comparison between median and mediolateral episiotomy. *British Journal of Obstetrics and Gynaecology* **87**, 408–12.

22. Ecker, J. et al. (1997). Is there a benefit to episiotomy at operative vaginal delivery? Observations over ten years in a stable population. *American Journal of Obstetrics and Gynecology* **176**, 411–14.

23. Prendiville, W.J., Elbourne, D., and McDonald, S. (2000). Active versus expectant management of the third stage of labour (Cochrane Review). In *The Cochrane Library* Issue 1. Oxford: Update Software.

24. Kettle, C. and Johanson, R.B. (2000). Absorbable synthetic versus catgut suture material for perineal repair (Cochrane Review). In *The Cochrane Library* Issue 1. Oxford: Update Software.

25. Larimore, W.L. and Cline, M.K. (2000). Keeping normal labor normal. *Clinics in Primary Care* **27**, 221–36.

26. World Health Organization. *Care in Normal Birth: A Practical Guide*. Report of a technical working group. WHO, 1999 (document can be obtained at: www.who.int/reproductive-health/publications/MSM_96_24/MSM_96_24_table_of_contents.en.html

8.9 Breastfeeding

Verity Livingstone

Breastfeeding is the ideal method of feeding and nurturing infants. The recommendation is to exclusively breastfeed for about the first 6 months followed by the timely introduction of table foods when the infant is neuro-developmentally ready to sit up, chew, and swallow without gagging. Child-led weaning should occur after the first year.[1]

Preparation for breastfeeding

The breastfeeding goals pre-natally are: to assist families make an informed choice about infant feeding; to prepare women cognitively and emotionally for breastfeeding; to identify and modify risk factors for lactation and breastfeeding; and to offer anticipatory guidance. Women should be screened for biological, psychological, and social risk factors that might interfere with lactation or breastfeeding. Clinical signs of successful mammogenesis include breast growth, increased breast sensitivity, and the production of a colostrum-like transudate by the end of pregnancy.

Maternal risk factors

- Anatomically abnormal nipples or breasts with insufficient glandular development.

- Breast surgery which interferes with lactiferous duct drainage.

- Endocrinopathies, including thyroid, pituitary, and ovarian dysfunction with relative infertility, may interfere with lactation.

- Chronic maternal illnesses may cause maternal fatigue.

- Women with physical disabilities need assistance with regard to safe, alternative nursing positions.

- Complications that may result in early maternal infant separation.

- Maternal infections such as hepatitis, human immunodeficiency virus (HIV), or cytomegalovirus may all be transmitted to the infant in utero; the added viral load through breast milk is probably clinically insignificant. In industrial countries, it is prudent to advise HIV or HTLV-1 positive women not to breastfeed.

- Women who abuse substances should be informed about the risks and counselled about abstinence. The risks of contaminated breast milk and the risks of artificial feeding must be weighed against the benefits of human milk.

- Previous unsuccessful breastfeeding may herald future problems.

- Previous or chronic psychiatric disorders including depression may recur in the postpartum period and interfere with maternal parenting abilities.

Infant risk factors

Several infant factors interfere with lactation and breastfeeding. They include prematurity, illness, early maternal/infant separation, oral/palatine abnormalities and sucking, swallowing or breathing disorders, and galactosaemia.

Psychological and social risk factors

Many factors influence a woman's choice of feeding methods including beliefs, attitude, knowledge, and skills. Women need to be provided with accurate information and support for their decision. The goal is to foster a positive emotional environment among family, friends, and community.[2]

Pre-natal breast examination

After reviewing the maternal history, perform a careful breast examination. The breasts should have enlarged by at least one or two bra cup sizes. Variations in breast appearance or asymmetry may indicate glandular insufficiency. Scars give clues to potential glandular, ductal, or nerve disruption. Gently pinch the areola to assess its elasticity and graspability. The action of sucking by the infant helps to draw out the nipple and form a teat. True inverted nipples may impede correct latching and suckling. There is no evidence to support nipple preparation.

Establishing breastfeeding

Within 120 min after birth neonates start suckling. The secretory IgA in the colostrum acts as the first immunization. Frequent episodes of breast stimulation cause surges of prolactin and oxytocin that trigger lactation, and facilitate uterine contractions. The duration of lactation correlates inversely with the time of the first breast stimulation. When mothers and infants are separated, lack of prolactin surges fail to trigger and maintain lactation. Clinical signs of successful lactogenesis are the production of colostrum, and fullness of the breasts followed by copious milk within 48 h.[3] If frequent and efficient breastfeeding is not possible, the mother must be taught how to express her milk. About 100 min of short, frequent pumping per 24 h help maintain adequate prolactin levels.

Pre-lacteal and complementary feeds upset the process of lactogenesis by removing the neonate's hunger drive. Postpartum haemorrhage with pituitary ischaemia or retained placental products may impair lactogenesis. Reduction mammoplasty results in lactiferous duct outlet obstruction and lactation failure.

UNICEF and the World Health Organization launched the global Baby Friendly Hospital Initiative in 1992 which outlines 10 simple steps designed to promote, support, and protect breastfeeding.[4,5]

Breastfeeding depends on careful positioning and attachment and an intact suckling ability of the infant. Infants suckle instinctively, mothers must be taught (Fig. 1).

- *Positioning*: The mother should sit comfortably with her arms and back supported and her feet raised on a small stool. Place the unswaddled baby on a pillow, facing the uncovered breast, tummy to tummy. The

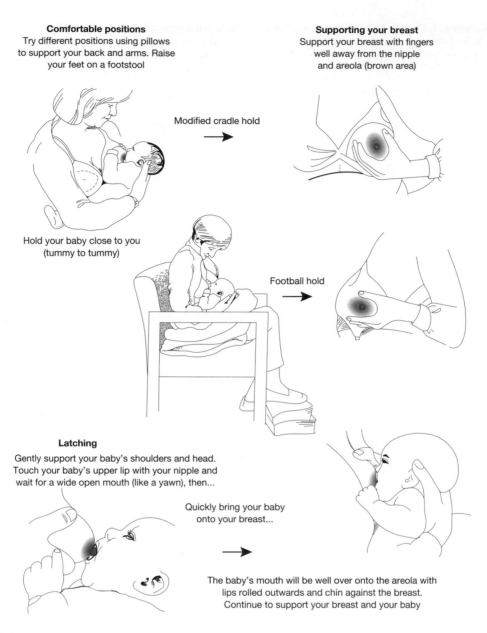

Comfortable positions
Try different positions using pillows
to support your back and arms. Raise
your feet on a footstool

Supporting your breast
Support your breast with fingers
well away from the nipple
and areola (brown area)

Modified cradle hold

Hold your baby close to you
(tummy to tummy)

Football hold

Latching
Gently support your baby's shoulders and head.
Touch your baby's upper lip with your nipple and
wait for a wide open mouth (like a yawn), then...

Quickly bring your baby
onto your breast...

The baby's mouth will be well over onto the areola with
lips rolled outwards and chin against the breast.
Continue to support your breast and your baby

Fig. 1 Breastfeeding techniques.

baby's arms should wrap around the breast. Cup the breast forming an oval that matches the shape of the mouth. Support the baby's head and shoulders.

- *Attachment:* Brush the nipple against the baby's upper lip and wait until he roots and gapes. Quickly draw the baby forward well over the nipple and on to the areola. The lips should be flanged and placed well behind the nipple base. The chin is extended into the breast. The mother must sandwich her breast and support the baby's head and shoulders, throughout the feed.

- *Suckling:* The infant draws the nipple and the areola tissue to the junction of the hard and soft palate and initiates suckling in a co-ordinated manner. A fixed, retracted, or engorged nipple or a large, well-defined nipple may interfere with grasping and result in sore nipples. Poor neonate suckling technique either because of a mechanical inability to grasp the areola correctly or because of a suck, swallow, or breathing disorder leads to inefficient milk transfer and poor weight gain. Retrognathia, cleft lip or palate, an uncoordinated, weak, fluttering or bunched-up tongue may

interfere with effective sucking dynamics. Ankyloglossia (tongue-tie) is an important cause of suckling difficulties. The nipple often becomes traumatized and sore. A simple frenotomy should be done when clinically indicated.

Initially, the infant drinks drops of colostrum. This rapidly increases to about 100 ml per feed. Infants should feed according to their cues, about 8–10 times per day. The duration varies between mother–infant pairs because the rate of milk transfer is not uniform. Infants recognize satiation and spontaneously stop suckling. Most feeds are complete within 30–40 min. The infant should remain at the first breast until the rate of flow of milk is no longer sufficient to satisfy the infant then offer the second breast.

Hospital discharge planning

Discharge planning allows early identification of breastfeeding problems. All mothers should be taught the signs of successful breastfeeding and instructed to call for advice if they have concerns. If an infant has lost more than 7 per cent of the birth weight or if the mother–infant pair has known risk factors, delay discharge or arrange early community follow-up. All mothers and infants should be reassessed within 1 week of birth.

Common postpartum problems

Not enough milk

Neonates lose less than 10 per cent of birth weight and start gaining weight within a few days and should regain birth weight in the second week. If the mother is having difficulties breastfeeding or if the infant's weight is more than 7 per cent below birth weight, perform a clinical assessment to identify causes of inadequate breastfeeding.[6] This includes taking a maternal, infant, and breastfeeding history and performing a maternal and infant examination. Observe breastfeeding to assess positioning, latching, suckling, and swallowing. An accurate test feed followed by pumping to estimate residual breast milk is helpful when assessing maternal milk yield and infant milk intake. Take care when using standard office scales due to their unreliability. Consider all causes of infant failure to thrive. Neonatal hypernatremic dehydration is a serious consequence of breastfeeding malnutrition. It is difficult to detect clinically, if the weight loss is greater than 10 per cent, obtain serum electrolytes.[7]

In broad terms, management includes avoiding the precipitating factors, stimulating lactation by correcting the breastfeeding technique, and increasing the frequency and duration of breastfeeding. Pumping after feeds and galactogues including metoclopramide and domeperidome 10–20 mg qid can effectively augment lactation. Some neonates will require complementary feeds using expressed breast milk or formula. Reassure mothers that partial breastfeeding or mixed feeding is still beneficial.

Too much milk

Milk stasis, blocked ducts, deep radiating breast pain, lactiferous duct colic, inflammatory mastitis, infectious mastitis, and breast abscess are common problems. Clinical experience has shown that most mothers experiencing any or all of these symptoms have large, thriving infants, and do not drain both breasts regularly. These symptoms and signs are consequences of a high rate of milk synthesis combined with milk retention due to incomplete breast drainage and possibly infection.

White spot

Mothers complain of sharp, 'knife-like' cramps or shooting pains deep in the breast, often between feeds. A small white spot visible on the nipple represents oedematous epithelium blocking the nipple pore and milk flow. A small white granule of caseinous milk precipitate may also cause lactiferous ductal obstruction. Outlet obstruction causes ductal cramping or colic due to increased retrograde pressure and myoepithelium smooth muscle contractions. Gentle abrasion or probing can remove the epithelium skin and relieve the obstruction. Occasionally, a small calculus or granule will pop out suddenly, relieving the obstruction. Occasionally, breastfeeding is ineffective at removing the thickened inspissated milk and manual or mechanical expression may be necessary. Show the mother how to firmly compress her breast with a cupped hand, squeezing gently towards the nipple whilst feeding or pumping, in order to dislodge the milk or calculus.

Milk stasis

A firm, lumpy, slightly tender quadrant in the breast signifies milk stasis. Over time, if this area is not drained, cytokines from the milk seep into the interstitial tissue causing an inflammatory mastitis. Inflammatory mastitis occurs within 12–24 h of milk blockage. Improved milk drainage will resolve the situation quickly.

Cellulitis

When there is a breach in the mucus membrane such as a cracked nipple, superficial skin contaminants such as *Staphylococcus aureus*, or *beta-haemolytic streptococcus* can lead to a spreading cellulitis with superficial erythema.

Acute mastitis

Breast pain and erythema associated with flu-like symptoms and fever are characteristic of infectious mastitis. A high rate of milk synthesis combined with continuous, poor drainage of a segment of the breast may result in the stagnant milk becoming secondarily infected with common skin pathogens via an ascending lactiferous duct infection leading to acute adenitis. Most mothers present with general malaise, chills or sweats, but others only have localized symptoms and signs of inflammation. In clinical practice, treatment is empirical. Common bacterial pathogens include *S. aureus, Escherichia coli,* group A *beta-haemolytic Streptococcus* with occasional *Streptococcus faecalis,* and *Klebsiella pneumonia.* Antibiotics of choice include penicillinase-resistant penicillins such as dicloxacillin, or erythromycin, cephalosporins, sulfonamides, and clindamycin. A 10–14-day course is required. The breast milk excretion of these antibiotics is minimal and it is considered safe to continue to breastfeed. Clinical improvement is usually seen within 24–48 h; the erythema subsides, the fever decreases, and breast pain improves.

Chronic mastitis

Chronic mastitis may be due to *re-infection* or a *relapsed* infection. Re-infection occurs sporadically due to exposure to a new pathogen, commonly transmitted from the infant. A relapsed infection occurs shortly after completion of therapy; it signifies inadequate primary treatment and failed eradication of the pathogen. Stricture formation in the duct may impair drainage and a deep nidus of infection leads to contaminated residual milk.

Breast abscess

Inadequately treated mastitis and ongoing milk retention can develop into a breast abscess. A high fever with chills and general malaise, associated with a firm, well-demarcated, tender, fluctuating mass, usually with erythema of the skin, indicates abscess formation, though in some rare instances systemic symptoms may be absent. Ultrasonography of the breast and needle aspiration under local anaesthesia are useful diagnostic techniques to identify collections of fluid or pus and distinguish mastitis from a galactocele or inflammatory breast cancer. An abscess requires incision and drainage under local or general anaesthesia. The incision should be radial, not circumferential, to minimize duct severance. Insert a large drain and irrigate daily until the cavity closes. Apply the dressings such that the infant can continue to breastfeed and/or the mother can express her milk. Regular drainage prevents further milk stasis and maintains lactation.[8]

Management goals

Correct breastfeeding techniques, improving milk drainage, and avoiding missed feeds are the sine qua non of treatment. Alternating positions allows thorough drainage of all segments and prevents milk stasis. Breastfeeding should start on the fullest breast and remain until all areas feel soft. Remaining at one breast allows a higher fat intake that often satiates the infant for a longer period and decreases the hunger drive. The second breast remains full and reduces milk synthesis. In some cases, bilateral breastfeeding with partial drainage reduces lactation more effectively. Sleeping through the night, returning to work, the introduction of bottles or table foods, and weaning are all periods when breastfeeds may be missed. Areas of breast lumpiness or caking that persist after breastfeeding may indicate milk stasis or a blocked duct. Thorough expression of this residual milk should relieve the situation and prevent secondary complications. Continue breastfeeding but if a mother must abruptly wean, use a lactation suppressant such as bromocriptine 2.5 mg bid for 14 days.

Sore nipples

When nipple pain, excoriations, dermatitis, or ulceration continue despite careful breastfeeding technique, a dermatological approach is required to elucidate the cause.

Nipple trauma

Tongue friction or gum compression, due to inappropriate latch, can cause trauma and result in superficial skin abrasions and painful nipples. Repositioning can have a dramatic effect and instantaneously remove the pain and discomfort. If necessary, stop breastfeeding and pump for 48–72 h to allow healing to occur.

Chapped nipples

Dry, cracked nipples may be chapped due to loss of the moisture barrier in the stratum corneum because of constant wet and dry exposure combined with nipple friction. Moisturisers and emollients such as USP modified anhydrous lanolin applied to the nipples and areola after each feed are cheap and effective. A mild corticosteroid ointment may help to decrease the inflammation.

Impetigo of the nipple

Sore nipples associated with skin breakage including cracks, fissures, and ulceration have a high chance of being contaminated with microorganisms. The clinical findings on the nipple and areola of local erythema, excoriations, purulent exudates, and tenderness are suspicious of impetigo vulgaris due to coagulase-positive *S. aureus*, and group A *beta-haemolytic streptococcus*.[9] The standard treatment for impetigo, includes careful washing with soap and water to remove crusting. Topical antibiotic ointments such as fusidic acid or 2 per cent mupuric acid help in conjunction with systemic penicillinase-resistant antibiotics, such as dicloxacillin, a cephalosporin, or erythromycin in penicillin-allergic patients. Treatment should continue for 7–10 days until the skin is fully healed. The source of the infection is often from the infant's oropharyngeal or opthalmic flora. In persistent or recurrent infections, it is necessary to treat the infant concurrently.

Candidiasis dermatitis

Suspect candidiasis when persistent nipple symptoms such as a burning sensation on light touch, and severe nipple pain during feeds, are combined with minimal objective findings on the nipple. Typical signs include a superficial erythema on the nipple and areola, or a dry, flaky dermatitis with clear demarcated edges over the areola. Clinical examination of the infant is mandatory because *Candida albicans* is passed from the infant's oropharynx to the mother's nipple. With persistent or atypical pain and dermatitis, culture the nipples and obtain skin scraping to determine a fungal infection.

The management includes careful hygiene, and antifungal creams such as nystatin, clotrimazole, miconazole, or 2 per cent ketoconazole. Apply the creams to the nipple and areola before and after each breastfeed for 10–14 days. In addition, treat other sites of candidiasis in both mother and infant, simultaneously. Oral thrush in the infant should be treated conscienciously with an oral antifungal agent after each feed. Carefully paint the oral cavity with 2 per cent miconazole gel or mycostatin suspension 100 000 U/g liquid and then insert 0.5 ml of mycostatin suspension into the mouth by dropper for 14 days. Oral fluconazole 3 mg/kg od for 14 days or oral ketoconazole 5 mg/kg/day for 7 days in approved for oropharyngeal candidiasis in newborns. Gentian violet 0.5–1 per cent aqueous solution is cheap and effective if used sparingly under medical supervision. Daily painting of the infants' mouth and mothers' nipples for about 5–7 days is usually sufficient. Excessive use may cause oral ulceration. Avoid or sterilize foreign objects contaminated with yeast, including soothers and rubber nipples, to prevent re-infection.

Vasospasm or Raynauds phenomenon

Vasospasm or Raynauds phenomenon of the nipple presents as a blanching of the nipple tip and severe pain and discomfort radiating through the breast after feeds and between feeds. Repetitive trauma to the nipple combined with local inflammation or infection and air cooling, trigger a characteristic painful vasospastic response. Correcting the latch and alternating breastfeeding positions throughout the feed will prevent ongoing nipple trauma. Avoid cold and apply warmth to the nipples to reduce the spasms and treat local infections aggressively.

Health professionals will be expected to take a leadership role in the promotion, protection, and support of breastfeeding.

Key points

1. Pre-natal lactation assessments, anticipatory guidance, early detection, and diagnosis combined with correct management of lactation prevents premature termination of breastfeeding.

2. A delay in early inititation of breastfeeding may result in subsequent lactation insufficiency.

3. Measure serum electrolytes if there is a significant weight loss in a breastfed neonate because signs of hypernatraemic dehydration may be absent.

4. Persistent sore nipples, excoriations, dermatitis, or ulcerations are pathological and need a dermatological evaluation.

References

1. *Breastfeeding and the Use of Human Milk*. American Academy of Pediatrics Policy Statement. 1997 http:/www.aap.org/policy/re9729.html.

2. **Riodan, J.M.** (1997). The cost of not breastfeeding: a commentary. *Journal of Human Lactation* **13** (2), 93.

3. Infant feeding: the physiological basis. *Science Journal of the World Health Organization*, bulletin supplement to Vol. 65, 19–40, 1989.

4. **WHO/UNICEF.** *Protecting, Promoting and Supporting Breastfeeding: The Special Role of Maternity Services*. Geneva: World Health Organization, 1989. http:/www.unicef.org/newsline/tensteps.htm.

5. **Perez-Escamilla, R., Pollitt, E., Lonnerdal, B., and Dewey, K.G.** (1994). Infant feeding policies in maternity wards and their effect on breastfeeding success: an analytical overview. *American Journal of Public Health* **84** (1), 89–97.

6. **Livingstone, V.H.** (1995). Breastfeeding kinetics. A problem-solving approach to breastfeeding difficulties, Vol. 78. In *Behavioural and Metabolic Aspects of Breastfeeding* (ed. A.P. Simopoulos, J.E. Dutra de Oliveira, and I.D. Desai), pp. 28–54. World Review of Nutrition and Dietetics. Basel: Karger.

7. **Livingstone, V.H., Willis, C.E., Abdul-Warren, L.O., Thiessen, P., and Lockitch, G.** (2001). Neonatal hypernatremic dehydration associated with breastfeeding malnutrition: a retrospective survey. *Canadian Medical Association Journal* **162** (5), 647–52.

8. **WHO.** *Mastitis: Causes and Management*. Department of Child and Adolescent Health and Development. Geneva: World Health Organization, 2000. WHO/FCH/CAH/00.13.

9. **Livingstone, V.H. and Stringer, L.J.** (1999). The treatment of staphylococcus aureus infected sore nipples: a randomised comparative study. *Journal of Human Lactation* **15** (3), 241–6.

Further reading

Lawrence, R.A. and Lawrence, R.M. *Breastfeeding: A Guide for the Medical Profession* 5th edn. St Louis Mo: Mosby Inc., 1999.

Breastfeeding (2001). Part 2: The Management of Breastfeeding. *Pediatric Clinics of North America*. Philadelphia PA: WB Saunders Co. A Harcourt Health Sciences Company, 2001, Vol. 48, Issue 2.

Hale, T.W. *Medications and Mother's Milk* 7th edn. Amillo TX: Pharmasoft Medical Publishing, 1998. http:/neonatal.ttuhsc.edu/lact/index.html.

Websites

Academy of Breastfeeding Medicine: www.bfmed.org

Lactation Education Resources: www.LERon-line.com

La Leche League International: www.lalecheleague.org

Livingstone, V.H. and Miller, B. The Art of Successful Breastfeeding—A Video Guide for Health Professionals, 1997. www.breastfeeding1.com

8.10 Feeding problems in infants and young children

David G. Riddell

Introduction

A mother's instinctive primary objectives are to nourish (love and feed) and protect her infant. Success in the first is measured by weight gain and an infant's contentedness. Routine advice concerning breastfeeding, selection of a formula, provision of supplements to avoid deficiencies, and the later introduction of solids, is easy for the parent to follow. Yet, we still commonly find infants with iron deficiency and even rickets. Excessive crying, regurgitation, changing bowel habits, and changes seen with progression of infant development create parental anxieties. These anxieties often focus on infant feedings. The practitioner may be required to spend considerable time exploring feeding and family issues.

Routine feeding advice

Breastfeeding is ideal, but after breast milk (see Chapter 8.9) formula is the preferred milk for infants under 1 year of age. Doctors' opinions are often not involved in the initial selection of a formula, and they are consulted mainly when problems arise. Fortunately, formula composition is very strictly controlled and all proprietary formulas are nutritionally adequate.

Selection of a formula

Primary formulas

The first-line formula for an infant should be an iron-fortified cow milk formula; the sugar should be lactose. Several varieties of formula fit into this category, all having a different type of protein component: a casein predominant formula, a whey predominant formula, and a whey protein formula with part of the protein content broken down into polypeptides. Cost and marketing often determine a parent's selection. To further compound the selection process, some of the above formulas will also have varieties of their formula available without iron, some without lactose, some for the older infant, some pre-thickened for the regurgitating infant, some with long chain fatty acids for the developing brain, and all of the above possibly available in ready to feed, liquid concentrate, and powdered forms.

Secondary formulas

Soy formulas

These do not contain animal protein and do not have lactose as the sugar. They may be used in cases of cow milk allergy, lactose intolerance (a very uncommon condition in infancy), and where parents do not wish their infant to have animal protein.

Specialty formulas

One should consider specialist referral before adventuring into using these products.

- Calorie enriched formulas—often used in failure to thrive conditions where fluid balance is a concern, for example, heart failure.
- Protein hydrolysate formulas—for example, for milk allergy.
- Elemental formulas—for example, for short bowel syndrome.
- Other more disease-specific formulas.

Other milks

For the infant under 1 year of age, any other type of milk, aside from breast milk and formula, is inferior and may be problematic.

- The use of any animal milk in unpasturized form should be avoided because of the risk of infection.
- An evaporated milk mixture needs to be carefully constituted to give adequate protein.
- Because of their high solute load, high protein content, and the association of occult gastrointestinal blood loss in infants under 6 months of age, whole cow's milk and goat's milk should not be used until after 9 months of age. Both milks need to be vitamin D fortified.
- Skimmed and partially skimmed milks should not be used until after 1 year of age because of uncertainties with caloric and essential fatty acid supply.

Introduction of solids

Four to six months of age is the time to introduce solids. There are a number of reasons for this. Development of lip and tongue control will now allow the infant to manipulate food within the oropharynx. Changes in taste and texture will lead to better acceptance of new foods later in the first year. In addition, iron stores have been depleted by 4 months of age and another source of iron is required. The methods available to introduce solids are diverse and heavily influenced by parental beliefs and attitudes.

Supplements

Nutritional supplements are only given to infants to prevent specific diseases caused by lack of nutrients in the milk. We recognize breast milk is low in vitamin D and iron. All formulas provide adequate vitamin D but some may be low in iron.

Vitamin K

Haemorrhagic disease of the newborn (early and late) is a deficiency disease secondary to a transient lack of vitamin K. The incidence is greater in breast-fed than in bottle-fed infants. It is prevented by the early administration of one dose of 1 mg of vitamin K. Intramuscular vitamin K is preferred as it is the most effective form. When the oral route is used, a second dose at 2 weeks and a third at 6–8 weeks of age helps prevent a delayed haemorrhagic condition occurring at about 1 month of age or beyond. The complexity of the oral regime adds to the problem.

Vitamin D

Nutritional rickets should not be considered a disease of the past. There are only a few natural sources of vitamin D; sunlight, certain fish oils, and egg yolk. All milk, including breast milk, needs fortification to supply adequate vitamin D. North of 50° latitude (applicable to the southern hemisphere also—although the population living south of 50° latitude is very small), the November to February sun is not strong enough to hydroxylate vitamin D in the skin. In addition, other geographic pockets are low in the amount of sunlight received at certain times of the year.

Although it does not require much sunlight exposure to make adequate vitamin D, there are other influences:

◆ The darker the skin, the more the suns rays are blocked by melanin.

◆ As the ozone is depleted and the melanoma rate increases, infants and children are being kept covered in clothing and sun block.

◆ Environmental smog has been shown to reduce vitamin D hydroxylation. It also keeps individuals indoors.

◆ Social customs may leave pregnant women with low vitamin D levels, increasing the risk of early rickets in their infants.

The age of onset of rickets may even be in foetal life if the mother is severely vitamin D depleted. Often, it is not until the second half of the first year that rickets becomes clinically apparent and the presentation may be quite variable. Developmental delay or failure to thrive may be warning signs, but it is the many bony changes that should lead to the diagnosis. These include: flared long bones, the 'rachitic rosary' which describes the enlargement of the costochondral junctions, frontal bossing, short stature, and bowed legs. Classical radiological features confirm this. A low serum calcium, low phosphate, and high alkaline phosphatase, along with normal renal and liver function, will support the diagnosis of nutritional rickets. A diagnosis or even suspicion of rickets is justification for specialist referral.

Prevention of rickets is the mandate of the family doctor. This will start with adequate supplementation of the mother during pregnancy and lactation if she is at risk. The infant requires at least 200 IU (5 µg) daily. This will be obtained in formula but the breast-fed baby should be supplemented unless the geographic area provides sufficient sun exposure.

Iron

This is a very common deficiency problem in the infant and young child. The incidence varies between 5 and 30 per cent in children 1–2 years of age, depending upon the population surveyed. Iron deficiency produces changes and alterations in many aspects of metabolism. It is the detrimental effect on cognitive and behavioural development that provides the impetus for prevention of iron deficiency. The cognitive impairment may not respond to subsequent iron treatment, suggesting that once the brain is affected, the damage is permanent. Non-cognitive changes due to iron deficiency in young children include short attention span, unhappiness, increased fearfulness, and increased body tension. Iron deficient infants may have lower scores in both motor and behaviour areas on infant development scales. There are many symptoms and signs attributable to iron deficiency; their non-specificity makes it a challenge to diagnose iron deficiency in the young child.

All natural milk is low in iron. Breast milk iron is absorbed very well but the total amount of iron is too low to maintain a positive balance for the infant beyond 4–6 months of age. Only iron fortified formulas are designed to provide this. Thus, for all infants beyond 4–6 months of age, there should be an external source of iron in the diet.

There are many ways to help prevent the prevalent problem of iron deficiency:

◆ in the premature infant, supplement with iron by 2 months of age;

◆ if exclusive breastfeeding is continued beyond 6 months of age, add an iron supplement;

◆ if formula feeding, use a formula with added iron;

◆ use infant cereals that are iron fortified from 4 months of age;

◆ introduce other iron-rich foods (meats) by 6–8 months.

It becomes more difficult to ensure iron adequacy as the child gets older. A dietary history should alert the physician to a potential problem but estimating iron intake from a dietary history is time consuming and inaccurate. For a quick dietary assessment of iron adequacy, consider instead the history of just the child's milk intake. This assessment is more difficult in the breast-fed baby where milk intake has to be estimated from feeding patterns and times (and interest in other foods). An infant up until 1 year of age will generally consume 80–100 kcal/kg daily. As the milk volume increases, the caloric intake from other foods decreases, thus reducing any other source of iron. To assess:

◆ Ask about the type of milk used.

◆ Make sure it is the average milk intake over 24 h.

   ■ 30 oz (~900 ml) non-iron-containing milk = 600 kcal = potential iron deficiency;

   ■ 40 oz (~1200 ml) non-iron-containing milk = 800 kcal = some degree of iron deficiency;

   ■ 50 oz (~1500 ml) non-iron-containing milk = 1000 kcal (total caloric needs) = moderate + iron deficiency.

◆ The longer the intake of milk at higher levels, the greater the deficiency.

The simplest means of diagnosis of iron deficiency is a blood count and red cell smear; this will demonstrate hypochromia and microcytosis, although in certain populations thalassaemia may confuse the issue. Further studies such as serum iron, iron binding capacity, serum ferritin are more confirmatory of a specific diagnosis but add greatly to the cost of a simple diagnosis. Treatment of iron deficiency consists of dietary adjustment along with an appropriate iron supplement dependent upon the degree of iron deficiency. Elemental iron in doses of 2–6 mg/kg/day for a 2–3 month period will treat most deficiencies.

Feeding problems

Infantile colic

The term 'infantile colic' often provokes anxiety in parents. It implies some mysterious condition that will cause their baby great distress. It is a term and condition loosely applied by both lay and medical persons. The amount of time crying per day is the only measure used to differentiate the 'colicy' infant from the normal infant, with 3 h or more of crying per day as the differentiating crying time. This definition is not very practical for the practitioner because of the inaccuracy in defining infant crying times. What is important is the fact there are no other features (e.g. excessive gas, pulling up of legs when crying, severity of crying, etc.) that are helpful with this diagnosis. Thus, this condition applies to infants who cry excessively without any apparent cause. It is very common for the parent and practitioner to attribute the crying to feeding problems.

Incidence estimates of colic range widely from 10 to 50 per cent; a frequent diagnosis in any case. The aetiology is likewise vague; literature is divided into two major camps—behavioural and milk protein intolerance. In approaching this problem, the practitioner should cover areas that would point to a specific cause of the infants irritability, but also explore characteristics that suggest another diagnosis, such as:

◆ Short-term irritability suggesting infection, inguinal hernia, etc.

◆ Neurological problems that often produce infant irritability but may be difficult to recognize. The pregnancy, birth, and family histories are helpful.

◆ Drug withdrawal that will often produce other symptoms along with the irritability.

◆ Excessive regurgitation that produces pain from oesophagitis.

◆ Maternal depression that may result in abnormal maternal–infant interaction.

The history should also explore:

◆ crying characteristics such as time of day, association with feedings, response to cuddling;

◆ sleep patterns;

◆ feeding history along with a family history of food-related problems;

◆ dietary changes and treatments tried already.

In the physical exam:

◆ growth parameters should progress along a normal curve;

♦ abnormal breathing patterns may indicate respiratory or cardiovascular conditions;

♦ abdominal distension may indicate renal or intestinal disease;

♦ the neurological examination should assess muscle tone, basic reflexes, and infant responsiveness.

As all other problems are ruled out, one is then left with an otherwise normal infant who cries excessively and is causing parental distress. *This is infantile colic—a diagnosis of exclusion* based loosely on behavioural characteristics. The history will roughly identify three groups of such infants. These patterns of crying often do not develop till 2–3 weeks of age as the effects of the birthing process wear off.

(1) The largest group—and indeed one can find this pattern in almost all infants—are infants who have a 2–4 h fussy period every day. For many this occurs in the evening. The physician can often predict this time of fussiness by inquiring about the timing of foetal activity patterns; activity implying wakefulness. These infants do not often cause undue parental distress.

(2) A group of infants who are problematic are the wakeful infants, who have poorly established sleep patterns, and do not settle after eating. They are restless and are often over-responsive to both external and internal stimuli. They cry when they should otherwise be content. Crying sometimes does not respond to the parent's best efforts to settle the child. This can be very frustrating to parents. It often leads the parents to concerns about feeding, gas, and bowel movements. Breastfeeding mothers will worry about the adequacy or content of their breast milk, and formula-fed babies often have their formula switched. These are the babies with the classic '3 month colic'. Simple reassurance is not adequate as some infants in this group are vulnerable to being battered. The parent must be guided to an understanding of infant behaviour. Often, these infants will have been very active foetuses, with poorly developed sleep/wakeful times. Exploring this with the mother is helpful. Parents need to realize that the baby is not going to settle easily. Increased carrying of the infant rather than putting the baby into the crib following feeds may help somewhat. The parent should also be encouraged to avoid over-stimulating the baby. The breastfeeding mother should be encouraged to continue breastfeeding. These babies often give confusing hunger signals and may be more successfully fed by the clock, rather than by demand. Removal of dairy products from mother's diet occasionally helps. For formula-fed babies, if it is felt necessary to change the formula, a hypoallergenic formula should be used. Lactose-free formulas are of little use as it is rare for a baby to be lactose intolerant. Use of medication such as simethicon and gripe water (alcohol free) are commonly used and although they rarely make a difference, they cause few side-effects. Other medication such as antispasmotics, herbal teas, other herbal medication, and sedatives should be avoided. These babies are mainly demonstrating behavioural changes.

(3) This last group of babies is fortunately small as they are very difficult babies. The history of these infants does suggest pain and discomfort but the cause is not apparent. They cry excessively, they feed poorly, sometimes arching and pulling away from the nipple, but are hungry at the same time. Sleep is fretful. Sometimes they burst into crying for what parents claim is no reason at all. Milk allergy may occur with this type of baby and a hypoallergenic formula may be useful. The breastfeeding mother should continue to breastfeed but alter her own diet and avoid dairy products. These babies may well need to be referred to a specialist to look for occult problems such as gastro-oesophageal reflux.

Gastro-oesophageal reflux

When does regurgitation, commonly seen in infancy, change to a diagnosis of gastro-oesophageal reflux? Parents commonly view repeated regurgitation as a problem and seek advice for its treatment.

While the lower oesophageal sphincter (LES) might be explained to the parents as a muscular ring that keeps gastric contents from washing back into the oesophagus, the actual mechanism is complex and the abnormality causing gastro-oesophageal reflex is unclear. The LES actually consists of:

♦ a diffuse high-pressure zone (no morphological muscle sphincter has been identified);

♦ the intra-abdominal oesophagus, the length of which is important for preventing reflux;

♦ the angle of His which is the angle the oesophagus makes when joining the stomach.

Symptomatic reflux may result from abnormalities of the LES (anatomic and functional), delayed gastric emptying, and increased intra-abdominal pressure. Most babies do not seem to develop problems from repeatedly spitting up. However, a variety of symptoms may indicate that this is a problem:

♦ failure to thrive secondary to impaired caloric balance;

♦ oesophagitis pain manifested in the infant by excessive irritability;

♦ respiratory symptoms that may be very varied, from cough and hoarseness, to aspiration and bronchospasm;

♦ 'spells' which may be apnea, cyanotic episodes, arching, even an apparent life-threatening event.

The presence of the above symptoms may be related to reflux and should necessitate a referral to the appropriate specialist.

Prolonged milk feeding

Whether by breast or bottle, a large milk intake persisting beyond 9–10 months of age creates problems. The busy youngster, who prefers a quick drink of milk, may manipulate the unsuspecting parents to this style of intake. Some of the consequences of this include:

1. Iron deficiency—details mentioned previously.

2. Food refusal—the baby who prefers the breast or bottle above all else will become increasingly dependent upon milk to the exclusion of solid foods. The parent often feels trapped knowing the baby will refuse and fight eating solids but will happily drink milk. The more determined the baby's personality, the more the parents are overwhelmed. The reversal of milk dependence and the introduction of other foods comes only with the reduction of milk intake first. It may take a lot of reassurance for the parent to follow advice to significantly reduce the milk intake and to realize that the child will not starve (for very long anyway). Solids are offered at the same time but not forced. It is only the exceptional child who will not alter eating patterns.

3. Baby bottle(breast) tooth decay is still a very common problem but one that is totally preventable. The upper midline teeth are maximally involved. The pathologic process is related to the amount of time the teeth are exposed to sugar-containing fluids. Parents often do not think that milk is included in this category, especially breast milk. Early fluoride drops are not preventative. Limiting excessive exposure of the teeth to sugar is the only prevention.

Conclusion

This chapter has briefly touched on a few key issues in infant feeding. Social and emotional elements, family, and cultural influences often affect the success of prevention and treatment efforts regarding feeding problems. It is not uncommon for a physician to be competing with advice from family members. A good relationship and interaction between physician and parent in resolving feeding problems is often the critical ingredient to the successful resolution of the problem.

Further reading

Lucassen, P.L.B.J. et al. (1998). Effectiveness of treatments of infantile colic: systematic review. *British Medical Journal* **316**, 1563–9.

Cervisi, J. et al. (1991). Office management of the infant with colic. *Journal of Pediatric Health Care* **5**, 184–90.

Hill, D. and Hosking, C. (2000). Infantile colic and food hypersensitivity. *Journal of Pediatric Gastroenterology and Nutrition* **30** (Suppl. 1), S67–76.

Orenstein, S. (1999). Consultation with the specialist; gastroesophageal reflux. *Pediatrics in Review* **20** (1), 24–8.

Brown, P. (2000). Medical management of gastroesophageal reflux. *Current Opinion in Pediatrics* **12**, 247–50.

8.11 Postpartum care

Dwenda Kay Gjerdingen

The postpartum period: general health, mechanisms of illness

Childbirth is followed by a period of recovery, called the puerperium, which has traditionally been defined as the period from termination of labour to complete involution of the uterus, approximately 42 days in duration. It is recognized, however, that recovery from childbirth frequently involves more than just the reproductive organs and often lasts for more than 6 weeks.

The physical process of giving birth naturally impacts the reproductive organs, including the uterus, ovaries, vagina, perineum, and breasts, in a variety of ways. After delivery, the enlarged uterus gradually shrinks in size over a period of several weeks, and lacerations or surgical incisions of the birth canal begin to heal. These processes may be complicated, however, by problems such as haemorrhage, haematoma, or infection. Ovulation, which has been suppressed throughout pregnancy, does not usually resume until several weeks after delivery. The breasts also undergo dramatic changes after delivery, which can lead to engorgement and pain. Here too, infectious complications may ensue, giving rise to mastitis or abscess (see Chapter 8.9, Breastfeeding).

Post-delivery changes are not limited to the reproductive organs, however. Childbirth may affect other organ systems, either directly or indirectly. For example, haemorrhage can result in anaemia, fatigue, and dizziness. Birth trauma may affect the nearby urinary tract, producing urinary retention, and eventually stress incontinence. Childbirth is also accompanied by numerous endocrine changes, one of these being a drop in oestrogen levels, which may cause vaginal atrophy, dry skin, mood disturbances, hot flashes, and increased sweating. For many mothers, the added responsibility of infant care contributes to their fatigue and decreased sexual interest and activity. Return to employment may exacerbate this fatigue, produce breast-feeding irregularities, and consequently, engorgement and infection, and increase the risk of respiratory infections resulting from daycare exposures.

In addition to these physical problems, many mothers also experience postpartum psycho-social disorders, such as the 'blues', depression, psychosis, panic disorder, post-traumatic stress disorder, and marital or partner conflicts. It is likely that a variety of factors, such as hormone shifts, role changes, heightened work responsibilities, and fatigue contribute to these problems. Both physical and mental postpartum disorders may persist for months or longer; further, mothers commonly experience several postpartum disorders concurrently. Such persistent, compound problems can produce distress and even functional limitations. Therefore, it is important that parents be educated about potential post-delivery health and social changes, that they are monitored for health problems, and that postpartum disorders are quickly recognized and effectively treated.

Postpartum education and surveillance

Education about postpartum well-being should be provided on a continuum, and can be incorporated into pre-natal, postpartum, and well-child visits. During the pre-natal period, expectant parents should be asked about their infant feeding preferences, and mothers should be encouraged to breastfeed their newborns, if possible. Expectant parents should also be asked about their desire for contraception after delivery, and informed of their options. Couples should be encouraged to plan together their parental work leave, strategies for managing additional post-delivery family responsibilities, and techniques for nurturing their relationship after childbirth.

During their postpartum hospital stay, mothers' complications of childbirth are recognized by asking about pain and discomfort, monitoring their temperature, vital signs, lochia, and haemoglobin, and by examining their abdomen and perineum, as indicated. Breastfeeding mothers should be coached in feeding techniques (please see Chapter 8.9, Breastfeeding), and they should be instructed to inquire about the safety of any drugs that they wish to take during the breastfeeding period. Drugs that are contra-indicated for breastfeeding mothers include tetracycline, chloramphenicol, iodine-containing substances, ergot alkaloids, gold, combination oral contraceptives, lithium, recreational drugs, radiopharmaceuticals, and most antineoplastic agents. Drugs that should be used with caution include sulfonamides, metronidazole, salicylates, antihistamines, psychotropic drugs, phenobarbital, alcohol, nicotine, and large quantities of caffeine.

Prior to their discharge from the hospital, mothers should again be asked about their desire for contraception and treated accordingly. Contraceptives that could be used soon after delivery are barrier methods and medroxy-progesterone injection. To ensure that medroxyprogesterone is not administered inadvertently to a pregnant women, it should be given within 5 days of delivery to a non-breastfeeding woman, or within the first 6 weeks after delivery to a breastfeeding woman. To minimize the risk of thrombo-emboli, combination oral contraceptives should not be started until 4 weeks after delivery. Combination oral contraceptives should be avoided in nursing mothers, as they may decrease the mother's milk production and cause jaundice and breast enlargement in the infant. However, progesterone-only oral contraceptives, barrier methods of contraception, and intrauterine devices can be used in women who breastfeed. Intrauterine devices can be inserted after complete involution of the uterus, at approximately 6 weeks postpartum (see Chapter 8.3 for additional information on contraception).

Mothers are typically asked to schedule an office visit in the early postpartum period. During this visit, women should be questioned about their breastfeeding, sexual activity, contraceptive concerns, physical health, energy, mood, plans for return to work, and marital or partner relationship. In addition, a physical examination, which includes the thyroid, breasts, and pelvis, should be performed. This single postpartum office visit does not provide adequate opportunity to effectively screen for problems that may occur later. For example, symptoms of postpartum thyroiditis or depression may not become obvious until weeks or even months after the postpartum visit. Therefore, it is important that mothers are encouraged to report delayed symptoms, particularly those relating to mood or extreme fatigue, and that these symptoms are evaluated, as previously described. Well-child visits provide convenient opportunities to briefly question parents about their well-being, and that of other family members.

Mothers' postpartum problems: prevalence, aetiology, diagnosis, and management

Problems that may be experienced by mothers in the early and later postpartum periods, along with their prevalence, aetiology, diagnosis, and management are shown in Tables 1 and 2. Additional problems, not shown in these tables, that occur with increased frequency in the months after

Table 1 Early postpartum disorders (initial 2 weeks)

Condition (prevalence)[a]	Clinical issues: aetiology, symptoms and signs, and/or diagnosis	Management
Physical disorders		
Perineal or rectal pain (most women)	Aetiology: vaginal or perineal lacerations, episiotomy, haematoma, haemorrhoids Symptoms and signs: pain secondary to lacerations or episiotomies usually diminishes over time, but may worsen with sexual activity; pain due to haemorrhoids is often aggravated by bowel movements	For perineal or rectal pain: tub baths, witch hazel, cool compresses, non-steroidal anti-inflammatory drugs, narcotics; for haemorrhoids: stool softeners, Anusol haemorrhoidal ointment or suppositories
Iron-deficiency anaemia (very frequent)	Aetiology: pregnancy, intrapartum/postpartum haemorrhage, caesarean section Symptoms and signs: fatigue, weakness, pale skin colour, hypotension, tachycardia Diagnosis: early, ↓ haemoglobin, haematocrit; later, ↓ mean cell volume and ferritin	If mild to moderate: oral iron (ferrous sulfate); if severe: transfuse
Fever	Aetiology: atelectasis, pneumonia, wound or urinary tract infection, breast engorgement, endometritis, transfusion reaction, septic pelvic thrombophlebitis Symptoms and signs: temperature ≥38°C, or 100.4°F	Differentiate cause and treat accordingly
Caesarean wound (4%) or perineal wound infection	Aetiology: *Staphylococcus aureus*, group A or B streptococci, *S. epidermidis*, enterococci, anaerobes, *Escherichia coli*, *Klebsiella* sp., *Clostridium perfringens* Symptoms and signs: inflammation, discharge, wound dehiscence, fever Diagnosis: WBC and differential, wound culture	Cefoxitin or cefotetan or ticarcillin/clavulanate or ampicillin/sulbactam or 2nd or 3rd generation cefalosporin plus metronidazol; surgical debridement if *Clostridium perfringens* infection
Endometritis (2.6% after caesarean section, 0.2% after vaginal delivery)	Aetiology: Bacteroides, group A and B streptococci, enterobacteriaceae, and *C. trachomatis*; more frequent after surgical procedures (e.g. caesarean section) Diagnosis: fever plus one or more of the following symptoms within 5 days of delivery—uterine tenderness, foul smelling lochia, leukocytosis of >12 000 after excluding other sources of infection	Clindamycin + gentamycin, if no improvement within 48 h, add ampicillin or vancomycin (if penicillin allergic); or 2nd or 3rd generation cephalosporin; continue i.v. treatment until afebrile for 48 h and clinically improved, then discontinue (need not follow with oral antibiotics)
Urinary retention (2–18%)	Aetiology: effects of anaesthesia (related to caesarean section or labour analgesia), pregnancy-induced hypotonic bladder Diagnosis: absence of spontaneous urination within 6 h after delivery or removal of urinary catheter	Initial measures: ambulation, privacy, warm bath; subsequent measures—catheterization every few hours until spontaneous voiding, prophylactic antibiotics if repeat catheterizations are necessary
Delayed postpartum haemorrhage	Aetiology: abnormal involution of placental site, endometritis, retained placental fragments Symptoms and signs: excessive bleeding ≥24 h after delivery, ↓ haemoglobin	I.V. fluids; uterotonics (oxytocin, methylergonovine, prostaglandins); ultrasound if continued bleeding; if retained placental fragments, curettage
Mental disorders		
The 'Blues' (26–85%)	Aetiology: likely, hormonal fluctuations Symptoms and signs: sadness, tearfulness, episodes of crying, anxiety, insomnia, poor appetite, irritability; begins within first week, lasts for a few hours to a few days	Support, reassurance
Psychosis (0.01–0.02%)	Aetiology: history of psychosis, bipolar disorder; provoked by childbirth factors Symptoms and signs: incoherence, loosening of association, delusions, hallucinations, grossly disorganized or catatonic behaviour; onset within first 2 weeks postpartum	Hospitalize, antipsychotics (see Section 9, Mental health problems, for further information)

[a] Prevalence is not listed for disorders where postpartum prevalence is unknown.

delivery, but for which treatment is primarily reassurance, include: hair loss (peaks to a 20 per cent prevalence at 6 months postpartum), increased sweating (17 per cent prevalence at 1 month), acne (16 per cent at 1 month), dizziness (11 per cent at 1 month), and hot flashes (10 per cent at 1 month).[4]

Fathers' and siblings' post-delivery problems

Although fathers tend to have fewer post-delivery health concerns than mothers, they too may experience a variety of problems for several weeks after delivery, including fatigue, insufficient sleep, headaches, colds, irritability, restlessness, nervousness, difficulty concentrating, worries about the future, sexual concerns, depression, anxiety, psychosis, impulsive behavioural disorders, sexual deviancy, and problem drinking. More than 10 per cent of fathers experience a psychiatric disorder after the birth of a child,[5] and depression in fathers is thought to be associated with that in mothers.

The infant's siblings often show behavioural changes after its arrival. These include imitations of the infant, attention-seeking behaviours,

confrontations with the mother or infant, regression, anxiety behaviours, maturity, and independence. Negative behaviours tend to be more frequent with siblings of the same sex, and they may result, at least in part, from mothers' decreased interactions with the older child.

Parents' post-delivery social changes

In addition to the physical and mental changes previously discussed, parents also experience dramatic social changes after they give birth, particularly with a first-born child. Two important social changes are those related to parents' work roles and their marriage or partner relationship.

Work responsibilities

Parents' work responsibilities after childbirth increase dramatically, primarily as a result of their additional childcare responsibilities. First-time parents are often ill prepared for this change and feel overwhelmed when these new responsibilities are combined with their previous household and employment activities.

Many women who deliver infants enter or re-enter the workforce after they give birth, although the timing and rate of re-entry vary from country

Table 2 Later postpartum disorders

Condition (prevalence)[a]	Clinical issues: aetiology, symptoms and signs, and/or diagnosis	Management
Physical disorders		
Sexual problems (≥50%)	Aetiology: vaginal/perineal trauma, vaginal atrophy (due to ↓ oestrogen), fatigue, competing work and childcare responsibilities, marital declines Symptoms and signs: dyspareunia, decreased sexual desire, satisfaction, and activity	Avoid episiotomies, if possible; oestrogen creams for vaginal atrophy (non-breastfeeding women); lubricants; encourage good communication
Fatigue (43% at 1 month)	Aetiology: childbirth, sleep loss, work responsibilities, anaemia, thyroid disorder, depression or other mental disorder, cardiomyopathy Diagnosis: if severe—physical exam, haemoglobin, thyroid stimulating hormone	Rest, support, treat associated disorders
Respiratory infections (>40% at 3–12 months)	Aetiology: aggravated by return to employment, child in daycare Symptoms and signs: cough, nasal congestion, rhinorrhoea, facial or ear pain, sore throat	Infection-specific medical treatment, minimize child's exposures to infections (handwashing, number of children in daycare)
Vaginal discomfort (21% at 1 month)	Aetiology: episiotomy (mediolateral > midline), perineal trauma, mucosal atrophy (due to decreased oestrogen) Symptoms and signs: pain with or without intercourse	Avoid episiotomies, if possible; if episiotomy is necessary, and if either midline over mediolateral episiotomy is acceptable, favour midline
Urinary stress incontinence (6–29%)	Aetiology: childbirth trauma, loss of muscle tone; risk factors include vaginal delivery, grand multiparity, and obesity Symptoms and signs: incontinence associated with coughing or sneezing	Pelvic floor muscle exercises, surgical repair if severe
Thyroiditis (5%)	Aetiology: autoimmune process Symptoms and signs: hyperthyroid phase (1–3 month)—fatigue, palpitations, goitre; hypothyroid phase (3–6 months)—depression, cognitive impairment, goitre Diagnostic studies: hyperthyroidism—↓ TSH (thyroid stimulating hormone), ↑ T_4 (rarely ↑ T_3); hypothyroidism—↑ TSH, ↓ T_4, and ↑ antimicrosomal antibodies	Hyperthroid phase: beta-blockers if symptomatic Hypothyroid phase: levothyroxine, attempt to with draw at 12–18 months postpartum, observe long-term for permanent hypothyroidism (seen in 23%)
Carpal tunnel syndrome (1–10%)	Symptoms and signs: hand numbness and tingling, pain, thenar weakness and atrophy, positive Tinel's and Phalen's signs Diagnosis: abnormal nerve conduction	Early symptoms: rest, night-time splints, non-steroidal anti-inflammatory drugs, corticosteroid injection; severe or prolonged symptoms: surgery
Psycho-social disorders		
Marital/partner dissatisfaction (majority of couples)	Aetiology: contributing factors—heavy workload, little leisure time, and perceptions of unfairness in division of household labour and childcare Symptoms and signs: decreased cohesion, consensus, affectionate expression, general satisfaction, and sexual interest; may persist until children reach school age	Encourage effective communication, sharing of work responsibilities, and other mutual emotional and practical support; protect individual/couple leisure time; support groups; couple therapy
Depression (5–10%)	Aetiology: associated with poor social support (especially partner's emotional and practical support), marital conflict, fatigue, sleep loss, thyroid disease, poor maternal or infant health, multiple births, low socio-economic status, immigrant status, short work leaves, and longer working hours Diagnosis: symptoms include depressed mood, decreased interest or pleasure with most activities, fatigue, feelings of worthlessness or inappropriate guilt, decreased ability to think or concentrate, recurrent thoughts of death or suicide, and ↑ or ↓ appetite, sleep, and psychomotor activity. To investigate secondary causes of depression, check haemoglobin and thyroid stimulating hormone levels	Support, psychotherapy and/or antidepressant medication; if non-breastfeeding, first choice is SSRI (selective serotonin reuptake inhibitor); if breastfeeding, weight risks and benefits of drug therapy; preferred drugs for breastfeeding women: amitriptyline, nortriptyline, desipramine, clomipramine, and sertraline[1] (see Section 9, Mental health problems, for further information)
Panic disorder[a]	Aetiology: childbirth-related stressors; associated with alcohol and drug abuse, poor physical/mental health, suicide attempts, marital conflict, and financial problems[2] Symptoms and signs: palpitations, dizziness, dyspnea, nausea, sweating, chest pain or discomfort, feelings of unreality, fears of dying or 'going crazy'	Pharmacological agents (SSRIs) and cognitive-behavioural therapy (see Section 9, Mental health problems, for further information)
Post-traumatic stress disorder[a]	Aetiology: emergency caesarean section or other traumatic childbirth event Diagnosis: history of traumatic, threatening event; symptoms (present for >1 month) include persistent re-experience of the event through intrusive distressing recollections, dreams, feelings (e.g. hallucinations or dissociative flashbacks), intense psychological distress, or physiologic reactions to symbolic cues; persistent avoidance of stimuli associated with the trauma; and increased arousal[3]	SSRIs psychotherapy, and patient education; continue treatment for 12 months or longer; prevent by having structured stress debriefings as soon as possible after the trauma (see Section 9, Mental health problems, for further information)

[a] Prevalence is not listed for disorders where postpartum prevalence is unknown.

to country. There is also international variation in maternity/parental benefits offered to parents with infants. A European Union directive mandating a 3-month parental leave was made in 1998. In most countries, the benefit is 80–100 per cent of wages, and in many countries, both paid maternity and paternity leaves are granted. However, unpaid maternity/parental/family leaves are in effect in Australia, New Zealand, Europe and the United States.[6] In the United States, the Family and Medical Leave Act of 1993 allows for 12 weeks of unpaid leave; however, this applies only to firms with 50 or more employees. As a result, less than half of the US work force is covered by this federal policy, and many parents return to work early for financial reasons. On average, US mothers take approximately 11 weeks of leave, and fathers only a few days. Because of their added childcare responsibilities, women from the United States and other countries frequently reduce their paid work hours in order to accommodate the needs of their infants. Mothers' postpartum paid work activities may impact their mental health, as women who work part-time appear less anxious than their full-time counterparts, and those taking shorter maternity leaves (6 weeks or less) have a greater risk of depression than those with longer leaves.[7]

The marriage/partner relationship

In general, the birth of a baby is associated with declines in marital or partner satisfaction, and these declines often persist until the children reach school age. For some couples, disturbances in the partner relationship are minimal, while for others, they reach crisis proportions. Specific changes that have been observed in couples across the transition to parenthood, and that may contribute to partner dissatisfaction, include: less marital/partner interaction, decreased sexual interest and activity, movement to a more traditional division of labour, and greater dissatisfaction with the division of labour and finances.

Measures that may help to stabilize or strengthen the couple's relationship during this period of transition include: providing pre-natal education about common postpartum sexual and other relationship changes, keeping work responsibilities to a manageable level, pre-planning for additional postpartum work responsibilities (including partners' work distribution), allowing for individual and couple leisure time, encouraging open communication, and attending parent support groups and/or couple therapy, when indicated. Recognizing the importance of social support to individuals' and couples' well-being,[8] it is especially important that partners be encouraged to give each other ample emotional and practical support during this period.

Implications of postpartum health problems

Untreated or inadequately treated postpartum problems may have serious long-term health or social implications for individuals, couples, families, and the workplace. The potential physical consequences of untreated postpartum disorders are numerous. For example, untreated pelvic infections may threaten subsequent fertility, or worse, a woman's life. Breast symptoms or infections that are not promptly managed can result in early cessation of breastfeeding, with potential adverse effects on the infant's nutritional and immune status. Constipation may aggravate haemorrhoids that developed during pregnancy or childbirth, thereby producing significant pain, and at times requiring surgical intervention.

Long-term mental or social problems may also develop from untreated postpartum disorders. A traumatic birth experience, sometimes seen with emergency caesarean sections, for example, may lead to post-traumatic stress disorder if parents do not have opportunity to debrief after the experience. Both postpartum depression and postpartum thyroiditis can produce cognitive impairment, fatigue, and mood disturbances—symptoms that are distressing in themselves, but if allowed to progress may weaken vital relationships and work performance, with potentially serious social and economic consequences. Postpartum depression may also affect the infant's cognitive and emotional development and contribute to a child's subsequent behavioural and emotional problems. Post-delivery disturbances in the couple's relationship, though relatively common for first-time parents, may threaten the couple's long-term relationship if allowed to progress. Therefore, it is important to monitor parents not only for physical disorders, but also for postpartum mental and social disturbances. Careful screening and management of such disorders will pay large dividends for not only individual parents, but also for couples, children, and society as a whole.

Key points

- Recovery from childbirth frequently involves more than just the reproductive organs, and often continues for months.

- Education about postpartum well-being can be incorporated into pre-natal, postpartum, and well-child visits, and should include information about breastfeeding, contraception, postpartum work responsibilities, postpartum mood disorders, and the marriage or partner relationship.

- Longer paid working hours and shorter maternity leaves tend to be associated with greater mental distress for mothers.

- Recognizing the importance of social support to parents' well-being, partners should be encouraged to give each other consistent emotional and practical support after they give birth.

References

1. **Wisner, K.L., Perel, J.M., and Findling, R.L.** (1996). Antidepressant treatment during breast-feeding. *American Journal of Psychiatry* **153**, 1132–7.

2. **Beck, C.T.** (1998). Postpartum onset of panic disorder. *Image: Journal of Nursing Scholarship* **30**, 131–5.

3. **Reynolds, J.L.** (1997). Post-traumatic stress disorder after childbirth: the phenomenon of traumatic birth. *Canadian Medical Association Journal* **156**, 831–5.

4. **Gjerdingen, D.K., Froberg, D.G., Chaloner, K.M., and McGovern, P.M.** (1993). Changes in women's physical health during the first postpartum year. *Archives of Family Medicine* **2**, 277–83.

5. **Ballard, C. and Davies, R.** (1996). Postnatal depression in fathers. *International Review of Psychiatry* **8**, 65–71.

6. **Kamerman, S.B.** (2000). From maternity to parental leave policies: women's health, employment, and child and family well-being. *Journal of the American Medical Women's Association* **55**, 96–9.

7. **Hyde, J.S., Essex, M.J., Clark, R., Klein, M.H., and Byrd, J.E.** (1996). Parental leave: policy and research. *Journal of Social Issues* **52**, 91–109.

8. **Gjerdingen, D.K. and Chaloner, K.M.** (1994). The relationship of women's postpartum mental health to employment, childbirth, and social support. *Journal of Family Practice* **38**, 465–72.

Further reading

Appleby, L., Warner, R., Whitton, A., and Faragher, B. (1997). A controlled study of fluoxetine and cognitive–behavioural counselling in the treatment of postnatal depression. *British Medical Journal* **314**, 932–6. (This double-blind randomized controlled treatment trial found that both fluoxetine and cognitive–behavioural counselling were effective treatments for postpartum depression, but that there seemed to be no advantage in combining these treatments.)

Bigner, J.J. (1998). Childbirth and the newborn. In *Parent–Child Relations: An Introduction to Parenting*, pp. 215–26. Columbus OH: Merrill. (This chapter reviews the literature on the transition to parenthood.)

Steiner, M. (1998). Perinatal mood disorders: position paper. *Psychopharmacology Bulletin* **34**, 301–6. (This paper reviews the prevalence, possible aetiologies, clinical assessment, and treatment of three postpartum mental disorders: the blues, postpartum depression, and postpartum psychosis.)

8.12 Unwanted pregnancy and termination of pregnancy

Ellen Wiebe

Introduction

Primary care physicians everywhere deal with the effects of induced abortion in their patients whether or not they work in countries in which abortions are legal. For the majority of physicians who do not do abortions themselves, it is important to understand the context, the psychological aspects, and the recognition and management of complications of abortion. This chapter will also discuss specific techniques for medical abortions and manual vacuum aspiration first trimester abortions with para-cervical block.

Historical and international context

Abortion has been practised since ancient times and there are references to surgical and medical abortions thousands of years ago in Greece, China, and Rome. In the nineteenth century, the first European laws were passed against abortion and soon became widespread. In the first half of the twentieth century, only a few countries had legal abortion, but by 2000, two-thirds of the world's women lived in countries where abortion was legal and available for all or most women requesting it. Most developing nations do not have legal abortion with the notable exceptions of China and India.

The World Health Organization estimates that each year 20 million unsafe abortions are performed, 95 per cent of which are in developing countries,[1] and which lead to 13 per cent of all maternal mortality. Romania gave us a striking example of the effect of abortion laws. Between 1966 and 1989, Romania had very strict laws prohibiting abortion. In addition to over 11 000 women dying of unsafe abortions during those years, there was a high rate of gynaecological morbidity and a high rate of abandoned and handicapped children. In 1990, the maternal mortality rate due to abortion dropped from 545 to 180. In some developing countries, despite restrictive abortion laws, it is still possible for many women to obtain safe abortions.[2]

In North America, safe legal abortions have been widely available since the 1970s but increasing antiabortion violence has occurred. The murders of abortion providers and other attacks on abortion clinics and staff have made it difficult to provide abortions and this has interfered with women's access in some areas.

Prevalence

As shown by Figs 1 (pie graph of induced abortions by region) and 2 (line graph of abortions legal and illegal per 1000 women by region), abortion rates are not dependent on whether abortion is legal or not.[3] For example, the rates of abortion in Africa and Latin America are higher than in Western Europe. The rates are the highest in the former communist countries of Europe. In the United States, the rate of unintended pregnancy is approximately 49 per cent of all pregnancies. This is higher than the unintended pregnancy rate in Western Europe and is the main reason for the higher abortion rate in the United States. Unintended pregnancies are related to poverty and younger age. The high rate of abortion in Eastern European countries is largely due to lack of affordable contraception. In Sub-Saharan Africa, a combination of poverty and lack of contraception leads to the relatively high rates of abortion. In North America and Western Europe, the majority of women having abortions are unmarried while in Asia and Africa most are married with children.

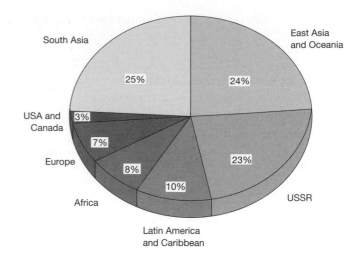

Fig. 1 Distribution of induced abortions by region, ca. 1990. [*Data from* Singh, S. and Henshaw, S. (1996). The incidence of abortion: a worldwide overview focusing on methodology and on Latin America. In *International Union for the Scientific Study of Population: Socio-cultural and Political Aspects of Abortion in a Changing World*. Belgium: Liege.]

Patient preparation

Primary care physicians are often involved in helping a woman make her choices around abortion. When counselling a woman in this situation, one needs to be non-judgemental and help her get the information she needs to make informed decisions. It is important that she has considered her options of continuing the pregnancy or terminating. The issues making it difficult for her may include religious beliefs, her relationship with her partner, guilt over her lack of contraception, sadness, and fear. These need to be explored. The emotional aspects are often more important to her than the physical ones. The most usual emotional reaction after an abortion is relief. The predictors of negative emotional reactions include previous depression, ambivalence about the decision, and the belief that abortion is murder.[4] She also needs help with choosing the best contraception to prevent any further unwanted pregnancies

The abortion procedures available in each area vary but may include medical abortions induced with methotrexate or mifepristone and misoprostol, surgical abortions with local or general anaesthesia in a clinic or hospital. Surgical abortions may be done with vacuum aspiration by suction machine or manually with a syringe and followed by curettage (D&C) or in the case of second trimester procedures, evacuation of foetal tissue (D&E). This chapter will discuss medical abortions and manual vacuum aspiration in more detail as these are often done by primary care physicians. When a woman is choosing between a medical and surgical abortion, it is helpful to let her know that surgical abortions are faster and more often complete and occur in the clinic or hospital while medical abortions take longer, involve medication side-effects, and cramping and bleeding that may occur at home. Women who prefer medical abortions say they are more natural, like a miscarriage, less invasive and the ones who abort at home say they like the privacy. Women who prefer surgical abortions say they prefer being in a clinic and the assurance that it is complete.

It is important that each woman facing an abortion is given detailed information about the procedure including the risks. An obstetrical history and a history of allergies, medical, and gynaecological conditions are important. Since abortions are very safe, there are no actual medical contra-indications to the procedure.[5] Women with Class III or IV heart disease, unstable epilepsy, uncontrolled diabetes, serious coagulopathies, and other serious medical conditions are best managed in a hospital with an anaesthetist present. Examination must include dating the

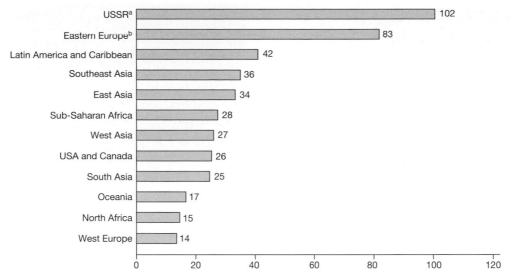

Fig. 2 Abortions (legal and illegal) per 1000 women age 15–44 by region, 1990. [*Data from* Singh, S. and Henshaw, S. (1996). The incidence of abortion: a worldwide overview focusing on methodology and on Latin America. In *International Union for the Scientific Study of Population: Socio-cultural and Political Aspects of Abortion in a Changing World*. Belgium: Liege. USSR data reported by Ministers of Health and Transport.]

pregnancy accurately. Most abortion providers give routine antibiotic pro-phylaxis to prevent endometritis but others give it only to high-risk women with a history of previous pelvic infection or multiple sex partners.

Surgical abortions

Most abortions world-wide are done by vacuum aspiration. It is important to assess the gestational age of the pregnancy accurately to plan the instruments and technique. The basic technique involves placing a speculum, cleansing the cervix, stabilizing the cervix with a tenaculum, using a para-cervical block with local anaesthesia, dilating the cervix, emptying the uterus with suction using a plastic suction catheter and suction machine, using a curette to check the uterus for retained tissue, re-suctioning, and removing the instruments. A manual vacuum aspiration is an inexpensive office procedure which can be used to complete an incomplete abortion (spontaneous or induced) or to perform a first trimester abortion and will be described in more detail.

Pain control

Abortion procedures are painful and require good pain management. In North America, most abortions are done with local anaesthesia with or without conscious sedation.[6] The most common practice is to use intravenous fentanyl and midazolam with a para-cervical block using lidocaine. The next most common is a para-cervical block with oral medications such as ibuprofen. Since the fundus is supplied with nerves that accompany the ovarian vessels, only the bottom two-thirds of the uterus is affected by a para-cervical block. The average worst pain level experienced by patients having first trimester abortions in a survey of National Abortion Federation clinics was between 4 and 5 on a scale from 0 to 10.[7] Good explanation and emotional support during the procedure help with pain control.

Para-cervical block

Clinicians use many different techniques of para-cervical block. The one described below is modified from one developed by Glick. For safety, it is

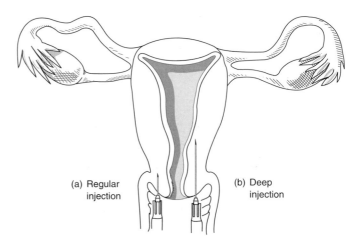

Fig. 3 Illustration of superficial (a) regular and (b) deep injections for paracervical block. [*From* Wiebe, E.R. (1992). Comparison of the efficacy of different local anaesthetics and techniques of local anaesthesia in therapeutic abortions. *American Journal of Obstetrics and Gynecology* **167**, 131–4. Reprinted with permission.]

important to use low-concentration, such as 1 or 0.5 per cent, lidocaine and use multiple injection sites. This prevents a bolus of intravenous injection which can cause toxic effects including death. For the same reason, it is important to stay below the total dose of 4.5 mg/kg or about 200 mg (20 ml of 1 per cent) and to monitor the patient for signs of toxicity such as visual disturbances, muscular twitching, and loss of consciousness[3] (Figs 3 and 4). Inject 1–2 cc of anaesthetic solution superficially into the tenaculum site at 12 o'clock. Gently grasp the cervix and inject 1–2 cc superficially to create blebs around the cervico-vaginal mucosa, using a total of about 10 cc to create a ring around the cervix. Move the tenaculum, without reclamping it, as needed for positioning. Inject the remaining 10 cc deeply into the lower uterine segment where the uterosacral ligaments attach. By pulling the cervix forward, one can see 'tenting' at the ligament attachment. Inject deeply using the full length of the 1.5-inch needle (Fig. 3) at 2, 3, and

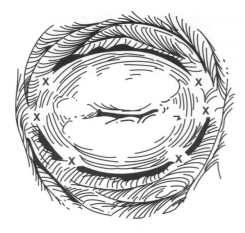

Fig. 4 Sites of injection for paracervical block using the Glick technique (see text for details). (*From* Paul, M., Lichtenberg, E.S., Borgatta, L., Grimes, D.A., and Stubblefield, P.G. A Clinician's Guide to Medical and Surgical Abortion. Philadelphia: Churchill Livingstone, 1998.)

between 4 and 5 o'clock on the one side and then at 10, 9, and between 7 and 8 o'clock on the other (Fig. 4). Aspirate before injecting and 'track' the injection by injecting as the needle goes in. One soon learns the amount of resistance present when the needle is correctly placed: if the needle is outside the uterus, there is no resistance; if the needle is too close to the internal os, there is more resistance than in the myometrium of the lower uterine segment.

Manual vacuum aspiration

Manual vacuum procedure can be used for abortion up to 12 weeks and to complete incomplete abortions. It is a suitable technique for primary care offices and emergency departments. The equipment needed (see Fig. 5) is inexpensive and widely available and includes a 60 cc locking syringe with plastic cannulas.

Procedure

Assess the gestational age of the pregnancy. Observe a 'no touch technique' so that the parts of the instruments which enter the uterus are sterile. Assess the size and position of the uterus. Insert the speculum and cleanse the cervix. Stabilize the cervix with a tenaculum and do the para-cervical block. Dilate the cervix if required using osmotic dilators, misoprostol or mechanical dilators such as Pratt dilators. By choosing a cannula which is slightly smaller in millimetres than the pregnancy is in weeks (e.g. 7 mm for 8 weeks), one often needs no dilation. Introduce the cannula, attach the syringe, and obtain suction. Evacuate the contents of the uterus by rotating the cannula and moving it back and forth within the uterine cavity. Ensure completion by noticing the gritty sensation of the empty uterus and checking the pregnancy tissue obtained.

Complications

The most common complications of surgical abortion are infection (0.5 per cent), retained products of conception (0.5 per cent), and haemorrhage (0.5 per cent). Ultrasound studies have shown that it is usual to have some retained clots and this can lead to cramps and heavy bleeding most commonly about 4–5 days after the procedure. Incomplete abortions which require re-aspiration cause haemorrhage or prolonged bleeding. Less common complications include failed attempted abortion (0.2 per cent), uterine injury (0.2 per cent), and anaesthetic complications. Case fatality rates in North America are less than 1 per 100 000 with 29 per cent of deaths

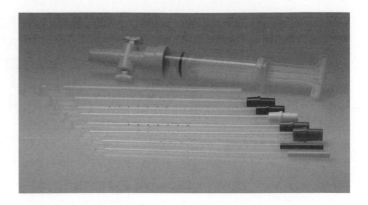

Fig. 5 The Ipas Manual vacuum aspiration device. © Ipas 2003. (Reproduced with permission.)

due to anaesthetics, 18 per cent to haemorrhage, 16 per cent infection, and 14 per cent due to embolism.[5]

Medical abortions

In the last decade of the twentieth century, about half a million women in Europe and millions of women in China had medical abortions using mifepristone followed by a prostaglandin. By the end of the century, many more countries had licenced mifepristone and others were using methotrexate with misoprostol to induce abortions. Mifepristone is an antiprogestin, competitively binding progesterone receptors. Methotrexate blocks the enzyme dihydrofolate reductase, inhibiting the production of reduced folates required for DNA synthesis primarily affecting rapidly dividing cells such as trophoblast. Misoprostol is a prostaglandin and when taken after mifepristone or methotrexate, causes bleeding and expulsion of the pregnancy.

Preparation

It is important that women planning a medical abortion understand that compared to a surgical abortion, there is a higher failure rate, that it takes longer, may involve drug side-effects, and there is usually more bleeding. The side-effects of all three drugs are similar and include nausea, vomiting, diarrhoea, headache, fever, and chills. There are no long-term side-effects at these doses. The women who chose medical abortions often say they prefer it because it is more natural, more private, and more like a natural miscarriage.

Protocols

Methotrexate and misoprostol can be used up to 7 weeks from the first day of the last menstrual period (LMP).[9,10] The usual dose of methotrexate is 50 mg/m² IM although doses of 50–75 mg IM or orally have also been used successfully. This is followed 4–7 days later by 800 μg misoprostol inserted vaginally. The misoprostol dose can be repeated several times on subsequent days. Mifepristone can be used up to 9 weeks and the usual dose is 600 mg followed 24–72 h later by 400 μg misoprostol orally.[11,12] Mifepristone has also been used successfully at doses of 100–200 mg followed by 800 μg misoprostol vaginally.

Complications

The most common problem with medical abortions is retained products requiring a surgical aspiration (2–5 per cent) and failure or continuing pregnancy (1 per cent).[5] Haemorrhage requiring transfusion is rare (0.02 per cent). The most worrisome problem is that methotrexate and misoprostol are teratogenic and so potentially, an abnormal child could be born from a failed procedure. It is crucial to counsel women in advance about this problem and to follow patients carefully to ensure that the abortion is complete.

Summary

Abortion is so common that every primary care physician frequently sees patients who have had abortions. It is important to help patients make the best choices and to be able to assess and manage complications.

References

1. World Health Organization, Maternal Health and Safe Motherhood programme. *Abortion: A Tabulation of Available Data on the Frequency and Mortality of Unsafe Abortion* 2nd edn. Geneva: World Health Organization, 1994.
2. Henshaw, S.K. (1990). Induced abortion: a world review, 1990. *Family Planning Perspectives* 22, 76–89.
3. Paul, M., Lichtenberg, E.S., Borgatta, L., Grimes, D.A., and Stubblefield, P.G. *A Clinician's Guide to Medical and Surgical Abortion.* Philadelphia: Churchill Livingstone, 1998.
4. Russo, N. and Zierk, K. (1992). Abortion, childbearing and women's well-being. *Professional Psychology* 23, 269–80.
5. Hakim-Elahi, E., Tovell, H.M., and Burnhill, M.S. (1990). Complications of first trimester abortion: a report of 170 000 cases. *Obstetrics and Gynecology* 76, 129–35.
6. Lichtenberg, E.S., Paul, M.E., and Saporta, V. *1997 Provider Clinical Survey; First Trimester Surgical Abortion Practice.* Washington DC: National Abortion Federation, 1997.
7. Rawling, M.J. and Wiebe, E.R. (1998). Pain control in abortion clinics. *International Journal of Gynecology and Obstetrics* 60, 293–5.
8. Westfall, J.M., Sophocles, A., Burggraf, H., and Ellis, S. (1998). Manual vacuum aspiration for first trimester abortion. *Archives of Family Medicine* 7, 559–62.
9. Wiebe, E.R. (1999). Oral methotrexate compared to injected methotrexate when used with misoprostol for abortion. *American Journal of Obstetrics and Gynecology* 181, 149–52.
10. Wiebe, E.R. (1997). Abortion induced with methotrexate and misoprostol: a comparison of various protocols. *Contraception* 55, 159–63.
11. Spitz, I., Bardin, C.W., Benton, L., and Robbins, A. (1998). Early pregnancy termination with mifepristone and misoprostol in the United States. *New England Journal of Medicine* 338, 1241–7.
12. Schaff, E.A., Fielding, S.L., Westhoff, C., Ellertson, C., Eisinger, S.H., Stadalius, L.S., and Fuller, L. (2000). Vaginal misoprostol administered 1, 2 or 3 days after mifepristone for early medical abortion: a randomized trial. *Journal of the American Medical Association* 284, 1948–53.

9

Mental health problems

9 Mental health problems

9.1 Depression

Tony Kendrick

Definitions of depression

Depressive symptoms are distributed continuously in the population (see Chapter 11.8 in Vol. 1), but when deciding whether or not to intervene, categorical definitions can be helpful.

Major depressive disorder

The diagnosis of depression requiring treatment in the United States is based on Diagnostic and Statistical Manual, 4th Version (DSM-IV) criteria.[1] These state that at least five of the following nine symptoms must be present to receive a diagnosis of major depression:

♦ depressed mood,

♦ markedly diminished interest or pleasure in almost all activities,

♦ significant weight loss/gain,

♦ insomnia/hypersomnia,

♦ psychomotor agitation/retardation,

♦ fatigue,

♦ feelings of worthlessness (guilt),

♦ impaired concentration,

♦ recurrent thoughts of death or suicide.

One of the symptoms must be depressed mood or loss of interest in usual activities. The symptoms should be present most of the day, nearly every day, for a minimum of 2 weeks, and must be accompanied by significant impairment of functioning.

The World Health Organization's International Classification of Diseases, 10th edition, (ICD-10) criteria for major depression are very similar to the DSM-IV.[2]

Other categories of depression

The term minor depression may be used to describe episodes which last for 2 weeks or more but in which fewer than five symptoms are present. Dysthymia is a term used to describe chronic low-grade depression and in ICD-10 requires that four or more depressive symptoms are present for at least 2 years.[2] Both dysthymia and minor depression are associated with significant morbidity and impairment of functioning. A fourth category, recurrent brief depression, may be applied where there are episodes of at least five depressive symptoms, like major depression, but which last less than 2 weeks (usually 1–3 days), recur at least 12 times a year, and impair the ability to function.

Whether or not antidepressant treatment is effective for minor depression has not been established with certainty in primary care. Two studies suggest it is no better than placebo for the milder forms,[3,4] but further research is needed. A placebo-controlled trial is currently being undertaken of the efficacy of selective serotonin reuptake inhibitors (SSRIs) and problem-solving therapy (see below) for minor depression and dysthymia in a primary care population in the United States.[5]

A recent systematic review and meta-analysis suggested that anti-depressant drug treatment is effective in the management of dysthymia, but the research studies analysed were conducted in secondary care settings.[6] Appropriate treatment strategies have not been identified for recurrent brief depression. There is, however, widespread agreement about the need to offer treatment for major depression (see below).

Epidemiology

Major depression is common, affecting more than 10 per cent of adults each year.[7] The life time prevalence is as high as 17 per cent and females have a much higher prevalence (21 per cent) than males (13 per cent). The commonest age of onset is from 20 to 40, but depression can start at any age. The point prevalence for major depressive disorder in Western industrialized nations is 2.3–3.2 per cent for men and 4.5–9.3 per cent for women.[8] Minor depression is around twice as common. The Office of National Statistics community survey of psychiatric morbidity in Great Britain found that around 14 per cent of adults aged 16–64 had some sort of mental health problem in the week prior to interview, including 7 per cent with mixed anxiety and depression.[9]

Presentation in primary care

In UK general practice studies, roughly 5 per cent of attenders are found to be suffering from major depression, and around another 15 per cent from some depressive symptoms.[10] Depression accounts for one in five general practice consultations, and around one-third of days lost from work due to ill health in the United Kingdom.

Causes of depression

Risk factors for depression are given in Fig. 1, which outlines a model of pathogenesis.

Primary care practitioners should be alert to the possibility of depression in the following groups of patients:

♦ those who have suffered recent unemployment, bereavement or divorce, financial difficulties, or housing problems;

♦ women with a recent childbirth (see Chapter 9.13), demanding child care, or menopausal symptoms;

♦ those who have been bereaved in the last 12 months, those who are caring for a disabled relative, and those who are living in residential care;

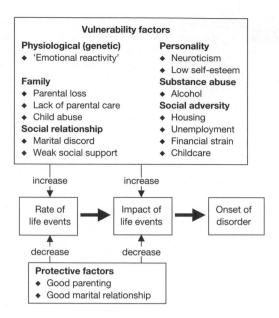

Fig. 1 Risk factors for depression, outlining a model of pathogenesis. (Model adapted from Goldberg, D. and Huxley, P. *Common Mental Disorders. A Bio-Social Model.* London: Routledge, 1992.)

- those who are suffering from a recent myocardial infarction or cerebrovascular accident, or malignancy;

- those with early dementia, Parkinson's disease, Huntington's disease, diabetes mellitus, chronic obstructive pulmonary disease, and chronic pain; and

- patients with multiple unexplained symptoms.

Diagnosis

Only around one-third to one-half of all cases of major depressive disorders are recognized by primary care practitioners.[8,10] Rates of detection are lower among patients in pre-paid health plans than those observed for patients in fee-for-service plans. Many patients consult with physical symptoms, which may explain why their depression goes unrecognized. While it is true that a proportion of the cases missed on a single occasion are subsequently recognized, and moreover that practitioners do recognize the large majority of patients with more severe depression, nevertheless there is clearly significant under-recognition of treatable depression in primary care.

It has been suggested that screening for depression should be conducted among primary care attenders. However, while there are a number of well-validated screening questionnaires available for use in research, using them to screen systematically for depression cannot be recommended at this time. The natural history of the disorder is not well described in primary care, and it has not been convincingly demonstrated that identifying cases through questionnaires leads to an improved outcome.

Diagnosis rests on the primary care practitioner being alert to non-verbal or verbal patient cues of depression. It has been demonstrated that relevant psycho-social health problems are more likely to be dealt with in longer consultations.[11] Higher detection rates are associated with greater knowledge about the symptoms of depression and available treatments, showing interest and concern and asking about the home, work, and family, giving more eye contact, listening and not interrupting, asking open-ended questions initially, asking about feelings, and making empathic comments.

Sleep problems (see Chapter 9.9) and fatigue (see Chapter 9.8) are symptoms with a relatively high positive predictive value for the presence of depression, and any patient presenting with these problems should be asked about the other symptoms of major depression.

Differential diagnosis

This will include other causes of tiredness, including anaemia, hypothyroidism, and chronic renal or hepatic problems (see Chapter 9.8). The presence of co-existing anxiety symptoms should be sought, and enquiry made about substance misuse including alcohol (see Chapters 9.4 and 9.5). Older women in particular should be screened for hypothyroidism, which has been found to be present in as many as 10 per cent of women over 50 and can present as a mood disturbance. A full blood count should be considered in patients presenting with fatigue, to exclude anaemia (see Chapter 9.8).

Principles of management

Antidepressant medication and focused psychological therapies have been shown to be effective for major depression in primary care. Antidepressants are recommended as first line treatment, as they are likely to be most cost-effective compared to psychological treatment.[12] Research studies have consistently shown, however, that drug treatment is inadequate in dosage, duration, or both, in the majority of cases of depression treated, when compared to recommendations in clinical practice guidelines. In major depression only about one-third of patients receive recommended treatment with antidepressants.

This is cause for concern because there is good evidence that treatment is indicated for major depressive disorder. Less severe levels of depression may not require either antidepressant drugs or specific psychological therapies, and the primary care practitioner should adopt a watchful waiting approach. Drug treatment should be considered if patients have enough symptoms for long enough to fulfil criteria for major depression, and significantly impaired functioning, even if there seems to be an understandable cause for the depression, such as social problems or physical health problems.

The US Agency for Health Care Policy Research (AHCPR) guidelines state that 'some patients who meet the criteria for major depressive disorder, but have a very mild condition…, may wait for a re-evaluation of their condition in 1–2 weeks before starting treatment, since some 15 or 25 per cent (or higher) of these patients respond to supportive care from the practitioner'.[13] For this reason, it is probably best practice not to prescribe antidepressants at the consultation when depression is first diagnosed, except perhaps where the patient has had a previous depression which responded well to drug treatment, and is requesting another course of treatment.

UK guidelines still recommend tricyclics as first-line treatment, because they are effective and cheaper than newer drugs. However, titration up to the recommended dosages may not be possible due to drowsiness and anticholinergic side-effects in many cases. Consequently, lower doses are often given, but these may not be superior to placebo. Newer drugs such as the SSRIs do not need to be titrated upwards like tricyclics and can be started at a therapeutic dose, but they are still more expensive than the older drugs, even though some of them are now coming off patent.

It has been suggested that the SSRIs may in fact be more cost-effective, as they may be better tolerated and therefore prevent the more costly complications of depression, including referrals and admissions. However, meta-analyses of trials comparing the two groups for their efficacy and discontinuation rates have found no overall difference in efficacy and only small absolute differences (around 3 per cent) in dropout rates. Furthermore, the advantage for SSRIs holds only against the older more toxic compounds (amitryptiline and imipramine) and not the newer tricyclics or tricyclic-related drugs. The SSRIs do have different side-effect profiles, however, and are less cardiotoxic and safer in overdose, and so can be recommended as first line treatment where side-effects are likely to be a problem or where there is a clear suicide risk.

A number of antidepressants which are neither tricyclic-related nor SSRIs have been developed more recently, including venlafaxine, mirtazapine, nefazodone, and reboxetine. Expert reviews of these newer drugs suggest they are all as effective as the tricyclics and SSRIs, but differ in their side-effect profiles and, being more expensive, can be recommended only as second choice agents. Whatever the choice of drug, it should be prescribed at a therapeutic dose where possible (consult formularies) or a lower dose if the patient has responded to this previously.

Psychological treatment

Referral for psychological treatment is indicated if the depression is mild to moderate, medication is unsuitable or the patient declines, the depression seems closely related to interpersonal or social problems, or the patient requests psychological treatment (see Chapter 9.10). Medication should still be considered either as an adjunct or an alternative to psychological treatment, particularly if patients do not respond within 6–12 weeks.

There is good evidence for the efficacy of structured treatments given by trained therapists, including cognitive–behavioural therapy (CBT) and problem-solving therapy (PST), when compared to usual care. In mild to moderate depression CBT, when given by trained therapists over 15–20 sessions, has been shown to be as effective as antidepressant treatment. Studies of shorter courses of cognitive therapy are needed in primary care, as this may be more cost-effective. Problem-solving has been developed in UK primary care as a six-session treatment which is also very structured, and can be delivered by primary care professionals after a short training. The combination of problem solving with antidepressant medication was found to be no more effective than either treatment alone. There is increasing evidence in the United Kingdom that brief counselling provided by experienced counsellors may be of value in depression, in getting patients better more quickly, and that the overall costs are no greater than treatment by the general practitioner alone.

All these psychological treatments are, however, underprovided in UK primary care (see Chapter 9.10 for a fuller discussion of psychological therapies).

Assessment of suicide risk

Suicidal ideas should be sought out routinely in every depressed patient. Asking about suicide does not increase the risk of self-harm. Patients may be asked if they have felt so bad they wished they were dead. If they answer yes to this, a further question should be asked about whether they have considered ending their life. If they answer yes to this, then enquiries should be made into any specific plans they have to carry out suicide, such as obtaining a weapon, collecting tablets, writing suicide notes, or putting their affairs in order. Patients who have specific suicidal ideas and plans should be referred to a psychiatrist urgently and may need to be admitted to hospital (see Chapter 9.3 for a fuller discussion of suicide risk assessment and management).

Assertive management

In the United States, evidence of undertreatment of major depression has stimulated new approaches to improve its management through the development of clinical practice guidelines and assertive initiatives to implement them. The US AHCPR guidelines[8,13] are similar to the UK guidelines, but go further in their recommendations about the frequency of follow-up and indications for referral.

Several controlled trials of reorganizing primary care to deliver the AHCPR-recommended evidence-based treatments more consistently and effectively have shown significantly improved outcomes in major depression over a period of up to 1 year.[14–16] The details differ between studies but all have included patient and doctor education, training or placing more specialized mental health care workers in primary care, the establishment of a depression case register, active case management and assertive outreach to those who fail to attend for follow-up, and integration of secondary care input for advice, shared care, or active management. Some have concentrated only on improving drug treatment while others have also improved access to effective therapy, such as CBT and PST. Such interventions work even among patients with persistent symptoms after 8 weeks of usual treatment, a group with a high risk of chronicity. Economic analysis of the trials suggests lower costs per case successfully treated than for usual care. Research is needed to evaluate such approaches in countries with different health care systems, where patients may be more reluctant to see specialist mental health care professionals.

Follow-up

The patient should be seen within the first 2 weeks after prescribing antidepressant drugs, as this is the time when the drug is beginning to work, and side-effects may need to be discussed and concordance with the medication encouraged.

Patients who respond to medication should be continued at the same dose for 4–9 months after they have recovered, to avoid early relapse.[13] Concordance with medication is improved by advising the patient that they need to take the medication for at least 2–3 weeks before they will notice any effect, that they should continue to take the medication even once they start to feel better, and giving specific instructions about what to do if they experience side-effects. It is particularly important to emphasize to patients that antidepressants are not addictive, as this misconception is held by a large proportion of the population.

If the patient has shown no response to an initial antidepressant by 6 weeks, then this should be changed to a second antidepressant in a different class. If the second antidepressant fails to resolve the symptoms referral to a psychiatrist is indicated after a further 6 weeks.

Referral

Referral is recommended in the UK consensus guidelines[10] in the following circumstances:

♦ where there is uncertainty about the diagnosis, for example, a possible psychosis;

♦ for advice about management, for example, failure to respond to two courses to antidepressants;

♦ for hospital investigations, for example, a brain scan to check for organic disease;

♦ suicidal or violent behaviour or serious self-neglect; and

♦ where there are co-existing problems such as substance misuse or eating disorder.

Referral may take place occasionally as a result of pressure from the patient or their family, or to reinforce the general practitioner's advice.

Long-term and continuing care

Depression is now recognized to be a relapsing life-long condition, which recurs in 80–90 per cent of those who experience a first episode.[7] Long-term follow-up studies in secondary care settings suggest a rate of chronicity of between 10 and 25 per cent, and some patients recover only incompletely from each new episode. It has been estimated that each new episode of recurrent depression conveys an additional 10–15 per cent risk of chronicity. In primary care, few long-term follow-up studies have been done. One long-term cohort study in the Netherlands suggested that the prognosis was better than for patients seen in secondary care. Recurrence of depression occurred in around 40 per cent of patients over a 10-year period.[17]

Patients should be considered for maintenance treatment if they have had three or more episodes of major depressive disorder, or two episodes and other circumstances which make recurrence more likely, including a family history of bipolar disorder; history of recurrence within 1 year; family history of recurrent major depression; onset before age 20; or severe life-threatening episodes.[13]

Most studies of longer-term treatment for the prevention of recurrent depression demonstrate benefit from all classes of antidepressants, with relapse rates of around 20 per cent compared to 40 per cent on placebo. The choice usually depends on what has produced acute benefit in a particular patient. The decision about maintenance will also depend on the severity of the episodes, their impact on the person's life and career, and the person's willingness to commit themselves to long-term treatment. Psychiatric referral may be valuable in deciding whether or not to continue treatment.

Implications for primary care and the public health

The total costs of depressive disorders in the United States were estimated in the early 1990s to be around \$12.6 billion for direct treatment.[18] Kind and Sorensen estimated the direct costs of depression in the United Kingdom in the early 1990s to be around £417 million, including £165 million for hospital admissions, £125 million for general practice attendance, and £14 million for costs of social services.[19] Antidepressant drugs alone cost the NHS around £100 million per year, prescriptions having increased steadily through the 1990s. The indirect costs of depression to the nation as a whole in terms of lost productivity have been estimated as around \$24 billion in the United States and £3 billion in the United Kingdom.

Depressed patients consult more frequently, receive more prescriptions for physical as well as mental health problems, undergo more physical investigations, and receive more non-psychiatric referrals and admissions to hospital.[20] Therefore, although treating depression is costly, the correct diagnosis of those with missed depression might in fact save significant resources.

There is some evidence of an increase in prevalence of depression in the last 20 years, and not just in the West. Depression is predicted by the World Health Organization and World Bank to become the second leading world health problem after ischaemic heart disease, in terms of disability adjusted life years, by the year 2020. The significance of depression as a public health problem therefore needs to be taken more seriously, in terms of greater education of the public about the problem and what can be done about it, significantly increasing the amount of undergraduate and post-graduate education of health professionals which is dedicated to depression, significant increases in the resources available to treat depression, and increased funding for research into this relatively neglected condition.

Key points

- ◆ Depression should be sought in patients with recent stressful life events, including childbirth and life-threatening or disabling physical illness, and always kept in mind where there is a previous history, or strong family history.

- ◆ There is good evidence that antidepressant treatment, or psychological treatments, are indicated for patients with major depressive disorder, and practitioners should know how to make that diagnosis.

- ◆ Minor depression may recover without treatment and practitioners should adopt a policy of watchful waiting and offering support.

- ◆ Suicidal ideas should be sought actively among all patients with depression.

- ◆ Specialist referral is indicated where treatment with two 6-week courses of antidepressants or psychological therapies has been unsuccessful, or where the patient is contemplating a specific suicide attempt, or is so disabled they cannot remain at home, or where long-term treatment to prevent relapse is being considered.

References

1. **American Psychiatric Association**. *Diagnostic and Statistical Manual of Mental Disorders: DSM-IV*. Washington DC: APA, 1994.

2. **World Health Organization**. *The ICD-10 Classification of Mental and Behavioural Disorders*. Geneva: WHO, 1993.

3. **Paykel, E.S., Hollyman, J.A., Freeling, P., and Sedgwick, P.** (1988). Predictors of therapeutic benefit from amitriptyline in mild depression: a general practice placebo-controlled trial. *Journal of Affective Disorders* **14**, 83–95.

4. **Katon, W.** et al. (1995). Collaborative management to achieve treatment guidelines. Impact on depression in primary care. *Journal of the American Medical Association* **273**, 1026–31.

5. **Barrett, J.E.** et al. (1999). The treatment effectiveness project. A comparison of the effectiveness of paroxetine, problem-solving therapy, and placebo in the treatment of minor depression and dysthymia in primary care patients: background and research plan. *General Hospital Psychiatry* **21**, 260–73.

6. **de Lima, M.S., Hotoph, M., and Wessely, S.** (1999). The efficacy of drug treatments for dysthymia: a systematic review and meta-analysis. *Psychological Medicine* **29**, 1273–89.

7. **Kessler, R.C.** et al. (1994). Lifetime and 12-month prevalence of DSM-III-R psychiatric disorders in the United States. *Archives of General Psychiatry* **51**, 8–19.

8. **AHCPR Depression Guideline Panel**. *Depression in Primary Care: Volume 1. Detection and Diagnosis. Clinical Practice Guideline, Number 5*. Rockville MD: US Department of Health and Human Services, Public Health Service, Agency for Health Care Policy and Research, 1993.

9. **Mason, P. and Wilkinson, G.** (1996). The prevalence of psychiatric morbidity OPCS Survey of Psychiatric Morbidity in Great Britain. *British Journal of Psychiatry* **168**, 1–3.

10. **Paykel, E.S. and Priest, R.G.** (1992). Recognition and management of depression in general practice: consensus statement. *British Medical Journal* **305**, 1198–202.

11. **Howie, J., Porter, A., Heaney, D.J., and Hopton, J.L.** (1991). Long to short consultation ratio: a proxy measure of quality of care for general practice. *British Journal of General Practice* **41**, 48–54.

12. **Anderson, I.M., Nutt, D.J., and Deakin, J.F.W.** (2000). Evidence-based guidelines for treating depressive disorders with antidepressants: a revision of the 1993 British Association for Psychopharmacology guidelines. *Journal of Psychopharmacology* **14**, 3–20.

13. **AHCPR Depression Guideline Panel**. *Depression in Primary Care: Volume 2. Treatment of Major Depression. Clinical Practice Guideline, Number 5*. Rockville MD: US Department of Health and Human Services, Public Health Service, Agency for Health Care Policy and Research, 1993.

14. **Katon, W.** et al. (1999). Stepped collaborative care for primary care patients with persistent symptoms of depression, a randomized trial. *Archives of General Psychiatry* **56**, 1109–15.

15. **Wells, K.B.** et al. (2000). Impact of disseminating Quality Improvement Programs for depression in managed primary care. *Journal of the American Medical Association* **283**, 212–20.

16. **Simon, G.E., von Korff, M., Rutter, C., and Wagner, E.** (2000). Randomised trial of monitoring, feedback, and management of care by telephone to improve treatment of depression in primary care. *British Medical Journal* **320**, 550–4.

17. **van Weel-Baumgarten, E., van den Bosch, W., van den Hoogen, H., and Zitman, F.G.** (1998). Ten year follow-up of depression after diagnosis in general practice. *British Journal of General Practice* **48**, 1643–6.

18. **Greenberg, P.E.** et al. (1993). Depression: a neglected major illness. *Journal of Clinical Psychiatry* **54**, 419–24.

19. **Kind, P. and Sorensen, J.** (1993). The costs of depression. *International Clinical Psychopharmacology* **7**, 191–5.

20. **Kendrick, T.** et al. (2001). Hampshire Depression Project: changes in the process of care and cost consequences. *British Journal of General Practice* **51**, 911–13.

Further reading

AHCPR Depression Guideline Panel. *Depression in Primary Care: Volume 1. Detection and Diagnosis. Clinical Practice Guideline, Number 5.* Rockville MD: US Department of Health and Human Services, Public Health Service, Agency for Health Care Policy and Research, 1993. (A fully referenced and justified guideline for the detection and diagnosis of depression in primary care.)

AHCPR Depression Guideline Panel. *Depression in Primary Care: Volume 2. Treatment of Major Depression. Clinical Practice Guideline, Number 5.* Rockville MD: US Department of Health and Human Services, Public Health Service, Agency for Health Care Policy and Research, 1993. (A fully referenced and justified guideline for the management of depression in primary care, including drug treatment and psychological therapies.)

Anderson, I.M., Nutt, D.J., and Deakin, J.F.W. (2000). Evidence-based guidelines for treating depressive disorders with antidepressants: a revision of the 1993 British Association for Psychopharmacology guidelines. *Journal of Psychopharmacology* **14**, 3–20. (The most up to date, well-referenced, and authoritative guidelines for the treatment of depression in the United Kingdom.)

Paykel, E.S. and Priest, R.G. (1992). Recognition and management of depression in general practice: consensus statement. *British Medical Journal* **305**, 1198–202. (An important consensus statement, including aspects of detection and referral.)

Wells, K.B. et al. (2000). Impact of disseminating Quality Improvement Programs for depression in managed primary care. *Journal of the American Medical Association* **283**, 212–20. (Evidence that an assertive approach to the treatment of major depression can be successfully disseminated across a number of primary care settings.)

9.2 Anxiety

Marilyn A. Craven and Richard P. Swinson

Prevalence, co-morbidity, and social costs

Anxiety disorders are common in the general population and in the primary care setting. The US National Comorbidity Survey found a 12-month prevalence rate of 17.21 per cent for anxiety disorders in the general population, a rate higher than for mood or substance use disorders.[1] The World Health Organization multinational study found that 10.2 per cent of 25 000 adult primary care patients had diagnosable anxiety disorders[2] and that anxiety symptoms were the principal reason for consultation in 4.6 per cent of visits.[3] Co-morbidity with depression, substance abuse, and other mental disorders is high,[2,4] and functional impairment in patients with untreated anxiety disorders is a major burden.[5,6] Rates of impairment may equal or exceed those found in chronic diseases such as diabetes or congestive heart failure.[7]

Recognition in primary care

Recognition and treatment rates for anxiety disorders tend to be low. A US study found that only 44 per cent of anxious patients were recognized and treated,[7] and in the WHO study, physicians identified anxiety syndromes in only 60.5 per cent of cases, half of whom received psychotropic drugs, and 35.6 per cent of whom were offered counselling.[3]

Presentation and assessment of anxiety disorders

Anxiety is a normal part of everyday life. Individual tolerance for anxiety and its physical manifestations varies greatly across people and time. Anxiety is abnormal when it is out of proportion to precipitants in severity, duration, or the adverse effects it has on physical health or function.

Anxiety symptoms present in three spheres

1. *Cognitive symptoms:* excessive worrying and apprehension, indecision, poor concentration, fears of going crazy, losing control, or dying, and intrusive unpleasant thoughts.

2. *Physical symptoms:* shakiness or tremor, dizziness or lightheadedness, weakness, sweating, muscle tension, palpitations, shortness of breath, sensations of choking, chest discomfort, abdominal discomfort, nausea, diarrhoea, flushing or chills, and numbness or tingling sensations.

3. *Behavioural symptoms:* avoidance of situations causing the anxiety, development of behaviours to permit the individual to cope with the feared situation, and rituals and compulsions (e.g. handwashing, checking, ordering).

Different constellations of these symptoms and behaviours combine in each of the diagnosable anxiety disorders. Table 1 contains a series of screening questions which will help to identify patients who may have an anxiety disorder. If the patient answers 'yes' to any of these questions, ask the patient what thoughts he or she is having when the anxiety peaks—this will help narrow the diagnosis—and then continue with the follow-up questions. To make a definitive diagnosis, refer to the full criteria for the anxiety disorders listed in the *Diagnostic and Statistical Manual of Mental Disorders, 4th Edition* (DSM-IV)[8] and in the *International Classification of Diseases, Tenth Edition* (ICD-10).[9]

Ruling out physical and drug-related factors

Anxiety disorders should not be diagnosed if a physical disorder can account for the patient's symptoms. Many medical conditions cause symptoms which may be confused with anxiety. These include hyperthyroidism, hypoglycaemia, arrhythmias, asthma and COPD, pulmonary embolism, hyperparathyroidism, silent myocardial infarction, pneumonia and other infections, vitamin B12 deficiency, seizure disorders, and phaeochromocytoma (very rare).

For patients with new onset anxiety, particularly the elderly, a physical examination and basic laboratory investigations should be carried out. Physical examination should focus on the body system(s) where the patient is most symptomatic (e.g. cardiac and respiratory). Subsequent investigation should be guided by history, physical findings and any known medical conditions.

While somatic symptoms may indicate underlying medical illness, the greater the number of physical symptoms, the more likely an anxiety or mood disorder is present.[10] A family history of anxiety disorders should also raise the index of suspicion for anxiety being a factor. On the other hand, anxiety disorders rarely present *de novo* in mid or late life.

Drugs can also cause anxiety symptoms. Caffeine is the commonest anxiogenic drug. More than two cups of coffee or tea, or cola-containing beverages a day can be problematic. Particularly sensitive patients should eliminate it from their diet altogether. Nicotine can exacerbate anxiety. Alcohol, frequently used by anxious patients to deal with social situations, to 'unwind', or to get to sleep at night, may cause insomnia or withdrawal symptoms indistinguishable from worsening anxiety. Other drugs to consider are sympathomimetics, stimulants, steroids, some antihypertensives, and some non-steroidal anti-inflammatory drugs.[11] Selective serotonin

Table 1 Screening questions for anxiety disorders (Adapted from ref. 14)

Do you ever have sudden unexpected episodes of severe anxiety? (Panic disorder)
Patients with panic disorder are often exquisitely sensitive to physiological manifestations of anxiety and may interpret these as evidence of impending serious illness
    Ask about the symptoms experienced, the frequency of the episodes and worry about having another attack
    Ask about avoidance of places or situations in which the attack occurred

Are there any situations you have to avoid? (Phobias)
Patients with specific phobias think about escape when they encounter the cue
    Ask specifically about insects, heights, dogs, enclosed spaces, blood, needles, etc.

Patients with social phobias fear the probability of negative evaluation by others
    Ask about level of comfort attending parties, meeting new people, dealing with authority figures, speaking in public, using public washrooms, writing or eating
       in front of others
    Ask about degree of avoidance and impairment

Do you have a need to repeat actions? (Obsessive compulsive disorder)
Patients with compulsions may be plagued with doubt (Did I really turn off the stove, lock the door, turn off my computer, etc.), or with thoughts of catastrophe if a special ritual is
    missed or actions do not follow a certain order, or they may fear that they have been contaminated
    Ask about handwashing, repeated checking, a need to do things in a set, unvaried order, and the amount of time each day spent in these activities

Do you have repeated unpleasant thoughts? (Obsessive compulsive disorder)
Patients with obsessive thoughts experience intrusive, unpleasant thoughts
    Ask about distressing, intrusive, repetitive thoughts or mental images that are uncontrollable
    Ask about the amount of time each day the thoughts are present

Do you worry a lot? (Generalized anxiety disorder)
Patients with GAD will endorse worrying about 'everything' for as long as they can remember
    Ask for a list of current worries and how long they have been a worrier

Have you been exposed to any severely traumatic events (Post-traumatic stress disorder)
Patients with PTSD are afraid to remember the event
    Ask about flashbacks, nightmares, sudden floods of memories

---

reuptake inhibitors (SSRIs) can also trigger or exacerbate anxiety symptoms, particularly early in treatment. Non-prescription drugs such as amphetamines, cocaine, and cannabis are frequently associated with anxiety.

Principles of treatment

A number of treatment principles and strategies apply to all the anxiety disorders:

◆ Emphasize the importance of not avoiding locations where traumatic events or panic attacks took place. *Avoidance reinforces fear and anxiety.*

◆ Encourage patients to tolerate the unpleasant feeling states of anxiety and reassure them that the feelings will gradually diminish. *Tolerating the internal feeling state is an important first step in recovery.*

◆ Symptom diaries are useful for defining the nature and severity of symptoms, and for identifying triggers. Keeping a daily diary keeps patients involved in their treatment and helps the physician assess motivation for change.

◆ Do not assume that your patient needs time off work or school. Encourage normal role functioning as much as possible.

◆ Be alert to the possibility of co-morbid major depression and treat with an antidepressant.

◆ Ideally, try cognitive–behavioural therapy (CBT) before pharmacotherapy. CBT and medication are both effective in many of the anxiety disorders, but the effects of CBT tend to persist longer.[12] Exceptions are very ill patients, patients with associated depression, and those not psychologically minded or non-compliant. Pharmacotherapy is appropriate for these patients. CBT may be added as the patient improves.

◆ If you are not comfortable providing CBT yourself, refer to someone experienced in anxiety disorders. Pharmacotherapy can be started if there is likely to be a significant delay in accessing CBT, but it may reduce motivation for psychological treatments.

◆ Deal with lifestyle issues such as work-related stress, and encourage appropriate nutrition, exercise, and relaxation strategies. Identify and address relationship problems.

◆ Eliminate caffeine and reduce or eliminate alcohol. Warn heavy caffeine consumers about withdrawal headaches.

◆ Teach sleep hygiene. Encourage a regular bed time, the avoidance of late meals, reduced alcohol, and use relaxation exercises, gentle stretching exercises, and non-stimulating reading.

◆ For new onset disorders, do not rush to intervene. Many patients who have recently experienced a traumatic event respond well to talking about the event, and to reassurance that symptoms are likely to improve. If more is needed, ask the patient to keep a symptom diary for a week or two and schedule a return visit for review. In many cases, significant improvement is likely.

◆ Involve family members or a close friend in therapy whenever possible. They can help reinforce the treatment plan and provide emotional support.

◆ Familiarize yourself with local support groups. They can be very useful adjuncts to therapy.

◆ Keep a list of self-help materials in the office. Many self-help books have workbooks or exercises for the patient to do (for a list of references, see DIRECT-Anxiety Information Centre at www.PsychDirect.com).

Treatment approaches for individual disorders

Panic disorder

Panic attacks are sudden, unexpected episodes of severe anxiety which, at some point, have occurred 'out of the blue', and are not attributed to a recognizable stressor. At least four of the following occur: palpitations or rapid heart beat, sweating, shortness of breath, chest pain or discomfort,

Table 2 Drugs used in the management of anxiety disorders

Drug	Indication(s)[a]	Dosage
Benzodiazepines	PD, PDA, GAD	
Alprazolam		PD, PDA: 0.25 mg TID–QID, up to 1 mg QID
Clonazepam		0.25–0.5 mg BID
Tricyclic antidepressants	PD, PDA, PTSD, GAD, SP	
Desipramine		75–300 mg/day
Imipramine		75–300 mg/day
Clomipramine	OCD	75–225 mg/day
Selective serotonin reuptake inhibitors	PD, PDA, OCD, PTSD, SP	
Citalopram		20–60 mg/day
Fluoxetine		20–80 mg/day
Fluvoxamine		150–300 mg/day
Paroxetine		20–60 mg/day
Sertraline		50–200 mg/day
Serotonin–norepinephrine reuptake inhibitors	GAD	
Venlafaxine		37.5–225 mg/day
Monoamine oxidase inhibitors	PD, PDA, OCD (refractory)	
Phenelzine		45–90 mg/day
Tranylcypromine		20–60 mg/day
Reversible inhibitors of monoamine oxidase-A	SP	
Moclobemide		300–600 mg/day
Azapirones	GAD	
Buspirone		5 mg BID–TID, up to 60 mg/day
Other	SP (specific task anxiety)	
Propranolol		10 mg, 30 min before task

[a] PD, panic disorder; PDA, panic disorder with agoraphobia; GAD, generalized anxiety disorder; OCD, obsessive compulsive disorder; PTSD, post-traumatic stress disorder; SP, social phobia.

nausea or abdominal distress, shakiness, dizziness, chills or hot flushes, paresthesias, and fear of going crazy, losing control or dying. The attacks start abruptly, escalate rapidly, and peak within 10 min. Panic attacks can occur at night and wake the patient from sleep, and can become attached to specific situations or places, so that these situations act as triggers.

Panic attacks are not in themselves a disorder. Thirty per cent of young adults will experience panic attacks.[13] They should be considered abnormal only if at least one panic attack has been followed by a month of worry about having another panic attack or what the consequences of the attack might be, or if they have caused significant changes in behaviour (usually avoidance).

Treatment of panic disorder begins with education and reassurance that the attacks are not dangerous. This is followed by an explanation of the basic pathophysiology of panic and how adrenaline produces the symptoms experienced. Patients should be encouraged to do two things: go back to the place where the panic occurred as soon as possible; and try to stimulate a panic attack in the physician's office by hyperventilating until some or all of the panic symptoms appear. Practice at home leads to tolerance of the symptoms and the lessening of fear of attacks.

Untreated panic may lead to agoraphobia, a fear of being in places where escape would be difficult or embarrassing if a panic attack were to occur. Situations often avoided include crowded places such as malls, theatres, restaurants, public transportation, and line-ups in supermarkets. Treatment of agoraphobia should address the panic attacks, but must also focus on exposure to the feared situation. Typically, in a behavioural approach, the patient and physician draw up a hierarchy of difficult situations ('Going to the mall when it's crowded' to 'travelling by train to visit my sister') and then gradually expose the person to the feared situations. Excellent resources now exist to assist physicians in developing and implementing treatment plans for patients with agoraphobia and other phobias (for a list of references, see DIRECT-Anxiety Information Centre at www. PsychDirect.com).

If you decide to use medication to treat panic symptoms, selective serotonin reuptake inhibitors are the first line drugs of choice (see Table 2). A transient increase in agitation or anxiety may occur: start with the smallest dose available. Increase the dose slowly until full antidepressant doses have been achieved. SSRIs may take 4–6 weeks to have an effect and up to 12 weeks for full effect. Treatment with SSRIs should continue for at least 1 year.[15] At that time, if the patient has been symptom free, try tapering slowly. If symptoms recur, re-start medication, but also reconsider implementing CBT.

Social phobia

Social phobia is an excessive fear of any social situation in which the individual may be scrutinized by others. The individual fears being the focus of attention, is afraid of acting in a way which will be embarrassing, and anticipates being judged negatively by others. The fear may be generalized to almost any social situation, or may be limited to specific situations such as public speaking or performing in public. Panic attacks associated with these situations are common and the individual is likely to be highly sensitive to any outward manifestations of anxiety, convinced that everyone is noticing his or her blushing, tremor, or shaking voice. Individuals with social phobia frequently avoid social situations altogether or endure them with great difficulty. Social shyness is common, but the diagnosis of social phobia should be made if the anxiety interferes significantly with social, school or occupational functioning.

The preferred treatment for social phobia is CBT, with an emphasis on exposure therapy. Group therapy and social skills training may also be helpful. Medication also works well, but is likely to be needed longterm. The SSRIs are the first-line drugs of choice. Start at low doses and titrate to full antidepressant doses slowly. Beta-blockers can be used in patients with circumscribed performance anxiety (e.g. public speaking or musical performance). These drugs can be given 1–2 h ahead of a single performance or on a regular basis for frequent performers. Clonazepam, 0.5–2 mg BID, given on a regular basis, is also effective in treating generalized social phobia, but has the disadvantages of producing dependence. It may cause cognitive impairment in some individuals. Relapse after stopping medications is common.

Specific phobia

Patients with specific phobias tend to request treatment only if the phobias are impairing their ability to function. An office worker who is afraid of elevators may ask for help only when his office is moved from the third floor to the 19th floor of his building. The patient is aware that his or her fear is excessive and may be ashamed of the 'weakness' it implies. A sympathetic, non-judgemental attitude is essential. Patients with specific phobias may develop panic attacks triggered by exposure to the feared situation or object.

Graduated exposure is the treatment of choice for specific phobias and is very effective. This usually takes from two to eight sessions and may begin with imagining the feared stimulus, looking at pictures, or simply talking about it. In a series of carefully graded steps, the patient learns to tolerate closer exposure to the stimulus. Self-help manuals, particularly in combination with physician support, can work for patients with mild phobias (e.g. able to tolerate the feared situation with discomfort, or avoids only intermittently). Those with more severe phobic responses are likely to need therapist-guided treatment. Medications are generally not indicated except for phobias which are rarely encountered (e.g. infrequent air travel, some medical tests) and which can be predicted. In these situations, pre-treatment with a benzodiazepine may be appropriate.

Obsessive compulsive disorder

Obsessive compulsive disorder (OCD) is characterized by obsessive thoughts and/or compulsive behaviours. Obsessive thoughts are intrusive, unwanted, and unpleasant thoughts or images. They are *not* ruminative worry about actual events or problems in the patient's life. Common obsessive preoccupations are fears of contamination, pathological doubt (e.g. about whether the door was locked, stove turned off), an excessive need for symmetry and orderliness, fears of behaving aggressively, fears of behaving in a sexually inappropriate or violent way. To cope with their obsessive preoccupations, patients frequently develop rituals to neutralize them or magically prevent some feared outcome. Common examples are excessive handwashing, repeated checking, counting, praying, or performing daily activities in a set, rigidly controlled order. The behaviours gradually become less effective in neutralizing the anxiety caused by the obsessive thoughts or images, and the patient develops more and more extensive, elaborate, or time-consuming compulsions. If obsessions or compulsions occupy more than 1 h a day, are distressing to the patient, or interfere with normal functioning, a diagnosis of OCD should be made.

Treatment of mild to moderate OCD should focus on exposure to the feared situation and the prevention of the rituals. As the patient 'sits with' the anxiety, without performing the compulsion, the anxiety peaks and diminishes. Repeated practice will gradually convince the patient that he or she can cope with the anxiety in more adaptive ways, without the 'help' of the compulsive behaviours. For patients with moderate to severe OCD, adjunctive medication may be necessary. First-line drugs are SSRIs, or clomipramine (a strongly serotonergic cyclic antidepressant). Treatment of moderate or severe OCD is probably best carried out by mental health professionals who are experienced in this disorder.

Post-traumatic stress disorder

A full discussion can be found in Chapter 9.12.

Generalized anxiety disorder

Generalized anxiety disorder is a chronic condition in which patients worry excessively, over long periods (>6 months) about multiple aspects of their lives. They frequently identify themselves as 'worriers' and are likely to have difficulty remembering a time when they were worry-free. Symptoms follow a waxing and waning course, often worsening in response to external stressors. Patients report feeling overwhelmed by their worries, and have difficulty controlling them. They constantly feel tense or 'uptight', or 'shaky inside' are easily fatigued, frequently have difficulty sleeping, and complain of irritability, muscle tension, and difficulties with concentration. Co-morbidity with depression or substance abuse is common.

Generalized anxiety disorder often requires long-term treatment, with increased support and intervention when external stressors are present. Cognitive–behavioural approaches have a significant advantage over medication. Cognitive restructuring, in which patients are taught to identify, challenge and consider alternatives to their anxious thoughts has been proven effective, alone or with relaxation exercises. Patients who are misusing alcohol or substances to cope with their anxiety should be referred for specific treatment. For patients who do not respond to CBT, or during particularly stressful periods, medication may be neccessary. First-line drugs are venlafaxine or paroxetine. Other SSRIs or buspirone can be effective. Benzodiazepines may work if prescribed on a regular basis, but carry real risks of dependence and problems with over-use. If they are used to help patients cope with an external stressor, they should be used at the lowest effective dose, and for short periods only.

Key points

- Anxiety disorders are very common, accounting for 4.6% of all primary care visits.
- Depression, substance abuse, and significant functional morbidity frequently accompany anxiety disorders.
- Physical and drug causes of anxiety symptoms should be ruled out.
- Psychotherapy and medication are both effective.
- Key psychotherapeutic strategies: discourage avoidance of anxiety-producing stiuations and encourage patients to tolerate anxiety symptoms until they diminish.
- Treat co-morbid major depression and substance abuse.

References

1. **Kessler, R.C.** et al. (1994). Lifetime and 12-month prevalence of DSM-III-R psychiatric disorders in the United States. *Archives of General Psychiatry* **51**, 8–19.
2. **Sartorius, N.** et al. (1996). Depression comorbid with anxiety: results from the WHO study on Psychological Disorders in Primary Health Care. *British Journal of Psychiatry* **168** (Suppl. 30), 38–43.
3. **Weiller, E.** et al. (1998). Prevalence and recognition of anxiety syndromes in five European primary care settings. A report from the WHO study on Psychological Problems in Primary Care. *British Journal of Psychiatry* **173** (Suppl. 34), 18–23.
4. **Nisenson, L.G.** et al. (1998). The nature and prevalence of anxiety disorders in primary care. *General Hospital Psychiatry* **20**, 21–8.
5. **Ormel, J.** et al. (1994). Common mental disorders and disability across cultures. Results from the WHO collaborative study on Psychological Problems in General Health Care. *Journal of the American Medical Association* **272** (22), 1741–8.
6. **Leon, A.C., Portera, L., and Weissman, M.M.** (1995). The social costs of anxiety disorders. *British Journal of Psychiatry* **166** (Suppl. 27), 19–22.

7. Fifer, S.K. et al. (1994). Untreated anxiety among adult primary care patients in a health maintenance organization. *Archives of General Psychiatry* **51**, 740–50.

8. **American Psychiatric Association**. *Diagnostic and Statistical Manual of Mental Disorders* 4th edn. Washington DC: American Psychiatric Association, 1994.

9. **World Health Organization**. *International Classification of Diseases* 10th edn. Geneva: WHO, 1992.

10. Kroenke, K. et al. (1994). Physical symptoms in primary care. Predictors of psychiatric disorders and functional impairment. *Archives of Family Medicine* **3**, 774–9.

11. **The Medical Letter, Inc.** (1998). Some drugs that cause psychiatric symptoms. *The Medical Letter on Drugs and Therapeutics* **40**, 21–4.

12. Antony, M.M. and Swinson, R.P. *Anxiety Disorders and their Treatment. A Critical Review of the Evidence-Based Literature*. Ottawa: Health Canada, Minister of Supply and Services Canada, 1996.

13. Norton, G.R., Dorward, J., and Cox, B.J. (1986). Factors associated with panic attacks in nonclinical subjects. *Behavior Therapy* **17**, 239–52.

14. Swinson, R.P. (2000). Anxiety disorders. In *Therapeutic Choices* 3rd edn. (ed. J. Gray), pp. 7–15. Ottawa: Canadian Pharmacists Association.

15. **American Psychiatric Assocation** (1998). Practice guideline for the treatment of patients with panic disorder. *American Journal of Psychiatry* **155** (Suppl. 5), 1–34.

Table 1 Suicide rates (per 100 000 persons per year) in selected countries (the most recent year available)

Countries with the highest suicide rates		Countries with lower suicide rates	
Lithuania	48.2	Czech Republic	15.4
Estonia	39.2	Germany	15.1
Latvia	38.9	Poland	14.4
Russian Federation	38.6	Sweden	14.3
Hungary	32.9	Canada	13.5
Ukraine	31.2	Rumania	12.8
Slovenia	31.0	Australia	12.5
Finland	27.6	United States	11.9
Croatia	22.8	Netherlands	9.8
Switzerland	21.6	India	9.7
France	20.6	Italy	8.4
Cuba	20.3	Spain	8.1
Austria	20.1	United Kingtom	7.1
Belgium	18.9	Brazil	3.6
Bulgaria	17.5	Greece	3.5
China (mainland)	16.1	Egypt	0.1

9.3 Suicide and attempted suicide

André Tylee and Zoltan Rihmer

Epidemiology, pattern of the problem in the community, and international differences

Suicide is among the most tragic events of human life, causing serious psychological distress among the relatives as well as great economic burden for society. Globally, around one million deaths from suicide are recorded every year, and the number of suicide attempts is estimated to be 10–15 million per year.[1] Suicide is a major cause of years of life lost and, therefore, suicide prevention is receiving increasing attention.

The highest national suicide rates (per 100 000 persons per year) have always been recorded in Europe (Hungary, Denmark, Austria, Germany, Finland, Lithuania, Estonia, Latvia, Russia, etc.), as have the lowest national suicide rates (Greece, the United Kingdom, Italy, Spain)[2] (Table 1).

Reasons for great differences between national suicide rates have not been sufficiently explained. Geographic, climatic, socio-cultural, religious, and economic differences can be taken into account, but the accuracy of the registration of suicide, the availability of lethal methods, and the availability as well as the level of the social/health care system should also be considered.

In the last 10–15 years, the suicide rates of several Western/Nordic European countries as well as that of Hungary have decreased substantially. Although the reasons for these favourable changes are not exactly known, better care of psychiatric patients may be one of the contributing factors.[3,4]

The very high suicide mortality of several post-communist countries cannot be fully explained either by the former political–economic system, nor by recent changes in this respect, since several post-communist countries (e.g. Rumania, Poland, Bulgaria, etc.) have always had a relatively low suicide rate. On the other hand, after the political changes in eastern Europe, the national suicide rates have either increased or not changed markedly, Hungary remaining the only country in which the suicide rate has dropped markedly in the last 15 years.[4]

Suicide mortality shows a clear gender difference: with the exception of some countries (especially China and India), two-thirds to three-fourths of suicide victims in the world are male. This may be a consequence, at least, in part, of the fact that males use violent methods (e.g. hanging, shooting, jumping) much more frequently, while females more often take overdoses or self-poison.[1,2,5,6]

Suicide rates, in general, are higher in urban than rural areas, while spring/early summer is the season of the highest and winter of the lowest incidence of suicide.[1,2,5] Suicide rates increase with age in both genders, although a marked increase in suicide mortality among young males in the United States and the United Kingdom has also been reported recently.[1,2]

In contrast to committed (fatal) suicide, in the case of attempted (non-fatal) suicide, the sex distribution is the opposite: more than two-thirds of suicide attempters are females and the most commonly used method is overdose.[2,5] The lifetime history of one or more suicide attempt(s) in the general population of Europe, North America, and Australia is 2–4 per cent, while the rate of attempted/committed is estimated to be about 10–15 : 1, but this ratio shows a decreasing tendency with age.[2]

Since the term 'attempted suicide' is imprecise (as many attempters do not actually wish to die), there have been some other terms introduced over the years such as 'parasuicide', 'deliberate self-harm', 'deliberate self-poisoning', etc. Suicide completers and attempters do not constitute two absolutely distinct populations, for 30–40 per cent of suicide victims have made at least one attempt previously.[1,2,6] Therefore, all suicide attempts, even though the method is far from lethal, should be taken seriously.

Possible causes and associated features

Suicidal behaviour is not a normal response to the levels of stress experienced by most people. Almost all the people who kill themselves have a diagnosable mental disorder, and this is often in combination with other

Table 2 Hierarchical classification of suicide risk factors

Psychiatric (primary) risk factors
Major psychiatric illness (depression, schizophrenia, substance-use disorders)
  Hopelessness, insomnia, agitation
  Co-morbid anxiety and/or personality disorder, serious medical illness
Previous suicide attempt
Communication of suicide intent/wish to die
Family history of suicide
Decreased/disregulated central serotonergic activity,[a] low serum cholesterol

Psycho-social (secondary) risk factors
Early negative life events (parental loss, separation, etc.)
Living alone, isolation (divorce, widowhood, etc.)
Unemployment, major financial problems
Severe acute stressors (actual negative life events, etc.)

Demographic (tertiary) risk factors
Male gender
Adolescence (males), old age (females)
Vulnerable intervals (spring/early summer), pre-menstrual period
Minority groups (relatives of suicide victims, immigrants, victims of war or
  natural disasters, prison residents, farmers, etc.)

[a] No peripheral biological marker that can be used routinely in everyday practice is available at present.

Table 3 Clinical characteristics helping the diagnosis of depression in medically ill patients

Family history of depression/mania
Family history of suicide
Previous depressive/hypomanic/manic episodes (good response to antidepressants in the past)
Previous suicide attempts
Seasonal fluctuation (not motivated by the course of medical illness)
Diurnal variation (worse in the morning)
Self-blaming, guilt, psychotic features

major risk factors. More than 90 per cent of suicide victims have one or more major psychiatric illnesses at the time of their death, and the most common diagnoses are major depressive episode (59–87 per cent), schizophrenia (8–12 per cent), and substance-use disorders (8–12 per cent).[1,2,6] Personality disorder or serious medical illness itself as the main (or only) diagnosis in suicide victims is relatively rare, although both are quite commonly present as a co-morbid diagnosis. The suicide mortality of patients with severe or terminal medical illness increases only in the presence of co-morbid depressive disorder.[1,2,6]

As most psychiatric patients do not take their own lives, major psychiatric illness itself is a necessary, but not sufficient, condition to explain the suicidal act. Suicide is a complex human behaviour with many causes and several biological and psycho-social components. Suicide is also associated with a number of risk factors with varying prognostic utility. The hierarchical classification of suicide risk factors[6] are presented in Table 2.

Although the statistical relationship between the different demographic (e.g. gender, age, etc.) and psycho-social (e.g. unemployment, living alone, etc.) risk factors and suicidal behaviour is well documented,[2,5,6] they have a very limited value in predicting suicide in individual cases. Psychiatric risk factors (e.g. depression with previous suicide attempt) are the strongest and clinically most useful predictors of suicide, particularly if psycho-social and demographic risk factors are also present. Hopelessness, insomnia, agitation, and a high level of anxiety also increase the risk of suicide.[1,2,6]

In contrast to the numerous risk factors, only few circumstances are known to have a protective effect against suicide. Besides good family and social support, pregnancy, being in the *postpartum* period, having a large number of children, and holding strong religious beliefs seem to provide some sort of protection.[6] A significant proportion of suicide victims contact their family physicians and other physicians some days, weeks, or months before their deaths.[6,7] Early detection and adequate treatment of mental disorder as well as the identification of those patients with a high suicide risk are very important in suicide prevention.

How common is presentation in primary care and impact

Suicide attempts and committed suicide are relatively rare in family practice. In a given region, where the suicide rate is 10 per 100 000, only every one-fifth of the 50 GPs of a district of a population of 100 000 will see one committed suicide a year. Using the rate of 15:1 for attempted: committed suicide—each GP will have approximately two to four persons with a suicide attempt per annum. However, major psychiatric disorders (particularly depression) as potential risk factors for suicide are much more common in family practice. Ninety per cent of people with mental health problems are seen and treated solely by GPs and the point-prevalence of major depressive disorders in family practice is between 5 and 15 per cent. It is very difficult often to recognize depression in primary care when the patients have concomitant physical illness[8] or when they do not mention their depression at the beginning of the consultation.[8] From a recent European community survey in six countries, around half of all people with depression did not consult their GPs and of those who did with major depression only around one-third were treated with antidepressants.[9] Despite a national consensus statement on the treatment of depression in England,[10] and a plethora of depression guidelines produced as a result, it still remains the case that many people do not present their depression to their GP or return for second or subsequent consultations. Many people stated in a public opinion poll in England that they would want counselling if they became depressed and they would be a lot less likely to want medication, with a majority stating that pills are addictive.[11] The importance of the family physicians in suicide prevention is underlined by the fact that 35–60 per cent of suicide victims contact their GPs 4 weeks, and 15–40 per cent 1 week before their deaths.[7] The rate of accurate diagnosis and appropriate treatment in such cases is disturbingly low,[1–3,6] but many patients consulted for other reasons.

Since the majority of depressed suicide victims with previous medical contact do not communicate directly their suicidal intent, the physician should focus on indirect signals or correlates like depression and other suicide risk factors. Physicians need a high index of suspicion.

The results of a Swedish study conducted on the island of Gotland showed that the clinical picture of suicidal, depressed men is often masked by aggressive, impulsive, and abusive behaviour, and that these men are better known to legal and social welfare agencies than to their GPs.[12] GPs tend to be more accustomed to identifying depression and managing it in women rather than men. Men who are depressed tend to act out and resort to alcohol[13] and it may be that they hide their distress more from their primary care workers. Women for a variety of reasons are more accustomed to being in the primary care setting and may find it easier to disclose their distress. It may be harder for men to continue to attend primary care settings.

The diagnosis of depression is sometimes difficult in medical patients, since many symptoms (e.g. anorexia, fatigue, weight loss, etc.) are common to both. Some of the characteristics that help make a diagnosis of depression in medically ill patients are listed in Table 3.

Concomitant depression increases the morbidity and mortality from medical illness, and patients with simultaneous medical disorder and depression are less compliant with treatment and take longer time to recover than non-depressed medical patients. Since severe physical illness in depressed patients serves often as a precipitating factor of suicidal act, medical treatment of somatic illness is also an important factor in suicide prevention.[1]

Assessment, risk management, and referral

In the Gotland study, GPs on the island received postgraduate training on the recognition and treatment of depression and there was an associated reduction in the suicide rate in the 2 years following the intervention.[8] The island population was small, there were few GPs, and a very few baseline suicides, no control group, and the change in suicide numbers could have been a chance finding. However, the results excited a lot of interest in the possibility of a link between postgraduate training using clinical guidelines on GP recognition and treatment of depression and patient outcome. It was, however, unclear whether the Gotland GPs were representative of GPs elsewhere. When this link was tested, with a larger sample and a control group, it was not demonstrated in Hampshire in the United Kingdom.[14]

It remains open to debate whether or not suicide is preventable through actions taken in primary care. The completed act is so rare among the patients of any one GP and the known risk factors are so non-specific. This is an area that needs more research.

Every nurse or doctor generalist who acts as first point of contact for patients should, however, be able to undertake a suicide risk assessment and know what to do if the patient has suicidal ideation or intent within or outside of surgery hours. Knowing the arrangements for crisis care out of hours as well as within surgery hours eases some of the stress that can occur when faced with a suicidal patient in a busy clinic. It is best to ask a hierarchy of questions. First, the patient needs to be asked more general questions about how they are managing and how they see the future, whether they can see that things could improve or not. More specific questions then need to be tailored to the answers to the earlier questions about helplessness and hopelessness. These need to cover whether the person has thought that life is not worth living or has ideas about harming themselves or putting an end to it all. They need to then be asked whether they have already planned or rehearsed a method. They may have tried and failed to kill themselves already. Patients do respond to such questioning and are not made more suicidal by discussing it. Rather, it is likely to be a relief to tell someone for the first time about the bottle of pills they are carrying around 'just in case things get worse' or the fact that they have been to the edge of the railway platform already. GPs can indicate to the suicidal patient that suicidal ideas and actions will disappear on recovery from depression (or even earlier). Many patients of one of the authors (Z.R.) find this beneficial as they had thought they were alone or unique in their suicidal ideas. Many suicidal ideas are fleeting, so it is worth checking whether the thoughts pass through or whether they stick. It is often surprising that people least expected to have suicidal thoughts readily disclose them on enquiry. Self-destructive behaviour usually does not occur in the very early stages of the depression and this often allows some time to make a precise diagnosis. Leaflets, posters, and fliers left in the waiting room indicating the main symptoms of depression may prompt people to ask for help. The Samaritans (i.e. befriender organizations for the suicidal), contact telephone numbers, and now Internet web addresses can be displayed as can details of other depression support groups such as Depression Alliance in the United Kingdom.

One of the authors (A.T.) is currently piloting with colleagues and the Charlie Waller Memorial Trust an open-access nurse-led service for the depressed and suicidal registered with a practice in Lambeth, South London. Charlie Waller was a young man who killed himself when depressed in London and this new service, jointly funded with London Region in his memory, whereby people can telephone the nurse for advice or an assessment, is being evaluated to see whether improved access improves outcome.

It is important to remember that certain patients may be at higher risk of suicide and that the index of suspicion for risk assessment should be correspondingly high. This would include people just discharged from psychiatric inpatient treatment, people with severe major depression, people newly diagnosed with schizophrenia who are recovering, people with agitation, anxiety, or panic attacks, people abusing alcohol or drugs, people with severe borderline personality disorder, etc. In practice, many people have more than one of these diagnoses (e.g. severe depression and alcohol/drug abuse).

If medication is prescribed, care is needed to ensure that drugs are used that are least toxic in overdose and that if toxicity could occur, only small amounts are given at a time (although this does not prevent someone from stock-piling their tablets). All patients with significant depression should be treated, whether or not they are suicidal, as decision to treat is mainly based on overall severity and interference with function (see Chapter 9.1).

Past suicide attempts increase risk, so it is important to take a history as well as determining the severity of any past attempts or deliberate self-harm. It may be that some people need to feel they are in a trusting doctor–patient relationship before they can communicate their suicidal intent and apart from consultation and communication skills, there needs to be good continuity of care. Davenport and colleagues[15] found that doctors vary in their ability to encourage non-verbal and vocal cues of emotional distress.

Two recent suicides in the general practice of one of the authors (A.T.) were middle-aged men who had reassured both their psychiatrist and the author's GP partners that it was safe to allow them home and that they had no suicidal intent. A potentially useful learning tool, which requires study, is for whole practice teams to review the circumstances leading up to any suicides in a positive way. Because suicide is such a rare event, research into this type of intervention, however, is unlikely to be completed as so many practitioners would be needed to be exposed to the intervention to ensure the study was properly powered. One thing is certain from speaking to many GP colleagues over the years about this subject, GPs can readily recall their patients over decades who have killed themselves with little prompting. Because such recall can arouse emotions in the doctors, training sessions on this subject need to make allowance for the possibility that the doctor will become distressed. One of the authors (A.T.) always teaches with a Samaritan or counsellor for this reason. Suicide prediction is an imprecise science in spite of our knowledge of risk factors and risk assessment. It is still hard to predict, considering that the average GP will only see a suicide every 3–5 years yet have a hundred or so people with major depression at any one time.

People at high risk for suicide usually need to be referred for urgent assessment by mental health services with a view to inpatient care. Such a decision will require considerable discussion and shared decision-making with the patient and carer(s). Suicidal intent usually requires referral. It may be necessary after discussion with a patient to remove possible means of suicide (e.g. firearms, medications, etc.) and arrange constant supervision. Supervision and constant checking may even be necessary in hospital and still is no guarantee of prevention.

Conclusions, controversy, public health measures, and areas for future research

Suicide is a rare event, but whilst it is hard to predict and prevent, such efforts are obviously worthwhile. GPs need to accept this reality and maintain a high index of suspicion, paying attention to risk factors. It is probably crucial to be available and provide continuity of care to those at risk and take suicide risk histories when appropriate, perhaps repeatedly. Some would say that suicide is an act that is often societally determined and that it is a basic human right to be able to end one's life. This may sometimes be the case, but the medical profession is duty bound to seek out psychiatric illness and treat it accordingly. Most people who killed themselves were suffering from a psychiatric disorder on psychological autopsy.

It is possible that an approach that communicates willingness to recognize, assess, and manage depressive illness helps prevent progression to suicidal intent in some people, although research is needed to see if this is so.

The recent failure to link guideline training to GP change in behaviour[10] has already been highlighted. In this study, the GPs only recognized

36 per cent of those with possible major depression (HAD-D score 8+) and only 15 per cent of patients received a therapeutic dose of antidepressants for 4 months or more and this remained so after the intervention.[11] Interestingly, most patients in this study recovered within 6 months despite having not received a therapeutic dose of an antidepressant, which calls the guidelines into question for many people seen in primary care.

Regarding public health measures, reducing the access to available methods can help reduce suicide rate (e.g. gas supply, access to high places, packaging and dispensing of paracetamol, etc.). We have yet to see whether the recent stress suffered by farmers in England and Wales by the foot and mouth epidemic has compounded their propensity to be an occupational group with one of the highest suicide rates in the United kingdom, with around one farmer taking his/her life every week for the last decade. There have been several initiatives by organizations such as the Samaritans and the National Farmers Union in the United Kingdom attempting to prevent suicide in farmers in recent years and the effect of these need to be evaluated. These initiatives represent a public health approach to prevention by occupational group. Recent concern about suicides in the prison population has led in the United Kingdom to greater awareness and training for prison staff and the preparation of educational material (Dr Rachel Jenkins, personal communication).

In summary, the main aspects of suicide prevention in people with mental health problems in primary care are likely to be:

♦ the identification of high-risk groups;

♦ prompt recognition and management of depression;

♦ reduced access to methods of suicide;

♦ referral for inpatient care when necessary.

One of the biggest challenges is to reduce stigma and encourage young men, in particular, to see primary care as a place to go for help, when depressed. Primary care needs to be more accessible and have the capacity to cope with those who are depressed and suicidal. This has huge workforce and training implications for many health care systems around the world.

Key points

♦ Although suicide and attempted suicide are relatively rare events, depression, the major cause of suicide, is common in primary care.

♦ Up to 60% and 40% respectively of suicide victims contact their GPs 4 weeks and 1 week before the death. Many attenders consult for other reasons.

♦ Many people do not readily present depression or suicidal ideas or intent in primary care, so a high index of suspicion is needed, especially in high-risk groups.

♦ There is some evidence that mental health training for GPs may be linked to the reduction of depressive suicides.

References

1. Wasserman, D. *Suicide. An Unnecessary Death*. London: Martin Dunitz Ltd., 2000.
2. Hawton, K. and van Heeringen, C., ed. *International Handbook of Suicide and Attempted Suicide*. Chichester: John Wiley and Sons, 2000.
3. Isacsson, G. (2000). Suicide prevention—a medical breakthrough? *Acta Psychiatrica Scandinavia* 102, 113–17.
4. Rihmer, Z., Belsō, N., and Kalmár, S. (2001). Antidepressants and suicide prevention in Hungary. *Acta Psychiatrica Scandinavica* 103, 238.
5. Gelder, M., Gath, D., and Mayou, R. *Oxford Textbook of Psychiatry*. Oxford: Oxford University Press, 1989.
6. Rihmer, Z. (1996). Strategies of suicide prevention: focus on health care. *Journal of Affective Disorders* 39, 83–91.
7. Pirkis, J. and Burgess, P. (1998). Suicide and recency of health care contacts. *British Journal of Psychiatry* 173, 462–74.
8. Tylee, A. (1999). Depression in the community: physician and patient perspective. *Journal of Clinical Psychiatry* 60 (Suppl. 7), 12–16.
9. Tylee, A. et al. (1999). DEPRES II (Depression research in European society II): a patient survey of the symptoms, disability and current management of depression in the community. *International Clinical Psychopharmacology* 14, 139–51.
10. Paykel, E.S., Tylee, A., Wright, A. et al. (1997). The Defeat Depression Campaign. Psychiatry in the public arena. *American Journal of Psychiatry* 154, 59–65.
11. Priest, R.G., Vize, C., Roberts, A., Roberts, M., and Tylee, A. (1996). Lay people's attitudes to treatment of depression: results of opinion poll for Defeat Depression Campaign just before its launch. *British Medical Journal* 313, 858–9.
12. Rutz, W. et al. (1997). Prevention of depression and suicide by education and medication: impact on male suicidality. An update from the Gotland study. *International Journal of Psychiatry in the Clinical Practice* 1, 39–46.
13. Angst, J., Gamma, A., Gastpar, M., Lepin, J.-P., Mendlewicz, J., and Tylee, A. (2002). Gender differences in depression. Epidemiological findings from the European DEPRES I AND II studies. *European Archives of Psychiatry and Clinical Neuroscience* 252, 201–9.
14. Kendrick, T., Stevens, L., Bryant, A., Goddard, J., Stevens, A., Raftery, J., and Thompson, C. (2001). Hampshire Depression Project: changes in the management of depressed patients and cost consequences. *British Journal of General Practice* 51(472), 911–13.
15. Davenport, S., Goldberg, D., and Millar, T. (1987). How psychiatric disorders are missed during medical consultations. *Lancet* 2 (8556), 439–40.

Further reading

The Hawton and van Heeringen handbook of suicide and attempted suicide as cited above is the most comprehensive text on the subject and has a chapter on primary care.

Andersen, U.A. et al. (2001). Contacts to the healthcare system prior to suicide: a comprehensive analysis using registers for general and psychiatric hospital admissions, contacts to general practitioners and practising specialists and drug prescriptions. *Acta Psychiatrica Scandinavica* 102, 126–34. (Data on 472 suicide victims in a Danish county shows that two-thirds of the suicides did visit their GP within the last 4 weeks before death and in comparison with general population, suicides visited their doctors three times more frequently. This study clearly shows the role and possibilities of GPs in suicide prevention.)

Appleby, L. et al. (1999). Aftercare and clinical characteristics of people with mental illness who commit suicide: a case-control study. *Lancet* 353, 1397–400. (It is well known that the suicide risk of psychiatric patients is especially high after hospital discharge. This study shows that lacking or reduced aftercare is among the main contributing factors to this.)

Partonen, T. et al. (1999). Association of low serum total cholesterol with major depression and suicide. *British Journal of Psychiatry* 175, 259–62. (Several recent studies reported on an association between low total serum cholesterol and suicide. The paper presents the most recent 5–8 years follow-up data in a community sample of almost 30 000 men aged 50–69 years.)

Rihmer, Z., Rutz, W., and Barsi, J. (1993). Suicide rate, prevalence of diagnosed depression and prevalence of working physicians in Hungary. *Acta Psychiatrica Scandinavica* 88, 391–4. (This Hungarian study shows that the more working doctors per 100 000 inhabitants, the better is the recognition of depression and the lower is the suicide rate of the given region, suggesting that not only psychiatrists but also all working doctors have a role in suicide prevention.)

9.4 **Drug misuse and dependence**

Clare Gerada and Jane Haywood

Introduction

Drug use touches every area of society, every social class, and all ages. The consequences of use are manifold and affect the individual user, their families, and society. Increasingly, health professionals have to deal with the medical, social, and psychological problems associated with drug use.

No drug is without harm, though some are more harmful than others. For some drugs the damage is predominantly a consequence of its illegality (such as becoming involved in violent crime), for others of the problems associated with long-term use, such as cancer of the lung with cigarettes. Some drugs are safe in moderation, causing problems with excess use, such as alcohol. So prevalent is drug misuse and so pervasive the problems associated with it, that it must be considered as part of any differential diagnosis in any clinical area.

In all cases, attracting a person into treatment reduces the harm that the drug can cause to them, and to society. Primary care is ideally sited to attract drug users early in their drug-using career and to make effective interventions. This chapter will focus on the illicit drugs, namely opiates (heroin), stimulants (cocaine, amphetamines), and cannabis.

Dependence

Not every one who uses drugs will go on to problematic use. Like alcohol use (though unlike tobacco), drug use ranges, though not always in a linear fashion, from experimental to occasional use, to regular recreational use, problematic use, and at the end of the spectrum dependent use.

Epidemiology

It is not known how many people use illicit drugs. In the United Kingdom, official figures of those presenting to treatment services were kept up to 1996 with the Home Office 'addicts index' replaced with a voluntary monitoring system called the Regional Drug Misuse Data Base. Using the Home Office figures, nearly 40 000 drug users were notified to the Home Office (1995)—an increase on the previous year by about 10 per cent. Heroin has always been the most common drug of addiction under this reporting system, accounting for 25 000, nearly two-thirds of all notifications. In the United States of America, around 6 per cent of Americans over 12 years old have taken an illicit drug in the previous month.[1]

Drug users come from diverse backgrounds and to simplify the causes does no justice to the complex interplay between environmental and individual factors. Drug use is both a cause of and result of social exclusion. Drug use is more common in young people. It is linked to social deprivation and school failure and more likely to be found in children with inconsistent parenting. The ability of a drug to produce a central effect and in particular, its ability to induce pleasure or euphoria is a very important factor in perpetuating its use. Other drug-related factors that determine whether a drug is used are its cost, legality, availability, and ability to cause dependence. In the United Kingdom, the price of heroin has not changed in real terms in the last 30 years, making it a cheap source of pleasure. Coupled with its wide availability and ability to cause dependence, it is hardly surprising that we are seeing an increasing number of young people using it (Fig. 1).

Drug related
- Cost (cheaper the more used)
- Availability (increase in availability increases the use)
- Ability to cause euphoria (little abuse of substances that cause no euphoric or hedonistic effect)
- Legality (tends to be prohibitive as one gets older)
- Fashion (i.e. designer drugs, trends of use)
- Ease of use, e.g. route of use (would determine first use)
- 'Advertising' (i.e. cigarettes, alcohol)

Individual
- Sex (men more than women)
- Age (younger more than older)
- Education (protective)
- Genetic predisposition (can also be protective, e.g. Chinese inability to metabolize alcohol)
- Cigarette use before the age of 12 years
- High psychological distress, e.g. depression, anxiety
- Personality disorder
- High level of use amongst friends
- Past history of physical or sexual abuse
- Childhood neglect
- Behavioural disturbances in childhood
- Poor academic achievement
- Unemployment

Environment (not a simple interplay)
- Poor housing, homeless
- Deprived neighbourhoods
- Lack of family cohesion
- Cultural and economic influences (e.g. adherence to strong faith is protective)
- Criminal sanction for use

Fig. 1 Factors that influence the use of illicit drugs.

Consequences of drug use

The complications of drug use are dependent on a number of factors relating to the drug itself, the context in and route by which it is taken and the underlying health of the user. Overall, drug users are more likely to die than an age-matched group, due to overdose, accident, and deliberate injury and infection. Up to 70 per cent of long-term injecting drug users are hepatitis C positive with estimates that at least 20 per cent of these will develop serious liver disease as a long-term complication.

The pharmacology of the drug will influence its direct effects and side-effects, both in normal doses and in overdose. For example, opiates can cause acute toxic effects including respiratory depression, coma, and even death. There are very few acute effects of tobacco use (except perhaps nausea and vomiting in the naive user) yet its long-term harmful effect is well known. Polydrug use is very common—for example, heroin mixed with cocaine or heroin regularly taken with benzodiazepines. Drug interactions can be unpredictable and idiosyncratic when substances are taken in high dosages in people with pre-existing medical problems (e.g. renal, liver, and cardiac disorders). The route of drug use is very important in determining the harm it may cause to the user. Complications are more pronounced, prevalent, and dangerous if drugs are taken through the intravenous route. Other factors determining the harm a drug can cause are related to the problems associated with a drug-using lifestyle. Frequent changes of addresses, reluctance on the part of many health professionals to engage with drug users, poverty, poor diet, and poor housing all contribute to the general illhealth frequently found in this population (Fig. 2).

The drug used
Nature of the drug, and its pharmacological effects
Purity of the drug (toxic contaminants and inert contaminants)

The route of administration
Intravenous (needle sharing, adulterants, increase risk of overdose, blood-borne viruses)
Smoked/inhaled
Oral

The individual
Tolerance
Individual variation
Physical factors
Illness
Intention

Fig. 2 Factors which influence the risk associated with drug use.

Presentation in primary care

Requests for prescriptions for drugs with potential for abuse, including opiate analgesics and tranquillizers, may raise concerns about possible drug misuse, especially where these requests are made out of hours, and the doctor is not the person's usual medical attendant. Suggestive symptoms and signs include unexplained constipation or diarrhoea, marked constriction or dilatation of the pupil, puncture marks, and scars over injection sites. Behavioural clues include unaccountable drowsiness, elation, or restlessness, an apparent loss of interest in personal appearance or work, and a history of offences to obtain money. Additional information should be sought from the patient's previous doctor, where appropriate (see Chapter 11.8, Vol. 1).

Specific substances

Cannabis

This is the most used illegal drug in Europe and North America, with substantial increases in use over the 1990s. At least 45 million Europeans (18 per cent of those aged 15–64 years) have tried cannabis at least once, and 15 million in the past 12 months. Heavy and regular cannabis users can consume more than five 'joints' per day using around $\frac{1}{2}$ oz of cannabis per week. Since 1991, there has been a continuous rise in cannabis use amongst American adolescents. Nearly one in 20 (4.9 per cent) of high-school seniors use it daily, while young peoples disapproval of the drug declines.[2]

Cannabis use is not without risk. When taken in high concentrations it can produce hallucinations, and in susceptible individuals psychosis and amotivational syndrome. Long-term use can cause other problems related to mixing the drug with tobacco and smoking—for example, oral and lung cancers, or to the combined effects of alcohol and cannabis. Cannabis use has been linked to fatalities from road traffic accidents, suggesting that the sedative effects can be dangerous for an individual in charge of a vehicle.[3] Nevertheless, of all illicit substances, cannabis is probably the least harmful and some countries, notably the Netherlands, are advocating removing its illegal status completely.

Health effects of cannabis

Acute

 ◆ Impairment of individuals' ability to learn and carry out tasks such as operating machinery or driving.

Chronic

 ◆ Damage to mental functioning—especially in prolonged heavy users.

 ◆ Development of cannabis dependence syndrome.

 ◆ Exacerbation of schizophrenia in affected people.

 ◆ Respiratory damage.

 ◆ Increased risk of bronchitis.

Heroin and other opiates (e.g. methadone, opium, pethidine)

Heroin use worldwide has increased year on year over the last few decades, with evidence that the age of first use is becoming younger. Heroin can be taken by any route, though the preferred routes are smoking (chasing the dragon) and injecting (fixing). Heroin causes an immediate 'rush' or high, with the effect as the feeling of being in 'cocooned warmth with intense security'. These sensations are explained by the ability of heroin to combine with opiate-like receptors in the brain. A dependent user may use up to 1 g–$1\frac{1}{2}$ g/day—costing around £60–100 (US$90–150) per day. The drug is frequently 'cut' or diluted at source and sold in this less pure form. These cutting agents include paracetamol, talc, or in some cases brick dust. Purity can, therefore, vary according to the dealer from 20 to 60 per cent. Fatalities can occur when the purity is unexpectedly high or when the drug is cut.

Deaths from acute causes, such as respiratory depression, are not uncommon. The mortality rate of heroin users is 14[4] to 32[5] times that of an age-matched population. Amongst heroin users, 9 per cent of a study sample reported at least one serious overdose and 43 per cent had witnessed an overdose in the previous 12 months.[6]

Continual use of heroin leads to tolerance and dependence, so that the individual requires larger and larger doses to produce the same effects. Abstinence results in withdrawal symptoms, which although described as 'not any more severe as the flu', can be extremely uncomfortable. Insomnia is perhaps the worst effect of prolonged withdrawal. Many of the complications of heroin use are related less to the drug itself than to the lifestyle associated with problem use, or dependence (e.g. involvement in crime, prostitution, poor housing, few social networks outside the drug using set) and to complications associated with its route of use—especially injecting drug use. Heroin use in pregnancy is associated with low birth weight and neonatal addiction. However, many of the complications of use are related to compounding factors such as concomitant cigarette smoking and poor general health. Encouraging women into treatment (be that antenatal or drug treatment) produces positive outcomes.

Other opiates and opioids (e.g. coproxamol, pethidine, dihydrocodeine)

Any opiate drug can be subject to abuse. The prescriber must always be aware of the dangers of diversion of medication prescribed for pain relief, symptom control, or palliative care.

Benzodiazepine drugs [e.g. diazepam (Valium), temazepam, and other tranquillizers]

Benzodiazepines have been prescribed less since the 1970s. However, in some age groups the use of these drugs is very prevalent. In the United States, an estimated 2 million adults aged 65 years and older are addicted to or at risk of addiction to sleeping medications or tranquillizers. Health care professionals are especially at risk from prescription drug abuse. Though most people use these drugs for legitimate and prescribed reasons, there is widespread illicit use, particularly amongst those who also use heroin. Some drug users use benzodiazepines with other drugs to boost the effects, or to help them to 'come down' from drugs that make them feel high. Overdose causes drowsiness and respiratory depression. Benzodiazepine use with other drugs such as heroin and/or alcohol can be dangerous, and overdose in these situations can cause death. Withdrawal can vary from mild anxiety and sleep disturbance to a severe state of fear and confusion. There is a risk of fits if a person stops these drugs after regular long-term use. The health risks of benzodiazepines are mainly those associated with dependence and overdose, as well as the effects on concentration and coordination. Before their removal, temazepam capsules ran the risk of being injected, with consequent loss of digits.

Stimulants (e.g. amphetamines, cocaine, ecstasy)

Amphetamines and ecstasy are the second most commonly used drugs of abuse in Europe. Amphetamine is generally bought as a white powder (amphetamine sulfate) or as tablets called dexamphetamine ('dexies'). It is usually taken by mouth, inhaled, or rubbed into the gums; some grind the tablets and inject them. Cocaine makes the user excited, happy, and energetic, and in less need of food and sleep. Other effects include anxiety, paranoia, and aggression. Amphetamine causes a rise in blood pressure. Overdose of amphetamine with other drugs can be very dangerous. High doses of amphetamine on its own can cause a distressing state of anxiety and panic. When used in high doses, amphetamine can also cause a psychotic illness, which closely resembles schizophrenia. This usually resolves gradually after the person stops taking amphetamine, but psychiatric treatment may be needed. Regular users may experience depression and sleep disturbance when they stop.

Cocaine

Cocaine comes in many different forms, though mostly it is bought as a white powder. It is usually sniffed or 'snorted' but can also be injected. 'Crack' is a form of cocaine treated to make lumps called 'rocks', which can be smoked in a pipe or heated to make vapour that can be inhaled. The effects are very similar to those of amphetamine, but may happen more quickly as a powerful 'rush' (within seconds) and wear off more quickly (few minutes). The problematic effects are also similar to those of amphetamine. Occasionally, the sudden rise in blood pressure caused by cocaine can lead to a stroke and myocardial infarction. Like amphetamine, cocaine can often be stopped safely without any clear withdrawal symptoms, but regular users may experience agitation, depression, and sleep problems. As cocaine lasts such a short time in the body, many cocaine users experience a brief but very unpleasant 'comedown' after use, with a severe feeling of depression. Increasing numbers of young people are using cocaine—both in its powder (snortable) and rock (smoking) forms. The most recent British Crime Survey showed a rise in the proportion of young people trying cocaine powder—with data for 1998 showing a 300 per cent increase on the previous 2 years.[7] In the rest of Europe and in North America cocaine use is increasing, particularly, amongst young socially active groups.

Ecstasy

This drug is known chemically as 3,4 methylenedioxy-methampethamine, or MMDA. It is a hallucinogenic amphetamine. The effects normally begin 30–60 min after ingestion and peak after 2–4 h, though the effects can last several hours. As with many drugs, the effects are influenced by the mood of the taker, the amount taken, and the circumstances in which it is ingested. Physical effects include sweating, dry mouth, raised blood pressure and hyperthermia, tachycardia, dilated pupils, increased energy, and loss of appetite. Users also report feeling warm, relaxed, and more energetic. There are high risks of hypertension, asthma, liver, and renal damage and MMDA can cause symptoms similar to neuroleptic malignant syndrome. Deaths have been reported and are thought to be related to hyperthermia and dehydration.

Role of the primary care team

Primary care is ideally suited to build up a therapeutic relationship and provide care to patients with chronic relapsing conditions, such as drug misuse. The family doctor is more able to access social, medical, and psychiatric information with their intimate knowledge of the patient spanning years and more able to use this knowledge to most effect, especially when trying to maintain them in treatment. Treatment should include the provision of general medical care and evidence-based effective interventions, which in many cases means the provision of medication

for treatment of withdrawal or for longer-term detoxification or maintenance.

There is no denying, however, that drug users are not on the whole welcomed by many doctors. They are often seen as difficult patients to treat, as time consuming (which they are—with attendance rates ten times an age-matched population). Coupled with lack of training in treating these patients, doctors are often reluctant to take them on for care.

Why primary care?

◆ Best placed to intervene early.

◆ Able to provide holistic longitudinal care to the patient and their family.

◆ Patients prefer care by general practitioners.[8,9]

◆ Drug users have high morbidity and mortality rates.

◆ Treatment in general practice is at least as good as specialist care for uncomplicated patients.

◆ Treatment works.[10]

Management

It is beyond the scope of this chapter to give a detailed appraisal of all the treatment options available. The reader is guided to documents such as the Drug Misuse Guidelines produced in the United Kingdom[11] or the guidelines written by the US Department of Health and Human Services.[12] Broadly, treatment options fall into three categories: pharmacological (symptomatic, substitution, maintenance), physical (immunization, advice regarding safer drug use), and social (help with housing, financial advice).

Treatment options available in primary care vary across different countries. In Europe, primary care doctors can offer a range of substitution treatment including methadone. However, in the United States, primary care practitioners tend to restrict themselves to identifying, screening, and referring patients with substance misuse disorders for further assessment or treatment. They are able to offer brief interventions to patients with milder or less-entrenched substance misuse problems.

Whilst each individual in treatment will have specific long- and short-term goals, all treatment programmes, whether in Europe or America,[13] have similar generalized goals, these are to:

1. reduce substance misuse or achieve abstinence;

2. enable the person to maximize aspects of their life functioning, such as education, employment, and social relationships;

3. prevent or reduce the frequency and severity of relapse.

Every contact with a drug user must be seen as an opportunity to nudge that patient forward into an illicit-drug-free state—making improvements in other areas of their life en-route. Evidence shows that the longer a patient is engaged with services the better the outcome in a range of parameters (financial, social, employment, physical, and continuing drug use).

Harm minimization advice

Health professionals are vital in their harm reduction role and there is evidence to show that brief intervention in primary care is effective in the prevention of the harm associated with drug using.[14] Every contact with a drug user must be seen as an opportunity of reducing the harm associated with drug use and of increasing the chance of that individual, in time, becoming drug free.

Minimum harm-reduction interventions in primary care should include safer injecting advice (including overdose prevention and action), observation of injecting sites, offering viral screening (hepatitis C, B, and HIV), hepatitis B vaccination, safer sex advice, and up-to-date information about pharmacy needle exchange schemes and local drug agency information.

Brief interventions

Brief interventions are inexpensive effective treatments that can be delivered in any primary care setting. At least one follow-up visit is recommended but the number and frequency of sessions depends on the severity of the problems and the individuals response to treatment.

Critical components of brief intervention include:

1. give feedback about screening results, including the risks involved;

2. inform the patient about safe consumption limits and advise about change;

3. assess the patients readiness for change;

4. negotiate goals and strategies for change;

5. arrange follow-up.

Substitution treatment

Substitution treatment first appeared in the late 1960s in response to the emerging opiate problem. Treatment varies across the world and is related to legislation, prescribing practice, and overall organization of services (primary, secondary, and NGO) across different countries. There is good evidence that substitution treatment works, including methadone maintenance.[15] Methadone is perhaps the most commonly used drug for opiate substitution. It is a long-acting synthetic opioid used to treat opiate addiction. Though an effective treatment, it is also not without risks. Methadone has a narrow therapeutic index, meaning that the margin between overdose and effective dose is small. Care must be taken in assessing the patient, confirming the diagnosis of opiate dependence (history, examination, and urine drug screen), before starting the patient on this drug. Increasingly, dose assessment (or dose titration) is used by specialist units and shared care services to ensure that the patient is started on a safe dose that is increased in small increments until a steady state is achieved. In an opiate-naive user or in a person taking other depressant drugs such as alcohol or benzodiazepines, methadone, even in low doses, can be fatal. Methadone is used in the treatment of opiate addiction either in the short-term as a detoxification or more often as a maintenance treatment. Long-term replacement of heroin with high-dose methadone (50 mg/ml or above), coupled with psycho-social interventions, has been shown to prevent illicit drug use (and hence criminal activity), improve employment prospects, and reduce the health risks of continuing drug use (including needle sharing). Compliance can be improved by daily dispensing and supervised ingestion.

Other substitute treatments available (in particular, buprenorphine)

This drug is new to the British market, though has been used in Europe and America for a number of years. Being a partial agonist and antagonist, it is considered safer in overdose than methadone. There is evidence that it is a useful tool in the treatment of heroin abuse, and is most effective for those individuals with high psycho-social functioning (Fig. 3).

General principles of treatment are:

♦ clinicians must work within their level of competence;

♦ confirm the diagnosis of drug misuse (assessment, examination, urine testing);

♦ ensure that care is taken to reduce diversion onto the illicit market (daily dispensing) and reduce the risks to the patient (dose assessment) and the doctor (work within a shared care environment).

Individual practice policy may include: type and formulation of substitute medication, maximum daily dose, frequency of pick-up, frequency of urine testing, frequency of review, etc. The dispensing pharmacist should be included in discussions and their active participation recognized.

Doctors must never feel pressurized to prescribe potentially lethal substitute drugs before undertaking an adequate assessment, which must include an assessment of past and current drug use, route of use, complications associated with use, and the patient's expectations of treatment (Fig. 4).

Conclusion

In society, a significant number of young people will invariably 'experiment' with drugs without problems. However, regular use may result in dependence and the need to access treatment for problem use. Primary care is readily placed to offer appropriate management. Due to an increase in the frequency of substance misuse problems, access to secondary care treatment can prove difficult due to long waiting times, for example. Primary care is ideally placed for the early detection and management of substance misuse.

Substitution substance	Characteristics of the substances	Countries reporting using the substances
Buprenorphine	Very long acting agonist–antagonist opioid	Belgium, Denmark, France, Italy, Austria, UK
Dihydrocodeine	Short acting semi-synthetic, weak agonistic opioid	Belgium, Luxembourg, Germany
Heroin	Short acting, strong agonistic opiate	Netherlands, UK
LAAM	Very long acting synthetic agonistic opioid	Denmark, Germany, Spain, Portugal
Mephenon	Long acting synthetic agonistic opiate	Luxembourg
Methadone	Long acting synthetic agonistic opiates	All EU member countries
Slow-release morphine	Long acting agonistic opiate	Austria

Fig. 3 Substitution substances used in EU.[16]

Purpose	Treatment goal	Examples
Detoxification	Enable patients to be safely withdrawn from their drug of dependency	Clonidine, lofexidine, methadone, buprenorphine in opiate addiction
Relapse prevention	Block reinforcing effects of opiates	Naltrexone, methadone, buprenorphine
	Treat underlying or drug induced psychopathology that may cause relapse of drug use	Antidepressants
Opioid maintenance	Reduce the medical and social health risks of heroin use	Methadone, buprenorphine

Fig. 4 Different uses of psychopharmacology in the treatment of drug dependency.

Key points

♦ Always be aware of drug misuse as part of your differential diagnosis.

♦ Before undertaking substitute prescribing, take a good history, examine for confirmatory signs of drug misuse, carry out urine analysis, and seek advice on prescribing regimes.

♦ Treatment works.

References

1. **Substance Abuse and Mental Health Services Administration, Office of Applied Studies** (1996). Any illicit drug use. In *National Household Survey on Drug Abuse, Advance Report No 18*. Rockville MD: Substance Abuse and Mental Health Services Administration.

2. **Johnston, L.D., O'Malley, P.M., and Bachman, J.G.** *National Survey Results on Drug Use from the Monitoring the Future Study, 1975–1995. Volume 1: Secondary School Students.* NIH Pub. No 97–4139. Rockville MD: National Institute on Drug Abuse, 1996.

3. **Williams, A.G.** et al. (1985). Drugs in fatally injured young male drivers. *Public Health Report* **100**, 19–25.

4. **Oppenheimer, E., Tobutt, C., Taylor, C., and Andrew, T.** (1994). Death and survival in a cohort of heroin addicts from London clinics: a 22-year follow up study. *Addiction* **89**, 1299–308.

5. **Esklid, A., Magnus, P., Samuelsen, S.O., Sohlberg, C., and Kittelsen, P.** (1993). Differences in mortality rates and causes of death between HIV-positive and HIV-negative intravenous drug users. *International Journal of Epidemiology* **22** (1), 315–20.

6. **Gossop, M.** et al. (1996). Frequency of nonfatal heroin overdose—survey of heroin users recruited in non-clinical settings. *British Medical Journal* **313**, 402.

7. **Ramsey, M. and Partridge, S.** *Drug Misuse Declared in 1998: Results from the British Crime Survey.* London: Home Office, 1999.

8. **Telfer, I. and Cludlow, C.** (1990). Heroin misusers: what they think of their general practitioners. *British Journal of Addiction* **85**, 137–40.

9. **Hindler, C.** et al. (1996). Characteristics of drug misusers and their perceptions of general practice care. *British Journal of General Practitioners* **46**, 149–52.

10. **Farrell, M.** et al. (1994). Methadone maintenance treatment in opiate dependence: a review. *British Medical Journal* **309**, 997–1001.

11. **Drug Misuse and Dependence—Guidelines on Clinical Management.** Department of Health, The Scottish Office Department of Health, Welsh Office Department of Health and Social Services, Northern Ireland, 1999.

12. **US Department of Health and Human Services/Substance Abuse and Mental Health Services Administration**. *A Guide to Substance Services for Primary Care Clinicians. Treatment Improvement Protocol* Series 24, 1998.

13. **American Psychiatric Association.** *Practice Guidelines for Treatment of Patients with Substance Use Disorders: Alcohol, Cocaine, Opioids.* Washington DC: American Psychiatric Association, 1995.

14. **Smitten, G.V.** (1996). Has the United Kingdom averted an epidemic of HIV-1 infection among drug injectors? *Addiction* **91** (8), 1085–8.

15. **Gossop, M.** et al. (1999). Methadone treatment practices and outcome for opiate addicts treated in drug clinics and in general practice: results from the National Treatment Outcome Research Study. *British Journal of General Practice* **49**, 31–4.

16. **European Monitoring Centre for Drugs and Drug Addiction**, 2000 (www.emcdda.org).

Recommended website

www.doh.gov.uk/drugs/index.htm

Further reading

Gerada, C.A. (1998). Drugs of dependence—illicit drugs. In *ABC of Mental Health* (ed. T. Davies and T. Craig), pp. 39–45. London: BMJ Books.

Ghodse, H. *Drugs and Addictive Behaviour: A Guide to Treatment.* Oxford: Blackwell Science, 1995.

Tackling Drugs to Build a Better Britain: The Government's Ten-year Strategy for Tackling Drug Misuse. London: The Stationery Office, 1998 (Cm 3945).

Preston, A., ed. (1996). *The Methadone Briefing.* Dorchester: West Dorset Community Alcohol and Drugs Advisory Service.

9.5 Alcohol misuse and primary care

Clare Gerada and Jo Betterton

Introduction

Alcohol contributes to physical, emotional, and social problems. Primary care is ideally placed to identify many of those affected by problem drinking, as problem drinkers are more likely to consult[1] there is ample opportunity for general practitioners (GPs) and others in primary care to identify them and intervene. GPs' abilities to detect and manage patients' alcohol problems are a central part of their role as generalist clinicians.

Extent of the problem[2,3]

Overall

Most people drink alcohol, with only 10 per cent of the population identifying themselves as teetotal. In the United Kingdom, 'at-risk drinking' levels (defined as over 14 units/week for women and over 21 units/week for men) are rising, with 28 per cent of men and 11 per cent of women drinking at levels that cause harm. 'Problem drinking' (defined as drinking that causes serious problems to the drinker, their family or social network, or to society) is present in around 1–2 per cent of the population. In most primary care samples, around 10–30 per cent of patients are found to have hazardous alcohol consumption, though only a small proportion of these will have been recognized.

International examples of alcohol consumption[4]

♦ A high level of alcohol consumption is a feature of Australian life where each Australian on average drinks 7.9 l of absolute alcohol per year, and where one-fourth of Australian men and 12 per cent of women report usually drinking more than four drinks per drinking session.[5]

♦ Belgium is traditionally a beer drinking country, where average consumption in 1993 was 110.5 l per person. Special beers from Belgium contain more alcohol (from 6 to 13 per cent) and have become increasingly more popular across the world.

♦ Hungarian drinking has increased considerably over recent years with an estimated 12 per cent of the population misusing alcohol. The indications of increased consumption include a four and a half times increase in alcohol-related deaths, a doubling of road traffic accidents where alcohol is implicated, and a fivefold increase in mortality from cirrhosis.

- Italy, historically, has high levels of alcohol consumption and is the European nation that has recorded the highest decrease in consumption over the last decade. This appears to be due to sociocultural modifications such as the internationalization of consumer habits (i.e. drinking beers and spirits as well as wine), changes in family structure, and the nature of employment, which has evolved from primarily physical labour to work that requires attention and accuracy. In the last 30 years, eating habits have changed, with at least one main meal taken outside the home in situations where one eats more quickly and where wine is usually not served, or is of poor quality.

- France had a tradition of giving a quarter of a litre of wine every day to the soldiers during the 4 years of the First World War. Consumption per capita population has increased continuously throughout the twentieth century and France now has the highest level of alcohol consumption in the world.

- Nearly one-fourth of Americans say their drinking 'has been a cause of trouble in their family' and an estimated 53 per cent of Americans of 18 years or older have a family history of alcoholism in their first- or second-degree relatives.[6]

Factors affecting use

In most countries, alcohol consumption has increased throughout the second half of the twentieth century. The increase is probably related to a number of factors, amongst them:

- increase in personal wealth amongst all groups, but especially in the young and amongst women;
- greater acceptance by women and young men;
- lower real price of alcohol;
- marketing by the drinks industry targeted at specific groups;
- commercialization of leisure;
- stress of modern life.

Epidemiology

Age

Drinking is increasing amongst the young: in the 16–24-year-old age group 37 per cent of men and 23 per cent of women regularly drink twice the recommended levels. Drinking in younger age groups is limited by lack of purchasing power; nevertheless, research shows that the age at which young people start drinking is falling across Europe. In the United Kingdom, among 11–15 year olds the number drinking at least once a week rose from 13 per cent in 1988 to 20 per cent in 1996. As well as contributing to exclusion from school, increased risky sexual behaviour, and possible longer-term health complications, children under the age of 10 run the risk of alcoholic poisoning, as the liver is not yet mature enough to metabolize alcohol.

Sex

Women drink less than men, total consumption varying between one-third and one-fifth of men's consumption. However, consumption by women is rising and surveys in the United Kingdom show that average weekly drinking amongst women has increased from 5.4 to 6.3 units. The change in women's drinking habits can be attributed to a combination of increasing purchasing power, working and socializing in the work place, the convergence of female and male recreational activity, greater acceptance of drinking by women, and increased availability outside traditional pubs or bars into supermarkets. Women weigh less than men on average and, taking physiological differences between men and women into account, along with possible increased vulnerability to tissue damage at equivalent doses to men, it is advisable that women should drink less than men.

Alcohol and pregnancy

There is conflicting evidence whether drinking during pregnancy has the potential to harm the foetus. Most studies have been conducted on animals and where done on humans the difficulties in interpreting the results in the presence of a number of confounding variables has proved very difficult. Nevertheless, there is general agreement that ethanol has the potential to induce the following effects: abortion, foetal growth retardation, facial and other dysmorphologies, and impaired post-natal physical and mental development. The advice given by the Department of Health[7] is that pregnant women should never become intoxicated and should reduce their intake to 1–2 units per week, while the Royal College of Obstetricians and Gynecologists in the United Kingdom recommends no more than one standard drink per day.

The full spectrum of physical and mental handicaps known as foetal alcohol syndrome[8] is seen only in the offspring of alcohol-dependent women. This is characterized by growth deficiency of prenatal onset, characteristic facial dysmorphology, and central nervous system involvement with developmental delay.

Alcohol and young people

Drinking by young children raises obvious concerns about its social desirability and the adequacy of supervision by parents and carers. Parents and carers of children who do drink should try to ensure that these children are aware of the dangers and that it is only consumed in moderate and safe quantities for their age group with reference to their physical development.

High-risk groups

The British Medical Association estimates that one in 15 doctors suffer from alcohol dependence. There is no reason to believe that other health professionals have lower levels.[9] Other high-risk groups include journalists, publicans, and those working in the media. About one-third of homeless people have an alcohol problem.

Units

The unit is 8 g or 10 cl of pure alcohol and is generally recognized as a bar measure of:

- half a pint of normal strength beer or lager;
- one glass of wine;
- one glass of sherry;
- one measure of spirit.

Safe or recommended weekly limits of consumption are 21 units for men and 14 units for women. These units should be spread across the week rather than consumed in one go. It is also advised that drinkers abstain for 1 or 2 days after a heavy alcohol intake.

Harmful effects of alcohol

The consumption of alcohol, both in the short and long-term, is associated with a range of different types of mortality, morbidity, and social problems. It is difficult to estimate the number of deaths caused by alcohol. Estimates in the United Kingdom vary from 5000 to 40 000 deaths per year, the range reflecting a number of methodological problems in separating direct and indirect factors.

A useful framework for conceptualizing the harm associated with alcohol (and drug use) involves the four-L model:

- *Liver*—health problems (liver damage, anaemia, neurological and central nervous system problems, psychiatric complications).
- *Lover* (domestic violence, family breakdown, loss of friends).
- *Livelihood* (job loss, debt, lack of interest in leisure).
- *Law* (being arrested for drunk driving, disorderly conduct).

An alternative way is to look at the short- and long-term problems associated with alcohol, such as:

1. Short-term effects and drunkenness: mostly related to single episodes of intoxication, for example, association with domestic violence, road traffic accidents, violent crime, child neglect, and abuse.

2. Longer-term effects including cirrhosis of the liver, cancer (upper aerodigestive tract, liver), hypertension, foetal alcohol syndrome, and association with a range of mental illness (depression, suicide) and neurological disorders.

Risks

Amongst all populations there is a spectrum of risk from social drinking to at-risk consumption to problem drinking and on to dependence. The effects follow a J-shaped curve of harm, with little or no harm at low and moderate levels of drinking (there is good evidence that moderate drinking (1–3 units, particularly of red wine) per week is protective against coronary heart disease, especially in post-menopausal women and men over 50 years) but the risks to health increasing rapidly with levels above recommended amounts.

Costs to health care

Alcohol is probably second only to tobacco as the major cause of death in most countries. Certainly, in the United Kingdom, one in six people attending accident and emergency departments have alcohol-related problems or injuries, rising to eight out of 10 at peak times, for example, weekends. At these times, around half of all patients admitted into hospital have an alcohol-related injury. Three per cent of all cancers are due to alcohol consumption, notably oesophageal and oral cancers, and there is also a link with breast cancer. In 11 per cent of cases the main cause of hypertension in men is alcohol consumption. More than one in five men and one in six women admit to having unprotected sexual intercourse after drinking too much.

What can be done in primary care to identify problem drinking?

The primary care physician is central to the effective identification and treatment of alcohol problems.[10,11] However, despite the prevalence of problems relating to heavy alcohol intake presenting to GPs, they often fail to make the association. Among American family physicians, only 19 per cent were able to correctly diagnose an alcohol problem presented in computer simulations.[12] Even when recognized, the ability of primary care physicians to address their patients' alcohol problems has been found to be poor. Similarly, Australian GPs' detection of patients' alcohol problems have been demonstrated to be poor, with less than 28 per cent of heavy drinkers identified by their family doctors.[13]

Beware

At the very least, GPs and primary care staff should be aware of the high prevalence of alcohol problems and have a high index of suspicion when seeing patients with conditions ranging from hypertension, anxiety, and depression, to upper gastrointestinal problems.

Asking about drinking patterns should become part of most consultations.

Screening[14]

Screening all patients for potential alcohol misuse will reveal a much higher number of patients with either problematic or potentially problematic drinking histories. The AUDIT questionnaire has a high accuracy rate (see below).

Screening tools

Alcohol Use Disorder Identification Test questionnaire[15]

This questionnaire has been validated by WHO—with high sensitivity and specificity. It can be self-competed or administered in 2–4 min. A score of 5 or above suggests that the patient may have, or be at risk from developing, an alcohol-related problem (Table 1).

Assessment

Not all patients with drinking problems are dependent on alcohol. Treatment must start with an assessment of the drinking pattern, how much is drunk in an average day and over an average 3-month period, the type of drink, the context, and whether there are symptoms of dependent drinking.

Drinking history

- Consumption over past 3 months.
- Typical day's drinking pattern.
- Frequency of drinking.

Table 1 AUDIT questionnaire[15]

Alcohol screening questions	Score				
	0	1	2	3	4
How often do you have a drink containing alcohol?	Never	Monthly or less	Two to four times a month	Two to three times a week	Four or more times a week
How many drinks containing alcohol do you have on a typical day when you are drinking?	1 or 2	3 or 4	5 or 6	7 or 8	10 or more
How often during the last year have you found that you were not able to stop drinking once you started?	Never	Less than monthly	Monthly	Weekly	Daily or almost daily
How often in the last year have you failed to do what was normally expected of you because of drinking?	Never	Less than monthly	Monthly	Weekly	Daily or almost daily
Has a close relative or other health worker been concerned about your drinking or suggested you cut down?	No		Yes, but not in the last year		Yes, during the last year

- Maximum in 1 day.
- Severity of dependence (morning drinking to stop shakes, past evidence of failure to control drinking).
- Alcohol-related physical, emotional, and special problems.
- Consider liver function tests, full blood count.
- Consider using a screening tool—such as the AUDIT questionnaire.

Symptoms of dependence

- Craving.
- Withdrawal symptoms after a period of abstinence. This may manifest itself as the 'early morning shakes', morning nausea and vomiting, or a generalized anxiety state.
- Stereotypic drinking, that is, drinking pattern follows the same routine irrespective of the social or other context.
- Compulsion to drink.

Brief intervention

Primary care professionals should never underestimate the power of their advice. There is good evidence that brief and minimum interventions, amounting to just a few minutes of giving advice, can produce significant reductions in harmful drinking patterns. Brief intervention by a GP has been shown to reduce consumption, especially in men, by as much as 20 per cent.[16]

Brief intervention involves the following:

F	feedback	assessment and evaluation of the problem
R	responsibility	emphasizing that drinking is by choice
A	advice	explicit advice on changing drinking behaviour
M	menu	offering alternative goals and strategies
E	empathy	the role of the counsellor is important
S	self-efficacy	instilling optimism that the chosen goals can be achieved

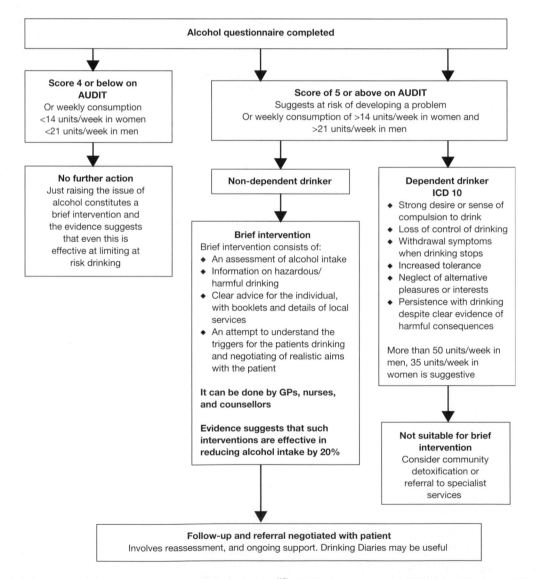

Fig. 1 Guideline for brief intervention following completion of AUDIT questionnaire.[19] (*MARG—Implementing Clinical Effectiveness Programme 1999—Primary Care Guideline for Brief Intervention in Alcohol for Moderate, Non-dependent Drinkers.*)

Harm minimization interventions include advising where drinking should be avoided, these include:

* before or during driving;
* before swimming;
* generally, before or during active physical sport;
* before working or in the work place when appropriate functioning would be adversely affected by alcohol;
* when taking medication, where alcohol is contra-indicated.

Pharmacological treatments for alcohol dependence

Different guidelines and protocols are available to guide the clinician regarding pharmacological treatment of withdrawal and detoxification (Fig. 1):[17,18]

* Briefly, having made a diagnosis of dependence the clinician must determine whether it is safe and practical to detoxify the patient in the community or whether a referral to a specialist or inpatient unit is the preferred option.

Detoxification

For patients who are physically dependent on alcohol, planned detoxification may be appropriate, once it is established that the patient fulfils the following criteria:

* no history of fits;
* not a suicide risk;
* has social support;
* no significant polydrug misuse;
* not dependent on benzodiazepines.

A withdrawal plan should be started if the patient is sober enough to agree to the plan and understands the principles involved. Daily assessment and the support of a carer should be seen as prerequisites for most patients.

In the United Kingdom, chlordiazepoxide is the recommended choice of medication although other benzodiazepines can be used. Chlormethiazole is not recommended due to its potential for dependence and abuse.

The following regime has been recommended in the United Kingdom Clinical Guidelines. Dosages and length of treatment will vary according to patient factors and the severity of dependence. This regime is for guidance only. It is strongly recommended that the clinician *seek expert advice before undertaking a community detoxification.* Deaths from overdose, especially if benzodiazepines are taken with alcohol, are not uncommon. To improve safety the medication should be dispensed daily, or involve family or other supporters. Ideally, the patient should be seen daily for the first 5 days and again at the end of the detoxification period. Abstinence should be confirmed before each daily dose for the first 3 days.

Days 1 and 2	20–30 mg of chlordiazepoxide four times daily;
Days 3 and 4	15 mg four times daily;
Day 5	10 mg four times daily;
Day 6	10 mg twice daily;
Day 7	10 mg at night.

It is useful to prescribe oral vitamin B complex or vitamin B1 (thiamine) 50 mg BD for 3 weeks to help recovery in thiamine levels.

Abstinence

Two specific therapies are licensed for use with dependent drinkers, to help them maintain abstinence in the face of craving. Both should be combined with alcohol-focused counselling.

Disulfiram

This drug has been used for many years, though there are few controlled trials of its use. There is evidence that it can reduce the frequency of drinking sessions, but no evidence of enhanced abstinence overall. There is also some evidence to suggest that supervised disulfiram is more effective than unsupervised prescription. Disulfiram works by altering the metabolism of alcohol and increases the level of acetaldehyde in the body, causing discomfort. It appears to be most effective with patients who are motivated to abstain, have good non-drinking social networks, and someone to encourage and support them in taking it regularly.

Acamprosate

This drug has been demonstrated in clinical trials to be an effective treatment in reducing drinking frequency and craving, with some evidence of enhanced abstinence overall. It also seems to be effective in reducing relapse when combined with a psycho-social programme. Treatment outcomes where abstinence is an original goal are high if treatment continues for 1 year or longer.

Naltrexone

Although this drug is predominantly used in opiate addiction, there is some evidence that naltrexone is effective in reducing drinking frequency and relapse rates in alcohol dependency. It is most effective when used as an adjunct to psycho-social treatments including cognitive–behaviour therapy.

> The process of recovery is likely to involve many relapses. Do not give up. Each attempt must be seen as being on the road to achieving the ultimate goal of abstinence. Carry on with a non-confrontational approach. Learning does occur and treatment does work—eventually.

Non-pharmacological treatments for alcohol dependence

The most common international self-help group is Alcoholics Anonymous (AA) and employs a '12-step' disease model. The programme aims for abstinence and works on the concept that alcoholism is a disease and that the individual is powerless to control his/her drinking. By following the clearly defined 12-step programme, individuals can lead a productive alcohol-free life. The first step is admitting that you are powerless to control your drinking and believe in spiritual support to overcome the problem. Although there are few controlled trials there are numerous anecdotal reports attesting to its effectiveness. It appears to work best for those individuals who accept higher levels of authority, have greater severity of alcohol dependency, and lower level of education and psychopathology.

The majority of counselling services work on a social-learning theory principle. This is based on the concept that individuals learn to behave, think, and feel in a certain way, and that the individual needs to learn new ways of managing 'trigger' situations. This approach can work for either controlled drinking or abstinence.[20]

Conclusion

Alcohol consumption is a rapidly growing problem and primary care physicians are ideally placed to address the issue. Research comparing responses to various treatment options demonstrates that it is the strength of the relationship with the professional that has the greatest impact on the eventual outcome. Primary care doctors and nurses already have the skills to develop and sustain this type of relationship and, therefore, can expect positive results when working with problem drinkers. It is essential that primary health care providers increase their awareness of non-dependent as well as dependent drinkers, and promote healthier drinking messages widely, to reduce problems in the longer term.

Key points

- At-risk drinking thresholds are 14 units per week for women and 21 for men.

- Around 10–30% of patients in primary care report hazardous consumption, but only a small proportion are identified.

- Screening will reveal a much higher number of patients at risk—the AUDIT questionnaire has a high accuracy rate.

- Brief intervention by a family doctor can reduce consumption by as much as 20%.

- Family doctors can detoxify some patients in the community, while others should be admitted.

- Two specific drugs are licensed to help dependent drinkers abstain.

- Alcoholics Anonymous works well for some dependent drinkers.

References

1. **Deehan, A.** et al. (1998). Low detection rates, negative attitudes and the failure to meet 'Health of the Nation' targets. *Drug and Alcohol Review* **17** (3), 249–58.

2. **Statistical Bulletin**. *Statistics on Alcohol: 1976 Onwards*. Bulletin 1999/24. ISBN 1 84182 090 3 (www.statisitcs.gov.uk).

3. *Britains Ruin? Alcohol Concern*. Waterbridge House, 32–36 Loman Street, London SE1 OEE (www.alcoholconcern.org.uk).

4. **World Health Organization**. *Alcohol, Drugs and Tobacco Programme*. EUR/HFA target 12, 1998 (www.who.dk).

5. *Statistics on Drug Abuse in Australia*. Canberra: Australian Government Publishing Services, Commonwealth Department of Human Services and Health, 1992.

6. **American Psychiatric Association**. *Diagnostic and Statistical Manual of Mental Disorders* 4th edn. Washington DC: American Psychiatric Association, 1994.

7. *Sensible Drinking. The Report of an Inter-Departmental Working Group*. London: HMSO, December 1995.

8. **Plant, M., Sullivan, F.M., Guerri, C., and Abel, E.L.** (1992). In *Health Issues Related to Alcohol Consumption* (ed. P.M. Verchuren), pp. 245–62. ILSI Europe.

9. **The British Doctors' and Dentists Group**. 0207487 4445. Or 020 7252 316 776. (This is an independent professional self-help organization for doctors and dentists who are alcoholic or drug dependent. Individual groups meet monthly across the United Kingdom and Republic of Ireland; there are also family support meetings. All enquiries are dealt with in the strictest confidence.)

10. **Clement, S.** (1986). The identification of alcohol related problems by general practitioners. *British Journal of Addictions* **81**, 257–64.

11. **Heather, N.** (1996). The public health and brief interventions for excessive alcohol consumption: the British experience. *Addictive Behaviours* **21**, 857–68.

12. **Brown, R.L.** et al. (1987). Diagnosis of alcoholism in a simulated patient encounter by primary care physicians. *Journal of Family Practice* **25**, 259–64.

13. **Reid, A.L.A.** et al. (1986). Detection of patients with high alcohol intake by general practitioners. *British Medical Journal* **293**, 735–7.

14. *Guidelines for the Management of Alcohol Problems in Primary Care and General Psychiatry—UK Alcohol Forum* 2nd edn. April 2001 (www.ukalcoholforum.org).

15. **Saunders, J.** et al. (1993). Development of the alcohol use disorder identification test (AUDIT): WHO Collaborative Project on Early Detection of Persons with Harmful Alcohol Consumption—11. *Addiction* **88**, 791–804.

16. **Bien, T., Miller, W., and Tonigan, J.** (1993). Brief interventions for alcohol problems: a review. *Addiction* **88**, 315–36.

17. *Drug Misuse and Dependence—Guidelines on Clinical Management*. Department of Health, The Scottish Office Department of Health, Welsh Office, 1999 (www.doh.gov.uk).

18. **American Psychiatric Association**. *Practice Guidelines for Treatment of Patients with Substance Use Disorders: Alcohol, Cocaine, Opioids*. Washington DC: American Psychiatric Association, 1995.

19. *Implementing Clinical Effectiveness Programme 1999*. Lambeth Southwark and Lewisham Health Authority. Multi-professional Audit Research Group (marg@kcl.ac.uk).

20. Project MATCH: rational and methods for a multisite clinical trial matching patients to alcoholism treatment—alcoholism. *Clinical and Experimental Research* **7** (6), 1130–45.

Further reading

Department of Health. *Sensible Drinking*. The report of an Inter-Department Working Group, December 1995.

9.6 Eating disorders
Doris Young

Dieting and concerns about body weight are very common amongst today's young people.[1] However, what is more worrying is that a proportion of these young people especially women will become obsessively preoccupied with dieting and slimness and continue on to develop eating disorders, namely anorexia nervosa and bulimia nervosa.

Anorexia nervosa is a syndrome that usually begins in adolescence, characterized by a relentless pursuit of thinness, resulting in weight loss and a refusal to maintain a normal body weight. *Bulimia nervosa* tends to have a later onset, affecting older teens and young women. The main difference between the two types of eating disorders is that anorexia nervosa sufferers, generally restrict their food intake, exercise more rigidly with a marked decrease in weight whereas sufferers from bulimia nervosa often maintain a normal body weight and can sometimes even be overweight. Their weight fluctuates as they binge in response to hunger and then vomit, purge, and/or diet. There are specific criteria that define each of these disorders according to Diagnostic Statistical Manual (DSM) IV (Table 1) and new features of the criteria are that both anorexia nervosa and bulimia nervosa have restricting and binge eating /purging sub-types.[2]

Epidemiology

In Western cultures, 0.5 per cent of young women have anorexia nervosa and 2 per cent have bulimia nervosa at some time.[3] However, the prevalence of bulimic behaviours is estimated to be much higher, up to 10–20 per cent in young women because the condition is difficult to detect. The highest incidence of anorexia nervosa is in females aged 15–19 and bulimia nervosa in those aged 20–24, with women at least 10 times more commonly affected than men. Although eating disorders are typically considered diseases of upper middle class Caucasians, recent studies show that these disorders affect other ethnic groups and social classes.[4] Those women whose occupation values thinness such as modelling, ballet, and gymnastics are particularly prone.

Table 1 Key clinical features of anorexia nervosa and bulimia nervosa (Diagnostic criteria summarized from DSM-IV. Criteria for anorexia/bulimia nervosa published in the American Psychiatric Association Press)

Anorexia nervosa
Refusal to maintain appropriate weight for age and height (<85%)
Pervasive fear of becoming fat or gain weight despite current underweight status
Significant distortion of perceived body size or body shape
Amenorrhoea (in post-menarchal females)

(Subtypes: restricting type and binge eating/purging type)

Bulimia nervosa
Recurrent episodes of binge eating
Behaviour to compensate for binge eating (e.g. vomiting, use of diuretics and/or laxatives)
Binge eating and compensatory behaviours occur over time (at least 3 months)
Excessive concern about weight or body shape

(Subtypes: purging type and non-purging type)

A review of *outcomes* studies reported that over 20 years, 50 per cent of anorexia nervosa sufferers make a good recovery, 30 per cent fair, and 20 per cent have poor outcomes with most remaining impaired in social and physical functioning.[5] Mortality rates of 10–15 per cent have been reported, the highest of any psychiatric disorder.[6] The outcome of bulimia nervosa is less well described, with 70 per cent of sufferers regaining or maintaining weight with reasonable stability.

The *aetiology* of eating disorders is not clear. It is certainly multifactorial with biological and genetic predispositions. There is also a hormonal causation attributed to a hypothalamic defect in causing amenorrhoea and inappropriate satiety control.

Sufferers often have extremely low self-esteem and feel ineffective. They tend to be perfectionists and overachievers with obsessive–compulsive traits. About 50–75 per cent of them also have an association with other psychiatric diagnoses including an estimated 25 per cent lifetime prevalence of obsessive–compulsive disorder, and a 50–75 per cent prevalence of dysthymia.[7] Additional factors associated with developing bulimia nervosa include a history of childhood sexual abuse, psychoactive substance abuse or dependence, and a family history of alcoholism or depression. Family communication characteristics such as blurring of boundaries and over-identification have also been implicated in the causation of eating disorders.

Presentation and history

Detecting the abnormal dieter

There is a great deal of experimental eating disorder behaviour in young women. The following questions regarding weight can be included in a routine interview with the young person to detect abnormal dieting behaviour:

- What do you think of your current weight?
- How do you maintain your weight?
- What is your ideal weight?
- Are you on any special diet?

This can be followed by another recently developed screening tool, the SCOFF questionnaire to screen for eating disorders:[8]

- Do you make yourself *S*ick because you feel uncomfortably full?
- Do you worry you have lost *C*ontrol over how much you eat?
- Have you recently lost more than *O*ne stone (14 lb or 6.4 kg) in a 3-month period?

- Do you believe yourself to be *F*at when others say you are too thin?
- Would you say *F*ood dominates your life?

Presentation

In anorexia nervosa, a typical presentation in primary care would involve a teenage female, reluctantly brought in by her mother because of excessive weight loss through dieting. Though not markedly overweight, the teenager may have been teased about being 'fat' and starting dieting. Once weight loss commences, she became increasingly fearful of weight gain and pursued lower and lower weight goals by exerting control over food intake. Many sufferers hold negative attitudes towards their own bodies and perceive their hips or thighs as 'big' even when emaciated. In males, health and physical fitness are more of an issue than appearance. In contrast to other physical illnesses there is no reported lethargy. On the contrary, there is excessive exercising and hyperactivity. Amenorrhoea is very common and often precedes marked weight loss. Constipation is also a common problem unless there is laxative abuse. Psychological symptoms such as poor concentration, headache, and irritability can also be present.

In bulimia nervosa, sufferers are much harder to detect as they are often of normal weight. They may self-refer as they feel guilty over their binge eating and self-induced vomiting habits and fear losing control. Irregular menses sometimes is also a concern. Anxiety and depression are often present with or without an associated history of past sexual abuse. Indeed, a retrospective review of clinic records showed that eating disorder patients present to their GPs more often for psychological problems than for physical complaints before the actual diagnosis of eating disorder was made.[9] In both groups, a history of preoccupation with food is present and episodes of restrictive dieting and bingeing followed by self-induced vomiting or laxative use will confirm the diagnosis.

In addition to the dieting and physical history, the primary care practitioner also needs to explore the developmental and psycho-social context in which the young person functions. Relevant enquiries include current social interactions with friends, family conflict around the theme of eating, changes in intimate relationships, self-confidence, and school achievement. Patients whose self-esteem and control rest solely on body weight are likely to need longer-term treatment.

Differential diagnoses

It is unlikely that a slim adolescent girl who has absent or irregular menses and who achieves thinness by dieting, self-induced vomiting, and excessive exercise will have a disorder other than anorexia nervosa or bulimia nervosa. For a male adolescent, more effort is needed to exclude other organic causes of weight loss given the lower incidence of eating disorders. In presentations that are not clear, one must consider other diagnoses that could cause weight loss and amenorrhoea.

Conditions that result in *weight loss* are:

- hyperthyroidism,
- adrenal insufficiency,
- gastrointestinal disturbances (e.g. Crohn's disease),
- psychiatric illness such as depression and schizophrenia,
- malignancy, and
- diabetes mellitus.

  Cause of *amenorrhoea* include:

- craniopharyngioma, and
- prolactinoma.

In young males presenting with weight loss, inflammatory bowel disease should be excluded before making a diagnosis of an eating disorder.

Physical examination

In the early stages of the disorder, there are usually no abnormal physical findings. In later stages of anorexia nervosa, physical findings such as the following are the direct result of starvation:

- loss of subcutaneous fat;
- sunken eyes, inelastic and dry skin with a yellow hue;
- decreased body temperature, pulse, and blood pressure;
- fine lanugo hair may appear particularly on the limbs.

In bulimia sufferers, menstrual irregularities are common. Their weight can be normal or even slightly above average. Callus on fingers from self-induced vomiting and the development of parotitis and dental enamel erosion can occur due to the constant presence of gastric juice in the mouth from vomiting.

In severe cases, hypokalaemia can cause cardiac arrhythmias, muscle weakness and muscle twitching.

Investigations

Laboratory tests are only required to exclude other diagnoses rather than as an aid to the diagnosis of anorexia nervosa or bulimia nervosa. Only a limited number of investigations are required for the assessment of a patient presenting with a suspected eating disorder. These include:

- urea and electrolytes;
- liver function tests and amylase;
- full blood count and differential;
- ESR; and
- thyroid function tests.

Even in extreme weight loss, the biochemistry can be normal with the exception of serum potassium levels, which may be low if self-induced vomiting or laxative and diuretic abuse are present. Urea may be raised due to dehydration and serum amylase elevated in chronic vomiting. Surprisingly, anaemia is not usual. Occasionally a normochromic normocytic anaemia is found and despite the presence of leucopaenia, there is no increased incidence of infections. A raised ESR points to an organic cause. A low triiodothyronine can be due to starvation. All the hormonal changes are reversible with improved nutrition and weight gain although restoration of the hypothalamic–pituitary–ovarian axis may be delayed. In long-standing sufferers, bone densitometry may be useful to monitor bone mass loss.

Principles of treatment

Randomized controlled trials of the treatment of eating disorders are few and far between. Treasure and Schmidt[10] reviewed the efficacy of different forms of treatment for anorexia nervosa and bulimia nervosa and concluded that not all patients require intensive treatments. In bulimia nervosa, a low intensity treatment is adequate initially to explore the patient's readiness to change. Cognitive–behavioural therapy (CBT) seems to be especially beneficial in treating bulimia nervosa. Key features include developing a partnership with the patient and giving them access to specialist knowledge through self-help manuals. The use of pharmacological agents has a limited place in the treatment of eating disorders. They are often used as adjuncts to psychotherapy. In controlled trials, the antidepressant, fluoxetine was shown to reduce food craving, pathologic eating, vomiting, and depression in patients with bulimia. There is also evidence to suggest that it prevents relapse in patients with anorexia nervosa.[11]

Management in primary care varies according to the duration and severity of the eating disorders. For early presentation and mild cases, the primary care practitioner should instigate the following first-line management:

- Establish rapport and engage the patient to forge a therapeutic alliance. This is vital as the patient is often brought in by her parents against her will.
- Address healthy eating patterns and maintain regular exercise. Often the sufferer needs some reinforcement regarding her nutritional needs.
- Explain normal weight for height and age. Calculations and explanations of the significance of BMIs are also helpful in reassuring them that their weight gain does not mean they will be fat.
- Use food diaries to identify triggers for food bingeing/abstinence. This is particularly useful for bulimia nervosa and bingeing eaters who can then avoid triggers.
- Discuss drug use and abuse if appropriate.
- Set short-term weight gains goals and reinforce successes—aim at BMI of 20, for those under 16 years; their target weight should be the 25th centile of the age–weight chart.

Depending on the counselling skills of the primary care practitioner, referral to mental health specialists is indicated in those with severe depression and suicidal ideation. Sufferers from bulimia nervosa rarely need admission to hospital. Even if hospital admission is indicated, it is usually brief for refeeding and in crisis situations. Indications for hospital admission are:

- Failure to progress despite a well-designed and delivered ambulatory care programme;
- Presence of severe depression, psychosis and suicidal risk;
- Family crisis;
- Marked decrease in weight with bradycardia, postural hypotension, and electrolyte imbalance.

Long-term and continuing care

Concerns about body weight and body image are rising in the community especially amongst young women. Prevention strategies for eating/dieting disorders include:

- Decrease the media's promotion and community's emphasis on thinness as 'attractiveness'.
- Increase awareness of weight concerns amongst young people attending primary care services to detect abnormal dieters.
- Raise awareness of mental health and well-being in young people to detect psychiatric co-morbidities.
- Public health education for appropriate nutrition and exercise for young women.

Implications of the problem

Eating disorders are costly to society in terms of lost lives and productivity of a group of young high achievers. So much is still unknown about the aetiology of the conditions and the effectiveness of various forms of treatment. Not enough evidence exists to guide attempts to match patients to different treatment programmes and the cost effectiveness of antidepressants, CBT, and other self-help programmes are still unknown. In primary care, we need prospective studies to identify those symptoms with the strongest association with eating disorders and psychological pathology in order to initiate early referral to mental health services.

Key points

- Detect the abnormal dieter.

- Exclude other causes for weight loss and amenorrhoea in young women.

- Food restriction and binge eating/purging sub-types exist in anorexia nervosa and bulimia nervosa.

- Treatment involves a multidisciplinary team to regain weight, self-esteem, and control of their lives.

- Drug treatment is rarely appropriate.

- CBT is useful in bulimia nervosa and family therapy in younger age groups.

References

1. **Patton, G.** et al. (1997). Adolescent dieting: healthy weight control or borderline eating disorder? *Journal of Child Psychology and Psychiatry* **38**, 299–306.

2. **American Psychiatric Association**. *Diagnostic and Statistical Manual of Mental Disorders* 4 edn. (DSM-IV). Washington DC: American Psychiatric Press, 1994.

3. **Hsu, L.K.G.** (1996). Epidemiology of the eating disorders. *Psychiatric Clinics of North America* **19**, 681–700.

4. **Robinson, T.N.** et al. (1996). Ethnicity and body dissatisfaction: are Hispanics and Asian women at increased risk for eating disorders? *Journal of Adolescent Health* **19**, 384–93.

5. **Herzog, D.B., Nussbaum, K.M., and Marmor, A.K.** (1996). Co-morbidity and outcome in eating disorders. *Psychiatric Clinics of North America* **19**, 843–59.

6. **Ratnasuriya, R.H.** et al. (1991). Anorexia nervosa: outcome and prognostic factors after 20 years. *British Journal of Psychiatry* **158**, 495–502.

7. **Halmi, K.A.** et al. (1991). Co-morbidity of psychiatric diagnoses in anorexia nervosa. *Archives of General Psychiatry* **48**, 712–18.

8. **Morgan, J.F., Reid, F., and Lacey, J.H.** (1999). The SCOFF questionnaire: assessment of a new screening tool for eating disorders. *British Medical Journal* **319**, 1467–8.

9. **Ogg, E.C.** et al. (1997). General practice consultation patterns preceding diagnosis of eating disorders. *International Journal of Eating Disorders* **22**, 89–93.

10. **Treasure, J. and Schmidt, U.** (1999). Beyond effectiveness and efficiency lies quality in services for eating disorders. *European Eating Disorders Review* **7**, 162–78.

11. **Fluoxetine Bulimia Nervosa Collaborative Study Group** (1992). Fluoxetine in the treatment of bulimia nervosa. *Archives of General Psychiatry* **49**, 139–47.

Further reading

Walsh, J.M., Wheat, M., and Freund, K. (2000). Detection, evaluation and treatment of eating disorders. *Journal of General Internal Medicine* **15**, 577–90. (A comprehensive update review of eating disorders for general clinicians.)

9.7 Psychiatric emergencies

Mary-Lynn Watson and Douglas E. Sinclair

A psychiatric emergency is defined as the sudden occurrence of abnormal behaviour that appears to be psychiatric in origin. This may be the result of a psychiatric illness or a medical illness presenting with psychiatric features[1] and may increase the potential for harm to self or others. The incidence of psychiatric emergencies in an urban emergency department has been found to be 4–10 per cent of all visits.[2] Knowledge of a general approach to these emergencies is important as these patients may do harm to themselves or to others.

Initial evaluation and management

The relatively high incidence of psychiatric emergencies mandates an approach to the initial evaluation of these patients. The first rule of initial evaluation is to protect the patient, other patients, and staff from harm. For patients who are very agitated, this may require a secluded area, absence of potential weapons, as well as subdued lighting in some cases. The availability of an alarm system for offices, an escape route, cell phone for home visits as well as continuing contact with support staff such as police or other members of the community will help prevent unnecessary risk to the physician assessing the patient.

The initial questions to ask when called on to assess a patient presenting with a psychiatric emergency include:

1. Is it safe for the patient to be assessed in your facility?
   (i) threatening or violent?
   (ii) intrusive?

2. Is the problem organic, functional, or a combination?
   (i) is the patient intoxicated?
   (ii) is there an underlying medical condition?
   (iii) previous history of psychiatric condition?
   (iv) vital signs stable?

3. Is the patient psychotic?
   (i) able to differentiate between fantasy and reality?
   (ii) able to focus on what you are saying?
   (iii) overtly responding to distorted thoughts or perception?

4. Is the patient suicidal or homicidal?
   (i) direct questioning is important in this assessment
   (ii) is this associated with psychosis?
   (iii) is there any evidence of substance ingestion?

5. To what degree is the patient capable of self-care?
   (i) is the patient unkempt?
   (ii) is there obvious malnourishment or dehydration?
   (iii) is there evidence of exposure to the elements?
   (iv) disorientation or confusion?
   (v) is there risk of harm to self or others?[3,4]

A general approach to assessing each of these questions involves:

- developing a rapport with the patient;

- gently and calmly listening to the patient and trying to establish trust;

- trying to provide a soothing environment for patient assessment;

- avoiding potential physical confrontation;

- consideration of chemical and or physical restraint to protect from harm.

Suicide risk

If you feel the patient may be managed as an outpatient, it is important to consider first the risk of suicide. Many studies have shown that certain patient characteristics are associated with an increased risk of suicide. The factors most commonly associated with this increased suicidal risk include:

- presence of a mood disorder,
- age over 45 years,
- Caucasian,
- living alone,
- having a chronic illness,
- male gender,
- previous attempt.[5]

There are, however, many other factors which may help to predict suicide risk. Please refer to Chapter 9.3 for a more detailed discussion of suicide.

History and physical exam

In general, obtaining the history from a patient with a psychiatric emergency may present a challenge. A collateral history from relatives, friends, and neighbours while maintaining patient confidentiality may be of great importance.

History should include:

- onset of the symptoms;
- previous medical and psychiatric history;
- a list of current prescribed medications, over-the-counter medications, as well as drugs of abuse;
- a careful social history may also be very helpful in elucidating any areas of concern, including social and work-related stresses;
- consideration of any other life stresses that may have precipitated the patient's presentation at the time.

Physical exam must include an evaluation for any underlying medical condition, which may present as a psychiatric emergency. The exam must include:

- vital signs including temperature, pulse, blood pressure, and oxygen saturation, as well as bedside glucometer reading;
- any evidence of trauma;
- breath odour, that is, ketones, alcohol, or solvents;
- puncture marks.

Laboratory investigations should be aimed at ruling out metabolic abnormalities which may masquerade as psychiatric illnesses. For most patients in whom an underlying medical illness cannot be excluded, this should include:

- complete blood count;
- electrolytes;
- glucose;
- blood alcohol;
- liver profile if known substance abuser;
- urea, creatinine, chest X-ray, urinalysis, and consideration of computerized tomography if the patient is elderly with a first presentation of psychiatric illness.[3]

A complete list of medical problems, which may present as psychiatric emergencies, is very extensive; however, there are some conditions that are more frequently encountered. These include:

- hypoglycaemia,
- infection,
- hypoxia,
- thyroid disease,
- uraemia,
- acute alcohol withdrawal,
- subdural haematoma,
- acute substance ingestion.

A careful examination and judicious use of laboratory screening may help prevent misdiagnosis of an underlying medical condition.

One of the most difficult patient populations to assess in the emergency situation is the patient with a known psychiatric condition who presents seeking care for a medical condition. These patients may be known to their caregivers and easily dismissed as frequent users of health services. They may also have difficulty expressing their physical symptoms and may describe their complaints in a very odd fashion that must be carefully considered by the caregivers before too easily dismissing this group of patients. Significant medical conditions may be missed under these circumstances and the health care workers must be vigilant to avoid such pitfalls.

The differentiation of organic versus functional psychiatric presentations may be somewhat challenging. There are, however, certain clues in both the history and physical exam that may be useful in differentiating between these underlying causes.

- Organic
  - abrupt onset,
  - tremor, ataxia,
  - visual hallucinations,
  - disorientation,
  - brief episodes of lucid behaviour,
  - greater than 40 years of age,
  - abnormal physical findings,
  - no previous history.
- Functional
  - gradual onset,
  - rocking, posturing,
  - auditory hallucinations,
  - oriented,
  - continuous abnormal behaviour,
  - less than 40 years of age,
  - normal physical exam,
  - previous history.[6]

Mental state assessment

After the patient has been carefully screened for a medical abnormality that may be contributing to, or directly causing the patient's symptoms, a careful mental state assessment may be undertaken. This should include:

- appearance and behaviour,
- affect,
- orientation,
- language use and understanding,
- memory,
- thought content,
- perceptual abnormalities,
- judgement.[7]

In the acute situation, this may be shortened to include only generalizations related to general appearance and use of language, content and gross memory.

Diagnosis suggested by abnormalities in the above include:

- delirium, dementia, and amnesia;
- substance abuse disorders;
- mental disorders due to underlying medical conditions;
- schizophrenia and other psychotic disorders;
- mood disorders;
- anxiety disorders;
- somatoform disorders;
- factitious disorders;
- dissociative disorders;
- eating disorders;
- adjustment disorders.[8]

Delirium

Delirium is an acute transient disturbance in consciousness that represents a change in the patient's ability to focus attention on tasks. There may also be a change in the patient's level of consciousness or orientation. In addition, agitation may occur, as well as depressed activity and perceptual abnormalities such as visual hallucinations that may lead to increased fearfulness.[9]

The diagnosis and treatment of this disorder is a true emergency and there must be consideration of underlying medical conditions that may present as delirium. Acute neurologic conditions such as infections, stroke, seizures, or trauma may present as acute delirium. Metabolic disorders, hypoxia, toxins, drugs such as steroids and antiparkisonian medications, infectious processes particularly respiratory or urinary tract or endocrinopathies should also be considered in the evaluation of the acutely delusional patient. These associated conditions frequently result in the manifestaion of symptoms over several hours rather than weeks or months.

Management of delirium must ensure safety for the patient and all others involved. If the patient is unwilling to be hospitalized for further assessment and treatment, the issue of competency must be evaluated. Medications such as haloperidol may be needed in a low dose but generally caution should be used, as further assessment of the patient may be difficult and therefore admission to hospital is indicated. The use of benzodiazepines may result in disinhibition and may render the situation more difficult.[9]

Dementia

Dementia is characterized by the presence of multiple cognitive defects that include memory impairment as well as aphasia, apraxia, agnosia, or impairment of executive functioning. There may also be poor judgement as well as other psychiatric symptoms such as delusions or hallucinations.[7]

The emergency evaluation of the patient who appears demented may be extremely difficult. The individual may present due to deterioration and may not have had a previous diagnosis or evaluation. The increased incidence of underlying medical conditions may also contribute to the diagnostic dilemma. A careful physical and mental status examination as well as laboratory investigation, is required in this group to avoid a misdiagnosis.

The treatment consists of correcting any underlying contributing factors as well as decreasing any environmental stimuli that may worsen the symptoms. Psychotic features may be treated as described below. Safety for the patient, as well as family members, must be ensured.

Acute psychosis

Psychosis is characterized by the inability to distinguish reality from delusions, hallucinations, or paranoia. As in other disorders, the elimination of an underlying medical condition that is contributing or causing the symptom is necessary. These include neurologic abnormalities such as infections, intoxication or hypoxia, as well as metabolic disorders and medications[9] including drugs of misuse such as amphetamines.

Psychosis may be the presenting symptom of schizophrenia, bipolar disorder, depression, and schizoaffective disorder.[9] The assessment of the patient that presents with an acute psychosis should include a careful physical examination as well as a mental status examination and laboratory investigations which should try to confirm there is no underlying medical abnormality presenting with a psychotic episode.

Antipsychotic medications are indicated in the treatment of this symptom and typically this includes haloperidol. Prophylaxis to prevent an acute dystonic reaction may be considered as this could be detrimental to the relationship with the paranoid or acutely agitated patient. Procyclidine 5 mg po BID or TID prophylactically must be considered in this situation.

Mood disorders

This group of psychiatric diagnoses represents a large portion of the emergency assessments in the health care setting. They are characterized by a prominent persistent mood that is either depressed or elevated. These symptoms cause a significant amount of stress to the patient and affect the patient at all levels of functioning.[7]

As with other conditions, the evaluation of the patient who presents with a mood disorder must include the exclusion of an underlying medical condition which may be causing or contributing to the disturbance. Most notable is the presence of hypo- or hyperthyroidism. A complete physical examination and lab testing may prevent the misdiagnosis of this population. Treatment for this group of disorders is aimed at the long-term control of the presenting symptoms with consideration of the complications of specific medications. Patients presenting with this group of disorders, as well as all acute psychiatric disorders, must be evaluated with respect to their suicide risk prior to decisions concerning disposition.

Emergency medications

For acute delirium, delusions, or hallucinations, consider the use of an antipsychotic such as haloperidol. This may be given orally, intramuscularly or intravenously at a dose of 0.5–5 mg. The use of respiridone by mouth may also be considered at a dose of 0.5–2.0 mg. This has been associated with fewer incidences of Parkinsonian side-effects.[10]

The patient who presents with marked agitation may be safely sedated with lorazepam in a dose of 1–2 mg by mouth, intramuscularly, or intravenously. The advantage of lorazepam is that it has a shorter duration of action, as well as freedom from the other side-effects associated with haloperidol.

Medication side-effects may be divided into various categories based on the class of drug used. The two major classes that may produce profound adverse reactions are neuroleptics and selective serotonin re-uptake inhibitors (SSRIs).

Neuroleptic side-effects may include:

1. Acute dystonias—may respond to benztropine 1–2 mg po or IV, or to diphenhydramine 50–100 mg po or IV.

2. Akathesias—may respond to propranalol 10 mg po or to benztropine 1–2 mg po or IV.

3. Parkinson's syndrome—adjust drug dose.

4. Anticholinergic effects—discontinue drug or give physostigmine 1–2 mg IV emergently only.

5. Cardiovascular-hypotension—IV fluids.

6. Neuroleptic malignant syndrome:

    (i) uncommon idiosyncratic reaction,

    (ii) rigidity, fever, tachycardia, diaphoresis, abnormal blood pressure,

    (iii) confusional state, rise in CPK, WBC, and LFTs,

    (iv) twenty per cent mortality rate,

    (v) discontinue medication, consider benzodiazepines or dantrolene, as well as blood pressure therapy as required.[10]

SSRI side-effects may include:

1. Serotonin syndrome—CNS or GI irritability (usually when combined with other drugs and treated by discontinuing the combination).

2. SSRI discontinuation syndrome—occurs within several days of stopping the drug (presents as flu-like symptoms and treated by restarting the medication).[11]

Special populations

The elderly

The elderly most commonly present to the emergency physician with medically related rather than psychiatric problems. It has been estimated that approximately 5 per cent of visits to the emergency department are related to purely psychiatric complaints.[12] Patients over the age of 65 years are more likely to present with delirium, dementia, medication side-effects, physical illness presenting as a psychiatric problem, depression, and alcohol abuse-related problems.[1]

Delirium in the elderly may be related to medications and the patient taking polypharmacy is particularly vulnerable. Physical illness, as well as drug withdrawal, should also be included in the list of potential causes.

Dementia is generally related to a multi-infarct picture or Alzheimer's disease. However, there is also a list of reversible causes that should be considered which includes depression, endocrine diseases, normal pressure hydrocephalus, subdural haematoma, and alcohol abuse (See Chapter 16.5).

Many medications have been implicated in the new onset of psychiatric complaints in the elderly. They are more at risk for difficulties due to underlying renal and hepatic disease and therefore the metabolism of various medications may be altered in this population. As well, the incidence of underlying illness in the elderly may result in behavioural abnormalities secondary to electrolyte abnormalities, vascular insufficiency, and chronic hypoxia.[12]

Children and adolescents

Children and adolescents with psychiatric complaints usually present for assessment due to the intervention of an adult rather than independently.[13] In this group, the most common psychiatric emergency is suicidal ideation or attempt. The management of the child or adolescent who presents with this complaint must include an evaluation of the family dynamics and quality of the various relationships within this group.

Aggressive behaviour as well as agitation or violence may lead to the presentation of the child or adolescent to the physician. When presented with a patient who exhibits these behaviours, the safety of the family, as well as the patient, must be considered and a careful history and evaluation, including homicidal ideation, must be obtained.[13]

Psychosis is an uncommon diagnosis in young children; however, a history may indicate a long course of pre-morbid changes that have not been recognized until the child is an adolescent.[14] It is particularly important to rule out medical and neurologic disorders and drug use prior to making the diagnosis of a functional psychosis.

Somewhat more common in the young population is the presentation of physical abuse or sexual abuse as a psychiatric emergency. It is important to consider these situations in the complete assessment of the child and adolescent in your facility. The assurance of a safe environment for both the evaluation and treatment of these patients is of paramount importance.

Disposition

If, after a careful assessment, it is felt that a patient may be released and followed as an outpatient, several conditions must be met. These have been described as a 'No Harm Contract' and include:

1. The patient must not be imminently suicidal.

2. The patient must be medically stable.

3. The patient and the family must agree to return as needed.

4. The patient must not be intoxicated, delirious, or demented.

5. Potentially lethal methods of self-harm must be removed.

6. The underlying psychiatric disorder must be diagnosed and appropriate treatment must be arranged.

7. Acute precipitants to the crisis must be addressed.

8. The physician must believe that the patient and the family will follow recommendations.

9. The patient's caregivers must be in support of the plan.[8]

The importance of meeting these objectives prior to discharge of a patient must be understood for the protection of the patient as well as other members of the family and community.

Key points

Five principles may characterize the general approach to the patient presenting with a psychiatric emergency:

1. Maintain a safe and comfortable environment.

2. Obtain a clear and complete history of the presenting complaint.

3. Consider underlying medical illnesses that may contribute to or present as psychiatric illnesses.

4. Be prepared for medication side-effects and know their treatment.

5. Carry out suicide risk assessment in all patients presenting with psychiatric emergencies.

References

1. Fauman, B. (2000). General approach to the psychiatric patient in the emergency department. In *Kaplan and Sadock's Comprehensive Textbook of Psychiatry* (ed. B. Sadock and V. Sadock), pp. 2808–15. Philadelphia PA: Lippincott Williams and Wilkins.

2. Oyewumbi, L., Odejide, O., and Kazarian, S. (1992). Psychiatric emergency services in a Canadian city: I. prevalence and patterns of use. *Canadian Journal of Psychiatry* **37**, 91–5.

3. Fauman, B. (2000). Other psychiatric emergencies. In *Kaplan and Sadock's Comprehensive Textbook of Psychiatry* (ed. B. Sadock and V. Sadock), pp. 2040–46. Philadelphia PA: Lippincott Williams and Wilkins.

4. Meyers, J. and Stein, S. (2000). The psychiatric interview in the emergency department. *Emergency Medical Clinics of North America* **18** (2), 173–83.

5. Hall, R., Platt, D., and Hall, R. (1999). Suicide risk assessment: a review of risk factors for suicide in 100 patients who made severe suicide attempts. *Psychosomatics* **40** (1), 18–27.

6. Williams, E. and Moore Shepherd, S. (2000). Medical clearance of psychiatric patients. *Emergency Medical Clinics of North America* **18** (2), 185–98.

7. Lagomasino, I., Daly, R., and Stoudemire, A. (1999). Medical assessment of patients presenting with psychiatric symptoms in the emergency setting. *The Psychiatric Clinics of North America* **22** (4), 819–50.

8. Rund, D. and Hutzler, J. *Emergency Psychiatry*. St Louis MO: The CV Mosby Company, 1983, pp. 69–70.

9. Riba, M. and Glick, R. (1997). Acute psychiatric disorders in primary care. In *Acute Care Psychiatry, Diagnosis and Treatment* (ed. L. Sederer and A. Rothschild), pp. 67–79. Baltimore MD: Williams and Wilkins.

10. Kennedy, G., Onuogu, E., and Lowinger, R. (1999). Psychiatric emergencies: rapid response and life-saving therapies. *Geriatrics* **54** (9), 38–46.

11. Grady, T., Sederer, L., and Rothschild, A. (1997). Depression. In *Acute Care Psychiatry, Diagnosis and Treatment* (ed. L. Sederer and A. Rothschild), pp. 83–121. Baltimore MD: Williams and Wilkins.

12. Tueth, M. (1994). Diagnosing psychiatric emergencies in the elderly. *American Journal of Emergency Medicine* **12** (3), 364–9.

13. Halamandaris, P. and Royster Anderson, T. (1999). Children and adolescents in the psychiatric emergency setting. *The Psychiatric Clinics of North America* **22** (4), 865–74.

14. Tomb, D. (1996). Child psychiatry emergencies. In *Child and Adolescent Psychiatry: A Comprehensive Textbook* (ed. M. Lewis), pp. 929–34. Baltimore MD: Williams and Wilkins.

9.8 Fatigue

Leone Ridsdale

Epidemiology

Tiredness is one of the symptoms with the highest prevalence in the community, and surveys find that up to a third of the population report this as being a recent health problem.[1] It is at least twice as common in women, and particularly those with young children. This symptom is equally prevalent in different social classes and in different countries. Without treatment the symptoms may remit and relapse in a similar way to other chronic conditions like depression. Whilst recognizing that the severity and duration of fatigue forms a continuum, researchers working in specialist care have generated various consensus criteria for chronic fatigue syndrome (CFS). If the fatigue is disabling, lasts at least 6 months, is unexplained by other medical or psychological conditions, and is associated with a specified number of additional symptoms, it is defined as CFS. The prevalence of CFS in the community has been estimated as ranging from 0.01 to 0.7 per cent.[2]

Service use

Although fatigue is common, the ratio of episodes reported in the community to consultations in primary care is 400 to one.[1] This is a good example of the iceberg phenomenon. The frequency with which fatigue is recorded as a reason for consulting depends to a certain extent on whether it is defined as a presenting symptom only, or as a presenting and/or supporting symptom. In British general practice, approximately 12 patients per 1000 reported fatigue as the most important reason for their consultation in 1 year.[1] When fatigue was counted as a presenting or supporting symptom, approximately 75 patients per 1000 consulted for fatigue.[1] Patients who do consult for fatigue tend to consult their doctors more frequently.[3] This consulting behaviour is not necessarily for fatigue. Frequent attendance has been related to the patient's self-reported symptoms of psychological distress.[3]

Approximately 98 per cent of patients presenting with tiredness are managed in primary care, with the remainder referred to specialists.[1]

Causes

Particular physical causes depend on age and gender. In young women, fatigue may be the presenting symptom of anaemia or pregnancy. In young people of both sexes, it may be the presenting feature of infectious mononucleosis or some other infection. Among older people, fatigue is more

Box 1 Causes of fatigue[4]

> 20–30% physical
> 40–50% psycho-social
> 20–40% mixed or unknown

commonly associated with circulatory disorders or prescribed drugs, for example, an antihypertensive medication. Occasionally, fatigue may be an early symptom of endocrine problems, such as thyroid disease or diabetes, or even cancer.[5]

So far as psycho-social causes are concerned, fatigue is a somatic symptom of depression, and three-quarters of patients who present with fatigue report symptoms of psychological distress.[5] Patients with prolonged fatigue, of more than 3 months duration, are more likely to have psychological symptoms and prior psychological problems.[5]

In primary care, it is likely that some patients who present with fatigue will have primarily social causes. The evidence that the highest prevalence is in women with children under 6 supports this hypothesis. Some patients will be found to have a working day which is long and difficult to organize, with ineffective boundaries between home and work. Some patients have extremely demanding occupations, and are highly demanding in the expectations they make of themselves. For these people, fatigue is not so much the chaff of living, but an occupational hazard of their chosen style of life.

How to make a diagnosis

The history, examination, and investigations will depend on age and gender. In young women, it is worth enquiring about menorrhagia or a missed period, and in both sexes about symptoms of infection. Amongst middle aged and elderly people, enquiry should be made with regard to symptoms of circulatory disorders such as chest or calf pain, fatigue on exertion, and shortness of breath. All prescribed drugs should be inquired about, particularly antihypertensives. Bearing in mind endocrine disease or malignancy, patients should be asked if they have experienced heat or cold intolerance, palpitations, polydypsia or polyuria, or weight loss.

As fatigue is a feature of depression, patients need to be asked about changes in appetite, weight, sleep, and ability to concentrate. Clearly positive responses do not exclude either organic or social causes. Direct questions about whether someone has been more depressed or sad than usual, or lost their enjoyment in their usual interests can elicit useful information, or be the first move in a continuing debate. It is important also to ask patients about their own ideas and concerns. The majority of patients believe the cause of their symptom is physical, although at the same time they may acknowledge some psychological concerns.[4] This information is important in predicting the natural history and in negotiating about management.

The examination is important, not least because patients believe their symptoms to be physical. Hypotheses which appear to have a higher probability on history will be more likely to be tested on examination, and more likely to be found positive. For example, a woman with menorrhagia will need the conjunctiva examined, and a young person with infection warrants inspection of their throat and glands. In an older person with chest pain or palpitations, examination of their blood pressure and vascular system is indicated. In a person with suspected hypothyroidism, their skin, hair, voice, thyroid, and pulse will be examined. Where depression is suspected, it is worth enquiring about the patient's previous psychological history and assessing their current affective state. The history and physical examination will yield a physical diagnosis in approximately 10 per cent of patients.[5]

Further investigations will depend again on age and gender, with young patients a blood count, monospot test and pregnancy test are the investigations with the highest yield.[5] With middle aged and elderly people, in addition to doing a haemoglobin and plasma viscosity, urea and electrolytes, glucose, and thyroid-stimulating hormone levels should be tested (Box 2). Any specific hypothesis raised by the history or examination can be explored through tests. A small proportion of patients are likely to be referred, either through their own preference or that of the doctor. The specialist chosen will depend partially on the particular history, examination and

Box 2   Abnormal results of laboratory tests in a group of 210 patients with fatigue[5]

Test	% abnormal
Haemoglobin	5
White blood cell count	4
Erythrocyte sedimentation rate/plasma viscosity	8
Urea	9
Electrolytes	2
Glucose	2
Thyroid-stimulating hormone	4
Monospot	10

Approximately one-third of these results, when taken with other information, were judged as clinically important by the doctor

investigative findings, and partly on the expertise available in the area. People with fatigue have been referred to internal medicine, infectious disease, neurology, and psychiatry clinics. The options should be discussed with the patient, with a plan made about their continuing care after the referral.

Principles of management

(a) *A safe generalist approach* will involve identifying the common and treatable causes of fatigue and also being alert to unusual causes, such as endocrine and malignant disease. This will be balanced with an ability to resist repeated investigations and referrals when the probability of a new diagnosis becomes increasingly low. If the patient appears to be depressed or somatizing, the doctor should not interpret these as diagnoses of exclusion or 'waste basket' diagnoses. Doctors and patients can perceive psychological diagnoses as being subjective, stigmatizing and contentious. However, as pharmacological and psychological interventions are both effective in alleviating symptoms,[1] doctors and patients need to discuss them, and acknowledge uncertainty with an open mind.

(b) *More specific management.* Physical causes like anaemia, thyroid disorder, and diabetes have specific treatments which are outlined in other sections of this text. There is some evidence that there is a specific fatigue syndrome which follows after glandular fever.[2] Knowing this occurs is helpful for patients. However, there is no evidence that bed-rest helps, and a gradual return to usual activity should be encouraged. Where patients complain of fatigue on anti-hypertensive drugs for example, it is worth changing them as this is likely to improve adherence. Some antiepilepsy drugs such as phenytoin and carbamazapine are associated with significant fatigue, about which patients are less inclined to complain. Enquiry about this and their desire to change to, for example, valproate or lamotrigine where this is appropriate, may lead to improvements in performance from a cognitive and occupational perspective.

Patients with primarily psycho-social causes for their fatigue are much more challenging. When patients present with fatigue of more than 3 months, and common physical causes have been excluded, there is evidence that approximately 70–75 per cent of patients will still have symptoms of fatigue 6 months later.[6] When patients have been offered six sessions of counselling or cognitive–behavioural therapy, approximately one-half of them were better and one half still had fatigue 6 months later.[6] Patients who acknowledge a psychological component to their fatigue symptoms at the outset,[7] and who express affect (their feelings) during therapy are more likely to have a positive outcome, regardless of the treatment.[8] Graded exercise provided by physiotherapists or exercise therapists will also benefit patients with fatigue in primary care.

Continuing care

Fatigue is a long-term problem, as when patients consult with fatigue of more than 2 weeks duration, about 60 per cent of them will still have significant symptomatology 6 months later.[5] Though patients who consult for this attend their doctors twice as frequently as other patients, it would seem that these consultations are not necessarily for fatigue, but for other symptoms, which may be associated with psychological distress.[3] A long duration of symptoms when the patient first consults, a history of psychological illness, and the belief that the symptom is physical, are all associated with persistence of symptoms.[7] A more proactive approach in primary care may prevent the patient from feeling as though their doctor is not interested, with ensuing strain in the doctor–patient relationship.

A booklet on fatigue and self-management has been shown to be of more benefit in terms of symptom resolution than usual care.[8] Patients who recognize they have co-morbid psychological problems could be referred to counsellors or cognitive–behavioural therapists depending on availability and cost. Patients with strong physical attributions may respond better to graded exercise.[9] Doctors who provide continuing care are best placed to judge the appropriateness of health care seeking behaviour, and sometimes to challenge reiterated demands for specialist referral and investigation, where this process seems more likely to increase anxiety than to solve the problem. Gask et al. have a technique of teaching doctors to reattribute symptoms.[10]

The implications of the problem

The symptom of fatigue clearly has important occupational, quality of life and psychological implications, and it is sometimes difficult to tease out cause and effect. When general practitioners have provided a sick note for fatigue, this has been associated with a poor subsequent outcome.[11] It is difficult to say whether this poor outcome was due to the prior severity of the condition, or to the GP giving support to sick role behaviour. Quality of life is impaired and this has been used as an outcome in most interventional studies. The role of depression as a cause, co-morbidity, or consequence of fatigue has been the subject of debate. Fatigue and low mood are associated in healthy adults,[12] but a fatiguing illness does not necessarily cause depression. It has been shown, for example, that patients with fatigue in association with neurological illness such as myasthenia gravis are significantly less likely to have depression than patients with CFS.[13]

The poorly understood nature, chronic course, and disabling consequences of chronic fatigue suggest a condition with potentially high health care costs, both in terms of help-seeking behaviour by patients, and a wide range of treatment responses by health care providers. There are economic consequences by loss or impaired ability to work, and by the opportunity costs associated with the provision of informal care giving. For example, one study in the United States that surveyed unemployment status and service use among chronically fatigued patients, revealed considerably increased rates of self-reported work disability (compared with the general population) and a high level of consultation with a range of allopathic and homeopathic health care providers.[14,15]

A study from the United Kingdom estimated that the cost of treatment and health care, plus patient and family costs for people consulting with fatigue of more than 3 months was approximately £4000 per year in 1999. Only 10–15 per cent of costs were due to treatment and health care, with the remaining 85–90 per cent attributed to days off work and informal care giving. When fatigue is more severe, the burden to the economy is proportionally greater. In Australia, the overall economic impact of chronic fatigue syndrome has been estimated at approximately Aus$ 60 million (1990 prices), at an average cost of approximately Aus$ 10 000 per case, resulting primarily from an estimated 50 per cent reduction in the employment rate following the onset of the illness.[14]

Scientific uncertainty and the uncertainty surrounding individual clinical cases has been associated with controversy, and fatigue being perceived as a heart-sink complaint. There is evidence from hospital outpatient studies that both cognitive–behavioural therapy and graded exercise are beneficial for patients with CFS.[2] More trials are needed in primary care to test the cost-effectiveness of these complex interventions together with other treatments such as counselling and graded exercise. In this context, it will be appropriate to ask questions about the 'dosage' necessary for different levels of fatigue severity, the characteristics of patients which predict outcome, the duration and timing of interventions. A more difficult question in complex interventions is: what are the 'active ingredients' in the intervention that are associated with beneficial effects? These are important questions which will require qualitative as well as quantitative research.

Key points

1. Fatigue is common in the community and in primary care.

2. Without treatment, most patients' symptoms become chronic.

3. Physical causes can be found and treated in a quarter of patients.

4. Most patients believe the cause is physical, but three-quarters also report symptoms of psychological distress.

5. Patients who acknowledge emotional distress are likely to improve with treatments including counselling, and cognitive–behaviour therapy.

References

1. Ridsdale, L. (1995). A critical appraisal of the literature on tiredness. In *Evidence-Based General Practice* Chapter 14 (ed. L. Ridsdale). London: WB Saunders Company Ltd.

2. Ramirez, G. et al. *Defining and Managing Chronic Fatigue Syndrome.* Rockville MD: Agency for Healthcare Research and Quality. Evidence Report/Technology Assessment, No. 42, 2001 (http://www.ahrq.gov/clinic/cfsinv.htm).

3. Ridsdale, L., Mandalia, S., and the General Practice Fatigue Group (1999). Tiredness as a ticket of entry: the roles of patients' beliefs and psychological symptoms in explaining frequent attendance. *Scandinavian Journal of Primary Care* 17, 72–4.

4. Ridsdale, L. et al. (1994). Patients who consult with tiredness: frequency of consultation, perceived causes of tiredness and its association with psychological distress. *British Journal of General Practice* 44, 413–16.

5. Ridsdale, L. et al. (1993). Patients with fatigue in general practice: a prospective study. *British Medical Journal* 307, 103–6.

6. Ridsdale, L. et al. (2001). Chronic fatigue in general practice: is counselling as good as cognitive behaviour therapy? A UK randomised trial. *British Journal of General Practice* 51, 19–24.

7. Chalder, T., Wallace, P., and Wessely, S. (1997). Self-help treatment of chronic fatigue in the community: a randomized controlled trial. *British Journal of Health Psychology* 2, 189–97.

8. Godfrey, E. et al. Investigating the 'active ingredients' of cognitive behaviour therapy and counselling for patients with chronic fatigue in primary care: an analysis of process and baseline predictors. *British Journal of Clinical Psychology* (in press).

9. Chalder, T. et al. (2003). Predictors of outcome in a fatigued population in primary care. *Psychological Medicine* 33, 283–7.

10. Gask, L. et al. (1991). Training general practitioners to teach psychiatric interviewing skills: an evaluation of group training. *Medical Education* 25, 444–51.

11. Cope, H., David, A., Pelosi, A., and Mann, A. (1994). Predictors of chronic 'postviral' fatigue. *Lancet* 344, 864–8.

12. Wood, C. and Magnello, M.E. (1992). Diurnal changes in perceptions of energy and mood. *Journal of the Royal Society of Medicine* 85, 191–4.

13. Wessely, S. and Powell, R. (1989). Fatigue syndromes: a comparison of chronic 'postviral' fatigue with neuromuscular and affective disorders. *Journal of Neurology, Neurosurgery, and Psychiatry* 52, 940–8.

14. Chisholm, D. et al. (2001). Chronic fatigue in general practice: economic evaluation of counselling versus cognitive behaviour therapy. *British Journal of General Practice* 51, 15–18.

15. McCrone, P. et al. (2003). The economic cost of chronic fatigue and chronic fatigue syndrome in UK primary care. *Psychological Medicine* 33, 253–7.

9.9 Sleep disorders

Arie Knuistingh Neven and M.P. Springer

Introduction

People who suffer from insomnia complain that it is difficult to fall or remain asleep, and that sleep is neither refreshing nor restorative.[1] Sleep quality is a personal, subjective experience. When a person sleeps poorly it does not always imply that he has a sleep disorder. The patient not only complains about bad sleep but also about performance during the day. A sleep disorder is a 24-h problem. Fatigue, sleepiness, irritability, and lack of concentration during the waking hours are integral parts of a sleep disorder.[2]

Bad sleep is mostly a symptom of some underlying condition. In order to find its possible cause, physicians should know something about the mechanisms of sleep disturbances and its most common causes. Identifying the possible underlying condition(s) is of utmost importance for the treatment of a sleep disorder. However, in some patients insomnia may be the basic problem rather than a symptom of some other disease.[3] There are a number of cases of insomnia which are not due to another sleep disorder, mental or physical illness, or the effect of medication.[3]

In this chapter, we propose a 'best approach' to sleeping problems in general practice based on a consensus protocol developed at the Department of General Practice of the Leiden University Medical Centre and applied in the Standard 'Insomnia and Hypnotics' of the Dutch College of General Practitioners (NHG).[4,5]

Frequency of bad sleep

Sleep disturbances are frequently encountered in general practice. In a survey performed by the Dutch Institute for Primary Healthcare Research, bad sleep was one of the 10 most common complaints in general practice. Another Dutch survey (using a questionnaire) demonstrated that 30 per cent of the adults in a sample of the population were not satisfied with their sleep; 18 per cent had mild sleep disturbances and 12 per cent reported serious sleep disturbances. Most of the complaints about sleep concerned lack of sleep or its poor quality. In these cases, the sleep disturbance is termed insomnia. Many studies have shown that only 10–15 per cent of patients with insomnia visit their doctor for that problem and in most cases it is presented as a secondary complaint. Insomnia is more prevalent among women and occurs more frequently with advancing age. About 20 per cent of the sufferers from insomnia state they have been bad sleepers from complaining of insomnia every day. Over 80 per cent of the patients visiting a GP for insomnia are treated with hypnotics. Consequently at any time 4 per cent of the adult population are taking hypnotics and in the elderly this may be as high as 10 per cent. Of those patients who take hypnotics, about 50 per cent take them every night.[6]

Classification of sleep disorders

To cope with sleep disturbances it is helpful to use a practical classification of sleep disorders. In 1990, the American Sleep Disorders Association published the International Classification of Sleep Disorders (ICSD).[7] It provides a general view on the subject. However, it has no practical value in the context of general practice. As far back as 1983, however, a more useful manual for the evaluation of insomnia was produced by a Consensus Development Conference.[8] Its starting point was the expected duration of an episode of insomnia. Three categories were distinguished:

1. Transient insomnia (duration of 1–3 days). Examples: jet-lag, hospital admission, examination stress.

2. Short-term insomnia (duration 1–3 weeks): emotional problems as a major initiator. Examples: death of a close relative, divorce, loss of job, and confrontation with a malignant disease.

3. Long-term insomnia (duration more than 3 weeks): many possible causes; difficult to analyse. Examples: chronic physical disorders, shift work, depression, chronic stress, conditioning of the sleep disturbance.

As a starting point for the development of the NHG-Standard 'Insomnia and Hypnotics' the manual of the Consensus Development Conference was used. Transient insomnia, however, is a condition rarely presented to physicians and it was therefore removed from the classification. Instead, the chronic use of hypnotics was added, because this is probably the most common cause of disturbed sleep. Thus, three major groups of sleeping disturbances are distinguished:

1. recent sleep problems: shorter than 3 weeks;

2. extended sleep problems: longer than 3 weeks; and

3. chronic use of hypnotics.

The diagnostic part of the management strategy of insomnia consists of detailed history taking. Physical examination is only necessary in case of a suspected sleep apnoea syndrome, to see whether there are predisposing factors for sleep apnoea and if there is any cardiovascular or pulmonary damage caused by the recurrent nightly apnoea periods. In the case of periodic leg movements (PLM) laboratory screening for anaemia, iron deficiency, and folic acid deficiency may be useful.

When the doctor fails to find a good explanation for the insomnia a sleep–wake diary may be helpful. In the diary the patient reports the sleep–wake schedule, major daytime activities and activities preceding bedtime over a period of 2 weeks. All patients with a suspected sleep apnoea syndrome should be referred to a centre for sleep disorders for further analysis. Other indications for referral to a centre for sleep disorders could be suspected PLM and failure to find a cause for the insomnia. The consecutive diagnostic and therapeutic steps are discussed in the next part.

Diagnosis

Evaluation of a sleeping problem starts with collecting some general information by means of history taking: what kind of sleeping problem does the patient have, when did it start, does the patient know a cause, are there other complaints, what kind of medication is used?

The second step is trying to decide if the sleeping problems can be regarded as true insomnia. We only talk about insomnia if a patient also complains about sleepiness, tiredness, and lack of concentration during the daytime hours. If there is a sleeping complaint without complaints during the daytime, we use the term 'pseudo-insomnia'. Pseudo-insomnia is found in normally short sleepers, in elderly people spreading out their sleeping hours over the day (naps) and people going to bed earlier than their biological clock dictates.

Insomnia may be classified as short-term insomnia (up to 3 weeks) or long-term insomnia (longer than 3 weeks). The period of 3 weeks has been chosen since negative conditioning is a perpetuating factor for sleep problems. Sleep itself and the sleeping circumstances will gradually become connected with negative feelings about sleeping behaviour. The patient becomes anxious simply by thinking about sleep or by being confronted with sleep-circumstances such as bed and bedroom.[2] Patients taking hypnotics every night for over 3 months need a specific approach and are therefore considered as a special group.

Short-term insomnia is commonly caused by physical disorders, disturbances of the sleep–wake schedule (e.g. jet-lag), and stressful life events. Of these three issues, stressful life events are the most common, causing over 65 per cent of all short-term insomnias.[4]

In case of long-term insomnia, the diagnosis is often difficult. Most patients do no longer know the original cause of their insomnia and in many cases there is more than one possible cause. Important causes for long-term insomnia that should be considered separately from the conditioning factor are chronic physical illness, depression, side-effects of medication, the use or abuse of alcohol, caffeine and nicotine, PLM, and the sleep apnoea syndrome.

Often, patients using hypnotics only do so in order to avoid discomfort. The cause of the sleeping problem that started the chronic use of hypnotics has often been long forgotten. After four weeks of continuous use the body adapts to the effect of benzodiazepines, and sleep quality often returns to the previous level. Because the patients expects to sleep badly without the hypnotic, there is probably also some sort of conditioning. This is enhanced by withdrawal effects after discontinuation of the hypnotic. Withdrawal effects may be anxiety, rebound-insomnia, tremor, and autonomic nervous complaints such as sweating, palpitation, dizziness, and nausea.

Treatment

The aims of treating sleep disorders are solving the complaint, preventing development of a conditioned insomnia and avoiding the chronic use of hypnotics. The central issue in treating sleeping problems is information about sleep (Table 1) and advice to improve sleep hygiene (Table 2). When it is possible to treat the cause of a sleeping problem this must, of course, take precedence. Depressions, for example, responds well to antidepressants (see Chapter 9.1). Physical disorders may be treated symptomatically or may even be cured. Pharmacological causes can be eliminated by reducing or stopping the agent causing the insomnia. Sleep apnoea needs specialized examination and, if possible, therapy.

The best indication for prescribing hypnotics is an acute stressful life event, for example, death of a relative, divorce, or loss of a job. When hypnotics are prescribed, some rules should be adhered to prevent their chronic use (Table 3). Benzodiazepines and non-benzodiazepine hypnotics with a short half-life (like temazepam and zolpidem respectively) are the

Table 1 Information about sleep

Information should be given to the patient about

1. Function of sleep, minor effect on health of insomnia
2. Sleep cycles, SWS/REM-sleep, normal duration of sleep
3. Biological clock, relation between sleep and temperature curve
4. Age-related changes in sleeping pattern: the elderly sleep more superficially, frequently wake up and often sleep shorter
5. Daytime naps influence night-time sleep

Table 2 Advices for sleep hygiene

1. Establish regular bedtimes, especially wake-up times
2. Not going to bed until sleepy
3. Not staying in bed unless asleep
4. Reserve the evening hours for leisure activities and relaxation
5. Avoid daytime naps
6. Avoid caffeine, alcohol, and nicotine
7. Create favourable conditions for sleep

Table 3 Guidelines for use of hypnotics

1. Use only benzodiazepines (like temazepam) or non-benzodiazepines (like zolpidem) with a short half-life
2. Prescribe maximal 10 tablets on a first occasion
3. Make a contract with the patient about the maximum duration of use with no extend longer than 4 weeks
4. Inform the patient about effects, side-effects, and dependency
5. Benzodiazepines have altered effects and pharmacokinetics in the elderly, the dosage should be adjusted (half of the usual adult dosage)
6. Benzodiazepines interact with alcohol and other psychotropics
7. Sleep apnoea is an absolute contra-indication for hypnotics

Table 4 Guidelines for stopping chronic use of benzodiazepines

1. Explanation of the effects of benzodiazepines, information about withdrawal effects (rebound-insomnia!)
2. Slow reduction of dose:
   after 1 month to 1/4 of dosage
   the rest within 2–3 months
3. Sleep hygiene
4. Relaxation techniques
5. Frequent evaluations (1 or 2 weeks)
6. Provide sympathetic support and motivation

preferred medication. Patients should be monitored continuously, restrict their daily hypnotic intake to the shortest possible period and not exceed a treatment period beyond four weeks or use their hypnotics according to an intermittent pattern. For long-term treatment of insomniacs, intermittent use of hypnotics is advisable, as this may benefit patients and prevent the development of dependency.[1] However, studies in the long-term treatment of chronic insomnia, as randomized, double-blind, parallel groups, placebo-controlled trials of the efficacy of the medication beyond 35 days are not available.

Information about sleep is useful in cases of conditioned insomnia, as well as advice to improve sleep hygiene and knowledge of methods to reverse the conditional habit. Relaxation therapy and sleeping courses can often be initiated by the GP. Behavioural treatment may be given by social workers, psychologists, or GPs. However, the main problem with behavioural therapies is that they are not readily available in routine medical practice. It has often been mentioned that effective but simple treatment techniques should be known to every physician, in particular the GP.[9] Sleep hygiene advice comprises some basic elements of behavioural treatment such as stimulus control and sleep restriction.

Discontinuation of the chronic use of sleeping pills can only be successful if the user is motivated to stop the habit. Information about possible withdrawal effects, improving sleep hygiene, and starting behavioural treatment, combined with a slow reduction of the dose of hypnotics, are essential issues when trying to stop its chronic use (Table 4).

There is a controversy about the long-term treatment of insomnia with benzodiazepine receptor agonist hypnotics.[10,11] Little controlled evidence on the benefits and drawbacks of benzodiazepine hypnotics is available. Therefore, a new paradigm for a rational treatment of insomnia, including implementation of simple behavioural techniques and a restrictive prescription of hypnotics for short-term use as well as for long-term use, is needed.[12]

Key points

1. Sleep disturbances are essentially a primary care problem.

2. Detailed history-taking is the most important diagnostic instrument in evaluating sleeping problems.

3. Information about the function of sleep, the causes of insomnia, and what can be done to improve sleep are preferable.

4. Benzodiazepine and non-benzodiazepine hypnotics are not the first choice when treating insomnia; they are currently the best available option with restriction of duration and daily intake, or an intermittent pattern.

5. Effective non-drug treatments for insomnia are sleep hygiene, comprising elements of behavioural treatment, and relaxation therapy.

6. Conditioned insomnia and chronic use of hypnotics can be prevented if sleeping problems have been evaluated properly and treated adequately.

References

1. Hajak, G. (2000). Insomnia in primary care. *Sleep* **23**, S54–63.
2. Buysse, D.J. and Reynolds, C.F. (1990). Insomnia. In *Handbook of Sleep Disorders* (ed. M.J. Thorpy), pp. 375–433. New York: Marcel Dekker Inc.
3. Hauri, P. (2000). Primary insomnia. In *Principles and Practice of Sleep Medicine* 3rd edn. (ed. M.H. Kryger, T. Roth, and W.C. Dement), pp. 633–9. Philadelphia PA: WB Saunders Company.
4. Eijkelenboom, P.R., Springer, M.P., and Dekker, F.W. (1992). The Leiden Sleep Protocol (in Dutch). *Huisarts Wetenschap* **35**, 465–9.
5. Knuistingh Neven, A. et al. (1999). NHG-Standard insomnia and hypnotics. In *NHG-Standards for General Practitioners I* (in Dutch) (ed. R.M.M. Geijer). Utrecht: Dutch College of General Practi-tioners (NHG).
6. Dunbar, G., Perera, M.H., and Jenner, F.A. (1989). Pattern of benzo-diazepine use in Great Britain as measured by a general practice survey. *British Journal of Psychiatry* **155**, 836–41.
7. The International Classification of Sleep Disorders, Thorpy, M.J., chairman. *Diagnostic and Coding Manual*. Rochester MN: American Sleep Disorders Association, 1990.
8. National Institutes of Health. *Drugs and Insomnia. Consensus Development Conference Summary* Vol. 4. Bethesda MD: NIH. Office of Medical Applications of Research, 1983.
9. Morin, C.M., Colecchi, C., Stone, J., Sood, R., and Brink, D. (1999). Behavioral and pharmacological therapies for late-life insomnia; a randomized controlled trial. *Journal of the American Medical Association* **281**, 991–9.
10. Kramer, M. (2000). Hypnotic medication in the treatment of chronic insomnia: non nocere! Doesn't anyone care? *Sleep Medicine Reviews* **4**, 529–41.
11. Kripke, D.F. (2000). Chronic hypnotic use: deadly risks, doubtful benefit. *Sleep Medicine Reviews* **4**, 5–20.
12. Buysse, D.J. (2000). Rational pharmacotherapy for insomnia: time for a new paradigm. *Sleep Medicine Reviews* **4**, 521–7.

Further reading

Hajak, G. (2000). Insomnia in primary care. *Sleep* **23**, S54–63.
Buysse, D.J. (2000). Rational pharmacotherapy for insomnia: time for a new paradigm. *Sleep Medicine Reviews* **4**, 521–7. (These articles provide a recent overview of sleep disorders in general practice.)

9.10 Psychological treatments for mental health problems
Lawrence Mynors-Wallis

Introduction

There is a large and increasing demand for the provision of psychological treatments within primary care. There are many reasons for this. There is an increasing awareness amongst the public of both the presence and significance of psychological symptoms, which is accompanied by the expectation of treatment. When weighing up the options between medication and a psychological treatment, the public choice is clearly in favour of a psychological intervention. Rightly or wrongly, patients are wary of the risks of dependence and the possibilities of side-effects if they take psychotropic medication. In addition, many patients conceptualize their psychological distress as resulting from psycho-social factors and hence wish to have a treatment directed at what they perceive as being the cause of their symptoms.

The availability of psychological treatments within primary care will vary enormously both between and within different health care systems. Cultural differences will also have a profound influence on help-seeking behaviour for psychological distress and the acceptability of a psychological treatment.

Mental health problems in primary care cover the full range of disorders from brief, transient distress, often in response to an adverse life event, to severe and enduring mental illness. Similarly, there is a range of potential psychological treatments that could be available in primary care from long-term specialist interventions to simple techniques provided within a general consultation. This chapter will focus on treatments that are feasible in primary care for those disorders that are mostly treated without specialist referral. The chapter is in three parts. Firstly, there is a description of the range of psychological treatments available in primary care. Secondly, there is a discussion of the general principles of using psychological treatments. Finally, there is a description of the use of psychological treatments in primary care for specific disorders.

Psychological treatments available in primary care

There are a broad range of psychological treatments that could be offered in primary care, although in practice, treatment options are often strictly limited by the availability of suitably trained therapists. It is helpful to consider four levels of possible psychological treatments within primary care (Fig. 1).

♦ *Level one* consists of self-help treatments and bibliotherapy (advising people to read written material). Although this level could be strictly

viewed as a community, rather than a primary care intervention, it is often the case that primary care staff direct patients to relevant self-help groups and literature. Self-help materials are available for a range of psychological disorders, in particular, anxiety disorders, depressive disorders, eating disorders, and the management of stress-related symptoms. Research evidence suggests that such interventions may help the milder of such disorders. A well-organized practice could bring together self-help materials and the availability of local self-help groups as a resource for both patients and primary care staff.

♦ *Level two* is the provision of brief psychological treatments within the routine consultation. Such interventions may include advice, reassurance and support, together with more specific techniques such as activity scheduling and brief interventions for alcohol disorders. There is some evidence that a positive consultation: giving a diagnosis and telling the patient that they will get better in a few days might be more beneficial than a 'negative' consultation in which no firm assurance is given.[1]

♦ *Level three* are those primary care psychological treatments that are, or could be, routinely given by members of the primary care team, for example, counsellors, nurses, doctors. These are relatively brief treatments (often six to eight sessions) and include counselling, and problem-solving treatment.

Counselling

The term counselling can be a confusing one. Counselling may be used to describe the provision of direct advice and information about risk, as in health promotion. The term may also be used to describe the provision of almost any psychological treatment. In the United Kingdom, counsellors are widely available in primary care with over 80 per cent of primary care groups having provision for practice-based counselling.[2] These counsellors come from a variety of backgrounds and often provide an eclectic range of interventions in a pragmatic attempt to help their clients. Although there is no unitary model of counselling, four core features have been identified, common to all forms of counselling: the relationship between the client and the counsellor, information giving, emotional release, and the examination of the client's situation and potential solutions.[3] Models of counselling will differ in the extent that they are unstructured and reflective, or focused and active. Patient satisfaction with counselling is usually high.

Problem-solving treatment

Problem-solving treatment is a brief, structured psychological intervention. The treatment shares with other cognitive–behavioural treatments, a focus on the here and now, rather than a dwelling on past experiences and regrets. The treatment involves an active collaboration between patient and therapist with the patient taking an increasingly active role in the planning of treatment and the implementing of activities between treatment sessions. There are seven stages to the treatment (Fig. 2).

♦ *Level four* are those specialist psychological treatments delivered by experienced therapists, often clinical psychologists. The best evaluated and most widely available treatment is cognitive–behaviour therapy (CBT), which is effective for a range of psychological disorders. Other specialist psychological treatments include but are not limited to interpersonal

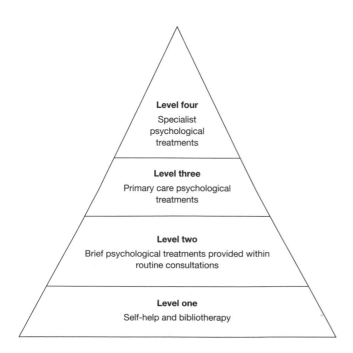

Fig. 1 Psychological treatments within primary care.

Stage 1: Explanation of treatment and its rationale, formulation of problem list
Stage 2: Clarification and definition of a chosen problem
Stage 3: Setting achievable goals
Stage 4: Generating solutions
Stage 5: Choice of preferred solution
Stage 6: Implementation of the preferred solution
Stage 7: Evaluation

Fig. 2 Stages of problem-solving treatment.

psychotherapy, brief dynamic therapies, and couple therapy. These treatments could be provided within primary care but are more often provided from specialist mental health services or voluntary agencies.

Cognitive–behaviour therapy

CBT helps patients to understand how their psychological symptoms have developed. A link is made between the patient's thoughts and beliefs, their emotional reactions and their behaviour. Cognitive techniques such as challenging negative, maladaptive thoughts, and behavioural techniques such as activity scheduling and behavioural experiments are used with the aim of relieving symptoms. Although much of the evidence base is derived from patients in non-primary care settings, studies within primary care support the use of CBT as an effective treatment for many conditions.

Interpersonal psychotherapy (IPT)

IPT has been most thoroughly evaluated as a treatment for depressive disorders but has also been shown to be of value for other psychological disorders including eating disorders. The aims of treatment are the clarification and resolution of one or more of the following interpersonal difficulties:

◆ bereavement and loss;

◆ interpersonal disputes;

◆ role transitions;

◆ interpersonal deficits.

A briefer form of IPT has been evaluated for use by nurses in primary care: interpersonal counselling.[4] A self-help guide is also available.[5]

Brief dynamic therapy

The goal of brief dynamic therapy is to resolve core conflicts based on personality and situation variables. It is argued that long-standing patterns of behaviour can be reversed through a time-limited psychotherapy that employs all the essential types of interpretation found in psychoanalysis. There is some evidence that patients with anxious and depressive symptoms benefit from such an approach.[6]

Couple therapy

Conflict with one's partner is a common, stressful life event. Where relationship problems are identified there is evidence that couple therapy is effective in reducing psychological symptoms.[7] One simple technique from couple therapy that might be used in primary care is reciprocity negotiation. Each partner moves from listing their complaints to vocalizing a specific behaviour or task that they wish the other to do, for example, I want you to pick the kids up from school once a week and in return I will let you watch the football once a week without moaning.

General principles of using psychological treatments

There are some broad principles to consider when using a psychological treatment. These need to be taken into account alongside the evidence about the efficacy of specific treatments for specific conditions.

The principles set out below are drawn from the *Clinical Practice Guideline: Treatment Choice in Psychological Therapies and Counselling* produced by the Department of Health:[8]

1. A psychological therapy should be routinely considered as a treatment option when assessing mental health problems. There is strong research evidence of the potential benefit of psychological treatments to individuals with a wide range of mental health problems.

2. In considering psychological therapies, more severe or complex mental health problems should receive a secondary, specialist assessment.

3. Effectiveness of all types of therapy depends on the patient and the therapist forming a good working relationship. This principle is important in decisions by GPs and their patients about the option of psychological therapy, because 'therapeutic alliance' is the single best predictor of benefit. A good working relationship in therapy does not necessarily mean the absence of conflict or difficulty, but a fundamental agreement on the goals and tasks of therapy and some level of commitment to the relationship. If this is lacking, the therapy is less likely to be helpful.

4. Therapies of fewer than eight sessions are unlikely to be optimally effective for most moderate to severe mental health problems. Often 16 sessions or more are required for symptomatic relief, and longer therapies may be required to achieve lasting improvement in social and personality functioning. In primary care, the less severe psychological problems may benefit from briefer therapies.

5. The patient's age, sex, social class, or ethnic group are, in general, not important factors in choice of therapy and should not determine access to therapies. Ethnic and cultural identity should be respected by referral to culturally sensitive therapists.

6. Patient preference should inform treatment choice, particularly where the research evidence does not indicate a clear choice of therapy.

7. The skill and experience of the therapist should also be taken into account. More complex problems, and those where patients are poorly motivated, require the more skilful therapist.

Psychological treatments for specific presenting problems

Depressive disorders

There are three presentations of patients with depressive symptoms in primary care. Patients with major depression (low mood plus four key symptoms), patients with a milder depression (recent onset and less severe than major depression), and patients with dysthymia (chronic, low-grade depression of 2 years or more duration). The evidence supporting the use of psychological treatments depends on the presentation. For patients with mild depression, education, reassurance, and support (level two interventions) plus watchful waiting is appropriate. Many such disorders will resolve with time and changing life's circumstances. There is no evidence that patients with dysthymia respond to psychological treatments (although they may respond to a course of antidepressants).

In the treatment of major depression, however, although medication is both convenient and effective, a psychological treatment may be the first-line treatment in certain circumstances: (i) the depression is of moderate severity or less; (ii) the symptoms are not chronic or psychotic; (iii) patient preference; (iv) medication contra-indicated; and (v) there is available a trained and competent therapist. For major depression, both level three and four interventions have been shown to be of value in randomized controlled trials.

Cognitive–behaviour therapy

CBT for depression is based on a cognitive model in which the patient's early experiences lead to certain core beliefs, for example, 'I'm not a nice person'. These core beliefs result in dysfunctional assumptions, for example, 'I must please people all the time'. Associated with these underlying assumptions are negative automatic thoughts, for example 'My friend has not telephoned—nobody likes me'. A stressful life event may precipitate a downward spiral in which the negative thoughts result in low mood and the symptoms of depression. As the patient becomes more depressed, more negative automatic thoughts occur. In treatment, the patient is taught to understand the nature and impact of negative automatic thoughts, to identify, and then challenge them. Behavioural tasks are set to counter both the thoughts and also the underpinning, dysfunctional assumptions.

CBT requires trained, experienced therapists. Treatment for depression has been evaluated in treatments of up to 20 sessions over 12–16 weeks.

There is good evidence for effectiveness. In a meta-analysis of 48 trials of patients with mild/moderate depression,[9] CBT was compared with other treatments. Compared with waiting list or placebo, the average patient receiving CBT was 29 per cent better (effect size 0.82, $p < 0.001$). Compared with antidepressants, the average patient receiving CBT was 15 per cent better (effect size 0.38, $p < 0.001$). Compared with a mixed bag of other psychological treatments, the average patient receiving CBT was 10 per cent better (effect size 0.24, $p < 0.01$). In primary care studies, CBT has been shown to be both effective and feasible.

Problem-solving treatment

Three studies have evaluated the effectiveness of problem-solving treatment for major depression in primary care. In the first study,[10] 91 patients with major depression from primary care were randomly allocated to problem-solving treatment, amitriptyline, or a placebo treatment involving both drug and psychological placebos. All treatments were given in six sessions over 12 weeks. At 6 and 12 weeks, problem-solving treatment was as effective in treating depression as amitriptyline, and significantly more effective than the placebo treatment. A second study[11] sought to answer two further questions. Firstly, is the combination of problem-solving treatment and antidepressant medication more effective than either treatment alone? Secondly, can the problem-solving treatment be delivered as effectively by suitably trained practice nurses as by GPs? One hundred and fifty-one patients were randomly allocated to receive problem-solving treatment from a GP, problem-solving treatment from a practice nurse, antidepressant medication alone from a GP, or the combination of problem-solving treatment and antidepressant medication. The results from this study at 6, 12, and 52 weeks indicated that there were no significant differences between any of the four treatment groups, providing further support for problem-solving treatment as an effective treatment for depressive disorders in primary care. A third study of problem-solving treatment in a depressed community sample[12] compared problem-solving treatment with an educational intervention and a control group. At 6 months, 59 per cent of patients who had received problem-solving treatment were recovered compared with 43 per cent of controls. Problem-solving treatment was more acceptable to patients than the educational intervention.

Counselling

For patients with mild to moderate depressive disorders, there is now evidence from two randomized controlled trials that counselling is an effective treatment. Non-directive counselling was shown at 4 months to be as effective as cognitive–behaviour therapy (both up to 12 sessions) for 464 primary care patients with depression and mixed anxiety and depression, and more effective than GP treatment as usual.[13] Generic counselling was as effective as antidepressant medication in a trial of 323 patients with mild/moderate depression in primary care.[14] Both these studies allowed for patient preference as an alternative to randomization. Neither found a significant difference between patients allocated to treatment following randomization and those able to choose treatment.

A randomized controlled trial of counselling by health visitors, trained in an eight-session intervention for post-natal depression found it to be of benefit compared with GP usual treatment;[15] 69 per cent of the treatment group had fully recovered at the end of treatment compared with 38 per cent of the control group. Also in mothers with post-natal depression, six sessions of CBT-based counselling by health visitors was more effective than one session and equally effective as fluoxetine.[16]

Other psychological treatments

Other psychological treatments have been shown to be effective for major depressive disorders, in particular, interpersonal therapy, behaviour therapy, short-term psychodynamic therapy, and couple therapy. There is little direct evidence from primary care populations for these treatments although there is no reason to suppose they would not be effective. The essence of effective psychological treatments for depressive disorders would seem to be an experienced therapist, delivering a time-limited structured treatment, focusing on problems in the here and now, for a motivated patient.

Anxiety disorders

Brief psychological treatments

A range of simple interventions may be used to treat anxiety disorders in primary care. Common sense suggests that information and reassurance are important: the appropriate explanation of physical symptoms, reassurance about the absence of physical illness, and the use of self-help leaflets to reinforce advice. There are then a range of simple psychological interventions that may be of help although there is little direct evidence of their value within a primary care consultation.

Advice about breathing

Hyperventilation may precipitate anxiety and is often a maintaining factor. Patients often describe the taking of deep breaths as a way of coping and then give a convincing demonstration of hyperventilation. Asking a patient to breathe quickly and shallowly for 30 s can often convincingly demonstrate the relationship between breathing and anxiety symptoms.

Patients can be given the following advice about slow breathing:

- breath in for 4 s and out for 4 s, pause for 4 s before breathing again;
- practice for 20 min morning and night (5–10 min is better than nothing);
- use before and after situations that make you anxious;
- regularly check and slow down breathing throughout the day.

Distraction

Worrying thoughts lead to anxious symptoms, which in turn often worsen worrying thoughts. Distraction is a method that can be used to empty the mind of worrying thoughts and replace them with neutral thoughts. Patients are asked to describe in detail to themselves a picture, a view, a story, or think of a relaxing image, for example, the seashore, lake, mountains. Patients should be advised to save up worries for a circumscribed 'worry time' each day—not just before bedtime.

Relaxation

There are a range of relaxation techniques although little formal evidence for effectiveness. Progressive muscle relaxation is popular. Patients are taught (often from a tape) to tense and then relax specific muscle groups. Patients learn to recognize when they are tense and to then counter this with relaxation. The technique is easily learnt and at the very least is a form of distraction—it is probably most effective when combined with exposure.

Simple exposure

Avoiding feared situations is an important factor in a large number of anxiety disorders. Each time a situation is avoided, the idea is further strengthened in an individual's mind that they would have been overwhelmed by anxiety. Patients should be advised to face the feared situation and remain in it until either the anxiety subsides, or until they can convince themselves that being in a situation will not lead to them losing control or being unable to deal with the anxiety. Patients should be encouraged to repeatedly place themselves in the feared situation.

Brief counselling

Many patients who disclose psycho-social problems receive 'brief counselling'. A study of recent onset anxiety disorders in Oxfordshire primary care showed that 'brief counselling' by the GP was as effective as anxiolytic medication. Brief counselling included: explanation of the nature of any symptoms and why they had occurred, exploration of underlying personal or other problems and ways of dealing with them, and reasons for not prescribing drugs if appropriate. Both groups improved with time, the 'brief counselling' did not result in longer consultations or more frequent follow-up than anxiolytic prescribing.[17]

Cognitive–behaviour therapy

The content of CBT for anxiety disorders varies according to the different conditions. Patients may be taught to identify triggers to their anxiety, for example, a chest muscle twinge may lead to a panic via a distorted cognitive belief that this is a heart attack. In treatment sessions and by behavioural experiments, the patient is helped to overcome the negative cognitions. In anxiety disorders, often a vicious circle is established which the patient needs to recognize and be helped to overcome. In the example of the muscle twinge this causes worry which leads to physical symptoms of anxiety (including a racing heart, hyperventilation, and dizziness), these physical symptoms then reinforce the worry about a heart attack.

CBT is probably the treatment of choice for panic disorder and agoraphobia. In a large meta-analysis,[18] the combination of CBT with exposure was shown to have an effect size of 1.79 for panic and 1.22 for agoraphobia. CBT is less effective for the treatment of generalized anxiety, although equivalent to medication. Social phobia and obsessive compulsive disorders also benefit from CBT techniques.

Emotional disorders

In primary care, psychological disorders do not necessarily fit into the simple diagnostic categories of anxiety and depression. Many patients present with both depressive and anxious symptoms—emotional disorders. These disorders may or may not fulfil the diagnostic criteria for specific disorders. Although many of these disorders resolve quickly, a significant proportion of patients develop chronic conditions with significant clinical and social morbidity. Hence, treatment studies have been undertaken in primary care to determine whether specific treatments are of benefit over and above GP usual care.

Problem-solving treatment

In a study of problem-solving treatment given by trained community nurses, patients with emotional disorders of at least 1 month duration were referred by their GPs.[19] These patients were randomly allocated, to either problem-solving treatment given by a trained nurse therapist or to treatment as usual from their GP. Although there was no difference in symptom scores between the two groups at 8 or 26 weeks, patients who had received problem-solving treatment had significantly less disability days and days off work.

Counselling

Many studies of counselling have recruited a broad range of patients with a variety of psychological disorders, most commonly patients with anxiety, depression, and stress-related disorders. These studies have taken as outcome measures symptom reduction, prescribing rates, patient satisfaction. A well-designed randomized controlled trial of 136 patients in North London found that counselling (1–12 sessions) was of no benefit in terms symptom reduction over routine GP care;[20] however, patients were more satisfied with help received from the counsellors. Similarly, a randomized controlled trial from Bristol of 162 patients comparing counselling (up to six sessions) with usual GP care found that both groups improved equally with time.[21] Although smaller studies and uncontrolled studies have showed symptomatic benefit and high levels of patient satisfaction, current evidence does not support counselling for non-specific emotional disorders.

Alcohol disorders

Brief psychological treatments

Brief interventions by GPs have been shown to be of benefit for non-dependent problem drinkers, both in reducing the weekly number of drinks and number of drinking binges.[22] Brief counselling around a simple mnemonic FRAMES (Feedback, Responsibility, Advice, Menu of options, Empathy, and Self-efficacy) could be feasibly applied during a routine primary care consultation (see Fig. 3 and Chapter 9.5).

Feedback
'Have you considered that your difficulties (e.g. sexual) may be related to use of alcohol?'

Responsibility
'Only you can decide. Why don't you see what happens if you cut down for a couple of weeks?'

Advice
'I recommend that you stop drinking and see if that improves the situation'.
- Counting the number of drinks and timing how long it takes to finish; put the glass down between drinking.
- Sipping rather than gulping.
- Using non-alcoholic spacers, e.g. buy yourself a non-alcoholic drink when it is 'your round'.
- Eating before and during drinking (this reduces appetite and slows alcohol absorption)
- Avoid salty food whilst drinking (it is a thirst stimulant)
- Use low alcohol drinks
- Have drink free days

Menu of options
'I appreciate you may not be able to manage this but if you find it hard going then our counsellor may be able to help. We could also arrange for you to attend the local self-help group'.

Empathy
'I know this must be hard for you because the wine helps you to relax and I am concerned by the amount of stress in your life'.

Self-efficacy
'Considering this has been going on such a long time it's good that you have asked for help. Your own determination will help you get through'.

Fig. 3 Brief counselling for alcohol use in primary care.

Ensuring the patient feels understood
- Why has the patient consulted?
  - ? symptom relief
  - ? diagnostic test and reassurance
- Identification of the relevant stressors including fear of illness
- Brief focused physical evaluation to reassure the patient that a medical problem is not being overlooked

Changing the agenda
Consider depression, alcohol, substance misuse

Making the link
- Reassurance that there is no physical disease requiring medical treatment
- An explanation linking stress and distress to the physical symptoms

Further management
Appropriate management of the underlying stressors or depressive disorder:
- Consider a problem-solving approach
- Encourage exercise and enjoyable activities
- Written information about stress

Fig. 4 Management of acute somatic symptoms. (Adapted from ref. 23.)

Somatic disorders

Medically unexplained symptoms are common in primary care. They are often associated with depression, anxiety or, substance misuse. The GP has a key role in ensuring that patients with medically unexplained symptoms do not have unnecessary investigations or receive potentially harmful interventions.

Brief psychological interventions

A simple explanation may be necessary to explain how emotional stress can cause and worsen physical symptoms. In turn, the worry about these physical symptoms may then worsen emotional stress. More detailed advice about the management of acute somatic symptoms is given in Fig. 4.

Counselling

Counselling was as effective as CBT (both up to six sessions) in a group of 160 patients with chronic fatigue in primary care.[24]

Conclusion

This review has had to be selective as to the psychological treatments reviewed and the diagnostic groups considered. The emphasis has been on those treatments feasible and generally available in primary care, with a focus on the most common disorders. The range of psychological treatments available has been highlighted in order to aid the appropriate targeting of treatments. The role of what a GP can offer within a normal consultation has been emphasized although clear evidence for such interventions is often not available. For the more specific psychological treatments, randomized controlled trials evidence has been reviewed, focusing particularly on trials done in primary care.

References

1. **Thomas, K.B.** (1987). General practice consultations: is there any point in being positive? *British Medical Journal* **294**, 1200–2.

2. **Anon** (2000). Counselling in general practice. *Drugs and Therapeutics Bulletin* **38**, 49–52.

3. **Hobbs, M. and Saunders, D.** (2000). Counselling. In *New Oxford Textbook of Psychiatry* (ed. M.G. Gelder, J.J. Lopez-Ibor, and N.C. Andreasen). Oxford: Oxford University Press.

4. **Klerman, G.L.** et al. (1987). Efficacy of a brief psychosocial intervention for symptoms of stress and distress among patients in primary care. *Medical Care* **25**, 1078–88.

5. **Holden, J.M., Sagovsky, R., and Cox, J.** (1989). Counselling in a general practice setting: controlled study of health visitor intervention in the treatment of postnatal depression. *British Medical Journal* **298**, 223–6.

6. **Shapiro, D.A., Barkham, M., Hardy, G.E., and Morrison, L.A.** (1990). The second Sheffield psychology project. *British Journal of Medical Psychology* **63**, 97–108.

7. **Leff, J., Vearnals, S., Brewin, C.R., Wolff, G., Alexander, B., Asen, E., Dayson, D., Jones, E., Chisholm, D., and Everitt, B.** (2000). The London depression intervention trial. Randomised controlled trial of anti-depressants versus couple therapy in the treatment and maintenance of people with depression living with a partner: clinical outcome and costs. *British Journal of Psychiatry* **177**, 95–100.

8. **Department of Health.** *Evidence Based Clinical Practice Guideline: Treatment Choice in Psychological Therapies and Counselling.* London: Department of Health Publications, 2001.

9. **Gloaguen, V.** et al. (1998). A meta-analysis of the effects of cognitive therapy in depressed patients. *Journal of Affective Disorders* **49**, 59–72.

10. **Mynors-Wallis, L.M., Gath, D.H., Lloyd-Thomas, A.R., and Tomlinson, D.** (1995). Randomised controlled trial comparing problem-solving treatment with amitriptyline and placebo for major depression in primary care. *British Medical Journal* **310**, 441–5.

11. **Mynors-Wallis, L.M., Gath, D.H., Day, A., and Baker, F.A.** (2000). Randomised controlled trial of problem-solving treatment, antidepressant medication and combined treatment for major depression in primary care. *British Medical Journal* **320**, 26–31.

12. **Dowrick, C.** et al. (2000). Problem-solving treatment and group psycho-education for depression: multicentre randomised controlled trial. *British Medical Journal* **321**, 1450–4.

13. **Ward, E., King, M., Lloyd, M., Bower, P., Sibbald, B., Farrelly, S., Gabbay, M., Tarrier, N., and Addington-Hall, J.** (2000). Randomised controlled trial of non-directive counselling, cognitive behaviour therapy and usual general practitioner care for patients with depression. *British Medical Journal* **321**, 1383–8.

14. **Bedi, N.** et al. (2000). Assessing effectiveness of treatment of depression in primary care partially randomised preference trial. *British Journal of Psychiatry* **177**, 317–19.

15. **Weissman, M.M.** *Mastering Depression: A Patient Guide to Interpersonal Psychotherapy.* Albany NY: Graywind Publications, 1985.

16. **Appleby, L., Warner, R., Whitton, A., and Faragher, B.** (1997). A controlled study of fluoxetine and cognitive behavioural counselling in the treatment of postnatal depression. *British Medical Journal* **314**, 932–6.

17. **Catalan, J., Gath, D., Edmonds, G., and Ennis, J.** (1984). The effect of non-prescribing of anxiolytics in general practice. *British Journal of Psychiatry* **144**, 593–602.

18. **Van Balkom, A.J., Bakker, A., Spinhoven, P., Blaauw, B.M., Smeenk, S., and Ruesink, B.** (1997). A meta-analysis of the treatment of panic disorder with or without agoraphobia. *Journal of Nervous and Mental Disease* **185**, 510–16.

19. **Mynors-Wallis, L.M., Gath, D., Davies, I., Gray, A., and Barbour, F.** (1997). A randomised controlled trial and cost analysis of problem-solving treatment given by community nurses for emotional disorders in primary care. *British Journal of Psychiatry* **170**, 113–19.

20. **Friedli, K.** et al. (1997). Randomised controlled assessment of non-directive psychotherapy versus routine GP care. *Lancet* **350**, 1662–5.

21. **Harvey, I., Nelson, S.J., Lyons, R.A., Unwin, C., Monaghan, S., and Peters, T.J.** (1988). A randomised controlled trial and economic evaluation of counselling. *British Journal of General Practice* **48**, 1043–8.

22. **Fleming, M.F.** et al. (1998). Brief advice reduced drinking in non-dependent problem drinkers. *Journal of the American Medical Association* **277**, 1039–45.

23. **Goldberg, R.J., Hovack, D.H., and Gask, L.** (1992). The recognition and management of somatisation. *Psychosomatics* **33**, 55–61.

24. **Ridsdale, L., Godfrey, E., Chalder, T., Seed, P., King, M., Wallace, P., and Wessely, S.** (2001). Chronic fatigue in general practice: is counselling as good as cognitive behavioural therapy. *British Journal of General Practice* **51**, 19–24.

Further reading

Mynors-Wallis, L., Moore, M., Hollingberry, T., and Maguire, J. *Shared Care in Mental Health.* Oxford: Oxford University Press, 2002. (Provides practical details of the psychological and pharmacological management of common mental health problems seen in primary care.)

Cognitive behaviour therapy (Chapter 6.3.2). In *New Oxford Textbook of Psychiatry* (ed. M.G. Gelder, J.J. Lopez-Ibor, and N.C. Andreasen). Oxford: Oxford University Press, 2000. (Excellent accounts of the theory and practice of CBT for anxiety disorders, eating disorders, depressive disorders, and schizophrenia.)

9.11 Adult survivors of sexual abuse

Shelley Rechner

Childhood sexual abuse (CSA) is a serious health and social problem. Since the late 1970s, political activists, researchers, clinicians, and the general public have increased our awareness of this significant health problem. However, many primary care clinicians in practice today have received little or no formal education about CSA yet are faced with caring for survivors on a daily basis. Issues such as definition, prevalence, and sequelae of CSA will be covered in this chapter. Risk factors for abuse will be outlined and suggestions for facilitating disclosures will be offered. Strategies for generalist care of survivors and referrals for specialist care will be discussed.

Definition

Clinicians and researchers have been struggling over the past 20 years to define precisely what is meant by CSA. That is, what types of childhood sexual experiences could have long-lasting negative effects on a person's psychological, emotional, and spiritual self? Child sexual abuse encompasses both contact and non-contact behaviours. It may involve either violent or seductive forms of abuse. For many children, the latter is the most confusing to deal with. The perpetrator may be a trusted authority figure, even a loved parent. The abuse may be the only close physical or emotional attention received so that a survivor may never consider what happened to him or her as abuse. Still other children may be 'groomed' or drugged into submission by strangers, family, and friends.

Non-contact abuse is defined by acts such as exhibitionism or being forced or lured into viewing pornography. Contact abuse may involve behaviours such as touching the perpetrators' genitals, the child being touched, oral sexual contact, masturbation of either child or perpetrator, and forcible and non-forcible anal, vaginal, and oral penetration. Any of these behaviours can have long-lasting negative consequences both in childhood and later in adult life so that the clinician would be wise to use this broader definition of abuse.

Some researchers exclude non-contact forms of abuse when attempting to quantify prevalence rates or to study significant sequelae of abuse. Others attempt to distinguish consensual same-age sexual-exploration experiences from the more damaging events where either the ages or social power between victim and perpetrator imply that consent cannot be given. The clinician is reminded that sexual experiences with others only a few years older than the victim can cause long-lasting harm, especially if threat or intimidation has been used. Many clinicians have adopted the research definitions to facilitate clarity in communications with patients and peers. The simplest definitions seem to be the most useful for both settings and include questions such as:

When you were growing up did any adult ever do any of these things to you against your will . . .

Exposed themselves to you more than once?

Threatened to have sex with you?

Touched the sex part of your body?

Tried to have sex with you or sexually attacked you?[1]

Questions like this have been used extensively to facilitate study respondents to disclose and could also be adapted to help to identify a history of child sexual abuse in the clinical setting.

Epidemiology

Although many studies were initially conducted in the United States, United Kingdom, Canada, Australia, New Zealand, and Sweden, reports have since been published from all over the world including: Costa Rica, El Salvador, France, Malaysia, South Africa, and Taiwan. Prevalence rates vary depending upon the methodology used and population studied. Estimates range from 62 per cent in an all-female population surveyed to 12.8 per cent for women[2] and 4.3 per cent men.[1] These latter figures are regarded as the best estimate to date because this was the largest general population surveyed (over 9000 respondents). Higher prevalence rates are found in studies in which:

- non-contact was included in the definition;
- the researcher defined that the experiences were abuse;
- the respondent was interviewed; and
- there was a higher response rate.

Although the clinician needs to be aware that child sexual abuse can and does occur in any ethnic or socio-economic status (SES) group, there are certainly some groups where social factors affect prevalence rates. Poverty, racial discrimination, and social disruption such as war and family fragmentation may increase the risk that a child may not be as protected as his/her peers in more favourable settings. Also, child sexual abuse can occur at any age. Estimates for the onset of child sexual abuse range between ages 8 and 10 years.

Who abuses?

When asked about their abusers, the vast majority of both male and female survivors report male perpetrators. Fergusson's study of more than 1000 boys and girls, followed for 18 years in New Zealand, reported a 94 per cent rate of male perpetrators.[3] There are a small but clinically significant number of females who abuse; their victims may be of either sex. The preponderance of victims are female but Macmillan's estimates of 3.9 per cent for males remind the reader that boys are vulnerable to abuse as well. Clinicians probably fail to identify many male survivors due to stereotyping males as being able to 'fend off assaults regardless of age or power'.[4] Family members, friends, or acquaintances and strangers all have been reported to be abuser(s) by survivors of both sexes.

Risk factors for abuse

Fergusson identified five risk factors for child sexual abuse: female gender of the victim, marital conflict, poor parental attachment, paternal overprotection, parental alcohol problems, and possibly low maternal education.[3] In other studies, low SES is associated with risk for child sexual abuse, but this does not appear to be as strong a risk factor for sexual as for physical abuse. There is some inconsistency in the literature as to whether the presence of a step-parent appears to be a risk factor for CSA. A useful guideline for the clinician is to keep the level of vulnerability of the child in mind. For example, how closely supervised is the child? Is he/she left with unreliable caregivers or how safe is the route to school? Would factors of race, SES, or disability render the child more vulnerable because she/he might not disclose or not be believed if he/she reported to an authority?

Much of sexual abuse is hidden from parents, clinicians, and authorities. Perpetrators lie to, or threaten children in order to keep their crime a secret. Children may be afraid, ashamed or do not really understand the implication of the abuse and thus do not report it. Rates of disclosure vary. Some early data about disclosure to family physicians suggested that many patients felt uncomfortable in discussing this with their practitioners. However, this may be changing as both patients and practitioners recognize the prevalence of CSA and feel more comfort in discussing the issue in a clinical setting.

Diagnosis

MacMillan's conservative estimates suggest that one in eight women and one in 25 men in the population have suffered an unwanted sexual act in childhood.[1] Thus, is the primary care clinician aware if he/she sees many survivors in a busy day? Does he/she need to identify every survivor in the practice at intake or during specific clinical presentations? Several studies have attempted to measure the frequency and presentation of survivors in primary care settings. Consecutive patients presenting for routine health maintenance care were asked about a variety of symptoms and health problems and whether they suffered a CSA.[5–7] Many survivors, unless asked directly, do not disclose their sexual abuse history to their clinician. Thus, a highly prevalent condition often remains unknown to the primary care practitioner. To date, there is no consensus as to whether every patient's CSA experiences needs to be 'diagnosed' or whether this should be considered in specific clinical situations where the abuse appears to be causing some problem for the adult survivor.

Adult sequelae

One of the most striking consequences of child sexual abuse can be the psychiatric condition known as post-traumatic stress disorder (PTSD). Although this condition occurs as the result of many other traumatic events, as discussed in the following chapter, many PTSD patients will report childhood sexual abuse. Only a proportion of survivors will exhibit the full clinical diagnosis of PTSD but many suffer some aspects of it, as will be described below. PTSD includes the following characteristics:

◆ the patient has experienced a traumatic event(s);

◆ the event is persistently re-experienced;

for example, through flashbacks (a sense of reliving the event), dreams, or can be triggered by similar situations/anniversaries, etc.,

◆ avoidance of stimuli associated with the trauma or numbing;

◆ increased arousal.

More severe sexual abuse (contact versus non-contact, penetration versus non-penetration) and concomitant other abuses (physical abuse and/or neglect) are associated with a higher rate of PTSD.

Survivors may present with many different symptoms of PTSD. Some symptoms may be with the survivor for much of his or her life. Others may be 'triggered' by specific situations that remind or re-traumatize. Among the commonest manifestations of PTSD suffered are nightmares and flashbacks. These may disrupt much of the survivor's daily life. Sleep, sex, employment, education, birthing, or parenting can all be affected. Medical examinations (vaginal, rectal, and even oral) can be traumatic if the touch reminds the survivor of the prior abuse. Specific times of the year, for example, religious or cultural holidays may prove to trigger a flood of memories and increase symptoms for the adult whose abuse occurred at these times. Some survivors find parenting a child who reaches the age when the parent's abuse started particularly difficult. External traumatic events such as a car crash, political, or marital violence can cause intense distress as well.

The 'avoidance of stimuli' aspect of PTSD is characterized by many survivors' failure to attend for routine health examinations even in the face of serious situations such as prolonged rectal bleeding or a highly abnormal Pap test. Other survivors may appear to be under-achieving or have severely restricted their life experiences as a means of avoiding traumatic situations. The last part of the DSM diagnosis for PTSD describes the state of 'increased arousal' that many survivors exhibit. This may manifest as the patient who startles with even the most careful touch or appears 'hyper-vigilant' to everything in the clinical setting. Physiologic experiments suggest that this state of hyperarousal persists long after the other aspects of the PTSD diagnosis have left.[8]

Although many survivors do not appear to fit the classic diagnosis of PTSD, many suffer health problems that appear to be associated with a history of CSA. A list of conditions for which there is a statistically significant increased rate of survivors as compared to non-abused controls is found in Table 1. Research on sequelae of child sexual abuse reveals associations rather than direct cause and effect. Thus, there are many factors in a child's growing years, which might mitigate the traumatic effects of CSA such as, a loving parental figure, success at school or with peers, early identification and intervention when the abuse is disclosed, etc.

The clinician may immediately recognize some of the conditions in Table 1 as logical sequelae of CSA. For example, depression or sexual dysfunction may often be consequences for an adult who had no control over his or her body as a child. Other problems such as functional GI and GU disorders are more clearly understood when one considers what the patient's symptoms might mean. For example, the patient with retching and nausea may be suffering body memories of intrusions such as oral rape. Other problems that appear less obviously related to CSA include chronic pain, addictions, and eating disorders. Sandra Butler has described the concept of 'self-soothing' behaviours to help reframe such self-destructive behaviours such as drinking, drugging, or overeating as ways that the survivor uses to cope with flashbacks, anxiety, and depression resulting from CSA.[9] Some listed

Table 1 Possible sequelae of child sexual abuse

Behavioural problems
    e.g. self-injury, driving while intoxicated, or not wearing seat-belts, risky
    sexual behaviour, higher number of lifetime sexual partners, sexually
    transmitted infections and PID, criminal behaviours, e.g. prostitution
Academic and vocational problems

Substance abuse, smoking
Eating disorders, morbid obesity
Not exercising

Poor self-esteem, depression
Suicidal ideas and behaviours, PTSD, and borderline personality disorder

Sexual dysfunction
Pregnancy prior to age 19, pregnant more than five times

Psychosomatic disorders
Chronic pain and fibromyalgia, headaches, greater number of pain meds
GI/GU, especially functional disorders
Surgical evaluation of pelvic pain

Non-compliance with invasive testing
Greater: symptom reporting, health care utilization, number of lifetime surgeries
    including surgical evaluation of pelvic pain

sequelae, such as higher numbers of sexual partners, pregnancies prior to age 19, etc. are clearly specific to the nation in which the data are collected and may not have as much relevance in cultures with much different norms. However, the international literature is more striking for similarities than differences. For example, Taiwanese survivors reported 'similar traumatic symptoms between Chinese survivors and their American counterparts'.[10]

Facilitating disclosure

The reader may be wondering which of his or her patients might be a survivor and ask how could one make the diagnosis? Facilitating disclosure is often no more complicated than a caring clinician considering the possibility and asking a question. One can use either an open-ended question such as 'In your childhood did anyone ever touch you in a sexual way that you did not want?' Or one could use a qualifier such as: 'Some people who have (your symptoms) have had an unwanted sexual experience in their childhood. Could this have been the case for you?' The clinician should adapt the wording to the level of understanding of the patient being asked.

One of the most important factors in helping a patient to disclose is to remain as calm and accepting as possible. Before exploring these issues with patients, the clinician may wish to read first person accounts about child sexual abuse.[11] This could provide the opportunity to experience one's own reactions in private and be prepared for emotionally powerful information in the consulting room. Disclosure can be quite traumatic. A survivor may suffer fear, shame, or embarrassment when describing the abuse. The clinician is cautioned to avoid probing into detail, to even consider limiting the extent of initial disclosure until the patient's psychological safety is assured. The clinician who is able to listen empathetically to the patient's narrative is immensely helpful to the patient.

Making a referral

Many clinicians upon hearing a disclosure may wish to immediately refer the patient along to someone with more clinical experience with survivors. However, one needs to be cautious about assuming every disclosure requires instant action. After a disclosure, the clinician could acknowledge how difficult it must have been for the patient to trust him or her with such important information. One could state that the patient is not alone—that many others have suffered such experiences. Some patients may have a strong sense of regret or fear about telling a professional, so it can be helpful to say that learning about the patient's past has helped to understand them better, not to regard them in a negative way.

The clinical situation in which the disclosure was made may dictate the next step of management. If the survivor was seeking therapy for problems arising from the sexual abuse issues, then the clinician may wish to refer for specialist care to psychiatric nurses, psychiatrists, psychologists, social workers, or front-line workers in rape crisis units. The clinician needs to consider accessibility, expertise, and funding of these various specialists in one's community before making a referral. In other situations, a crisis such as a referral for specialist medical or surgical care may have led to consideration of CSA experiences. For example, consider the patient who discloses when faced with an upcoming colonoscopy. One could help the survivor to explore what aspects of the procedure will be most difficult to undergo. Would a trusted friend or family member accompanying the patient make the procedure easier or less threatening? Would the gender of the specialist doing the procedure matter? Would a phone call ahead to the colonoscopy unit to prepare them for the patient help? Scrupulous attention to confidentiality and consent from the patient for release of information is essential to maintain the patient's trust.

In summary, the primary care clinician is uniquely placed to help these patients. Anticipating that he/she is already caring for survivors, one can teach oneself and colleagues about child sexual abuse. Caring for survivors involves the same management principles as other clinical situations: knowledge, respect, caring, and flexibility. What seems to distinguish effective care of survivors is an imaginative anticipation of what symptoms might mean and what situations might be difficult for a survivor to endure. This is truly a creative aspect of primary care and it is greatly rewarding for the clinician, especially since many will be involved with these patients over the long-term.

Conclusions

There is still much work to be done to help clinicians to care for survivors of sexual abuse. More research is needed in developing countries, where current treatment models may not be relevant or culturally appropriate or where war and famine add to the trauma suffered. Over the last 25 years, developed countries have seen rapidly rising numbers of disclosures, probably as a result of political movements such as feminism, greater clinical awareness, and the development of programmes to assist the diagnosis and treatment of children who have been sexually abused. Sadly, however, the prevalence of CSA appears to be fairly stable. Despite our ability to diagnose it more often, we seem unable to reduce how frequently it occurs.

Identification and treatment of boys and adult male survivors remains a challenge. Research is needed to identify the factors that cause perpetrators to abuse, to offer effective treatment for offenders and to ultimately prevent abuse from occurring. Bridging the gap between the forensic literature on offenders and the clinical literature on survivors may offer solutions for identification and treatment of perpetrators. More likely, the answers as to what causes CSA will have to be sought beyond clinical settings and will challenge each society to reconsider how it views violence, pornography, and the rights of children.

Key points

- Child sexual abuse may involve contact or non-contact (exhibitionism) unwanted or exploitative sexual contact.

- The most conservative estimates suggest that one in eight women and one in 25 men have experienced an unwanted sexual act in childhood.

- The sexual abuse survivor may present to the primary care clinician with a wide variety of sequelae of their abuse including post-traumatic stress disorder.

- The primary care clinician is uniquely situated to assist in facilitating disclosure of CSA and he/she can do so through simple, sensitive history-taking.

- Referral to specialist care is not automatically required and is guided by the patient's needs and symptoms.

References

1. MacMillan, H. et al. (1997). Prevalence of child physical and sexual abuse in the community: results from the Ontario health supplement. *Journal of the American Medical Association* **278**, No. 2, 131–5.

2. Wyatt, G. (1985). The sexual abuse of Afro-American and white-American women in childhood. *Child Abuse and Neglect* **9**, 507–19.

3. Fergusson, D., Lynskey, M., and Horwood, J. (1996). Childhood sexual abuse and psychiatric disorder in young adulthood: I. prevalence of sexual abuse and factors associated with sexual abuse. *Journal of American Academy of Child Adolescent Psychiatry* **34**, 1355–64.

4. Gold, S. et al. (1998). Abuse characteristics among childhood sexual abuse survivors in therapy: A gender comparison. *Child Abuse and Neglect* **22**, 1005–12.

5. Walch, A. and Broadhead, E. (1992). Prevalence of lifetime sexual victimization among female patients. *The Journal of Family Practice* **35**, 511–16.

6. Lechner, M. et al. (1993). Self-reported medical problems of adult female survivors of childhood sexual abuse. *The Journal of Family Practice* **36**, 633–8.

7. Felitti, V. (1991). Long-term medical consequences of incest, rape and molestation. *Southern Medical Journal* **84**, 328–31.

8. Orr, S. et al. (1998). Psychophysiologic assessment of women with post-traumatic stress disorder resulting from childhood sexual abuse. *Journal of Consulting and Clinical Psychology* **66**, 906–13.

9. Butler, S. *Conspiracy of Silence: The Trauma of Incest*. California: Volcano Press, 1985.

10. Tsun-yin, E. L. (1998). Sexual abuse among Chinese survivors. *Child Abuse and Neglect* **22**, 1013–26.

11. Bass, E. and Davis, L. *Courage to Heal*. New York: Harper and Row, 1988.

Further reading

Laws, A. (1993). Does a history of sexual abuse in childhood play a role in women's medical problems? A review. *Journal of Women's Health* **2**, 165–72.

Holmes, W. (1998). Sexual abuse of boys. *Journal of American Medical Association* **280**, 1855–62.

Bala, M. (1994). Caring for adult survivors of child sexual abuse. Issues for family physicians. *Canadian Family Physician* **40**, 925–31.

9.12 Post-traumatic stress disorder

Derek Summerfield

Psychological responses to trauma and adversity have probably always been with us, but there is no doubt that interest in the subject has increased dramatically in recent years, as part of a general humanitarian concern with the plight of victims. One sign of this was the introduction of a new condition, post-traumatic stress disorder (PTSD), into the Bible of psychiatric classification, the Diagnostic and Statistical Manual (DSM) of the American Psychiatric Association, in 1980. However, it is a term not without problems.

Brief history

It is worth a brief discussion of the origins of PTSD in order to understand the uses, but also the limitations, of the diagnosis. A central assumption behind psychiatric diagnosis is that disease has an objective existence in the world, discovered or not, and is independent of the gaze of psychiatrists or anyone else. In fact, the emergence and official recognition of almost all psychiatric categories was shaped not just by trends in medical thinking but also by socio-cultural and sometimes political variables. PTSD is a legacy of the US war in Vietnam, a product of the post-war fortunes of the frequently conscripted men who served there. They came home to find that their nation, and even their families, were disowning their own guilt for the war and blaming them instead. This reception—more rejection than acknowledgement—may have been a prime factor in the incubation of the well publicized difficulties, including antisocial behaviour, which some had in readjusting to peacetime roles. Those attracting psychiatric attention acquired diagnoses like anxiety states, depression, substance abuse, personality disorder, and schizophrenia, later to be supplanted by PTSD.

The early proponents of PTSD were part of the antiwar movement in the United States, and were angered that military psychiatry was serving the interests of the army rather than those of soldier-patients. They lobbied hard for veterans to receive specialized medical care organized around a new and distinctive diagnosis: PTSD, the successor to older formulations like battle fatigue or war neurosis. PTSD shifted the focus of attention from the details of an individual soldier's background and psyche to the fundamentally traumatogenic nature of war itself. This was a considerable transformation: Vietnam veterans were to be seen not as perpetrators or offenders, but as traumatized—by roles thrust on them by the US military. PTSD gave some of them legitimated victimhood, moral exculpation and a disability pension through a doctor-attested sick role.[1]

In the last two decades the utilization of PTSD has gone far beyond the problems of Vietnam veterans. The medicalization of life has been a major cultural trend in Western societies in this century, and one recent facet of this has been the spectacular rise of 'trauma'—whether as idiom of distress or as clinical formulation (PTSD). The conflation of distress with 'trauma' increasingly has a naturalistic feel, part of everyday descriptions of life's vicissitudes. So too with the term 'stress', which many British GPs now put on sick certificates for employers where previously they put 'anxiety and depression'.

A striking development has been the globalization of PTSD by humanitarian programmes addressing war-affected peoples anywhere. It is promoted as a universalistic basis for capturing and addressing the impact of events like war and atrocity—whatever the background culture, current situation, and the subjective meaning brought to bear by survivors. For some this carries the danger of reducing the misery and horror of war to a technical issue, tailored to Western mental health approaches (see below).

Epidemiology

These cultural trends must raise queries about epidemiological studies which assume that capturing the prevalence of PTSD is similar to capturing the prevalence of, say, tuberculosis. It is not surprising that studies in the United States—there are few data of this kind from elsewhere—have yielded widely differing prevalence rates: between 1 and 7.8 per cent[2,3] with Australian and German data at the low end of the spectrum. Given that rates of exposure to traumatic events is no lower in Australia than the United States, for example, it suggests once again that most traumatic events are not followed by PTSD, and that many cultural variables may determine rates of illness.

So called 'co-morbidity' also presents problems. All studies agree that most cases of PTSD also fulfil criteria for other psychiatric disorders, such as depression or anxiety. For these and other reasons it is difficult to obtain reliable data on presentation rates in primary care settings and referral rates to specialist services.

Causative factors for PTSD

The most obvious cause for PTSD is being exposed to trauma. But what trauma? Originally framed as applying only to extreme experiences like war or disaster, which few would expect to encounter in a normal life, PTSD has come to be associated with a growing list of relatively commonplace events: an accident, a mugging, a difficult labour (with healthy baby), verbal sexual harrassment, or the shock of receiving (incorrect) bad news from a doctor—though the diagnosis was checked and rescinded shortly afterwards. Increasingly, the workplace in Britain is being portrayed as traumatogenic even for those just doing their job: paramedics attending road accidents, police constables on duty at disasters, and even employees caught up in what they would once have described as a straightforward dispute with management, are all seeking compensation for PTSD or for not being offered counselling. The most recent reformulation of PTSD, in the 4th edition of DSM, makes it easier to qualify by widening the definition of traumatic stressors to include the experience of hearing the news that something bad has happened to someone close. Second hand shocks now count.

There is one further problem with the label of PTSD. Psychiatric diagnoses are usually descriptive, not aetiological—think about depression or schizophrenia. This is because psychiatric disorders are almost invariably multifactorial. Likewise PTSD. However, the very term PTSD itself seems to (falsely) suggest that the cause of PTSD is the trauma alone. Doctors need to remember that PTSD is no different from any other psychiatric disorder, and giving the diagnosis must not distract from a consideration of the many factors pre- and post-trauma which may have contributed. Indeed, studies of those exposed to a range of man-made and natural events have consistently found that pre-event factors account for more of the variance in PTSD symptoms than do event characteristics. These factors include the tendency to respond to life experiences with negative emotion (trait neuroticism), an externalizing emotion-focused coping style, a previous psychiatric history, level of intelligence, and social support.[4]

The diagnosis of PTSD

PTSD is classified in DSM and ICD as a protracted response—generally arising within 6 months and lasting at least 1 month—to an experience of an exceptionally threatening or catastrophic nature. Some cases are noted as following a chronic course over years, and 'late onset' PTSD is also recognized by some authorities, but studies suggest this is unusual, and is more likely to reflect late presentation than true delay.

Core features include:

1. Episodes of distressing or intrusive *recollections* of the traumatic event (sometimes labelled 'flashbacks' or 're-experiencing') during the day or in sleep.

2. *Avoidance* of situations reminiscent of the event, and *sensitivity* to cues associated with the event.

3. *Diminished interest* in significant activities, emotional numbness, or detachment from other people.

4. Persistent symptoms of *increased autonomic arousal* include a disturbed sleep pattern, irritability, difficulty in mental concentration, being easily startled, and unusually vigilant.

Sudden episodes of fear, panic, or aggression triggered by stimuli associated with the original event are also described, but acknowledged to be rare. Far more common is anxiety and depression, and also excessive use of alcohol or drugs. Thoughts of self-harm are also not unknown.

Like many psychiatric diagnoses, PTSD is not an 'all or nothing' phenomenon. There is no simple cut-off between normal and abnormal distress after trauma, any more than there is a simple cut-off between normal and abnormal depression. The criterial features are basically subjective and the diagnosis can be made in the absence of significant, objective dysfunction. PTSD supposedly represents a distinct category of psychopathology but is largely grounded in phenomena common both to other psychiatric diagnoses and to normally unhappy people—concerning mood, anxiety-based features, sleep pattern, etc. The objectification of distress, or suffering per se may mean simply reifying the contents of subjective consciousness—this risks being clinically meaningless, a pseudocondition.

As far as differential diagnosis is concerned, an acute stress reaction is a transient disorder (a few hours or days) following a highly aversive event. Symptoms may include an initial state of daze, disorientation, and inability to comprehend stimuli, followed by withdrawal or by agitation and overactivity. An adjustment disorder may arise after a stressful life event or significant life change, usually within 1 month and lasting up to 6 months. Social dysfunction accompanies the manifestations of distress. Lastly, there is a diagnostic overlap with anxiety and depressive disorders, as noted above.

There has been considerable investment into isolating a psycho-biological marker for PTSD, but no distinctive finding has emerged. Although some psycho-biological abnormalities have been shown, none is specific enough to help in diagnosis. Once again, in this respect PTSD is no different from most other psychiatric categories.

PTSD and culture

PTSD is not the only psychiatric category which clearly demonstrates the problem of separating out medicopsychological facts from social values and expectations. What constitutes 'psychology' or 'mental health' are social products. Collectively held beliefs about a particular negative experience are not just potent influences but carry an element of self-fulfilling prophecy for individual victims, who will largely organize what they feel, say, do and expect of the future, to fit prevailing expectations and categories. Underpinning all this is the concept of a person held by the particular culture at that point in time. This embodies prescriptions for questions like: how much or what kind of adversity can a life face and still be 'normal'; what is reasonable risk; when is fatalism appropriate and when a sense of grievance; what is acceptable behaviour at a time of crisis, including expressions of distress, and modes of help-seeking and restitution. In Britain, for example, personhood has traditionally invoked notions of stoicism and understatement—the 'stiff upper lip'.

Primary care settings are certainly one place to witness the tension between these older ideas, which centre on resilience and composure, and what is emerging today. In Western societies an expressive, psychologically minded, individualism is increasingly salient, as is the promotion of personal rights and the language of entitlement. Moreover, there is waning belief in the comfort of religion and in the benevolence of authority. For good or ill, an individualistic rights-conscious culture can foster a sense of personal injury and grievance, and thus a need for restitution, in encounters in daily life that were once experienced as misfortune rather than injustice. PTSD is *the* diagnosis for an age of privatized disenchantment.[5]

Today, there is often more social utility attached to expressions of victimhood than to survivorhood, perhaps the reverse of earlier times. Once it becomes a cultural option to frame 'distress' as a psychiatric condition, people will choose this if there is more to gain in presenting as medicalized victim than as feisty survivor.

In international terms, the key question is whether Western psychiatric taxonomies and categories like PTSD can be assumed to have universal validity, or are merely the product of one among many ethnopsychiatries. Every culture has its own traditions and interpretations of the world which determine psycho-social norms, including expressions of distress and modes of help-seeking. Presentations by people from non-Western cultures may 'fit' poorly with what is familiar to primary care staff. DSM and ICD are held to represent universal knowledge but their categories only represent phenomenological constellations and are not necessarily scientifically validated as entities in the natural world. They are Western cultural documents whose contents evolve as Western thinking evolves. PTSD, like anorexia nervosa, might yet be a Western culture-bound syndrome.

A psychiatric diagnosis is primarily a way of seeing, a style of reasoning, and (particularly relevant to PTSD) a means of persuasion: it is not at all times a disease with a life of its own. In the West—though often not in other cultures—positivism and instrumental reasoning are privileged modes of persuasion: in order to show that you have been wronged, you seek to show that you were not just hurt but impaired. In Western countries, PTSD can for some become a means by which people seek doctor-attested victim status, with its associated moral high ground, in pursuit of recognition and compensation. As an editorial in the *American Journal of Psychiatry* put it dryly, it was rare to find a psychiatric diagnosis that anyone liked to have, but PTSD was one.[6]

Prevention

Short of not being exposed to traumatic events, very little if anything has been shown to prevent the occurrence of post-trauma psychiatric injury. So called 'debriefing' has been promoted as a form of trauma counselling which, conducted immediately after a violent event, may prevent later mental disorders (in particular PTSD). A review of what studies exist of one-off trauma counselling could find no evidence for these claims, and a recent trial with victims of serious traffic accidents in Britain found that subjects were slower than controls to get back to normal on both subjective and objective measures.[7,8] The vast majority of those caught up in a public disaster manage their shock and grief within their own personal networks and, for example, crisis counselling services set up by mental health professionals in the days after 11 September 2001 in New York found that they had little to do. The absence of mass panic in the evacuation of the World Trade Centre reminds us that people are more resilient than we given them credit for.

Management

Most people exposed to trauma do not show psychological disturbance, or if they do, can still be expected to improve over time.

Clinical assessment must take account of the fact that the impact of a traumatic event is centrally shaped by what it means to that person, or comes to mean. No psychiatric model captures this active conceptualizing, which will include appraisal of whether the event is seen in wider society as one subject to restitution, including compensation. It is this which distinguishes the shock of a road accident from, say, being made redundant at work: post-redundancy PTSD officially does not exist.

Clinical assessment should include the potential contribution of pre- and post-trauma variables, like a history of contact with mental health services or other indication of pre-existing vulnerability like alcohol problems, and current family or work pressures.

When the patient is foreign (like an asylum-seeker), primary care staff need to have some awareness of the cross-cultural and cross-situational factors that may shape the way distress is articulated. A professional approach must be taken to the provision of interpreter services.

Management should involve a series of 'stepped' approaches. Simple reassurance may be all that is necessary. Failing that basic measures such as sleep hygiene (since sleep is a very frequent casualty of the immediate trauma reaction) should be tried. There is also a place for short-term medication if sleep is seriously disturbed.

If it appears that simple measures have not worked, and that spontaneous resolution appears unlikely (either because of the passage of time or the presence of numerous risk factors) more active management may be required. Management has essentially been either pharmacotherapy or talk therapy, typically aimed at catharsis through emotional ventilation. In the experience of the author, cases of clinical severity diagnosable as PTSD can almost always be co-diagnosed as depressive disorder and merit a trial of antidepressants. No conclusions can be drawn as to the claims of one class of antidepressant over another.

Recent studies have confirmed that cognitive–behavioural techniques and cognitive–behaviour therapy (CBT) is effective, even if hard to obtain. A recent meta-analysis of 61 treatment–outcome trials for PTSD showed that talk therapies were in general more effective than medication, and had lower dropout rates.[9]

In Western countries, there has been a trend for the establishment of specialist traumatic stress clinics, with patients being referred on from primary care. Those who have been through certain kinds of experiences—like rape or childhood sexual abuse—are often seen as self-evident candidates for referral. PTSD can be too simplistic a concept to explain the difficulties such patients may have. Broader ways of understanding do better.

Specialist PTSD services are available in some areas as a 'last resort' for complex cases. However, the efficacy of complex interventions remains unproven, and there are examples from the United States and Israel in which such services may assist in generating dependency. For example, in the United States, PTSD clinics for Vietnam veterans have been run for 20 years by the Veterans Administration and there is now some disillusionment about the results. Some critics suggest that the system has generated many professional PTSD cases still no nearer to 'recovery'.[10] There are reminders here for doctors to take a rigorous approach to the power to award sick roles which society confers on them, not least with a disease category with low specificity like PTSD. To do otherwise may promote abnormal illness behaviour and prolong psycho-social disability.

When PTSD cases are tied in with a medico-legal argument, outcomes will shaped by factors beyond the reach of the clinic. 'Recovery' from PTSD, in advance of a legal settlement, may be problematic.

Social factors in recovery from war

Looking worldwide, the other major realm concerns survivors of war or atrocity, many of whom have become asylum-seekers in Western countries where primary medical care services are a key point of reference at the outset. As mentioned above, the rise of trauma programmes addressing 'post-traumatic stress' shows the danger of looking at war with a gaze borrowed from a psychiatric clinic. To characterize the misery of war as psycho-pathology is to apply a paradigm that transforms the social into the biopsychomedical. Even consultants to WHO and UNICEF have made expansive claims, in former Yugoslavia and Rwanda, for instance, that hundreds of thousands of people needed professional assistance for their PTSD, and that early intervention would avert the later onset of mental problems and new cycles of violence. The assumption was also that there is basically one universal human response to traumatic events, captured by Western psychological frameworks, and that all victims did better if they emotionally ventilated/'worked through' their experiences. There is little basis for any of this, no more so in Westernized former Yugoslavia than in Rwanda, and the detached introspection of counselling (the assumed antidote) is of course especially alien to those from non-Western cosmologies and ontologies.[11,12]

Whilst we must acknowledge the paucity of reliable studies, it does not seem that the psychiatric fall-out of war, torture, or other atrocity, and refugeedom, affects more than a tiny majority of those exposed (some of whom had demonstrated pre-trauma vulnerabilities). My own clinical experience over many years with this group is consistent with this. Northern Ireland presents an interesting case since it has been one war zone where

comprehensive health records have been maintained. Over the past 30 years there is no evidence of a significant impact on referral rates to mental health services.[13]

The secondary consequences of violent conflict—on family, social, and economic life—are important predictors of psychological outcomes in tortured political activists.[14] In Iraqi asylum-seekers in London, poor social support was more closely related to depression than was a history of torture.[15] People do well or not as a function of their capacity to rebuild social networks and viable ways of life. Thus, employment rates may say more about recovery from the trauma of war than do PTSD prevalence rates.

Some implications

This paper has sought to illuminate some core medical aspects of PTSD, and also to point to their dynamic interplay with social and cultural trends and expectations. Some cases of PTSD do have clinically significant dysfunction but the poor specificity of its diagnostic criteria means many false positives. It might be timely for the mental health professions to review the epistemological status of PTSD as a disease entity, whether it has sufficient robustness and explanatory power for the diverse uses to which it is now being put. We should also not lose sight of the fact that PTSD is not the only psychiatric condition to arise after trauma, nor even the most common, and that the tried and tested categories of anxiety and depression should never be overlooked.

The trend in Western societies to portray the work place as a potentially traumatogenic environment even for those just doing their ordinary job, of 'post-traumatic stress' as an occupational hazard akin to pneumoconiosis in miners, begs socio-moral questions meriting the widest possible debate. Are there societal limits to the medicalization of life?

Key points

1. Psychological trauma is not like physical trauma: people do not passively register the impact of external forces (unlike a leg hit by a bullet) but engage with them in an active and social way.

2. People are more resilient than we think—most people exposed to trauma do not develop psychiatric disorder. So called 'debriefing' does not prevent subsequent disorder.

3. PTSD diagnostic criteria may distinguish poorly between normal distress and pathological distress. Distress or suffering per se is not psycho-pathology. Look for evidence of significant, persistent global dysfunction.

4. Clinical assessment should include pre- and post-trauma factors, for example, prior psychiatric history, current family or work stressors, etc.

5. Simple measures promoting natural recovery are all that are needed for most. In those who fail to recover, antidepressants and/or CBT have a role.

6. PTSD is a Western way of thinking about trauma—care should be taken before applying the same criteria to other cultures.

References

1. **Young, A.** *The Harmony of Illusions: Inventing Posttraumatic Stress Disorder.* New Jersey: Princeton University Press, 1995.

2. **Helzer, J., Robins, L., and McEvoy, L.** (1987). Post-traumatic stress disorder in the general population. *New England Journal of Medicine* **317**, 1630–4.

3. Kessler, R., Sonnega, A., Bromet, E., Hughes, H., and Nelson, C. (1995). Post-traumatic stress disorder in the national comorbidity survey. *Archives of General Psychiatry* **52**, 1048–60.

4. Bowman, M. (1999). Individual differences in post-traumatic distress: problems with the DSM-IV model. *Canadian Journal of Psychiatry* **44**, 21–32.

5. Summerfield, D. (2001). The invention of post-traumatic stress disorder and the social usefulness of a psychiatric category. *British Medical Journal* **322**, 95–8.

6. Andreason, N. (1995). Post-traumatic stress disorder: Psychology, biology and the Manichean war between false dichotomies. *American Journal of Psychiatry* **152**, 963–5.

7. Wessely, S., Rose, S., and Bisson, J. (1998). A systematic review of brief psychological interventions (debriefing) for the treatment of immediate trauma-related symptoms and the prevention of post-traumatic stress disorder (Cochrane Review). In *The Cochrane Library* Issue 2. Oxford: Update Software.

8. Mayou, R., Ehlers, A., and Hobbs, M. (2000). Psychological debriefing for road traffic victims. Three year follow-up of a randomised controlled trial. *British Journal of Psychiatry* **176**, 589–93.

9. Van Etten, M. and Taylor, S. (1998). Comparative efficacy of treatments for post-traumatic stress disorder: a meta-analysis. *Clinical Psychology and Psychotherapy* **5**, 126–44.

10. Shephard, B. *A War of Nerves. Soldiers and Psychiatrists 1914–94*. London: Jonathan Cape, 2000, pp. 385–99.

11. Summerfield, D. (1999). A critique of seven assumptions behind psychological trauma programmes in war-affected areas. *Social Science & Medicine* **48**, 1449–62.

12. Bracken, P. (1998). Hidden agendas: deconstructing post-traumatic stress disorder. In *Rethinking the Trauma of War* (ed. P. Bracken and C. Petty), pp. 38–59. New York: Free Association Books.

13. Loughrey, G. (1997). Civil violence. In *Psychological Trauma: A Developmental Approach* (ed. D. Black, M. Newman, J. Harris-Hendriks, and G. Mezey), pp. 156–60. London: Gaskell.

14. Basoglu, M., Paker, M., Ozmen, E., Tasdemir, O., and Sahin, D. (1994). Factors related to long-term traumatic stress in survivors of torture in Turkey. *Journal of the American Medical Association* **272**, 357–63.

15. Gorst-Unsworth, C. and Goldenberg, E. (1998). Psychological sequelae of torture and organised violence suffered by refugees from Iraq. Trauma-related factors compared to social factors in exile. *British Journal of Psychiatry* **172**, 90–4.

9.13 Post-natal depression

Deborah J. Sharp

Introduction

Post-natal depression is a term that is used to describe a variety of emotional disorders that occur in women following childbirth. However, it is most useful to reserve it for the specific depressive illness that affects between 10 and 15 per cent of women in the first year after birth.[1] It must be distinguished from the 'baby blues' which affects as many as 50 per cent of women in the first week after childbirth. The blues are characterized by tearfulness and emotional lability, usually responds to simple reassurance and is likely to have a hormonal aetiology.[2] In a very few instances, it may herald the onset of a much rarer disorder, puerperal psychosis. This serious illness affects only one to two women per 1000 in the first month after childbirth. It is a florid disorder which may manifest itself with signs of either mania or depression. Alternatively, there may be overt psychotic phenomena with disordered thinking, paranoia, and confusion, and women may have the idea of harming themselves or the baby. Again it is likely to have a hormonal aetiology, possibly with some genetic component and is seen more often in younger women, primiparae and women with a personal or family history of psychosis. It is usually best treated in a specialized mother and baby unit and responds well to treatment with major tranquillizers and antidepressants, although occasionally ECT is required.[3]

Classification

Post-natal depression is thus defined as a non-psychotic depressive disorder meeting standardized diagnostic criteria for a minor or major depressive disorder beginning in, or extending into the post-natal period.[4] However, it is not clearly or explicitly defined as such in either of the two major classifications of psychiatric disorder, ICD-10 and DSM-IV. Both classifications code mental disorders associated with the puerperium according to the presenting psychiatric disorder, with a second code F53 (ICD-10) or a specifier 'with postpartum onset' (DSM-IV) applied for disorders presenting in the first 6 weeks or first 4 weeks after delivery, respectively. A diagnosis of post-natal depression usually requires that a woman experiences dysphoric mood along with several other symptoms such as sleep, appetite or psychomotor disturbance, fatigue, excessive guilt, and occasionally, suicidal thoughts. Typically symptoms must be present for a minimum amount of time (at least 2 weeks) and must result in some impairment in the woman's functioning.

Epidemiology

The absence of post-natal depression from the major classification systems in part represents the underlying uncertainty as to the existence of a specific entity called 'post-natal depression'. There are still unanswered questions as to whether there is an increased relative risk of depression within a given time after delivery, what these time limits might be, whether there are any characteristic clinical features that distinguish post-natal depression from any other kind of depression and whether aside from the coincidence with childbirth, there are any other pathognomonic aetiological factors associated with depression beginning after childbirth.

A meta-analysis of 59 studies (including 12 810 women, mainly from First World countries) found an average prevalence of post-natal depression of 13 per cent (95 per cent CI 12.3–13.4).[5] This meta-analysis included studies in which the diagnosis was made using validated psychiatric interviews and self-report questionnaires. The prevalence varies depending on the method of assessment, the differing inclusion criteria for the studies and the length of the follow-up. The incidence is highest in the first 3 months postpartum and the peak time of onset is in the first 4–6 weeks.

A series of controlled studies designed to answer the question as to whether there is a specific association between non-psychotic depression and childbirth have not unequivocally provided evidence of a significantly increased rate of depression following childbirth compared with a variety of different control groups.[6] However, when one considers the specific timing of cases of depression, there does seem to be a clustering effect within the first 3–6 months postpartum. What is clear, is that very few of these women are recognized as 'cases' in primary care, especially by doctors, and even fewer are seen in secondary care. In terms of severity, post-natal depression sits somewhere between the blues and puerperal psychosis, but from a public health perspective, due to its high prevalence it is probably the most important adverse psychological outcome of childbirth. One index of the severity of depression is the length of the episode. The average length of episodes of post-natal depression seems to be of at least several months duration, although the range is wide with episodes as short as 3–4 weeks, but also as long as 12 months or more.[6]

The most recent controversy surrounding post-natal depression concerns the timing of its onset and the question as to whether it is an extension of antenatal depression or a totally different entity. Recent studies reveal an equally high or higher level of antenatal depression and problems with recall bias in retrospective interview-based studies call into question the supremacy of post-natal depression over antenatal depression in terms of predicting adverse sequelae for mother and child.[7]

There are varying reports of the prevalence of post-natal depression in different ethnic groups.[8] There are studies which show that women are protected in some cultures from post-natal depression whilst they maintain their socio-cultural practices, but others show the same prevalence in very diverse countries. It may be that 'depression' is a Western construct of a disease not culturally recognized in other parts of the world. Women may be at greater risk after immigration when it is not so easy to maintain their usual rituals around the time of childbirth. For example, the attention from families and social networks after birth seems to preclude Chinese women from experiencing post-natal depression as experienced in the West.[9] Chalmers similarly describes abundant traditional social support for mothers in rural Southern Africa. This contrasts with urban black mothers' experiences where only nurses are birth companions with the possible consequence of not only post-natal depression but also obstetric complications.[10] When considering the three main post-natal syndromes there appears to be a lower incidence of the blues in Japan. Most research has been carried out in North America and Western Europe, but studies in Uganda, South Africa, and India reveal very little non-psychotic disorder after childbirth. However, methodology is vital and the seminal study of Cox[11] found Ugandan mothers depressed at the same rates as in the United Kingdom. Similar rates have been found in comparing Australian, Dutch, and Italian mothers; Greek and English mothers, and an incidence rate of 9.2 per cent in Chilean mothers.[8] Thus, there seem to be no major differences in the few cross-cultural comparisons that have been undertaken.

Presentation in primary care

In terms of its presentation and detection in primary care, post-natal depression is no different to depression occurring at other times in a woman's life, in that only around 50 per cent of cases are detected by primary care professionals in routine clinical practice.[12] Depression occurring after childbirth may show a symptom pattern different to depression occurring at other times in a woman's life. Pitt argued in his seminal study[13] that depression occurring after childbirth was 'atypical', by which he meant that there was a preponderance of neurotic symptoms such as anxiety, irritability or phobias, which tended to overshadow more classical depressive symptoms. However, a plethora of subsequent studies have failed to convince that post-natal depression is indeed atypical in terms of its phenomenology. In fact, post-natal depression is very typical of the depressive disorders seen in primary care as opposed to specialist psychiatric practice. It is to some extent the very wide variation in symptomatology which makes it difficult to diagnose, especially since some women are not aware or do not wish to believe that the symptoms from which they are suffering are due to depression.

However, even if the level of symptomatology some of these women are experiencing is not sufficient to reach the threshold demanded by the rigid diagnostic schedules, the distress caused to them is serious enough in its own right to merit attention from primary care professionals. Furthermore, there is now evidence that depressive disorders postpartum do not simply have an impact on the mother, but also on her partner, family, and friends, and most importantly, her baby. The major consequence to a woman of post-natal depression is the risk of future depression and thus her ability to function in her roles as mother, partner, friend and at work. Equally important is the impact on infant development which persists well beyond the mother's recovery. Early mother–infant interaction may be impaired and long-term prospective studies have shown impairment in cognitive and emotional development, social adjustment and in boys, behavioural problems still present in the early school years.[14]

Clinical features of post-natal depression

Thus, the clinical features of post-natal depression are primarily those of a neurotic depression. Low mood varies and is often worse later in the day—often exacerbated by tiredness. The invariable irritability can be particularly worrying for women with older children, who fear that these feelings might put their ability to care for these children safely in jeopardy. Sleep disturbance is common including initial insomnia or early waking, and in particular difficulty in returning to sleep after getting up for the baby. Tiredness and tearfulness contribute to a general feeling of inadequacy. Poor concentration and loss of appetite may be present, and loss of libido is often profound which may damage an already strained marital relationship. Vague physical symptoms such as headache, backache, and vaginal discharge, for which no cause can be found, are common. In a few women, obsessional thoughts about harming the baby are present and in a minority of women, suicide may be contemplated.

Causes

Synthesizing the research evidence on the possible causes of post-natal depression has to contend with a large number of methodological inconsistencies. Most important amongst these are the means of classifying the depression, the severity of the disorder, the timing of the disorder, and small sample sizes compounded by poor statistical analyses. However, in line with depression occurring at any other time, the classification of likely causes follows a logical sequence. It is well known that depression has a genetic component and a positive family history has often been found. In addition, since all emotional and behavioural phenomena tend to be recurrent, postnatal depression occurs more often in women with a previous history of depression, puerperal or otherwise, during pregnancy, as well as in those with a family history of depression.

Since the correlates of the blues and puerperal psychosis are likely to be hormonal, a biological basis for post-natal depression has been widely sought. However, no definite links with progesterone, oestrogen, cortisol, or prolactin have been found. Several investigators have pursued a possible relationship between thyroid dysfunction and depressive symptomatology postpartum, but the number of women included in these studies is small and as yet no definite conclusions reached. In addition, several studies have investigated possible continuities between menstrual disorders and post-natal depression based on the assumption that similar types of hormonal dysfunction might be responsible for both, but no such association has consistently been found.

Childbirth itself is a stressful physical event leading to a search for associations between the physical morbidity of pregnancy, the circumstances of the delivery, and subsequent post-natal depression. The relationships are inconsistent with some studies finding less mood disturbance in women with more pregnancy and delivery complications rather than the more expected result of an increase.[6]

Adverse life events, which are associated with depression outside the puerperium, might also increase the risk of depression after delivery. Several studies have indeed shown that higher levels of stressful life events during pregnancy and after delivery are associated with an increased risk of post-natal depression. Difficult personal relationships are an important factor, especially that of the woman and her partner. Many women with post-natal depression report a poor marital relationship after delivery but more importantly, a poor marital relationship during pregnancy is often an antecedent of post-natal depression. The evidence as to whether a woman's relationship with her parents, especially her mother, is an aetiological factor is equivocal. In general settings, social support from spouse, family and friends during times of stress is thought to help reduce the likelihood of depression and in general this finding is confirmed in studies of post-natal depression.

Diagnosis

Early detection of post-natal depression requires awareness on the part of all those in close contact with the mother. This includes partner, family, and friends who may be the first to notice that something is wrong.

Of all the groups of people with depressive illness, women with post-natal depression should be the easiest to identify. They are in regular and frequent contact with the primary health care team throughout pregnancy and the first post-natal year. The opportunity should be taken to identify those women at high risk (see above) and monitor their progress carefully. In addition, it should be possible to use the post-natal examination at about 6 weeks postpartum, or the first immunization visit for the baby at about 8 weeks, to screen all women for post-natal depression (see below).

General practitioners, as well as health visitors and midwives, need to be alert to a mother's emotional state and not concentrate solely on mother and baby's physical needs. They should be able to distinguish the symptoms of depression from normal postpartum adjustment such as the blues and be able to assess their severity and impact on mother and baby. In practice, the diagnosis of post-natal depression is frequently missed.[12] This is in part due to the fact that women are reluctant to seek help for their symptoms, some believing they are normal or understandable and in part because the professionals lack the specific skills to make the diagnosis.

An effective clinical approach requires a full mental state examination, exploring the symptoms and their impact on the woman in terms of her personality and circumstances. It is necessary to explore her relationships with her partner, baby and other children, and to establish what support is available to her. In addition, it is useful to review the events of the pregnancy and delivery, and enquire about feeding difficulties and any physical morbidity. The diagnosis of post-natal depression is not difficult if a standardized approach is utilized.

An aid to diagnosis is to use a screening instrument as it is clear that this disorder occurs in a particular segment of the population at a defined time. The Edinburgh Postnatal Depression Scale (EPDS)[15] is a screening instrument which offers the potential to identify women who are sufficiently depressed to require active management. The EPDS is a 10-item self-report questionnaire, validated for use at 6–8 weeks postpartum in research settings. It has not yet been formally validated in a UK primary care service setting. Women generally find the EPDS acceptable and understand its purpose. On its own, however, the EPDS is not sufficient to make the diagnosis of post-natal depression, which requires a clinical interview.

Management of post-natal depression

There is clear evidence from a number of studies that there are effective treatments for post-natal depression. A trusting relationship between the woman and her carer is vital and may be critical in determining her willingness to accept her diagnosis and thus treatment. Effective treatments basically comprise a choice of either psychological therapies or antidepressants.

There is good evidence for the effectiveness and acceptability of health visitor counselling.[16] An early study in the United Kingdom showed a significant reduction in depression in a group of women who received eight weekly visits of non-directive counselling compared with a control group. A smaller trial in Sweden found a similar result. A third study assessed one or six sessions of cognitive–behaviour therapy (CBT) with either fluoxetine or placebo and found at the end of 12 weeks that fluoxetine was superior to placebo, and six sessions of CBT better than one session in securing improvement. This latter is also the only controlled trial of antidepressant treatment for post-natal depression.[16] Non-directive counselling, CBT, and interpersonal psychotherapy have also been compared with usual care in a randomized trial. All therapies were superior to placebo and improvement was maintained over 18 months.[17] A different form of one to one therapy for post-natal depression, home visits from a post-natal support worker, has recently been evaluated but although women valued the service, there was no evidence of any health benefit at 6 weeks or 6 months follow-up, and the service was more expensive than routine care.[18]

Other potentially helpful therapies include peer group support, contact with those voluntary organizations dedicated to the welfare of new mothers, and discussions with carers around lifestyle issues such as healthy eating, taking regular physical exercise, and taking 'time out'.

Whilst there has only been one randomized trial of antidepressants, there is no reason to believe that they should be less effective than for depression occurring at any other time, although many women with post-natal depression are unwilling to take antidepressants and prefer a psychological approach. However, in women who fail to respond to counselling or have a severe depressive illness, antidepressant therapy is indicated. All antidepressants are secreted in breast milk, but only very small amounts are found in the plasma of breastfed infants, and there is no evidence that women should stop breastfeeding whilst taking a tricyclic or SSRI.

A Cochrane Review[19] has found that there is no place for synthetic progestogens in the prevention or treatment of post-natal depression. The role of natural progesterone has yet to be evaluated in a randomized controlled trial. Oestrogen therapy may be of modest value at a late stage of post-natal depression.

Prevention of post-natal depression

Given the prevalence of post-natal depression and its adverse sequelae, there has been a good deal of interest in preventive strategies.[20] There is, however, limited evidence that primary prevention is either possible or cost effective. Interventions during pregnancy, at delivery and in the early puerperium focusing on psycho-social support have been inconsistent in terms of reducing the incidence of post-natal depression. In practice, primary prevention means identification of high-risk women and possibly their partners being targeted by midwives and health visitors for extra support.

The role of secondary prevention, which mainly comprises early detection and treatment, has been covered earlier, but these results are only valid in the research setting. Implementing a secondary prevention strategy would require better training of primary care professionals and the routine use of a screening instrument, such as the EPDS. This strategy is now part of the National Service Framework for Mental Health.[21]

Post-natal depression outside the United Kingdom

The issues surrounding the detection and management of post-natal depression are also of concern to countries other than the United Kingdom. The meta-analysis of the rates and risks for post-natal depression[5] included studies from Western Europe, Scandinavia, North America, Australia and New Zealand, Chile, and Japan. A major influence on service provision for post-natal depression is the structure of the health care system. Thus, the strong primary care sector in the United Kingdom has to a large extent driven screening for post-natal depression by health visitors using the EPDS. In France, Italy, Austria, and Sweden their public health nurses, the equivalent of our health visitors, carry out hearing checks and do immunizations but do not screen for emotional disorders. In Sweden, the decision has been taken to set up a maternal screening programme for post-natal depression using psychologists working in the community.[22] There is a recent move by the National Department of Health in South Africa to develop policy guidelines for women's mental health, especially post-natal depression. And in New South Wales, Australia, an Integrated Perinatal Care programme aims to improve mental health in the broadest sense and uses the EPDS to screen for distress through pregnancy and the first post-natal year.

Conclusions

Post-natal depression affects around 70 000 women annually in the United Kingdom. Whilst it may be short lived in some women, it can become a chronic illness with the usual attendant adverse consequences of a chronic disorder. It can also have a major impact on the family, particularly the developing child. It is the timing of the depression that is critical, as this should enable earlier detection by health care professionals and there are known effective treatments. The major phenomenological issue as to whether post-natal depression is a distinct and unique illness remains to be clarified. Furthermore, the evidence base for both routine screening and the relative efficacy of psychological and pharmacological treatment needs to be strengthened.

Key points

- Differentiate from the 'blues' and puerperal psychosis.
- Consider post-natal depression even if low mood not pervasive.
- Assess safety of child.
- Involve health visitor and other primary care mental health professionals.
- Offer counselling/CBT and/or antidepressants.
- Consider routine screening with EPDS at 6 weeks.

References

1. **Kumar, R. and Robson, K.** (1984). A prospective study of emotional disorders in childbearing women. *British Journal of Psychiatry* **144**, 35–47.

2. **Stein, G.** (1982). The maternity blues. In *Motherhood and Mental Illness* (ed. I.F. Brockington and R. Kumar), pp. 119–54. New York: Academic Press.

3. **Kendell, R.E., McGuire, R.J., and Platz, C.** (1987). Epidemiology of puerperal psychoses. *British Journal of Psychiatry* **150**, 662–73.

4. **Cox, J.L., Murray, D., and Chapman, G.** (1993). A controlled study of the onset, duration and prevalence of postnatal depression. *British Journal of Psychiatry* **163**, 27–31.

5. **O'Hara, M.W. and Swan, A.M.** (1996). Rates and risk of postpartum depression—a meta-analysis. *International Review of Psychiatry* **8** (1), 37–54.

6. **Brockington, I.,** ed. *Motherhood and Mental Health* Chapter 3. A portfolio of postpartum disorders. Oxford: Oxford University Press, p. 135, 1996.

7. **Evans, J., Heron, J., Francomb, H., Oke, S., and Golding, J.** (2001). Cohort study of depressed mood during pregnancy and after childbirth. *British Medical Journal* **323**, 257–60.

8. **Kumar, R.** (1994). Postnatal mental illness: a transcultural perspective. *Social Psychiatry and Psychiatric Epidemiology* **29**, 250–64.

9. **Pillsbury, B.L.K.** (1978). 'Doing the month': confinement and convalescence of Chinese women after childbirth. *Social Science & Medicine* **12**, 11–22.

10. **Chalmers, B.** *African Birth: Childbirth in Cultural Transition.* River Club, South Africa: Berer Publications CC, 1990.

11. **Cox, L.** (1983). Postnatal depression: a comparison of Scottish and African women. *Social Psychiatry* **18**, 25–8.

12. **Hearn, G., Iliff, A., Jones, A., Ormiston, P., Parr, P., Rout, J., and Wardman, L.** (1998). Postnatal depression in the community. *British Journal of General Practice* **48**, 1064–6.

13. **Pitt, B.** (1968). 'A typical' depression following childbirth. *British Journal of Psychiatry* **114**, 1325–35.

14. **Murray, L. and Cooper, P.J.** (1997). Postpartum depression and child development. *Psychological Medicine* **27** (2), 253–60.

15. **Cox, J.L., Holden, J.M., and Sagovsky, R.** (1987). Detection of postnatal depression. Development of the 10 item Edinburgh Postnatal Depression Scale. *British Journal of Psychiatry* **150**, 782–6.

16. **Appleby, L., Koren, G., and Sharp, D.** (2000). Depression in pregnant and postnatal women: an evidence based approach to treatment in primary care. *British Journal of General Practice* **49**, 780–2.

17. **Cooper, J. and Murray, L.** (1997). The impact of psychological treatments of postpartum depression on maternal mood and infant development. In *Postpartum Depression and Child Development* (ed. L. Murray and P. Cooper), pp. 201–20. New York: The Guilford Press.

18. **Morrell, C.J., Spiby, H., Stewart, P., Walters, S., and Morgan, N.** (2000). Costs and effectiveness of community postnatal support workers: randomised controlled trial. *British Medical Journal* **321**, 593–8.

19. **Lawrie, T.A., Herxheimer, A., and Dalton, K.** (2001). Oestrogens and progesterones for preventing and treating postnatal depression (Cochrane Review). In *The Cochrane Library* Issue 3. Oxford: Update Software.

20. **Sharp, D.J.** (1996). The prevention of postnatal depression in primary care. In *The Prevention of Mental Illness in Primary Care* (ed. A. Kendrick, A. Tylee, and P. Freeling), pp. 57–73. Cambridge: Cambridge University Press.

21. **Department of Health.** *National Service Framework: Mental Health.* London: Department of Health, 1999.

22. **Wickberg, B.** (2000). The role of the Child Health Services in promoting mental health: an introduction. *Acta Paediatrica Supplement* **89** (434), 33–6.

10

Child health

10 Child health

10.1 Approach to the sick infant

Joe Kai

Introduction

The effective assessment of sick infants marks the epitome of primary medical care and the value of the generalist. Practitioners providing first contact care see many ill young children. They face the challenge of handling this large reactive workload in the community caringly and efficiently, while still picking out the minority of children with serious illness. As generalists they seek to avoid unnecessary treatment or referral. Yet, they must still leave parents feeling their concerns have been addressed and confident to deal with their child's illness.

All children in the first year of life will become unwell and will have acute symptoms from time to time. This includes approximately four to six episodes of acute infectious illness. In England and Wales, children aged 4 and under will be taken to their general practitioner an average of five times a year, and the consulting rate for minor illness is the highest of any patient age group.[1]

There are two key challenges for the primary care practitioner. The first is to identify the child who has serious or potentially life-threatening illness from the majority of children who have minor self-limiting problems. The second is being able to listen to parents' concerns and empower them to understand and manage their children's illness appropriately.

Causes of acute illness

Several factors predispose infants to develop acute illness. The commonest cause of acute illness is infection (see Table 1). Common and respiratory infections, otitis media, and fever are discussed in the following chapters in this section.

Neonates are particularly prone to infection either from the mother perinatally or from carers. Passive immunity resulting from maternal transfusion of IgG in the last trimester of pregnancy confers some protection to babies for 3–6 months. Premature babies are thus more vulnerable to infection.

Older infants usually acquire infectious illness through siblings and contact with other children. Other predisposing factors include impaired immune response due to malnutrition, malabsorption, chronic disease, or drugs (in particular steroids), and, more rarely, malignancy and congenital or acquired immune deficiency such as AIDS.

While infection is the commonest cause, other conditions may present as non-specific acute illness. These include the acute abdomen (e.g. intussusception or strangulated hernia), metabolic disorders such as hypoglycaemia, renal failure, the effects of drugs, and physical abuse in non-accidental injury (e.g. intracranial haemorrhage).

Table 1 Common infective causes of acute illness in infants

Respiratory infections
Upper respiratory tract infection
Influenza
Bronchiolitis
Pneumonia
Non-specific viral infections
Otitis media
Gastroenteritis
Viral exanthems (chickenpox, measles, rubella, etc.)
Urinary tract infection
Soft tissue infection
Meningitis
Meningococcal disease
Septic arthritis

Assessment of the sick infant

Detecting major illness in babies is difficult as they may show few, if any, specific symptoms or signs. Thus, it is crucial to approach the sick infant in a systematic way. Alongside careful history and physical examination, *observation* of the child is a key part of assessment. The outstanding features of serious acute illness in young babies are anorexia, impaired alertness, and floppiness.

History

In general, and in the absence of dehydration, a baby that is currently feeding well is unlikely to have major acute illness. Key points in the history should include:

- How is the baby feeding?
- Is there regular or persistent vomiting? (In addition to gastroenteritis, a non-specific feature of more serious acute illness such as urinary tract infection or meningitis.)
- Is there bile-stained vomiting? (Suggesting intestinal obstruction.)
- Is there persistent diarrhoea or blood in the stools?
- Is there a cry that is unusual? (High-pitched or moaning?)
- Has the baby been drowsy or lost interest in what is going on around him/her?
- What are the parents' beliefs and concerns about the illness?

The volume of consultations for sick children is not only time consuming but can become repetitive and frustrating for practitioners. In many consultations, early observation of the alert and smiling infant may easily lead to a potentially premature diagnosis of minor illness unlikely to require intervention. Nevertheless, methodical exclusion of serious illness should always be the first priority. While in the majority of instances it will remain clear the problem is minor, it is important to *be unhurried and listen to parents attentively.*

Parents may have particular beliefs or concerns about their child's illness, which are unfounded but understandable. For example, a parent whose child has an upper respiratory tract infection may fear that her baby's chesty cough places him in danger of choking to death in his sleep, or that his fever will escalate out of control causing brain damage.[2] Such *anxieties cannot be directly addressed if they are not exposed* by exploring them.

Although parents may be less able to assess the severity or cause of their child's illness, they know their child's normal behaviour and presentation better than anyone else. *A parent's assessment that their child is unwell demands respect.* For example, parents usually know the different cries their baby makes. If they are worried that she/he is in pain then this should be taken seriously.

Observation and examination

The infant is likely to be happier and more cooperative when held or on the parent's lap. It is helpful to precede one's approach by pretending to examine the parent or encouraging the child to play with your stethoscope before using it. Examination of the ears and throat may provoke more resistance and it is wiser to perform these last.

Observation

Assessment of movement and tone can be judged as appropriate against expected motor ability, noting, for example, if the baby is lying limply or if all limbs are active. Often, the most helpful way of assessing the degree of illness is *observing the extent of the child's interaction with his or her environment.*

◆ *What is the level of alertness?* Is the baby looking at you? Can the baby make sustained eye contact (after 4 weeks of age)? Is she/he looking around the room? On the other hand, is the child not interested in his surroundings or staring vacantly into space?

◆ *Is the baby responsive?* Is she/he smiling, reaching for things (your stethoscope or the pen you offer), playing with toys? Or is the child irritable? Most children can be consoled and will stop crying, at least temporarily, when the parent holds them. Significant illness may be more likely if crying continues, or is even made worse by being held.

Physical examination

Examination and its focus should be guided by the history, for example, seeking focal signs of infection. Key clinical points in examining the undressed infant include looking for:

◆ increased tension of the anterior fontanelle;

◆ dehydration (dry mouth, tachycardia, reduced skin turgor, sunken fontanelle and eyes);

◆ fever (rectal temperature is more accurate than axillary temperature);

◆ pallor, rash, or jaundice;

◆ intercostal or subcostal recession;

◆ tender abdomen or obstructed inguinal hernia.

Gauging illness severity

Rating scores are useful aids for evaluating illness severity. *Baby Check*[3] was originally designed to help parents assess whether a baby aged 6 months or less is significantly ill but it is also a helpful tool for practitioners. It uses items derived from a study of symptoms and signs in 1007 babies that were associated with moderate or serious illness.[4] Each item can be scored and the total score used to gauge if the baby is mildly, moderately, or seriously ill.[3] The main features of Baby Check are shown in Table 2.

The Acute Illness Observation Scales can be used to identify serious illness in *febrile* children.[5] They involve observing whether each of six items are normal, moderately impaired, or severely impaired. They include

Table 2 Features to consider in deciding the severity of acute systemic illness in a baby aged 6 months or less[3]

Item	Features to consider
In previous 24 h	
Vomiting	Regular or bile-stained?
Fluid intake	Volume reduced by a third or more?
Urine output	Fewer wet nappies/diapers than expected?
Blood in stool	Frank blood in stool?
Drowsiness	Abnormally drowsy most of the time?
Abnormal cry	Moaning or high pitched?
Examination	
Alertness	Less watchful? Less interested in environment?
Floppiness	Persistent and generalized?
Pallor	
Cyanosis of periphery	
Wheeze	Expiratory
Recession	Indrawing of intercostal or subcostal areas
Skin perfusion	Delay in reperfusion of big toe after squeezing?
Inguinal hernia	
Rash	Generalized? Purpuric?
Pyrexia	Rectal temperature >38.3

quality of cry, reaction to parent stimulation (effect on crying when held or jiggled), state variation (level of consciousness), colour, hydration, and response to social overtures. When *taken together* these items are predictive of serious illness.[5]

Brief practical guidance concerning the crying baby, breathing difficulty, meningitis, and meningococcal disease is provided below.

The crying baby

A baby presented because it is crying too much may have hunger, wind, a noisy temperament, or discomfort (e.g. soiled nappies/diapers, clothing, colic). Crying is often also attributed to teething. Crying that accompanies feeding and possetting (burping) may indicate reflux oesophagitis. Commonly, there may also be parental anxiety, family or other environmental stress in the home to which infants are sensitive. Assessing parental coping followed by explanation, reassurance, and support will be important.

If crying is of *acute onset or if the baby is unwell* (e.g. irritable and off feeds), the presence and severity of illness should be assessed as above, and organic causes excluded. These include any acute illness, commonly otitis media. Serious causes such as meningitis, injury, and intussusception (acute and severe paroxysmal crying with *marked pallor* in attacks, with or without blood in stool and palpable abdominal mass) should be considered.

Infantile colic is characterized by paroxysmal crying, a tense abdomen, and drawing up of the legs. The baby is usually only consoled by constant holding and carrying. It occurs in babies less than 3–4 months of age, typically in the evening. While traditionally thought to be intestinal in origin, its causes are uncertain. Parents should be reassured it resolves by 4 months old. They may require considerable support and sympathy. There is no convincing evidence for effective treatments or need to change infant formula milks if bottle-fed.

Breathing difficulty

Assuming the baby's nose is not blocked by a cold, the ability of a baby to take a feed is a useful guide to the existence of significant cardiac or respiratory compromise (e.g. due to bronchiolitis, pneumonia, or heart failure). Is the baby too breathless to suck normally or does she/he get tired quickly when feeding?

Peripheral cyanosis is common, with healthy babies' hands and feet going blue when cold. However, any central cyanosis with a blue tongue is always abnormal. Patterns of respiration in young healthy babies are surprisingly irregular when observed and vary, for example, with crying. In general, a respiratory rate of below 40 per minute is normal though may be higher if there is fever. A sustained tachypnoea over 50 per minute is abnormal particularly when accompanied by intercostal and subcostal recession, or the grunting common with pneumonia.

The rather coarse, added sounds of an upper respiratory tract infection transmitted to the lungs tend to differ from the more high pitched and persistent expiratory wheeze, or fine inspiratory crackles, that may reflect more significant respiratory illness or cardiac problem.

Meningitis

Meningitis should loom large in the differential diagnosis of any acutely ill child. The baby with meningitis is typically unhappy, febrile, and may be irritable or drowsy. There may be prolonged or high-pitched crying even when cuddled. Meningitis should be considered in any child under 1 year who has a seizure. In young babies, the classical neck stiffness of meningeal irritation is usually absent, and a bulging fontanelle is a late sign. Thus, any degree of tension of the anterior fontanelle should be sought. Observation of the baby's interaction and level of consciousness is the most helpful touchstone. Is the baby alert and interacting as described above?

Meningococcal disease

A non-blanching purpuric or petechial rash is the key clinical sign in diagnosing meningococcal disease. It may be scanty or generalized and is absent in 20 per cent of cases. The rash is more likely to be absent, or may actually be blanching and maculopapular, in the early stages of the disease. Ideally, all febrile children without obvious cause for fever should be fully undressed. This rash may be present in other illnesses. However, the key to diagnosis of this immediately life-threatening illness is to consider its possibility in the first place.

In those with meningococcal meningitis the likely abnormal features are of irritability, drowsiness, and decreased conscious level. However, in those with meningococcal septicaemia the child may appear alert and responsive until late in the illness. Seeking the early signs of circulatory shock (tachycardia, peripheral vasoconstriction with pallor, cool peripheries, and mottling) is key to recognition. If meningoccocal disease is suspected, children under 1 year should be given 300 mg of benzylpenicillin by intravenous or intramuscular injection before immediate transfer to hospital.

Principles of management

The majority of sick infants with minor illness can be managed in primary care by their parents given appropriate support, symptomatic advice, and reassurance. The investigation and management of common infections and fever are considered in the following chapters.

Where assessment suggests more serious illness there should be a low threshold for onward referral and specialist care. Infants are particularly at risk of systemic infection in the first month or two of life. They may deteriorate rapidly. There should be no hesitation in referring a sick neonate to hospital.

Where infants are assessed as having apparently minor and self-limiting illness, parents should be provided with advice about symptoms and signs that might suggest significant clinical change or deterioration. Practitioners should indicate a *readiness to reassess any ill baby promptly* where there is concern.

Empowering parents

Parents may have difficulty making sense of their child's illness. This can be due to inadequate information sharing by professionals (e.g. explaining 'it's just a virus'), and variations in professionals' behaviour (e.g. the inconsistent prescribing of antibiotics).[6] Parents' attempts to understand illness may be frustrated by disparity between their beliefs and expectations about illness (e.g. noisy breathing suggesting a lung infection requiring antibiotics) and professional decision-making about illness (e.g. lungs clear on auscultation suggesting self-limiting upper respiratory infection).[6] Major facets of management are being able to address parents' concerns, and to empower parents to understand and manage their children's illness appropriately.

Practitioners may do this by attending to the way they communicate with, and *listen to parents.*[6] This involves eliciting parents' concerns, beliefs, and understanding of the illness. *Sharing of appropriate information and explanation* can then be tailored to parents' particular needs. Practitioners should remember that what constitutes common technical knowledge for professionals may not be so readily accessible to parents.[2] Beyond *discussion with parents about their specific concerns* or the nature of an illness,[2] some parents may find scoring systems to help them gauge illness severity of considerable value.[7,8] The latter neither increase nor decrease demand for care.[9]

All parents worry about their children when they are ill. Moreover, parents and professionals alike worry about missing serious illness. Yet, it is easy to unintentionally undermine parents' confidence by suggesting their anxieties are unfounded. Rather, practitioners should *acknowledge and value parents' skills* in detecting their children are unwell and in providing the vast majority of children's health care without recourse to health services. When professional help is sought, the practitioner's aim is to *facilitate and empathize with parents' often-arduous task* rather than make parents feel guilty for consulting.

Finally, a history of frequent consultation may reflect the need to *address the parent's own health and well-being* rather than focus upon that of the child. New parents or mothers with several young children may need considerable support and opportunity to ventilate how they feel. They face the demands of parenting, chronic fatigue, and life and relationship transitions. In particular, practitioners should be alert to the possibility of maternal depressive illness.

A cornerstone of primary care

Consultations about ill infants are challenging in their imperative to identify serious illness, and in avoiding treating most encounters as mundane. They should be regarded both as a real test of clinical acumen and as an ideal opportunity to develop a supportive and continuing relationship with young families. This will pay dividends in addressing their future health needs. The systematic assessment of sick infants and empowering of parents is an indispensable and privileged role for the primary care generalist.

Key points

- Assess methodically.
- Observe the baby's alertness and interaction.
- Have a low threshold for referral, especially in younger infants.
- Be ready to re-assess promptly.
- Listen to parents and address their concerns.
- Empower and facilitate parents.

References

1. McCormick, A., Fleming, D., and Charlton, J. *Morbidity Statistics from General Practice. Fourth National Study 1991–1992.* London: Stationery Office, 1995.
2. Kai, J. (1996). What worries parents when their pre-school children are acutely ill and why? A qualitative study. *British Medical Journal* 313, 983–6.
3. Morley, C.J. et al. (1991). Baby Check: a scoring system to grade the severity of acute systemic illness in babies under 6 months old. *Archives of Disease in Childhood* 66, 100–6.
4. Morley, C.J. et al. (1991). Symptoms and signs in infants younger than 6 months of age correlated with the severity of their illness. *Pediatrics* 88, 1119–23.
5. McCarthy, P.L. et al. (1982). Observation scales to identify serious illness in febrile children. *Pediatrics* 70, 802–9.

6.   Kai, J. (1996). Parents' difficulties and information needs coping with acute illness in pre-school children: a qualitative study. *British Medical Journal* 313, 987–90.

7.   Thornton, A.J. et al. (1991). Field trials of the Baby Check score card: mothers scoring their babies at home. *Archives of Disease in Childhood* 66, 106–10.

8.   Kai, J. (1994). Baby Check in the inner city: use and value to parents. *Family Practice* 11, 245–50.

9.   Thomson, H. et al. (1999). Randomised controlled trial of effect of Baby Check on use of health services in first 6 months of life. *British Medical Journal* 318, 1740–4.

Further reading

Green, M., Haggerty, R., and Weitzman, M., ed. *Ambulatory Pediatrics.* Philadelphia: WB Saunders, 1999. (This text offers wide-ranging coverage of child health, and includes the Acute Illness Observation Scales referred to in this chapter.)

10.2 Childhood respiratory infections

George Rust, Yvonne Fry, and Kathi Earles

Introduction

The respiratory tract is the most common nidus of childhood infections. These infections may be localized anatomically to the upper respiratory tract (nose and paranasal sinuses, throat, and bronchial tubes) and the lower respiratory tract. Although these infections are often acute and self-limited viral syndromes, serious infections of the respiratory tract are a significant cause of hospitalizations and even deaths worldwide.

Acute viral syndromes of the upper respiratory tract

Rhinitis/laryngitis

Epidemiology, aetiology, and risk factors

Acute viral rhinitis, or the common cold, is one of the most frequently encountered infections in family medicine. Rhinovirus and coronavirus are common aetiologic agents. Because of genetic variations in the virus (rhinovirus alone has over 100 serotypes), infections do not confer immunity.

In addition to rhinitis, other self-limited upper respiratory viral infections can occur. For example, laryngitis usually occurs in children greater than 5 years old most commonly during the fall and winter months. It is usually viral in origin with parainfluenza 1 and 2, adenovirus, respiratory syncytial virus, and influenza being common.

Clinical presentation

Acute viral rhinitis typically presents with rhinorrhoea and nasal congestion, cough, 'scratchy' throat, and low-grade fever. Symptoms last 7–10 days, regardless of treatment, and nasal discharge frequently becomes mucopurulent (thicker and yellow-green) during the last few days of illness,

often leading to overdiagnosis of sinusitis or purulent rhinitis and overuse of antibiotics.

The patient with laryngitis presents with a 2–3-day history of cough, rhinorrhoea, and a low-grade fever. Hoarseness subsequently develops due to inflammatory oedema of the vocal cords and subglottic tissue. The clinical course is usually mild and the patient recovers without incident in 3–7 days.

Treatment

Management is largely supportive. Humidified air may provide comfort. Various non-prescription formulations are marketed for symptom relief, with little evidence of benefit. Antimicrobial agents are not indicated.

Children who have a history of asthma exacerbations associated with viral respiratory infections may require some increase in their anti-inflammatory regimen, such as increasing their dose of inhaled steroids or using short-course oral prednisolone or injectable decadron.

Prevention

Prevention efforts include effective hand washing, hygiene, and the avoidance of sick contacts in susceptible children.

Acute bronchitis

Epidemiology, aetiology, and risk factors

Acute bronchitis in children is most commonly due to respiratory syncytial virus or parainfluenza, and less frequently, adenovirus and rhinovirus. Secondary bacterial infections may follow with *Streptococcus pneumoniae*, *Moraxella catarrhalis*, and *Haemophilus influenzae*.

Clinical presentation

Clinically, children with acute bronchitis develop a dry and hacking cough that often progresses to a productive cough with purulent sputum. Patients may have a low-grade fever and complain of shortness of breath, low substernal or anterior chest pain. Physical findings may include signs of nasopharyngitis, conjunctival injection, and rhinitis. Auscultation often reveals course breath sounds, rales, and high-pitched rhonchi, which resemble wheezing.

Patients with repeated episodes of acute bronchitis should be evaluated for respiratory anomalies, including foreign bodies, ciliary disorders, bronchiectasis, tuberculosis, immune deficiencies, allergies, sinusitis, tonsillitis, and cystic fibrosis.

Treatment

Most patients with acute bronchitis recover uneventfully without any treatment. Supportive measures such as antipyretics, fluid, and cough suppressants may provide temporary relief. Antibiotics are generally not indicated.

Laryngotracheobronchitis (croup)

Epidemiology, aetiology, and risk factors

Laryngotracheobronchitis, or croup, is common in children between the ages of 6 months and 3 years, especially during the autumn and winter months in northern climates. The organisms that cause croup (usually parainfluenza 1 and 2, but also respiratory syncytial virus, echovirus, adenovirus, and influenza) are spread via respiratory droplets or through direct contact from contaminated fomites.

Clinical presentation

The clinical manifestation of croup, which can be very alarming to parents, are attributed to the inflammation and oedema of the hypopharynx and the narrowing of the subglottic region. Children frequently present with rhinorrhoea, low-grade fever, and cough. The character of the cough changes to a 'barky' sound within 2–3 days. The patient may also develop inspiratory stridor, and suprasternal and subcostal retractions. PA view on X-ray may reveal a long tapered area of narrowing, narrowest just below the vocal cords ('steeple sign'). Most patients experience a mild course with symptoms worsening at night due to airway drying from mouth breathing necessitated by nasal congestion.

Viral croup must be differentiated from epiglottitis (see below), caused by *H. influenzae*, in which oral examination prior to airway stabilization may lead to a potentially life-threatening airway obstruction.

Treatment

Patients with mild illness respond well to home care with supportive therapy, humidified air via a vaporizer, nebulizer or the steam from a shower and parental reassurance. Symptoms usually resolve within 3–7 days. A small percentage of patients progress to moderate to severe respiratory distress as evidenced by the development of inspiratory and expiratory stridor, nasal flaring, and wheezing. In these patients, oral examination is contra-indicated until the airway is secure.

Patients who require additional treatment are best treated in the hospital. Systemic corticosteroids provide significant benefit in hospitalized patients, as do aerosolized racemic epinephrine, and cool mist administration. The benefits of racemic epinephrine are short lived and are followed by a rebound effect. Hospitalized patients may require treatments every 20 min along with continuous mist therapy and supplemental oxygen. If symptoms do not improve or persist for greater than 1 week, laryngoscopy may be performed. A sudden deterioration marked by the development of a high fever, severe respiratory distress, and leukocytosis suggest a complicating bacterial tracheitis, which is a potentially life-threatening condition.

Bacterial infections of the upper respiratory tract

Sinusitis

Epidemiology, aetiology, and risk factors

Sinusitis is part of a continuum of respiratory illnesses including viral rhino-sinusitis, acute bacterial sinusitis, and chronic bacterial sinusitis. Approximately 30 per cent of the population will eventually have a diagnosis of sinusitis. In the United States alone there are 16 million office visits yearly for this disease process, and it is the fifth most common diagnosis leading to a prescribed medication.

The most common aetiology is bacterial overgrowth of the sinus due to impaired sinus drainage when the sinus ostia become inflamed or swollen due to upper respiratory infections, allergic rhinitis, and inhaled irritants such as tobacco smoke. Concomitant involvement of the middle ear (otitis media) and sinuses (sinusitis) is also common.

The most common bacterial causes are *S. pneumonia, H. influenza, M. catarrhalis, S. pyogenes, Staphylococcus aureus,* and, increasingly, *Chlamydia pneumonia.* Aerobic organisms predominate in the acute disease process (<3 weeks), while anaerobes are more common in chronic infections (≥6 weeks).

Clinical presentation

Children less than 12 years of age tend to present with rhinitis and cough, especially noted when lying down. They may also complain of sore throat and fever. Approximately 10 per cent of colds in children are followed by sinusitis. Adolescents complain of headache, facial pain, tenderness, and oedema. Other symptoms for both age groups include loss of smell and taste, halitosis (bad breath), aches and malaise, and green or purulent rhinorrhoea or post-nasal drip.

One may consider sinusitis as a diagnosis if the patient has upper respiratory infection symptoms for greater than 14 days, or earlier if the child presents with a high temperature (>39°C), purulent rhinitis, periorbital swelling, and headache.

Sinus X-rays are not diagnostically sensitive in sinusitis. Classical sinus X-rays showing air-fluid levels, mucosal thickening, and opacified sinuses occur in less than half of cases. Diagnosis is made based on history and physical examination, although there is significant discordance between X-ray findings, CT scan, and clinical diagnosis. In persistent cases, a CT scan may be conducted to rule out less common diagnoses or extension of infection. Flexible rhinolaryngoscopy allows for observation of the actual sinus openings. If the patient is immunocompromised, resistant to treatment, or has a life-threatening illness, the most accurate way to obtain a culture is by sinus aspiration with direct antral puncture.

Treatment

Antibiotics are frequently prescribed empirically, although several large controlled studies have failed to demonstrate benefit of antibiotic therapy in acute, uncomplicated sinusitis. This may reflect difficulties in case definition and diagnosis. If the clinical course does not improve, a change in antibiotic therapy to cover resistant organisms may be indicated.

Antibiotic therapy is empirically chosen to cover *S. pneumoniae* (30–40 per cent) non-typeable *H. influenzae* (20 per cent), and *M. catarrhalis* (20 per cent). Therapy includes initial treatment with amoxicillin, or amoxicillin-clavulanate. Cotrimoxazole (trimethoprim-sulfa) or erythromycin-sulfasoxazole may be used for penicillin-allergic patients. Newer macrolide antibiotics such as azithromycin or later-generation ephalosporins such as cefuroxime or ceftriaxone may be used in resistant cases. Treatment should continue until the patient is asymptomatic for at least 7 days (average treatment is 10–14 days).

Potential (though rare) complications include orbital cellulitis or abscess, optic neuritis, periorbital cellulitis, meningitis and associated cavernous/saggital sinus thrombosis, epi/subdural abscess and osteomyelitis.

Pharyngitis and peritonsillar infections

Epidemiology, aetiology, and risk factors

Pharyngitis by definition includes tonsillitis, tonsillopharyngitis, and nasopharyngitis. Pharyngitis or tonsillopharyngitis accounts for 5 per cent of paediatric office visits, with peak incidence in fall and winter months. It is rare in patients under 1 year of age, and is predominately observed in the 5–8-year age group. Incubation is from 1 to 5 days and spread is due to airborne transmission through oral and nasal secretions, hand-to-hand contact, or fomites. The natural history is spontaneous recovery.

Group A beta-haemolytic *S. pyogenes* is the predominant organism, causing pharyngitis in 15–20 per cent of affected school-aged children. If treatment of streptococcal pharyngitis is not adequate, 0.3 per cent (up to 3 per cent in epidemics) develop rheumatic fever, and as many as 15 per cent of cases may develop glomerulonephritis. The most common viral aetiologies are rhinovirus, adenovirus, coxsackie, and echovirus type A (enteroviruses). The latter two cause vesicular, ulcerated lesions on anterior tonsillar or soft palate and are associated with temperatures greater than 38.5°C. Coxsackie A 16 (and B) viruses are the aetiology of hand–foot–mouth disease, and present with ulcers on the oral mucosa (tongue, palate, anterior tonsillar pillars) with high temperatures.

Epstein–Barr (EB) virus causes the clinical syndrome of mononucleosis, in which pharyngitis is a prominent feature. However, these patients also may have hepatosplenomegaly, more diffuse lymphadenopathy, temperature elevation, and profound fatigue. Herpes simplex virus presents with gingivostomatitis (anterior oropharynx) with ulcerative white/yellow plaques on an erythematous base. Symptoms persist for 7–10 days.

Other causes of pharyngitis include *Neisseria gonorrhoea* and *C. trachomatis* in sexually active or abused adolescents or children. Finally, pharyngitis may be caused by any one of a long list of other pathogens, including Groups B, C, F, and G beta-haemolytic streptococci, *Corynebacterium diphtheria, Mycoplasma pneumonia, Yersinia enterolitica, Francisella tularensis, Candida albicans,* and *Coxiella burnetti.*

Clinical presentation

Patients with pharyngitis typically present with sore throat and fever. Because of the potential for disabling complications related to streptococcal pharyngitis, it is essential to differentiate between viral and bacterial aetiologies. Both present with throat pain, fever, and erythema of the tonsils and pharynx, but viral infections typically demonstrate more rhinorrhoea or conjunctivitis. Exudative lesions are present in viral and bacterial infections, while viral infections tend more towards follicular and ulcerative lesions. There are four key findings that make a diagnosis of bacterial strep throat more likely. A presumptive diagnosis of streptococcal pharyngitis may be made if three or four factors are present during a season when strep infections are common in the local community:

1. temperature greater than 38.5°C;

2. tonsillar exudates;

3. tender anterior cervical lymphadenopathy; and

4. absence of rhinorrhoea or other viral upper respiratory symptoms.

Diagnosis

Laboratory work-up consists of an in-office rapid strep antigen test, although these can be falsely negative. A throat culture should be performed for confirmation if the strep screen is negative and no treatment is given. If the throat culture is also negative, but clinical complications require confirmation of streptococcal infection, then ASO and anti-DNAase B titres may be performed. To screen for mononucleosis, one may perform a heterophil agglutination test, although this is more often falsely negative in younger children. EB viral antibody titres may also be performed, along with a complete blood count with differential, looking for lymphocytosis (50–60 per cent) and greater than 10 per cent atypical lymphocytes.

Treatment

Comfort treatment includes hydration and pain relief. Antibiotic treatment of streptococcal pharyngitis may reduce symptoms by less than a day, but is essential for preventing rheumatic fever and other complications. Penicillin V is the drug of choice for streptococcal pharyngitis, and may be given twice or three times daily. Ten days of treatment is mandatory to prevent non-suppurative (acute rheumatic fever, acute glomerulonephritis) and suppurative complications (peritonsillar abscess, otitis media, sinusitis, cervical adenitis, toxic shock). Intramuscular benzathine penicillin is an alternative. Patients with penicillin allergy may be treated with erythromycin or an oral cephalosporin. Specialist referral is indicated for peritonsillar abscess, retropharyngeal abscess, epiglottitis, and pharyngeal tumours or trauma. Controversy remains over indications for tonsillectomy.

Complications

Suppurative complications of tonsillopharyngitis include peritonsillar abscesses, lateral pharyngeal abscesses, and retropharyngeal abscesses. Peritonsillar abscesses are the most common.

The majority of cases in children occur in those less than 6 years old, and 50 per cent of those occur among infants less than 12 months of age. Retropharyngeal infections occur ten times more often than lateral pharyngeal infections in children. Lateral pharyngeal abscesses occur more often in older children.

The bacterial causes of peritonsillar abscess include alpha and gamma group A haemolytic streptococci, *S. aureus*, and oral anaerobes. Retropharyngeal abscesses result from dental abscesses, traumatic perforations (endotracheal intubation, endoscopy, and foreign bodies), and bacterial extension from the lateral pharyngeal spaces. Lateral peritonsillar abscesses result from oral infections (dental, tongue, parotid gland), pharyngitis, otitis media, and mastoiditis.

Signs and symptoms include fever, sore throat, drooling, tachypnoea, toxic appearance, decreased neck motion, poor oral intake, muffled ('hot potato') voices, stridor (50 per cent), torticollis, dysphagia, and restlessness. Peritonsillar abscesses are not associated with significant neck masses, while retropharyngeal and lateral pharyngeal abscesses are.

Complete blood count may show increased bands and segmented neutrophils. Needle aspiration may be both diagnostic (gram stain and culture) and therapeutic. Most cases of peritonsillar abscess will resolve with needle aspiration and antibiotics alone. Some experts allow for a second needle aspiration in cases with persistent fluctuance the following day, or

one may proceed to surgical incision and drainage. The imaging study of choice is CT scan of the neck, although clinical diagnosis is usually apparent.

Initial therapy is antibiotics, empirically chosen to cover beta-lactamase producing organisms, until culture results are available. Treatment is for 10–14 days.

Hospitalization may be indicated to observe for upper airway obstruction, sepsis, or resultant respiratory distress. Some children may require intubation to maintain patency of their airway while incising and draining a large abscess. Complications if treatment is delayed include severe upper airway obstruction, abscess rupture into the airway leading to asphyxiation, pneumonia, empyema, or pulmonary abscess, septic pulmonary emboli, cranial nerve palsies, or Horner's syndrome.

Epiglottitis

Epidemiology, aetiology, and risk factors

Prior to the introduction of HIB vaccine in the mid-1980s, epiglottitis was usually caused by deep tissue infection with *H. influenzae* type B and occurred most commonly in children aged 2–7, although adolescents and young adults could also be affected. In areas of the world where HIB vaccination is the norm, cases of epiglottitis have declined significantly. Causative agents now include non-typeable *H. influenzae*, as well as various streptococcal species, *S. aureus*, *Neisseria meningitidis*, *Klebsiella pneumonia*, and even Candida species or viruses.

Clinical manifestations

Symptoms begin with fever and sore throat. Over several hours, a child may begin to appear quite ill or anxious, classically drooling, and leaning forward to maintain their airway. The voice may be muffled, and there is respiratory stridor. The presentation may initially be confused with viral croup, but the child with epiglottitis is usually older, lacks the barking cough of croup, and often appears quite toxic with fairly rapid clinical deterioration.

Diagnosis

Clinical signs and symptoms lead to a presumptive diagnosis of epiglottitis. No other studies, including visual inspection of the airway or blood tests, should be undertaken unless the airway is secure, or the child is in a controlled operating room environment. Lateral soft tissue X-rays of the neck may be taken with the child sitting upright if the child has an ambiguous presentation, but only if the child is accompanied by a health professional capable of performing a potentially difficult intubation. In epiglottitis, the lateral films will show the classic 'thumb sign' of an enlarged epiglottis, and perhaps hypopharyngeal dilatation. Once the airway is secured, blood cultures and throat swabs may be taken, and a search for other foci of infection (meningitis, pneumonia, etc.) may be undertaken. A non-specific leukocytosis with left shift is typically present. Rapid latex agglutination tests of blood or urine may confirm infection with *H. influenzae* before culture results are available. Mortality rates may be as high as 15 per cent if diagnosis and control of the airway are delayed.

Treatment

Securing the airway is the most urgent treatment priority. In most cases, the child should be taken directly to the operating room, and intubated in the sitting position either by direct laryngoscopy or by fibreoptic nasolaryngoscopy. Once secured, then intravenous antibiotics may be started with coverage targeting *H. influenzae*. Combined treatment with ampicillin and chloramphenicol is the traditional regimen, although ceftriaxone or cefotaxime may be used as single agents. Rapid improvement with antibiotics is typical. Careful monitoring to prevent accidental extubation is essential.

Prevention

HIB vaccination has resulted in dramatic reductions in this disease in many countries. However, once a case is identified, antibiotic prophylaxis with rifampin is required for household contacts of all ages in households in which young children are present. Rifampin is 95 per cent effective in eliminating the carrier state.

Infections of the lower respiratory tract

Bronchiolitis

Epidemiology, aetiology, and risk factors

Acute bronchiolitis usually occurs during the fall and winter months. Children less than 2 years of age are most commonly affected, with a mean age of 6 months. Approximately 50 per cent of children experience acute bronchiolitis during the first 2 years of life. By the age of 3 years, 95 per cent of children demonstrate evidence of previous infection. Boys are affected more frequently than girls. Infants with family members who smoke in the household are more susceptible. Respiratory syncytial virus is the most commonly isolated organism, but other organisms, including adenovirus, parainfluenza, influenza, and rhinovirus, have been isolated.

Clinical presentation

Infants with bronchiolitis present with cough, sneezing, rhinitis, and low-grade fever, followed by dyspnoea and irritability. Physical examination reveals a tachypnoeic infant with a hyperexpanded chest and nasal flaring. Auscultation reveals wheezing and crackles with a prolonged expiratory phase. Air trapping, peribronchial thickening, atelectasis, and infiltrates may be present on the chest X-ray. Hypoxaemia results from ventilation and perfusion mismatching. Most patients recover without incident, but young infants, premature infants, and children with chronic disease are at special risk. Approximately 5 per cent of patients with acute bronchiolitis will require hospitalization due to severe respiratory distress.

Indications for hospitalization of children with bronchiolitis include age less than 6 months of age, hypoxaemia (PaO_2 <60 mmHg or oxygen saturation <92 per cent), rapid deterioration, apnoeic episodes, inability to tolerate oral feeding, or social concerns.

Treatment

Management of infants with mild disease may occur at home using antipyretics, fluids, and oral or aerosolized beta-2 agonists in selected patients. Hospitalized infants should receive supplemental humidified oxygen to maintain PaO_2 between 70 and 90 mmHg. Aerosolized bronchodilators, including aerosolized epinephrine, have proven benefit in a selected group of patients. Hospitalized patients may also benefit from parenteral fluids to counteract the dehydrating affect of tachypnoea. Infants with an underlying lung disorder or congenital heart disorder could be considered for administration of a specific antiviral agent, such as aerosolized ribavirin, but a meta-analysis of eight randomized controlled trials found no significant benefit. Intubation and mechanical ventilation are required to treat apnoea and respiratory failure.

Complications

Most children with acute bronchiolitis have an excellent prognosis, but those with underlying pulmonary disease, prematurity, or heart disease may be more prone to complications. Complications include respiratory failure, apnoea, atelectasis, pneumothorax, pneumomediastinum, and secondary bacterial infection.

Prevention

In a small group of infants with underlying lung disease, heart disease, or low birth weight, monthly RSV hyperimmune gamma globulin has been proven to offer some protection from severe disease. Antibiotics are indicated in secondary bacterial infection.

Pneumonia

Epidemiology, aetiology, and risk factors

Pneumonia is defined as inflammation of the pulmonary tissue with consolidation of the alveolar spaces. The most common causative organisms in children are viral, especially respiratory syncytial virus. Viral URI or bronchiolitis may also precede the onset of a bacterial pneumonia. Bacterial pathogens are responsible for only 10–30 per cent of all cases of infectious paediatric pneumonia. *S. pneumoniae* is the most common bacterial cause of childhood pneumonia, although this may soon decrease with new recommendations for universal pneumococcal vaccination. *H. influenzae* type B pneumonia is associated with bacteraemia and other deep tissue infections such as meningitis, arthritis, and cellulitis. *S. aureus* causes an aggressive pneumonia which may be preceded by a staphylococcal skin infection or by viral illnesses such as varicella (chickenpox) or measles. It is frequently accompanied by acute respiratory failure, empyema, and pneumatocoeles.

Young infants between the ages of 1 and 3 months may present with afebrile pneumonia caused by environmentally or congenitally acquired organisms such as *C. trachomatis*, *Ureaplasma urealyticum*, and cytomegalovirus (CMV). Children with immune deficiencies may present with opportunistic organisms including *Pneumocystis carinii*, gram negative enteric bacteria, anaerobes, mycobacteria, and fungi.

Clinical manifestations

Malaise, cough, chest pain, tachypnoea, and retractions are common to both viral and bacterial causes of pneumonia. Viral pneumonias are usually associated with a non-toxic appearance, low-grade fever, wheezing, cough, and stridor.

Bacterial pneumonias have the clinical presentation of a sicker-appearing child with a high fever, chills, cough, and dyspnoea. Physical findings once consolidation occurs include decreased breath sounds, dullness to percussion, and egophony on the affected side. Occasionally, the earliest diagnostic clue may be tachypnoea out of proportion to the level of fever. The white blood cell count is often elevated (>15 000) with a predominance of neutrophils.

Diagnosis

Cases of pneumonia are often diagnosed presumptively based on the clinical presentation and perhaps an X-ray. Chest X-ray findings in viral pneumonias include patchy or streaky, often bilateral, interstitial patterns and hyperinflation of the lungs. Bacterial pneumonias show classic lobar consolidation and alveolar infiltrates, although X-ray findings typically lag behind the clinical course by 1–2 days, and may be completely normal on day one. Pleural effusions may also be seen.

Sputum gram stain and culture are commonly performed, but have a low yield. Some bacterial agents may be identified via antigen detection from blood samples. *M. pneumoniae* may be diagnosed with a positive cold agglutinin test of peripheral blood. Invasive procedures such as bronchoalveolar lavage, lung aspiration, and bronchoscopy are reserved for special circumstances, such as diagnosing pneumonia in the immunocompromised host.

Treatment

Although most cases of pneumonia may be managed in the outpatient setting, infants with neonatal or congenital pneumonia less than 2 months of age should be considered for hospitalization and intravenous antibiotics. Indications for hospitalization in any patient include failure to respond or tolerate oral antibiotics, moderate to severe respiratory distress, significant deficit in oxygenation (A-a O_2 gradient), more than one area of lobar-consolidation, empyema, immunosupression, abscess formation, pneumatocoele, or underlying cardiopulmonary disease. Treatment of neonatal pneumonia should target group B streptococci, as well as gram-negative organisms such as *E. coli*. Older children with suspected bacterial pneumonia should be treated with antibiotics that provide appropriate coverage for *H. influenzae* and *S. pneumoniae* such as amoxicillin-clavulanate, cefuroxime, ceftriaxone, or azithromycin. Pneumonia in children greater than age 5 years should also include coverage for *M. pneumoniae*, using antibiotics such as erythromycin or clarithromycin. When symptoms reoccur or persist for greater than 1 month, further evaluation for an underlying condition should be undertaken (tuberculosis skin test, serum immunoglobulin, bronchoscopy, barium swallow, and sweat chloride test).

Prevention

Heptavalent pneumococcal vaccine is now recommended for all children younger than age 2, and for children age 2–5 with underlying lung disease or other chronic conditions such as HIV, heart failure, or sickle cell disease, as well as children with recurrent otitis media, children in group day care, and children in higher-risk socio-economic or ethnic groups. Influenza vaccine is also indicated for children with risk factors for pneumonia.

Tuberculosis

Epidemiology, aetiology, and risk factors

In many parts of the world, tuberculosis (TB) is one of the most common causes of fatal respiratory infection among children. Worldwide in 1990, there were 1.3 million new cases of TB among children, and as many as 450 000 deaths. In North America, TB rates rose during the decade of the 1980s, but since 1992 rates have declined by roughly one-third.

The most important risk factor for childhood TB is living in a household with an adult who has active TB. Twenty to 50 per cent of children who have household exposure will develop infections themselves. In addition, children who are born in countries with high endemic rates of TB are at risk, as are children with HIV infection or other immune deficits.

TB is caused by airborne exposure to the organism *Mycobacterium tuberculosis*, usually via contact with other infected individuals. Pulmonary TB is the most common form, although extrapulmonary forms (meningitis, peritonitis, renal, etc.) may occur in very young children (age 0–4), high-endemic populations, and in patients with impaired immunity.

Clinical manifestations

TB is a life-threatening infection in children. Children aged 0–4 are especially susceptible to haematogenous spread of the infection, such as TB meningitis and miliary TB. For typical pulmonary tuberculosis, symptoms include cough, fever, wheezing, and weight loss or failure to gain weight. Physical findings other than weight loss are scarce, but may include wheezes, rales, or signs of consolidation in the affected lung field.

Diagnosis

Skin testing is still the best method of testing for exposure to the tuberculosis organism. Intradermal testing with 5 Tuberculin Units (0.1 ml) of purified protein derivative (PPD) is more accurate than multiprong tine testing. Interpretation depends on the patient's risk of disease. Children with a history of direct exposure to active cases of TB, or with impaired immunity such as HIV, should be considered to have a positive test if the area of induration is greater than 5 mm at 48–72 h. Most other children should be considered positive with induration greater than 10 mm. Very low risk children (age greater than 5 years, no history of exposure, normal immune system, and low rates of TB in the surrounding population) would be considered positive with induration greater than 15 mm. Children vaccinated with BCG vaccine may still be accurately tested with PPD.

For children with symptoms, or with a positive PPD, a chest X-ray and sputum cultures for acid-fast bacilli (AFB) are required. Typical chest X-ray findings include hilar or mediastinal lymphadenopathy, patchy infiltrates, apical scarring, and pleural effusions. Cavitary lesions are less common in younger children. Disseminated miliary TB may show typical 'millet-seed' granulomas scattered diffusely throughout the lung fields.

Sputum cultures may be difficult to obtain from children, even using induced sputum techniques. Less than 20 per cent of children have a positive AFB smear from sputum, although three consecutive morning gastric aspirates may yield positive results in up to half of infected children. Polymerase chain reaction (PCR) techniques may detect TB in sputum samples or gastric aspirates, but the method is expensive, requires meticulous technique, and is subject to cross-contamination. Therefore, clinical diagnosis is often based on history of exposure, clinical signs, and chest X-ray findings. Because of the increasing frequency of multiply drug resistant TB, it is essential to find the index adult case and to obtain sputum cultures and drug sensitivities from that individual to guide therapy for the child with negative cultures but active disease.

Treatment

Treatment of active pulmonary tuberculosis requires a multidrug regimen for 6–12 months. Ethambutol is not recommended for children whose visual acuity can not be monitored. For uncomplicated pulmonary tuberculosis, a short-course protocol of four drugs for the first 2 months and two drugs for the next 4 months is effective. In some settings, directly observed therapy may reduce treatment failures due to non-compliance.

Prevention

The most important elements of prevention are screening for exposure, detection, and follow-up of active cases, and prophylaxis of infected but clinically asymptomatic individuals. Children with a positive PPD but no symptoms and a negative chest X-ray should be treated with isoniazid (INH) daily for 9 months.

Key points

- Patients with repeated episodes of acute bronchitis should be evaluated for respiratory anomalies, including foreign bodies, ciliary disorders, bronchiectasis, tuberculosis, immune deficiencies, allergies, sinusitis, tonsillitis, and cystic fibrosis.

- Viral croup must be differentiated from epiglottitis, caused by *H. influenzae*, in which oral examination prior to airway stabilization may lead to a potentially life-threatening airway obstruction.

- Sinusitis is common, and should be considered as a diagnosis when nasal congestion or rhinitis (especially with prolonged greenish nasal discharge) continues for an extended period of more than 10 days, even in infants. Sinus X-rays are not diagnostically sensitive in sinusitis.

- Antibiotic treatment of streptococcal pharyngitis may reduce symptoms by less than a day, but is essential for preventing rheumatic fever and other complications.

- Rule out retropharyngeal abscess in children with history of sore throat and fever, who present with torticollis, muffled speech, 'hot potato' voice, uvular deviation, neck swelling, drooling, and dyspnoea. Similar symptoms with *stridor* in a sick-appearing child also suggest the possibility of epiglottitis, a childhood emergency.

- Indications for hospitalization of children with bronchiolitis include age less than 6 months of age, hypoxaemia (PaO_2 <60 mmHg or oxygen saturation <92%), rapid deterioration, apnoeic episodes, inability to tolerate oral feeding, or social concerns.

- PPD testing is an effective screening tool for exposure to tuberculosis, even in children who have received BCG vaccination.

- In infants and young children, sputum AFB smears and cultures plus gastric aspirates each morning for 3 days may yield the diagnosis only 50% of the time. Other cases may need to be treated presumptively, based on exposure, symptoms, and chest X-ray.

Further reading

Acute viral upper respiratory syndromes

Vesa, S., Kleemola, M., Blomqvist, S., Takala, A., Kilpi, T., and Hovi, T. (2001). Epidemiology of documented viral respiratory infections and acute otitis media in a cohort of children followed from two to twenty-four months of age. *The Pediatric Infectious Disease Journal* **20** (6), 574–81.

Gupta, R., Sachdev, H.P., and Shah, D. (2000). Evaluation of the WHO/UNICEF algorithm for integrated management of childhood illness between the ages of one week to two months. *Indian Pediatrics* **37** (4), 383–90.

Greenes, D.S. and Harper, M.B. (1999). Low risk of bacteremia in febrile children with recognizable viral syndromes. *The Pediatric Infectious Disease Journal* **18** (3), 258–61.

Sinusitis

Nash, D. and Wald, E. (2001). Sinusitis. *Pediatrics in Review* **22** (4), 111–17.

American Academy of Pediatrics. Subcommittee on Management of Sinusitis and Committee on Quality Improvement (2001). Clinical practice guideline: management of sinusitis. *Pediatrics* **108** (3), 798–808.

Shrum, K.M., Grogg, S.E., Barton, P., Shaw, H.H., and Dyer, R.R. (2001). Sinusitis in children: the importance of diagnosis and treatment. *Journal of the American Osteopathic Association* **101** (Suppl. 5), S8–13.

Goldberg, A.N., Oroszlan, G., and Anderson, T.D. (2001). Complications of frontal sinusitis and their management. *Otolaryngologic Clinics of North America* **34** (1), 211–25.

Pharyngitis

Hayes, C.S. and Williamson, H., Jr. (2001). Management of group A beta-hemolytic streptococcal pharyngitis. *American Family Physician* **63** (8), 1557–64.

Gerber, M.A. and Tanz, R.R. (2001). New approaches to the treatment of group A streptococcal pharyngitis. *Current Opinion in Pediatrics* **13** (1), 51–5.

Ebell, M.H., Smith, M.A., Barry, H.C., Ives, K., and Carey, M. (2000) The rational clinical examination. Does this patient have strep throat? *Journal of the American Medical Association* **284** (22), 2912–18.

Peritonsillar abscess

Schraff, S., McGinn, J.D., and Derkay, C.S. (2001). Peritonsillar abscess in children: a 10-year review of diagnosis and management. *International Journal of Pediatric Otolaryngology* **57** (3), 213–18.

Verghese, S.T. and Hannallah, R.S. (2001). Pediatric otolaryngologic emergencies. *Anesthesiology Clinics of North America* **19** (2), 237–56, vi.

Laryngotracheobronchitis (croup)

Klassen, T.P. (1999). Croup. A current perspective. *Pediatric Clinics of North America* **46** (6), 1167–78.

Leung, A.K. and Cho, H. (1999). Diagnosis of stridor in children. *American Family Physician* **60** (8), 2289–96.

Griffin, S., Ellis, S., Fitzgerald-Barron, A., Rose, J., and Egger, M. (2000). Nebulised steroid in the treatment of croup: a systematic review of randomised controlled trials. *British Journal of General Practice* **50** (451), 135–41.

Epiglottitis

Stroud, R.H. and Friedman, N.R. (2001). An update on inflammatory disorders of the pediatric airway: epiglottitis, croup, and tracheitis. *American Journal of Otolaryngology* **22** (4), 268–75.

Nakamura, H., Tanaka, H., Matsuda, A., Fukushima, E., and Hasegawa, M. (2001). Acute epiglottitis: a review of 80 patients. *Journal of Laryngology and Otology* **115** (1), 31–4.

Bronchiolitis

Panitch, H.B. (2001). Bronchiolitis in infants. *Current Opinion in Pediatrics* **13** (3), 256–60.

Perlstein, P.H., Kotagal, U.R., Schoettker, P.J., Atherton, H.D., Farrell, M.K., Gerhardt, W.E., and Alfaro, M.P. (2000). Sustaining the implementation of an evidence-based guideline for bronchiolitis. *Archives of Pediatric Adolescent Medicine* **154** (10), 1001–7.

Garrison, M.M., Christakis, D.A., Harvey, E., Cummings, P., and Davis, R.L. (2000). Systemic corticosteroids in infant bronchiolitis: A meta-analysis. *Pediatrics* **105** (4), E44.

Pneumonia

Cherian, T., Steinhoff, M.C., Simoes, E.A., and John, T.J. (1997). Clinical signs of acute lower respiratory tract infections in malnourished infants and children. *The Pediatric Infectious Diseases Journal* **16** (5), 490–4.

Gross, P.A. (2001). Vaccines for pneumonia and new antiviral therapies. *Medical Clinics of North America* **85** (6), 1531–44.

Swedish Consensus Group (2001). Management of infections caused by respiratory syncytial virus. *Scandinavian Journal of Infectious Diseases* **33** (5), 323–8.

Roson, B., Carratala, J., Dorca, J., Casanova, A., Manresa, F., and Gudiol, F. (2001). Etiology, reasons for hospitalization, risk classes, and outcomes of community-acquired pneumonia in patients hospitalized on the basis of conventional admission criteria. *Clinical Infectious Diseases* **33** (2), 158–65.

Zimmerman, R.K. (2001). Pneumococcal conjugate vaccine for young children. *American Family Physician* **63** (10), 1991–8.

Tuberculosis

Khan, E.A. and Starke, J.R. (1995). Diagnosis of tuberculosis in children: increased need for better methods. *Emerging Infectious Diseases* **1** (4), 115–23.

Voss, L.M., The Australasian Subgroup in Paediatric Infectious Disease of the Australasian Society for Infectious Diseases. The Australasian Paediatric Respiratory Group (2000). Management of tuberculosis in children. *Journal of Paediatrics and Child Health* **36** (6), 530–6.

Joint Tuberculosis Committee of the British Thoracic Society (1998). Chemotherapy and management of tuberculosis in the United Kingdom: recommendations 1998. *Thorax* **53** (7), 536–48.

10.3 Otitis media

William R. Phillips

Ear infections are the most common cause of doctor visits for sick children, sleepless nights for parents, and antibiotic prescriptions by primary care physicians. Otitis media is a common but not a simple problem. It presents clinical dilemmas, scientific questions, and public health concerns.

Otitis media is inflammation in the middle ear space. *Acute otitis media* (AOM) is an acute illness with pus in the middle ear and signs and symptoms of infection. *Otitis media with effusion* (OME) is the persistence of effusion without signs of infection for 3 months or more. It is also called serous or secretory otitis media, or glue ear. *Recurrent otitis media* is repeated episodes of AOM with documented resolution in the intervals. *Chronic suppurative otitis media* (CSOM) is persisting infection in the middle ear with perforation of the tympanic membrane (TM) and discharge (otorrhoea).

Epidemiology

Most children get ear infections: 10 per cent by 3 months, more than half by 3 years. More than one-third will have more than three episodes of AOM by age three. About one-third of children under age 3 visit their primary care physician each year for AOM. The incidence is highest between ages 6 and 15 months.

Paralleling the pattern of viral upper respiratory infections (URIs), AOM occurs more in the winter and spring and in children exposed to more children at home or at group day care. Increased incidence of AOM is associated with: age less than 2 years, exposure to cigarette smoke, craniofacial abnormalities, and possibly pacifier use and bottle feeding (especially in the prone position). AOM and CSOM are more common among indigenous peoples in several developed countries, perhaps due to poor nutrition, crowding, or immunologic factors.

In developed countries, AOM has a high incidence and a low mortality. Serious complications are rare, but a 1954 Swedish trial reported a 17 per cent rate of mastoiditis in AOM not treated with antibiotics. The WHO estimates that 51 000 children under 5 die each year in developing countries from complications of AOM.

OME affects up to 80 per cent of children by age 10 years. Between ages 2 and 4 years 5 per cent of children at any time have OME with bilateral hearing loss for over 3 months. Placement of tympanostomy tubes or grommets for OME is the most common surgical procedure performed on children in United States and United Kingdom.

Presentation in primary care

AOM is an acute illness that presents with abrupt onset of fever, ear pain, and other local and systemic signs of infection. It often follows a viral URI. Severe pain from pus under pressure against the TM may be suddenly relieved by spontaneous rupture and drainage.

For children in countries where antibiotic treatment is routine, AOM is the most common reason for illness visits to primary care physicians and the most common reason for prescription of antibiotics. In the United States, doctor visits for ear infections more than doubled from 1975 to 1990.

AOM in a newborn may be a sign of sepsis and requires careful evaluation and possibly hospital care.

OME is the chronic persistence of non-infected fluid in the middle ear and presents with problems with hearing, development, or behaviour, not usually with ear pain or fever. It may be found on routine examination or following AOM. Effusion persists for at least 1 month in half the children with treated and resolving AOM. The diagnosis of OME should be reserved for cases lasting at least 6 weeks.

CSOM presents with persistent ear discharge through a perforated TM and occurs in patients with a history of recurrent AOM. There is usually no pain, fever, or the local tenderness and swelling that suggest otitis externa.

Causes

Bacteria causing AOM are the same as those causing other acute infections of the respiratory tract: *Streptococcus pneumoniae* (40–50 per cent), *Haemophilus influenzae* (20–30 per cent), and *Moraxella catarrhalis* (10–15 per cent). Viruses are identified in about 20 per cent and no pathogen can be found in 30 per cent or more of cases. In children aged less than 2 months, the gram-negative bacteria *Escherichia coli* and *Klebsiella* and *Staphylococcus aureus* cause about 15 per cent of AOM. Cultures of the nose and throat do not reliably identify pathogens infecting the middle ear.

S. pneumoniae is the most common cause of AOM and the least likely to resolve without antibiotic treatment. Drug resistant *S. pneumoniae* (DRSP) is a growing concern in many areas where antibiotics are used as the initial treatment of AOM. Risk factors for resistant infections include age less than 2 years, antibiotic use within 3 months, and group day care.[1]

The pattern of causative organisms may evolve with increases in drug-resistant bacteria and the use of childhood immunizations against haemophilus and pneumococcus.

Diagnosis

Diagnosis of AOM requires evaluation of the child, not just the ear. The history is of sudden onset of fever and pain. In the young child, pain is often suggested by holding, pulling, or batting at the ear, and by waking at night crying. Non-specific signs of infection may be present: lethargy, irritability, anorexia, vomiting, or diarrhoea. AOM often follows URI. Ear discharge may be present if the TM has spontaneously ruptured and this often coincides with resolution of pain. Diagnosis of AOM requires seeing signs of acute infection in the middle ear space: the TM is red, opaque, has lost its light reflex, and bulges outward under pressure obscuring the landmarks and reducing its mobility. Mobility should be tested with the pneumatic otoscope and can be measured with tympanometry.

Many of the findings in AOM are not specific and cannot be relied upon to make the diagnosis. Viral respiratory tract infections can cause fever, fussiness, obstruction of the eustachian tube, and mild redness of the TM. Fever or crying during the examination can make the TM pink.

Diagnosis of OME requires time. Persisting middle ear effusion without signs of infection must be documented with pneumatic otoscopy or tympanometry, if available. Serous effusion in the middle ear space causes dullness, distortion, and decreased mobility of the TM. The TM might also show air-fluid levels or retraction with prominent bony landmarks.

Examining the ears of a small child requires skill and patience. The embrace of a confident parent is usually the best restraint, cradling the child's head against the parent's chest and restraining its arms. Optimum examination requires skilled use of a pneumatic otoscope with bright light and a good air seal between the speculum and the ear canal. Adequate examination may require removal of cerumen and discharge from the external ear canal. Examination tools and techniques are further discussed in Chapter 3.2.

Management

Acute otitis media

Various medical and surgical treatments have been used for AOM[2] (see also Chapter 3.2). Controversy focuses on the need for routine use of antibiotics, particularly in children older than 6 months with uncomplicated AOM. Antibiotics are routinely prescribed for AOM in most western nations. In the Netherlands, however, the usual practice is to treat symptoms and observe children without immediate antibiotic treatment unless they appear systemically ill.[3] Their protocol provides close observation without initial antibiotics for 24 h in children aged 6 months to 2 years and for 72 h in children over age 2 years. Antibiotics are prescribed if the child gets worse or if improvement does not occur during the observation period. This wait-and-see approach is accepted by practitioners and parents and produces comparable results with few complications.[4–6]

In contrast to placebo, initial treatment of AOM with antibiotics shows only modest benefits in meta-analyses of randomized trials.[7–10] Treated patients have no additional reduction of ear pain at 24 h, but about 28 per cent additional reduction at 2–7 days. Since about 80 per cent of AOM cases resolve spontaneously within that period, the absolute reduction is only about 5 per cent. About 17 children need to be treated with antibiotics to eliminate one child's pain after 2 days. It appears that in most cases, by the time the antibiotic works, the infection is getting better on its own. Early antibiotic treatment can reduce the development of bilateral infection, but has not been proven effective in reducing long-term hearing loss, recurrence of AOM, or complications.[11] With this information, parents can be given a choice between immediate antibiotic treatment and watchful waiting. Reducing the use of antibiotics can also help reduce the problem of antibiotic resistance.[12]

These trials come from industrialized nations. More aggressive initial treatment might be warranted in developing countries where children have less access to primary care, difficulty with close follow-up, or greater risk of serious complications from AOM.[13]

Just because a child does not get antibiotics does not mean she/he does not get care. Pyrexia and pain are the pressing problems. Paracetamol (acetaminophen) or non-steroidal anti-inflammatory drugs given in regular, full doses for age and weight improve comfort for patients and parents. Topical analgesic drops help relieve TM pain.

If antibiotic treatment is chosen, the first-line drug is amoxicillin. Concern about drug resistant *pneumococcus* has led to recommendations to increase the dosage from the usual (40–45 mg/kg/day) to a high-dose regimen (80–90 mg/kg/day) for those at risk of infection with resistant organisms, including day care attenders and recent antibiotic users.[1] For children with penicillin allergy, erythromycin and trimethoprim–sulfamethoxazole are alternatives for initial treatment if the risk of drug resistance is low. The standard duration is 10 days in children under age 2 and 5 days in older children without risk factors for complications. Shorter treatment is less effective and longer treatment shows no advantage but more side-effects.[14]

Treatment is considered a failure if specific signs and symptoms do not improve within 3 days. Second-line antibiotic choices include: amoxicillin–clavulanate, cefuroxime axetil, and intramuscular ceftriaxone. There are few studies testing the effectiveness of other oral antibiotics, particularly in the treatment of drug-resistant organisms. No oral antibiotic eradicates all AOM bacteria. The dose of amoxicillin given in the amoxycillin–clavulanate combination can be increased without increasing risk of the diarrhoea associated with clavulanate by using a new formulation or by adding amoxicillin.

Intramuscular injection of ceftriaxone assures full treatment (a single dose or a 3-day series), even in a child unwilling or unable to take oral medicine. *Pneumococcus* that is resistant to beta-lactam drugs is often resistant to trimethoprim/sulfamethoxazole and erythromycin or other macrolides. Thus, these drugs are not good second choices for AOM that has already failed treatment.

If the child with a treatment failure has recently had multiple courses of different antibiotics, a 3-day course of ceftriaxone or tympanocentesis for culture and susceptibility testing are appropriate steps.

Antihistamines and oral or topical decongestants are not effective in reducing pain or shortening illness.

Myringotomy does not add significantly to antibiotics for treatment of AOM, but can be considered for therapy if pain is severe or for culture if treatment fails. It is important in the treatment of mastoiditis. Tympanocentesis is a skill that can be mastered by the primary care physician but requires an excellent view of the TM and absolute restraint of the child; both are often difficult to achieve.

Referral should be considered for dangerous or unusual problems: suppurative complications such as mastoiditis, meningitis, cholesteatoma, persisting TM perforation, evidence of enlarged adenoids obstructing the eustachian tubes, and persisting hearing loss or delay in language development (see Chapter 3.2).

Otitis media with effusion

Treatment of OME has also been controversial, partly because of difficulty in diagnosis, high rates of spontaneous resolution, and unknown effects on the important long-term outcomes of hearing loss and language development.

At least 65 per cent of effusions clear within 3 months with no treatment. Antibiotic treatment can speed clearing of effusion but has little long-term benefit.[15–17] Evidence-based recommendations suggest treatment for children with documented effusion that persists for more than 3 months with bilateral hearing loss of at least 20 dB. At that point, either medical or surgical treatments become options. Medical treatment is with usual antibiotics for AOM. Antihistamines, decongestants, and steroids (oral or intra-nasal) add no proven long-term benefits.

Surgical treatment is myringotomy with placement of tympanostomy tubes (also called ventilation tubes or grommets), usually performed under general anaesthesia. Increasing doubt has been cast on this procedure. Tympanosclerosis is the major complication. Tubes usually stay in place for up to a year and fall out on their own.

Recurrent otitis media

Most children get repeated ear infections. If one episode resolves clinically and another occurs after an interval of 4 weeks or more, the management is the same as for the initial episode. Recurrent otitis media is defined as three documented and distinct episodes of AOM in 6 months or four episodes in 12 months. Prophylactic daily antibiotic treatment reduces the rate of recurrence in these children, but only by about one episode per year.[10,15] Sulfasoxizole is the first-line antibiotic, with amoxycillin, trimethoprim–sulfamethoxazole, or erythromycin as effective alternatives. Prophylactic antibiotics are given daily in reduced doses over a course of 6 months. Episodes of AOM that arise during a course of prophylactic antibiotic should be treated with full doses of a different drug. Tympanostomy tube placement may also help prevent recurrent otitis media and is another alternative to long-term antibiotic use. Adenoidectomy may help in the child over 4 years of age who has clear evidence of eustachian tube obstruction and recurrent otitis media. Concern about haemorrhage limits adenoidectomy in younger children or any added benefit from tonsillectomy.

Complications

AOM can lead to TM perforation, tympanosclerosis, recurrent or chronic otitis media, and hearing loss (see Chapter 3.2). Rarely, this local infection can spread by extension leading to mastoiditis, labyrinthitis, lateral sinus thrombosis, and infection of intracranial structures. Meningitis can develop from haematogenous spread, particularly in infants. When AOM and meningitis occur together, they both most likely came from a common upper respiratory source. AOM can develop into *recurrent otitis media* or CSOM. Side-effects (common) and complications (rare) of medical and surgical treatments must be considered adverse outcomes and weighed against the benefits of any intervention for ear infections.

OME can lead to long-term conductive hearing loss with adverse impact on a child's language development and learning but these outcomes have been hard to prove.

Continuing care

The debate about antibiotics for AOM is not between antibiotic treatment versus no treatment, but between initial antibiotic treatment versus initial observation with delayed antibiotics if needed. Reducing initial antibiotic treatment requires protocols for the close monitoring of these children and systems for their follow-up care.

No clear evidence dictates the plan for follow-up of the child with AOM. The high rate of resolution, with or without antibiotic treatment, suggests that cure is likely in children who show prompt clinical resolution. Re-examination of the TM is often suggested at 3–6 weeks after initial treatment. However, the TM may still appear pink and middle ear effusion is still present in about one-third of children at this point in the resolution of AOM and does not require treatment. It is important to distinguish the residual effusion AOM from the persistent effusion of OME. Delaying follow-up examination until 8 weeks may reduce unnecessary retreatment.

Some clinicians support home use of otoscopes to allow parents to check their child's TMs if they suspect ear infection. This involves parents in their children's care and may reduce unnecessary doctor visits. However, diagnosis of AOM requires more than spotting a red eardrum.

Although no trials prove the effectiveness of interventions in preventing AOM, reducing risk factors makes sense, if only for other benefits to patients and their families. Encourage breastfeeding. Discourage cigarette smoking. Consider reducing day care exposure to many other children. Treat allergies in children who have symptomatic congestion and recurrent AOM or OME.

Immunizations against childhood diseases, such as *H. influenza*, pneumococcus, and influenza, may offer some protection against AOM and its complications and reduce the use of antibiotics.

Implications

In treating ear infections, as in most quality primary medical care, there is room for judgement in selecting the management strategy to fit the individual patient. Diagnostic criteria are not absolute. Treatment effects are modest. If the physician uses a high threshold for the diagnosis of AOM—such as high fever, intense pain, and a red, bulging TM—then early treatment with antibiotics seems reasonable. If the diagnosis rests on findings of mild fever, fussiness, and a cloudy TM, then withholding antibiotic treatment may be more prudent. If most children are initially observed without antibiotics, then those who later require antibiotics may benefit from a longer course of treatment.

The current debate about the need for antibiotic treatment for most cases of AOM is important because it deals with one of the most common encounters between patient, parent, and primary care doctor. It will affect the most common rationale for prescribing antibiotics. It will also influence the emergence of drug resistant bacteria that cause common and serious illnesses in our patients and our communities.[12]

One important adverse effect of universal early treatment of AOM with antibiotics is that it leads parents to expect antibiotics for common, self-limited infections. Doctor visits that lead to prescriptions lead to more doctor visits.

Ear infections in children provide opportunities for the primary care physician to use time as a diagnostic and therapeutic tool, to customize the treatment to the patient, to consider patient/parent preferences, and to integrate these tasks through the use of clinical judgement.

Key points

1. Most children get AOM and most cases will resolve with or without immediate antibiotic therapy. Treatment of pain and fever ease suffering of patients and parents.

2. Initial antibiotic treatment may reduce symptoms in some children at 2–7 days but does not seem to improve long-term outcomes. No clinical characteristics identify those children whose illnesses will not resolve quickly and may benefit from early antibiotics.

3. If antibiotic therapy is elected for AOM, amoxycillin is still the best first choice. Consider a high-dose regimen if drug-resistant bacteria are a concern.

4. Middle ear effusion usually resolves spontaneously within 3–6 months. Treat OME only if it persists longer and is associated with hearing loss.

5. The most important long-term patient outcomes of ear infections, hearing loss, and impaired language development are difficult to assess. No specific treatment has proven effective in reducing these problems.

6. Management of AOM provides opportunities to individualize care, partner with parents in decision-making, and reduce unnecessary antibiotic use.

References

1. Dowell, S. et al. (1999). Acute otitis media: management and surveillance in an era of pneumococcal resistance—a report from Drug-resistance *Streptococcus pneumoniae* Therapeutic Working Group. *Pediatric Infectious Disease Journal* **18**, 1–9. (Discusses clinical questions on increasing drug resistance of common AOM pathogens. Recommends high-dose amoxycillin as first-line treatment.)

2. Berman, S. (1995). Current concepts: otitis media in children. *New England Journal of Medicine* **332**, 1560–5. (Clinical review on AOM and OME with algorithm of treatment options.)

3. Froom, J. et al. (1990). Diagnosis and antibiotic treatment of acute otitis media: report from International Primary Care Network. *British Medical Journal* **300**, 582–6. (Wide variation between countries in treatment of AOM suggests antibiotics may not be needed for all cases.)

4. van Buchem, F., Peeters, M., and van't Hof, M. (1985). Acute otitis media: a new treatment strategy. *British Medical Journal* **290**, 1033–7. (Netherlands experience with selective use of no antibiotics treatment for most cases of AOM.)

5. Froom, J. et al. (1997). Antimicrobials for acute otitis media? A review from the International Primary Care Network. *British Medical Journal* **315**, 98–102. (International primary care study on use of antibiotic treatment for AOM.)

6. Damoiseaux, R. et al. (1998). Antibiotic treatment of acute otitis media in children under 2 years of age: evidence based? *British Journal of General Practice* **48**, 1861–4. (Meta-analysis of RCTs of antibiotic treatment for AOM.)

7. Rosenfeld, R. et al. (1994). Clinical efficacy of antimicrobial drugs for acute otitis media: meta-analysis of 5400 children from thirty-three randomized trials. *Journal of Pediatrics* **124**, 355–67. (Large systematic review of RCTs of antibiotics in treatment of AOM.)

8. Glasziou, P., Del Mar, C., and Sanders, S. (2001). Antibiotics for acute otitis media in children (Cochrane review). In *The Cochrane Library* Issue 2. Oxford: Update Software. (Meta-analysis of RCTs of antibiotics for AOM.)

9. Little, P. et al. (2001). Pragmatic randomized controlled trial of two prescribing strategies for childhood acute otitis media. *British Medical Journal* **322**, 336–42. (Recent RCT of early antibiotics versus wait-and-see management, showing some benefit after 24 h.)

10. O'Neill, P. (2001). Acute otitis media. *Clinical Evidence* **5**, 181–8. (Systematic review on drug treatments for acute and recurrent otitis media.)

11. Marcy, M. et al. *Management of Acute Otitis Media. Evidence Report/Technology Assessment No. 15.* AHRQ Publication No. 01-E010. Rockville MD: Agency for Healthcare Research and Quality, 2001. (Review and meta-analyses of literature on treatment of AOM using explicit methods.)

12. Dowell, S. et al. (1998). Otitis media—principles of judicious use of antimicrobial agents for pediatric upper respiratory tract infections. *Pediatrics*, **101** (Suppl. 1), 165–71. (Literature review suggests evidence-based use of antibiotics to reduce antibiotic resistant infections.)

13. Berman, S. (1995). Otitis media in developing countries. *Pediatrics* **96**, 126–31. (Most studies may not apply to management and complication rates in the developing world.)

14. Kozyrskij, A. et al. (2001). Short course antibiotics for acute otitis media (Cochrane review). In *The Cochrane Library* Issue 2. Oxford: Update Software. (Meta-analysis of RCTs of brief antibiotic treatments for AOM.)

15. Williams, R. et al. (1993). Use of antibiotics in preventing recurrent acute otitis media and in treating otitis media with effusion. A meta-analytic attempt to resolve the brouhaha. *Journal of the American Medical Association* **270**, 1344–51. (Meta-analysis of RCTs of treatments for OME and recurrent AOM.)

16. Stool, S. et al. *Otitis Media With Effusion in Young Children. Clinical Practice Guideline No. 12.* AHCPR Publication No. 94-0622. Rockville MD: Agency for Health Care Policy and Research, 1994. (Evidence-based clinical practice guideline on OME using explicit methods.)

17. Williamson, I. (2001). Otitis media with effusion. *Clinical Evidence* **5**, 359–66. (Systematic review on drug, surgical, and preventive interventions for OME.)

10.4 Fever and common childhood infections

Walter W. Rosser

Introduction

Fever in a child has always been a source of anxiety to parents, health care workers and to a lesser extent, physicians. Acute fever in a child is usually a symptom of bacterial or viral infection although there is a long list of other causes of elevated temperature. A child's temperature is considered elevated if the rectal temperature is greater than 38°C or oral temperature is greater than 37.5°C.

Fever as a symptom is generally harmless but the anxiety generated in parents by a child's fever has been called 'fever phobia' by some paediatricians. One survey found up to 94 per cent of parents feared that fever could lead to the death of their child. Anxiety is generated in parents because the child with a fever tends to appear and behave as if they are unwell. Most parents believe that the fever itself can cause brain damage or nerve damage. One of a parent's worst fears is the onset of febrile seizures, which many believe are life-threatening for their child. Given this level of anxiety, it is not surprising that there is evidence of extensive overuse and inappropriate use of health care providers, the health care system, and antipyretic medication in children.[1,2]

In contrast with parental beliefs, there is an ongoing debate in the medical community questioning the need for antipyretic treatment, since pyrexia is a sign of a healthy immune response to infection. There is some evidence that an elevated temperature facilitates the immune response. The debate is based on animal studies that have found that when fever is controlled with antipyretics the mortality in infected animals rises.[3] In the absence of human studies, the debate over the desirability of fever control is likely to continue.

The principal reason to treat the fever is to make the child more comfortable. Studies have found that only two-thirds of parents properly measured the correct amount of fever medication to give the child and less than one-third actually gave the correct dose.[4] This suggests that primary care givers need to pay more attention to instructing parents on correct dosage of antipyretic medication. Providing parents with specific written guidelines for the correct dosage may assist.

Determining the cause of fever

Newborn to 2 years

A baby with a fever is the most common reason for a child being brought to see a primary care provider either in an emergency room, surgery, or office. The duration of the fever and the temperatures measured and the accuracy of the reports need to be noted. A low-grade temperature (orally under 39°C) is usually caused by a viral infection of the upper respiratory tract. Higher temperatures are more likely to be caused by bacterial infections. Any primary care provider assessing a febrile child should conduct a complete physical examination. Specific foci of the examination should include assessment of the eardrums and pharynx, which combined account for the most common cause of fever in children under 5. Otitis media is not as simply detected as the majority of physicians assume (see Chapter 10.3). Detecting the likely aetiology and most appropriate management of pharyngitis in a child can be assisted by use of a sore throat score (see Chapter 10.2).

The chest should be observed for evidence of in-drawing. The physician should auscultate the baby's chest to detect evidence of infections. The most common causes of lower respiratory infections in the under 2 age group are broncheolitis (rhonchi), pneumonia (rales), or a consolidation (absence of respiratory sounds). A chest X-ray can improve the accuracy of diagnosis if any of these abnormalities are observed (see Chapter 10.2).

Urinary tract infections are an important cause of fever in babies under 2. The diagnosis of urinary tract infection can be confirmed by several techniques of urine collection. Using a urine bag to catch the specimen is the simplest method but risks contamination and false positive results in up to 16 per cent of specimens. Clean catch urine samples require a parent or someone to wait and attempt to catch the urine sample whenever it comes. This method has a very low false positive rate but requires patience and dexterity at catching.[5] More invasive methods include catheterization and suprapubic aspiration, depend on the skills and experience of the person performing the test.

Immediate assessment of a urine specimen is best performed by microscopy. Detection of bacteria by a skilled microscopist is the best predictor of the presence of a urinary tract infection. Dipstick urine testing lacks the specificity and sensitivity to give one confidence in the results.[6] Cultures should be performed to confirm the diagnosis and identify the infecting organism, and if appropriate its antibiotic sensitivity profile, but are of little value in making an acute diagnosis when determining the cause of a fever.

An important part of every assessment of a febrile child is the ruling out of the possibility of meningitis. Although the prevalence of meningitis has declined with extensive use of haemophilus vaccine, early diagnosis of meningitis remains very important in reducing the adverse effects of this devastating infectious disease. Physical examination to detect evidence of neck stiffness is an essential when examining any febrile baby but in children under 18 months becomes progressively less reliable with younger age. Infants under the age of 1 year, in whom there is any suspicion of meningitis deserve a lumbar puncture for early diagnosis.

Pyrexia of unknown origin: failure to detect a cause of fever in a child after physical assessment presents a dilemma for the physician. Management is determined in part by the age of the infant.

Infants less than 2 years old

Pyrexia of unknown origin has a long differential diagnosis and requires extensive investigation. Many clinicians believe that an infant with a persistently high fever and no detectable cause deserves blood cultures to detect the possibility of septicaemia and a white blood cell count. Studies have been carried out to determine the predictive value of the clinical assessment of children with fever of unknown origin. If a child has some abnormal physical findings and looks ill, they have up to a 75 per cent risk of septicaemia or serious infection. If they have abnormal physical findings but do not appear ill or toxic the risk of serious illness drops to less than 25 per cent.[7]

There is considerable debate as to whether physicians should use broad-spectrum antibiotics in infants with high fever of unknown origin prior to determining the type of bacteria and source of the infection. The alternative of the physician treating the symptom of fever, while investigating for the source of the infection and identifying the infecting agent is questionable. Studies have found that only 1.6 per cent of children with a fever of unknown origin actually have a septicaemia that justifies hospitalization and aggressive antibiotic therapy.[8] Kramer and Shapiro reviewed guidelines and meta-analysis that recommended immediate aggressive antibiotic treatment when no cause for fever in infants was found. Their finding was that studies on which widely used recommendations were based were methodologically flawed. Since true septicaemia is rare, they recommended no investigations in the febrile child with PUO who did not appear toxic, but close monitoring and at least daily reassessment. If the child appears toxic they should be hospitalized and monitored with cautious use of antibiotics.[9] In rural areas where this is not possible paediatric advice should be sought.

Children over the age of 2

The most common source of febrile illness in children over the age of 2 is the ears and upper respiratory tract. Children in this age group that are in day care may experience as many as one episode of upper respiratory tract infection per month as the spread of viral and bacterial infections in day care centres is very difficult to control.[8] Since the child is old enough to indicate that they have pain in a specific area and is also old enough to co-operate with collection of urine specimens, the difficulties experienced with the under 2 age group no longer persist. Detection of meningitis does not present the same problems as in babies where the assessment of pain and stiffness is more challenging. As the Eustachian tube opening into the naso-pharynx increase in size, obstruction that leads to frequent episodes of otitis media in those under 5 declines. History-taking from the patient becomes easier and the difficulties of detecting the source of fever experienced in those under 2 diminish.

Managing fever

Given the parental concern about fever which is based more on perception than actual risks, it is not surprising that both parents and primary care givers feel compelled to control the fever and will be reassured (possibly falsely) when the temperature approaches normal. The traditional drug for fever control was ASA, but concerns about the linkage with Reye's syndrome has seen ASA for control of infant and child fever abandoned in the 1980s. Acetaminophen (paracetamol), with its long history of safety and efficacy, has replaced ASA as the drug of choice for fever control. Over the past decade, ibuprofen has come into use for children over the age of 2 for fever control. A number of studies have found that children and adults given ASA or acetaminophen for URI actually shed the viruses for several days more than the control group and remain unwell for at least one more day.[10] Trials with ibuprofen did not find the same delayed effect. Ibuprofen carries a slightly higher rate of adverse gastrointestinal reactions compared to acetaminophen but both drugs have similar effects in temperature control.[11]

It is important to remember that the purpose of treating a child with a fever is to make the child more comfortable through lowering the temperature rather than lowering the temperature to prevent adverse effects of fever. For the comfort of the child under 2, The Canadian Taskforce found strong evidence and made a strong recommendation for using the correct dose of acetaminophen.[11] For children over 2, there is the same level of evidence supporting benefit from both ibuprofen and acetaminophen. Both drugs have a similar safety profile. An older strategy for managing a febrile child is to sponge with tepid (slightly above room temperature) water. The same task force found strong evidence but made only a moderate strength recommendation that tepid bathing adds to the comfort or lowers the fever of the child.[12]

Febrile convulsions

One of the major sources of anxiety when a child suffers from a fever is the thought of febrile convulsions. Febrile convulsions are the most common seizures at any age and peak in incidence between 18 and 22 months. By definition, the child must have both a fever and a true seizure to be diagnosed as having a febrile seizure. Most children completely recover within 1 or 2 h from the seizure and suffer no sequelae. Although most parents believe that their child is going to die when seizing, the risk of death is very low. Follow-up studies have found there is only a 2–4 per cent risk of a child who suffer a febrile seizure becoming epileptic.

Following a first febrile seizure, children have a 30–40 per cent risk of another seizure when they develop a subsequent fever.[13] Children at highest risk for recurrent febrile seizures are those whose first seizure occurred at a relatively low temperature, have a family history of febrile seizures, were under 14 months when the first seizure occurred, and had a short duration of illness when the first seizure occurred.[14]

The acute management of a febrile seizure is to end the seizing as soon as possible. In the office setting this is best achieved by inserting a syringe without needle into the child's rectum and injecting 0.5 mg/kg of

diazepam. The seizure usually stops within 1 or 2 min of the injection; the long half-life of diazepam reduces the risk of recurrence.

Once the child has stopped seizing, there should be no residual neurological signs. All children under 1 year of age should undergo a lumbar puncture (LP) to rule out meningitis, given the low predictive value of neurological signs in this age group. Children older than 1 with residual neurological signs should also undergo an LP. The yield in these two groups of an LP positive for meningitis is only 15 per cent but the benefits of early detection of meningitis justify the procedure.[15]

Once the child has recovered without any residual neurological findings or evidence of meningitis from the LP, there is no evidence that further investigations will be helpful.[15] Appropriate management of the infection or cause of the fever should proceed. Investigations such as testing the white blood cell count or the blood sugar or creatinine are of little value. An EEG, CT scans, or MRI scans have no demonstrated value in investigating an uncomplicated febrile seizure. Once the appropriate dose of diazepam has been absorbed and the cause of the fever treated, the risk of recurrence in the next 24–48 h is low and there are no further investigations or treatments that require hospitalization.

The biggest problem in this situation is the reassurance of parents terrified by having observed the seizure and fearing for the life of their child. There is no evidence that admitting the child to hospital to reassure the parents has any benefit. The primary caregiver's problem in this situation will be to reassure the parents that the child is best cared for at home. The physician might help in the process of reassurance by seeing the child within 24–48 h although there is no specific indication for such a visit. Unfortunately there is no support that rigorous use of antipyretic medication at the first sign of the next fever prevents subsequent febrile seizures.[16] The drugs used for prophylaxis have been phenobarbitol and valproic acid. Studies have found significant side-effects from both drugs and clinically insignificant benefit so they are not recommended. The peak age for febrile seizures is 14–18 months and they do not occur after 5 years. The first sign of epilepsy is a seizure in the absence of fever.

Key points

- Ninety-four per cent of parents fear that a fever in their child could lead to death.

- The most important reason to lower a child's temperature is to make them more comfortable.

- Parental education and reassurance are essential in proper fever management.

- Only 1.6% of children with a fever of unknown origin have septicaemia justifying hospitalization and extensive antibiotic use.

- There is no evidence that any treatment to prevent recurrent febrile seizures is effective.

References

1. Schmitt, B.D. (1980). Fever phobia. Misconceptions of parents about fevers. *American Journal of Diseases in Children* **134**, 176–81.

2. Kramer, M.S., Naimark, L., and Leduc, D.G. (1985). Parental fever phobia and its correlates. *Pediatrics* **75**, 1110–13.

3. Kluger, M.J., Ringler, D.H., and Anver, M.R. (1975). Fever and survival. *Science* **188**, 166–8.

4. Weinkle, D.A. (1997). Over the counter medications. Do parents give what they intend to give? *Archives of Pediatric and Adolescent Medicine* **151**, 645–6.

5. Boehm, J.J. and Haynes, J.L. (1966). Bacteriology of 'mid stream' catch urines. Studies in newborns. *American Journal of Diseases in Children* **111**, 366–9.

6. Kramer, M., Tange, S., Drummond, K., and Mills, E. (1994). Urine testing in young febrile children. A risk benefit analysis. *Journal of Pediatrics* **125**, 6–13.

7. McCarthy, P.L. et al. (1985). Predictive value of abnormal physical examination findings in ill appearing and well appearing febrile children. *Pediatrics* **76**, 16–172.

8. Glezen, W.P. (1991). Viral respiratory infections. *Pediatric Annals* **20**, 407–12.

9. Kramer, M.S. and Shapiro, E.D. (1997). Is expectant antibiotic treatment effective? *Paediatrics* **100**, 128–34.

10. Graham, M.H. et al. (1990). Adverse effects of aspirin, acetaminophen, and ibuprofen on immune function, viral shedding, and clinical status in rhinovirus infected volunteers. *Journal of Infectious Diseases* **162**, 1277–82.

11. Autert, E. et al. (1994). Comparative efficacy and tolerance of ibuprofen syrup and acetaminophen syrup in children with pyrexia associated with infectious diseases and treated with antibiotics. *European Journal of Clinical Pharmacology* **46**, 197–201.

12. Sharber, J. (1997). The efficacy of tepid bathing to reduce fever in young children. *American Journal of Emergency Medicine* **15**, 188–92.

13. Berg, A.T. et al. (1992). Predictors of recurrent febrile seizures: a prospective study of the circumstances surrounding the initial febrile seizure. *New England Journal of Medicine* **327**, 1122–7.

14. Gerber, M.A. and Berliner, B.C. (1981). The child with a simple febrile seizure. Appropriate diagnostic evaluation. *American Journal of Diseases in Children* **135**, 431–3.

15. Rutter, M. and Smales, O.R.C. (1977). Role of routine investigations in children presenting with their first febrile convulsion. *Archives of Disease in Childhood* **52**, 188–91.

16. Van Stuijvenberg, M. et al. (1998). Randomized controlled trial of ibruprofen syrup administered during febrile illness to prevent febrile seizure recurrences. *Pediatrics* **102**, 51e.

Further reading

McCarthy, P.L. et al. (1985). Predictive value of abnormal physical examination findings in ill appearing and well appearing febrile children. *Pediatrics* **76**, 16–172.

Berg, A.T. et al. (1992). Predictors of recurrent febrile seizures: a prospective study of the circumstances surrounding the initial febrile seizure. *New England Journal of Medicine* **327**, 1122–7.

van Stuijvenberg, M. et al. (1998). Randomized controlled trial of ibruprofen syrup administered during febrile illness to prevent febrile seizure recurrences. *Pediatrics* **102**, 51e.

Kramer, M.S., Naimark, L., and Leduc, D.G. (1985). Parental fever phobia and its correlates. *Pediatrics* **75**, 1110–13.

Feldman, W. *Evidence Based Pediatrics*. London: BC Decker Hamilton, 2000.

10.5 Failure to thrive

Lakshmi Kolagotla and Deborah A. Frank

Introduction

Failure to thrive (FTT) is an imprecise term that describes children who are unable to maintain normal growth rates for their age and gender.[1] It is impossible to estimate the true prevalence of FTT because there is no standard definition. In clinical practice, a diagnosis of FTT is made when a child's weight crosses two or more major percentiles on a standardized growth grid, remains persistently below the third or fifth percentile, or is less than 80 per cent of median weight for age.[2]

Usually, FTT is caused by a complex interaction of environmental and medical factors that results in inadequate caloric intake and subsequent malnutrition. Malnutrition can occur when children are not offered sufficient nutrients, ingest inadequate amounts of offered nutrients, do not retain ingested nutrients, or have pathologically increased metabolic demands that outstrip ingested nutrients. The current approach to the treatment of FTT is based on correcting the factors contributing to malnutrition and providing treatment for the complications of malnutrition including growth delay, impaired immunity, and deficits in cognitive and social development.

Historical perspective

Historically, FTT was dichotomized into 'organic' or 'non-organic' categories. Cases with underlying medical conditions were labelled 'organic'. 'Non-organic' FTT was attributed to parental neglect and was referred to as 'maternal deprivation syndrome'.[3]

Although FTT was first described in institutionalized children, clinicians eventually came to recognize that FTT could occur in intact families as well.[4] Whitten et al.[5] were the first to provide evidence that the 'maternal deprivation syndrome' was not caused by psychological factors alone. They demonstrated that maternally deprived infants developed growth failure because they were not sufficiently fed. More useful than the organic/non-organic dichotomy is the modern model of FTT in which a variety of factors interact to cause malnutrition and growth failure.

Risk factors

Poverty is the single most important risk factor for FTT, exerting its effects from the pre-natal period onwards. Maternal undernutrition before and during the pregnancy and other risk factors associated with poverty such as infection, tobacco use, and poor pre-natal care are strong predictors of low birth weight. Formerly, low birth weight infants comprised from 10 to 40 per cent of children hospitalized for FTT in several studies. Impoverished infants and children are at greater risk for infections that can interfere with growth. Families living in poverty may be less able to meet the emotional needs of their children, as they struggle to provide basic necessities. Children living in these stressful conditions may be less capable of engaging affective responses from their parents. Primary prevention of FTT must ensure that all families with children are able to meet basic material needs.[6]

FTT may be a manifestation of family dysfunction and can occur even in the presence of adequate material resources. Families of children with FTT tend to have higher levels of stress and fewer social supports regardless of income level. Family conflict has been associated with slow growth in children.[7]

FTT can also result when the *primary caretaker* is unable to perceive or act upon the cues provided by the infant. However, the majority of research thus far has focused only on maternal risk factors. In one study, FTT mothers tended to be less receptive to feeding cues from their child and were more likely to terminate feedings arbitrarily.[8] FTT mothers tend to have higher rates of depression and substance abuse disorders,[9] which can interfere with the ability to perceive and respond to the child's needs. History of abuse as an adult or child can also affect a mother's ability to interact appropriately with her children. Maternal history of sexual or physical abuse is positively correlated with FTT in the child.

Physical and mental impairments in the primary caretaker also can play an important role in FTT. Parental ill health can drain the nurturing resources of the well parent and can impair the ill parent's ability to be an effective caretaker. Mentally retarded parents may require monitoring and support to adequately care for their children and may benefit from placement with their children in a group home or from the services of a parent aide.

Children may also have characteristics that put them at greater risk for growth failure. Not surprisingly, children who have difficulty communicating, are less engaging, or require extra care are more likely to develop FTT. They are also more likely to have delays in motor and verbal development at diagnosis though it is difficult to ascertain whether these delays and behavioural difficulties precede growth failure or result from malnutrition.

Aetiology

The differential diagnosis of FTT encompasses every serious illness of infancy and childhood. Even for children with chronic medical conditions, such as congenital heart disease or cystic fibrosis, environmental and nutritional factors can still play a significant role. The more subtle organic aetiologies of FTT must also be considered in the evaluation of growth failure. Children with oral motor deficits may have difficulty maintaining adequate caloric intake because of difficulty in chewing. Children with large tonsils or adenoids can develop obstructive sleep apnoea, which has been associated with FTT. Poor dentition can make eating a painful experience leading to limited solid intake. Similarly, food allergies can be associated with unpleasant sensations of flushing or pruritus and lead to overgeneralized avoidance of foods by either child or caregiver.

FTT can also occur when parents place unnecessary restrictions on the child's diet when parents incorrectly diagnose food allergy or intolerance, adhere to strict vegan or macrobiotic diets, or have excessive concerns about obesity and heart disease.

In most cases, FTT results from an interaction of environmental and medical factors and *not* from intentional maltreatment. However, FTT can be a presentation of two specific types of child abuse, Munchausen syndrome-by-proxy (MSBP) and hyperphagic short stature (HSS). In MSBP, children are poisoned to induce vomiting or diarrhoea that can lead to growth failure. In HSS, or psycho-social dwarfism, children from stressful, frequently abusive, households develop growth deficiency. These children exhibit bizarre eating behaviours such as gorging, foraging through garbage for food, stealing and hoarding food. Since, these syndromes can have catastrophic and even fatal consequences, it is imperative that these children are diagnosed and placed in a safe environment without delay.

Evaluation

A thorough history and physical examination will provide important clues to the aetiology of FTT. Suggested aetiologies can then be confirmed or rejected through focused laboratory testing. The history should be obtained from both parents, if available. It is *impossible* to perform a complete evaluation without the input of the primary caretaker, who may not be the biological parent. The physician should take care to place the caretakers at ease and to foster a trusting, collaborative relationship.

History

The history should contain the following components: pre-natal and birth, post-natal, family, developmental, nutritional, social, and a complete review of systems. A complete review of systems will highlight diagnoses that need further exploration. The history will also be helpful in creating a medical, nutritional, and developmental plan for the child.

The pre-natal history should include information about pregnancy course, including in utero exposure to toxins, infections, and physical abuse, and the infant's gestational age, weight, length, and head circumference at birth and perinatal complications. Premature infants should be assessed using the corrected age for the first 3 years of life. The corrected age is calculated by adding the chronologic age to the gestational age and then subtracting 40 weeks.

Intrauterine growth retardation (IUGR) is diagnosed when the birth weight is lower than expected for the gestational age. Asymmetric IUGR among infants whose weight is disproportionately lower than their length and head circumference usually indicates less prolonged exposure to stress. These infants are capable of catch-up growth if provided adequate nutrition. In symmetric IUGR, the weight, length, and head circumference are all depressed. Symmetric IUGR is associated with congenital infections, genetic syndromes, and foetal toxin exposure.

Numerous legal and illegal substances have been associated with IUGR. Foetal exposure to tobacco or cocaine can cause low birth weight but does not limit the capacity for post-natal growth. In contrast, infants with foetal alcohol syndrome are born with low birth weight and will have ongoing growth failure often associated with neural, motor and other developmental deficits. These children will gain weight with continual support and monitoring but will often remain microcephalic and short for age.

The post-natal history should include information about immunizations, chronic and recurrent self-limited illnesses, past surgical procedures, medications, and allergies. A history of recurrent infections can indicate an underlying primary or secondary immunodeficiency. It is important to obtain a complete medication history since many medicines can suppress the child's appetite.

The review of systems should focus on factors that can interfere with intake, absorption, and utilization of nutrients. For example, a history of recurrent rash can suggest eczema and possible food allergy or a history of vomiting can indicate gastro-oesophageal reflux.

It is especially important to obtain the family history from both parents if possible. A family tree is helpful in highlighting miscarriages, neonatal demise, and consanguinity, alerting the clinician to the possibility of a hereditary disorder. It will also uncover any serious medical conditions in other members of the family. Serious illnesses in a child's grandparents, parents, or siblings can be stressful and bring about family dysfunction.

Parental height and weight can be helpful in evaluating the nutritional status of the parents and in estimating the growth potential of the child. Parental undernutrition can be associated with financial need or in the financially secure family, an undiagnosed illness, or eating disorder. Parental heights should be used with care in estimating the child's growth potential since chronically undernourished adults may not have reached their true potential stature. A history of delayed onset of puberty in either parent can be useful in diagnosing constitutional growth delay.

The developmental history should focus on details of current and past development. A loss of milestones can indicate a serious and degenerative disorder. A thorough developmental evaluation should be arranged for all children with signs of developmental delay.

The nutritional evaluation should include details about diet, feeding environment, and meal frequency. The clinician should enquire about types and portions of foods, including liquids, that are offered and ingested throughout the day. Information should be obtained about who feeds the child, where the child is fed, and how long it takes the child to eat a typical meal. A 24-h recall is helpful in establishing the number and timing of meals, snacks, and liquid. A child who sips on a bottle or juice cup or eats small amounts of solids all day is said to be 'grazing'. 'Grazing' and intake of large quantities of liquids with poor nutritional value, such as tea, carbonated beverages, juice, or water, can interfere with appetite and contribute to FTT.

The nutritional evaluation should also include a direct observation of a feeding interaction in the home environment if possible. This will be useful in evaluating the caretaker's knowledge of appropriate foods and portion sizes, ability to use effective feeding techniques, and the affective tone of the feeding environment. Direct observation also allows the clinician to assess the caretaker's ability to recognize and respond to the infant's cues, the infant's oral motor development, and reciprocal caretaker–infant interactions.

The clinician or a social worker should elicit information about adequacy of finances, including access to public funds for food and availability of subsidized housing for low-income families. Poor families often live in substandard housing conditions and may not have facilities for proper food preparation or storage. The social history should also include details about other aspects of the child's environment that can impact on the family's ability to nourish the child, including substance abuse, psychiatric or medical illness, homelessness, family discord, and availability of a support system. It is important to ask tactfully about a history of child abuse, domestic violence, restraining orders, and involvement of child protective services.

Physical examination

A complete physical exam should be performed, paying particular attention to signs associated with suspected aetiologies. For example, subtle dysmorphisms suggest a genetic syndrome. All children must have an accurate measurement of the weight, length, and head circumference. All measurements are performed with the child *fully* unclothed and serial measurements should be made using the same instruments to ensure validity of gains or losses.[10] The anthropometric measurements should be plotted on a standard growth curve to assess the degree of malnutrition.

Laboratory

Untargeted laboratory testing has limited diagnostic yield in the evaluation of FTT.[11,12] All children, however, should receive a complete blood count, urinalysis, and, in areas of endemic risk, a lead level. The urinalysis is useful in identifying urinary tract infection, renal tubular acidosis, and ruling out Type 1 diabetes. A bone age is helpful in children who are older than 1 year of age and whose weight is less than the fifth percentile and weight for height is greater than the 10th percentile. Children with familial short stature will have a bone age equal to their chronologic age while those with nutritional or endocrine deficiency will have a delayed bone age.[10] Seriously malnourished children should be evaluated for electrolyte abnormalities, acidosis, and dehydration, and for decreased serum albumin. In addition, these children should be evaluated for rickets with serum calcium, phosphorous, and alkaline phosphatase levels. Further laboratory investigation should be tailored to each case, including screening for HIV and cystic fibrosis in children at demographic risk.

Treatment

The goals of therapy are to correct the growth deficiency and to provide a supportive environment to diminish the effects of malnutrition on development and behaviour. An outpatient multidisciplinary team approach is preferred. The team consists of a consulting paediatrician, a social worker, a nutritionist, and a developmental specialist. Each member of the team evaluates the child and family independently and a case-specific treatment plan is implemented. The team follows the child closely and home visits are made if possible.[13]

The consulting paediatrician provides medical expertise and acts as a liaison for the primary care physician and referral services. Since these children are at greater risk for recurrent infection, the child should receive all required immunizations and additional vaccines such as the conjugate pneumococcal vaccine and yearly influenza vaccine. Clinicians should have a lower threshold for initiating antibiotics for suspected bacterial illnesses such as otitis media, sinusitis, or pharyngitis since malnourished children are relatively immunocompromised.

These children often require referral to numerous specialty services. However, referrals should be limited to only a few at a time so that the family does not become overwhelmed.

The social worker should help families apply for public sources of income, housing, food, and other subsistence support. A home visit is helpful in assessing the family living conditions. Efforts should be made to help families living in substandard housing conditions relocate to better housing if available. Children exposed to ongoing domestic violence or child abuse should be identified and referred to child protective agencies. Families and children in immediate danger should be placed in domestic violence

shelters or foster homes. Finally, caretakers who are impaired physically or mentally should receive the appropriate evaluation, treatment, and extra assistance in caring for themselves and their child.

The nutritionist should devise a concrete dietary plan based on the initial evaluation and home visit if possible. Often, modification of the frequency and timing of meals, offering whole milk, formula, or breastmilk after solids and limiting juice intake to 4 oz. or less per day, while omitting soda, tea, and water, will result in marked improvements in growth. The nutritionist should teach parents about effective feeding techniques and about age-appropriate foods and portions. The feeding environment should be discussed and a high chair provided for infants and toddlers. Children who fail to gain weight with these interventions and those with increased caloric requirements will benefit from nutritional supplements.

Malnutrition places children at risk for developmental and behavioural deficits. Children with FTT should be placed in intellectually supportive environments to ameliorate the effects of malnutrition on development.[14] Daycare and pre-school providers can be helpful in providing extra support during meals and ensuring that the child receives nutritional supplements, as well as developmental stimulation.

Though the majority of FTT can be treated on an outpatient basis, hospitalization is required for severely malnourished children and children who fail to gain weight in the outpatient setting. Children with severe malnutrition may require intravenous fluids for dehydration.

Observation in the hospital may be useful in helping to monitor caloric intake and to assess caretaker–child interaction. However, some children will eat even less in the unfamiliar setting of the hospital. Short-term nasogastric alimentation may sometimes be required. Surgical gastrostomy placement has been useful in promoting weight gain in children with FTT, but should, in general, be limited to severely handicapped or mentally impaired children who do not have long-term potential for self-feeding. It can be extremely difficult to wean children from gastrostomy tube feeds and may require behavioural therapy or another hospitalization.

Outcome

Untreated malnutrition can have long-term consequences on physical and cognitive development. Infants with FTT are more likely to be shorter and weightless than peers into late childhood.[15] Early studies showed that these children were more likely to have ongoing cognitive and behavioural deficits when compared to peers.[15,16] More recent studies controlling for demographic variables have produced conflicting results,[16] illustrating that environment interacts with the child's nutritional status and other illnesses to play an important role in predicting intellectual outcome.[17]

Key points

1. The proximal aetiology of most cases of FTT is malnutrition.

2. The dichotomization of FTT into organic and non-organic categories is now obsolete.

3. FTT arises from the interaction of a variety factors including caretaker factors, infant factors, and environmental factors.

4. A thorough history and physical examination are of utmost importance in the evaluation of the child with growth failure.

5. Successful treatment of the child with failure to thrive cannot occur without the cooperation and involvement of the primary caretaker(s).

References

1. **Zenel, J.A.** (1997). Failure to thrive: a general pediatrician's perspective. *Pediatrics in Review* **8** (11), 371.

2. Frank, D.A., Drotar D., Cook J., Kasper D., and Bleiker, J. (2001). Failure to thrive. In *Child Abuse: Medical Diagnosis and Management* (ed. R. Reese), pp. 307–38. Baltimore: Lippincott Williams and Wilkins.

3. Glaser, K. and Eisenberg, L. (1956). Maternal deprivation. *Pediatrics* 18, 626.

4. Coleman, R.W. and Provence, S. (1957). Environmental retardation in infants living in families. *Pediatrics* 19, 285.

5. Whitten, C.F., Pettit, M.G., and Fischoff, J. (1969). Evidence that growth failure from maternal deprivation is secondary to under-eating. *Journal of the American Medical Association* 209, 1675.

6. Frank, D.A., Allen, D., and Brown, J.L. (1985). Primary prevention of failure to thrive: social policy implications. In *New Directions in Failure to Thrive* (ed. D. Drotar), pp. 337–58. New York: Plenum Press.

7. Montgomery, S.M., Bartley, M.J., and Wilkinson, R.G. (1997). Family conflict and slow growth. *Archives of Disease in Childhood* 77 (4), 326.

8. Drotar, D. et al. (1990). Maternal interactional behavior with nonorganic failure-to-thrive infants: a case comparison study. *Child Abuse and Neglect* 14, 41.

9. Polan, H.J. et al. (1991). Psychopathology in mothers of children with failure to thrive. *Infant Mental Health Journal* 12 (1), 55.

10. Frank, D.A. (1999). Failure to thrive. In *Ambulatory Pediatric Care* 3rd edn. (ed. R. Dershowitz), pp. 903–7. Philadelphia: Lippincott-Raven.

11. Berwick, D.M., Levy, J.C., and Kleinerman, R. (1982). Failure to thrive: diagnostic yield of hospitalization. *Archives of Disease in Childhood* 57, 347.

12. Sills, R.H. (1978). Failure to thrive—the role of clinical and laboratory evaluation. *American Journal of Diseases in Children* 132, 967.

13. Bithoney, W.G. et al. (1989). Prospective evaluation of weight gain in both nonorganic and organic failure-to-thrive children: an outpatient trial of a multidisciplinary team intervention strategy. *Developmental and Behavioral Pediatrics* 10 (1), 27.

14. Brietmeyer, B.J. and Ramey, C.T. (1986). Biological nonoptimality and quality of postnatal environment as co-determinants of intellectual development. *Child Development* 57 (5), 1151.

15. Drewett, R.F., Corbett, S.S., and Wright, C.M. (1999). Cognitive and educational attainment at school age of children who failed to thrive in infancy: a population-based study. *Journal of Child Psychology and Psychiatry* 40 (4), 551.

16. Glaser, H.H., Heagarty, M.C., Bullard, D.M., and Pivchik, B.A. (1980). Physical and psychological development in children with early failure to thrive. *Journal of Pediatrics* 73, 690.

17. Drotar, D. and Sturm, L. (1988). Prediction of intellectual development in young children with early histories of nonorganic failure-to-thrive. *Journal of Pediatric Psychology* 13, 281.

Further reading

Frank, D.A., Drotar, D., Cook, J., Kasper, D., and Bleiker, J. (2001). Failure to thrive. In *Child Abuse: Medical Diagnosis and Management* (ed. R. Reese), pp. 307–38. Baltimore: Lippincott Williams and Wilkins.

Frank, D.A. (1999). Failure to thrive. In *Ambulatory Pediatric Care* 3rd edn. (ed. R. Dershowitz), pp. 903–7. Philadelphia: Lippincott-Raven.

Sills, R.H. (1978). Failure to thrive—the role of clinical and laboratory evaluation. *American Journal of Diseases in Children* 132, 967.

Berwick, D.M., Levy, J.C., and Kleinerman, R. (1982). Failure to thrive: diagnostic yield of hospitalization. *Archives of Disease in Childhood* 57, 347.

Zenel, J.A. (1997). Failure to thrive: a general pediatrician's perspective. *Pediatrics Review* 8 (11), 371.

10.6 Anticipatory guidance and prevention

Walter W. Rosser

As a child grows from baby to toddler to pre-school and school-aged, the risks of injury and the importance of early detection of problems changes. This chapter will deal with anticipatory guidance according to four age groups and focus on the strength of evidence supporting physician or primary care provider interventions that reduce risks and improve health outcomes.

There is accumulating evidence that physician advice in isolation from the community has minimal impact. A concerted effort by physicians and other primary care providers with community agencies and service organizations to promote child safety is essential. Working with the community to advocate for laws to improve child safety (i.e. auto-restraint systems) achieves major improvements in child safety. Evidence supporting statements or interventions is classified according to the criteria used by the Canadian Task Force on the Periodic Health Examination.[1]

Newborn (birth to 1 year)

Screening

Number of well baby physician visits in the first year of life

The number of well baby visits recommended in the first year of life is a source of controversy. The American Academy of Pediatrics recommends 10 well baby visits in the first 2 years of life. The Canadian Pediatric Association recommends five visits in the first year of life. Gilbert et al. conducted a trial in Canada to determine if there was a difference in child and parental outcomes when well babies had five or 10 visits in the first 2 years. They found no difference in outcomes between the two groups, although those randomized to the five-visit group averaged seven visits during the 2 years as did those in the 10-visit group.[2]

The current practice of discharging mother and newborn from birthing facilities within 24–48 h of birth has prompted concern that a visit within 5–7 days of discharge is also needed. However, there is no evidence supporting this practice.

Screening for physical and psychological development

Simple assessment by physicians of the approximate stage of development of the child according to age specific guidelines is a fair way of detecting children with delayed development. Routine use of instruments, like the Denver Development Screening Test, have not been shown to be beneficial.[3] Routinely measuring height, weight, and head circumference provide little assistance in detecting developmental delay.[4]

Although there is no randomized controlled trial demonstrating benefit from early detection of strabismus or amblyopia, most clinicians agree that early detection and correction prevents visual impairment. The red reflex in the eye should be assessed to detect congenital cataracts at all early well baby visits. The light reflex from the cornea and the patch test should be used routinely to assess the alignment of the eyes.

The parents or grandparent's observations of a child's response to noise is the best screening test for hearing impairment. Evidence does not support the use of neonatal auditory brain stem response measurement as a screening test.[5]

Early detection of developmental dysplasia of the hip is best done using Barlow's and Ortolani's tests at every well baby visit. Barlow's test is done by exerting longitudinal pressure on the two adducted hips to detect abnormal movement in the joint. Ortolani's test is by abducting the hip; a 'clunk' is felt as the dislocated hip is reduced. Early detection and appropriate treatment of hip dysplasia prevents subsequent disability. The skill of the clinician in performing these manoeuvres influences their positive predictive value (see Chapter 10.8).

Routine testing of haemoglobin levels in infants remains controversial. Many clinicians believe that all children at high risk for iron deficiency (children living at or below the poverty level, premature, or low birth weight infants, and infants fed only non-iron fortified formulas) should have a haemoglobin test at 9–12 months of age.[6]

Anticipatory guidance

Although the primary care practitioner may find the list of effective counselling strategies long, some time should be spent at each well baby visit providing counselling. Excellent materials are available on the internet and from local health departments. Parents will be overwhelmed with safety information if they receive everything on the first well baby visit. Ideally the physician or other provider should plan to discuss two or three issues on each well baby visit (Table 1). When contemplating the time needed for counselling in a busy practice, remember that the evidence demonstrates that 2 or 3 min of carefully structured counselling during well baby visits is more effective at improving babies' health than time spent on physical assessment. Use of a check list or flow sheet on the medical record, to track and assure that priority preventive topics are discussed, can improve efficiency.[7]

Since injuries are the most common causes of death and morbidity in children, preventive counselling should emphasize child safety. Children under 1 year of age are completely dependent on parents for their safety. The primary caregiver's relationship with the parents provides an important opportunity to facilitate developing a safe environment for the child.

Restraint in an automobile is the first step in creating a safe environment for the newborn. It is beneficial to counsel parents about proper baby care restraints during pre-natal care and assisting with seat restraints at the time of newborn hospital discharge. Providing loans or financial assistance to purchase approved baby seats is effective. Brief counselling during well baby visits promoting auto restraint systems and babies riding in the back seat is effective.[8] Programmes run by community service clubs to promote proper child restraint combined with enforcement of laws requiring restraints for babies has reduced the auto injury rate.

Children under 1 year of age are at risk for falls usually from modest heights such as beds or change tables. There is evidence that providing parents with information about preventing falls at well baby visits reduces the number of injuries.[9]

Burns and scalds are the third most common cause of injury in children under 1 year of age. The temperature of the hot water supply should be below 130°F or 54.4°C. Counselling parents to check the hot water temperature and be aware of risks around fires or stoves has been beneficial. Reinforcing the need for continuous supervision when bathing is important to prevent drowning in the under 1 age group.

Babies after the age of 5–6 months begin to grab anything within reach and put it into their mouths. Parents need to be alerted to prevent access to small coins, buttons, or anything smaller than 2 cm in diameter to prevent choking.

Children from 1 to 5 years old
Screening

The ideal number of visits for children in this age group is unknown. Many clinicians suggest annual well child visits. There is little evidence of benefit from annual visits as screening becomes less important with age while child safety concerns increase in importance.

Parental concerns about child development often result in the use of instruments like the Denver Developmental Screening Test even though they have not been found to be helpful. The recommendation is that each concern raised by parents should be dealt with by reassurance or as a diagnostic problem.

Table 1 Anticipatory guidance and prevention: newborn (birth to 1 year)

Frequency	Screening to prevent	Intervention	Quality of evidence	Strength of recommendation
First four to five well baby visits	Detection of developmental abnormalities	Clinical assessment for abnormalities	I	A
Each well baby visit	Developmental delay	Clinical assessment for developmental delay	II-2	B
Every well baby visit	Failure to thrive or obesity	Measuring height, weight, and head circumference	II-2	B
Every well baby visit	Decreased visual acuity or amblyopia or strabismus	Testing of eyes for opacity and fusion	II-1	B
Early well baby visits	Early detection of impaired hearing	Brainstem evoked response	II-2	C
All well baby visits	Developmental dysplasia of the hip	Examining hip with Ortolani's or Barlow's manoeuvre	II-1	B
Injury prevention in newborn to 1 year of age				
During pre-natal care and the first three well baby visits	Injury in automobiles	Counselling at pre-natal and well baby visits for car seat use	I	A
During one or two well baby visits	Injury in automobiles	Counselling to prevent front seat riding	I	A
First well baby visit	House fire injury	Counselling to install smoke alarms	I	A
		Counselling about home fire safety	I	A
Visits around 6–9 months	Electrical injury	Counselling about outlet covers and electrical safety	I	A
First well baby visit	Scalds from hot water	Counselling for lower hot water tank temperature and other scald prevention	I	A
Second and third well baby visits	Prevention of falls	Counselling about approved safe cribs, stair guards, and not purchasing walkers	I	A

Strength of recommendation: A, recommended; B, recommended with reservations; C, does not make a difference; D, some evidence of causing harm; E, good evidence of causing harm.

Quality of evidence: Level 1, good quality RCTs supporting evidence; Level 2, no RCTs but good quality evidence from other trials; Level 3, opinion.

Height and weight are measured on a regular basis although growth and weight gain may be sporadic after the age of 1. The increasing incidence of obesity in children is a concern yet there remains little evidence of long-term benefit from diet or nutrition counselling for parents of pre-school children.[4]

There is one study that found that visual acuity testing of preschool children using a modified Snellen chart reduced vision problems in school.[10]

Hearing problems in pre-school children in the absence of congenital hearing deficiency are likely due to chronic otitis media, thus hearing assessment should be considered for pre-school children only if there is fluid behind the eardrum.

Although urinalysis is performed on most medical visits, there is no evidence of benefit from early detection of renal disease or urinary tract infection. False positive results cause anxiety and unnecessary tests.[11] The problem for clinicians is to persuade parents that the physician is competent and thorough in the absence of urine testing.

The routine Mantoux skin test for tuberculosis is not recommended for children in developed countries except in populations at increased risk. Testing of high-risk groups of children known to have been exposed to tuberculosis is recommended.[12]

Anticipatory guidance

The list of effective counselling topics seems lengthy, however the use of structured short messages with supportive print material is practical and effective.

As the child becomes more mobile and physically stronger during the first and second year of life, the types of risk change. Falls from windows and down stairs are more dangerous. The toddler can pull pots from the stove, touch hot elements, or stick objects into electrical plugs (Table 2). The risk of drowning in ponds, streams, and swimming pools increases.

Poisoning results from the ability to open cupboards or drawers. Auto-restraint becomes difficult as the mobile child resists.

The risk of poisoning can be reduced, by counselling parents about the use of cupboard locks where toxic or hazardous substances are stored. Parental instruction on first aid procedures for poisoning improves child outcomes.[9]

Counselling parents to use stair gates and window guards reduces the risk of falls.

Many physicians believe that baby walkers should be banned, but removing their wheels provides an alternative. Counselling parents about the inherent danger of walkers is effective.

Children aged 5 and older
Screening

The issue of the ideal frequency of well child visits in this age group remains unanswered. The medical recommendation is for annual visits. Teenaged children have increasing reluctance to attend their primary health care provider, especially if the provider cares for other family members. Adolescents often seek medical assistance at birth control or STD clinics.

Screening for height, weight, vision, and hearing in this age group is not considered of value unless there is a complaint from the child or the school. Questions about school performance, emotional, and psychological development and behaviour may require reassurance or referral for psychology or child psychiatry evaluation.

During visits for children over 6, blood pressure should be measured on three different occasions using a small cuff that covers no more than two-thirds of the upper right arm (Table 3). If blood pressure is consistently elevated (from tables of normal blood pressure) then investigation is indicated. Two-thirds of children at a child hypertension clinic with elevated blood pressure were found to have a renal cause, 10 per cent another physical cause

Table 2 Anticipatory guidance and prevention: age 1–5 years

Frequency of action	To prevent	Intervention	Quality of evidence	Strength of recommendation
Age 2	Developmental delay	Denver developmental test	II-2, II-3	C
All well child visits	Abnormal growth	Measure height and weight	II-2	B
On visits where child is over weight	Obesity	Counselling about diet and nutrition	II-2	C
Pre-school visits	Problems with visual acuity	Modified Snellen chart assessment	II-1	B
Pre-school visits	Hearing problems	Pure tone audiometry	II-1, II-2	D
Pre-school visits	Renal disease Urinary tract infections	Dipstick urinalysis in asymptomatic children	II-2 II-1	D E
Pre-school visits	Early detection of tuberculosis	Mantoux skin test	II-2	E
Visits after 1 year of age	Automobile injuries	Counselling about auto restraint and seat belt use	I	B
Visit around 2 years of age	House fire injury	Counselling about smoke alarms and house fire safety	I	A
Visits at 1 year or before child becomes mobile	Electrical injury	Counselling about outlet covers and electrical safety	I	A
Visit when child becomes mobile	Scalding	Counselling about stove dangers and hot water tank temperature	I	A
Visits when the child becomes mobile	Poisoning	Counselling about cupboard locks and proper storage of hazardous materials; also counselling on first aid for poisoning	I	A
Visits when the child becomes mobile	Falls	Counselling about window guards and latches, gates for stairs	I	A

Strength of recommendation: A, recommended; B, recommended with reservations; C, does not make a difference; D, some evidence of causing harm; E, good evidence of causing harm.

Quality of evidence: Level 1, good quality RCTs supporting evidence; Level 2, no RCTs but good quality evidence from other trials; Level 3, opinion.

Table 3 Anticipatory guidance and prevention: age 5 years or older

Age when intervention is recommended	To prevent	Intervention	Quality of evidence	Recommendation
Between 6 and teenaged years	Adverse effects of high blood pressure in early adulthood	Measure blood pressure	II-3	B
Between 10 and 14 years	Scoliosis	Adams forward-bending test	II-2	B
Any visit	Renal disease	Urine dipstick	II-2	D
Any visit	Asymptomatic infection	Urine dipstick for WBC	I, II-1	E
Any visit	Auto injury	Counselling about seat belt use	II-2	B
Any visit after child begins to ride a bicycle	Prevent injury	Counselling on helmet use	I	C
Any visit after child begins to ride a bicycle	Prevent head injury	Counselling and provision of a subsidized helmet	I	A

Strength of recommendation: A, recommended; B, recommended with reservations; C, does not make a difference; D, some evidence of causing harm; E, good evidence of causing harm.

Quality of evidence: Level 1, good quality RCTs supporting evidence; Level 2, no RCTs but good quality evidence from other trials; Level 3, opinion.

and 25 per cent essential hypertension. Early detection of hypertension can prevent cardiovascular problems and hypertension-related mortality.[13]

Routine screening for anaemia, haemoglobinopathies, and tuberculosis are not appropriate. Screening for renal disease or infections by urinalysis is not effective.

Anticipatory guidance

Road accidents are the main cause of death and injury. More than half of these injuries occur when the child is a passenger in a car. Injuries from bicycles and as pedestrians have their highest incidence in 14-year-old boys. Interventions in the physician's office to prevent pedestrian injuries have not been evaluated. Effective prevention involves intersection engineering and public and school campaigns to increase safety knowledge. Legislation to enforce safe driving practices and consideration of pedestrians by vehicle drivers is important. Safety regulations involving the operation of school buses are important in school age child safety. If safety legislation is inadequate, physicians should become child health advocates.

Automobile restraint counselling in the primary care office setting diminishes in value as the child becomes older, stronger, and more independent. Strictly enforced seat belt laws with stiff fines for non-compliance represent the most effective strategy to improve auto-restraint of children in this age group.

Development of bicycle lanes and bicycle paths separated from roadways are community strategies that reduce bicycle injuries. Intensive education programmes in schools or the community about bicycle safety for children are important since the under-14 age group accounts for 40 per cent of injuries and mortality from bicycles.

Trials assessing the effect of counselling children or parents on visits to an office or emergency room after bicycle-related injuries do not result in parents purchasing more bicycle helmets. Offers to subsidize the cost of bicycle helmets had minimal effect.[14]

Teenagers

Screening and anticipatory guidance

There are only two screening procedures to consider in adolescents. Blood pressure assessment is recommended on three occasions over several years as outlined for those over 6. The other procedure is to screen for scoliosis in children between the ages of 10 and 16 using the Adams forward-bending test. Although there is considerable controversy about benefits of treatment, this procedure is recommended.

Anticipatory guidance in children in their teens is influenced by the rapid increase in risk-taking behaviour. After intensive school campaigns against smoking, surveys estimate that 85 per cent of children under 16 have tried to smoke at least once resulting in 25–30 per cent becoming smokers in North America. In some countries, the numbers are considerably higher. A similar but less dramatic pattern exists with alcohol consumption, and illicit drug use. Most of the power to reduce the societal loss generated by teenaged risk-taking behaviour is not in the physician's office but through legislation. Raising the price of cigarettes, making birth control clinics more accessible, and introducing graduated licensing laws slows the uptake of risk-taking behaviour. Given the failure of many efforts at counselling of teenaged children, the physician's role, other than to educate teenagers about the potential consequences of their choices, is limited. Physicians and primary health care providers should continue to advocate for appropriate safety legislation.

Key points

- Seven well baby visits in the first 2 years of life should be planned.
- Preventive screening in the first year of life should focus on detection of congenital anomalies that can be corrected and prevent life-long disability.
- One to 3 minutes should be spent on each well baby visit promoting injury prevention facilitated with written material.
- For 2–5-year-old children, injury prevention involving motor vehicles, drowning, falls, or burns predominate.
- Advocacy promoting raising the price of cigarettes and the driving age are the most effective preventive strategies for adolescents.

References

1. **The Canadian Task Force on the Periodic Health Examination.** *Canadian Guide to Clinical Preventive Health Care.* Ottawa: Canada Communications Group, 1994.
2. **Gilbert, J., Feldman, W., and Siegal, L.** (1984). How many well baby visits are necessary in the first two years of life? *Canadian Medical Association Journal* **130**, 857–61.
3. **Glascoe, F., Martin, E., and Humphrey, S.** (1990). A comparative review of developmental screening tests. *Pediatrics* **86**, 547–54.
4. **US Preventive Services Task Force.** *Guide to Clinical Preventive Services: Report of the US Preventive Services Task Force* 2nd edn. Baltimore MD: Williams and Wilkins, 1996, pp. 219–29.
5. **Bachmann, K.R. and Arvedson, J.C.** (1998). Early identification and intervention for children who are hearing impaired. *Pediatric in Review* **19** (5), 155–65.

6. American Academy of Pediatrics CoPAoCaFH (1995). Recommendations for preventive pediatric health care. *Pediatrics* **96**, 373–4.

7. Panagiotou, L., Rourke, L.L., Rourke, J.T., Wakefield, J.G., and Winfield, D. (1998). Evidence based well baby care. Part 2. Education and advice section of the next generation of the Rourke baby record. *Canadian Family Physician* **44**, 568–72.

8. Berger, L.R., Saunders, S., Armitage, K., and Schauer, L. (1984). Promoting the use of car safety devices for infants. An intensive health education approach. *Pediatrics* **74**, 16–19.

9. Clamp, M. and Kendrick, D. (1998). A randomized controlled trial of general practitioner safety advice for families with children under five years. *British Medical Journal* **316**, 1576–9.

10. Feldman, W., Milner, R., Sackett, B., and Gilbert, S. (1980). Effects of pre school screening for vision and hearing on prevalence of vision and hearing problems 6–12 months later. *Lancet* **2**, 1014–16.

11. O'Mara, L.M., Issacs, S., and Chambers, L.W. (1992). Follow-up of participants in a pre school hearing screening program in child care centers. *Canadian Journal of Public Health* **83**, 373–8.

12. Canadian Pediatric Society IdaIC (1994). Childhood tuberculosis: current concepts in diagnosis. *Canadian Journal of Pediatrics* **1**, 97–100.

13. Gillman, M. and Ellison, R. (1993). Childhood prevention of essential hypertension. *Pediatric Clinics of North America* **40**, 179–94.

14. Cushman, R., James, W., and Waclawik, H. (1991). Physicians promoting bicycle helmets for children: a randomized trial. *American Journal of Public Health* **81**, 1044–6.

Further reading

Clamp, M. and Kendrick, D. (1998). A randomized controlled trial of General Practitioner safety advice for families with children under five years. *British Medical Journal* **316**, 1576–9.

Panagiotou, L., Rourke, L.L., Rourke, J.T., Wakefield, J.G., and Winfield, D. (1998). Evidence based well baby care. Part 2. Education and advice section of the next generation of the Rourke baby record. *Canadian Family Physician* **44**, 568–72.

US Preventive Services Task Force. *Guide to Clinical Preventive Service: Report of the US Preventive Service Task Force* 2nd edn. Baltimore MD: Williams and Wilkins, 1996, pp. 219–29.

Feldman, W. *Evidence Based Pediatrics*. London: BC Decker Hamilton, 2000.

10.7 Disorders of growth

Lewis C. Rose

Immunization and antibiotics have made childhood safer from infections. Now the doctor must place more emphasis on prevention of disease and early detection of treatable problems. Changes from the expected growth pattern provide important information about the health of the child and may give the first warning of a growth disorder. The record of a child's growth is most useful when it is started at birth and continues until growth is complete. If deviations occur, their nature, rapidity, and age of onset help to establish their significance.[1]

Measurement

A child less than 2 years old should be weighed without clothing. Older children can be weighed wearing light clothing without shoes. The practice of weighing an adult holding the child and then subtracting the weight of the adult is too inaccurate for medical use.

Before the age of 3, the head–heel length should be determined with the child lying stretched on a measuring board. It is inadequate to mark the infant's head and the heel positions on the paper of the examination table, then measuring the distance between the marks. After the third birthday, the height can be measured with the child standing without shoes with the heels touching a wall. A flat object is placed horizontally on the head, and the child is invited to push it up the wall without raising the heels. A mark is made where the flat object touches the wall and the distance measured to the floor. The steel measuring bar and hinged head-arm attached to a weighing scale can be used for older children.

Head size is measured with a tape stretched around the largest circumference of the head from the occipital to the frontal prominences. If the child is struggling, this measurement should be repeated two or three times. Older children whose head growth has always been normal do not need to have their head circumference plotted.

Errors of measurement and recording are quite common. Whenever there is an unexpected finding, the physician should recheck all the measurements independently. Anomalies that persist through two or more visits are more likely to be important than those seen just once.

The World Health Organization has approved printed standard growth curves. If the doctor uses these to record the progress of each child, a disorder of growth can be detected earlier and more easily. Within the standard curves, lines highlight the 95th, 90th, 75th, 50th, 25th, 10th, and 5th percentiles to be expected of normal children as they grow older.

Growth curves require thoughtful interpretation. The growth curves used in most doctors' offices in the United States are based on data collected from a large group of white children in Yellow Springs, Ohio, as part of the Fels Longitudinal Study, and published in 1979. They may not represent the whole truth in the twenty-first century, or when used in other settings. They illustrate the wide range of normal that exists in any group. To be tracking close to the 50th percentile is not more normal than to be following the 20th percentile, it is just more common. Parents are interested to see how their child is doing compared with a 'normal' child of the same age. They may be disappointed to see their child appearing at the 10th percentile, or pleased to see their child above the 90th percentile. The doctor must explain the meaning of these findings so that the parents will understand why they are useful.

The curves also show the period of very rapid relative growth during the first 3 months of age, slowing of growth between the ages of 6 and 9 years, and accelerated growth of puberty between 10 and 15 years of age. More recent studies remind us that what was true of the population of Ohio in the 1970s may no longer be true today and is not exactly true for other populations in other locations.[2,3] For growth curves to be meaningful, the measurements must be taken carefully and consistently.

Normal growth

When normal growth is occurring, the child's parameters usually will be in proportion. If a small boy is on the 20th percentile for height, usually he also will be close to the 20th percentile for weight and head circumference. When rechecked later, he will have grown in all directions, and his weight, height, and head circumference will remain at the 20th percentile for his new age. In babies who start with a low birth weight, there is often, but not always, a gradual catch up or change towards or beyond the mean.[4–7] Traditionally, children are measured when seen for their immunizations, at 2 weeks, 2 months, 4 months, 6 months, 12 months, and 15 months, and once each year thereafter. Babies under 1 year change quickly and as the need for intervention is much more urgent, growth parameters that appear abnormal should be rechecked within 1 or 2 weeks. As the child gets older, the interval to recheck can be longer.

Generalized growth acceleration

This child will be growing faster than expected, crossing the percentile lines in an upward direction. The parents are often pleased, believing this to be evidence of their good care. Because any child may grow at varying speeds, such acceleration may be transient and normal.[8] It also occurs normally during the puberty growth spurt. If the acceleration persists, and the child is not adolescent, then an excessive food intake is most likely. Hypothyroidism, cortisol excess, and other endocrine problems may cause weight gain, but not usually a proportional increase in height. An endocrine work-up is indicated in doubtful cases.

Generalized growth retardation

In this case, the graphs of all three of the child's measurements will drop below the previous percentile lines; for example, a boy, having been at about the 50th percentile for height and weight, drops to the 40th, and then the 25th line. Because head growth is very slow after 2 years of age, older children with generalized growth retardation will exhibit little or no change in the head curve. Untreated juvenile diabetes will slow growth, or cause weight loss, but its onset is usually sudden and dramatic. This diagnosis does not depend on the growth curves. Usually, a generalized slowing of growth should trigger investigations for endocrine disease, such as hypothyroidism, panhypopituitarism, diabetes insipidus, human growth hormone (HGR) deficiency, or tissue resistance to HGR. General debilitating diseases such as congenital or acquired heart disease, chronic pulmonary disease, renal failure, or chronic infections may cause this growth retardation. Severe malnutrition in infancy may be a cause, but while the level of under-nutrition seen in highly developed nations may cause a change in the weight curve, it is unlikely to affect the height or head circumference curves. Stunting of growth in the first 2 years of life has been shown to be associated with school absenteeism and poor performance in cognitive tests. These problems are probably caused by the same factors, including poverty, chronic infections, overcrowding, and family disruption that cause the stunting. Any intervention should not address nutrition alone, but all these factors.[9,10]

Stable disproportion

This occurs when one or two parameters are inconsistent with another, but the inconsistency remains constant. For example, some children are always overweight. In such a case, the child's height and head circumference follow the 50th percentile through many visits, but the weight is always at or beyond the 80th percentile. This is childhood obesity. Observation of other family members may show that high-calorie diets are usual in that household, and discussion of diet and exercise may help the entire family.

Disproportionate head growth can be due to several causes. Hydrocephalus is discussed below under *Increasing head circumference*. Achondroplasia slows the growth of the limbs and facial bones, leaving a disproportional large calvarium. If the disproportion of the head remains stable, and no signs or symptoms of neurological disease can be found at subsequent visits, then the child may normally have a large head. If some of the relatives have large heads the cause may be genetic rather than acquired.

Stable disproportion of stature

Some children are always tall or short for age. The family of origin may share these characteristics. There is a guideline that suggests that a boy will be 6.2 cm (2.5 in) taller, and a girl will be 6.2 cm (2.5 in) shorter than the average of the height of the mother and father. This is confounded by the general increase in stature that has occurred with successive generations. A short child may always have a short stature relative to the weight and head circumference, but continue steadily along the same height percentile line. Many of the causes of generalized slow growth may first be noticed as short stature. Hormonal causes should be ruled out. X-ray of representative epiphyses will reveal the child's bone age. If the bone age is normal, the child has genetic short stature and the adult stature will be appropriate for the

child's genetic forebears. If the bone age is delayed, the child has constitutional short stature and can be expected to grow to normal adult height eventually. In both these cases there is nothing to be gained by further investigation or attempts at treatment. Many normal variations in adult bodily habitus first appear as stable disproportions in childhood.[11,12]

Unstable disproportion

In this case, one parameter becomes more and more out of line with the others. This is the most ominous finding (see Fig. 1).

Increasing weight out of proportion to height

This may be due to:

◆ Endocrine disorders

  ▪ cortisol excess (Cushing's disease),

  ▪ hypothyroidism,

  ▪ thalamic or pituitary disorders,

  ▪ syndrome X (insulin resistance, hypertension, obesity).

◆ Genetic disorders

  ▪ Down syndrome,

  ▪ Lawrence–Moon–Biedl syndrome,

  ▪ Prader–Willi syndrome.

◆ Psycho-social factors

  ▪ family eating habits,

  ▪ depression.

When weight is increasing more rapidly than the height or head circumference, the most common reason is obesity. Post-pubertal girls may be pregnant. Certain groups such as adolescents of American-Indian or Mexican descent may have Type 2 diabetes. Fluid retention may mimic weight gain. Investigations should depend on the clinical findings, but may include urinalysis for protein and blood chemistry.[13]

Lagging weight

This may be due to:

◆ under-nutrition,

◆ failure of a major organ system, especially GI, renal, pulmonary, cardiovascular,

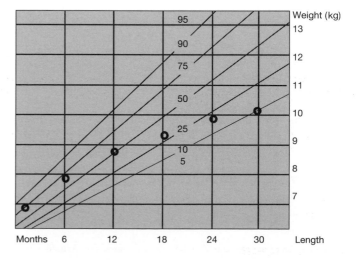

Fig. 1 Unstable disproportion. The child's weight has dropped from the 75th to the 10th percentile.

- diabetes,
- hypothyroidism,
- iron deficiency,
- lead intoxication,
- inborn errors of metabolism,
- zinc deficiency,
- malignancy,
- immune deficiencies,
- HIV infection,
- psycho-social deprivation,
- child abuse.

The abused, neglected, malnourished child may continue to grow taller while the weight remains stationary or increases only very slowly. In older children and adolescents, there may be smoking, alcohol or drug abuse, anorexia nervosa, or other psychiatric or behavioural problems. With so many possibilities a careful history taken from one or more adults, and directly from the child interviewed alone, may help to shorten the list. This topic is dealt with more fully in the chapter on failure to thrive (Chapter 10.5).[14]

Increasing height

This may be due to:

- growth hormone excess, spontaneous or from hormone abuse,
- Klinefelter syndrome,
- XXY-syndrome,
- Marfan syndrome,
- acromegaly,
- homocysteinuria,
- hyperthyroidism.

A disproportional increase in height may occur normally during puberty as the child grows out of pre-pubertal fat. Hormone assays and X-rays of the skull may be useful.

Lagging height

This may be due to:

- growth hormone deficiency,
- hypothyroidism,
- chronic anaemia,
- chromosomal disorders (e.g. Turner's syndrome),
- failure of a major organ system especially GI, renal, pulmonary, cardiovascular,
- skeletal dysplasia/rickets,
- psycho-social deprivation.

A child whose height growth slows while the weight continues to increase may have just completed adolescence, and come from short heavy parents. Otherwise, investigation for growth hormone deficiency or resistance, diabetes insipidus, or premature fusion of the epiphyses is warranted.

Increasing head circumference

This may be due to:

- hydrocephalus
  - primary,
  - secondary to associated CNS disease such as Arnold–Chiari malformation.
- megalencephaly

  - primary,
  - secondary to associated CNS disease such as neurofibromatosis or tuberous sclerosis,
  - secondary to metabolic storage disease such as Krabbe disease.

If the infant head is increasing more rapidly than the height and weight, then hydrocephalus may be the cause, requiring urgent evaluation. A CT of the spine may show spina bifida occulta. Referral to a neurosurgeon is mandatory.

Lagging head circumference

This may be due to:

- craniosynostosis
- prenatal insult
  - maternal drug or alcohol abuse,
  - maternal infection,
  - complications of pregnancy/birth.
- Chromosome defects.

A child with craniosynostosis (tower skull) has premature closure of the cranial sutures. The fontanels will close clinically well before the first birthday. X-rays of the skull show fusion of the sutures and MRI may show the loss of brain volume. Prompt referral for surgical separation of the bones of the calvarium is required to prevent loss of intellect.

Conclusion

If there are good records of a child's growth, and health professionals who understand their importance, growth disorders can be suspected and investigated early. Often the child and parents can be reassured that nature is taking its normal course. Sometimes focused investigation of a growth abnormality will reveal a curable disorder that might have been devastating if left untreated.

Key points

- There are very wide variations in normal growth.
- Normal growth rates are not constant, but vary from week to week, and from age to age.
- Parents may not raise the question of an unusual growth pattern in their child.
- Regularly plotting the child's height, weight, and head circumference on a standardized chart is the best way to confirm that growth is normal.
- Regularly plotting the child's height, weight, and head circumference on a standardized chart is most sure to reveal deviations from normal early enough for intervention.

References

1. Leglre, J.D. and Rose, L.C. (1999). Assessment of abnormal growth curves. *American Family Physician* **59** (4), 784–6.
2. Martins, S.J. and Menezes, R.C. (1997). A mathematical approach for estimating reference values for weight-for age, weight-for-height, and height-for age. *Growth, Development and Aging* **61** (1), 3–10.
3. Binns, H., Senturia, Y.D., LeBailly, S., Donovan, M., and Christoffel, K.K. (1996). Growth of Chicago area infants 1985 through 1987. Not what the reference curves predict. *Archives of Pediatric and Adolescent Medicine* **150** (8), 842–9.

4. Guo, S.S., Roche, A.F., Chumlea, W.C., Casey, P.H., and Moore, W.M. (1997). Changes in weight, recumbent length, and head circumference for pre-term low-birth-weight infants during the first three years of life using gestation adjusted ages. *Early Human Development* **47** (3), 305–25.

5. Karlberg, J., Albertsson-Wickland, E., Baber, F.M., Low, L.C., and Yeung, C.Y. (1996). Born small for gestational age: consequences for growth. *Acta Paediatrica Supplement* **417**, 8–13.

6. Eriksson, J.G. et al. (1999). Catch-up growth in childhood, and death from coronary heart disease: a longitudinal study. *British Medical Journal* **318**, 427–31.

7. Strauss, R.S. and Dietz, W.H. (1998). Growth and development of term children born with low birth weight: effects of genetic and environmental factors. *Journal of Pediatrics* **133** (1), 67–72.

8. Hermanussen, M. et al. (1998). Periodic changes of short term growth velocity (mini growth spurts) in human growth. *Annals of Human Biology* **15**, 103–9.

9. Mendez, M. and Adair, L. (1999). Severity and timing of stunting in the first two years of life affect performance on cognitive tests in late childhood. *Journal of Nutrition* **129**, 1555–62.

10. Polychronakos, C. et al. (1988). Transient growth deceleration in normal short children. *European Journal of Pediatrics* **147**, 582–3.

11. Zachmann, M. (1978). Diagnosis of treatable types of short and tall stature. *Postgraduate Medical Journal* **54**, 121–9.

12. Mahoney, C.P. (1987). Evaluation the child with short stature. *Pediatric Clinics of North America* **34**, 825–49.

13. Brook, C.C.D. (1982). The fat child. In *Growth and Assessment in Childhood and Adolescence*, pp. 96–111. Oxford: Blackwell Scientific Publications.

14. Bithoney, W.G. et al. (1992). Failure to thrive/growth deficiency. *Pediatrics in Review* **13**, 453–60.

Further reading

Legler, J.D. and Rose, L.C. (1998). Assessment of abnormal growth curves. *American Family Physician* **58** (1), 153–8.

Binns, H., Senturia, Y.D., LeBailly, S., Donovan, M., and Christoffel, K.K. (1996). Growth of Chicago area infants 1985 through 1987. Not what the reference curves predict. *Archives of Pediatric and Adolescent Medicine* **150** (8), 842–9.

Guo, S.S., Roche, A.F., Chumlea, W.C., Casey, P.H., and Moore, W.M. (1997). Changes in weight, recumbent length, and head circumference for pre-term low-birth-weight infants during the first three years of life using gestation adjusted ages. *Early Human Development* **47** (3), 305–25.

Strauss, R.S. and Dietz, W.H. (1998). Growth and development of term children born with low birth weight: effects of genetic and environmental factors. *Journal of Pediatrics* **133** (1), 67–72.

Zachmann, M. (1978). Diagnosis of treatable types of short and tall stature. *Postgraduate Medical Journal* **54**, 121–9.

10.8 The child with a limp

Robert B. Salter

In this era of complex diagnostic methods, much useful information can still be obtained simply by observing patients, especially the way in which they walk. The patient's gait is an essential part of the physical examination. Indeed, important diagnoses often go undetected because the busy physician, seeing large numbers of children, has failed to have them walk back and forth in such a way that he or she can actually analyse their gaits.

Table 1 A classification of the causes of limp in childhood

1. Painful conditions
   (a) Trauma
   (b) Inflammation
   (c) Avascular necrosis of epiphyses
   (d) Certain neoplasms

2. Neurologic disorders
   (a) Flaccid paralysis
   (b) Spastic paralysis
   (c) Ataxia

3. Muscular disorders
   (a) Muscular dystrophy
   (b) Myodystrophia foetalis (amyoplasia)
   (c) Ischaemic muscle contracture (Volkmann)

4. Joint disorders
   (a) Stiffness (fibrous and bony ankylosis)
   (b) Contracture
   (c) Instability (subluxation and dislocation), developmental displacement of the hip

5. Bony deformity
   (a) Leg length discrepancy
   (b) Developmental coxa vara
   (c) Adolescent coxa vara (slipped capital femoral epiphysis)
   (d) Genu valgum
   (e) Torsional deformities of the lower extremities

6. Functional states
   (a) Hysteria

7. Mimicry

A 'walkway' of 20–30 ft is ideal, but a well-lit corridor or hallway will suffice, provided the patient is ensured privacy.

Normal gait consists of a series of rhythmic, well-coordinated, painless movements of the lower extremities and the pelvis. The gait of a normal child varies considerably during the growing years from the toddler phase through childhood and adolescence to adult life.

Although the variations of normal gait in children are innumerable, it is usually obvious, when a child is actually *limping*. Parents are acutely aware of any limp in their children. Consequently they consult their physician early to find out *why* their child is limping and *what* can be *done* about it. Therefore, the physician must be able to analyse the child's gait accurately so that pertinent investigations may be carried out, the correct diagnosis made, and treatment instituted. Some limps are almost pathognomonic of a specific disorder, but often the limp is but one physical sign that necessitates carefully evaluating the child's symptoms, eliciting other physical signs and, when indicated, investigating further by diagnostic imaging and laboratory examination.

Classifying the causes of limp in childhood provides a framework upon which the differential diagnosis of the limp can be built (Table 1).

Painful conditions

A child who experiences pain on walking usually has the good sense to limit such activity. The gait resulting from pain is a protective limp (antalgic gait, literally 'against pain') characterized by placing the foot down gently on the affected side, taking a shorter step with the affected extremity and then rapidly shifting the weight back to the normal extremity. Fortunately, the child of walking age can localize the pain, but the possibility of referred pain must be considered—especially pain in the knee referred from the hip, and pain in the hip referred from the spine or lower part of the abdomen.

Trauma

The traumatic causes of painful limp include skin irritation from ill-fitting shoes; lacerations and foreign bodies in the feet; ligamentous strains and sprains; muscle tears; fatigue fractures and undisplaced fractures, especially 'toddlers fractures' of the tibia.

Inflammation

Any inflammatory process in the lower extremities, lumbosacral spine, and even in the lower portion of the abdomen will result in a painful limp. The commonest inflammatory conditions in children causing a painful limp are idiopathic monarticular synovitis (especially in the hip joint), acute rheumatic fever, rheumatoid arthritis, acute osteomyelitis, and septic arthritis.

Avascular necrosis of epiphyses

Several epiphyses in the lower extremities may undergo avascular necrosis with a resultant painful limp during the early course of the condition. Avascular necrosis (or 'osteochondritis') may affect the head of the second metatarsal (Freiberg's syndrome), the tarsal navicular (Köhler's), the calcaneal apophysis (Sever's), the tibial tuberosity (Osgood–Schlatter's) or the head of the femur (Legg–Perthe's). Osteochondritis dissecans in the ankle, knee, or hip will also produce a painful limp. These diagnoses are readily confirmed by diagnostic imaging.

Neoplasm

A painful limp may be one of the first manifestations of a malignant bone tumour, such as an osteogenic sarcoma or Ewing's sarcoma, or secondary deposits of neuroblastoma, and even leukaemia. Benign tumours less frequently cause a painful limp with the exception of an osteoid osteoma (especially when it is situated close to a joint).

Neurologic disorders

The varieties of limp caused by neurologic disorders are as numerous as the number of disorders themselves plus the degree of involvement in each. The principle is that, in a child with such a disorder, carefully observing the limp and analysing the muscle actions involved should stimulate the clinician to conduct a complete neurologic examination in order to make the diagnosis.

Flaccid paralysis

The more striking examples of flaccid paralytic gaits are the drop-foot gait associated with paralysed dorsiflexors of the ankle; the calcaneous gait with no push-off, due to paralysed calf muscles; and the gluteal limp with shift of the trunk toward the affected side with paralysed hip abductors. Neurologic examination, including testing muscle groups, will differentiate between spina bifida, peripheral nerve lesions, and other less common neurologic disorders associated with flaccid paralysis.

Spastic paralysis

The child with spasticity of the lower extremities has poor voluntary control of the involved muscle groups combined with a hyperactive stretch reflex, so that the gait is poorly coordinated, stiff, and jerky. Severe involvement is readily diagnosed but there are many lesser degrees of either brain or spinal cord damage. Indeed, mild spastic hemiplegia and mild spastic diplegia frequently go undiagnosed for the first few years of life primarily because the clinician has failed to observe the child walking. The limp due to spastic paralysis becomes more obvious when the child is asked to walk quickly or to run, at which time it will be observed that the heel does not touch the floor, the hip and the knee tend to remain flexed, and the thigh is adducted and internally rotated. With hemiplegia, even of mild degree, observing the affected arm on the same side will suggest the diagnosis immediately.

Further investigation will be required to determine the site and pathologic nature of the underlying lesion in the brain or spinal cord.

Ataxia

The ataxic child walks with an unsteady, uncertain, hesitating limp and a rather broad base. It is usually obvious that the child's balance is disturbed, particularly in the ataxic form of cerebral palsy.

Muscular disorders

The abnormal gaits associated with muscle disorders are due to contracture and weakness. In muscular dystrophy (a sex-linked disorder that affects only boys) the contracture of the calf muscles, if severe, causes the child to walk up on his toes; if less severe, the contracture causes him to walk with his feet turned outward and in valgus. Owing to hip flexion contracture and weakness of the spinal muscles, the child walks with an exaggerated lumbar lordosis. A positive Gower's sign is diagnostic. (The child has to use his hands to push on his knees to help himself rise from the floor to a standing position.) In myodystrophia foetalis (amyoplasia) and Volkmann's ischaemic contracture, the abnormal gait is due to muscle contracture and resultant limitation of joint movement.

Joint disorders

Joint disorders of the lower extremity include those in which the joint is stiff, as in fibrous and bony ankylosis, those in which a given movement of the joint is restricted by a joint contracture, and those in which the joint is unstable, as in subluxation and dislocation.

Joint stiffness or contracture

When one of the major joints of the lower extremity is either completely stiff or limited in its range of movements by contracture, careful analysis of the resultant limp will usually indicate that the involved joint is not moving through its normal range. If the hip is stiff in abduction, the affected leg will seem too long; if it is stiff in adduction or excessive flexion, the affected leg will seem too short.

Joint instability

The classic example of joint instability in the lower extremity in childhood is congenital dislocation or subluxation of the hip, now referred to as 'developmental displacement of the hip' (DDH). When the child's weight is transmitted to the dislocated hip, the already shortened extremity is still further shortened by the associated telescoping, and the pelvis dips down on the affected side. When the opposite foot is lifted from the ground, a second factor, ineffectual action of the hip abductors, comes into play, producing a drop of the pelvis on the opposite side and a compensatory shift of the trunk to the same side, that is, the Trendelenburg limp. The ineffectual action of the abductor muscles is due to the fact that there is no fulcrum upon which they may act. If the dislocation is bilateral, the child walks with a waddle.

Instability of the subtalar joint is seen in the congenital hypermobile type of flatfoot. The foot appears relatively normal until weight is put on it, when the heel assumes a valgus position and the longitudinal arch becomes flattened. Such a child demonstrates some loss of the normal spring in the gait and resultant difficulty in running well.

Bony deformity
Leg length discrepancy

Discrepancies from 0.5 to 1 in (1.2–2.5 cm) depending on the size of the child are easily masked in the gait, but greater discrepancies are associated with the trunk leaning to the affected side (secondary to downward tilt of the pelvis) each time the shorter extremity is placed on the floor during walking. The child also takes a shorter step with the shorter leg and may attempt to compensate for the discrepancy by walking on tiptoe on the shorter side and by keeping the knee flexed on the longer side. The shorter leg is not always the abnormal leg, for example, overgrowth of the longer leg due to neurofibromatosis or congenital arteriovenous malformations.

Developmental and adolescent coxa vara

In developmental coxa vara, the femoral neck-shaft angle is more acute than normal; the greater trochanter is closer to the pelvic brim, and the normal resting length of the hip abductors is decreased. Consequently, the child walks with a Trendelenburg limp as described in the section on instability of the hip.

In adolescent coxa vara (slipped capital femoral epiphysis), there is not only a more acute femoral neck shaft angle, but also an external rotational deformity of the femur at the epiphyseal plate so that the child walks with a Trendelenburg gait and also with the involved lower extremity externally rotated from the hip.

Genu valgum

A child with bilateral genu valgum (knock knees) walks rather awkwardly because the knees tend to rub as they pass one another. Bilateral genu varum (bow legs), on the other hand, is not usually associated with a limp.

Torsional deformities of the lower extremities

Internal torsion of the tibia or femur, or both, results in a toeing-in gait which, when severe, may cause the child to trip frequently. It is more of an awkward gait than a limp. The normal degree of internal tibial torsion present in the newborn usually corrects spontaneously, but in some children it persists or even becomes exaggerated.

Functional states

Although functional states are not often manifest in the gait, a child may limp with the condition of hysteria. The limp is likely to be most noticeable when the child is aware of being observed, and it may be absent when the child feels that no one is watching. The hysterical limp is usually both bizarre and histrionic. Furthermore, it does not fit any known pattern of abnormal gait.

Mimicry

Occasionally, a child will consciously, or subconsciously, mimic the limp of another member of the family, a playmate, or some other person in the neighbourhood, to the extent that it temporarily becomes a habit.

Investigation of limp

An accurate history will often provide extremely useful information as to the cause of the limp. Carefully analysing the limp with the child, suitably clad in underwear or a bathing suit will further narrow the differential diagnosis. A general physical examination should usually precede examination of the lower extremities, and the latter should include inspection, palpation, range of joint movements, leg length measurements, and neurologic examination. Finally, diagnostic imaging and laboratory examinations may be required to make an accurate diagnosis of the underlying condition responsible for the limp.

Conclusions

Limp is a cardinal physical sign of considerable diagnostic importance. It is more appropriate to be cognizant of the causes of limp and to be capable of arriving at a logical diagnosis by careful investigation rather than to make a 'spot' diagnosis from the limp alone, for the latter often indicates cleverness rather than wisdom. The family physician/general practitioner needs to be aware of the potential significance of the limp and if unsure of the aetiology should seek the help of an orthopaedic surgeon.

Key points

- ◆ Important diagnoses often go undetected because the physician fails to have children walk back and forth for gait analysis.

- ◆ An accurate history will often provide extremely useful information as to the cause of the limp.

- ◆ A general physical examination should precede examination of the lower extremities, and the latter should include inspection, palpation, range of joint movements, leg length measurements, and neurologic examination.

- ◆ The gait resulting from pain is a protective limp characterized by placing the foot down gently on the affected side, taking a shorter step with the affected extremity and then rapidly shifting the weight back to the normal extremity.

- ◆ The abnormal gaits associated with muscle disorders are due to contractures and weakness; joint disorders include those in which the joint is stiff, those in which a given movement of the joint is restricted, and those in which the joint is unstable.

Further reading

Staheli, L.T. (1992). Limp. In *Fundamentals of Pediatric Orthopedics*, pp. 4.2–4.3. New York: Raven Press.

Flynn, J.M. and Widmenn, R.F. (2001). The limping child: evaluation and diagnosis. *Journal of the American Academy of Orthopaedic Surgeons* **9**(2), 89–98.

Salter, R.B. (1968). Gait disturbances and limp in childhood. In *Ambulatory Pediatrics* (ed. M. Green and R.S. Haggerty), pp. 232–6. Philadelphia PA: WB Saunders.

10.9 Developmental delay

Julie Lumeng and Steven Parker

Introduction

Developmental disabilities are common. The worldwide population prevalence of mental retardation is estimated at 1–3 per cent and cerebral palsy at 0.2–0.3 per cent. Developmental disabilities are not easily described in terms of *incidence* (i.e. the occurrence of new cases in a specified time period), since the diagnosis is complex and often is revealed over time. Therefore, prevalence figures are more appropriately applied to the discussion of developmental delays. International differences in the prevalence of developmental disabilities appear to be small, although data collection is difficult. Within nations, developmental disabilities tend to be more common in rural communities and those of lower socio-economic status.

The natural history of a developmental disability varies with severity. Severe mental retardation and cerebral palsy are unusual, but more easily

Table 1 Differential diagnosis of developmental delay

Congenital
Cerebral malformation
Chromosomal abnormality
Degenerative neurological disorders
Hearing or vision deficit
Hypothyroidism
Inborn errors of metabolism
Foetal alcohol syndrome
Teratogenic exposure

Perinatal/Pre-natal
Birth or intrauterine trauma
Infection
Ischaemic event
Kernicterus
Prematurity

Environmental
Abuse and neglect
Extreme poverty
Lead poisoning
Nutritional and/or vitamin deficiency

Post-natal illness
Head trauma
Meningitis
Obstructive sleep apnoea
Recurrent otitis media
Seizure disorder

identifiable early in life. These conditions are due to static insults that will have significant and long-lasting impacts on lifetime functioning. In contrast, the prognostic significance of early mild developmental delays is not clear. Early motor delays, for example, may represent a marker for subtle neurologic dysfunction, manifesting in later childhood as learning disabilities or as cognitive delays. Alternatively, they may simply represent a transient immaturity of the motor system. As will be discussed later in this chapter, mild developmental delays are remarkably amenable to educational and psycho-social interventions. For this reason, early identification and treatment is an essential task for the primary care provider.

The primary care provider is often the first, if not only, professional to see a young child with a developmental delay. In a typical practice, approximately 2–3 per cent of children will not have normal acquisition of motor milestones. Of those infants, an estimated 15–20 per cent will have a significant neuromotor diagnosis. In addition, 5–10 per cent of toddlers in a typical practice will have a delay in language or cognitive skills. On the average, physicians initially make the diagnosis of mental retardation at a mean age of 39 months and of cerebral palsy at 10 months. This delay in diagnosis affords less time for intervention services.

Most cases of developmental delay, especially mild developmental delay, have no identifiable aetiology. The most common diagnoses for cases with identifiable causes are Fragile X, Down syndrome, and foetal alcohol syndrome, which together account for about one-third of all identifiable causes of developmental delay. The differential diagnosis of developmental delay is listed in Table 1.

Diagnosis

Development is generally divided into several domains, which may include: (i) visual motor/fine motor; (ii) gross motor; (iii) socio-emotional; (iv) cognitive; and (v) language. When a child's best performance of tasks in a particular domain on a standardized developmental test falls more than two standard deviations below the mean for other children of the same age, a developmental delay is highly suspect. Performance at this level indicates that the child cannot yet perform a skill that 98 per cent of his or her peers of the same age can.

The primary care provider basically has four options to identify a child with a developmental delay:

1. *Developmental assessment:* A comprehensive assessment using standardized instruments with proven validity and reliability can be performed. Unfortunately, this is often impractical in the office setting due to the length of time needed to complete such an evaluation and the level of training required to do so accurately.

2. *Developmental screening:* A less comprehensive assessment intended to identify children falling outside the normal range and requiring more in-depth evaluation can be performed. The physician can use one of the many commonly available developmental screening tests, such as the Denver Developmental Assessment, or the Clinical Linguistic and Auditory Milestone Scale (CLAMS)/Clinical Adaptive Test (CAT). In choosing a good screening test, one should look for a test with high sensitivity (able to detect nearly all children with the problem) and high specificity (able to accurately identify children without problems). In addition, the test should have high content validity (able to measure what it purports to measure), and high test–retest reliability and inter-rater reliability (able to give similar results when given multiple times). Unfortunately, recent research has shown that the developmental screens used in clinical practice lack many of these attributes. In addition, these screens require an amount of time and precision that is unavailable in the standard office practice, and the temperament and state of the child on the particular day of the visit can have a significant impact on performance. Indeed, past research has documented the infrequent use of developmental screening tests by primary care providers in clinical practice.

3. *Screening questionnaires:* Parents can be provided with one of the commonly available developmental screening questionnaires, which they complete while waiting to be seen in the office. The physician can then use this information to perform targeted developmental testing. Parental concern is extremely accurate. One study demonstrated that relying on parental report had a sensitivity of 80 per cent, specificity of 94 per cent, positive predictive value of 76 per cent, and negative predictive value of 95 per cent.[1] Because 20–25 per cent of parents, however, will not recognize their child's delay, the clinician cannot rely exclusively on this method.

4. *Developmental surveillance:* An abundance of research suggests that when paediatric providers incorporate parental data and clinical impressions, accuracy in detecting developmental delay increases. Developmental surveillance, therefore, makes systematic use of clinical information and combines it, when needed, with standardized screening. Indeed, this is the approach currently practiced by the majority of primary care paediatric providers. Developmental surveillance is defined as: 'a flexible, continuous process whereby knowledgeable professionals perform skilled observations of children during the provision of health care'.[2] To perform developmental surveillance, the physician should: (i) elicit parents' concerns; (ii) obtain a relevant developmental and behavioural history; (iii) observe the child's skills in the office, possibly using an informal collection of age-appropriate tasks selected from various developmental schedules; (iv) perform a physical examination; and (v) share opinions and concerns with other relevant professionals, such as teachers. The strength of developmental surveillance is that it recognizes the many psycho-social and biological factors contributing to development, and aims to address them simultaneously.

In performing developmental surveillance at each well child visit, some 'red flags' that should alert the physician to the need for additional investigation are listed in Table 2.

Information about a child with a potential developmental delay should be gathered as one would with any thorough medical history. It is often effective to begin by asking the parent, 'Do you have any concerns about your child's development?' Risk factors for developmental delay are additive, and therefore a comprehensive social, family, and medical history is

Table 2 'Red flags' at each well child visit that should prompt further investigation

2 months	Inability to lift head, smile, or respond to noise
4 months	Inability to grasp rattle, no vocalizations
6 months	Inability to roll over or reach for toy
9 months	Inability to sit without support or self-feed finger food
12 months	Unable to stand briefly unsupported, no jabbering
15 months	No words
18 months	Not walking
24 months	Unable to remove clothing or combine two words; vocabulary <50 words
Any age	Loss of previously attained milestones

Table 3 Additional features of the standard history and physical in the child with developmental delay

History of present illness
Has your child lost skills he previously had?
Does your child frequently vomit, appear lethargic, or have an unusual body odour?
Does your child snore?
Has your child had difficulties with growth?

Past medical history
Has your child ever had a head injury, or hit her head so hard that she passed out?
Has your child ever had lead poisoning, seizures, or meningitis?
Has your child had his hearing and vision tested?

Social history
Some families I see have difficulties having enough money at the end of the month. Is this a concern for your family?

Family history
Have there been any children in your extended family who died in early childhood?
Is there anyone in your extended family who had difficulty in school? Did not graduate from high school? Had trouble learning to read? Had mental retardation?
Is there any history in your family of mental health concerns, such as anxiety or depression?

Physical examination
Growth parameters, including head circumference
Dysmorphic features, including minor anomalies
Skin findings consistent with a neurocutaneous disorder
Evaluation of primitive reflexes, postural responses, and motor milestones

essential. Certain additional helpful questions in the history and components to note in the physical examination deserve special mention, and are listed in Table 3.

Testing and referral

History and physical examination should guide laboratory and radiological investigations. For example, a metabolic evaluation is only indicated if the history includes lethargy, vomiting, loss of milestones, or a positive family history. Neuroimaging is only necessary for an unexpected change in behaviour, head circumference, motor status, cognitive abilities, neurologic examination, or seizure frequency. Although seizures are common in children with developmental delay, there is little evidence that seizures are a common aetiology of aggression, tantrums, or behaviour dysfunction. Thus, electroencephalogram is rarely indicated. Tests to be considered in the evaluation of developmental delay are listed in Table 4.

Table 4 Tests to be considered in the work-up of developmental delay

Complete blood count
Electroencephalogram
Hearing test
Vision test
High resolution chromosomes
Fragile X
Subtelomeric FISH (fluorescent in situ hybridization)
Screening for human immunodeficiency virus
Metabolic screening: serum electrolytes, pyruvate, lactate, ammonia, glucose, pH, urine amino acids, urine organic acids
Neuroimaging
Thyroid function studies

Studies show that primary care physicians *underidentify* developmental delays, even when using the best available screening tests rigorously. Therefore, when in doubt about a child's developmental status, the best policy is early referral. Where to refer will depend largely on the available resources. In many centres, however, there are multidisciplinary teams consisting of developmental paediatricians, physical, occupational, and speech therapists, psychologists, and social workers. For the child with dysmorphic features or an abnormal chromosomal screen, a geneticist is indicated. For the child with episodes of lethargy, vomiting, and loss of milestones, an urgent evaluation by a specialist in metabolic disease is needed. The child with developmental delay and seizures would benefit from a referral to a neurologist. All children with language delay should be referred to an audiologist for a thorough hearing evaluation. For the child with mild developmental delay, no other associated symptoms or concerning history, and all of the appropriate therapeutic interventions in place, referral is not indicated.

Treatment

The differential diagnosis of developmental delay is deep and broad, and the vast majority of aetiologies do not have any known treatment. It is essential, however, that the practitioner recognize early and accurately the small number of treatable conditions that can lead to developmental delay. These include: hearing loss, vision loss, galactosaemia, fructosaemia, hypoglycaemia, lead intoxication, hypothyroidism, phenylketonuria, maternal phenylketonuria, maple syrup urine disease, recurrent otitis media, malnutrition, Menkes disease, and Lesch–Nyhan syndrome.

Although the remainder of the causes of developmental delay do not have medical treatments, early therapeutic services have proven efficacy. Underlying biological conditions are not changed, but children are helped to reach their potentials. This is particularly true for children from socially disadvantaged backgrounds. There is also strong evidence for short-term benefits to intelligence and long-term benefits for school completion, job satisfaction, and social adjustment for children with developmental delays due to environmental risk. Early intervention involves a multifaceted approach consisting of: (i) educational interventions such as speech therapy, physical therapy, and occupational therapy; (ii) social interventions, such as addressing difficulties with resources and parental stress; and (iii) behavioural interventions, such as addressing parenting behaviours that may adversely affect development. Programmes that involve parents, promote normal development, and combine both home and centre-based interventions are the most successful.

There are detailed health supervision guidelines for individuals with specific conditions, such as Down syndrome, myelomeningocoele, and many genetic syndromes. These are beyond the scope of this chapter, but can be reviewed in the texts recommended for further reading.

Long-term and continuing care

Primary care providers are in a unique position to help children with developmental delay reach their potentials. Because biologic and social risk factors compound one another, the primary care provider can intervene at many points to enhance development. For instance, the physician may be involved in the treatment of conditions associated with developmental delay, such as hyperactivity or drooling, and in assuring that routine preventive care and health education is obtained. The physician should also remain in contact with other practitioners, including therapists, psychologists, and teachers, and assist families in advocating for appropriate services as needs change over time. In addition, although referral to specialists improves health and longevity in many of these children, it also often results in the duplication or absence of services, and a lack of communication between multiple care providers. The result can be an increased burden on an already overwhelmed family. Children with developmental delays are also at higher risk for behavioural and emotional problems including aggression, self-injurious behaviour, inappropriate social behaviour, and sleep disorders. An additional critical role for families affected by a genetic disorder, is adequate education and counselling to support informed decision-making related to family planning. For these reasons, the primary provider's role in coordinating care and providing a 'medical home' for the family is crucial. The physician should be prepared either to help families manage these problems, or to provide a referral to the appropriate specialist.

Until research provides greater understanding of the aetiologies of developmental delay, primary prevention is difficult. Previous public health successes in this area have included screening for lead poisoning and iron-deficiency anaemia, recommending folic acid for the prevention of neural tube defects, iodized salt for the treatment of hypothyroidism, bicycle helmets, seat belts, and newborn screening programmes for metabolic diseases.

Having a child with a developmental delay has been shown to be very stressful for families. The diagnosis of a developmental disability evokes a complicated grief reaction, which is a lifelong process. Emotional needs of the well siblings may be neglected as the family focuses on the disabled child. The primary care provider can play a key role in helping families become strong advocates for their child, and cope with the stresses involved in caring for a child with a disability.

Key points

1. Developmental delays are common in clinical practice. The primary care provider is the first to identify most developmental delays.

2. Identification of developmental delays is best accomplished in the setting of a busy practice through a combination of history, observation, and intermittent formal screening measures.

3. No standard diagnostic tests are indicated for all children with developmental delays. A careful history and physical examination directs further work-up and referral.

4. Early, multidisciplinary, comprehensive intervention is effective in modifying the outcome of developmental delays.

5. Biological, social, environmental, and emotional risk factors are cumulative in affecting developmental delays. A comprehensive approach to all risk factors is essential.

6. Having a child with a developmental delay is an ongoing stress for families. The primary care provider is in a key position to advocate for appropriate services for children and families.

References

1. Glascoe, F.P. and Dworkin, P.H. (1995). The role of parents in the detection of developmental and behavioral problems. *Pediatrics* **95** (6), 829–36.
2. Glascoe, F.P., Altemeier, W.A., and MacLean, W.E. (1989). The importance of parents' concerns about their child's development. *American Journal of Diseases of Children* **143**, 955–8.

Further reading

Dixon, S.D. and Stein, M.T. *Encounters with Children: Pediatric Behavior and Development.* St Louis MO: Harcourt Health Sciences, 2000, pp. 1–666. (Fundamental concepts of child development presented in an age-based, clinically useful format.)

Parker, S.P. and Zuckerman, B. *Behavioral and Developmental Pediatrics: A Handbook for Primary Care.* London: Little, Brown, and Co, 1995, pp. 1–447. (Common developmental and behavioural concerns encountered in primary care with succinct descriptions of aetiology, work-up, and treatment.)

10.10 Sleep disorders in children

James F. Pagel

Sleep in childhood is the best sleep, both quantitatively and qualitatively, which most of us ever experience, yet sleep disorders are common and sometimes dangerous in children. In clinical practice, most complaints pertaining to the child's sleep come from the parent—the one losing the most sleep.

Sleeplessness

When children lose sleep at night, they make it up during the daytime. The sleepless child is likely to have late bedtimes or early wakings, frequent or long wakings and insufficient napping with associated changes in mood, behaviour, and attentional abilities. These symptoms may present as parental stress and anger, and altered bedtime interactions.

In evaluating the sleepless child, it is important to take a careful and detailed history. The most useful information comes from a precise description of the child's usual sleep and waking patterns on typical nights, not the extremes. Parental response and interaction to the child including use of aids to sleep (such as bottles, pacifiers, toys, and lullabies) should be explored. Bedtime routines, including naps, and a sleep diary to visualize variables affecting sleep and waking schedules should be documented in detail. In addition to a standard history, review of systems and physical examination, a thorough paediatric sleep history should include a description of the child's peer interactions, school performance, home and social tensions, and the physical layout of the child's site of sleeping.

Most sleep complaints in children result from behavioural and circadian issues rather than being the result of medical or physiological dysfunction. Common behavioural sleep problems include sleep onset association disorder, excessive nighttime feedings, limit-setting sleep disorder, and sleep-related fear.

Sleep onset association disorder

A child must learn to fall asleep under the same circumstances that will be present when he wakes during the night. Children who become used to falling asleep while being held, rocked, or using a pacifier may not be able to fall asleep on their own without the re-establishment of these associations. Treatment involves educating the parents: teaching parents that awakenings during the night are normal, that associations with falling asleep are learned and present at all ages, and that new sleep associations can be easily taught. In a child more than 5 months of age, behavioural treatment works well for sleep association disorder. Behavioural treatment for paediatric sleeplessness is based on a stimulus response protocol alternating comforting with increased times for the child of sleeping alone. The parent should place the child in the crib and leave the room returning to comfort the crying child after several minutes. This comforting should be verbal and the parent would stay in the room only briefly—not until the child falls asleep. The parent should gradually increase times between comforting episodes until eventually the child falls asleep. The usual response time is three to five nights. If symptoms persist, consider that instructions are not being followed, that co-existing problems exist (e.g. anxiety), that more time is needed (a few more nights), or that another diagnosis exists affecting the child's ability to sleep (e.g. inappropriate sleep schedule).

Excessive nighttime feedings

By 2–3 months of age, most normal full-term infants require no more than a single feeding in the middle of the night, and by 5–6 months even that requirement disappears. The symptoms of excessive nighttime feeding disorder include breast or bottle feedings required for a return to sleep, resulting in conditioned hunger in the child and multiple wakings. The digestion and metabolism of food raises body temperature and results in a cascade of biological functions that disrupt sleep. As a result, the newborn sleep pattern is maintained, rotating around wakings and feedings spread across the 24-h day. Although this diagnosis can reflect severe childhood sleep disturbance, it is often one of the easiest to treat. Nocturnal feedings can be tapered with decreased food amounts and increased time between feedings until nocturnal feedings are no longer required.

Limit-setting sleep disorder

Once a child learns to climb out of a crib, his or her control boundary shifts away from a simple physical barrier. In its first attempt to assert control, the child may leave the bedroom repeatedly, making a series of demands on the parents to stall or refuse bedtime. Treatment emphasizes limit-setting on the part of the parents. The setting of sleep-related limits should include and may improve the setting of daytime limits. A consistent scheduled bedtime must be developed and set, not re-negotiated night to night. Use of gate can help a 2- or 3-year-old child stay in his/her own room. A reward system involving stickers or tokens can provide positive reinforcement. These 'star charts' can be developed as creative solutions to improve communication between the parent and child.

Sleep-related fears

Sleep-related fears may be rational (clear cause) or irrational (monsters) and some may be part of normal developmental separation anxiety. Bedtime-related fears are often best treated by setting consistent and appropriate limits, schedule adjustment, and positive reinforcement (star charts). The child can be asked to describe what might alleviate the insecurity. For the child with major fears, co-sleeping with the parent in the bedroom may be a good starting place. Sometimes that is enough to break the cycle of anxiety, and after several weeks the child becomes confident enough to let the parent leave. If a high level of fear persists as a manifestation of primary anxiety disorder, professional counselling may be required.

Circadian sleep disorders

Sleep cycles are controlled by our biologic clock, set by light exposure which controls times of sleepiness and times of waking. Circadian sleep disorders result from a mismatch between the endogenous rhythm of sleep and alertness and the desired or expected schedule. An advanced sleep phase presents as the tendency to fall asleep earlier than others, associated with the complaint of late afternoon and evening daytime fatigue. A delayed sleep phase is more common in adolescents. Symptoms include an inability to fall asleep at night, difficulty waking in the morning, and daytime fatigue followed by arousal in the evening. Sleep phase can be altered with bright light therapy either in the evening (advance-phase disorder) or the morning (delayed-phase disorder). Naps should be eliminated in the attempt to gradually normalize sleep and waking times, along with the adolescent's frequent 'weekend recovery' sleeps.

When sleep schedules are inconsistent, disrupted, and unpredictable, an irregular sleep schedule disorder can develop. Satisfactory sleep patterns can emerge with the normalizing of sleeping patterns and appropriate napping. Without realizing it, parents can enforce a bedtime schedule to match their own sleeping expectations or desires. A child's bedtime should match the child's actual time of sleep.

Parasomnias

Parasomnias are undesirable behaviours or experiences that occur during sleep. Parasomnias are classified according to their sleep stage association. The arousal disorders are associated with arousal from deep sleep (stages 3 and 4). REM sleep associated parasomnias occur on arousal from REM sleep. Other parasomnias such as bruxism, periodic limb movement disorder, and restless leg syndrome occur during wake/sleep transitions or are not clearly associated with particular sleep stages.

Arousal disorders

The arousal disorders are characterized by either partial or complete arousal from deep sleep. Sleep walking, confusional arousals, and sleep terrors are the most common of these disorders. Arousal disorders are exacerbated by sleep deprivation, sleep fragmentation, and psychological factors including anxiety and stress. All share the clinical characteristics: occurrence in the first half of the night, confusion/autonomic behaviour, difficulty waking from the event, fragmented imagery, rapid return to sleep, and amnesia for the event.

Sleep walking (somnambulism) is most frequently characterized as quiet wandering around the home. Somnambulism is not usually associated with injury. Surprisingly complex behaviours can occur—the child can be seen negotiating obstacles and carrying out seemingly purposeful tasks, as well as some inappropriate behaviours, such as urination. Most spells are brief (5–15 min). During a confusional arousal, the child may seem to be awake, if not considerably confused. The child may cry, yell, moan, or speak in unintelligible sentences and may or may not recognize the parental figure. A 'blood-curdling' scream and autonomic discharge accompanies the more extreme form of confusional arousal, the sleep terror (Table 1).

The primary treatment for the parasomnias is parental education and environmental protection for the child (e.g. these children should not sleep in bunk beds and may require closures on the bedroom door). All parasomnias become unusual with the onset of adolescence, with few of these children maintaining symptoms into adulthood. If nocturnal njuries occur, polysomnography is required to definitively characterize the parasomnia and rule out seizure activity.

REM sleep associated disorders—nightmares

In childhood, nightmares are by far the most common REM sleep associated disorder. Nightmares (more than twice a week) affect 20–40 per cent of children between 5 and 12 years of age. They typically occur during the last third of the night, and often include bizarre, complex, action-packed dreams involving many associations. The child is often fully alert following the dream and easily comforted though return to sleep may be delayed. The child's reaction to the dream is generally an emotional outpouring rather than the autonomic discharge seen in the sleep terror. Nightmares in children do not usually reflect underlying psychopathology, but if

Table 1 Nightmares and night terrors: distinguishing characteristics

Night terror	Nightmare
Associated with arousals from deep sleep (stages 3 and 4)	Associated with REM sleep
Intense: vocalizations (blood curdling scream), fright, somnambulism, autonomic discharge	Intense: vocalizations, fright, motility autonomic discharge
Sparse mental content—amnesia	Elaborate mental content—less amnesia
Difficulty in arousing individual	Often associated with arousals from sleep
More likely to occur early in the night	More likely to occur late in the night
Unusual—in childhood only 2–4% affected	Very common in children—40–50% affected
Not associated with pathology in children	Usually reflects no pathology in children, associated with PTSD and other psychiatric illness
Exacerbation by sleep deprivation, sleep fragmentation, and psychological factors	Exacerbation by sleep fragmentation, psychological factors, development and medical/psychiatric illness

Table 2 Differential diagnosis for the sleepy child

Sleep disorders	Medical/psychiatric
Sleep-disordered breathing	Drugs
Insufficient sleep	Depression
Poor sleep hygiene	Trauma
Narcolepsy	Infections
Delayed sleep phase	CNS abnormalities
Periodic limb-movement disorder	Hypothyroidism
Idiopathic hypersomnia	Sequale of CNS trauma

nightmares are frequent, persistent, or result in daytime dysfunction, medical or psychological evaluation may be indicated. Treatment can be as simple as explanation and reassurance, or sleep hygiene. When severe, behavioural therapies have been shown to be very effective in the elimination or reduction of nightmares in both children and adults.

Sleep–wake transition disorders—the rhythmic movement disorders

The sleep–wake transition disorders occur during transitions between sleep states, or on arousal to and from sleep. These disorders include the rhythmic movement disorders, sleep starts, and somniloquy (sleep talking). The rhythmic movement disorders include body-rocking, body-rolling, and head banging and range from mild to severe in intensity. These behaviours can occur in up to two-thirds of normal children, more frequently in males than females at a 4 : 1 ratio. They tend to extinguish with time, and disappear by age 4 in 90 per cent of cases. These children should be protected from possible injury. Sometimes volitional reproduction of the movements using a rocker or waterbed can help to extinguish the activity. In severe cases, benzodiazepines, carbamazepine, and antihistamines have been of benefit. If the symptoms are severe, persistent, and include injuries, other disorders associated with rhythmic movement should be considered (e.g. autism, seizures).

Other parasomnias—bruxism, periodic limb movement disorder, and restless leg syndrome

Bruxism is the repetitive grinding of teeth during sleep. It occurs in up to 50 per cent of children, and is most common in stage 2 sleep. It is exacerbated by stress. Bruxism usually begins in late childhood or early adolescence. If necessary, a mouth guard can be used to minimize trauma to the teeth and jaw.

Periodic limb movement disorder (PLMD) consists of stereotypical limb movements (usually the lower extremities) that often result in arousals. Because of this, PLMD can fragment sleep and result in daytime sleepiness. Some children will complain of limb cramps ('growing pains'). Restless legs syndrome (RLS) may occur in association with PLMD and is generally described as 'crawly' sensations in the legs and the inability to keep the legs still. RLS like PLMD can result in insomnia. A familiar pattern may be found for both disorders. When treatment is necessary due to complaints of insomnia or daytime sleepiness, benzodiazepines (clonazepam and lorazepam) can reduce movements and arousals.

The sleepy child

The sleepy child presents differently than the sleepy adult. Sleepiness in children results in poor attention, the failure to complete tasks, and/or staring spells. The sleepy child often has restless, irritable, impulsive, or hyperactive behaviour that can lead to misdiagnosis of attention deficit disorder (ADD), depression, learning disability, conduct disorder or obsessive compulsive disorder (Table 2).

Narcolepsy

The symptoms of narcolepsy most commonly present between 11 and 15 years of age. Children with narcolepsy are often described as 'long sleepers', spending longer times in sleep and napping. In addition to sleepiness, narcolepsy is associated with symptoms of cataplexy (a sudden loss of muscle tone brought on by strong emotion), sleep paralysis, and hypnagogic hallucinations (dream-like imagery at sleep onset). Narcoleptic children are often considered as lazy or slow, and may describe social isolation and academic difficulties. Unfortunately, the diagnosis of narcolepsy is rarely made until adulthood.

The sleep laboratory evaluation of narcolepsy includes both polysomnography and multiple sleep latency testing. The testing diagnostic criteria for narcolepsy include short latencies to sleep onset and REM onset sleep periods. HLA typing can be used to rule out or support a clinically suggested diagnosis of narcolepsy. Few normative data exist for children and diagnostic testing must be considered as supportive data for clinical impressions.

Treatment of narcolepsy in the child includes education of patient, parent, and academic environments. It is critical to aid the child and parents in establishing realistic schedules and goals, in avoiding alcohol, in limiting driving times. Scheduled napping is often useful. The child's activities should be coordinated with times of peak functioning. It is also necessary to monitor the child for drug abuse and depression. Adolescents sometimes use recreational stimulants (cocaine and meth-amphetamine) to induce alertness. The pharmacologic treatment of narcolepsy involves the use of stimulant medications to modify sleepiness (methylphenidate, dextroamphetamine, and modafinil). Associated symptoms of cataplexy often respond to the stimulants; however, adjunctive use of antidepressants might be required.

Respiratory sleep disorders
Obstructive sleep apnoea (OSA) in children

OSA is a common disorder in adults that is most likely under-diagnosed in children. Seven to 20 per cent of children snore frequently. Current best

Table 3 Symptoms of obstructive sleep apnoea

Nocturnal symptoms	Diurnal symptoms
Loud snoring	Daytime sleepiness (inattentiveness, irritability, and hyperactivity)
Snorting/gasping/apnoeic pauses	Behavioural/school problems (impulsivity and aggressiveness)
Restless sleep	Difficulty waking in morning
Diaphoresis	Morning headaches
Abnormal sleeping position	Nasal congestion
Secondary enuresis	Mouth breathing

estimates suggest the 1–3 per cent of pre-school children have significant OSA. The peak age for paediatric OSA is from 2 to 5 years, corresponding directly with the ages of peak adenotonsilar hypertrophy. Risk factors include adenotonsilar hypertrophy, craniofacial abnormalities, Down syndrome, obesity, and neurologic disorders characterized by decreased muscle tone. Physical examination is often normal, with severity of OSA not consistently related to degree of tonsillar hypertrophy. Symptoms occur during sleep and during waking (Table 3).

A sleep study (polysomnography) is generally required to confirm the diagnosis of OSA when it is suspected on clinical grounds. The polysomnographic findings in childhood OSA differ from adults to children. Children have fewer and shorter apnoeic events [a respiratory disturbance index (RDI) of more than 5 is considered abnormal] and significant O_2 desaturation with their apnoeic events. The child with OSA also has fewer cortical arousals and tends to preserve sleep architecture. Treatment options for OSA include: weight loss if obese, nasal continuous positive airway pressure, and surgery (adenotonsillectomy is usually highly effective in children with adenotonsillar hypertrophy).

Sudden infant death syndrome (SIDS)

SIDS is the sudden death of any infant or young child that is unexplained by the child's history or a through post-mortem examination. SIDS is the most common cause of post-neonatal infant death [2500 deaths per year, 1 per 1000 live births (USA 1998)]. Risk factors include prematurity (18 per cent), a previous apparent life-threatening event (ALTE) (7 per cent), and subsequent siblings of SIDS victims (1 per cent). The vast majority of infants succumbing to SIDS have no known predisposing causes. Incidence of SIDS is increased in males (60 per cent), and occurs most often in winter, among lower socio-economic groups, and among children whose parents smoke. Infants at risk for SIDS may have decreased respiratory drive, decreased arousal response, and an increase in obstructive apnoeas. Polysomnography, however, has not generally been useful in predicting which infants may be at risk for SIDS.

A primary risk factor for SIDS is sleeping in the prone position. Campaigns led by the public health officials of several different countries to encourage parents to place their newborns to sleep in the supine position have led to decreases of at least 50 per cent in SIDS deaths in those countries. The relative risk of sleeping in the prone position for SIDS is several times the risk of sleeping supine or laterally. However, the actual risk of SIDS when placing an infant to sleep in the prone position is still extremely low.

In children who have experienced an ALTE, a full work-up is indicated including laboratory testing: CBC, electrolytes, chest X-ray, ECG, and physiologic monitoring during sleep. Predisposing causes can be elicited in 60 per cent of patients, with gastrointestinal reflux the most common (28 per cent). A cardiorespiratory home monitor is often used to alert caregivers to events. Caregivers should be taught CPR, and home monitoring continued until no true alarms have been experienced for at least 2 months.

Key points

- Common behavioural sleep problems include sleep onset association disorder, excessive nighttime feedings, limit-setting sleep disorder, and sleep-related fear.
- The parasomnias are undesirable behaviours or experiences that occur during sleep. The arousal disorders are associated with rousal from deep sleep (stages 3 and 4). REM sleep associated parasomnias occur on arousal from REM sleep.
- Sleepiness in children results in poor attention, the failure to complete tasks, and staring spells. The sleepy child often has restless, irritable, impulsive, or hyperactive behaviour that can lead to misdiagnosis of attention-deficit disorder (ADD), depression, learning disability, conduct disorder, or obsessive compulsive disorder.
- Obstructive sleep apnoea (OSA) is a common disorder in adults that is most likely under-diagnosed in children. Current best estimates suggest the 1–3% of pre-school children have significant OSA.
- The vast majority of infants succumbing to SIDS have no known predisposing causes. The relative risk of sleeping in the prone position for SIDS is several times the risk of sleeping supine or laterally.

References

1. American Academy of Pediatrics Task Force on Infant Positioning and SIDS (1992). *Pediatrics* **89** (6 Pt 1), 1120–6.
2. Goldberg, R., Ferber, R., Pagel, J., and Sheldon, S. (2000). Non-respiratory sleep disorders in children. In *An Educational Slide Set from the American Academy of Sleep Medicine* (ed. L.J. Brooks). Rochester MN: AASM.
3. Goldberg, R., Marcus, C., and Owens, J. (2000). Respiratory sleep disorders in children. In *An Educational Slide Set from the American Academy of Sleep Medicine* (ed. L.J. Brooks). Rochester MN: AASM.
4. Ferber, R. and Kryger, M., ed. *Principles and Practice of Sleep Medicine in the Child*. Philadelphia: WB Saunders Company, 1995.
5. National Institutes of Health Consensus Development Conference on Infantile Apnoea and Home Monitoring, 29 September to 1 October 1986, Consensus Statement. *Pediatrics* 1987 **79** (2), 292–9.
6. Sheldon, S.H., Spire, J.P., and Levy, H.B. *Pediatric Sleep Medicine*. Philadelphia: WB Saunders Company, 1992.

10.11 Behaviour problems in children

Graham J. Reid

People notice what children do. Parents love to talk about the latest things their children are up to. But parents, teachers, and other adults also notice when children* do things that are problematic or distressing. Problems with children's overt behaviours result in referrals by teachers or others, or

---

* Unless otherwise noted, the term children will be used to refer to all ages less than 18 years.

parents seeking help, more often than when children are shy, withdrawn, sad, or anxious. There is no accepted definition of behaviour problems. Behaviour problems include difficulties with aggression, bedtimes, crying, or psychiatric disorders (e.g. conduct disorder). This chapter discusses issues in assessment and approaches to treatment, emergence of behaviour problems, and a template for interventions with behaviour problems followed by a discussion of specific behaviour problems for infants, pre-school-age and school-age children, and adolescents.

Prevalence and identification of behaviour problems

Without a clear definition, prevalence data for behaviour problems overall are not available. About one out of every five pre-school- and school-age children and adolescents has a clinically significant psychosocial problem.[1] The prevalence in primary care settings is identical. Without treatment, 50 per cent of children with psychosocial problems have problems into adolescence or adulthood.

When physicians identify a child as having a behaviour problem they are usually correct (i.e. high sensitivity); however, physicians do not dentify the majority of children with such problems (i.e. low specificity). Physician's failure to ask, and parents' or adolescents' failure to mention psychosocial concerns, contribute to this problem. However, when parents *do* mention concerns, half of the time physicians give no response or only passively acknowledge parents' concerns.

Screening questionnaires for psychosocial problems in primary care settings are rarely used. Eliciting concerns is a valid screening method. However, screening should be undertaken only with a careful assessment of available interventions. Asking about behavioural problems implies that treatments are available. Due to lack of community resources, waiting lists, etc., options for referral are often limited. In such situations, physicians should be willing and able to provide the treatment themselves.

Physicians' treatment of behaviour problems

Only a handful of studies have tested the effectiveness of physicians' interventions for children's behavioural, psychosocial, or psychiatric problems in primary care settings.[2] Overall, physician interventions tended not to be effective. Interventions by other members of a primary care team (health visitors, psychologists, social workers) have found positive effects. This is a dilemma. Despite that lack of demonstrated treatment efficacy or effectiveness, parents and adolescents turn to physicians for help with behavioural problems. Physicians could consider building a team that includes individuals skilled in treating behaviour problems.

Issues in assessment and approaches to treatment

Physicians' advice is often based on their own parenting. However, what worked for the physicians might not work for their patients due to differences in their children and personal, family, and community resources. Many parents try non-conventional treatments such as elimination diets and vitamin and herbal remedies. No diet or other alternative treatments have demonstrated efficacy for behaviour problems. Such situations can be handled by acknowledging these treatments as evidence of parents' love and concern, informing parents that these 'treatments' are often not without risk, and discussing if parents wish to invest their resources (time and money) in an unproved treatment or one with demonstrated success.

Emergence of behaviour problems

Research has shown that behaviour problems are determined through the interaction of risk and protective factors at the child, parent, family, and community/environmental levels (see Table 1). The likelihood of developing

Table 1 Risk and protective factors related to the development of behavioural and psycho-social problems at the individual, parent/family, and community/neighbourhood levels

	Risk factors	Protective factors
Individual level	Pre-natal exposure to drugs, tobacco, or alcohol	Positive parenting
	Low birth weight	Secure attachment
	Difficult temperament	History of competence, social competence
	Male sex	Intelligence, cognitive ability, reading skills
	Medical condition	Internal locus of control
	Genetic vulnerability to psychopathology	Optimism
	Racial[a] minority	Planning for the future
	Early onset of behaviour problems	Self-esteem, self-efficacy, self-understanding
Parental/family level	Parental psychopathology (especially maternal depression) or criminality	Advanced maternal education
	Younger maternal age	Maternal employment
	Lower parental education	Paternal involvement in childcare
	Child separation from parents	Social support
	Family stress and experiencing stressful life events	
	Single parenthood	
	Poor home environment	
	Poverty	
	Marital distress	
Community/environmental level	Living in a violent or economically poor community/neighbourhood	Church involvement
	Belonging to a deviant peer group	Positive relationship with a non-custodial adult
		Participation in extracurricular activities and the community
		Taking responsibility in the home or job
		Extrafamilial support for mother

[a] Race is a characteristic of the individual but its relation to psychopathology operates mainly through interactions within the community.

problems increases exponentially as the number of risk factors increase. Protective factors reduce the impact of risk factors. The presence of risk factors signals the need for greater attention to psychosocial issues while awareness of protective factors can act as a template for intervention regardless of the specific problem.

A template for providing interventions for child behaviour problems in primary care

Regardless of the specifics of a behaviour problem, physicians can advise parents on ways to enhance protective factors. For example, help parents identify and strengthen areas of competence in their children; foster the idea that 'no-one is good at everything but everyone is good at something'. Reading to and with children facilitates language and reading skills. At the family level, paternal involvement and giving children age-appropriate chores can be encouraged. Also, help increase parents' and children's connections within the community.

Some effective parenting strategies are applicable to all types of child behaviour problems. Have regular family routines (e.g. eating meals together, stable bedtimes, set curfews, regular times and locations for homework) and rituals (e.g. celebrating birthdays, weekly family game or movie night). Parental knowledge (e.g. what television shows their children watch, what Internet sites they access) and active involvement (e.g. who are their children's friends, knowing the whereabouts of adolescents) in their children's lives are protective.

Specific behaviour problems

The most common behaviour problems and those that parents frequently ask physicians for advice during each developmental stage are discussed. The Zero-to-Three,[3] DSM-IV,[4] and DSM-PC[5] diagnostic systems provide details for specific disorders for children.

Infants

Feeding problems (e.g. refusal to eat, not hungry at mealtimes) occur in 5–25 per cent of infants. Feeding problems are determined by the infant's ability to self-regulate, oral-motor functioning, development, history of feeding problems and environmental factors related to parent–child interactions. About half of the infants with feeding problems will continue to have problems by age 2 as well as adverse developmental and psychosocial outcomes. Monitoring of feeding problems and growth, and anticipatory guidance are warranted, although data on their effectiveness is limited. Books on breastfeeding, feeding, and nutrition may be of interest. Failure to thrive, the extreme result of feeding problems in infancy, is discussed in Chapter 10.5 and more detail about feeding problems is provided in Chapter 8.10.

Colic—intense periods of crying and fussiness lasting 3 or more hours a day, at least 3 days a week, for 3 weeks in a healthy infant—occurs in 5–20 per cent of infants. Colic is likely due to either gastrointestinal problems (e.g. immaturity, gastro-oesophageal reflux) or allergic reactions (e.g. cow's milk). Problems with parent–child interactions may continue once colic has subsided. Frequent regurgitation, apnoea, cyanosis, fever, respiratory difficulties, failure to gain weight, or neurological abnormalities warrants further investigation. (see also Ch 8.10).

Changes in diet have positive effects. Colic is reduced when breastfeeding mothers eat a hypoallergenic diet (milk, egg, wheat, nut product free) or when infants are given hypoallergenic (whey hydrolysate) or soy formula. Lactase or fibre-enriched formulas and sucrose treatments are not effective. Increased carrying of the infant and car ride stimulation is not effective. Behavioural parent training and reducing infant stimulation do have positive effects.[6] Pharmacological treatments are not recommended.

Pre-school-age children

Problems with sleeping and eating behaviours, toilet training, and discipline are the predominant areas of concern among parents of young children. Chapter 10.10 discusses sleep problems.

Eating or mealtime behaviour problems (e.g. refusal to eat, picky eater) occur in 20–30 per cent of young children. Children's eating problems are fairly persistent and may be linked to later behaviour problems. One study found eating problems during infancy (<12 months) continued to age 10 years in 85 per cent of these children.

Brief parent training or a problem-specific booklet has resulted in 50–80 per cent decreases in inappropriate mealtime behaviour in the two studies that have been conducted on this topic. The following advice for parents might be helpful:

- General advice
  - mealtimes should be free of distractions (e.g. television),
  - do not make multiple meals for different family members,
  - make mealtimes pleasant by talking about the day, etc.,
  - mealtimes should last 20–30 min after which food should be removed.
- Between meals
  - offer healthy snacks,
  - do not allow snacks shortly after a meal that was not eaten,
  - have set time for snacks and meals.
- Getting children to eat
  - initial refusal of new foods is normal,
  - children must taste new foods multiple (8–15) times before they will accept it,
  - provide small portions and allow seconds when child finishes what has been given,
  - do not coax, nag, or force a child to eat,
  - praise good eating,
  - reinforce good eating with activities not with preferred foods (e.g. sweets, desserts).
- Mealtime behaviour
  - respond to inappropriate behaviour (e.g. spitting food, getting up from the table multiple times) as with any other inappropriate behaviour (e.g. one warning followed by time out).

Disruptive behaviour problems (e.g. non-compliance, aggression, poor impulse regulation) occur in 10–17 per cent of children. Many parents and professionals view the 'terrible twos' as a normal developmental phase. However, 50 per cent of pre-school children have these behaviour problems years later and 5–8 per cent have chronic, unremitting problems into adulthood. Early aggressive and oppositional behaviour and poor impulse control are consistent predictors of conduct disorder and delinquency. Children with poor impulse control, lack of empathy, and attention problems should be monitored for development of ADHD (see Chapter 10.12) and language problems and learning disabilities (see Chapter 10.12). Early language problems are a risk factor for developing oppositional problems and co-occurrence has poorer prognosis. The first presentation may be a mother concerned with temper tantrums in her 2–3-year-old. Such concerns should not be dismissed and follow-up is needed.

General advice to parents can include: reduce situational factors likely to trigger child outbursts (e.g. fatigue, hunger, transitioning between activities), establish daily routines, praise appropriate behaviour, ignore negative behaviour, label the child's emotional state, use distraction and redirection, and time out. Discuss parent's needs to manage their own emotional reactions. Connecting parents with community parenting resources is the next step. Self-administered parenting interventions via videotape[7] or specific problem booklets (e.g. interrupting, tantrums) are more effective

(45–55 per cent success) than no treatment (25–30 per cent) but somewhat less effective than treatment administered by a mental-health professional. Children with multiple risk factors should be referred early to more intensive programmes given high risk for ongoing problems and efficacy of early intervention.

School-age children

Encopresis. Almost all children are toilet trained (independent, volitional bowel and bladder control) by age 4 years. However, at least 20 per cent of children demonstrate non-retentive encopresis or stool toileting refusal (regular bowel movements in diapers or pants but not toilet). Toilet refusal contributes to retentive encopresis (i.e. chronic faecal soiling at age 4 years or older) and chronic constipation (i.e. <3 stools/week), which affects 3 per cent of pre-school-age children and 1–2 per cent of school-age children. Most of these children have painful, hard stools and withholding before age 2.5 years. An acute problem with defaecation (e.g. pain) may lead to chronic constipation.

Positive approaches to toileting success and early detection and intervention by primary care physicians are recommended. There are guidelines for both non-retentive[8] and retentive encopresis.[9] History should include stool patterns, constipation and soiling, diet, appetite changes, medication, urinary symptoms, and family history. Abdominal, rectal, and neurological examinations should be included in the physical. Organic factors account for about 1 per cent of cases of non-retentive and 5 per cent of retentive encopresis. Rectal examination should be conducted with caution, appropriate explanation, and preparation to minimize trauma and pain.

Treatment for both types of encopresis is the same with the addition of disimpaction as the first step for retentive encopresis. Disimpaction can be achieved orally: mineral oil—15–30 ml/year of age per day for 3 days or Bisacodyl tablet every day or twice daily. Oral methods are preferred over enemas to minimize additional rectal trauma and pain. Children may accept mineral oil more easily if well mixed with flavoured pudding. Treatment should last at least 6 months with diet change lasting at least a year and include:

1. Behavioural training: (a) regular toilet sitting (three to four times per day for 5–10 min); (b) record all stool passage (time, amount, location); (c) reinforce stool production; and (d) avoid embarrassment or punishment.

2. Diet: (a) daily fibre intake of child's year of age plus 5 g; (b) adequate fluids (1 l/day); (c) restrict constipating foods.

3. Oral medications (for children 6 months or older): (a) mineral oil, magnesium salts, or lactulose: 1–3 mg/kg per day; (b) Senna syrup: 1–5 years = 5 ml daily; >5 years = 10 ml daily.

4. Follow-up for treatment compliance, avoiding reimpaction.

If treatment non-compliance occurs the child should be referred to a behavioural specialist. The addition of behavioural components and/or biofeedback provided by a specialist increases cure rates from about 50 per cent to 75–80 per cent.[10]

Enuresis is defined as urination in bed or clothes in a child older than 5 years, at least twice per week (DSM-IV) or twice per month under age 7 years and once a month over age 7 years (ICD-10), for 3 or more consecutive months—or when wetting results in significant distress or impairment. Enuresis may be nocturnal, diurnal, or both and may be primary (urinary continence never established) or secondary (occurrence after urinary continence established). Organic factors should be ruled out. Prevalence at age 5 years is 7–12 per cent for boys and 3–9 per cent for girls; at age 10 it is 7 per cent for boys and 3–5 per cent for girls and by age 15 it is 1 per cent or less. The spontaneous resolution rate is about 16 per cent per year. Anticipatory guidance with toileting may be preventive.

Enuresis may be related to toilet training problems. Nocturnal enuresis is often considered a problem of maturational delay. There is a strong genetic component with 60–80 per cent of first-degree relatives affected. Bed-wetting occurs when bladder capacity is reached at all stages of sleep not just in 'deep' sleep. Day wetting may present as urge incontinence, dysfunctional voiding associated with paradoxical contraction of the urethral sphincter, or voiding postponement. The first two types have associated urine flow abnormalities. Diurnal enuresis is often associated with urinary tract infections. Enuresis is not associated with higher levels of psychopathology but is related to lower perceived social competence; behaviour problems may occur in children over age 10.

Clinical interview should include medical, developmental and family history, toilet training experiences, psychosocial stressors, and behavioural description of wetting. Assessment includes physical examination, urine culture and urinalysis, and urodynamic testing if warranted.

Behavioural treatments should be used first for both day and night wetting.[11,12] Urine alarms designed to wake the child when urine comes in contact with a pad are used with a variety of behavioural treatments (e.g. overlearning, retention control training) and achieve 75–80 per cent success within 2–3 months.[13] Relapse rates are 10–40 per cent depending on treatment intensity. Drop out rates are high.

Desmopressin and imipramine are more effective than placebo but relapse rates after discontinuation are nine times greater than with the urine alarm. Desmopressin may be warranted for short-term treatments (e.g. camp, sleep over); imipramine has more side-effects. Oxybutinin has been shown effective with urge incontinence.

Behavioural treatments are effective but compliance can be a problem. Consider referral to a behavioural specialist especially if there are child oppositional or parent/family problems, which predict poorer outcomes. If intensive supervision by the physician or referral is not possible, no treatment is a viable option rather than having the child/family become frustrated with treatment, leading to more problems. Parents should maintain a neutral attitude toward wet beds, avoid punishment, praise dry beds, use appropriate protection for the bed, and ensure the child is bathed and clean in the morning.

Adolescents

Conduct disorder is characterized by significant and persistent violations of rules and the rights of others including aggression, property destruction, theft, truancy, etc. Adolescents with conduct disorder frequently show a lack of empathy and fail to appreciate the seriousness of their behaviour. Problems across settings (i.e. home, school, work) are common. Engaging in other risky behaviour (e.g. substance use, early sexual activity) and delinquency is common. Girls use more indirect and verbal forms of aggression (alienation, ostracism). Conduct disorder is less prevalent among older children (boys 3–5 per cent; girls 1–4 per cent) than adolescents (boys 5–10 per cent; girls 2–8 per cent) and much more common among boys than girls (3–5 : 1).[14] Adolescent-onset has a better prognosis than when conduct disorder develops out of childhood oppositional-defiant behaviour. Prognosis for girls is worse than for boys. Co-morbidity of conduct and mood problems has a poorer prognosis.

With adolescent-onset conduct problems of mild severity, advice and guidance for parents may be helpful. Re-establishing a positive parent–adolescent relationship is a good first step, to be followed by development and consistent enforcement of reasonable, clear, behavioural expectations. Connecting the adolescent with positive role models in the community should be encouraged as parents themselves often have problems. Searight et al.[15] offer practical suggestions that would be most appropriate for pre-teens and younger adolescents:

◆ Assess severity and refer for treatment with a sub-specialist as needed.

◆ Treat co-morbid substance abuse first.

◆ Describe the likely long-term prognosis without intervention to caregiver.

◆ Structure children's activities and implement consistent behaviour guidelines.

◆ Emphasize parental monitoring of children's activities (where they are, who they are with).

◆ Encourage the enforcement of curfews.

◆ Encourage children's involvement in structured and supervised peer activities (e.g. organized sports, Scouting).

◆ Discuss and demonstrate clear and specific parental communication techniques.

◆ Help caregivers establish appropriate rewards for desirable behaviour.

◆ Help establish realistic, clearly communicated consequences for non-compliance.

◆ Help establish daily routine of child-directed play activity with parent(s).

◆ Consider pharmaco-therapy for children who are highly aggressive or impulsive, or both, or those with mood disorder.

Adolescents with more than mild problems, problems of longer duration, or older adolescents should be referred for comprehensive treatment involving the adolescent, family, school, peers, etc. This is necessary and effective. Individual treatment is generally ineffective.

Health risk behaviours

A recent survey of high school students in the United States found in the previous 30 days 35 per cent had smoked cigarettes, 50 per cent had drunk alcohol, 33 per cent had ridden with a driver who had been drinking alcohol and 26.7 per cent had used marijuana. Obesity, eating disorders, and suicide are covered in Chapters 9.3, 9.4, and 9.5, respectively. Adolescents often engage in more than one health risk behaviour and adolescents engaging in risky behaviour often have mental health problems and poor academic achievement.

Adolescents view physicians as sources of information on health behaviour. They are reluctant but willing to discuss health behaviours with physicians. Confidentiality concerns can be overcome with explicit reassurance. Physicians report screening 65–98 per cent of adolescents for health risk behaviours (i.e. alcohol, drugs, smoking, sexual behaviours) while 55–70 per cent of adolescents report being asked about risk behaviours and 40–60 per cent report receiving counselling for these behaviours.

The effectiveness of physicians' interventions for risk behaviours has not been well documented. One UK study found that 60 per cent of adolescents who smoked regularly agreed to quit after counselling by their primary care physician or nurse; follow-up data were not obtained. An open-label trial found that nicotine patch and brief counselling for adolescent regular smokers reduced smoking rates. The five As are recommended for smoking interventions in primary care: *ask* patients about tobacco use, *advise* them to quit, *assess* willingness to quit, *assist* in attempting to quit, and *arrange* follow-up.[16] The effectiveness of this approach with adolescents is unknown.

References

1. **US Department of Health and Human Services.** *Mental Health: A Report of the Surgeon General.* Rockville MD: US Department of Health and Human Services, Substance Abuse and Mental Health Services Administration, Center for Mental Health Services, National Institutes of Health, National Institute of Mental Health, 1999.

2. Bower, P., Garralda, E., Kramer, T., Harrington, R., and Sibbald, B. (2001). The treatment of child and adolescent mental health problems in primary care: a systematic review. *Family Practice* **18**, 373–82.

3. **Zero-to-Three.** *Diagnostic Classification 0–3: Diagnostic Classification of Mental Health and Developmental Disorders in Infancy and Early Childhood.* Washington DC. Zero to Three: National Centre for Infants, Toddlers, and Families, 1994.

4. **American Psychiatric Association.** *DSM-IV: Diagnostic and Statistical Manual of Mental Disorders.* Washington DC: American Psychiatric Association, 1994.

5. **American Academy of Pedatrics.** *Classification of Child and Adolescent Mental Diagnoses in Primary Care: Diagnostic and Statistical Manual for Primary Care (DSM-PC).* Elk Grove IL: American Academy of Pediatrics, 1996.

6. Garrison, M.M. and Christakis, D.A. (2000). A systematic review of treatments for infant colic. *Pediatrics* **106**, 184–90.

7. Webster-Stratton, C. (1994). Advancing videotape parent training: a comparison study. *Journal of Consulting and Clinical Psychology* **62**, 583–93.

8. Kuhn, B.R., Marcus, B.A., and Pitner, S.L. (1999). Treatment guidelines for primary nonretentive encopresis and stool toileting refusal. *American Family Physician* **59**, 2171–6.

9. Felt, B., Wise, C.G., Olson, A., Kochlar, P., Marcus, S., and Coran, A. (1999). Guideline for the management of pediatric idiopathic constipation and soiling. *Archives of Pediatric and Adolescent Medicine* **153**, 380–5.

10. McGrath, M.L., Mellon, M.W., and Murphy, L. (2000). Empirically supported treatments in pediatric psychology: constipation and encopresis. *Journal of Pediatric Psychology* **25**, 225–54.

11. von Gontard, A. (1998). Day and night wetting in children: a paediatric and child psychiatric perspective. *Journal of Child Psychology and Psychiatry* **39**, 439–51.

12. **Community Paediatrics Committee Canadian Paediatric Society** (1997). Enuresis. *Paediatrics and Child Health* **2**, 419–21.

13. Mellon, M.W. and McGrath, M.L. (2000). Empirically supported treatments in pediatric psychology: nocturnal enuresis. *Journal of Pediatric Psychology* **25**, 193–214.

14. **American Academy of Child and Adolescent Psychiatry** (1997). AACAP official action: practice parameters for the assessment and treatment of children and adolescents with conduct disorder. *Journal of the American Academy of Child and Adolescent Psychiatry* **36**, 122–39.

15. Searight, H.R., Rottnek, F., and Abby, S.L. (2001). Conduct disorder: diagnosis and treatment in primary care. *American Family Physician* **63**, 1579–88.

16. Fiore, M.C. et al. *Treating Tobacco Use and Dependence: Clinical Practice Guideline.* Rockville MD: US Department of Health and Human Services. Public Health Service, 2000.

10.12 School issues

Debra M. Phillips

Introduction

A physician who cares for the young patient has to become involved with their patient's school system. The family physician needs to know the school system and team members, applicable laws, testing interpretation, diagnosis and management of school-specific problems, and referral mechanisms. The physician can serve as a trained observer that follows the patient for their lifetime and can effectively interface with the school system as an advocate for their patient.

More extensive involvement occurs when the physician is the school's medical advisor. The medical advisor physician role requires a special commitment which includes becoming involved with such issues as health curriculum, policy and procedures dealing with violence, drugs, and sex education.

School readiness and early intervention

School failure is a major concern in most countries. For instance, 7–10 per cent of children in the United States experience substantive school failure and drop out before completing high school.[1] Validated screening tools are recommended but most physicians depend on clinical judgement rather than screening tools. This detects fewer than 30 per cent of children with impairments.[1] Systematically eliciting parental concern about

Table 1 Normal pattern of speech development (adapted from ref. 4, p. 41; 6, 7)

Age	Achievement
1–6 months	Coos in response to voice
6–9 months	Babbling
10–11 months	Imitation of sounds; says 'mama/dada' without meaning
12 months	Says 'mama/dada' with meaning; often imitates two- and three-syllable words
13–15 months	Vocabulary of four to seven words in addition to jargon; <20% of speech understood by strangers
16–18 months	Vocabulary of 10 words; some echolalia and extensive jargon; 20–25% of speech understood by strangers
19–21 months	Vocabulary of 20 words; 50% of speech understood by strangers
22–24 months	Vocabulary >50 words; two-word phrases; dropping out of jargon; 60–70% of speech understood by strangers
2–2.5 years	Vocabulary of 400 words, including names; two- to three-word phrases; use of pronouns; diminishing echolalia; 75% of speech understood by strangers
2.5–3 years	Use of plurals and past tense; knows age and sex; counts three objects correctly; three to five words per sentence; 80–90% of speech understood by strangers
3–4 years	Three to six words per sentence; asks questions, converses, relates experiences, tells stories; almost all speech understood by strangers
4–5 years	Receptive skills: Understands four-element commands; links past and present events Expressive skills: Six to eight words per sentence; names four colours; counts 10 pennies correctly. 2700 word vocabulary; defines simple words; auxiliary verbs: 'has, had'; conversationally mature; 'how and why' questions in response to others; articulation: 'b, k, g, f'; five word sentences; 'normalizes' irregular verbs and nouns
5–6 years	Receptive skills: Understands five element comments; can follow a story without pictures; enjoys jokes and riddles; can comprehend two meanings of word Expressive skills: Correct use of all parts of speech: vocabulary 5000 words; articulation 'y, ng, d' six-word sentences; corrects own errors in speech; can use logic in recounting story plots
6–7 years	Receptive skills: Asks for motivation and explanation of events; understands time intervals (month, seasons); right and left differences Expressive skills: Articulation: 'l, r, t, sh, ch, dr, cl, bl, gl, cr' has formal (adult) speech patterns
7–8 years	Receptive skills: Can use language alone to tell a story sequentially; reasons using language Expressive skills: Articulation: 'v, th, j, s, z, tr, st, sl, sw, sp'
8–9 years	Articulation: 'th, sc, sh'

development is an important method of identifying infants and young children with developmental problems. Parental concerns about language, fine-motor, cognitive, and emotional–behavioural development are highly predictive of true problems.[2] Glascoe[3] has shown that by asking about developmental concerns systematically, the physician can screen for developmental delays as effectively as by using formal developmental screening tools that require developmental examination of the child.

The physician should perform vision testing or know that it is done by the school system. The most significant visual abnormalities develop before or around the time of school entry. Most infantile esotropia and extropia are caught before this age but accommodative esotropia is the result of excessive ocular convergence in farsighted children when they accommodate for near vision. Distant visual acuity of each eye separately is fairly sensitive and specific for these problems but specific testing such as with the Titmus Stereo Fly test improves the detection of accommodative strabismus.[4] At or soon after school entry, all children's hearing should be screened with pure-tone audiometry at 25 dB over at least three frequencies.

Language skills should be monitored at each visit with referral to a speech therapist for further evaluation if there is a problem. A child who is having problems with phonics and reading, even with a normal speech pattern, might benefit from a speech therapist evaluating the child for auditory discrimination[5] (Table 1).

School team members and responsibilities

Family physicians need to coordinate their efforts with many others involved in helping children reach their potentials. Table 2 defines the team members, their roles and responsibilities. The physician's role is to counsel the parents and child by explaining psycho-educational 'jargon', legal rights of student and family, special school programmes. The physician must present both the strengths and weaknesses of any treatment, and suggest behavioural management strategies. Medical assessment should include anticipatory guidance; assessment and treatment of underlying diseases and chronic conditions; pharmacological management when necessary; compiling and reviewing medical tests, psycho-educational tests, parent and teacher evaluation, and psycho-social reports; communicating with school personnel; and participating in multidisciplinary education planning.

Table 2 Multidisciplinary team members—their roles and responsibilities[10]

Team member	Roles and responsibilities
Family physician	Assesses child for medical problems that affect child's ability to learn Provides consultation with regard to medical condition or medication
Parents/guardians	Act as advocates for the child Provide historical, genetic, medical, and environmental information Manage child's behaviour at home
Child	Presents his or her unique perception of the problem
School psychologist	Administers and interprets academic and behavioural assessments Often serves as leader of multidisciplinary team
School teacher	Identifies specific behaviours that interfere with learning Implements curricular modifications and behavioural interventions
Special educator	Acts in a wide variety of roles—may assist with evaluation; designs and implements curriculum or behaviour modifications
School nurse	Dispenses medications prescribed by physicians Consults with teachers regarding effects of medication
School counsellor	Ensures that child is receiving appropriate education regardless of disabilities
School social worker	Acts in a wide variety of roles—may provide vocational, individual or family counselling Provides case management services to child and family
Speech and language specialist	Assesses child's ability to formulate, transmit or receive information; treats speech and language impairments
Medical specialist	Conducts specialized assessments on referral from family physician

Referral to other agencies/services as needed such as social skills training, parenting support groups, speech, physical rehabilitation and occupational therapies, along with monitoring of progress and updating of treatment plan should be integral to the care of the child. The school and other professionals should be notified when a change occurs that might require a change in strategy or treatment plan.[8,9] The physician should be familiar with the applicable laws of their country. The school administration should be able to supply the current laws and local interpretation.

Specific tests

The physician usually will rely on a school psychologist or a consultant to perform psychometric tests. However, the physician needs to have enough familiarity with psychometric tests to assess the appropriateness of the screening administered and the skill of the interpreter, much as the physician can evaluate the quality of the radiologist's interpretation. A cooperative dialogue with the tester will facilitate understanding how the test relates to the physician's patients. Rating scales, especially for attention, usually will be used when evaluating children for attention deficit/hyperactivity disorder. The physician should investigate which one the school's teachers are using. The most common are the Connor's Parent and Teacher Rating Scale and Child Behavior Checklist.

School problems

The family physician should be ready to help in treating or arranging treatment for learning disorders, emotional, and behavioural disorders, and in managing children with mental retardation or chronic illness to maximize their educational potential.

Learning disabilities are characterized by difficulties in the acquisition and use of listening, speaking, writing, reasoning, or computing. Estimates of the incidence of learning disorders range from 2 to 10 per cent (ref. 11, p. 70). Learning disabilities are 'not a single condition but a wide variety of specific disabilities that are presumed to stem from some dysfunction of the brain or central nervous systems'.[12] Family stresses such as marital discord, moves, poverty, or inadequate financial, housing, or other resources can exacerbate learning problems by causing a child to be preoccupied with these issues and less receptive to learning new facts and skills (ref. 11, p. 72). The criteria for diagnosing the different types of learning disabilities are in the DSM-IV diagnostic manual.[13] The family physician has a key role in identifying children likely to suffer from learning disabilities. However, usually the physician relies on the expertise of the school psychologist for diagnosing the learning disability and recommending appropriate interventions. The school system should undertake specific curricular and educational modifications to enhance student learning. Often a physician's interest will expedite this process. Occasionally children will be retained. When this occurs, the physician should advocate for a diagnosis and appropriate intervention. 'Retention without diagnosis is in effect gross institutional educational negligence and should never be condoned.'[14]

Emotional and behavioural disorders can impact school performance problems. It is estimated that 14–20 per cent of learners experience some form of behavioural disorder during their school years.[15] These problems can range from minor disturbances to dramatic symptoms displayed by children with oppositional defiant disorder or conduct disorder. Emotional problems in children are often overlooked or minimized as a reason for poor performance. The family physician must not fail to evaluate the child for the presence of an emotional or psychiatric disorder that might also contribute to school problems. If the physician determines an emotional or behavioural problem, referral and reciprocal communication to a social worker, counsellor, or other mental health professional is appropriate. Specific behavioural disorders, such as conduct disorder and oppositional defiant disorder are discussed in Chapter 10.11.

Mental retardation is characterized by significant cognitive impairments in intellectual functioning and adaptive life skills. 'Approximately 11.5 per cent of all students ages 6 to 21 with disabilities have mental retardation.'[8] A role of the family physician is to be supportive of the parents and to serve as an advocate for the patient. This may involve becoming familiar with educational laws and interfacing with school officials when needed. For example, in the United States, laws concerning least restrictive environments might influence the retention of the child in a neighbourhood school with personalized assistance.

Chronic illness impacts learning when students experience a sensory, physical, or other health-related impairment and may require specific modifications in educational programming. Those impairments include permanent medical conditions such as brain injury, autism, convulsive disorders, and cerebral palsy. Chronic illness also includes chronic or episodic medical condition that may interfere with school, for example, asthma, allergies, diabetes, repeated otitis media, thyroid disorders, or cancer. Candid discussion with the patient, parents, and teachers about what to expect from this condition or illness can be invaluable in preventing secondary reactionary emotional or behavioural problems.

Physical disabilities include hearing impairments, visual impairments, and orthopaedic problems affecting mobility through genetic or accidental injury. Obviously, most if not all other conditions will require physician assessment, diagnosis, and treatment in addition to classroom and curricular adaptations.

Attention deficit hyperactivity disorder/attention deficit disorder

Attention problems affect a child's ability to concentrate and learn. Situational stress, family discord or dysfunction, depression, anxiety, medication or drug use, and illness might be the cause for a child's apparent inability to attend. Attention Deficit Hyperactivity Disorder (ADHD), another reason for learning or behaviour problems in school, is pervasive and characterized by developmentally inappropriate degrees of inattention and impulsiveness with or without hyperactivity.

ADHD affects 3-5 per cent of American school-aged children. In Britain, where there is a more restrictive definition of ADHD, the prevalence rate is 0.1 per cent.[16] Diagnostic criteria of DSM-IV for ADHD require six or more features of inattention (often fails to give close attention to details; has difficulty sustaining attention; does not seem to listen; does not follow through on instructions and fails to finish schoolwork, chores or duties; has difficulty organizing tasks and activities; avoids tasks that require sustained mental effort (such as schoolwork or homework); loses things necessary for tasks or activities; is easily distracted by extraneous stimuli, is forgetful in daily activities) or six or more features of hyperactivity and impulsivity (often fidgets or squirms; leaves seat in classroom; inappropriately runs about or climbs excessively; has difficulty playing or engaging in leisure activities quietly; is 'on the go' or acts as if 'driven by a motor'; talks excessively; blurts out answers before questions have been completed; has difficulty awaiting turn; interrupts or intrudes on others) for at least 6 months that are maladaptive. Gordon[17] presents six 'guideposts' to an ADHD diagnosis, which may be helpful in determining whether a child meets criteria for this disorder. They include:

1. *Impulsivity:* Evidence of impulsive behaviour required, whether hyperactivity is present or not.

2. *Severity:* Symptoms are more frequent and severe than those usually seen in peers.

3. *Onset before 7 years of age:* DSM-IV requirement, reflecting the notion that ADHD is innate.

4. *Pervasiveness:* Symptoms present in at least two settings (e.g. home and school).

5. *Chronicity:* Symptoms present at least 6 months; child has 'always been this way'.

6. *Intentionality:* Unless comorbid with oppositional defiant disorder or conduct disorder, child exhibits remorse about behaviour and, despite best intentions, cannot seem to control behaviour without extreme effort.

An algorithm to help in the diagnosis of ADHD is given in Fig. 1.

If ADHD is diagnosed, a multidisciplinary approach including educational and behavioural interventions must be used in its treatment. Often,

the physician must decide if medications are to be used, recognizing that without appropriate educational interventions, parental involvement, and behaviour modification, medication will not serve the child well. Family physicians should be familiar with commonly used medications, standard monitoring guidelines for the medications and their side-effects. Some family physicians decide not to take a primary role in treating ADHD with medication and refer patients to a developmental paediatrician; however, they often will see the child for other problems and need to be aware of the medication and its effects. If located in a tertiary facility, the developmental paediatrician is not necessarily in the best position to monitor and intervene in the local school system. The family physician will need to maintain an active involvement.

Medication for ADHD

The stimulant medications for ADHD are the mainstay of treatment. Methylphenidate exists in immediate release, sustained release, extended release with an osmotic delivery system and biphasic formulation. Dextroamphetamine also exists in immediate release and sustained release. Pemoline (Cylert) generally should not be prescribed unless the physician is very familiar with the medication and its necessary monitoring. Second- and third-line medications are Clonidine (Catapress), Guanfacine (Tenex), Bupropion (Wellbutrin). The non-selective norepinephrine re-uptake blocker, desipramine, (Norpramin) has been used but has the potential to affect cardiac rhythm. A recently approved, nonstimulating medication that is a selective NE re-uptake blocker, a tomoxetine, has been shown to ameliorate ADHD symptoms. Medications under investigation also include Selegine (Eldepryl) and Modafinil (Provigil). As ADHD is often accompanied by comorbid disorders, SSRIs (Prozac, Zoloft, etc.) and mood stabilizers (lithium, depakote, tegretol) might also be prescribed by specialists. The more commonly used medications by primary care physicians are listed in Table 3.

Stimulant dosages are not weight dependent, so treatment should start with a low dose, titrated until the optimal effect is received with minimal side-effects. To minimize sleep disturbances, the last dose of an immediate release should be prescribed no more than 6 h prior to bedtime. Periodic assessment through rating scales, child, parental, and teacher reports will assist in adjusting dosages. The advantage of once daily dosing is to minimize school administration of medication. Reportedly, the osmostic delivery system gives a more level dosage of medicine. Methylphenidate is also available in a biphasic delivery system, a multiparticulate system in which individual beads of the drug are prepared with specific rate-controlling membranes providing a unique release profile. Continuous release beads and rapid release beads are placed in capsules. Capsules allow children that have not mastered the skill of pill swallowing to take the medication as a sprinkle. This medication reportedly attains peak levels quickly. If one medication

Table 3 Medications used in treating ADHD

Medication	Trade names	Timing
Methylphenidate, immediate release	Ritalin, generic	Daily, bid, tid
Methylphenidate, sustained release	Ritalin SR	Daily
Methylphenidate extended release (osmotic delivery system)	Concerta	Daily
Methylphenidate controlled delivery (biphasic pellet imbedded)	Metadate CD	Daily
Dextroamphetamine, immediate release	Dexedrin	Daily or bid
Dextroamphetamine spansules	Dexedrin spansules	Daily
Amphetamine in combination with dextroamphetamine	Adderall	bid
Amphetamine in combination with dextroamphetamine, extended release	Adderall XR	Daily
Atomoxetine HCL	Strattera	Daily or bid

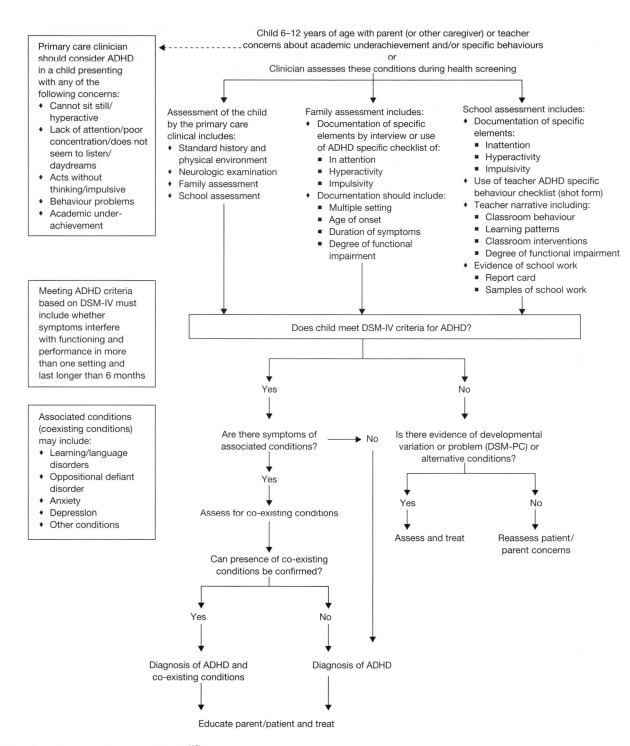

Fig. 1 Algorithm to help in the diagnosis of ADHD.[18]

does not have the desired effect and has been titrated appropriately, the physician should sequentially move to other stimulant medications. After two medication trials, the physician might consider referral for reassessment of the diagnosis and possibly other medication.

Side-effects

The most common side-effects of stimulants are decreased appetite, headache, stomachache, delayed sleep onset, jitteriness, and social withdrawal. Stimulant medication is relatively contra-indicated in children

with seizure disorders and should be initiated by a specialist. Approximately 15–30 per cent of children can experience motor tics while on stimulant medications. Most of these are transient. Having tics or developing them during treatment is not an absolute contraindication to the use of stimulant medications.[19] Growth delay has been clinically reported but no significant impairment of height attainment in adult life was found in a prospective follow-up study.[20] If a child has experienced appetite suppression with weight loss from treatment with a stimulant medication, then drug holidays on weekends and vacations may be helpful because appetite returns immediately when the medication is stopped.[21]

Conclusion

Educational teaching methods and teaching strategies are constantly changing, as are medical interventions. The physician that cares for children should develop a partnership with the education system while keeping abreast of the literature. While physicians will variably choose to be involved, they should at the very least be an advocate and know the appropriate referral resources.

The physician's role is to assist the child to stay as healthy as possible and to communicate with the school as to how the condition and any required medication affects the child's learning ability. Family physicians can monitor the process to assure that the school is responsive to the child's needs, can serve as an advocate for the child, and should monitor any medical interventions for impact on child's learning ability. Periodic contact with teachers is important as well as is providing parental support. Interfacing with the school system, parents and child is well worth the effort as the child's interaction with the school will forever impact their lives.

References

1. Glascoe, F.P. (2000). Early detection of developmental and behavioural problems. *Pediatrics in Review* **21** (8), 272–9.
2. Developmental Surveillance and Screening of Infants and Young Children (RE0062). American Academy of Pediatrics, http://www.aap.org/policy/re0062.html.
3. Glascoe, F.P. *Collaborating with Parents: Using Parents' Evaluation of Development Status to Detect and Address Developmental and Behavioral Problems in Children.* Nashville TN: Ellsworth and Vandermeer Press, 1998.
4. Nader, P., ed. *School Health: Policy and Practice.* Elk Grove Village IL: American Academy of Pediatrics, 1993.
5. Fox, M. and Mahoney, W. *Children with School Problems, A Physician's Manual.* Canadian Paediatric Society, 1998.
6. Leung, A.K.C. and Kao, C.P. (1999). Evaluation and management of the child with speech delay. *American Family Physician* 3121-34. http://www.aafp.org/afp/990600ap/3121.html.
7. Schwartz, E.R. (1990). Speech and language disorders. In *Pediatric Primary Care: A Problem Oriented Approach* (ed. M.W. Schwartz), pp. 696–700. St Louis: Mosby.
8. McInerny, T.K. (1995). Children who have difficulty in school: a primary pediatricians approach. *Pediatrics in Review* **16** (9), 325–32.
9. Dworkin, P.H. (1989). School failure. *Pediatrics in Review* **10** (10), 301–11.
10. Phillips, D., Longlett, S., Mulrine, C., Kruse, J., and Kewney, R. (1999). School problems and the family physician. *American Family Physician* **59** (10), 2816–24.
11. Wolraich, M.L., ed. *The Classification of Child and Adolescent Mental Diagnoses in Primary Care: Diagnostic and Statistical Manual for Primary Care (DSM-PC) Child and Adolescent Version.* Elk Grove Village IL: American Academy of Pediatrics, 1996.
12. Slavin, R.E., ed. *Educational Psychology* 5th edn. New York: Houghton Mifflin, 1997.
13. American Psychiatric Association. *Diagnostic and Statistical Manual of Mental Disorders* 4th edn. Text revision. Washington DC: American Psychiatric Association, 2000.
14. Accardo, P. The invisible disability: understanding learning disabilities in the context of health and education. Occasional Paper, National Health/Education Convention, 1996, p. 27.
15. Borich, G.D. and Tombari, M.L., ed. *Educational Psychology: A Contemporary Approach* 2nd edn. New York: Longman, 1997.
16. Esser, G., Schmidt, M.H., and Woerner, W. (1990). Epidemiology and course of psychiatric disorders in school-age children: results of a longitudinal study. *Journal of Child Psychology and Psychiatry* **31**, 243–63.
17. Gordon, M. *How to Operate an ADHD Clinic or Subspecialty Practice.* DeWitt NY: GSI Publications, 1995.
18. American Academy of Pediatrics (2000). Clinical Practice Guideline: diagnosis and evaluation of the child with attention deficit/hyperactivity disorder. *Pediatrics* **105**, 1158–70.
19. Gadow, K.D., Sverci, J., Sprafkin, J., Nolan, E.E., and Grossman, S. (1999). Long-term methylphenidate therapy in children with co-morbid attention-deficit hyperactivity disorder and chronic multiple tic disorder. *Archives of General Psychiatry* **56**, 330–6.
20. Mannuzza, S. et al. (1991). Hyperactive boys almost grown up. Replication of psychiatric status. *Archives of General Psychiatry* **48**, 77–83.
21. Adesman, A.R. and Morgan, A. (1999). Management of stimulant medications in children with attention-deficit/hyperactivity disorder. *Pediatric Clinics of North America* **46**, 945–63.

Further reading

Physician

Greydanus, D. and Wolraich, M., ed. *Behavioural Pediatrics.* New York: Springer-Verlag, 1992.

Classification of Child and Adolescent Mental Diagnoses in Primary Care. American Academy of Pediatrics, 1996.

Aylward, G. *Practitioner's Guide to Developmental and Psychological Testing.* New York: Plenum Publishing, 1994.

Fox, M. and Mahoney, W. *Children with School Problems, A Physician's Manual.* Canadian Paediatric Society, 1998.

Paasche, C.L., Gorrill, L., and Strom, B. *Children with Special Needs in Early Childhood Settings.* New York: Addison-Wesley Publishing Company, 1990.

Batshaw, M.L. and Perret, Y.M., ed. *Children with Disabilities: A Medical Primer.* Baltimore MD: Brooks, 1992.

Parker, S. and Zuckerman, B., ed. *Behavioral and Developmental Pediatrics: A Handbook for Primary Care.* Boston MA: Little Brown and Company, 1995.

Parent

Barkley, R.A. *Taking Charge of ADHD,* revised edition. New York: Guilford Press, 2000.

Silver, L.B. *The Misunderstood Child: Understanding and Coping with Your Child's Learning Disabilities.* Times Books, 1998.

Internet websites and organizations

Centers for Disease Control and Prevention, Division of Adolescent and School Health (DASH), http://www.cdc.gov/nccdphp/dash/.

American School Health Association, http://www.ashaweb.org/.

School Health Resources, http://www.schoolhealth.org/.

Children and Adults with Attention-Deficit/Hyperactivity Disorder, http://www.chadd.org.

Learning Disabilities Association of America, http://www.ldaamerica.org.

11

Neurological problems

11 Neurological problems

11.1 Headache and facial pain

John Murtagh

According to Cormack et al., 85 per cent of the population will have experienced headache within 1 year and 38 per cent will have had a headache within 2 weeks.[1]

In Denmark, a survey of 1000 people found that the lifetime prevalence of episodic tension headache was 66 per cent, of migraine 15 per cent, chronic tension headache 3 per cent, hangover 72 per cent, disorders of the nose and sinuses 15 per cent, and disorders of the neck 1 per cent.[2]

In the United States, a study based on telephone interviews of more than 12 000 people showed marked differences in the prevalence of migraine in individuals from various ethnic backgrounds.[3] The prevalence of those of European, African, and Asian origin were, respectively, 20, 16, and 9 per cent for women and 8, 7, and 4 per cent for men. Prevalence in men and women was roughly equal until puberty.

Five per cent of children suffer from migraine by the age of 11 years. A study of 617 Australian University students revealed that 8 per cent of men and 18 per cent of women had suffered from migraine.

A study of 3501 subjects in Greece in 1996 revealed that 19 per cent of men and 40 per cent of women suffered from headaches in the previous year.[4] Headaches were more frequent in lower social classes, in people with less education and in those between 45 and 64 years of age. Daily headache was present in 15 per cent of headache sufferers. There was a significant correlation with headaches and low mean temperature (Northern versus Southern Greece).

Presentation in general practice

Headache is certainly a common presenting problem in general practice. Excluding pregnancy, hypertension, immunization, and routine check-up it was the sixth most common presenting symptom in a morbidity study of Australian General Practice, representing two per 100 encounters.[5] A morbidity study in the United States indicated that the frequency of headache was less than the Australian study being the tenth most frequent symptom.

Prevalence of the types of headaches vary according to different medical settings with specialist practice invariably reporting a much higher incidence of vascular headache compared with general practice (e.g. 34 versus 13 per cent) while there is a similarity in frequency of presentation for tension-type headache.[6] General practice reports a higher level of mixed or undiagnosed headache (of the order of 15–20 per cent) and the 'other' category includes causes such as influenza, sinusitis, and trauma. Accident and emergency departments report a different spectrum with a predictably higher incidence of 'general medical', febrile illness, intracranial bleed, and raised intracranial pressure.

Causation of headache and facial pain

Common causes

The commonest cause of headache and facial pain presenting in general practice is acute respiratory infection. The most common causes of chronic daily headache are tension-type headache, so-called transformed migraine and combination headache. Dental disorders are the commonest cause of facial pain accounting for up to 90 per cent of pain in and about the face.[7] There is also a significant association with anxiety disorders and depressive illness.

Tension-type headache

Tension or muscle contraction headaches are typically a symmetrical tightness. They tend to last for hours and recur each day. They are often associated with cervical dysfunction and stress or tension, although a patient usually does not realize the headaches are associated with tension until it is pointed out. Seventy-five per cent of patients are female.[8]

Migraine

Migraine, or the 'sick headache', is derived from the Greek word meaning 'pain involving half the head'. It affects at least one person in 10, is more common in females and peaks between 20 and 50 years. There are various types of migraine with classic migraine (headache, vomiting, and aura) and common migraine (without the aura) being the best known.

Transformed migraine

This describes the progressive increase in frequency of migraine attacks until the headache recurs daily. The typical migraine features become modified so that the pattern resembles that of tension headache but with the unilateral situation of migraine. Overuse of analgesics are implicated.

Combination headache

General practitioners would recognize this pattern, which is typified by relatively constant pain lasting for many days and had a mix of components such as tension, migraine, depression, cervical dysfunction, and drug dependence. Neurologists may refer to these headaches as 'tension-vascular headache'.

Dental pain

Dental pain in the maxillary and mandibular regions of the face is caused by dental caries, impacted teeth, infected tooth sockets and dental roots (periapical and apical abscesses). Pain is usually confined to the affected tooth but it may be diffuse.

Sinusitis

Sinusitis which usually accompanies a generalized upper respiratory tract infection presents as a frontal or retro-orbital headache or with maxillary facial pain. There is usually tenderness to percussion over the affected sinuses.

Cervical neuralgia

Headache from neck disorders, often referred to as occipital neuralgia is often managed successfully by physical therapists. Pain from cervical structures can be referred retro-orbitally and over one-half of the head. The headache is often incorrectly diagnosed as migraine.[8]

Drug rebound headache

These headaches are usually associated with analgesic and ergotamine dependence of long standing. The headache is present on waking and typically persists throughout the day but fluctuates in intensity. Drug rebound headaches should be suspected in any patient who complains of a headache 'all day, every day'.

Serious causes not to be missed

For the acute 'thunderclap' headache it is vital not to miss subarachnoid haemorrhage or an enlarging aneurysm. Intracranial haemorrhage, especially involving cerebellar, intraventricular, and frontal lobe areas, needs to be considered. Benign intracranial hypertension also requires consideration especially in obese young women.

Acute 'thunderclap' headache

This is a sudden severe headache that can be caused by the following:

- *Enlarging aneurysm:* an enlarging aneurysm or vascular malformation can cause acute headache.
- *Subarachnoid haemorrhage (SAH):* the pain is typically occipital, localized at first, then generalized, and may vary in intensity.
- *Meningitis:* must be considered if the headache is generalized especially in the presence of malaise, fever, and neck stiffness. The ache which is constant and severe may begin abruptly.

Raised intracranial pressure

This should be considered with a progressive increasingly severe headache especially if it is associated with symptoms such as diplopia, mental changes, or impairment of consciousness. Typical features are generalized headache, usually worse in the morning, aggravated by abrupt changes in intracranial pressure such as coughing.

Consider an extradural haematoma if there has been a history of head injury in the past 24 hours. Also consider subdural haematoma which may take days or weeks to develop. Consider benign (idiopathic) intracranial hypertension in an obese young woman once a space-occupying lesion has been excluded. It may be precipitated by specific medications such as tetracyclines. Headache is an uncommon presenting symptom of a cerebral tumour but they can cause headache early if their situation displaces major vessels or obstructs the flow of CSF.

Giant cell (temporal) arteritis

Giant cell arteritis should be considered in a patient aged 55 or older who presents with headache for the first time. There is usually a persistent unilateral throbbing headache in the temporal region while pain in the jaw muscles on chewing (jaw claudication) and the generalized muscle and joint pains of polymyalgia rheumatica may provide clues to the diagnosis which is reinforced by an elevated ESR.

Carcinoma of facial and skull structures

Carcinoma of structures such as the nasopharynx, mouth, tonsils, sinuses, bone, and orbit can present with atypical chronic facial pain. Nasopharyngeal cancer spreads upwards to the base of the skull early.

Unusual 'neurological' causes

The following which include migraine variants and cranial nerve neuralgias need to be considered.

Cluster headache

Occurs in paroxysmal clusters of unilateral headaches that typically occur nightly (early morning 2–4 a.m.) for weeks or months at a time followed by months or years of freedom. The pain is usually retro-orbital and associated with redness and watering of the eye but no visual disturbances or vomiting. It occurs typically in males (6 : 1 ratio).

Facial migraine or 'lower half headache'

Migraine may rarely affect the face below the level of the eyes, causing pain in the area of the cheek and lower jaw. The pain is dull and throbbing and nausea and vomiting are commonly present.

Chronic paroxysmal hemicrania

In this episodic condition, there is headache and unilateral upper facial pain that can resemble chronic cluster headache but the duration is briefer (about 15 minutes) and it may recur many times a day. It usually responds dramatically to indomethacin.

Trigeminal neuralgia

Classical 'tic douloureux' is a severe stabbing pain usually affecting the second and third divisions of the trigeminal nerve. The brief paroxysms (typically 1–2 minutes) are often associated with trigger factors such as touching the nasolabial folds or chin, chewing or wind blowing in the face.

Glossopharyngeal neuralgia

This is a rare condition of the ninth cranial nerve causing paroxysms of severe lancinating pain in the back of the throat around the tonsillar fossa with radiation into the ear and ear canal.

Atypical facial pain

This is mainly a diagnosis of exclusion in which patients, usually middle aged women, complain of atypical diffuse deep seated 'boring' pain in the cheek—unilateral or bilateral—without conforming to a specific nerve distribution. They may respond to an antidepressant.

Herpes zoster

The nerve root pain of the pre-eruption phase and subsequent post-herpetic neuralgia which causes difficulty with diagnosis initially and then management needs to be borne in mind.

Other causes

There are a multiplicity of other causes such as temporomandibular joint dysfunction, eye disorders (glaucoma, iritis, refractive errors), depression, sleep apnoea, post head trauma, hypoglycaemia, Paget's disease and hypertension, which is an uncommon cause.

Making the diagnosis

It is important in general practice to develop a diagnostic protocol based around an appropriate history which in turn is based on sound knowledge of the important causes and their patterns of presentation.

The history

A full description of the pain including a pain analysis should be obtained.
The essentials include the following:

Length of headache history: hours, days, months, years?
Site: unilateral or bilateral, localized or diffuse?
Radiation: to the occiput, the vertex, face, eye, teeth, or other areas?
Quality: tightness or pressure, pulsatile, lancinating
Severity: debilitating or tolerable, effect on activities
Frequency: of recurrence
Duration: minutes, hours, days, weeks?
Onset or offset: abrupt or gradual, waking from sleep, time of day

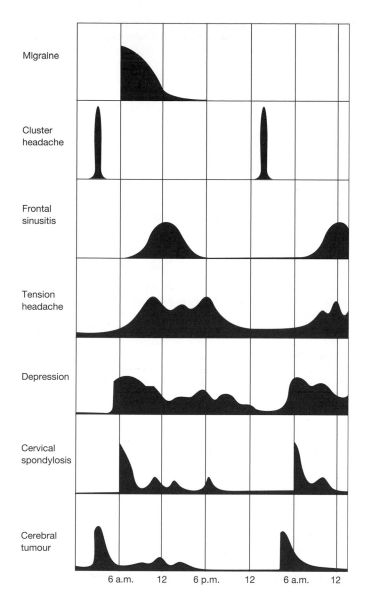

Fig. 1 Typical diurnal patterns of various causes of headache; the relative intensity of pain is plotted on the vertical axis. (Reprinted from: Murtagh, J. *General Practice*. Sydney: McGraw-Hill, 2001.)

Premonitory symptoms including aura

Precipitating factors: emotion, stress, alcohol, exercise, straining, hunger, others?

Relieving factors: relaxation, drugs, alcohol, food, sleep, complementary therapy?

Associated factors: nausea, vomiting, dizziness, problems with vision, teeth, nose, scalp?

Other aspects of the history should include past history (e.g. head injury, illness), family history (e.g. migraine), social history, psychological history, and drug use (alcohol, tobacco, other social drugs, analgesics, oral contraceptive pill).

As a diagnostic pointer, the author finds that plotting the fluctuation of headache during the day is very helpful (Fig. 1). It is useful to get the patient to plot on a prepared grid the relative intensity of the pain and the times of day (and night) that the pain is present or onsets.

It is important to consider red flags, that is, warning features of a serious illness (Table 1).

Table 1 Headache and facial pain: red flags (history)

Sudden onset
Severe and debilitating pain
Fever
Vomiting
Disturbed consciousness
Worse with bending or coughing
Maximum in morning
Neurological symptoms/signs
Young obese female? on medication
'New' in elderly, especially >50 years

Table 2 Headache and facial pain: red flags (examination)

Altered consciousness or cognition
Meningism
Abnormal vital signs: BP, temperature, respiration
Focal neurological signs including pupils, fundi, eye movement
Tender, poorly pulsatile cranial arteries

The physical examination

For the physical examination, it is appropriate to use the basic tools of the trade, namely the thermometer, sphygmomanometer, pen torch, and diagnostic set including the ophthalmoscope and the stethoscope. Record the basic parameters: temperature, pulse rate, blood pressure, and respiratory rate. Inspect the head, temporal arteries, and eyes. Areas to palpate include the temporal arteries, the facial and neck muscles, the cervical spine and sinuses, the teeth and temporomandibular joints. Search especially for signs of meningeal irritation and papilloedema.

A mental state examination is mandatory and includes looking for altered consciousness or cognition and assessment of mood, anxiety–tension–depression, and any mental changes. Neurological examination includes assessment of visual fields and acuity, reactions of the pupils and eye movements in addition to sensation and motor power in the face and limbs.

Consider significant signs that warn of a serious causation (Table 2).

Investigations

Investigations should be judiciously selected. A clear cut and long history of classical tension-type headache or migraine does not require investigation. Ordering complex imagery to reassure an anxious or demanding patient should be resisted.

An urgent CT scan is required for an acute severe headache. If normal but the index of suspicion of subarachnoid haemorrhage is high, a lumbar puncture should be performed after a time elapse of 12 h. CT scans will reveal 90–95 per cent of SAH if performed within 4–5 days. Other investigations including a full blood count and ESR, X-rays of sinuses, neck or teeth, or temporal artery biopsy may be required where dictated by the clinical features.

Principles of management

The basic cause must be treated by the appropriate means whether it be with antibiotics for an infective cause, dental or surgical intervention, antiepileptics such as carbamazepine for the neuralgias, indomethacin for facial migraine (lower half headache), exercises for cervical or temporomandibular dysfunction, prednisolone for temporal arteritis, antidepressants for depression or the various antimigrainous preparations for migraine. In all instances, the ideal general practice model of appropriate patient support, patient education, reassurance about the nature of a non-serious cause, preventive measures, and referral to a specialist where indicated should be followed.

Tension-type headache

The principle is to direct patients to modify their lifestyle and avoid tranquillizers and analgesics. The key is reassuring patient education followed by counselling. This includes advice on stress reduction, relaxation therapy, and yoga or meditation classes. If analgesics are needed, recommend milder ones such as aspirin or paracetamol. The antidepressant, amitriptyline, has proven usefulness in controlling chronic tension headache.

Migraine

Lifestyle factors and precipitating causes need to be assessed and addressed where appropriate. An important principle is to prescribe the simplest possible effective analgesic as early as possible. For example, some patients can be relieved adequately by taking paracetamol or resting quietly. However, in most cases it is recommended to prescribe an antiemetic such as metoclopramide or prochlorperazine followed by three soluble aspirin, or an ergotamine preparation or a triptan 10 minutes later.[1,3]

According to Lance, prophylactic therapy is required if migraine is recurring more than twice a month and not responding rapidly to acute therapy. Options include 5-HT2 antagonists (pizotifen, cyproheptadine, methysergide), β-blockers without any sympathomimetic activity (propranolol, timolol, metoprolol, atenolol), sodium valproate and selected antidepressants (tricyclics, phenelzine).

Explore the possibility of complementary therapies especially for severe chronic cases. Examples include stress reduction and related therapies, cervical mobilization and exercises, acupuncture, and special dietary modification.

Cluster headaches

Proven options to treat bouts of cluster headache are verapamil, lithium carbonate, methysergide, sodium valproate, corticosteroids (a short course), and ergotamine. Inhalation of 100 per cent oxygen for 15 minutes can terminate most attacks. Other options are sumatriptan SC injection, and dihydroergotamine plus metoclopramide by injection.

Long-term and continuing care

Strategies for long-term and continuing care include the following principles which the family doctor is ideally placed to supervise.

♦ Continuing support including regular review.

♦ Providing quality patient education material for specific conditions.

♦ Promote optimal lifestyle factors including nutritional advice, regular exercise, and relaxation.

♦ Avoidance of foodstuffs or drinks that may trigger migraine syndromes, for example, alcohol (especially red wine), chocolate, oranges, tomatoes, citrus fruits, cheeses.

♦ Avoidance or use in moderation of toxic products such as social drugs including alcohol and nicotine, analgesics, prescribed drugs.

♦ Modification of occupation factors such as undue stress, inhalation of toxic fumes, and excessive physical work especially affecting the spine.

♦ Regular dental checks.

♦ Self-treatment of a new onset upper respiratory infection early and vigorously with rest, simple analgesics, and inhalations.

Implications of the problems

The problem of headache particularly chronic recurrent headache has profound social and economic implications. As a common problem it causes individual suffering as well as public expense. For the individual sufferer there is loss of productivity, family and workplace stresses, and loss of self-esteem.

A study by Strang et al. on 'Reduced labor force participation among primary care patients with headaches'[9] concluded that the likelihood of reduced labour force participation among primary care patients with headaches was considerable and concentrated among the one in five patients with a poor long-term outcome. Furthermore, headache patients are at a social disadvantage in attaining occupational role stability such as younger women or poorly educated patients. They were more likely to report reduced labour force participation.

A Swedish study by Antonov and Isacson[10] indicated that both physical and mental work stress were strongly associated with frequent headaches among both men and women, being most common in the age group 25–44 years. Heavy mental work stress was most strongly associated with frequent headache among men and heavy physical work stress among women. The obvious recommendation was that improved working conditions could be one way of preventing headache, thereby decreasing individual suffering and employer as well as public expense.

According to figures released by the Australian Bureau of Statistics in its 1989–90 survey, the cost to Australia of migraine has been estimated as between 302 and 721 million dollars each year.

Key points

♦ The GP should always be alert for life-threatening causes of headache by considering carefully the so-called 'red flags'. Be surveillant for subarachnoid haemorrhage, an enlarging aneurysm, or meningitis (particularly meningococcal meningitis).

♦ Migraine affects at least 10% of the adult population and one-quarter of these patients require medical attention for their attacks at some stage. Be careful to avoid labelling SAH and drug-seeking patients as migraine attacks.[8]

♦ Cluster headache is quite different from migraine, both in terms of presentation and in terms of proper treatment.

♦ Many headaches previously considered to be tension are secondary to disorders of the neck, eyes, teeth, temporomandibular joints, or other structures.[8]

♦ For each migraine sufferer, an individual treatment plan including a migraine action plan should be devised.

♦ Hypertension is a rare cause of primary headache but blood pressure measurement should be taken in these patients particularly to reassure them.

♦ Analgesic dependence/abuse can transform episodic migraine or tension-type headache into chronic daily headache.

References

1. **Cormack, J., Marinker, M., and Morrell, D.** (1980). The patient complaining of headache. In *Practice*, p. 3.12. London: Kluwer Medical.
2. **Rasmussen, B.K.** (1995). Epidemiology of headache. *Cephalagia* **15**, 45–68.
3. **Stewart, W.F., Lipton, R.B., and Liberman, J.** (1996). Variation in migraine prevalence by race. *Neurology* **47**, 52–9.

4. **Mitsikostas, D.D.** et al. (1996). The prevalence of headache in Greece: correlation to latitude and climatological factors. *Headache* **36** (3), 168–73.

5. **Bridges-Webb, C.** et al. (1992). Morbidity and treatment in general practice in Australia 1990–1991. *Medical Journal of Australia* (Special Suppl.), S1–56.

6. **Fardy, H.J. and Harris, M.** (1993). Headache in general practice. *Medical Journal of Australia* **159**, 36–9.

7. **Gerschman, J.A. and Reade, P.C.** (1984). Orofacial pain. *Australian Family Physician* **13**, 14–24.

8. **Anthony, M.** (1996). Migraine and tension headache. In *MIMS Disease Index* 2nd edn., pp. 313–16. Sydney: IMS Publishing.

9. **Strang, P., Von Korff, M., and Galer, B.S.** (1998). Reduced labor force participation among primary care patients with headache. *Journal of General Internal Medicine* **13** (5), 296–302.

10. **Antonov, K. and Isacson, D.** (1997). Headache in Sweden: the importance of working conditions. *Headache* **37** (4), 228–34.

Further reading

Moulds, R.F.W. et al. *Therapeutic Guidelines: Neurology.* Melbourne: Therapeutic Guidelines Limited, 1997, pp. 52–8. (A comprehensive summary of headache syndromes with specific management guidelines.)

Lance, J.W. (2000). Headache and facial pain. *Medical Journal of Australia* **172**, 450–3. (An authoritative overview in the MJA's Practice Essentials series with excellent references. The main reference for this chapter.)

Murtagh, J. Headache (Chapter 55, pp. 515–31); Pain in the face (Chapter 48, pp. 487–95). In *General Practice.* Sydney: McGraw-Hill, 2001. (Detailed information relevant to general practice.)

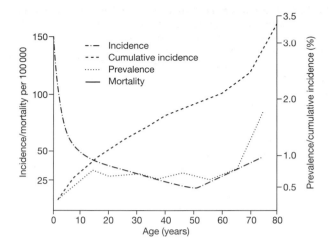

Fig. 1 Incidence, prevalence, and cumulative incidence rates for epilepsy in Rochester, Minnesota 1935–74. (Reproduced from Anderson et al.[1] with permission.)

which patients have been followed from the time of first presentation show that although the chance of recurrent seizures following a single seizure is relatively high (approximately 50–70 per cent risk in the following 2 years), the long-term prognosis is good.[2] A retrospective population-based study carried out in Rochester, Minnesota,[3] of patients registered with epilepsy who were followed up over many years, found that by 20 years from the onset, 76 per cent of patients had at least one 5-year period of complete freedom from seizures, and 70 per cent remained seizure-free. Approximately 50 per cent of the total were in a remission of at least 5 years and had been off all antiepileptic drugs for at least 5 years. The fact that in most studies the cumulative incidence of epilepsy is considerably higher than the prevalence confirms the fact that many people who have epilepsy at some time in their lives subsequently enter long-term remission.

11.2 Epilepsy

Leone Ridsdale and Yvonne Hart

The epidemiology of epilepsy

Incidence and prevalence

Epilepsy is the commonest serious neurological condition. Precise estimates of incidence and prevalence vary according to the definition (e.g. whether patients with single seizures are included), and are complicated by the difficulty in making a diagnosis. However, the annual incidence of epilepsy, defined as 'the tendency to recurrent unprovoked seizures' has usually been estimated at between 30 and 70 per 100 000. All age groups are affected, with a high incidence in the elderly, probably due to the effect of cerebrovascular disease (Fig. 1).[1] The incidence is also high in children, but falls in middle age.

The prevalence of active epilepsy has been estimated at between four and eight per 1000 people, in the developed world, though it may be higher in developing countries. The lifetime prevalence of seizures (the risk of having a non-febrile epileptic seizure at some point in an average lifetime) is around 2–5 per cent.

The natural history of epilepsy

Epilepsy has traditionally been viewed as a chronic condition starting in childhood and with only a small chance of remission. However, studies in

How common is epilepsy in primary care?

A general practitioner with 1500 patients will have about 10 patients on antiepileptic drugs, and one patient newly developing epilepsy each year. Of these, on average one patient will have seizures that are difficult to control, and three will have had a seizure in the past 6 months.[4]

General practitioners in the United Kingdom are generally less used to monitoring epilepsy than some other chronic conditions such as asthma and diabetes. On average a patient will discuss their epilepsy with their general practitioner once a year.[4] The average period since last consultation with a specialist is 5 years, though there is considerable variation.

What are the causes of epilepsy?

Most studies have identified an underlying cause for epilepsy in only about 50 per cent of cases or less. In the National General Practice Study of Epilepsy (NGPSE),[5] in which patients newly developing or diagnosed with epilepsy were studied, the probable aetiology could be identified in 41 per cent. The commonest cause overall was cerebrovascular disease, which was responsible for seizures in 15 per cent of patients. Cerebral tumour was present in 7 per cent, alcohol abuse in 6 per cent, a history of trauma in 3 per cent, and current or past infection in 2 per cent. Other causes, including perinatal injury, drugs, vaccination, tuberous sclerosis, and metabolic disorders were responsible in a small percentage of patients.

Table 1 International classification of epileptic seizures (simplified)

I Partial (focal, local) seizures
A Simple partial seizures (consciousness not impaired)
B Complex partial seizures (with impairment of consciousness)
C Partial seizures secondarily generalized
II Generalized seizures (convulsive or non-convulsive)
A Absence seizures (formerly 'petit mal')
B Myoclonic seizures
C Clonic seizures
D Tonic seizures
E Tonic–clonic seizures (formerly 'grand mal')
F Atonic seizures
III Unclassified epileptic seizures

Seizure types

The proportion of patients with generalized and partial seizure types is dependent on the age at which the epilepsy develops. In the NGPSE, encompassing patients of all ages, 39 per cent of patients had generalized seizures, with neither clinical nor EEG evidence of focal onset. Fifty-two per cent had partial or secondarily generalized seizures, while in 9 per cent the seizures were unclassifiable. Generalized seizures are more common in children than in adults.

The classification of epilepsy

Systems for classifying epilepsy vary slightly. A simple version is shown in Table 1.

Broadly speaking, the classification divides seizures into two groups: partial seizures, in which the clinical and/or electrographic features indicate that the onset is limited to a particular part of one cerebral hemisphere, and generalized seizures, in which involvement of both hemispheres (usually with immediate loss of awareness) occurs from the onset. The first presentation of generalized seizures is commonly, though not exclusively, in childhood or adolescence. 'Unclassified' epileptic seizures are usually those about which there is insufficient information to classify them into one of the other groups.

This classification is of practical use in guiding drug treatment: for example, ethosuximide is helpful in the treatment of absence seizures but not other seizure types, while in children with generalized tonic–clonic seizures in addition to absences, sodium valproate would be the drug of choice.

Two important syndromes arising in childhood or adolescence are benign epilepsy of childhood with centrotemporal spikes (BECCTS) (sometimes known as benign Rolandic epilepsy), and juvenile myoclonic epilepsy. BECCTS causes 10–15 per cent of childhood epilepsy, and usually develops between the ages of 5 and 10 years. The presentation is commonly with simple partial seizures, often affecting the face, and occasionally progressing to become complex partial or secondarily generalized seizures which occur particularly at night. The interictal EEG is characteristic. The importance of recognizing this syndrome is that it has a good prognosis, with complete remission of seizures by the time of puberty, and treatment may not always be necessary.

Juvenile myoclonic epilepsy (JME), like BECCTS, is common, probably being responsible for 5–10 per cent of cases of epilepsy. It usually starts between the ages of 12 and 19 years, the patients experiencing myoclonic jerks, usually occurring soon after awakening, and commonly associated with generalized tonic–clonic seizures. The seizures are usually easily controlled with sodium valproate, but if this is withdrawn, relapse occurs in most patients.

The diagnosis of epilepsy

The diagnosis of epilepsy carries serious social and medical implications, and is perhaps the most important part of epilepsy management. The differential diagnosis of epilepsy depends to a considerable extent on the seizure type. For simple partial seizures, it includes migraine or transient ischaemic attacks, while the commonest differential diagnoses for seizures involving loss of consciousness are syncope and 'non-epileptic seizures' (previously known as 'pseudoseizures'). The diagnosis of most medical problems can be made on the history alone, and this is particularly true in epilepsy, with its paroxysmal nature, in which interictal examination and investigations may be entirely normal. It is crucial to obtain an eye-witness description in addition to the patient's own account, and the general practitioner should encourage an observer to accompany the patient to the hospital consultation.

Differentiation of seizures from syncope

A detailed history is crucial to making an accurate diagnosis. Important aspects include the circumstances of the episode of loss of consciousness, precipitating factors, the nature of the attack itself, and the description of the post-ictal phase. These are exemplified in the differentiation of seizures from syncope. Contrary to popular belief, syncope may cause stiffening of the body, twitching of the limbs, and occasional incontinence, and such symptoms should not be considered pathognomonic of epilepsy. The history should initially concentrate on attempting to identify a precipitating factor for syncope, such as standing for long periods, particularly if the ambient temperature is hot, pain, strong emotion, micturition, diarrhoea, and vomiting. Secondly, it is uncommon for syncope to occur without some warning symptoms, usually including some combination of nausea, blurred vision, light-headedness, and a sensation of muffled hearing (the epigastric sensation which may occur in temporal lobe epilepsy needs to be distinguished from the nausea heralding syncope). While syncope is often accompanied by pallor and sweating, cyanosis is usual in the early stages of generalized tonic–clonic seizures. The actual duration of the loss of consciousness in syncope usually amounts to a few seconds (generally <20) only; it may, however, be longer if the patient is supported in the upright position after fainting, so that adequate cerebral circulation cannot be re-established and a provoked seizure ensues, or if the patient sustains a head injury in the course of fainting causing a concussive seizure. Except in such complicated cases, the post-ictal phase following syncope does not involve prolonged drowsiness and confusion, and recovery is generally rapid, though the patient may feel a sense of malaise for some time. Tongue-biting suggests the occurrence of a seizure.

Other important aspects of the history

The previous medical history may indicate possible causes of epilepsy or alternative diagnoses. Thus, a history of birth injury, prolonged febrile seizures, significant head injury, meningitis, encephalitis, or a family history of epilepsy may indicate a specific cause for epilepsy. Enquiries should also be made about intake of alcohol and drugs. On the other hand, a history of cardiac disease could suggest a dysrhythmia as a cause for blackouts, while a history of previous somatisation disorder, for example, might raise the possibility of non-epileptic attacks.

Although the history is likely to provide the diagnosis in the majority of cases, a brief neurological examination (including examination of fundi) and general examination (to include measurement of blood pressure and examination of the heart) should be carried out.

At this point, the diagnosis may be clear, and if it is syncope, reassurance of the patient all that is required. Other investigations such as routine ECG, echocardiogram, or 24-h ECG monitoring may be indicated by the history. If the diagnosis at this stage appears most likely to be a seizure, the patient should be advised regarding safety precautions (including being told not to drive) and referred to a neurologist or other specialist with an interest in epilepsy.

Referral and investigations

For the specialist, as for the family doctor, the most important aspect of the consultation is the history, since epilepsy remains essentially a clinical

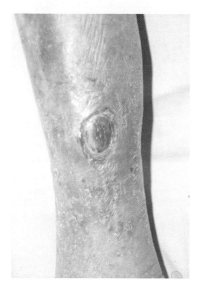

Plate 1 Arterial leg ulcer with 'punched out' appearance and muscle in the base.

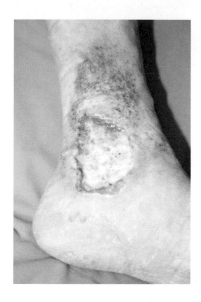

Plate 2 Mixed venous ischaemic ulcer. Past history of recurrent venous ulceration, on examination poor palpable pedal pulses and unable to tolerate compression.

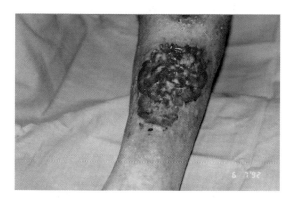

Plate 3 Large hypergranulating ulcer present for over 2 years. Biopsy revealed squamous cell carcinoma.

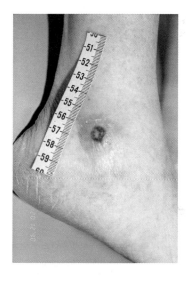

Plate 4 Classical lateral malleolus pressure ulcer.

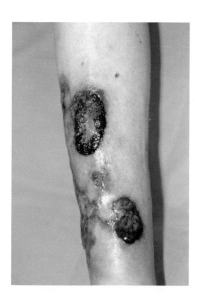

Plate 5 Painful vasculitic ulcer with rapidly extending necrotic border and evidence of palpable purpura.

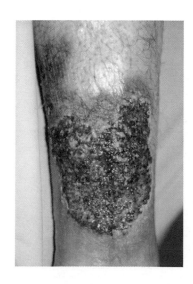

Plate 6 Pyoderma gangrenosum. One of four bilateral painful ulcers. All healed rapidly with oral corticosteroids.

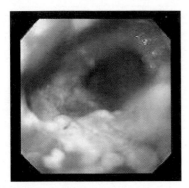

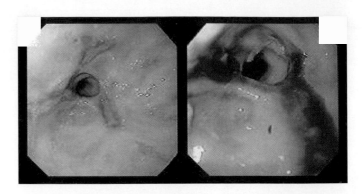

Plate 7 Adenocarcinoma arising in Barrett's epithelium.

Plate 8 Benign stricture before and after dilatation.

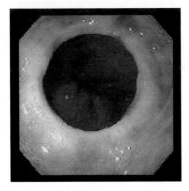

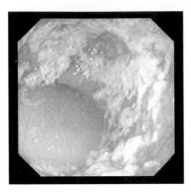

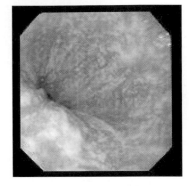

Plate 9 Shatzki ring.

Plate 10 Achalasia showing dilated oesophagus with fluid level.

Plate 11 Oesophageal candida.

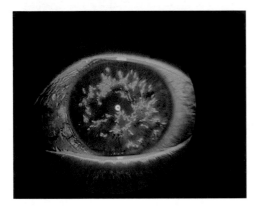

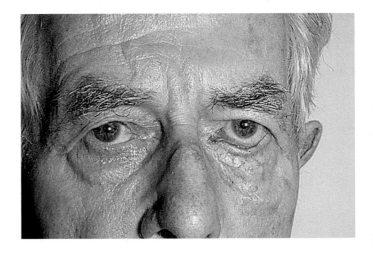

Plate 12 Corneal damage from dendritic ulcer (stained with fluorescein and viewed with blue light). [Source: Marsh and Easty in *Oxford Textbook of Ophthalmology* (ed. Easty and Sparrow), Oxford University Press, 1999.]

Plate 13 Ectropion and poor eye closure due to Bell's palsy. [Source: Ellingham and Ellingham in *Oxford Textbook of Ophthalmology* (ed. Easty and Sparrow), Oxford University Press, 1999.]

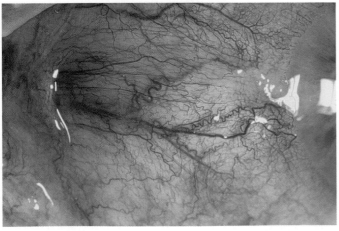

Plate 14 Scleritis showing dilation of deep vessels and bluish discoloration from scleral thinning. [Source: de la Meza and Foster in *Oxford Textbook of Ophthalmology* (ed. Easty and Sparrow), Oxford University Press, 1999.]

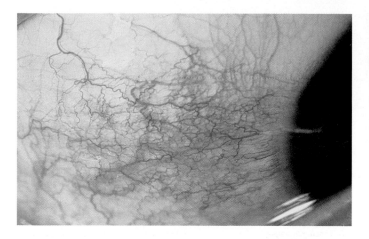

Plate 15 Episcleritis showing dilatation of superficial vessels only. [Source: de la Meza and Foster in *Oxford Textbook of Ophthalmology* (ed. Easty and Sparrow), Oxford University Press, 1999.]

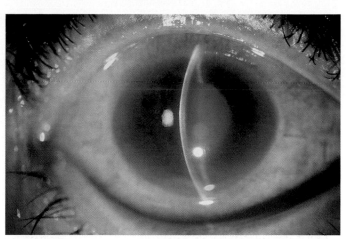

Plate 16 Acute glaucoma showing red eye, corneal oedema, and fixed oval pupil (white flare from slit lamp reflects shallow anterior chamber). [Source: Kitazawa and Yamamoto in *Oxford Textbook of Ophthalmology* (ed. Easty and Sparrow), Oxford University Press, 1999.]

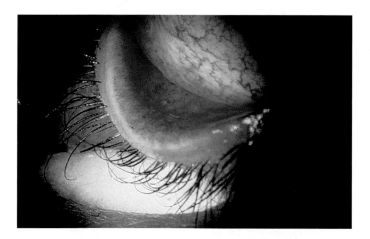

Plate 17 Acute follicular conjunctivitis caused by adenovirus serotype 8. [Source: Hodge and Smdlin in *Oxford Textbook of Ophthalmology* (ed. Easty and Sparrow), Oxford University Press, 1999.]

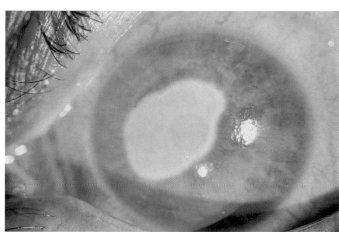

Plate 18 Corneal abrasion (stained with fluorescein). [Source: Pfister in *Oxford Textbook of Ophthalmology* (ed. Easty and Sparrow), Oxford University Press, 1999.]

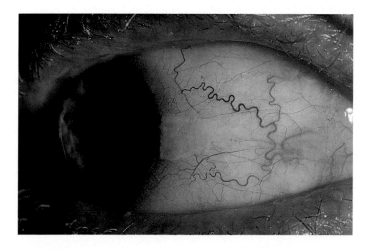

Plate 19 A pingueculum (an innocent fatty lump on the sclera). [Source: Larkin in *Oxford Textbook of Ophthalmology* (ed. Easty and Sparrow), Oxford University Press, 1999.]

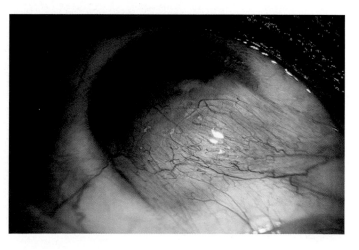

Plate 20 A pterygium (in this case extending onto cornea and requiring excision). [Source: Larkin in *Oxford Textbook of Ophthalmology* (ed. Easty and Sparrow), Oxford University Press, 1999.]

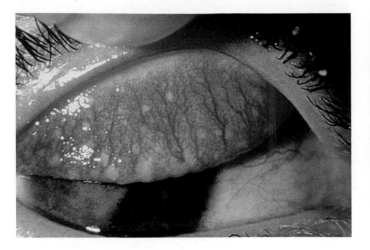

Plate 21 Trachoma conjunctivitis showing characteristic white-yellow follicles. [Source: Taylor and Vajpayee in *Oxford Textbook of Ophthalmology* (ed. Easty and Sparrow), Oxford University Press, 1999.]

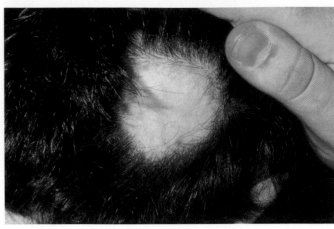

Plate 22 Patches of non-scarring alopecia.

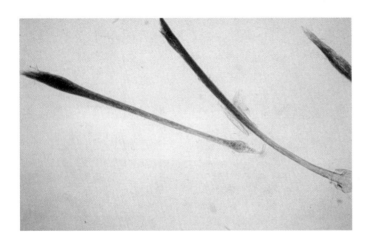

Plate 23 'Exclamation mark' hairs in alopecia areata.

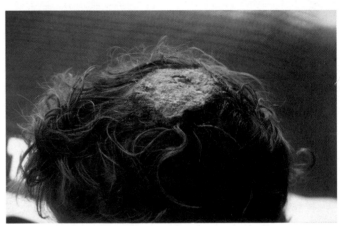

Plate 24 Kerions in *Tinea capitis* infection.

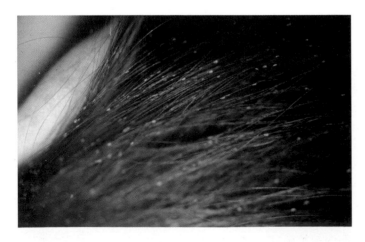

Plate 25 Nits in *Pediculosis capitis* infestation.

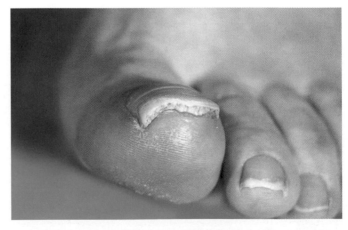

Plate 26 Onychomycosis (fungal infection) of the nail.

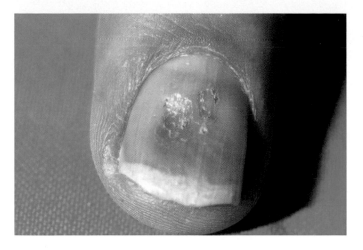

Plate 27 Nail showing psoriasis.

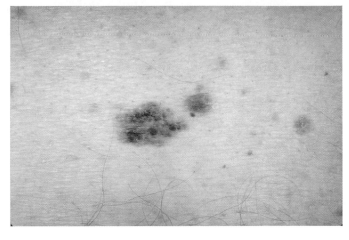

Plate 28 Atypical mole (dysplastic naevus).

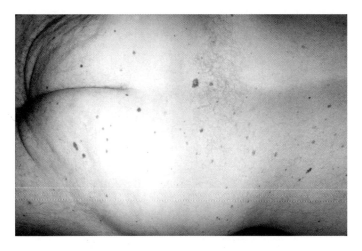

Plate 29 Atypical mole syndrome. Notice the presence of multiple naevi on the relatively sun protected area of the buttocks.

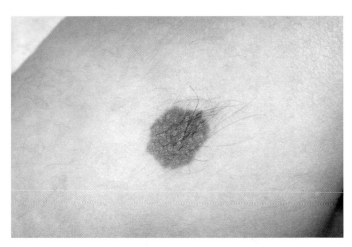

Plate 30 Medium-sized congenital melanocytic naevus.

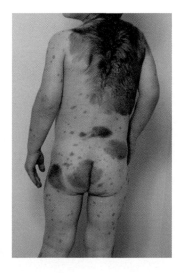

Plate 31 This patient with a large congenital naevus on the back and with multiple satellite naevi is at high risk for developing neurocutaneous melanocytosis.

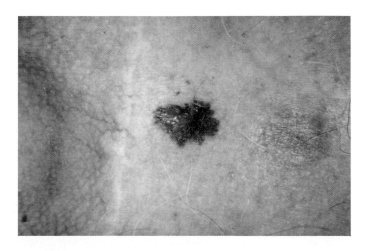

Plate 32 Malignant melanoma demonstrating some of the 'ABCD' features of melanoma.

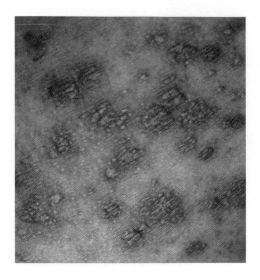

Plate 33 An eczematous rash or lichen simplex chronicus.

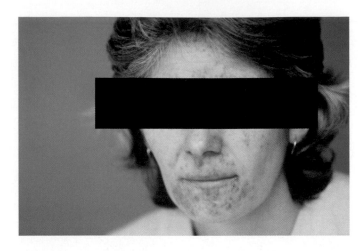

Plate 34 Rosacea characterized by papules and papulopustules on the face.

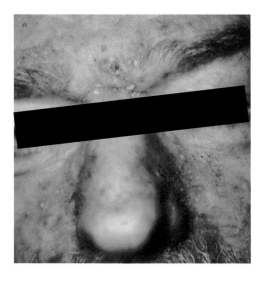

Plate 35 Seborrhoeic dermatitis present as greasy scales.

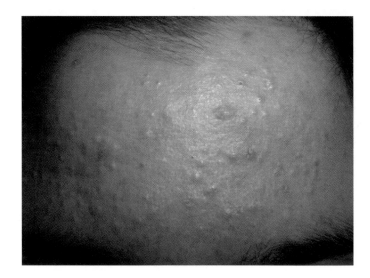

Plate 36 Mild acne, demonstrating both closed and open comedones. This photograph was supplied by Dr Chris Baker.

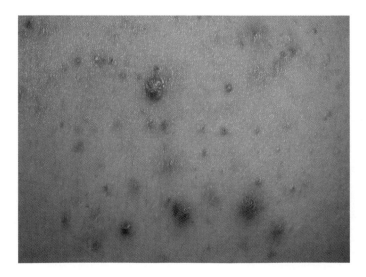

Plate 37 Severe acne showing papules, pustules, and cysts. This photograph was supplied by Dr Chris Baker.

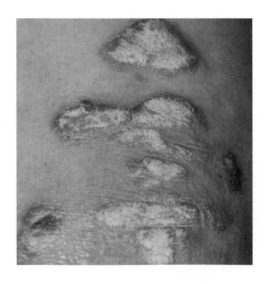

Plate 38 Psoriasis plaques are thick, red, and scaly. The borders of the lesions are usually very sharp.

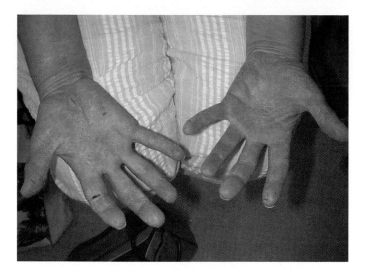

Plate 39 Acute form of atopic dermatitis.

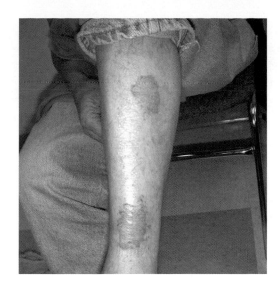

Plate 40 Coin-shaped ('nummular' or 'discoid') lesions on the leg.

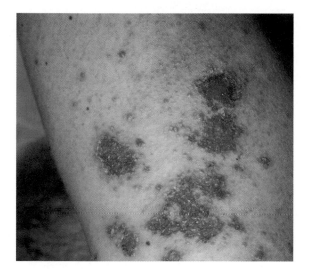

Plate 41 Non-bullous form of impetigo characterized by crusts.

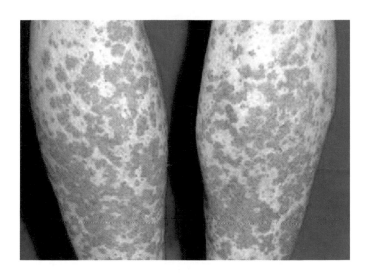

Plate 43 Leukocytoclastic vasculitis of calves.

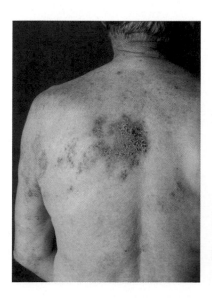

Plate 42 Typical case of shingles affecting the T2 dermatome on the left side.

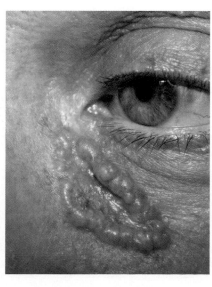

Plate 44 Nodular basal cell carcinoma showing a raised border, smooth pearly surface, and telangiectasias.

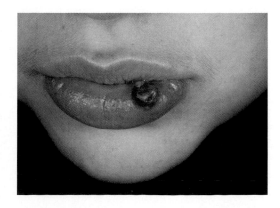

Plate 45 Erythematous friable papule indicating diagnosis of pyogenic granulomas.

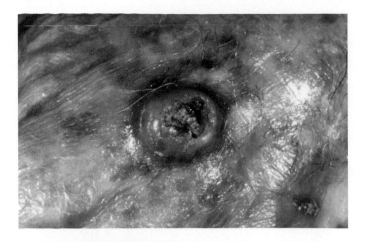

Plate 46 Keratoacanthoma is a dome-shaped nodule with a central keratotic core.

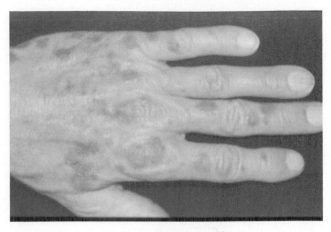

Plate 47 A photosensitive patient having sharply demarcated eruptions, small papules coalescing to plaques, and small vesicles.

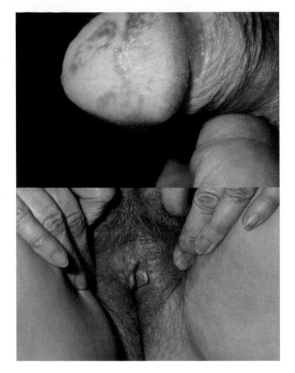

Plate 48 Lichen sclerosus.

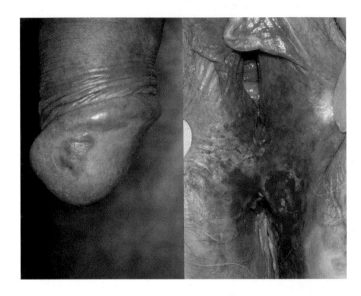

Plate 50 Intraepithelial neoplasia.

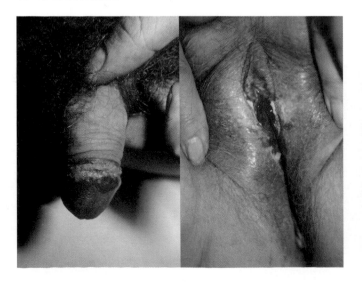

Plate 49 Lichen planus.

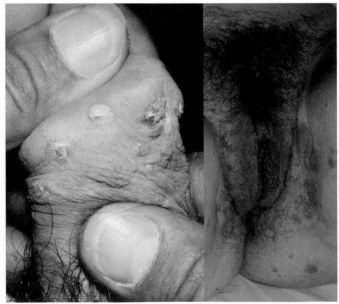

Plate 51 Genital psoriasis.

diagnosis. However, subsequent investigation including an EEG and neuroimaging, in most cases an MRI or CT scan of the head, may well be undertaken.

EEG

The EEG is of limited use in making the diagnosis of epilepsy, unless by chance a seizure is recorded in the course of the investigation. Only about 35 per cent of patients with established epilepsy consistently show epileptic abnormalities on their EEG, a further 50 per cent will sometimes do so (particularly if provocative measures such as sleep deprivation are employed), and in the remainder, the interictal EEG never shows epileptic activity. In patients who have had a single seizure, the proportion with frankly epileptic abnormalities is even lower, and so a normal EEG cannot be used to rule out a diagnosis of epilepsy. Where such epileptic abnormalities are seen, however, this provides strong evidence in favour of epilepsy, since such activity only occurs in about 0.5 per cent of the general population. The EEG is helpful in classifying the type of epilepsy, and in identifying the site of onset of focal epilepsy in patients with intractable epilepsy in whom surgery is being considered. The percentage of people with epileptic abnormalities in the absence of epilepsy is higher in those taking certain drugs (particularly psychotropic medication) and in the relatives of people with epilepsy.

Neuroimaging

Neuroimaging is an essential part of the investigation in nearly all adults developing seizures. It has been argued that it may be unnecessary in the very elderly, in whom the cause may already be apparent (e.g. following a stroke) and in whom even the discovery of a tumour might not influence clinical management. However, in these instances a scan may still be valuable in allowing informed counselling of the patient, particularly regarding prognosis, or excluding other causes of 'stroke'.

CT scanning facilities are now widely available and these scans are sufficient to identify many causes of epilepsy (including the majority of tumours and strokes). MRI scans are more sensitive to many abnormalities underlying epilepsy (e.g. mesial temporal sclerosis, neuronal migration defects, encephalitic changes, and some tumours), and are the investigation of choice. Even if they are not readily available for all patients, they should be carried out in those patients not responding quickly to medical treatment, or in whom surgery is considered.

The principles of management

In the United Kingdom, it is common practice to wait until the patient has had at least two seizures before medication is begun, except where there are other factors (e.g. a structural lesion such as a brain tumour) making recurrence more likely. Treatment should not be started unless the diagnosis is clear, since medication is likely to be continued for several years and may well have adverse effects. 'Trials of therapy' should be avoided.

Around 70 per cent of patients starting treatment quickly achieve good seizure control, and only a few, perhaps 10–15 per cent of the total, benefit from combination therapy with two (or rarely more) drugs. When the decision to initiate treatment has been taken, the patient should be started on a first-line drug for the seizure type(s), at a low dose to minimize the risk of adverse effects. The dose should be gradually increased until seizure control is achieved, or until evidence of toxicity occurs. Measurement of serum drug levels is unnecessary in the majority of cases, but may be useful when using phenytoin, which has non-linear pharmacokinetics, and occasionally in other circumstances, for example, when poor compliance is suspected, in cases of status epilepticus, in patients with learning difficulties, in patients with symptoms which may or may not be due to drug toxicity, and in some patients with other medical conditions (particularly those affecting hepatic or renal function) or concomitant medication causing drug interactions. For partial onset seizures, carbamazepine or sodium valproate are commonly used first-line drugs. Phenytoin is commonly used for such seizure-types in the United States, though it tends to be used as a second-line drug in the United Kingdom. Lamotrigine and oxcarbazepine are also licensed for use as monotherapy in such seizures, but are generally more expensive than the older drugs and are commonly used as second-line agents. Other second-line treatments for partial-onset seizures include topiramate, levetiracetam, gabapentin, clobazam, clonazepam, acetazolamide, tiagabine and phenobarbitone.

Sodium valproate is an effective treatment for generalized tonic–clonic seizures, myoclonus and absence seizures and is thus a drug of first choice in idiopathic generalized epilepsy. Ethosuximide is also a useful treatment for absence seizures and clonazepam for myoclonus. Topiramate and lamotrigine are licensed for use in primary generalized tonic–clonic seizures. Carbamazepine and phenytoin may be helpful in the management of generalized tonic–clonic seizures but can worsen absence epilepsy. Adverse effects of drugs include acute toxic effects (e.g. unsteadiness and blurred vision occurring with excess of carbamazepine or lamotrigine), chronic toxic effects (e.g. gum hyperplasia with phenytoin or hair loss with sodium valproate), acute idiosyncratic reactions, and teratogenicity.

It is generally accepted that treatment should usually be continued for 2 or more years before drug withdrawal is attempted. A study carried out by the MRC Anti-epileptic Drug Withdrawal Study Group (1991),[2] in which patients seizure-free for at least 2 years were randomized to either slow withdrawal or medication or continuing medication suggested that the risk of recurrence following withdrawal of medication was around 40 per cent, with most relapses occurring in the first 2 years. An increased risk of recurrence was found in patients aged over 16 years, those taking more than one antiepileptic drug, those with a history of seizures after starting antiepileptic drugs, a history of tonic–clonic or myoclonic seizures, or an abnormal EEG in the previous year.

Long-term and continuing care

Informing patients about epilepsy and the management of risks

The way in which patients manage information in another neurological disease, Parkinson's disease, has been described by Pinder.[6] She felt that patients' responses fell into three groups:

1. *Seekers:* those patients who actively sought to discover what was likely to happen. This task involved sustained research from medical and lay sources.

2. *Weavers:* those patients whose needs for information fluctuated. Sometimes they felt able to assimilate additional facts; at other times they preferred not to know.

3. *Avoiders:* those patients who deliberately chose not to find out the implications, the anxiety of not knowing was preferable to the risk of having their private, often unacknowledged, fears about the illness confirmed.

Pinder found this model useful in classifying patients' responses during the evolution of Parkinson's disease, but clearly this model may apply more widely. A patient's receptivity to information and their consequent ability to manage their condition, which are cognitive and behavioural processes, depend to a certain extent on a resolution of their emotional response to the condition which was described above. The ability to seek and apply information to their disease management will also depend on the patient's educational level. We found that school leaving qualifications were associated with patients' knowledge of their epilepsy, with those with no qualifications knowing significantly less about their condition.[7,8] Doctors and nurses need first to establish what the patient knows in order to add to this information appropriately. If this learner-centred style is not adopted it is likely that there will be a downward spiral by which those who are already socially disadvantaged get less help which might enable them to manage their condition and cope.

The diagnosis

It is important for the patient to understand, and in the long run accept, that they have been diagnosed with one of a variety of conditions that are grouped under an overall title of the epilepsies. This does not necessarily mean that they are the same as other patients who have been given this label, as there are many ways in which the disorder presents. It is useful at this point to check out their understanding of the tests they have undertaken and to emphasize that this is a clinical diagnosis. Some patients who are still in denial or bargaining mode may use reports that their brain scan or EEG were normal to justify their belief that they do not have epilepsy. The patient's own ideas and concerns about the diagnosis need to be known in order to engage in a fruitful exchange about this.

Seizure management

Epilepsy can be very frightening for relatives, and it is important that they are educated about the acute management of seizures. This includes ensuring that the patient is not in immediate danger (e.g. from a fire), allowing the seizure to take its course, then turning the patient in the recovery position. Prolonged recurrent seizures may require hospital treatment.

Other lifestyle risk management includes advice on moderate alcohol intake and sufficient sleep. This is particularly difficult for young adults, especially men, as taken in conjunction with the loss of a driving licence it may curtail their social life considerably, or lead them to intermittently disregarding advice and losing epilepsy control. At the two extremes are patients who become quite socially isolated, and others that want to participate socially, and experience an enormous amount of peer pressure, for example, to drink, which may result in loss of epilepsy control. Epilepsy is associated with a two to three times increased risk of sudden death and this occurs particularly in young men in the context of alcohol. Domestic risks include cooking and having a bath. There is an increased risk of burns in patients with epilepsy, so advice on this is important. Risk may also occur in the context of a seizure whilst bathing alone, so showers are preferable to baths.

The medication

Patients frequently complain that they have not been told about drug side-effects[4] and interactions, for example, with contraceptives. It seems remarkable that other patients who take continuing medication such as contraceptives get detailed information provided by the pharmaceutical company, whilst patients who are on equally long-term medications, such as antiepileptic drugs may have received little written information, either from the doctor or the pharmaceutical supplier. Many, if not the majority of patients have experienced some side-effects, such as sedation or gum hypertrophy and many have tried stopping their drugs. This is not irrational in view of the fact that they may have experienced no seizures whilst they continued to experience adverse effects from their medication. Had the medication withdrawal been gradual, this patient-led strategy might have been successful. However, lack of knowledge or advice on the subject may lead to patients stopping drugs abruptly with a recurrence of their epileptic attacks. Accurate advice on prognosis at the outset and systematic follow-up may trigger patients to reconsult when they are in remission, before gradually reducing their antiepileptic medication.

Driving

Driving regulations vary from country to country, but most impose some restriction on people with epilepsy. In the United Kingdom, people with epilepsy must have been seizure-free for at least 1 year before becoming eligible to drive: the definition of 'seizure' includes myoclonus and other minor seizures such as simple partial seizures. Those patients experiencing seizures only during sleep must have been established in this pattern for at least 3 years before driving is permitted. The onus is on the patient to inform their insurers and the driving license authority.

Contraception and pregnancy

Certain antiepileptic drugs, including phenytoin, carbamazepine, oxcarbazepine, topirimate, and barbiturates, induce liver enzymes. Women on these drugs need to have a higher dose of oestradiol (usually at least 50 μg, and sometimes more) in their contraceptive pill. The presence of breakthrough bleeding suggests that the dose of oestrodiol may be ineffective.

Much research is currently being undertaken into the role of the various different antiepileptic drugs in causing teratogenicity. Women with epilepsy on antiepileptic drugs have a two to three times risk of malformations in their offspring. In one study of women with epilepsy, more than 50 per cent of pregnancies were unplanned.[9] It is therefore important that advice about contraception, pregnancy, and teratogenicity is given at the time of diagnosis or when the patient first reaches sexual maturity. They should be advised of the need to review their medication beforehand, to try to reduce the number of drugs and dosage if possible, and to take folic acid 5 mg daily for 3 months prior to pregnancy and during the first trimester. Patients on enzyme-inducing drugs should also take vitamin K1 (phytomenadione) 10–20 mg daily for the last month of pregnancy, and the baby should receive vitamin K 1 mg intramuscularly at birth, to reduce the risk of haemorrhagic disease of the newborn.

The implications of the problem

The psycho-social impact of epilepsy and its management

The diagnosis of epilepsy can cause considerable psychological distress, which needs to be addressed proactively by the general practitioner and/or nurse. Information may have been provided in specialist care, but if the patient was at this stage denying, anxious or bargaining about the diagnosis they may have taken very little of it in, and they may not be able to do so until they have emotionally 'made sense' of the diagnosis in the context of their own lives. Frequently, the diagnosis leads to a profound loss of confidence. Compared to other patients with epilepsy, those who had experienced an attack in the prior 6 months are three times more likely to have high depression scores and a perception that they are stigmatized.[10] Some patients may actually become depressed as a consequence of their illness and if this is not addressed it may contribute to a decline in their coping in terms of employment, relationships and drug taking. A sequence of losses may then worsen the depressive symptoms. Awareness of this possibility and monitoring of patients, particularly those with more frequent seizures, may identify those in need of supportive psychotherapy or antidepressants.

Psychiatric illness and epilepsy

Depression not uncommonly occurs in association with epilepsy, and requires appropriate treatment. Although theoretically most antidepressant agents can worsen epilepsy, in the authors' experience this is only rarely a practical problem. Serotonin re-uptake inhibitors are less epileptogenic than some older drugs. Alternatively, non-drug treatments may be considered. Patients with bipolar affective disorder (manic depression) may also experience more seizures when they are treated with lithium, and carbamazepine may be a useful alternative.

The team and their possible roles

A general practitioner will have approximately one patient newly diagnosed with epilepsy each year and this person may benefit from information and support either from the doctor or another suitably trained person.

Whilst a check-list approach to teaching and learning seems reductive, it is one way to increase the chance that patients are offered the information they need to manage a complex condition. Without a systematic approach general practitioners cannot satisfy their own criteria for providing evidence of advice having been given on basic topics like driving, drug compliance and side-effects, alcohol, and self-help groups.[4] A nurse with appropriate training can significantly improve the level of advice given to patients with epilepsy and recorded in the notes.[11] Advice given in clinics run by a nurse in general practice or specialist care is a satisfactory form of management from the point of view of patients.

References

1. Anderson, V.E., Hauser, W.A., and Rich, S.S. (1986). Genetic heterogeneity in the epilepsies. *Advances in Neurology* **44**, 59.

2. Medical Research Council, Anti-Epileptic Drug Withdrawal Study Group (1991). Randomised study of anti-epileptic drug withdrawal in patients in remission. *Lancet* **337**, 1175–80.

3. Annegers, J.F., Hauser, W.A., and Elveback, L.R. (1979). Remission of seizures and relapse in patients with epilepsy. *Epilepsia* **20**, 729–37.

4. Ridsdale, L. et al. (1996). Epilepsy monitoring and advice recorded: general practitioners' views, current practice and patients' preferences. *British Journal of General Practice* **46**, 11–14.

5. Hart, Y.M. et al. (1990). National General Practice Study of Epilepsy: recurrence after a first seizure. *Lancet* **336**, 1271–4.

6. Pinder, R. *The Management of Chronic Disease: Patient and Doctor Perspectives on Parkinson's Disease.* Basingstoke: MacMillan Press, 1990.

7. Ridsdale, L., Kwan, I., and Cryer, C. (1999). The effect of a special nurse on patients' knowledge of epilepsy and their emotional state. *British Journal of General Practice* **49**, 285–9.

8. Ridsdale, L., Kwan, I., and Cryer, C. (2000). Newly diagnosed epilepsy: can a nurse specialist help? A randomized controlled trial. *Epilepsia* **41** (8), 1014–19.

9. Fairgreave, S.D. et al. (2000). Population based, prospective study of the care of women with epilepsy in pregnancy. *British Medical Journal* **321**, 674–5.

10. Ridsdale, L. et al. (1996). Epilepsy in general practice: patients' psychological symptoms and their perception of stigma. *British Journal of General Practice* **46**, 365–6.

11. Ridsdale, L. et al. (1997). The effect of nurse run clinics for patients with epilepsy in general practice. *British Medical Journal* **314**, 120–2.

11.3 Movement disorders

Christopher Ward and Brian Hurwitz

General issues in diagnosis and management

Definition of movement disorders: a primary care perspective

A primary care-oriented definition of movement disorders is hard to achieve. Neurologists use the term to describe specific syndromes causing involuntary movements and abnormalities of muscle tone.[1] Though such conditions are rare—comprising only 50 per 7000 consultations annually by the average UK GP[2]—together they are an important cause of distress and disability.

Movement disorders as defined in neurology exclude a wider range of neurological deficits which we shall term 'disorders of movement'. In primary care, a broad view encompassing all types of tremors, involuntary movements and abnormal patterns of posture and voluntary movement offers the best framework within which to consider diagnosis, especially in the early stages of presentation. Parkinson's disease (PD), first characterized by a London GP,[3] is the paradigm syndrome, being the most frequent cause of complex disability.[4] In common with several other conditions in this group of movement disorders, PD also causes cognitive and behavioural impairments.

Clinical management should be sensitive to psychological aspects of movement disorders and to the social stigma which frequently attaches to these conditions. Certain symptoms are open to misinterpretation by the public: bradykinesia can be perceived as stupidity, involuntary movements (tremor, chorea, and tics) as nervousness, ataxia as drunkenness, tics and dystonia as histrionic behaviour. Although medical management of these conditions is generally less than curative, many patients benefit from correct medical diagnosis and from consequent contact with patient support groups.

Prevalence of important movement disorders

Parkinson's disease is the most important of the severely disabling movement disorders. It has a prevalence of 1.6 per 1000,[5] generating some 15 consultations per year in UK primary care. Essential tremor is the most prevalent of the classic movement disorders followed by focal and segmental dystonias, such as writer's cramp and spasmodic torticollis. Huntington's disease (HD) is much less common, other progressive syndromes being very rarely encountered by family practitioners. The wider group of disorders of movement will not be discussed in any detail in this chapter.

Classification and diagnosis of movement disorders

Good clinical management of these conditions depends on recognizing the significance of subtle clinical features which may emerge only after many consultations. We devote less attention here to the distinction *between* these diseases—since they are mostly too rare to be diagnosed definitively without neurological advice and are well described in textbooks of neurology—but devote more attention instead to the recognition and description of disordered movements.

Clinical varieties of disordered movement and tone

The following notes supplement Table 1, which offers a schematic algorithm to assist in classification and identification of involuntary movements.

Tremors, oscillations, and ataxias

Tremor is a rhythmical oscillation of the extremities or head (titubation). A fine rapid physiological tremor (8–12 Hz) is often associated with anxiety. Essential-type tremor (ET) is of larger amplitude than physiological tremor, is not quite so rapid, becomes more obvious during voluntary actions and while hands are outstretched, and in severer cases can occur at rest. The reverse is true of parkinsonian tremor, which is slower (4–6 Hz) than ET. PD tremor is more complex in form (discussed below), occurs at rest, and although action may suppress the tremor it frequently does not. *Clonus* is an oscillation due to hyper-reflexia caused by an upper motor neurone syndrome. Clinically it is brought out by muscle stretch. When provoked by a trivial stimulus clonus can resemble spontaneous tremor, typically of the foot.

Ataxia disrupts the timing and coordination of voluntary movements. In cerebellar ataxia, deviations from a desired trajectory become more severe the more that greater accuracy of movement is required, as seen in intention tremor. Where the trunk is involved the gait is broad-based. Most ataxias are attributed to cerebellar damage, but brainstem lesions also cause the condition. Loss of joint sensation in the limbs may cause sensory ataxia, which is characterized by obvious worsening when patients close their eyes. The term ataxia should not be used for unsteadiness due to labyrinthine and vestibular damage which are frequently distinguished by subjective symptoms such as dizziness, nausea, and vertigo and which do not occur in cerebellar ataxia.

Jerks and spasms

In form, *myoclonus* is the most abrupt and the simplest of all involuntary movements and occurs most commonly as benign nocturnal myoclonus. Chorea, tics, dystonias, and athetosis form a group of involuntary movements which can occur in various combinations following damage to the basal ganglia. *Chorea* is a spontaneous, brief movement which flits unpredictably from one body part to another and is often mistaken for fleeting fidgets, gestures, or grimaces. *Tics* are brief, stereotyped movements recurring at irregular intervals in specific parts of the body, producing recognizable actions such as sniffs, coughs, or shoulder-shrugs. They should be distinguished from *stereotypies*, repetitive 'habit movements' sometimes of a ritual quality seen in people with severe learning disabilities or progressive dementia. *Automatisms* are movements (e.g. lip-smacking) occurring during partial seizures and do not fall strictly within the movement disorder group.

Dystonia is a sustained muscle contraction producing postural changes which are sustained for at least a few seconds. Focal dystonia involves a single body part, segmental dystonia a body region such as the face and neck, while torsion dystonia is generalized. Dystonic postural deformities are often spasmodic but can also be sustained. In cerebral palsy, it is not always clear whether deformities are dystonic or spastic in nature. Some dystonias, such as writer's cramp, are highly task-specific. *Athetosis* is a sinuous movement which disturbs the maintenance of bodily postures.

Muscle hypertonia

Increased tone is termed rigidity and is a hallmark of extrapyramidal impairments. *Rigidity*, a sign rather than a symptom, is best elicited with the patient relaxed and distracted. All forms of pathological hypertonia tend to increase in one limb whilst the opposite limb is voluntarily active. When tremor is inconspicuous, cogwheel rigidity provides additional evidence of parkinsonism. Lead pipe rigidity is so called to contrast it with spasticity, where the amount of resistance varies with the rapidity of muscle stretch. Gegenhalten (go/stop resistance) describes resistance to movement of a limb rather than a muscle, and is neither as consistent as leadpipe and cogwheel rigidity, nor as velocity-dependent as spasticity. Dystonia is another cause of variable or sustained resistance to passive movement.

A practical approach to identifying involuntary movements

Table 1 suggests a diagnostic approach to involuntary movements, including those not conventionally classed by neurologists 'movement disorders'.

It is useful to divide involuntary movements into those which are spontaneous and those which are induced. Most tremors and jerks are essentially spontaneous, occurring in any situation during waking hours. Some posturally related movements can seem spontaneous but are reduced or suppressed when muscles fully relax (usually only possible when supine). Dystonia can be specific to one or a few particular actions; apraxias will affect all classes of purposive action.

The speed of phenomena allows some involuntary movements to be distinguished from one another. Another distinction is between simple or complex movements. Parkinsonian tremor is termed 'compound' because it involves groups of muscles which produce action-like movements, such as pill-rolling. By contrast, physiological tremor, milder forms of ET, cerebellar ataxic tremor, and clonus, are simple oscillations largely involving agonist-antagonist muscle pairs, typically producing predictable up-down or side-to-side movement of a single joint. Chorea, athetosis, dystonia, and tics, which like parkinsonism have an extrapyramidal basis, cause complex movements reminiscent of everyday actions.

Table 1 Classification of types of disordered movement

	Spontaneous? (NB: do not occur in sleep except where stated)	Induced or made worse by? (NB: most movements are worsened by stress)	Suppressible by? (NB: rarely suppressed voluntarily)	Speed	Number of muscle groups involved
Oscillations—tremor, clonus, ataxia					
Physiological tremor	Yes	Posture, action	Rest	Very rapid	Few
Essential tremor	Yes when severe	Posture, action	Rest	Relatively slow	Few
Parkinsonian tremor	Classical rest tremor	Posture, action	Action	Relatively slow	Many
Clonus	No	Muscle stretch	Relaxation; postural support	Relatively slow	Agonist/antagonist
Ataxia/ataxic tremor	No	Action	Rest	Slow	Agonist/antagonist
Continuous twitches or jerks					
Muscle fasciculation	Yes	Percussing muscle	No	Variable/slow	Variable
Myokymia	Yes	Nil	No	Rapid	Few
Hemifacial spasm	Yes (occurs in sleep)	Nil	No	Variable/slow	Single muscle group
Sporadic jerks/spasms					
Myoclonus	Yes (± in sleep)	Action (some types)	No	Rapid	One or few muscles
Chorea	Yes	Nil	No	Rapid	Gesture-like; few muscles
Tics	Yes	Nil	Voluntary effort	Relatively rapid	Resembles gesture or action
Athetosis	Yes	Nil	No	Relatively slow	Several muscles
Dystonia	Yes	Action (some types)	No	Relatively slow	One or few muscles
Spastic spasms	Yes (± in sleep)	Sensory stimuli; muscle stretch	Rest; postural support	Slow	One or two groups
Pseudoathetosis	No	Action, eyes closed	Visual control	Slow	Several muscles
Apraxia	No	Specific actions	No	N/A	N/A

Specific movement disorders

Diagnosis and management of specific disorders

In this section, we provide a brief survey of the principal syndromes and diseases which cause the movement impairments discussed above. Table 2 provides a condensed scheme for differential diagnosis.

In approaching the diagnosis of individual diseases we should first ask: what are the critical management decisions required in primary care? What is the penalty for delaying diagnosis? How will the initial approach to diagnosis and management affect the physical or psychological outcome?

Most people may lose little from delay in the diagnosis of PD since treatment does not affect disease progression, but early symptoms can be unpleasant and are controlled by treatment, and in older people there is a danger of reversible impairments being mistaken for 'senility' or 'arthritis'. Delaying diagnosis of PD in a young person can lead to irreversible life decisions, such as retirement, which effective drug treatment could have deferred. Similar considerations apply to other progressive, familial movement disorders, such as the hereditary ataxias. People with focal and segmental dystonias or with hemifacial spasm often have to endure many years of misdiagnosis before they benefit from botulinum toxin injections and other interventions.

Drug-induced movement disorders

Physiological tremor can be produced by centrally acting alpha- or beta-adrenergic drugs. Sodium valproate produces an essential-type tremor; other anticonvulsants and central nervous system depressants can cause non-specific ataxia. Non-specific tremor or ataxia can be due to alcohol intoxication or to a metabolic encephalopathy, ataxia being a long-term effect of CNS alcoholic intoxication (peripheral neuropathy so caused may also contribute to ataxia). Neuroleptics used as antipsychotics, tranquillizers, vestibular sedatives, or antiemetics in young adults occasionally trigger an acute dystonic reaction and often cause parkinsonism in older patients. Their long-term use can induce oromandibular dystonic movements (tardive dyskinesia), focal dystonias (such as tardive dystonia), and, occasionally, tics resembling Gilles de la Tourette syndrome ('Tourettism'). When used for PD, levodopa often induces choreo-athetoid dyskinesias.

Monosymptomatic movement disorders

Essential tremor can be confused with PD despite the paucity of additional features, such as slowness of movement. When ET is present throughout adult life, there is often a clear autosomal-dominant type family history.

Table 2 Differential diagnosis of conditions causing movement disorders

Specific condition (annual UK GP consultation rate per 10 000 population with condition as main reason for consulting[1])	Presenting symptoms	Major impairments	Distinguishing features	Often confused with
Essential tremor[a] (3.25)	Tremor	Tremor, very slow progression	Family history common	Parkinson's disease, drug-induced parkinsonism
Focal dystonias[a] (2.03)	Pain or spasm (e.g. writer's cramp)	Focal dystonic spasms, little or no progression	Geste antagonistique (torticollis) Action-induced (e.g. writer's cramp)	Psychogenic conditions
Generalized torsion dystonia (0.11)	Dystonia	Dystonia, progression	Family history	Psychogenic conditions
Progressive cerebellar ataxia[a] and spinocerebellar degenerations (1.65)	Gait ataxia	Impaired mobility, dexterity and speech	Additional signs in different syndromes: sensory loss; deafness; optic atrophy; dementia	Multiple sclerosis Alcohol related
Gilles de la Tourette syndrome (GTS)[a] (0.79)	Motor tics	Motor tics which can be suppressed briefly	Vocal tics; family history common	Benign non-GTS tics, 'habit-spasms'
Parkinson's disease[a] (41.19)	Tremor Limb stiffness Pain	Impaired dexterity, agility, speech, gait	Always: hypokinesia Usually: asymmetry; good response to levodopa	Other parkinsonian syndromes
Cortical Lewy Body dementia (NK)	Parkinsonism	Parkinsonism, hallucinations, dementia	Non-drug-induced hallucinations, dementia early in course	Parkinson's disease
Multi-system atrophy (Shy–Drager) (NK)	Parkinsonism and/or ataxia	Bulbar signs, poor mobility, speech, autonomic dysfunctions (± dementia)	Autonomic symptoms	Parkinson's disease
Progressive supranuclear palsy (Steele–Richardson) (NK)	Parkinsonism	Bulbar signs, poor mobility, speech, dementia	Impaired vertical eye movements Extensor neck rigidity	Parkinson's disease
Huntington's disease (1.13)	Chorea Psychiatric symptoms	Involuntary movements, poor balance, speech, cognition; altered mood and behaviour	Family history	Other dementias; Parkinson's disease
Wilson's disease (<0.01)	Tremor Decline in school performance	Tremor, dystonia, poor mobility + speech	Recessive inheritance; liver involvement; Keyser–Fleischer rings	Essential tremor; dystonias; Parkinson's disease

[a] Conditions can be mimicked iatrogenically by drugs (see text).

NK = not known.

Although termed 'benign', ET can slowly progress, causing considerable social and physical disabilities. About half of patients notice definite improvement with alcohol (which can sometimes lead to dependence). The simplest treatment is propranolol but drug treatments are generally not very effective.

Parkinsonian syndromes

Parkinsonism is a syndrome with several causes in addition to idiopathic PD. Slowness of movement (termed hypokinesia, bradykinesia, or akinesia) is its hallmark, but the diagnosis cannot be made without coexisting parkinsonian tremor or extrapyramidal muscle rigidity. Impairment of postural reflexes contributes to the tendency to fall either 'like a felled log' or backwards in stuttering steps (retropulsion), and is now commonly regarded as a fourth cardinal feature, along with bradykinesia, tremor, and rigidity.

Parkinson's disease is the commonest cause of parkinsonism. Typically beginning unilaterally, PD often remains asymmetrical throughout its course. Deceptively, the very earliest symptoms can be focal pain. Apart from tremor, the symptoms most sensitive to the presence of progressive parkinsonism include difficulty in getting out of a chair, difficulty turning in bed and smaller handwriting. In PD, parkinsonism predominates at presentation (bradykinesia, blank facial expression) and also remains predominant throughout the course. Non-parkinsonian neurological features, such as ataxia or pyramidal signs, should not be ascribed to PD. Autonomic symptoms and dementia develop in some cases but are inconspicuous at presentation. Progressive deterioration in PD is inevitable, steady, and usually prolonged. Marked initial benefit from drug treatment is the rule, and subsequent levodopa-induced involuntary movements are more severe in PD than in other causes of parkinsonism. Specific cognitive deficits are characteristic in PD, progressive dementia in 20–30 per cent, with depression, anxiety, and sleep disorders being important causes of disability.

Differential diagnosis

Once drug-induced parkinsonism has been excluded, several less common parkinsonian syndromes should be considered. These are more likely where typical parkinsonian tremor is inconspicuous or absent, and where at onset there is symmetry of signs, hallucinations or dementia. An apparently typical case of PD, over time, may develop additional atypical features; at diagnosis, therefore, it is often best to be quite cautious about the diagnosis and prognosis and to explain that a number of possibilities may only be ruled out once the patient's condition has been monitored for some time. Non-PD syndromes tend to progress more rapidly and respond less well to drugs than does PD. Prominent autonomic symptoms suggest multisystem atrophy (Shy–Drager syndrome); failure of downward gaze of the eyes and extensor neck rigidity suggest progressive supranuclear palsy (Steele–Richardson syndrome). Dementia at onset, especially with visual hallucinations not due to drugs could signal cortical Lewy-body dementia. Diffuse cerebrovascular disease can produce a symmetrical akinetic-rigid syndrome affecting especially the gait; in such patients cognitive function is sometimes relatively preserved.

Parkinson's disease and parkinsonism are difficult diagnoses for family physicians to confirm. A cross-sectional survey of parkinsonism undertaken in 15 general practices found that among patients whose GP records contained a diagnosis of Parkinson's disease or parkinsonism made by GP and/or hospital consultant, and prescription of antiparkinsonian drugs, or mention of tremor after the age of 50, only 78 per cent on formal assessment were found to be suffering from parkinsonism.[6] We strongly recommend referral to a specialist who has an interest in PD and its related syndromes in order to confirm the diagnosis.

Management

In advanced PD, patients require a multiplicity of aids and therapies, including home adaptations, referral to speech, physio- and occupational therapy, day centres, and hospital outpatients. Drug treatment does not affect the course of disease and it is best to adopt a 'trial and error' approach in which good relationships with patients, carers, specialist physicians, and nurses are of paramount importance. The number of drugs recommended

Box 1 Role of community-based Parkinson's Disease Nurse Specialist

◆ Counselling and educating patients and carers about PD—in their homes, at health centres and GP clinics, in hospital outpatients, and on the telephone

◆ Provision of drug information to patients under the auspices of GPs and consultants

◆ Monitoring clinical well-being and response to treatment (minimum of two assessments per year), reporting to GPs and consultants where appropriate

◆ Instigating respite and day hospital care where appropriate; seeing patients in hospital if admitted, and liaising with hospital staff when discharged

◆ Assessing social security benefit entitlement

◆ Liaison with members of local multidisciplinary primary care teams for ongoing assessment and therapy where appropriate

should be kept as small as possible particularly because of the high risk of mental confusion. Nevertheless, for many patients at least two antiparkinsonian drugs are required. In the United Kingdom, the role of the Parkinson's Disease Nurse Specialists (PDNS) has developed over the past 10 years[7] (see Box 1). Community-based PDNSs have been shown to benefit subjective well-being of patients without increasing health care costs, but they have little overall influence on PD deterioration or mortality.[8]

Levodopa treatment

Response to the most effective drug, levodopa, often becomes erratic resulting in peak-dose choreo-athetoid movements, end-of-dose wearing off akinesia, unpredictable swings in mobility (the on–off syndrome) and other distressing symptoms, including painful dystonias and drug-related mood swings. These phenomena can emerge within 3–5 years of treatment, and are more frequent in younger patients. It is uncertain whether controlled-release levodopa preparations delay the onset of erratic response. One way of reducing the risk of complications is to use a less potent drug initially, such as selegiline, thereby delaying introduction of levodopa. The major peripheral unwanted effect of levodopa is nausea, but this usually responds to domperidone which may also improve levodopa-induced postural hypotension. Once response to levodopa begins to become erratic, several empirical manoeuvres are available: using smaller, more frequent levodopa doses, controlled-release levodopa alongside standard formulations; adding a drug which slows the catabolism of cerebral dopamine–entacapone or selegiline–adding or substituting a dopamine agonist.

Dopamine agonists

There is strong evidence that use of a dopamine agonist as initial treatment reduces the risk of erratic response to drug treatment or at least delays its onset. The relative merits of the growing list of dopamine agonists cannot be discussed definitively here, but all such drugs share certain characteristics: they are less potent than levodopa, more liable to cause peripheral side-effects (some of which can be improved with domperidone), and most importantly, they are more liable to cause hallucination, confusion or frank psychosis. To some extent, these complications occur with all antiparkinsonian drugs and can have serious untoward social and personal effects.

Drug treatment of other features of PD

Parkinson's disease is notable for a high incidence of depression which often responds to conventional drug treatment while anxiety is often more difficult to treat. Disturbed sleep sometimes responds to an antidepressant, and sometimes to changes in antiparkinsonian treatment (which may improve sleep through alleviating physical discomfort, or may worsen it by causing nocturnal agitation). Daytime somnolence appears occasionally to be a specific deficit in PD but can also be drug related; sleep attacks are an uncommon but important effect of drug treatment.

Huntington's disease

Huntington's disease comprises impairments in movement, behaviour, mood, and cognition.[9] Symptoms can develop as early as the first decade but typically begin in the fourth or fifth and progress over the next 10 years. HD is an autosomal dominant condition with full clinical expression (penetrance). Although the prevalence does not exceed 10 per 100 000 perhaps four times as many people are at 25 or 50 per cent risk of HD. Reliable DNA testing is available and requires to be handled carefully and sensitively: because test results are of profound significance to the family as well as the patient, pre-test counselling is essential.

A family history may or may not be clear at presentation. Most often a parent will have been affected, new mutations being very rare; but because the age of onset of HD is quite variable, the affected parent might have died without being diagnosed. Most individuals known to be at risk of HD are in no hurry for early diagnosis since there is no treatment as yet which influences long-term outcome. Moreover, early detection of HD can adversely affect insurance prospects. However, families are often unaware of HD and early detection in an index case will radically affect other family members who may wish to consider predictive testing as a guide to future life decisions. Specialist clinical genetic advice should be arranged.

Wilson's disease

Wilson's disease is a very rare, autosomal, recessive disorder of copper metabolism which can be treated effectively if diagnosed early. A typical presentation would be a teenager, or young adult, with declining educational performance and an incipient movement disorder such as a tremor (see Table 2).

Rehabilitative management in movement disorders

Assessment and monitoring

Two specific issues frequently encountered in movement disorders are especially relevant to assessment and monitoring. The first is *variability of disability*: erratic response to levodopa can cause people with PD to have devastating disabilities at one moment but virtually no deficits at another. Other movement disorders, such as the dystonias, are also notoriously variable in their effects. Rehabilitation should take account of both minimum and maximum abilities experienced day-to-day, and hour-to-hour. For these reasons, repeated assessments including occasional home-based evaluations can be helpful. A second reason for careful assessment and re-assessment is co-existent *multiple pathology*. Common symptoms, such as pain, dyspnoea, constipation, weight loss, and incontinence may be linked directly or indirectly (via medication effects, low mobility, poor diet) to the underlying movement disorder, but may often have other causes, too.

Principles of rehabilitative management

Medical care and rehabilitation should run in parallel during the successive phases of chronic and progressive disorders. Rehabilitation is an active, collaborative process directed towards goals relevant to individuals' daily lives.[10] For all movement disorders, and particularly for those which progress, a mainstay of rehabilitative management is an effective relationship between the patient, immediate family, GP, and community care agencies. Because movement disorders are uncommon, all parties in this relationship will need to educate themselves and each other. There are four phases to consider: (a) pre-diagnosis; (b) post-diagnosis; (c) evolving disability; and (d) end-stage. In each of these phases, patients and family usually require supportive counselling and information appropriate to their needs. There are four broad targets for intervention: *Prevention*, *Independence*, *Lifestyle*, and *Social resources* (PILS).

Prevention entails assessment and reduction of the risks of physical, psychological, and social complications and begins at the pre-diagnosis stage: a thorough response to initial symptoms and a well-supported diagnostic process will help to prevent development of morbid anxiety and potentially lifelong misconceptions about prognosis. A primary preventive task is to help people with movement disorders combat social prejudices. For example, if a tremor is being misinterpreted as nervousness in the workplace, information and counselling can avert premature retirement. Advice at diagnosis about practical issues, such as personal finances or housing, can prevent major problems developing prematurely, although insurance issues may be difficult to resolve, especially in HD.

As the patient enters the stage of evolving disabilities, a preventive agenda should be considered. Physical risks associated with parkinsonian syndromes, HD and ataxias include falls, skin sores, deformities of the spine and limbs, and nutritional problems (ABCD *A*ccidents, *B*roken skin, *C*ontractures, *D*iet). A history of falls should lead to review and home assessment by an occupational therapist. Seating and mattress should be the foci for measures to prevent skin problems and to discourage contractures. In all these conditions, loss of weight is the most common nutritional issue: among treatable causes of this are increased caloric demand, abnormal movements (a major issue in HD and occasionally also in the late stages of PD), dysphagia, and depression.

Interventions to promote *independence* can be directed at physical impairment: there is evidence for the efficacy of physiotherapy in PD (although not in HD). Occupational therapy can improve independence through a remedial programme and through adaptations to the physical environment. It is important to be aware that depression, anxiety, and impairments of communication and cognition can be potent sources of dependency, each suggesting different possible therapeutic approaches. The testimony of PD carers suggests that the physical difficulties experienced are easier to cope with than psychological impairments.

Lifestyle is not synonymous simply with physical independence but refers to a person's roles and aspirations—in the workplace and or family—and can be conserved in many disorders of movement for many years.[11–13] Primary care physicians are generally in better positions than hospital staff to understand what is meaningful to patients in these regards, and to institute supportive services which positively support lifestyle.

The fourth PILS category, *social resources*, is primarily an *aide memoire* to review the needs of family members and others. Prior to the stage of evolving disabilities, no-one is required to care *for* people with a condition such as PD or HD, but one or more relatives or friends are likely to care *about* them and will require information, education, and psychological support. In HD and other familial conditions, at-risk relatives are vicarious clients: they will suffer from insensitive handling of a relative's diagnosis, from misinformation about prognosis and genetic risks. Among physical resources, review of money and housing can be part of a forward-looking strategy which may become crucial during the stage of evolving disability; transport is another important consideration. As always, good rehabilitation and the best results depend on good communication and good sources of information.

Acknowledgements

Dr Guy Sawle kindly commented on a draft of this chapter and Debbie Hart extracted rates per 10 000 registered patients from Morbidity Statistics in General Practice, but responsibility for any errors rests with us. Professor Paul Dieppe, Dr Ted Cantrell, and Dr John Burn contributed to the development of the PILS scheme.

References

1. Marsden, C.D. and Fowler, T. *Clinical Neurology.* London: Arnold, 1998.
2. McCormick, A., Fleming, D., and Charlton, J. *Morbidity Statistics from General Practice.* Fourth National Study, 1991–1992. London: HMSO, 1995.

3. **Parkinson, J.** *The Shaking Palsy.* London: Sherwood, Nelly, and Jones, 1817. Facsimile reprint. London: Macmillan Magazines Ltd and Parkinson's Society, 1992.

4. **Mutch, W.J., Strudwick, A., Roy, S.K., and Downie, A.W.** (1986). Parkinson's disease: disability, review and management. *British Medical Journal* **293**, 675–7.

5. **Mutch, W.J., Digwall-Fordyce, I., Downie, A.W., Paterson, J.G., and Roy, S.K.** (1986). Parkinson's disease in a Scottish city. *British Medical Journal* **292**, 534–6.

6. **Schrag, A., Ben-Shlomo, Y., and Quinn, N.P.** (2000). Cross sectional prevalence survey of idiopathic Parkinson's disease and Parkinsonism in London. *British Medical Journal* **321**, 21–2.

7. **MacMahon, D.G. and Thomas, S.** (1998). Practical approach to quality of life in Parkinson's disease: the nurse's role. *Journal of Neurology* **245** (Suppl. 1), S19–22.

8. **Jarman, B., Hurwitz, B., Cook, A., Bajekal, M., and Lee, A.** (2002). The effects of community-based Parkinson's disease nurse specialists on health outcomes and costs: a randomised controlled trial. *British Medical Journal* **324**, 1072.

9. **Ward, C.D., Dennis, N.R., and McMillan, T.** (2003). Huntington's disease. In *Handbook of Neurological Rehabilitation* Chapter 40, 2nd edn. (ed. R. Greenwood, M.P. Barnes, T. McMillan, and C.D. Ward), pp. 553–66. Hove & New York: Psychology Press.

10. **Ward, C.D.** (2000). Rehabilitation in Parkinson's disease and parkinsonism. In *Parkinson's Disease and Parkinsonism in the Elderly* Chapter 16 (ed. J. Meara and W.C. Koller), pp. 165–84. Cambridge: Cambridge University Press.

11. **Drake, D. and Guillory, D.** (2001). Finding balance. *Lancet Supplement* **358**, S36.

12. **McMurray, S.E. and McMurray, C.T.** (2001). A sports star and a cook. *Lancet Supplement* **358**, S38.

13. **Harvey, D.** (2001). A disease that takes you unawares. *Lancet Supplement* **358**, S48.

11.4 Dizziness

Irwin Nazareth

Dizziness is an illusion of movement of oneself or the environment. There are several causes of dizziness that include vestibular, neurological, general medical, and psychological disorders. Vertigo, swimminess, giddiness, wooziness, lightheadedness, unsteadiness, and imbalance are some of the other common words used by people to describe this symptom.

Epidemiology

The prevalence of dizziness in a UK community sample has been estimated to be 233 per 1000 people between the ages of 18–64 years and half (109 per 1000) of these are handicapped by their symptoms.[1] In this point prevalence survey, about a quarter (26 per cent) reported a recent onset of the disorder (i.e. within the last 6 months), 44 per cent reported presence of the symptoms for 6 months to 5 years and 30 per cent presented a more chronic history (i.e. more than 5 years). A follow-up of this cohort at 18 months found that 47 per cent reported persistent symptoms, but only 29 per cent were more handicapped by them.[2] Similar cohort data from the United States, 1 year after an initial presentation of dizziness indicated that 45 per cent reported persistent symptoms and 11 per cent worsening of their condition.[3]

The prevalence of dizziness in people over 65 years in the United Kingdom is 30 per cent.[4] Lower prevalence rates of 24 per cent have been reported in people over 72 years of age in the United States.[5] Little is known about the occurrence of dizziness in childhood. Studies from Israel on children at a higher risk of the disorder (i.e. with a current history of otitis media or middle ear effusion) suggest that about 60 per cent of children have vertigo and dizziness.

How common is this presentation in primary care?

Consultation rates: Despite the high prevalence of the dizziness in the community, only 1 per cent of all consultations in British general practice[6] and 2 per cent in the United States have been associated with dizziness.[7]

In a small study conducted in three group practices in the United Kingdom, GPs were able to volunteer a diagnosis for only half of all the patients presenting with symptoms of dizziness. The most common provisional diagnostic categories were ENT (34 per cent), neurological (5 per cent), and cardiac (4 per cent). Most of these patients (84 per cent) were managed in primary care. The length of the presenting history and repeated attendance for the same problem were the chief factors that influenced the GPs' decision to refer to secondary care.[8] Patients with chronic symptoms of dizziness and the elderly who would benefit from specialist care were less often referred.

What are the possible causes?

Balance is maintained by an integration of vestibular, proprioceptive, and visual inputs that are modulated within the central nervous system. Impairments of primary sensory inputs or central pathology will lead to symptoms of dizziness. Normally symmetrical neural activity is generated by the vestibular receptors in each ear which sense linear and angular acceleration in the three planes of space. Vestibular damage (e.g. due to viral labyrnthitis) results in asymmetry of neural activity. Recovery eventually occurs leading to resolution of symptoms, as a result of central compensation or adaptation to the change in neural activity. Intermittent decompensation (due to other concurrent disease such as cold, influenza, and lack of sleep, etc.) or ongoing pathology within the labyrinth (e.g. Meniere's disease) produces recurrent dizziness. For example, in the elderly, a 'multisensory dizziness syndrome' can result from dysfunction of two or more sensory inputs (e.g. visual defects, arthritis, old injury to the labyrinth) combined with specific disorders of the central nervous system. The vertebro-basilar circulation supplies both peripheral and central vestibular systems and hence dysfunction at this level will lead to a mixed syndrome. Anaemia, hypoglycaemia, or hyperglycaemia due to inadequate oxygenation or metabolism within the vestibular nuclei and the peripheral vestibular receptors can also induce dizziness.

Differential diagnoses

Table 1 provides a fairly exhaustive list of the possible causes of dizziness and all these should be considered in the differential diagnoses. Anecdotal clinical experience suggests that vestibular dysfunction is the most common cause of dizziness in general practice. Half of all patients with dizziness in the community, however, have associated psychological dysfunction.[9,10] Psychological distress can cause dizziness through its central action. On the other hand, symptoms of dizziness are distressing to a person and can independently lead to psychological distress. Irrespective of causation, recognition and management of psychological disorders is an integral part of dealing with a person presenting with dizziness.

Table 1 Causes of dizziness

Mechanism	Example of causes
Otological	Vestibular neuronitis and acute labyrnthitis
	Ear infection—acute otitis media, cholesteomata and mastoiditis
	Benign positional vertigo
	Meniere's disease
Psychological	Anxiety
	Panic disorders
	Depression
Neurological	Cerebral
	Trauma
	Concussion
	Multiple sclerosis
	Vertiginous epilepsy
	Cerebello-pontine pathology
	Brain stem or cerebellar haemorrhage or infarction
	Opthalmoplegia with diploplia
	Acoustic neuroma
	Spinocerebellar atrophy
	Arnold Chiari type I malformations
	Tumours of brain stem and cerebellum
Haemodynamic	Haemotological
	Anaemia
	Cardiovascular
	Migraine
	Vetebro-basilar insufficiency
	Arrhythmias
	Postural hypotension

How to make a diagnosis

The important history and examination details are highlighted below:

History

The value of detailed history taking cannot be over emphasized. This should include the following:

Type of presentation

Clarification of the presentation is essential to ascertain that the person does suffer vertigo. Vertigo is an illusion of rotation that arises during the interaction between an individual and their environment. A major diagnostic clue is the duration of the vertigo: brief (<1 minute) episodes suggest benign paroxymal positional vertigo. Vertigo lasting hours is seen in migraine and Meniere's disease but when it lasts several days is usually due to vestibular neuritis. Almost all types of vertigo are aggravated by head movements and relieved by being still. If the dizziness does not have these features, either the person does not have vertigo or has mispresented the story. For example, unsteadiness due to osteoarthritis of the knees or peripheral neuropathy could be mistakenly interpreted as dizziness, as could transient lightheadedness of postural hypotension.

Precipitating factors

The next step is to ascertain whether the attacks are spontaneous or positional. Dizziness associated with a change in position is frequently due to benign postural vestibular dysfunction. Meniere's disease can cause spontaneous attacks of vertigo but in general practice, migraine is one diagnosis that should come to mind. Spontaneous episodes with loss of consciousness must be investigated for cardiac or neurological abnormalities. Loss of consciousness triggered by changes in posture (i.e. from lying to standing position) can be caused by orthostatic hypotension. Measurement

of blood glucose during an attack with a finger prick test is the most direct way of making a diagnosis of hypoglycaemia.

Duration of symptoms

The duration of the symptoms can also offer insights into the possible causes of dizziness as described below:

1. A single episode: for 3–4 days with total recovery over several weeks is suggestive of benign labyrinthine disorders such as viral labyrinthitis.

2. Recurrent episodes with associated headaches can occur following migraine.

3. Persistent symptoms for more than 6 weeks occur with uncompensated vestibular pathology or due to central vestibular dysfunction.

Other relevant symptoms

Other relevant symptoms must be sought and will assist diagnosis as follows:

1. Psychological symptoms: such as psychosomatic complaints (i.e. muscle tension, headaches, and fatigue) phobias, irritability, anxiety, and depression. However, it must be noted that psychological disorder is frequently co-morbid with physical disorders provoking dizziness and so the presence of psychological symptoms does not exclude a physical cause for dizziness.[9]

2. Pain in the neck might be present due to cervical pathology but it is important to ensure that those suffering from chronic dizziness may hold their head rigidly (consciously or unconsciously) to avoid precipitating positional symptoms, thus inducing secondary neck pain and stiffness. Usually neck symptoms are secondary to vestibular disorders or essentially unrelated to a vestibular disorder (e.g. arthritis).

3. Vetebro-basilar insufficiency (or more specifically vetebro-basilar transient ischaemic attacks) is usually associated with neurological symptoms and does not occur with vertigo alone.

4. Associated symptoms in the cochlea (deafness and tinnitus), cardiovascular (palpitations or chest pains), central nervous (numbness of weakness in face or limbs, slurred speech, diploplia), and endocrine systems (e.g. symptoms of diabetes or thyroid dysfunction) must also be sought.

Drug history

The relevance of a detailed drug history cannot be overemphasized. This is particularly important in the elderly who are often on several medications. Gentamycin is one of the drugs known to cause vestibular disorders (see below). Other drugs with effects on the central nervous systems, however, are also known to cause dizziness especially in the elderly.

Examination

The examination should include:

1. Ear: otoscopic examination for chronic otitis media can be done but it's value is limited, as the presence of a perilymph fistula will be missed.

2. Cardiovascular: to check for arrhythmia and for orthostatic hypotension. The latter is particularly important in the elderly on anti-hypertensive medication.

3. Visual: fundi, visual fields, visual acuity.

4. Eye movement examination is essential in people with balance problems. Examination of cranial nerves III, IV, and VI as well as testing for saccades or pursuit abnormalities. Abnormalities indicate neurological problems.

5. Identification of spontaneous and/or positional nystagmus is important. Nystagmus is a rhythmic oscillation of the eye that occurs

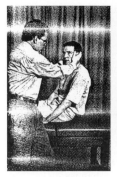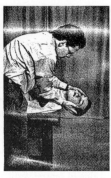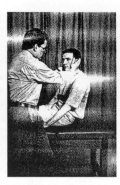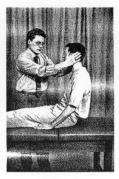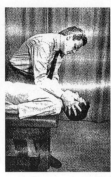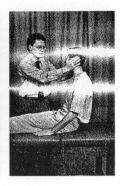

Fig. 1 Hallpike positional manoeuvre for diagnosis of benign positional vertigo. Patients must be warned that transient vertigo may develop in any position. Patients are instructed to keep their eyes open throughout and stare at the examiner's nose. In each position observe eyes closely for up to 30 seconds for development of nystagmus. This manoeuvre can be applied safely to patients with cervical spondylosis if the neck is not hyperextended. From left to right: Begin with patient sitting upright on a couch with head turned 45° to left to test left posterior canal. With head in this position, lie patient down rapidly until head is dependent. Return patient to upright position. Approach patient from the other side and rotate head to right to test right posterior canal. Lie patient down into opposite head hanging position. Return patient to upright. [Reproduced with permission from: Lempert, T., Gresty, M., and Bronstein, A. (1995). Benign positional vertigo: recognition and treatment. *British Medical Journal* **311**, 489–91.]

due to disorders of the vestibular labyrinth and/or the central vestibular–ocular pathways. In the most common form it is characterized by slow movements of the eye in one direction and a fast movement in the reverse direction. The latter is described as the beat direction of the nystagmus. The person is told to fix his/her gaze straight ahead and then asked to gaze upwards, downwards, right and left, to assess nystagmus. The person should hold their gaze in each of these positions for more than 5 seconds. Nystagmus occurring in the light is a sign of an acute vestibular disorder, a neurological disease or a congenital nystagmus. The latter is usually asymptomatic and patients may be aware that they have had nystagmus since childhood.

6. Hallpike's manoeuvre is described in Fig. 1. The person sits near one end of the examination couch and their head is turned to the right by 45°. The person is now rapidly moved backwards with the head over the couch (see Fig. 1). A positive test produces persistent nystagmus accompanied by dizziness. The test is then repeated with the head turned to the left. This test is positive in benign paroxysmal positional vertigo.

7. Romberg's test: ask the person to stand with his/her feet close together with his/her eyes open and then closed. Most people are unsteady with their eyes closed rather than open but if the patient falls or nearly falls the test is said to be positive. Romberg described this test in tabes dorsalis (i.e. spinal cord dorsal column disease) and this still holds true. However, in the very early stages of unilateral vestibular lesions, the person may fall in the direction of the lesion.

8. The head impulse tests: the person fixes his/her gaze to a distant object and the examiner turns his/her head by 15 degrees to one side and then to other side. The test is positive if the person cannot keep fixating at the target so that he/she has to make a voluntary rapid eye movement back to the target after the head is rotated. Total loss of vestibular function will produce a positive test. Although this is a good test, its execution and interpretation requires a lot of skill and hence it cannot readily be used in general practice settings.

9. Other central nervous system tests should include a brief examination of cerebellar functions and reflexes.

The three types of clinical presentation

The three presentations of dizziness can be linked to specific diagnoses.[11] These are described below.

The person who has had recurrent attacks of dizziness but is well when seen by the GP

Based on a detailed history and examination, the differential diagnosis of this presentation is as follows:

1. Benign paroxysmal positional vertigo is caused by stray otoconial particles within the duct of the posterior semicircular canals and is diagnosed by the Hallpike manoeuvre.

2. Migraine is a common and important diagnosis and must be searched for by taking a careful history.

3. Meniere's disease presents as recurrent spontaneous vertigo lasting for an hour or more. The pathophysiology of this condition is endolymphatic hypertension producing disabling attacks of vertigo, nausea, and vomiting together with frequent hearing loss and a low frequency tinnitus with a sense of fullness and blockage in the ear (that lasts for several days after subsidence of dizziness). The prevalence estimates of Meniere's disease range from 0.1 to 1 per cent of the population.

4. Panic and phobic attacks as the main cause of dizziness should be confirmed in the presence of psychological dysfunction and the absence of a presentation typical of vestibular or other medical disorders.

The patient who is experiencing a first ever attack of acute spontaneous vertigo

This is an acute presentation of intense spontaneous dizziness, nausea, and vomiting often encountered on a home visit. Acute labyrinthitis is the most common cause of such a presentation but an important differential diagnosis is cerebellar infarction. A meticulous history must be taken and a relevant examination conducted as described in the previous section. The differential diagnosis of the common syndromes are discussed below:

1. Acute vestibular neuritis presents with clinical symptoms similar to those experienced after a labyrinthectomy or vestibular neurectomy. There is horizontal–torsional spontaneous unidirectional nystagmus with the slow phases to the affected ear and quick phases to the unaffected side. Bidirectional nystagmus is not associated with this condition. Moreover, nystagmus is suppressed by visual fixation and hence could be missed if not specifically looked for. The head impulse test is positive. Lastly, although the person is unsteady, he/she can stand without support with the eyes open but will rotate towards the side of the lesion if asked to walk briskly on the spot with the eyes closed (positive Unterberger test).

Table 2 Exercise for dizziness, vertigo and imbalance

Exercise sheet used in controlled trial of exercise therapy for dizziness in primary care:[12] *exercises for dizziness, vertigo, and imbalance*
The process of getting over dizziness or vertigo is exactly the same as when a sailor gets his or her 'sealegs', or a dancer learns to spin around without getting dizzy. The only way that the balance system can overcome dizziness and imbalance is by practising the movements and situations, which cause dizziness. The aim of these exercises is to give your balance system all the practice it needs, at a time and place where you will not be distracted or put at risk.

The exercises listed below should be performed *twice a day*. Make sure you carry them out somewhere safe, where you will not bump into anything sharp or hard. At first, the exercises will probably make you feel a bit dizzy and sick, and you may experience some tiredness and headache. These feelings may last for a little while after you have done the exercises, or may even come on some time later. Do not worry about these feelings—they are a sign that the exercises are working. If the dizziness and sickness is really unpleasant, or is causing problems, then do the exercises more slowly and do fewer of them at first; as you recover you can gradually increase the number and speed of the exercises you do.

If the exercises seem to bring on any of the symptoms listed below (which is *very* unlikely), stop doing them at once and ring for help.

Stop doing the exercises if you experience:
Sharp, severe or prolonged pain in your neck, head, or ear
A sensation of fullness in the ear, deafness, or noises in the ear
Fainting, loss of consciousness, blacking out, double vision
Numbness, weakness, or tingling in your arms or legs

1. Sit upright with your legs out in front of you. Quickly lie straight down on your back. Wait for your symptoms to calm down, and then sit back up again. Repeat two or three times. *Advanced stage.* When you can do this exercise without dizziness, try it with your head turned first to the left and then to the right.

2. Sitting in a chair, bend forward and bring your head down halfway towards your knees. Wait for your symptoms to calm down, and then sit back up again. Repeat two or three times. *Advanced stage.* When you can do this exercise without dizziness, try it with your head turned first to the left and then to the right.

3. Sitting in a chair, quickly turn your head and eyes from left to right, five times in each direction, as if you were watching a tennis match. Try to focus on an object in each direction. Stop, wait for your symptoms to go away, and repeat three times. *Advanced stage.* When you can do this exercise without dizziness, try doing it while you are standing up.

4. Repeat the same exercise, but looking up and down instead of left and right. *Advanced stage.* When you can do this exercise without dizziness, try doing it while you are standing up.

5. Do exercise 3 with your eyes closed. (NB: Do *not* do this exercise standing up).

6. Do exercise 4 with your eyes closed. (NB: Do *not* do this exercise standing up).

7. Sit in a chair with one arm outstretched in front of you with your first finger pointing up. Stare at your finger and turn your head to left and right 10 times. Start slowly and gradually speed up. Repeat three times.

8. Repeat the same exercise, but hold your finger sideways and move your head up and down.

General balance training:
Go for a walk (include some stairs or hills if possible) or play a ball-game either for 5–10 min, 5 days a week, or for 15–30 min, 3 days a week

2. Cerebellar infarction: is a rare and severe condition and is the main differential diagnosis of acute vestibular neuritis. In cerebellar infanction:

(i) head impulse test is always negative;

(ii) nystagmus might be bilateral, vertical and is not suppressed by visual fixation;

(iii) the sufferer cannot stand without support.

The sequelae of this presentation are:

1. A person suffering from vestibular neuritis should recover spontaneously over a few weeks but risks developing more persistent positional symptoms due to inadequate compensation or subsequent attacks of BPPV. These can be treated by vestibular rehabilitation exercises (Table 2) or particle repositioning, respectively.

2. A person with a small infarct in their cerebellum may present with a vascular event elsewhere.

The person who is persistently off balance

This presentation is one of continuous and persistent dizziness while standing or walking. There are many possible causes for this presentation and it is often impossible to arrive at a single diagnosis, especially in older people. The chief differential diagnoses are:

1. Chronic uncompensated vertigo of labyrinthine origin is a multisensory disorder that presents either as chronic persistent or relapsing dizziness with evidence of peripheral vestibular dysfunction. Most sufferers have failure of cerebral compensation together with visual defects such as cataracts, musculoskeletal disorders, or associated general medical disorders such as hypertension or cerebrovascular diseases.

2. Chronic hyperventilation (overbreathing), often secondary to anxiety, causes dizziness, unsteadiness, and feeling of unreality. Symptoms include breathlessness, frequent sighing, gasping, or yawning. Hyperventilation can be confirmed if voluntary overbreathing for a minute or two reproduces the usual symptoms.

3. Bilateral loss of vestibular function is the most common *single cause*. When the person tries to stand with their eyes closed on a soft-yielding surface such as mattress they are likely to be unsteady (positive modified Romberg's test). Head impulse is positive for left, right, up and down movements. The most common cause of this disorder is gentamycin toxicity and this should be considered if imbalance occurs after a hospital admission.

4. Chronic central vertigo is a poorly understood condition and is found in approximately 20 per cent of people with multiple sclerosis. It is associated with abnormal eye movements (such as periodic alternating pendular nystagmus and microsaccadic oscillations) and other neurological pathology.

5. Rare syndromes: such as familial vestibulopathy (a rare inherited disorder), normal pressure hydrocephalus, posterior fossa tumours, and Parkinsonian syndromes.

Principles of management

Table 3 provides a management checklist for each of the three common presentations of dizziness.

Investigations and specialist referral

Most patients encountered in general practice suffer from brief acute transitory episodes of dizziness that do not require extensive investigation. The only investigations that can be done in general practice are routine blood tests to rule out general medical disorders. More specialized investigation can only be done by a specialist. Referral to secondary care should be considered in the following circumstances:

1. Persistent dizziness (that last more than 4–6 weeks) and in the absence of a general medical or neurological disorder.

2. In the first acute attack when the general practitioner is unable to differentiate between acute vestibular neuritis and cerebellar infarction.

3. Unilateral hearing loss (possible acoustic neuroma).

Table 3 Management check-list for people presenting with vertigo

Type of presentation	Possible causes	Management approach
Patients with repeated attacks of vertigo	Benign paroxysmal positional vertigo	Diagnosis—Hallpike manoeuvre positive Treatment—particle repositioning
	Meniere's disease	Diagnosis—history and signs Treatment—cinnarzine, betahistidine, surgery (vestibular ablation/neuronectomy)
	Panic/phobic attacks	Diagnosis—psychological assessment Treatment—psychological treatments
Patients with first ever attack of vertigo	Acute vestibular neuritis	Diagnosis—examination Treatment—prochloperazine, cinnarzine
	Cerebellar infarction	Diagnosis—examination Treatment—refer specialist
In patients who are off balance most of the time	Chronic vertigo of labyrinthine origin Chronic hyperventilation Bilateral loss of vestibular function Chronic central vertigo Rare syndromes (familial vestibulopathy, normal pressure hydrocephalus, posterior fossa tumour, progressive supranuclear palsy)	For all patients Diagnosis—history and examination Treatment—refer specialist

Patients with persistent dizziness or a suspected acoustic neuroma are best referred to an ENT specialist and all others to a neurologist. A detailed neuro-otological evaluation by a specialist will involve an assessment of auditory function and an evaluation of the cochlea and auditory nerve. Such investigations provide information about the peripheral and central vestibular pathways. If central vestibular dysfunction is suspected, useful diagnostic information will be obtained from a MRI scan.

Treatment

Treatment of the main clinical syndromes associated with dizziness is described below:

1. Benign positional vertigo of paroxysmal type is best treated with particle repositioning procedures (also referred to as Epley's manoeuvre). A number of studies have suggested an 80–90 per cent success rate with such procedures.[13] This procedure relieves the symptoms by removing otoconial particles from the semicircular canals. The procedure only takes a few minutes, is non-invasive and can be performed in primary care, but GPs will require special training on how to perform this manoeuvre.

2. The diagnosis of Meniere's disease should not be made lightly, and it is essential that a general practitioner refers all patients suspected with this condition to a specialist for confirmation of diagnosis. Dietary sodium restriction and even diuretic therapy have long since been considered effective treatments but there is no evidence from randomized controlled trials on the effectiveness of these management options. Betahistine has also been used for long-term management of the condition as it is believed to lower endolymphatic pressure. Controlled trials have demonstrated significant improvements in dizziness, imbalance and tinnitus, and effective prophylaxis of acute attacks early in the disease with this agent. There is, however, no evidence that any of these treatments modify the disease process. On the other hand, comparative studies of cinnavizine, a vestibular sedative with placebo and prochlorperazine in two double-blind trials suggest that the drug was more effective than placebo and as effective as prochlorperazine. However, vestibular sedatives should only be used for temporary symptom control and are not recommended for long-term use, as they retard central compensation.

Failure to respond to medical treatment will necessitate a referral to a specialist for surgical treatment such as saccus drainage procedures or more radical treatment such as ablation of the labyrinth, vestibular neuronectomy or vestibular ablation.

3. Phobia and panic attacks are best managed by a combination of relaxation exercises, breathing exercises, and cognitive and behavioural approaches. Appropriate drug therapy might be considered in cases of severe anxiety, panic, and agoraphobia. More evidence, however, is required on the application of such approaches to the management of dizziness in these patient groups.

4. Acute labyrinthitis often presents as an emergency and will require treatment with an antiemetic such as prochlorperazine (administered buccally, intramuscularly, or by suppository). This can be followed by a vestibular sedative such as cinnarizine 15 mg (dose adjustment will have to be made in the elderly) given every 8 hours until the attack subsides.

5. Chronic vertigo of labyrinthine origin is best managed by vestibular compensation exercises (Table 2). These are taught to the patient by a trained therapist and then practiced for 5–10 minutes a day, twice a day. The exercises initially provoke dizziness but with continued practice symptoms resolve over 6–12 weeks. Psychological treatments and support are also an essential aspect of management and include provision of information on the causes of vertigo and simple relaxation and breathing exercises.[14] Acute attacks can be treated by vestibular sedatives and antiemetics.

6. Acute hyperventilation is relieved by breathing for a minute or two into a paper bag. Patients should be taught how to reduce their respiration by breath holding for 10–40 seconds and paced breathing (one breath every 4–6 seconds).

Long-term and continuing care

Although dizziness is common in the community, few people consult their GP for this reason.[6,7] In the absence of clear management guidelines, GPs often find difficulty in assessing and managing such symptoms effectively, demonstrated by a community-based survey in which there was evidence of under-referral of patients with chronic symptoms of dizziness, particularly the elderly.[8] In people with symptoms of chronic dizziness, psychological distress often co-exists. Screening for common psychological symptoms such as anxiety, depression, phobias, or panic disorders could identify associated problems that can then be appropriately managed. It has been suggested that such approaches could alleviate symptoms of recurrent and troubling dizziness. Long-term management of people in general practice through information provision (on the causes of dizziness) and specific preventive strategies such as lifestyle changes and vestibular rehabilitation exercises are acceptable and feasible. More information, however, is required on the clinical effectiveness of such an approach.

Implications of the problem

Dizziness is an upsetting symptom and at least half of those affected by it report some handicap in their daily, social, or leisure activities. In most cases dizziness presents as an acute symptom. About 30 per cent of people with dizziness report a chronic recurrent and upsetting problem.[1] Functional disability is worse in people with bilateral vestibular dysfunction as compared with unilateral pathology. In the elderly, chronic dizziness is associated with risk of falling, experiencing syncope, worsening of depressive symptoms, poor self-rated health, and interference with social activities.[5] Quality of life is most likely to be affected by frequent long-term dizziness, nausea, and the feeling that the ground was distant or as though the person was walking on clouds.[15] Other factors such as personality traits and patients' capacity to cope with the symptoms, however, impair quality of life.

Further research

Until recently, most research on dizziness was conducted in secondary care. This chapter has described some of the studies from primary care. More research, in the primary care setting, is required on:

- the prevalence of dizziness in people below the age of 18 years;
- the spectrum of presentations in general practice and their causes;
- the clinical and cost effectiveness of care packages that include psychological and vestibular rehabilitation strategies.

Key points

- The point prevalence of dizziness in people between 18 and 65 years in the community is 233 per 1000.

- Despite this, only 1–2% of all general practice consultations are due to dizziness and the GP is able to make a definitive diagnosis in only half of all presentations.

- The most common presentation is a history of recurrent attacks of dizziness. The common clinical causes are benign paroxysmal vertigo (managed by particle repositioning manoeuvres), Meniere's disease (managed by drug therapy and surgery), and panic and phobic attacks (managed by psychological therapy).

- Another common presentation (often seen at a request for a home visit) is a person experiencing their first ever attack of acute vertigo with nausea and vomiting. Acute vestibular neuritis (treated by drugs) or cerebellar infarction (that requires referral) are the two most common causes.

- The least common and most troubling presentation is persistent dizziness due to chronic vertigo of labyrinthine origin, bilateral loss of vestibular function, chronic central vertigo and other rarer syndromes.

- Referral to a specialist must be considered in all patients with persistent dizziness and those with acute vertigo and vomiting where differentiation between acute vestibular neuritis and cerebellar infarction cannot be made.

References

1. Yardley, L., Owen, N., Nazareth, I., and Luxon, L. (1998). Prevalence and presentation of dizziness in a general practice community sample of working age people. *British Journal of General Practice* **48**, 1131–5.

2. Nazareth, I., Yardley, L., Owen, N., and Luxon, L. (1999). Outcome of symptoms of dizziness in a general practice community sample. *Family Practice* **16**, 616–18.

3. Kroeke, K., Lucas, C.A., Rosenberg, M.L., Scherokman, B., and Herbers, J.E. (1994). One outcome in patients with a chief complaint of dizziness. *Journal of General Internal Medicine* **9**, 684–9.

4. Colledge, N.R., Wilson, J.A., Macintyre, C.C.A., and MacLennan, W.J. (1994). The prevalence and characteristics of dizziness in an elderly community. *Age and Ageing* **7**, 1–8.

5. Tinette, M.E., Williams, C.S., and Gill, T.M. (2000). Dizziness among older adults: a possible geriatric syndrome. *Annals of Internal Medicine* **132**, 337–44.

6. Sloane, P.D. (1989). Dizziness in primary care. Results from the National Ambulatory Care Survey. *Family Practice* **29**, 33–8.

7. Office of Population Censuses and Surveys. *Morbidity Statistics from General Practice—Fourth National Study 1991–1992*. London: HMSO, 1995.

8. Bird, J.C., Beynon, G.J., Prevost, A.T., and Baguley, D.M. (1998). An analysis of referral patterns for dizziness in the primary care setting. *British Journal of General Practice* **48**, 1828–32.

9. Yardley, L., Burgeneay, J., Nazareth, I., and Luxon, L. (1998). Neuro-otological and psychiatric abnormalities in a community sample of people with dizziness: a blind controlled investigation. *Journal of Neurology, Neurosurgery and Psychiatry* **65**, 679–84.

10. Yardley, L., Nazareth, I., and Luxon, L. (1999). Psychiatric dysfunction and dizziness. *Lancet* **353**, 2069.

11. Halmagyi, G.M. and Cremer, P.D. (2000). Assessment and treatment of dizziness. *Journal of Neurology, Neurosurgery and Psychiatry* **68**, 129–36.

12. Yardley, L., Beech, S., Zander, L., Evans, T., and Weinman, J. (1998). A randomized controlled trial of exercise therapy for dizziness and vertigo in primary care. *British Journal of General Practice* **48**, 1136–40.

13. Beynon, G.J. (1997). A review of benign paroxymal positional vertigo by exercise therapy and by repositioning manoeuvres. *British Journal of Audiology* **31**, 11–26.

14. Yardley, L., Burgneay, J., Andersson, G., Owen, N., Nazareth, I., and Luxon, L. (1998). Feasibility and effectiveness of providing vestibular rehabilitation for dizzy patients in the community. *Clinical Otolaryngology* **23**, 442–8.

15. Mendel, B., Bergnius, J., and Langius, A. (1999). Dizziness symptom severity and impact on daily living as perceived by patients suffering from peripheral vestibular disorder. *Clinical Otolaryngology & Allied Sciences* **24**, 286–93.

Further reading

Luxon, L.M. and Davies, R.A., ed. *Handbook of Vestibular Rehabilitation*. London: Whurr, 1997. (Specifies the delivery of vestibular rehabilitation.)

Baloh, R.W. and Hamagyi, G.M., ed. *Disorders of the Vestibular System*. New York: Oxford University Press, 1996. (Details the causes of dizziness.)

Kerr, A.G. and Scott-Brown, W.G., ed. *Scott-Brown's Otolaryngology*. London: Butterworth-Heineman, 1996. (Provides an overview of the treatment of dizziness.)

11.5 Peripheral neuropathies

Martin Schwartz

Background

Although disorders of the peripheral nerves are frequently encountered in clinical practice, the exact incidence of peripheral neuropathy is not known. While diabetes and alcohol abuse are the commonest causes of peripheral neuropathy in developed countries, leprosy probably represents the commonest treatable cause of neuropathy worldwide. A wide range of other factors—hereditary, inflammatory, toxic, metabolic, and neoplastic—is involved in causing peripheral neuropathy, and infection with human immunodeficiency virus (HIV) is assuming increasing importance.

Epidemiology

Data on the incidence and prevalence of the peripheral neuropathies are scarce. The mononeuropathies, including the nerve entrapment syndromes, are seen at all ages, and while some of the generalized polyneuropathies are more common in older patients, possibly because of coexistent age-related neurological degeneration, peripheral nerve disorders are seen at all ages. Few reliable data are available on the effects of geography and ethnicity.

Causes and classifications of polyneuropathies

The polyneuropathies can be classified in a number of ways—acute or chronic, mononeuropathic or polyneuropathic, and motory or sensory, as well as considering the underlying aetiologies. The underlying pathogenesis includes Wallerian degeneration, secondary to nerve injury, primary axonal

Table 1 Peripheral neuropathies

Mononeuropathies	Generalized polyneuropathies

Cranial neuropathies
  Trigeminal neuralgia (painful neuropathy
    of the fifth cranial nerve)
  Bell's palsy (motor neuropathy of
    the seventh cranial nerve)
  Diabetic cranial neuropathies
    (e.g. occulomotor palsies)
	Hereditary
	  Charcot–Marie–Tooth
	  Refsum's and other rare
	    syndromes

Carpal tunnel syndrome	Metabolic
	  Diabetes
	  Alcohol
	  B12 and folate
	  Uraemia
	  Porphyria

Ulnar nerve entrapment	Infectious and post-infectious
	  HIV
	  Guillain–Barre
	  Lyme disease
	  Post-viral

Sciatic and femoral nerve entrapment	Toxic
	  Lead, thallium, mercury, arsenic
	  Organic chemicals
	  Animal and insect bites

Brachial plexus/thoracic outlet entrapment	Paraneoplastic (cancers, paraproteinaemias)
Mononeuritis multiplex (diabetes, polyarteritis nodosa, amyloidosis)	

degeneration, segmental demyelination, and primary disorders of sensory or motor cell bodies. The mononeuropathies affect single nerves and cause focal motor, sensory, or reflex changes. The commonest cause of the mononeuropathies are the entrapment syndromes,[1] although mononeuritis multiplex, which is a focal involvement of two or more nerves, is sometimes associated with a systemic disorder, such as diabetes mellitus or amyloidosis, and results in multiple peripheral nerve lesions. In addition, the cranial neuropathies are essentially mononeuropathies, and these include trigeminal neuralgia, Bell's palsy and the diabetic cranial neuropathies. The common underlying causes of peripheral neuropathy are shown in Table 1.

Mononeuropathies

The most common entrapment syndrome is *compression of the medial nerve in the carpal tunnel*, or carpal tunnel syndrome. This occurs most frequently in middle-aged women, when it is generally unaccompanied by disease, but it may also be a complication of pregnancy, hypothyroidism, acromegaly, or rheumatoid arthritis. The typical presentation includes pain, numbness and tingling in the thumb and fingers supplied by the median nerve, particularly on using the hand or at night time, when the patient may be woken from sleep. Objective sensory loss often accompanies these symptoms, and there may be weakness and wasting of abductor pollicis brevis and opponens pollicis muscles. The condition is sometimes bilateral.

Cubital tunnel syndrome represents a similar, but much less common, entrapment syndrome affecting the *ulnar nerve*. Causes include fracture deformities, arthritis and repetitive occupational or recreational trauma. There is often sensory loss in the fifth finger and half of the fourth finger, accompanied by wasting of the intrinsic muscles of the hand and, later, weakness of grip. Compression of the *radial nerve* is much less common, generally occurs in the axilla or the upper arm and may be seen with improperly used crutches or after prolonged pressure during sleep, known not inappropriately as the Saturday night palsy. Direct injury may also be involved. The cardinal symptom is wrist-drop; muscle wasting is rarely present and recovery usually occurs within 6–8 weeks.

The upper extremities may also be affected by a number of other entrapment syndromes, including *cervical radiculopathy* and myelopathy, *brachial plexus neuritis*, *thoracic outlet syndrome*, and *long thoracic nerve entrapment*. Cervical spine problems are discussed elsewhere in this book, but brachial plexus neuritis is a particularly difficult problem which, for some reason, often develops after immunization and produces severe shoulder and upper arm pain, followed by weakness. Recovery is generally full, but prolonged.

Thoracic outlet syndrome is usually due to the presence of a cervical rib or bony abnormality of the first rib. It presents as pain in the arm in certain positions, accompanied by colour changes in the hand and a pattern of sensory loss and weakness most pronounced in the fourth and fifth fingers. Deep tendon reflexes are generally preserved. The differential diagnosis includes Raynaud's phenomenon, ulnar nerve entrapment and brachial plexus involvement in cancer or fibrosis.

In the lower limb, entrapment syndromes include *lateral femoral cutaneous nerve compression, femoral neuropathy, sciatic nerve syndromes* and, often linked to these, lumbar disc syndromes.

When the lateral femoral cutaneous nerve of the thigh is compressed in the region of the anterior superior iliac spine and the insertion of the sartorious muscle, an unpleasant characteristic burning pain along the anterolateral and lateral aspects of the thigh develops, often exacerbated by standing or walking. This is often accompanied by sensory changes, but not by weakness or changes in reflexes, and is known as *meralgia paraesthetica*. Although the neuropathy usually regresses spontaneously, surgical release may be required.

Femoral nerve entrapment may occur in the inguinal region and from direct retroperitoneal compression by tumour or haematoma. However, the most common cause of this syndrome, which is often of surprisingly sudden onset, is nerve infarction, seen in diabetes and vasculitis. A combination of thigh pain, weakness, and sensory loss is often seen in diabetic femoral neuropathy.

The *sciatic nerve*, arising from the lumbosacral plexus (L4-S3) may be compressed by tumours within the pelvis or, more commonly, from prolonged sitting or lying on the buttocks. Gluteal abcess and misplaced buttock injections can also cause sciatic nerve injury. *Common peroneal compression* can also occur at the level of the fibular head, and is often seen in cachectic patients following prolonged bed rest, as well as in alcoholics.

Finally, it is important to distinguish these nerve compression syndromes from the much commoner *lumbar disc syndromes*, which produce a characteristic pattern of pain, weakness, and sensory changes, depending on the level of compression.

Generalized polyneuropathies

In these conditions, the lesion usually lies in the nerve cell body so that the first signs of disease are at the distal ends of the longest nerves, resulting in the typical picture of distal parasthesiae first affecting the feet, and, later, the hands—the so-called glove and stocking distribution. Sensory changes are often accompanied by distal weakness with diminished or absent tendon reflexes.

The range of causes of the generalized peripheral neuropathies is wide. Some are genetically determined and include the peripheral type of peroneal muscular atrophy, progressive hypertrophic polyneuritis and hereditary sensory neuropathies. Charcot–Marie–Tooth syndrome is an example of a range of hereditary sensory–motor neuropathies, with extremely complex underlying pathological and genetic mechanisms. Refsum's syndrome is a phytanic acid storage disease, leading to multiple neurological problems, including peripheral neuropathy, visual impairments, ataxia, impaired hearing and skin and bone changes. More commonly peripheral neuropathy is related to deficiencies of vitamins B6, B12, and to folate deficiency whilst, conversely, toxic peripheral neuropathies can be caused by a range of agents including, lead, arsenic, mercury, organic chemicals such as carbon tetrachloride, acrylamide, and analine dyes, and a large number of medications, including the Vinca alkaloids, phenytoin, and chloroquine.

Infections also play a role in causing the peripheral neuropathies. Leprosy is the most typical of these, but polyneuropathies may complicate infections such as influenza, measles, and typhoid fever, whilst some are directly due to exotoxins as in diphtheritic polyneuropathy and acute post-infective polyneuropathy, the Guillain–Barre syndrome. Connective tissue disorders, notably polyarteritis nodosa, rheumatoid arthritis, and giant cell arteritis, can cause polyneuropathy, whilst metabolic causes include diabetes, renal and hepatic failure, and acute intermittent porphyria. Carcinoma of the bronchus and other malignant diseases, including the paraproteinaemias, are associated with painful peripheral neuropathy.

The peripheral neuropathy of diabetes is often complex,[2] and includes distal, symmetrical, and mixed sensory–motor polyneuropathies, pure motor neuropathies, diabetic amyotrophy, sensory neuropathies and, often extremely disabling for patients, autonomic neuropathy, which can lead to impotence and autonomic diarrhoea and loss of bladder control.

The Guillain–Barre syndrome, acute post-infective polyneuropathy, classically follows an acute viral illness by 1–4 weeks. It often presents with pain in the back, frequently between the shoulder blades, with distal tingling of the limbs and progressive weakness which may become profound. In severe cases tetraparesis and respiratory failure can develop within hours of the initial symptoms. In others progression is slower, over a period of 1–2 weeks. Intensive supportive therapy may be required but the prognosis is ultimately good.

Presentation and diagnosis in primary care

Patients frequently consult primary care physicians because of focal numbness, tingling, weakness, pain, or combinations of these symptoms. Although, in general, major acute neurological illness is unlikely to be the underlying diagnosis, because peripheral neuropathy can signal the presence of a serious underlying disease it is important to try to arrive at an accurate diagnosis. However, this is often not possible, and as many as 50 per cent of patients referred to neurology specialists with symptoms of peripheral neuropathy do not receive a definitive diagnosis.[3,4]

The first step in diagnosis is to determine whether the patient does, indeed, have a peripheral neuropathy, or whether there is evidence of a more widespread disorder, such as motor neurone disease. Other conditions, such as syringomyelia, dorsal column disorders, such as tabes dorsalis, and myelopathies, as well as hysterical symptoms, can sometimes mimic a peripheral neuropathy.

It goes without saying that a full clinical history is essential. Indeed, the time course of the disorders may give important clues to the likely cause. The precise nature of the symptoms—are they motor, sensory, or mixed?—the patient's current and previous medical problems, as well as a detailed occupational history and system review are important too, as is a search in the history for symptoms suggestive of autonomic dysfunction or recent or underlying infection. Details of current medication and possible toxin exposure are essential, and information about dietary habits and alcohol must also be obtained.

In performing the neurological examination, the presence and distribution of weakness, the pattern of tendon reflexes and responses to pain, light touch, vibration, and propperception must all be measured. It is worth palpating relevant nerves in order to detect sites of compression or attachment, and also, of course, to look for evidence of muscle weakness and wasting.

The history and examination in a primary care setting are often sufficient to distinguish between a mononeuropathy and a polyneuropathy and, in the former case, to single out patients likely to have an entrapment syndrome. Where this has not been possible, or where a more widespread polyneuropathy of uncertain aetiology is identified, further investigations will be required.

Investigations

It is probably appropriate to arrange routine screening haematology and biochemistry tests, plus haemoglobin A1C and urinalysis, serum B12 and folate, and thyroid function tests. A number of possible underlying causes, including hepatic and renal dysfunction, diabetes, and vitamin deficiencies, may be identified by these simple investigations.

If no further clues emerge from these investigations, referral for further investigation is likely to be required, and will typically consist of electrodiagnostic studies, including nerve conduction and electromyography, which are undertaken to confirm the presence of a neuropathy, to differentiate axonal from demyelinating conditions and to differentiate myogenic from neurogenic causes of weakness.

Further sophisticated serological and genetic testing, biopsy and imaging techniques may also be required in the specialist setting.[5]

Management

The management of the peripheral neuropathies is closely related to the management of one of the many underlying conditions that can cause the problem and which may have significant implications for patients, such as diabetes, alcohol abuse and diabetic and renal disease. A clear explanation to patients, who may become very concerned about the extent of their medical problems, is essential.

The entrapment syndromes are, for the most part, approached conservatively, although evidence of cervical myelopathy, accompanied by significant X-ray changes, is an indication for specialist referral.

The brachial plexus and thoracic outlet syndromes may, likewise, require referral because of the need for complex imaging techniques and electro-physiological studies.

Carpal tunnel syndrome should generally be treated in primary care, although confirmatory electromyographic studies may sometimes be needed. Wrist splints and anti-inflammatory medications are the mainstay of treatment, although surgical relief is relatively straight forward and effective, and should be considered when symptoms persist.

Meralgia paraesthetica and femoral neuropathies are also likely to resolve without intervention, but the possibility of underlying systemic disease in all these conditions needs to be borne in mind.

Amongst the generalized peripheral neuropathies, urgent intervention is most important in patients with symptoms suggestive of Guillain–Barre syndrome, where hospital referral is required, particularly if symptoms are rapidly progressive.[6]

Hospital referral may also be required for some of the rarer, but potentially extremely dangerous, toxic causes of peripheral neuropathy, due to poisoning. Puffer fish and other large carnivorous tropical fish can cause poisoning leading to acute demyelination and painful paraesthesiae. The toxic agent is tetrodon, which is produced by puffer fish, and to which there is no known antidote. Neurotoxic spider bites from black widow spiders can also cause rapidly progressive neurological symptoms. Rat poisons that contain thallium salts can also produce a painful neuropathy which can be associated with other life-threatening symptoms. Tick-borne viral infections, particularly Lyme disease, are responsible for demyelinating peripheral neuropathies. Patients who appear to have a neurotoxic reaction to an unknown toxin (e.g. lead and arsenic) should also be referred for a specialist opinion.

The medical treatment of the peripheral neuropathies is, of course, the treatment of the underlying metabolic, nutritional, or endocrine disorder. Whilst correcting thyroid dysfunction or vitamin deficiency is relatively straight forward, more complex disorders such as diabetes or HIV infection demand more complex therapeutic approaches. There is evidence that tight diabetic control is associated with remission of some of the associated polyneuropathic symptoms.

In some patients, troublesome chronic neuropathic pain develops, which may be resistant to simple, moderate analgesics. A combination of tricyclic antidepressants with carbamazepine is often useful, and there is accumulating evidence that the anticonvulsant gabapentin is also efficacious.

Prevention

The scope for prevention of peripheral neuropathies is limited, although regular review and tight control of underlying metabolic disorders, such as diabetes, is likely to be important. A discussion of preconception genetic screening in the hereditary polyneuropathies is beyond the scope of this chapter.

Key points

- Peripheral neuropathies can be broadly divided into mononeuropathies, usually entrapment syndromes, and generalized neuropathies, which usually have an underlying systemic cause.

- Conservative treatment of the entrapment syndromes in primary care is appropriate, although specialist referral and surgical treatment may sometimes be required.

- The underlying cause of the generalized polyneuropathies should be sought, initially with simple investigations carried out in primary care, but often with the help of specialist referral.

- Some causes of peripheral neuropathy include potentially serious and life-threatening disorders.

References

1. Dowson, D.W. (1993). Entrapment neuropathies of the upper extremities. *New England Journal of Medicine* 329, 2013–18.
2. Partanen, J. et al. (1995). Natural history of peripheral neuropathy in patients with non-insulin dependent diabetes mellitus. *New England Journal of Medicine* 333, 89–94.
3. Dyck, P.J., Oviatt, K.E., and Lambert, E.H. (1981). Intensive evaluation of referred unclassified neuropathies yields improved diagnosis. *Annals of Neurology* 10, 222–6.
4. Thrush, D.C. (1992). Investigation of peripheral neuropathy. *British Journal of Hospital Medicine* 48, 13–22.
5. Gabriel, G.M. et al. (2000). Prospective study of the usefulness of sural nerve biopsy. *Journal of Neurology, Neurosurgery and Psychiatry* 69, 442–7.
6. Bolton, C.F. (1992). Neuropathies in the critical care unit. *British Journal of Hospital Medicine* 47, 358–60.

Further reading

Federico, P. et al. (2000). Multifocal motor neuropathy improved by IV IG. *Neurology* 55, 1256–62.
McLeod, J.G. (1992). Peripheral nerve lesions. *Medicine International* 100, 4191–7.
McLeod, J.G. *Inflammatory Neuropathies*. London: Boullion Tindall, 1994, p. 215.
Said, J. et al. (1988). The peripheral neuropathy of necrotising arteritis. *Annals of Neurology* 23, 461–5.
Swash, M. and Schwartz, M.S. *Neuromuscular Diseases*. London: Springer, 1997.

11.6 Progressive neurological illnesses: multiple sclerosis and amyotrophic lateral sclerosis

T. Jock Murray

Introduction

Many disorders of the nervous system are characterized by progression, and the practitioner needs to remember that evidence of progression demands urgent assessment and consultation to identify and manage the problem. Conditions such as multiple sclerosis (MS), amyotrophic lateral sclerosis (ALS), Alzheimer's disease, brain and spinal cord tumours, and general symptoms such as weakness, visual loss, memory loss, and speech difficulty are examples of conditions that require immediate investigation. In this chapter, MS and ALS are considered in detail.

Multiple sclerosis

Epidemiology

In temperate zones, there is a prevalence rate of one case of MS in 500 in the population, and an incidence rate of about five per 100 000. The usual age of onset is between 20 and 40, with an average age of onset at age 30. The disease is two to three times more common in women.

The most intriguing finding in the epidemiology of MS is the increasing prevalence at latitudes farthest from the equator, both north and south. It is a rare disease in tropical countries, but one of the more common serious neurological disorders in the northern United States, Canada, Great Britain, and Central Europe. Isolated areas of increased prevalence have been found in New England, the Orkney Islands, Washington State, Nova Scotia, and Alaska. It has been suggested from migration studies that the risk factor for MS is carried with the person if they move from an area of high incidence to one of low incidence. Conversely, if one moves from an area of low incidence to an area of high incidence, one takes on the greater risk of the new country, but this is age-related and seems to correspond to a critical age of 15 years, suggesting the presence of an environmental risk factor acquired around the age of puberty.

Pathology

Multiple sclerosis is a progressive neurological disorder of young adults characterized by recurrent or increasing signs and symptoms due to scattered plaques of demyelination in the white matter of the brain, brain stem, and spinal cord of the central nervous system. Although the disease was thought to be active only when symptoms recurred, we now know from MRI scans that the disease shows continuing activity even when the person is unaware of any change. A breakdown in the blood–brain barrier is associated with new patches of demyelination, and axonal damage is responsible for the eventual progression of disability.

Aetiology

Degenerative, vascular, biochemical, infectious, and allergic theories have been advanced to explain the aetiology of MS. Although a viral infection as an initiating event in a susceptible person has been a long-standing theory, no virus has been isolated consistently and there is only weak evidence for suspects such as Epstein–Barr and canine distemper viruses, measles, and herpes virus 6. Attempts to demonstrate a slow virus aetiology by transmission with a long incubation period have been unsuccessful. It is possible that different viruses may initiate a breakdown in the blood–brain barrier and subsequent demyelination in predisposed patients, as it was noted that MS populations have slightly elevated levels of antibody to various viruses when compared to groups of normals.

Many factors have been considered to explain the world distribution of MS, including temperature, solar radiation, local infections, diet, and other environmental factors, but none is convincing. It has been postulated that the disease originated in Central Europe, and that the world distribution corresponds to the areas to which these peoples migrated, taking a genetic defect with them.

Family history

About 20 per cent of patients with MS have a family history of this disorder which is strong evidence for genetic influences in MS. A first-degree relative of an MS patient has about a 2–5 per cent risk of developing the disease, about 10 times the risk in the normal population. In identical twins, the risk is one in three.

Course of the disease

Multiple sclerosis is classified according to the course of the disease. About 85 per cent of patients present with *relapsing–remitting* (RR) MS, with attacks of discrete motor, sensory, cerebellar, or visual symptoms that may fully or partially recover, followed by a variable period of remission. After many years most will show progression, entering the *secondary progressive* (SP) pattern of the disease. Patients with the *primary progressive* (PP) pattern of MS show a slow and gradual progressive worsening from the onset, without attacks. About 15 per cent of patients present with this pattern. This is more common in men, especially with later onset of the disease and is characterized by spastic legs and bladder involvement. MRI studies show less 'activity' and 'disease burden', and more axonal loss in PP than in the RR and SP patients. *Progressive–relapsing* MS has been characterized as a course that begins as primary progressive but the patient may later have one or more acute attack. This classification of MS applies to patients in their initial years. An interesting group of the RR patients seem to have little disability after 10 years, and are then termed *benign* MS because of their very slow course of progression. This group cannot be diagnosed early, although there are some predictive associations (sensory symptoms, few or no motor or cerebellar findings, female sex, early onset) and they still may have slow deterioration many years later. By 5 years following the onset of the disease, it usually is clear which pattern the patient is following. Although 85 per cent of patients begin as relapsing remitting, by 5 years half are transformed into relapsing–progressive MS.

Attacks in MS usually occur without any obvious precipitant, but two factors have been shown to be related to attacks—acute infections, and the 6-month postpartum period. Patients may blame the exacerbation on physical or emotional stressful events in the preceding week but there is little evidence that these are related. Pregnancy seems to have a protective effect with 70 per cent less than predicted events during this period, but with an equal increase in the number of events in the 6-month postpartum period.

Presenting clinical symptoms

The symptoms of MS are extremely varied, as the lesions can disrupt function in many areas of the white matter. A *monosymptomatic* onset occurs in about 40 per cent of cases, though other sites are affected within the nervous system over time, and the MRI may show scattered lesions when the patient is manifesting only one symptom. Such symptoms include numbness, diplopia, blurred vision, poor balance, and limb weakness. These symptoms may clear spontaneously only to be replaced in time by other relapses and combinations of symptoms which suggest a diagnosis of MS.

Involvement of the *pyramidal tract* anywhere along its course will result in spasticity with the characteristic findings of hyperreflexia, clonus, loss of abdominal reflexes, and extensor plantar responses, eventually developing into progressive limb weakness. *Cerebellar* involvement commonly produces nystagmus, incoordination, dysarthria, and ataxia. *Sensory tract* involvement causes numbness, tingling and other symptoms of sensory loss and abnormal sensations called dysaesthesias. Sensory symptoms are common at the onset and can have a distribution similar to that of peripheral neuropathy, but the reflexes are usually increased (in a neuropathy they are usually lost). Involvement of the *posterior columns* is often associated with a Lhermitte sign, which is a shock like electric sensation down the back or in the limbs with neck flexion.

Any of the *brainstem nuclei* may be involved, causing diplopia and mild facial numbness, weakness or fine rippling of the facial muscles (*myokymia*). Involvement of the vestibular system results in vertigo, nausea, and unsteadiness. It is common on examination to find nystagmus but one should particularly look for nystagmus, greater in the abducting eye and associated with poor adduction of the other eye. This 'internuclear ophthalmoplegia' results from a lesion in the medial longitudinal fasciculus (MLF) coordinating movements of all the oculomotor muscles. It is a common finding in MS and is almost diagnostic in young people, particularly when bilateral. Trigeminal neuralgia is mainly a disorder of the elderly, so when it occurs in someone under 45, MS should be suspected. When the optic nerves are affected there may be blurring, dimming, or loss of vision and alteration of visual fields. Acute optic neuritis is a common problem, presenting with pain on eye movement, blurring or loss of vision, altered visual fields or scotomas. Seventy-five per cent of people who present with an optic neuritis have or will later develop signs of MS.

Mental changes may occur, but obvious cognitive changes usually develop late and include complaints of poor concentration, difficulty with attention and slowness in learning new material. Euphoria was once said to be the most common emotional abnormality, but depression is more common. Grand mal *seizures* occur in about 6 per cent of MS patients during the course of the disease.

In the presence of bilateral corticospinal lesions, a *spastic bladder* is to be expected, with complaints of urgency, frequency, and incontinence. Such symptoms may actually be due to detrusor muscle or sphincter spasticity, dyssynergia of these, or some other change; a full urological assessment is required in order to choose appropriate therapy. *Impotence* occurs in about half of men with MS, usually in association with progressing spasticity. When this first occurs, a strong psychogenic reaction is common and both the physical and psychological aspects must be assessed and sensitively managed.

The patients' coping skills, their spirituality, attitude, and their support system are very important in determining how well they manage their MS and whether or not they can get on with their lives and responsibilities. It is not surprising to note anxiety and depression in the patient who develops new symptoms and realizes what this means for his/her life and future. Even numbness of a hand that could be minimized by many physicians has ominous meaning for the patient. Conversion symptoms may occur and may be hard to differentiate from another attack of demyelination.

Diagnosis

Multiple sclerosis is a diagnosis made clinically or by autopsy, but some tests provide supportive evidence for the presence of plaques of demyelination with accompanying immunological changes. MRI scans may show scattered lesions in the white matter as a result of inflammation with swelling and subsequent demyelination. The CSF may contain increased gamma-globulins and on electrophoresis show oligoclonal bands. Evoked potential tests may show slowing of conduction in the optic nerves, the auditory system or the posterior columns, but these are non-specific because impaired conduction may also be caused by other conditions.

Medical treatment

There is at present no specific cure for MS. Therapy is directed at the acute attacks, at the underlying disease mechanisms, and at the symptoms of the disease and its complications.

Acute attacks of MS, if they are impairing activities, mobility or vision, are treated with high doses of intravenous steroids, such as 1000 mg methylprednisolone infused over 30 minutes daily for 3 doses. This may hasten recovery but it is uncertain if recovery is better after such therapy.

In recent years, four new agents which can change the pattern of acute attacks and possibly the eventual outcome in the disease have been developed (interferon beta-1b, two versions of interferon beta-1a, and glatiramer acetate).

Interferon beta-1a (Avonex; Rebif), interferon beta-1b (Betaferon), and glatiramer acetate (Copaxone) can reduce the number and severity of attacks of MS and reduce the activity seen on MRI. Whether these agents will have a significant effect on the long-term progression of the disease remains to be seen. The rate of attacks is reduced by about one third, and their severity by about half, but attacks will still occur in many patients. Patients should be aware of the reasonable expectations for the treatment, or they will discontinue therapy. The drugs are all very expensive, and careful selection of cases is important (patients with primary progressive and late stage secondary progressive disease do not respond). All four drugs are administered by injection, either subcutaneous (Betaferon; Rebif; Copaxone) or intramuscular (Avonex). The most troublesome side-effects from the interferons are a 'flu-like' reaction soon after the injection and local injection site reactions. The flu-like symptoms can be managed by ibuprofen or acetaminophen, and in most they decrease and disappear within 2 months. Glatiramer acetate (Copaxone) has less side-effects than the interferons, although rashes, allergic reactions, and injection site reactions occur. An acute sensation of chest tightness can occur, although this is infrequent, benign and may not recur if the drug is continued.

Immunosuppressants such as cyclophosphamide, azothioprine, cyclosporin A, and methotrexate have been used to treat MS but produced unconvincing benefits and serious side-effects, and are now reserved only for rapidly progressing cases. Mitoxanthrone has recently been shown to reduce progression in patients with secondary progressive MS but there are concerns about the possibility of cardiac effects. Cladribine reduces the MRI 'lesion burden' although it has not yet been shown to have a clinical benefit.

Symptom management

Treating symptoms can provide comfort for many patients. Spasticity is the most disabling problem in MS, and is particularly difficult to manage. Baclofen and tizanidine are helpful in reducing the spasms, pain and associated aching. Unfortunately, when the spasticity is reduced the patient's function does not necessarily improve and some spasticity is necessary for support and movement of the weakened legs. Baclofen pumps inserted under the skin allow higher doses to be given directly into the intrathecal space. This is helpful in severe spasticity when the patient is having

difficulty staying mobile, but the procedure is complicated and expensive. Tizanidine is a recently introduced antispasticity agent which can be used alone (4 mg once to four times daily) or with baclofen. The use of cannabis for the treatment of spasticity is controversial; studies have shown that the patients felt better but all measures of their performance, such as balance, mobility, alertness, and concentration, were worse.

Cerebellar ataxia is another disabling feature of MS. Weighing of the wrists with 250–350 g increases inertia and reduces tremor slightly. A number of agents have been tried but the results are disappointing and the side-effects disturbing.

Many patients have noticed that a warm room, a humid day, sitting in front of a hot fire, or taking a hot bath causes an increase in symptoms. Conversely, treatment with ice packs, or getting into a cool swimming pool sometimes improves symptoms and allows the patient 2 or 3 h of painless increased mobility and strength, far outlasting the cooling effect of the ice or cold water. Cooling suits give some relief for the 60–80 per cent of MS patients that find this a troublesome symptom. The use of 4-aminopyridine and 3,4-aminopyridine in heat-sensitive patients is growing, although their place in therapy is uncertain, and the side-effects include dizziness and seizures.

A number of surgical procedures have been carried out for contractures, spasticity, and deformities in the advanced stages of the disease, and when the patient is bedridden.

Urological assessment is needed to clarify the type of bladder dysfunction when the MS patient begins to complain of frequency, urgency, or incontinence. Mild degrees of upper motor neuron bladder dysfunction may respond to anticholinergic drugs such as oxybutynin (Ditropan) or propantheline bromide (ProBanthine). Patients should try to schedule their fluid intake and activities in relation to bladder function. If necessary, with a more significantly spastic bladder with incontinence, a condom drainage system can be used. A catheter should be avoided if possible because of the dangers of infection but if a catheter has to be used, intermittent catheterization should be tried. In a few cases an indwelling catheter is needed. In the male, the penis should be taped to the abdominal wall to avoid a penile–scrotal junction fistula.

Inactivity predisposes to constipation, and MS patients should be on a high-fibre diet, with regular bran and adequate fluids. When constipation is a problem other agents may be needed such as psyllium hydrophilic colloid (Metamucil).

Impotence is common in males after years with pyramidal involvement from MS. Understanding and support are important. Sensory changes may also alter sexual responses and prevent orgasm in women. Oral sildenafil (Viagra) is likely to become the treatment of choice for impotence. Formerly, injection of papaverine into the penis with a fine needle was useful to produce satisfactory erections, and was reasonably well tolerated. Penile implants may also produce satisfactory results.

Pain is more common in MS than is often thought; symptomatic trigeminal neuralgia, muscle spasms, and dermal hyper- or dysaesthesias are examples. Carbamazepine (Tegretol) is effective for trigeminal neuralgia and other lancinating pains in MS, while spasms in the back and limbs are often relieved by local cooling, massage, hydrotherapy, and exercise. Limb spasms, trigeminal neuralgia, and other pains also respond to baclofen (Lioresal) clonazepam or gabapentin (Neurontin), each somewhat useful in those patients who cannot tolerate carbamazepine. Tricyclic drugs are also useful in chronic diffuse pain and transcutaneous electrical stimulation is helpful in those with muscular pains.

Fatigue is the most common complaint of MS patients, occurring in 80 per cent, and is their major complaint in 40 per cent of cases. It is an unusual fatigue, consisting of a feeling of inertia as if the subjects main spring had broken rather than increasing weakness with persisting muscular activity, and it can be very severe and disabling. Rest periods and naps may help, but the fatigue often continues despite adequate rest and good sleep. Amantadine (Symmetrel) 100 mg twice a day, helps about half of these patients, dramatically in some. In the long-term, many patients develop livido reticularis, though this is not a serious side-effect and it clears when the drug is stopped. Ritalin and Prozac have less effect but are sometimes useful. The new narcolepsy therapy Modafinil taken in low dose of 200 mg daily is helpful for fatigue in many MS patients.

Advice and support

Multiple sclerosis patients require education about their disease in order to gain confidence. Most have many unresolved conflicts and problems related to their families, income and future; many of these profound and long-standing frustrations can be resolved by a sensitive and understanding physician who will take the time to listen and to talk. Tranquillizers and antidepressants are effective when used in appropriate situations, but they should not be used to replace the personal impact of the physician. Patients often relate acute exacerbations to periods of physical or emotional strain. They cannot possibly avoid all of these situations but should recognize the importance of avoiding such stresses where possible and the family should understand this too.

Multiple sclerosis societies are active in North America and in Europe and chapters and support groups are to be found in most communities. They are able to provide information, expertise, companionship, reassurance, social benefits, and health care aids. As well as having an important function in research funding, these societies offer much for the MS patient, and we encourage our patients to contact them early, most easily through the internet.

Aids and appliances

Many aids are available to assist MS patients in overcoming problems, including prisms for double vision; adapted cutlery; canes and walkers for gait difficulty; braces for drop foot; wheelchairs and electric scooters for mobility in the community; lifts and special beds for those who are bedridden; and house, kitchen, and bath adaptions such as ramps, grab bars, shower seats, elevated toilet seats, and lowered kitchen counters and cabinet handles. Occupational therapists are important advisors on how to adapt the environment to copy with handicaps.

General health issues

Although MS is usually diagnosed by a neurologist, the general needs of an MS patient are best managed by a general doctor. People with MS do not experience *more* diseases than other people, but they do experience the *same* diseases as other people. People with MS also have the same health needs as everyone else; for a good self-image; for a positive approach to life; for laughter; for a balanced diet; for regular exercise; and for health maintenance.

Exercise is important for MS patients, but a few will note increasing symptoms and weakness when their body heat increases. An unusual symptom that rarely occurs is to have increased blurring of vision as the exercise continues, improving as the person cools off. MS patients do well with exercises in a swimming pool because the water cools the body, increasing their exercise tolerance.

Quality of life issues

The quality of life is altered for an MS patient early in the disease as the diagnosis brings with it concerns about health, employment, life plans, children, and future plans. Even before significant disability occurs, the quality of life suffers and continues to suffer as attacks occur and as disability increases. Quality of life is particularly affected by the presence of fatigue and signs of cognitive change. Many emotional changes may be seen, of which depression is the commonest, and it responds well to treatment.

Conclusions

Multiple scelrosis may not yet be curable but much can be done to improve the general health and outlook of the person, including recognizing the non-MS diseases and problems that can occur to MS people as they occur to others, as well as the complications of the disease and the treatments. A positive outlook, a generally healthy state, a good support system including an emphathetic physician who will stay with them through their course can improve the quality of life of every MS patient.

Key points

1. MS is characterized by recurrent attacks and progressive neurological symptoms and signs due to scattered lesions in the white matter of the brain, brainstem, and spinal cord.

2. Common features are sensory loss, weakness, optic neuritis, fatigue, bladder frequency and urgency, heat sensitivity, diplopia, vertigo, and gait and balance difficulty.

3. Management is directed at explanation and support, symptom management, rehabilitation, treatment of acute attacks, and therapies that may modify the course of the disease.

4. Acute attacks that are mild usually improve spontaneously, but more severe attacks may be treated with high-dose IV steroids.

5. The attacks of MS may be reduced in number and severity by interferons or glatiramer acetate. It remains to be determined if this alters the long-term progression of the disease.

Amyotrophic lateral sclerosis

In ALS (also called motor neuron disease), the anterior horn cells and corticospinal tracts are usually affected at many levels, although a few patients have clinical manifestations of involvement at only one level. It has clinical features of involvement of both the upper and lower motor neurons.

Classification

According to the pattern of involvement, different names have been employed for the motor neuron diseases, for example, *progressive muscular atrophy* (anterior horn cell degeneration only); *primary lateral sclerosis* (pyramidal tract degeneration only); *progressive bulbar palsy* (brainstem motor nuclear degeneration); and *pseudobulbar palsy*. The most common picture, however, is a mixture of these features, the patient having both upper and lower motor neuron signs and symptoms often with bulbar involvement as well, *amyotrophic lateral sclerosis*. Because the disease eventually generalizes to involve both upper and lower motor neurons at both cranial and spinal levels, many authors use the term ALS for all forms. At death, some patients who have had clinical evidence of degeneration at only one level may show pathological changes at other levels not evident clinically. The pathological features are primarily degeneration of motor cells in the spinal cord, brainstem and to a lesser extent the cerebral cortex, with secondary degeneration of pyramidal tracts.

Epidemiology

The incidence of ALS is two cases per 100 000. The onset is usually between the ages of 50 and 70 years and occurs twice as often in men. Although 95 per cent of cases are sporadic, 5 per cent have a familial basis, and a few cases can be associated with other diseases, especially malignancy. It accounts for one in 1000 deaths. An ALS-like syndrome (post-polio syndrome) sometimes occurs many years after an episode of poliomyelitis but this syndrome is unrelated, and is much more benign. An ALS syndrome with associated parkinsonism and dementia occurs on the island of Guam.

Clinical features

Most patients first notice weakness in their legs or arms, but they may also note that the muscles are getting smaller and that there are twitching movements in the muscles due to fasciculations. On examination, these patients have atrophy, weakness, and fasciculations in their limbs, indicating a lower motor neuron lesion, combined with hyperactive reflexes and Babinski signs. It is this combination of upper and lower motor neuron signs in all limbs that is the hallmark of ALS.

The course of the disease is variable, but the average life expectancy is 3.5 years from onset, and only 20 per cent survive over 5 years. To some extent, survival depends on the type of ALS but there is great variation even within the same type. In general, those with bulbar palsy have a more rapid course than those with primary lateral sclerosis, in whom the prognosis is better.

Diagnosis

Although the diagnosis is usually evident clinically, there are a few investigations that can be used to confirm the diagnosis or to rule out other diseases or associated disease. Nerve conduction studies yield results that are normal or only slightly slowed. EMG shows evidence of denervation and reduced numbers of motor unit potentials among which are giant units and polyphasic potentials, as well as fasciculations. Muscle biopsy will demonstrate the characteristic features of a neurogenic muscular atrophy but a biopsy is seldom needed, unless a condition such as inclusion body myositis is suspected.

Investigations should be undertaken to rule out underlying malignancy if there is any atypical feature on examination or investigation, such as marked slowing of motor nerve conduction velocities. Cervical myelopathy can look like ALS if cord compression is combined with root involvement. The lower motor neuron findings will be only in the arms, an important diagnostic feature, and this situation can be confirmed by imaging of the cervical cord, and using EMG to show fasciculations in the legs.

Management

Current management is supportive, as treatment of the underlying disease has been disappointing, despite some new agents that may make a slight difference in the course of the progression. Riluzole (Rilutek®), a glutamate blocking agent, has shown a statistical improvement in the rate of progression, but this is of minor clinical significance as the difference translates to a prolongation of death by 3 months or so. Despite its minor effect, the release of this drug, the first to make any difference in the disease, has had a much greater effect on the sense of hope for these patients, who have had little before. A number of other agents are under study, but none as yet has shown much promise. With such first steps, however, there is always the hope of the next.

Long-term care

Despite limited therapy for the underlying disease, the patient can be helped with some of the major problems. Aids such as foot braces and properly fitted wheelchairs allow for mobility despite the increasing weakness. Anticholinergic agents can dry secretions if there is difficulty swallowing saliva and drooling. The patient will decide how liquid the food should be, and how large the mouthfuls. Cricopharyngeal myotomy can be performed to aid swallowing.

Involuntary limb jerks and occasional cramps and aching can be reduced by phenytoin, carbamazepine, baclofen, and clonazepam in standard doses. Pain is not a common complaint. Difficulty with insomnia and problems turning in bed can be improved by special beds which can be leased or borrowed. Family and friends may organize a roster of people to sleep over, sparing the spouse from waking every 3 hours to turn the patient. The patient remains mentally alert, and as weakness increases, frustration and boredom become a problem. Occupational therapists can advise on a number of communication aids.

Occupational therapy assessment of mobility and posture can be arranged for the home environment, providing rails, hoists, or supports, eliminating stairs where possible, and advising on helpful devices for feeding, shaving, dressing, recreation, and ambulation. Posture may be improved with a collar, brace, or spring-loaded splints. Leg swelling can be helped by elevation and elastic stockings. Diuretics are not useful for this.

Constipation results from weak abdominal muscles, reduced activity, and often inadequate fluids. Increased fluids, bulk purgatives, laxatives, and enemas are helpful. Weight loss and cachexia characterize the late stages. Swallowing can be improved, but a nasogastric tube may become necessary when weakness and atrophy advances. Gastrostomy can be helpful.

Respiratory infections become a risk as chest movement is restricted and the patient is bedridden. When there are early signs of respiratory failure the patient may be made more comfortable, especially at night, by non-invasive positive pressure ventilation (NIPPV) methods such as bilevel positive air pressure (BiPAP). At some point a decision will have to be made about whether a tracheotomy and mechanical ventilation will be used to continue support. It is important not to embark on measures which will only prolong distress. With a tracheostomy and ventilator, the patient may have a year of passive, non-communicative existence, and that is the choice of some, but most do not wish this. It is crucial to determine if the patient is willing to accept this state well before it occurs, by means of early discussions and the drawing-up of a living will. The patient should appoint a trusted person to act with power of attorney on his or her behalf.

End-of-life care

Amyotrophic lateral sclerosis patients and their families have to come to grips with many end-of-life decisions. These include the need to get the many events in life in order, come to terms with relationships, and decide how future disabilities will be handled. Patients may raise the question of suicide or assisted suicide, and the physician should be comfortable in talking about these issues, and to call on others who may have more expertise and experience in discussing them. This is one of the many disorders when the primary care physician's role becomes one of coordination of the multidisciplinary team, accompanying the patient as an advisor and friend on the difficult road to the end.

Key points

1. ALS affects both the upper motor neurons (paralysis, hyperreflexia, Babinski signs) and lower motor neurons (paralysis, atrophy, fasciculations).

2. ALS is a progressive neurological disease with an average life expectancy of 3.5 years.

3. ALS management is of the weakness, difficulty with swallowing, respiration, and nutrition.

4. Physicians must assist in outlining the options and the need for decisions around end-of-life care.

Further reading

Multiple sclerosis

Reviews of all aspects of multiple sclerosis

Compston, A. et al. *McAlpine's Multiple Sclerosis* 3rd edn. Edinburgh: Churchill Livingstone, 1998.

Paty, D.W. and Ebers, G.C. (1998). Multiple sclerosis. In *Contemporary Neurology Series* Vol. 50. Philadelphia PA: F.A. Davis Co.

Practical clinical reviews

Holland, N.J., Murray, T.J., and Reingold, S.C. *Multiple Sclerosis: A Guide for the Newly Diagnosed*. New York: Demos Vermande, 1996.

Van den Noort, S. and Holland, N.J., ed. *Multiple Sclerosis in Clinical Practice*. New York: Demos, 1999.

Review of all treatments for MS including alternative therapies

Polman, C.H., Thompson, A., Murray, T.J., and McDonald, W.I. *Multiple Sclerosis: The Guide to Treatment and Management* 5th edn. New York: Demos, 2001.

Primary care management of MS patients

Halper, J. and Murray, T.J. (1999). Primary care needs of multiple sclerosis patients. In *Multiple Sclerosis in Clinical Practice* (ed. S. Van den Noort and N. Holland), pp. 115–24. New York: Demos.

Amyotrophic lateral sclerosis

Mitsumoto, H. and Norris, F.H., ed. *Amyotrophic Lateral Sclerosis: A Comprehensive Guide to Management.* New York: Demos Publications, 1994. (This review covers the full range of therapeutic efforts needed for ALS patients and their caregivers.)

Mitsumoto, H. et al. (1997). Motor neuron diseases. *CONTINUUM*, American Academy of Neurology **3**, 48–77. (A succinct review of the current understanding of ALS and its management.)

Mitsumoto, H., Chad, D.A., and Pioro, E.P. *Amyotrophic Lateral Sclerosis.* Philadelphia PA: F.A. Davis Co., 1996. (A comprehensive review of ALS.)

Rowland, L.P., ed. *Amyotrophic Lateral Sclerosis and other Motor Neurone Diseases.* New York: Raven Press, 1991. (A review of the neurological sciences and research as well as management of ALS.)

Websites

www.nmss.org.
www.infosci.org/MS-UK-MSSoc.
www.infosci.org/IFMSS/ifmsswel.html.
www.mssociety.ca.

Table 1 Glasgow Coma Scale

Eye Opening	
Nil	1
To pain	2
To speech	3
Spontaneous	4
Best motor response	
Nil	1
Abnormal extension	2
Abnormal flexion	3
Withdraws	4
Localizes	5
Obeys command	6
Best verbal response	
Nil	1
Incomprehensible sounds	2
Inappropriate words	3
Confused speech	4
Orientated	5

- ◆ Recorded as E + M + V (e.g. E4; M6; V5 = 15) (minimum = 3/maximum (alert) = 15)
- ◆ GCS of E2; M4; V2 or less is considered as coma
- ◆ Tracheostomy, endotracheal tube or facial injuries invalidate the verbal response

11.7 Coma

Katia Cikurel

In areas where ambulance services and hospital facilities are readily available, the primary care physician is not frequently involved with patients in coma. However, it is essential to have a working knowledge of the important and treatable differential diagnoses and to have an emergency management strategy, as coma is often the end point of many extremely serious diseases with high mortality.

Definition

Coma defines a state in which the patient is unrousable and unresponsive.[1] Various terms are applied to the progressive levels of impaired consciousness between the alert state and coma. These include inattention, confusion, lethargy, obtundation, and stupor, but each of these terms are not clearly defined and are subject to misinterpretation between observers. Coma can be more objectively assessed using the Glasgow Coma Scale (GCS) (Table 1), which provides a figure for three markers of consciousness—eye opening, motor, and verbal responses. However, it is most usefully used as a trend rather than a single figure at one point in time. The following discussion will be limited to the state of coma.

Epidemiology

Population-based data concerning the incidence of coma worldwide are sparse. A recent epidemiological study of children aged between 1 month and 16 years presenting with non-traumatic coma was carried out in the north of England.[2] The incidence in this age group was calculated to be 30.8 per 100 000, equivalent to 6.0 per 100 000 in the general population. Infection formed a high percentage of causes in this age group, although central nervous system (CNS) specific presentations increased with the age of the child.

In general, in adult populations, CNS-specific causes are more common. In a series of 500 patients presenting with coma, initially categorized as 'coma of unknown aetiology', the lesion responsible for the coma was eventually categorized as follows:[1]

1. diffuse cortical disorder—65 per cent;

2. supratentorial lesion (downward pressure on the reticular activating system)—20 per cent;

3. infratentorial lesion (involving reticular activating system)—13 per cent;

4. psychiatric—2 per cent;

Examples of conditions and lesions responsible for the categories listed above are given in Tables 2–4.

Worldwide, there are variations and for instance in areas where malaria, viral encephalitides and human immunodeficiency virus (HIV) are endemic, infectious causes will be more prevalent in an adult population than in urban communities, where drugs, metabolic aetiologies, and trauma often predominate.

Mortality figures are highly dependent on the aetiology and in the paediatric study outlined previously, mortality ranged between 3 and 84 per cent. With 12-month follow-up, the overall series mortality was 46 per cent. Worldwide, these figures are also highly dependent on the availability of relevant drugs and secondary medical facilities.

Causes of coma

Neuroanatomical basis of coma

Coma is caused by diffuse bilateral hemisphere dysfunction, failure of the ascending reticular activating system in the brainstem and its connections, or a combination of both. A unilateral hemisphere lesion does not cause coma unless there is secondary brainstem compression caused by herniation. The reticular formation has connections with the thalamus and

Table 2 Causes and clinical features of coma due to diffuse hemisphere dysfunction

Causes	Clinical features
Drug overdose/alcohol/toxins	Opiates—pin-point pupils; slow respiration Tricyclics—dilated pupils Alcohol—ethanolic fetor; Wernicke's encephalopathy Carbon monoxide poisoning—red skin colour
Hypoglycaemia/hyperglycaemia	Hypoglycaemia—known diabetic often; preceding confusion; tachycardia; clammy; tremulous; seizures Hyperglycaemia—dehydration; hyperventilation; ketotic fetor
Circulatory collapse/hypotensive injury/hypoxic injury	Cardiac (arrhythmia/myocardial infarction/cardiac arrest)—hypotension; tachycardia; rhythm disturbance; cardiac failure Respiratory arrest—stridor; respiratory compromise; ?drug ingestion Septicaemic shock—pyrexia; rigors; peripheral vasodilatation; signs of focal infection Hypovolaemia (blood loss/severe diarrhoea)—e.g. melaena; haematemesis; abdominal pain (ruptured aortic aneurysm); hypotension; dehydration Hypotensive drugs
Vascular brain injury	Subarachnoid haemorrhage—explosive onset headache; collapse; neck stiffness; subhyaloid haemorrhages; focal neurological signs if intracerebral extension of blood Hypertensive encephalopathy—hypertension; retinopathy; seizures
Systemic metabolic and endocrine abnormalities	Uraemia—sallow skin; uraemic fetor; hypertensive; anaemic; anuric Hepatic encephalopathy—jaundice; signs of portal hypertension; asterixis; hepatomegaly Hypocalcaemia—carpopedal spasm; muscle twitching Hypercalcaemia—polyuria; abdominal pain; vomiting Hypo/hyperkalaemia—arrhythmia; ileus; diabetes insipidus; muscle weakness Hypo/hypernatraemia—subacute onset; muscle twitches; dehydration Metabolic acidosis—hyperventilation Hypercapnoea—history of lung disease; pink puffer; bounding pulse; papilloedema; asterixis Chronic hypoxia causing cerebral oedema (rare) Hypoadrenalism—hypotension especially postural; abdominal pain; buccal and flexure hyperpigmentation Hypopituitarism—pallor; hairlessness; hypogonadism; hypoadrenalism features Hypothyroidism—rare cause of coma; dry, coarse facies; hypotension; bradycardia; hypothermia; slow relaxing reflexes
Hypothermia/hyperpyrexia	Measure temperature
Trauma (closed head injury)	Look for signs of trauma
Epilepsy	Following a generalized seizure—convulsive movements; incontinence; bitten tongue; period of cyanosis (NB: The 'coma' can be post-ictal or secondary to hypoxic brain injury)
Infections	Meningitis—headache, pyrexia, meningism; focal signs; seizures; maculopapular or purpuric rash (especially meningococcal) Encephalitis—altered behaviour; seizures; focal signs; pyrexia Cerebral malaria—endemic area; marked pyrexia, seizures; high mortality Septicaemia—cerebral and non-cerebral sources

Table 3 Causes and clinical features of coma due to infratentorial lesions

Causes	Clinical features
Vascular lesions	Brainstem *haemorrhage* (hypertensive; vascular malformation; aneursym) or *infarction* within the posterior circulation (embolic; vertebral dissection)
Structural lesion	Brainstem tumour, e.g. glioma
Metabolic	Wernicke's encephalopathy (deficiency of vitamin B1, thiamine) Eye signs—nystagmus, ophthalmoplegia; rarely fixed pupils Ataxia—gait, limbs and vestibular paralysis (absent caloric responses) Confusion/coma Hypothermia and hypotension (hypothalamic involvement—rare)
Infective	Brainstem encephalitis, e.g. Listeria or abscesses, tuberculomas
Trauma	Look for signs of trauma

Table 4 Causes and clinical features of coma due to supratentorial or cerebellar lesions

Causes	Clinical features
Vascular lesions	Intracerebral haemorrhage—collapse or history of headache and rising intracranial pressure; hypertensive; focal neurological signs Extradural haemorrhage—evidence of head injury; blood or CSF from nose or ear Infarction—(NB: anterior circulation strokes rarely cause coma)—the rare exceptions include a complete middle cerebral artery territory infarction with oedema and an infarction within the thalamus
Structural lesion	Any space occupying lesion with oedema and mass effect, e.g. glioma, metastasis, abscess, causing herniation—headache; signs of raised intracranial pressure; papilloedema (NB: often a late sign); focal and progressive neurological signs; seizures
Infection	Abscess (single or multiple)—sub-acute onset; headache; focal neurological signs; seizures; signs of source of infection elsewhere, e.g. ears, heart valves, sinuses
Trauma	Causing haemorrhage, contusion, penetrating injuries, and oedema

hypothalamus and therefore lesions of these structures can also produce alteration of consciousness. Whether a brainstem lesion will cause coma depends on the speed of onset and the size of the insult. Brainstem haemorrhage and infarction often cause coma, whereas multiple sclerosis and tumours involving the brainstem rarely do. The coma produced by drugs and metabolic diseases is often caused by depression of both the cortex and the reticular activating system.

Tables 2–4 outline the possible aetiological mechanisms of coma, by considering conditions which cause diffuse hemisphere dysfunction, brainstem (infratentorial) lesions which directly affect the reticular activating system and hemisphere (supratentorial) or cerebellar lesions which exert downward pressure on the reticular activating system.

Differential diagnosis

Certain conditions may mimic coma and need to be differentiated from it.

Locked-in syndrome

Locked-in syndrome is a condition in which the patient is aware, but cannot move or communicate except by vertical eye movements and blinking volitionally. It is caused by a lesion of the ventral pons and there is therefore preserved cortex and reticular formation. A state similar to locked-in syndrome may occasionally be seen in severe polyneuropathy, myasthenia gravis, and following neuromuscular blocking agents, but the history will help to differentiate them.

Persistent vegetative state

Following severe widespread cerebral damage, the patient has no cognitive function or awareness of the environment, despite a preserved sleep–wake cycle. There may be non-purposeful movements and spontaneous eye opening or eye movements.

Catatonia

The catatonic patient is mute with no volitional motor or emotional response to external stimuli. The maintenance of body posture, the ability to sit or stand, and waxy flexibility (holding bizarre postures for long periods) distinguishes this from coma. It is usually a psychiatric manifestation but can rarely be caused by frontal lobe damage or drugs.

Clinical approach to the comatose patient

The clinical approach to the comatose patient is summarized in Table 5.

The most important first step is to provide immediate cardiorespiratory resuscitation by assessing the airways, breathing, and circulation ('A, B, C'):

- *Airway*—clear the mouth and throat and establish an airway as necessary.

- *Breathing*—ensure the patient is breathing, if not begin external ventilation (mouth-to-mouth or intubate and bag, if available) and provide oxygen if possible.

- *Circulation*—ensure there is a cardiac output, otherwise begin external cardiac massage. If hypovolaemic, provide intravenous fluid, if available, preferably having taken a glucose measurement first. If there is circulatory failure, the potential cause needs to be pursued and managed.

Evaluation must be rapid and comprehensive. It should be undertaken while simultaneously taking steps to minimize further neurological damage.

Assessment must also comprise taking a history from relatives, friends or witnesses, and a search for identifying discs or cards, which are carried by individuals with diabetes mellitus, epilepsy, hypoadrenalism, and those taking corticosteroids. Patients may already be well known to the primary physician, or additional information may be available from practice notes. All this information will help to guide further action.

Table 5 Clinical assessment of coma

Cardiorespiratory status
Start cardiorespiratory resuscitation as necessary
General examination
Temperature (pyrexia, e.g. infection/hypothermia/circulatory failure)
Skin (rash, anaemia, jaundice, cyanosis)
Respiratory pattern (Cheyne–Stokes/Kussmaul/central neurogenic hyperventilation)
Fetor (ketosis, alcohol, fetor hepaticus)
Blood pressure (? septicaemic shock/postural change with Addison's)
Cardiac (arrhythmia)
Abdomen (? organomegaly)
Neurological examination (general status)
Response to external stimulus
Glasgow Coma Scale (verbal response, eye opening, motor response—see Table 1)
Meningism (stiff neck, Kernig's sign)
Brainstem function
Pupillary response
Ocular deviation
Spontaneous eye movements
Oculocephalic response (doll's eye manoeuvre)
Oculovestibular response (caloric response)
Fundoscopy (papilloedema, subhyaloid haemorrhage)
Corneal responses
Motor examination
Symmetrical or asymmetrical
Muscle tone
Decerebrate/decorticate posturing
Motor response to stimulus
Deep tendon reflexes
Plantars

Once cardiorespiratory stability has been achieved, emergency management includes correction of metabolic derangement, particularly glucose, (which should be administered with thiamine to prevent Wernicke's encephalopathy in susceptible individuals), control of seizures (e.g. rectal benzodiazepine), and specific treatments such as administration of naloxone in suspected opiate overdose or antibiotics in a patient with suspected bacterial meningitis. In all traumatic injuries the neck must be stabilized.

After many intracranial events, especially ischaemic and haemorrhagic, there is an accompanying rise in systemic blood pressure. This is often a protective mechanism for the brain and the usual recommendations are not to treat hypertension unless it is greater than 200/120 and then only cautiously.

A general and neurological examination should follow making an assessment of the level of coma using the Glasgow Coma Scale (Table 1).

General examination

Possible sources of the coma may be ascertained from general examination.

Temperature

Temperature may be raised in infection and hyperpyrexia. The patient may be hypothermic.

Skin

The patient may be jaundiced, cyanosed, have a purpuric rash, signs of trauma, needle marks, or have flexural skin pigmentation.

Fetor

The patient's breath might be ketotic (diabetic ketoacidosis) or alcoholic.

Respiratory pattern

Patterns of abnormal respiration may be helpful diagnostically.

◆ *Cheynes–Stokes respiration:* alternating hypo- and hyperventilation represents widespread hemispheric dysfunction and is often found in metabolic and drug-induced coma, or bilateral deep hemispheric lesions (thalamus or internal capsule).

◆ *Central neurogenic hyperventilation:* rapid, sustained breathing found in upper pontine lesions.

◆ *Kussmaul (acidotic) respiration:* deep, sighing hyperventilation seen mainly in ketoacidosis and salicylate overdose.

◆ *Apneustic respiration:* rapid breathing with pauses of 2–3 seconds occurring after inspiration. Found in lower pontine lesions.

Neurological examination: specific examination for the comatose patient

Response to external stimuli

The level of coma should be assessed using the Glasgow Coma Scale (Table 1), but the stimulus type should also be documented. The mechanisms to assess arousal include the voice, visual menace, and painful stimuli.

All patients should be asked to open their eyes and move the eyes from side to side and up and down. This is particularly important for the 'locked-in' patient who will be able to follow these commands but not make any other purposeful response.

The assessment of the motor response and eye opening in the comatose patient usually requires the administration of a painful stimulus, which should not cause injury. This can be administered by pressure over the supraorbital nerve to elicit facial grimace, which may be present when limb responses are diminished or by producing pressure over the nail-beds with a pen or tendon hammer laid horizontally across the nail. The degree and asymmetry of the response may help to localize the lesion and narrow the possible aetiological mechanisms, for example, a reduced response to nail-bed pressure in the right arm and leg is most likely to indicate a focal lesion within the left hemisphere.

Pupillary responses

If the visual pathways are intact, assessment of the pupillary responses may help to localize the site of the coma and may differentiate structural from metabolic and toxic causes. Enquire about previous eye surgery and use of eye drops, for example, pilocarpine for glaucoma, which will affect the assessment. Remember, also, that some drugs used for resuscitation, for example, atropine and adrenaline, will affect the pupillary responses.

A bright convergent light source is required such as a pen torch. An ophthalmoscope beam diverges the light source and is not as useful. However, an otoscope can provide both a convergent light source and useful magnification.

◆ *Bilateral pin-point fixed pupils*—pontine lesions (e.g. pontine haemorrhage) and opiates.

◆ *Bilateral mid-position fixed pupils*—midbrain lesions. The pupils may be slightly irregular.

◆ *Bilateral dilated, fixed pupils*—can occur in deep coma of any cause, especially coma due to barbiturate or mydriatic (e.g. tricyclic antidepressant) overdose and hypothermia, but are also a cardinal feature of brainstem death.

◆ *Bilateral mid-position or slightly dilated, reactive pupils*—occur in most metabolic and drug-induced comas except opiates and mydriatic drugs.

◆ *Unilateral dilated pupil*—this represents a neurosurgical emergency. It is usually caused by a supratentorial mass causing herniation of the uncus of the temporal lobe and indicates a third nerve palsy. It may be accompanied by deviation of the eye in a downward and lateral position.

Ocular movements

Ocular motility centres lie close to the brainstem regions responsible for arousal and the assessment of ocular movements provide a valuable guide to involvement of the brainstem in coma. Normal reflex eye movements imply that the pontomedullary junction to the level of the third nerve nucleus (oculomotor) in the midbrain is intact. In addition, the third nerve itself is susceptible to compression in herniation of the temporal lobe caused by an expanding supratentorial lesion and the sixth nerve may also be stretched producing a false localizing sign in raised intracranial pressure.

◆ *Oculocephalic reflex (doll's eye manoeuvre)*—this test must not be carried out in patients that may have instability of the cervical spine. On rotating the patient's head to the left and then to the right, the patients eyes should conjugately move to the opposite direction to the movement of the head when the brainstem is intact. An abnormal response, either absent or asymmetrical, implies brainstem involvement.

◆ *Oculovestibular reflex (caloric response)*—the tympanic membranes must be checked to be intact prior to carrying out this test. Ice-cold water is irrigated into each ear in turn. In the intact brainstem, this causes a slow conjugate deviation of the eyes towards the irrigated side. Absence or asymmetry indicates brainstem involvement.

Ocular deviation

The eyes may be conjugate or disconjugate and may be fixed or moving.

◆ *Resting position of the eyes*—on passively lifting the eyelids the resting position of the eyes should be noted.

   ■ Sustained conjugate lateral deviation—occurs *towards* the side of a destructive frontal lesion (i.e. the eyes look towards the normal limb). Irritative lesions, such as an epileptic focus, may cause conjugate deviation *away* from the lesion and may be the only sign in non-convulsive status epilepticus.

   ■ Unilateral downward and lateral displacement—indicates a third nerve palsy.

   ■ Disconjugate deviation—indicates a third or sixth nerve palsy or a brainstem lesion.

   ■ Skew deviation (one eye deviated upwards and the other downwards) is rare and indicates a cerebellar or brainstem lesion.

◆ *Spontaneous eye movement*

   ■ Purposeful movements—if these are present in an otherwise unresponsive patient, consider locked-in syndrome or pseudo-coma.

   ■ Roving eye movement—slow, conjugate, movements from side to side. These indicate that the third nerve connections are intact and usually occur in toxic, metabolic, and bilateral hemisphere causes of coma.

   ■ Ocular bobbing—these are sudden, brisk downward, conjugate jerks of the eyes, with a slow return to the mid-position. This occurs in acute pontine lesions.

Fundoscopic examination

Papilloedema (raised intracranial pressure), subhyaloid haemorrhage (subarachnoid haemorrhage) and hypertensive retinopathy should be looked for. The absence of papilloedema does not exclude raised intracranial pressure, as raised pressure needs to be established for some time before it develops.

Motor examination

Examination of the comatose patient should begin with assessment of the resting posture and spontaneous movements. If the eyes and head are deviated to the side *away* from limbs that are not spontaneously moving (i.e. a hemiparesis), this implies a large hemispheric lesion, whereas deviation of the eyes and head *towards* a hemiparetic side, indicates a pontine lesion.

- *Decerebrate posturing*—this refers to the *extensor* posture of the upper and lower limbs bilaterally, found in bilateral midbrain or pontine lesions.
- *Decorticate posturing*—this refers to the bilateral flexion of the upper limbs and extension of the lower limbs, usually due to upper brainstem lesions.

Unilateral decerebrate or decorticate posturing may be seen and indicate a unilateral lesion. The asymmetry provides localizing value.

- *Movement disorder*—tonic–clonic convulsions, epilepsia partialis continua (constant, repetitive jerking of a focal area usually due to focal seizure activity) and myoclonus may all be found in the comatose patient. Generalized myoclonic jerks are commonly found following anoxic/ ischaemic insult and in metabolic disorders. Seizures should be treated accordingly.
- *Meningism*—the presence of a stiff neck (lifting the patient by the head also lifts the shoulders, when severe) may indicate meningitis, meningeal irritation by blood or herniation of the cerebellar tonsils.
- *Asymmetrical motor responses*—asymmetry of muscle tone, response to painful stimuli, tendon jerks, and plantar responses may all be valuable in localization of structural lesions and in differentiation from metabolic and drug-induced causes that are usually symmetrical.

Further management

Table 6 gives guidelines for the emergency management of unexplained coma.

Following immediate resuscitation and preliminary treatment options, comatose patients should be transferred to hospital where further investigations, intensive monitoring and if necessary, ventilation is available. In some situations this may not be necessary, such as the known diabetic with hypoglycaemia that is successfully treated, or the patient who has regular seizures and regains consciousness.

If hospital admission is required, one must be aware that during transfer, continued monitoring of systemic and neurological status is required, with particular attention to the cardiorespiratory system, pupillary, and motor responses. Certain treatments may need to be repeated such as the use of naloxone in opiate overdose, (as the half-life of naloxone is shorter than most opiates), or mannitol for raised intracranial pressure.

Table 6 Emergency management of unexplained coma

Ensure adequate airway and respiration—provide ventilation as necessary with airway and/or provide oxygen or intubate if required and if possible

Support circulation—external compression if required/intravenous fluid

Administer naloxone if opiate overdose suspected (100–200 µg intravenously, repeated as necessary)

Administer flumazenil 200 µg intravenously if benzodiazepine overdose suspected and then 100 µg at 1-minute intervals (max. 1 mg)

Administer thiamine (100 mg intravenously) prior to giving glucose

Administer glucose, e.g. 50 ml of 50% glucose, if hypoglycaemia suspected

If raised intracranial pressure present: give mannitol +/− dexamethasone

Stop seizures if present with diazepam and if possible followed by phenytoin intravenously (1000 mg over 30–60 minutes watching for hypotension and cardiac arrhythmias)

If infection suspected, try and obtain appropriate cultures (not a lumbar puncture) and give appropriate antibiotics e.g. the antibiotic of choice for presumed meningitis will vary throughout the world depending on the most likely organisms and the local resistance patterns

Bring body temperature to normal

Prognosis

The prognosis following coma is highly dependent on the underlying cause, the depth of the coma, duration of coma and clinical signs.[3] In a study of 210 patients who presented following cerebral hypoxic–ischaemic injury, such as cardiac arrest, Levy et al.[4] found that patients with absent pupillary light reflexes at the onset never regained independent daily function. By contrast, the initial presence of pupillary light reflexes, despite poor response in other measures, was often found in patients who did regain independent functioning. However, when the cause of coma is unknown, and the use of miotic drugs is uncertain, such outcomes are much more difficult to predict.

Patients with coma caused by drug overdose often have a good prognosis, if properly supported, despite appearing deeply comatose with depressed brainstem reflexes. Metabolic causes of coma often have better outcomes than those with anoxic–ischaemic causes, and coma of cerebrovascular aetiology (haemorrhage and stroke) carries the worst prognosis.[5]

The only certain state from which recovery is not possible is *brain death* in which all brainstem reflexes are absent, the features of which are listed below. All must be present to diagnose brain death. There are some international variations with respect to whether an electroencephalogram (EEG) recording is used, the timings of repeated testing and the seniority and specialization of the doctors involved. The tests are usually carried out within a hospital setting. For instance, in the United Kingdom, the testing must be performed by two senior doctors a minimum of 24 h after the onset of coma and repeated after a number of hours.

- absent pupillary responses to light;
- absent oculocephalic reflexes (doll's eye manoeuvre);
- absent corneal reflexes;
- no grimace in response to facial pain;
- absent oculovestibular reflexes (caloric reflexes);
- absent gag reflex;
- absence of any respiratory effort, even after fully oxygenating patient and then allowing the pCO_2 to rise to at least 50 mmHg or 6.7 kPa.

Public health issues

The main public health issues surrounding the prevention and management of coma, concern the education of patients and their families with conditions such as diabetes and epilepsy, campaigns to reduce illicit drug use, and public awareness and application of first aid management of unconscious individuals and those having a cardiorespiratory arrest. Worldwide, local and government issues may arise, such as in malaria-ridden areas, the instigation of bioenvironmental controls[6,7] which may help to prevent cerebral malaria which is associated with a high mortality.

Key points

- Coma is a medical emergency.
- Immediate cardiorespiratory assessment ('ABC') and administer oxygen.
- Stabilize the cervical spine following trauma.
- Assess for potentially treatable causes and administer treatment— [e.g. hypoglycaemia (cover with thiamine), meningitis, seizures, opiate overdose, hypovolaemia, rising intracerebral pressure].
- Review cardiorespiratory and neurological status regularly and give further treatment as required.
- Organize emergency transfer to hospital.

References

1. Plum, F. and Posner, J.B. *The Diagnosis of Stupor and Coma* 3rd edn. Philadelphia PA: F.A. Davis.
2. Wong, C.P., Forsyth, R.J., Kelly, T.P., and Eyre, E.A. (2001). Incidence, aetiology and outcome of non-traumatic coma: a population based study. *Archives of Disease in Childhood* 84, 193–9.
3. Levy, D.E. et al. (1981). Prognosis in non-traumatic coma. *Annals of Internal Medicine* 94, 293–301.
4. Levy, D.E. et al. (1985). Predicting outcome from hypoxic–ischaemic coma. *Journal of the American Medical Association* 253, 1420–6.
5. Bates, D. (2001). The prognosis of medical coma. *Journal of Neurology, Neurosurgery and Psychiatry* 71 (Suppl.), 120–3.
6. Dua, V.K., Sharma, S.K., and Sharma, V.P. (1991). Bioenvironmental control of malaria at the Indian Drugs and Parmaceuticals Ltd., Rishikesh (U.P.). *Indian Journal of Malariology* 28, 227–35.
7. Victor, T.J. and Reuben, R. (2000). Effect of plant spacing on the population of mosquito immatures in rice fields in Madurai, south India. *Indian Journal of Malariology* 37, 18–26.

11.8 Meningitis and CNS infections

William Howlett

Acute bacterial meningitis

Meningitis is an inflammation of the pia and arachnoid meninges and the cerebrospinal fluid (CSF) that surrounds the brain and spinal cord. The main causes are viral and bacterial. Meningitis is classified as acute or chronic. Acute meningitis occurs within hours or days and is classified as aseptic which is mostly viral in origin or septic which is caused by bacteria. Chronic meningitis by definition persists for 4 or more weeks and is mainly caused by tuberculosis and fungal infection. The aim of this chapter is to provide an overview of acute bacterial meningitis and to give a brief account of some other main central nervous system (CNS) infections encountered in clinical practice.

Epidemiology

The main causes of acute bacterial meningitis are *Neisseria meningitidis*, *Streptococcus pneumoniae*, *Listeria monocytogenes*, and *Haemophilus influenzae* type b (Hib). Each year, there are over 2000 new cases of acute bacterial meningitis in England and Wales giving an annual incidence rate of approximately 5 per 100 000 (Table 1). Similar rates have been reported in Europe with somewhat lower rates in the United States.[1] The epidemiology of acute bacterial meningitis has changed markedly in the last decade with a 95 per cent decrease in the incidence of Hib meningitis and a 75 per cent decrease in the incidence of serogroup C meningococcal infection. This decrease is mainly due to the introduction of the conjugated Hib vaccine and more recently the meningococcal conjugated C vaccine. Prior to this Hib was responsible for almost half the total annual cases of meningitis and the mean age of onset was 15 months.[2] Hib now accounts for only 1–2 per cent of overall cases of meningitis and the mean age has increased to 25 years.

Table 1 The approximate annual incidence of CNS infections in England and Wales (pop. 51 million)

	New cases per 100 000 pop. per annum	Years between two cases in a list of 2000 patients
Viral meningitis	20	2.5
Viral encephalitis	5–10	10–5
Bacterial meningitis	5	10
Meningococcal disease	5	10
Herpes encephalitis	0.2	250
CNS tuberculosis	0.2	250

The annual incidence of meningococcal disease in England and Wales is also approximately 5 per 100 000. This figure includes both cases of septicaemia and meningitis. In England and Wales, meningococcal meningitis is the major cause of acute bacterial meningitis accounting for 60 per cent of overall cases giving an incidence rate of 2–3 per 100 000.[3] A lower incidence rate of 0.6 per 100 000 has been reported in the United States where it accounts for about 25 per cent of overall cases.[2] In England and Wales, pneumococcal meningitis accounts for 13 per cent of meningitis cases giving an incidence rate of 0.5 per 100 000. In contrast, an incidence rate of 1.1 per 100 000 has been reported in the United States where it is the most common cause of bacterial meningitis.[2] Listeria meningitis (8 per cent) is the third most common cause, an incidence rate of 0.2 per 100 000 has been reported in the United States.[2]

Frequency in primary care

The frequency of the main CNS infections in the general population and in family practice in England and Wales is presented in Table 1.

Aetiology

Neisseria meningitidis

Neisseria meningitidis is a gram-negative diplococcus and infection results in meningococcal disease. The term meningococcal disease includes meningitis alone (45 per cent), meningitis and septicaemia (45 per cent), and septicaemia alone (10 per cent). The incubation period is 2–7 days. The peak incidence is in children aged 1–24 months with a second peak in teenagers aged 15–19 years, together accounting for 70–80 per cent of all cases. Most infections are sporadic and occur in winter but outbreaks can occur in households and schools. Risk factors for infection include household contact, asplenism, influenza A, smoking in a household member, IgM, IgG and complement deficiencies, and travel to an endemic area. Meningococcus is classified into serogroups, including A, B, C, W135, and Y. Serogroup B is most common accounting for about two-thirds of cases and is on the increase. It occurs mostly in children and has no vaccine. Serogroup C mainly affects teenagers as clusters in schools and universities, causes most of the remaining cases and now has an effective vaccine. The incidence in this serogroup has rapidly declined since the introduction of a vaccine in 1999. Serogroup A is important worldwide causing large epidemics in Sub-Saharan Africa but is rare in Western countries. There are effective vaccines for serogroups A and C combined and more recently for the serogroup W135 which has occurred in pilgrims returning from Saudi Arabia. Serogroup Y is rare in the United Kingdom but common in North America.

Streptococcus pneumonia

Streptococcus pneumonia is a gram-positive coccus. The incubation period is unknown. It affects mainly adults but can affect all age groups especially infants aged 1–24 months and has a high mortality. The main source of infection is haematogenous from the respiratory tract. Risk factors for infection include basilar skull fractures, dural defects post-neurosurgery, chronic otitis media, sinusitis, asplenism, alcoholism, and chronic disease. A pneumococcal vaccine is recommended for those at increased risk and more recently for infants in the United States.

Listeria monocytogenes

Listeria meningitis is caused by *L. monocytogenes*, a small gram-positive rod that is commonly found in soil and water. The incubation period is 3–7 days. It can infect humans and animals and mainly leads to asymptomatic faecal excretion. Infection, however, can result in sepsis and meningitis. All age groups are affected but neonates, pregnant women, immunosuppressed, and the elderly are at increased risk. Sources of infection are contaminated vegetables, unpasteurized milk, soft cheeses, paté and chilled meats. The organism replicates at fridge temperatures and can survive heating up to 60°C. Prevention largely depends on adequate food hygiene, heating of chilled foods and avoidance of high-risk foods by those at risk.

Other less common causes of acute bacterial meningitis include Hib, *E. coli*, group B streptococcus, and *Staphylococcus aureus*.

Pathogenesis

With the exception of Listeria, all the main bacterial causes of meningitis colonize the nasopharynx of asymptomatic carriers. Colonization rates of around 10 per cent are common place with higher rates (20–50 per cent) in winter in children, young adults and case contacts. Spreads is by droplets or close physical contact with asymptomatic carriers (95 per cent) or occasionally direct from cases. Bacteria reach the meninges via the bloodstream or by direct invasion, and the presence of a polysaccharide capsule helps their survival in the blood stream. Clinical disease is rare and only occurs when there is septicaemia or penetration across the blood–brain barrier. The multiplication of bacteria in the CSF triggers a massive host immune response with release of inflammatory cytokines and accumulation of cells and exudate. This leads to a further breakdown in the blood–brain barrier with resultant cerebral oedema, raised intracranial pressure, cerebral thrombosis, and infarction.

Clinical diagnosis

The classical clinical features of acute bacterial meningitis are headache, fever, and neck stiffness. When this triad is accompanied by alteration in consiousness or seizures the diagnosis of meningitis is usually not in doubt. Other common presenting symptoms include photophobia, nausea, vomiting, backache, and lethargy. The finding of a haemorrhagic rash is strongly suggestive of meningococcal infection. Progression occurs in most cases over 1–3 days, a small number have an acute fulminant course lasting hours while a third group progress rapidly over 24 hours. The cardinal signs of meningitis are *neck stiffness, Kernig's and Brudzinski's signs*. These are usually elicited with the patient in the supine position and should be checked for in all suspected cases of meningitis. Neck stiffness is the most important sign and is present when the neck resists passive flexion to bring the chin on to the chest. It is found in about 90 per cent of adults and 60–80 per cent of children with meningitis. *Kernig's sign* is elicited by passively attempting to straighten the leg with the hip and knee flexed to more than 90°. In cases of meningitis, there is resistance and pain caused by spasm in the hamstrings as a result of stretching inflamed nerve roots. Forward flexing the neck elicits Brudzinski's sign, and in cases of meningitis, there is involuntary hip and knee flexion. This sign is elicited mainly in young children. These signs are present in most cases of established meningitis but are less likely in the very young and the elderly. In infants, the combination of fever, respiratory distress, irritability, crying, vomiting, drowsiness, and failure to feed may be the only findings. The association of bulging fontanel, neck retraction, and seizures should however suggest the diagnosis. In older children and adults, there may be backpain and myalgia in addition to the classic features. In the elderly, an alteration in level of consiousness and fever may be the only

Table 2 Presenting clinical features of meningococcal disease

Non-specific features	%	Major clinical features	%
Fever	71–100	Petechial/purpuric rash	48–71
Nausea/vomiting	34–69	Neck stiffness	71–79
Upper respiratory tract infection	10–27	Altered level of consciousness	65–91
Any rash	71–93	Seizures	4–21
Headache	34		

Based on review of five series of admission hospital records, Granier, et al. (1998). *British Journal of General Practice* **48**, 1167–71.

findings. Seizures occur in about one-third of patients typically in children and may be the presenting complaint. Focal neurological abnormalities and coma occur mainly as complications. There may also be evidence of infection outside the CNS or an underlying condition predisposing to meningitis. The main differential diagnosis in primary care includes viral meningitis, viral childhood exanthema, encephalitis, and subarachnoid haemorrhage.

Meningococcal disease

The main clinical features of meningococcal disease are outlined in Table 2. The onset is typically abrupt and disease develops in most patients over 24–48 h. The pathognomonic feature is the haemorrhagic rash, which is non-blanching and present in around 80 per cent of cases. About 10 per cent of cases have a maculopapular rash, which is non-haemorrhagic, erythematous, and blanching while the remainder have no rash at all. The rash of meningococcaemia may begin as a diffuse pink maculopapular rash in 20–25 per cent of children. It has a characteristic 'flea bitten' appearance on the limbs and trunk. Associated symptoms at this stage may be non-specific resembling influenza; and the diagnosis of meningitis is extremely difficult. In a matter of hours, a petechial and purpuric rash develops in about 80–90 per cent of children and 60–70 per cent of adults. This appears first as small flat red or purple spots over the trunk, buttocks or lower limbs before becoming more widely distributed on the arms and soles of feet. The lesions do not blanch under pressure and this can be confirmed by gentle pressure with a glass when the rash can be seen to persist. Parents are encouraged to use this '*tumbler test*'. A common error is failure to examine the concealed areas such as buttocks groins and axillae. In dark-skinned patients, the conjunctiva, palate, soles, and palms should be examined particularly. Pethechiae may later progress to larger confluent purpuric areas with central necrosis in a condition called purpura fulminans.

The clinical features of meningococcal septicaemia may vary from mildly symptomatic patients with positive blood cultures to acute fulminant infection, which is one of the most feared of all infections. Symptoms can progress rapidly from drowsiness and rash to circulatory failure, toxic shock, coma, and death within hours of onset. Complications include skin necrosis, serositis, gangrene, arthritis, and Waterhouse–Friderichson syndrome of adrenal failure.

Pneumococcal meningitis typically presents with marked meningism. It generally lacks a rash but pneumonia may be present. Patients tend to progresses rapidly in 24–48 hours to drowsiness, confusion, coma, and seizures. Listerial infection is frequently asymptomatic in the normal host but causes acute sepsis and meningitis in the neonate and a subacute meningitis in the at risk adult. Hib meningitis has a characteristic slow onset over several days often starting with fever or respiratory tract infection. The onset of drowsiness, vomiting, and convulsions in an infant in this setting may suggest the diagnosis.

Meningitis in primary care

The average doctor in primary care will encounter only one new case of acute bacterial meningitis every 10 years (Table 1). While the diagnosis of the classical case is relatively straightforward the main difficulty in primary care is discriminating between the rare patient with a life-threatening meningitis and the majority with similar symptoms but self-limiting viral illnesses.[4] Failure to make the correct diagnosis most often occurs in the early stages, in the young and elderly. Symptoms and signs that are strongly suggestive of meningitis in the hospital setting may be non-specific or be absent altogether in primary care. In one primary care study on patients presenting with new onset headache, only 0.4 per cent had meningitis,[5] whereas on average 2 per cent of the population consult their doctor annually for headache. Notably, about half the cases of meningitis are missed at the time of first examination mainly because of the absence of meningism and a rash.[6–9] The rash has been identified as one of the most important factors in primary care in the decision to refer to hospital.[10,11] Primary care doctors therefore need a high index of clinical suspicion and vigilance and need constantly to be aware of the possibility of meningitis. They need to examine for signs of meningitis in any ill or febrile patient particularly where the diagnosis is in doubt. Every effort should be made to revisit or recall 'sick patients' with puzzling findings especially if clinical deterioration or a rash develops or parents become concerned. There should also be a low threshold for using prophylactic antibiotics and hospital referral.

Key messages in primary care

> ◆ Half of all cases of acute bacterial meningitis are missed at first visit.
>
> ◆ The signs of meningitis may be absent in the early stages and in infants and the elderly.
>
> ◆ The characteristic haemorrhagic rash may be absent in meningococcal disease.
>
> ◆ The diagnosis of meningitis requires a high index of clinical suspicion.
>
> ◆ Doctors should re-examine febrile sick patients with puzzling symptoms and trust parents' instincts.
>
> ◆ The mainstay of management is early recognition, prompt antibiotics and urgent transfer to hospital.
>
> ◆ *Neisseria meningitidis* infection is the leading infectious cause of death in children and young adults.
>
> ◆ All children who recover should have a formal hearing test.

Outcome

Bacterial meningitis is the leading infectious disease cause of death in children and young adults in western countries. Nearly 20 per cent of patients with bacterial meningitis die and this figure has changed little in the last 20 years. Poor prognostic factors include coma, short duration of symptoms, lack of meningism, shock, extensive purpura, and seizures.[12] The overall mortality in meningococcal disease is 8–10 per cent. It ranges from 2 to 4 per cent in uncomplicated meningitis to over 20 per cent in septicaemia and 50 per cent in shock. By age group, mortality rate is lowest in those aged 5–9 years with higher rates in young children and teenagers. It reaches 40–50 per cent in neonates and the elderly. By organism, it ranges from 3 to 6 per cent in meningococcal and Hib infection to 15–20 per cent in *S. pneumonia* and *N. meningitidis*. Permanent neurologic deficits persist in 10–20 per cent of adults, 10–30 per cent of children, and 15–50 per cent of neonates. These include deafness, cranial nerve palsies, seizures, paralysis, cognitive impairment, and sometimes blindness. They are more common after *S. pneumococcus* and Hib infection.

Management

The mainstay of effective management of suspected meningitis is early recognition, immediate use of antibiotics and rapid referral to hospital.[13] Family practitioners are advised to carry benzylpenicillin in their bag at all times. There is evidence that preadmission parenteral penicillin reduces mortality in meningococcal disease. The aim is that all cases should have benzylpenicillin within 30 minutes of suspected diagnosis. The preferred route is intravenously or failing that intramuscularly. Recommended dosages are 300 mg for children under 1 year, 600 mg for children aged 1–9 years, and 1200 mg for children aged 10 years and adults. A history of anaphylaxis is a contraindication for penicillin but a history of a rash following penicillin is not. Alternative antibiotics include cefotaxime and ceftriaxone especially in countries with penicillin-resistant *S. pneumoniae*. Attention to airway, oxygen administration, and seizure control on route to hospital may also be necessary.

Prevention

Meningococcal disease is a notifiable disease. All suspected cases should be reported immediately to the Public Health Authority. Chemoprophylaxis is required for household contacts and close contacts of the index case within the previous 7 days.[13] Adults and children over 12 years should receive Rifampicin 600 mg orally twice daily for 2 days or Ciprofloxacin 500 mg orally as a single dose. For children 1–12 years use Rifampicin 10 mg/kg twice daily for 2 days or ceftriaxone 125 mg IM as a single dose. Infants require lower doses. Contacts of vaccine preventable strains should also be offered vaccination in addition to chemoprophylaxis. For Hib meningitis, Rifampicin 20 mg/kg daily (maximum 600 mg daily) as a single dose for 4 days is recommended for all household and nursery contacts when other children below age 4 years are present. Chemoprophylaxis is not recommended for those fully vaccinated against Hib. Chemprophylaxis is not usually indicated for close contacts of pneumococcal meningitis, however asplenic patients should receive long-term penicillin prophylaxis in addition to vaccine.

During the last decade we have witnessed the very effective primary prevention of Hib and *N. meningitidis* serogroup C meningitis. However, it should be noted that the overall incidence of meningitis has not declined and there are still no vaccines available against common causes of bacterial meningitis. There is also a dearth of community-based research on the early recognition and management of bacterial meningitis in primary care. Any future recommendations must include more research in these two key areas.

Other CNS infections

Viral meningitis

Viruses are the leading cause of meningitis worldwide and the commonest cause of meningitis encountered in primary care. Viral meningitis is usually a benign disease with less than 1000 cases reported annually in the United Kingdom. This is considered a gross underestimate as most cases go unreported (Table 1).[14] The overall annual incidence in the United Kingdom is estimated to be about 20 per 100 000. It is commonest in the age groups 0–1 years and 4–15 years but can affect all age groups. The *enteroviruses, echo and coxsackie* viruses account for over 90 per cent of cases. Other viruses include *arboviruses, adenoviruses,* and more recently, *HSV-2.* Young children are the usual source with spread via the faecal oral route within families. Outbreaks frequently occur in hospitals, nurseries, schools, and residential homes. It occurs throughout the year with a seasonal peak in summer. There may be a history of a viral like illness with rash. The onset can be acute or subacute with severe headache, photophobia and fever occur in most patients. Neck stiffness is frequently mild and only present in half the cases. Neurologic abnormalities are rare but febrile convulsions may occur in children. The illness can last over a week in children and longer in adults. The prognosis is generally excellent. Clinically, at onset it can be indistinguishable from bacterial meningitis and often requires provisional emergency antibiotics followed by prompt hospital referral. A lumbar puncture and CSF examination are usually diagnostic. Treatment is mainly symptomatic and mild cases can be observed at home and the diagnosis reviewed. Suspected *HSV-2* infection may be treated with acyclovir.

Viral encephalitis

Encephalitis is inflammation of the brain. It is predominantly a disease of children. The incidence of encephalitis ranges from 8 to 30 per 100 000 in children to approximately 5 per 100 000 in adults (Table 1).[14] The causes of encephalitis include the *epidemic viruses, enteroviruses* and the *arthropod-borne viruses. Herpes simplex type 1, (HSV1)* an endemic herpes virus is the most common sporadic cause of encephalitis in adults in Western countries. It occurs mostly in the over-50s, but can affect all age groups. Fewer than 100 cases are reported annually in the United Kingdom but this is considered an underestimate. Clinically HSV encephalitis usually begins as a non-specific febrile illness characterized by headache often unilateral, malaise, and altered mental status. Most patients go on to experience confusion, personality change, dysphasia, focal neurological findings and temporal lobe seizures. Symptoms typically evolve over several days and often take 2–3 weeks to reach their maximum severity. Suspected cases are transferred urgently to hospital and treated with intravenous acyclovir. The prognosis is particularly poor in coma. The case fatality rate in treated cases is around 20 per cent, in untreated cases it is 50–70 per cent. Morbidity is over 50 per cent and includes memory loss, cognitive impairment, and seizures.

Tuberculosis

Each year an estimated 8 million people worldwide develop clinical tuberculosis, of whom less than 1 per cent go on to develop CNS involvement. Tuberculous meningitis (TBM), tuberculoma, and spinal cord disease are the main clinical presentations. *Mycobacterium tuberculosis* is the main cause. One hundred to 200 cases of TBM are reported annually in England and Wales mostly in adults (Table 1). Risk factors include alcoholism, drug abuse, homelessness, malnutrition, and residence, or travel to endemic area and more recently HIV. TBM typically has a slow onset over 2–3 weeks presenting with chronic unrelenting headache, low-grade fever, tiredness, and mild meningism. Cranial nerve palsies, seizures and confusion develops in half the cases. Coma and death inevitably follow if left untreated. Rarely, the presentation is more acute over a few days. A history of TB exposure or disease is found in about half the cases. The diagnosis is confirmed by demonstrating mycobacterium in the CSF. The case fatality rate is 20–25 per cent. Morbidity (25–40 per cent) includes seizures, hydrocephalus, cranial nerve palsies and paralysis. Spinal cord disease results from spinal tuberculosis or Potts disease.

Brain abscess

Brain abscess is a focal pyogenic infection within the brain, subdural or epidural space. The majority are caused by bacteria including *Streptococcus viridans, S. aureus,* and *bacteroides fragilis.* In immunocompromised patients, toxoplasmosis and fungal infections are the main causes. Each year, approximately 200 cases are reported in the United Kingdom half of whom have a known risk factor. These include otitis media, mastoiditis, sinusitis, dental abscess, recent skull fracture or neurosurgery, bronchiectasis, cyanotic heart disease, and more recently, HIV. They are more common in males with the majority in the third or fourth decade. Over half the patients present with headache, fever, and focal neurological deficits. The fever is usually low grade and seizures occur in about a quarter of patients. The duration from onset to complications takes 1–2 weeks in half the cases. The main differential diagnosis is a brain tumour. The diagnosis is usually suggested by neuroimaging and occasionally by brain biopsy. Management is based on antibiotics, anticonvulsants and surgical drainage. The case fatality rate varies from 10 per cent in uncomplicated cases to 50 per cent in patients with coma. Morbidity is about 30 per cent and includes epilepsy and focal neurological deficits.

HIV

HIV disease and syphilis are worldwide venereal diseases caused by the *human immunodeficiency virus* and the spirochete *Treponema pallidum,* respectively. Neurosyphilis is now extremely rare in western countries and has largely been replaced by HIV disease as a cause of neurological disorders. Neurological disorders occur at all stages of HIV infection and about 10 per cent of AIDS patients will develop a major neurological disorder. These are caused mainly by opportunistic infections including *Toxoplasma gondii, Cryptococcus neoformans, Mycobacterium tuberculosis* and tumours including CNS lymphoma. The main clinical presentation is that of a space occupying lesion secondary to toxoplasmosis or lymphoma with headache, confusion, focal neurological deficit, or seizures evolving over 1–2 weeks. *Cryptococcus neoformans* and tuberculosis infection present mainly as chronic meningitis. Other presentations include retinitis caused by *cytomegalovirus* infection and shingles caused by *herpes zoster.* AIDS dementia complex develops in about a fifth of patients, mainly those with advanced disease. This is caused by direct HIV virus and is characterized by difficulty concentrating and remembering and general slowing of mental and motor tasks. Later, frank dementia may set in. The use of highly active antiretroviral treatment has decreased its severity. Peripheral manifestations occur in over half of AIDS patients. These include polyneuropathies, mononeuropathies, myelopathy and myopathy. The diagnosis of HIV is confirmed by serology.

References

1. **Bannister, B., Begg, N.T., and Gillespie, S.H.** (2000). Infections of the central nervous system. In *Infectious Diseases* 2nd edn. (ed. B. Bannister), pp. 301–31. Oxford: Blackwell Science. (An excellent textbook on CNS infections for clinicians.)

2. **Schuchat, A.** et al. (1997). Bacterial meningitis in the United States in 1995. *New England Journal of Medicine* **337**, 970–6. (An excellent study on bacterial meningitis in the United States.)

3. **MacDonald, B.K.** et al. (2000). The incidence and lifetime prevalence of neurological disorders in a prospective community-based study in the UK. *Brain* **123**, 665–76. (A good epidemiological study of neurological disorders in primary care.)

4. **Granier, S., Owen, P., and Stott, N.C.H.** (1998). Recognising meningococcal disease: the case for further research in primary care. *British Journal of General Practice* **48**, 1167–71. (An excellent review of meningococcal disease in primary care.)

5. **McWhinney, I.R.,** ed. *A Textbook of Family Medicine* 2nd edn. Oxford: Oxford University Press, 1997. (Essential reading for doctors in primary care.)

6. **Granier, S.** et al. (1998). Recognising meningococcal disease in primary care: qualitative study on how general practitioners process clinical and contextual information. *British Medical Journal* **316**, 276–9. (An important study on decision making in primary care.)

7. **Andersen, J.** et al. (1997). Acute meningococcal meningitis: analysis of features of the disease according to age of 255 patients. *Journal of Infection* **34**, 227–35. (A detailed hospital-based study.)

8. **Ragunathan, L.** et al. (2000). Clinical features, laboratory findings and management of meningococcal meningitis in England and Wales: report of a 1997 survey. *Journal of Infection* **40**, 74–9. (A detailed review of meningococcal meningitis.)

9. **Koorevaar, R.** et al. (1995). Patients with suspected meningitis: a study in general practice. *European Journal of General Practice* **1**, 21–3. (A prospective general practice study.)

10. **Riordan, F.A.I.** et al. (1996). Who spots the spots? Diagnosis and treatment of early meningococcal disease in children. *British Medical Journal* **313**, 1255–6. (A prospective primary care study on the rash.)

11. **Cartwright, K.** et al. (1992). Early treatment with parenteral penicillin in meningococcal disease. *British Medical Journal* **305**, 143–6. (A study on the use of early penicillin.)

12. **Aronin, S.I.** et al. (1998). Community-acquired bacterial meningitis: risk stratification for adverse clinical outcome and effect of antibiotic timing. *Annals of Internal Medicine* **129**, 862–9. (A detailed study on factors affecting outcome.)

13. **Begg, N.** et al. (1999). Consensus statement on diagnosis, investigation, treatment and prevention of bacterial meningitis in immunocompetent adults. *Journal of Infection* **39**, 1–15. (An excellent review of guidelines in bacterial meningitis.)

14. **Marra, C.M.** (1999). Central nervous system infections. *Neurologic Clinics* **17**, 4. (A detailed review of main CNS infections.)

12

Eye problems

12 Eye problems

12.1 Acute red eye

Theo Voorn

The incidence of disorders of redness of one or both eyes in general practice is about 40 per 1000 patients a year. The red eye is one of the most common ocular problems presenting in general practice and occurs in all age groups. The common causes of red eye are summarized in Fig. 1. The redness of the eye is caused by dilated blood vessels in the conjunctiva or episclera or by subconjunctival bleeding. In 75 per cent of the cases, the diagnosis is infectious or allergic conjunctivitis. Simple conjunctivitis is almost always simply treated with medication and seldom referred to a specialist. However, other causes of red eye include keratitis, iritis, and acute glaucoma—all of which are sight threatening and need urgent referral. The key to managing the red eye is therefore making a firm and safe diagnosis on the basis of the history, symptoms, and signs. Diagnostic uncertainty is an indication for urgent referral.

Taking the history

Establish whether the symptoms are present in one or both eyes and start always with three questions:

- Do you have *pain*? (It is important to differentiate between pain and itchiness or feelings of a foreign body.)
- Is your *vision* changed or reduced?
- Does *bright light* increase the *discomfort*?

The *absence* of these three symptoms effectively excludes serious disorders of the anterior eye chamber and the cornea. The presence of any of these symptoms does not confirm serious pathology but makes the investigator alert for the possibility.

Next ask about *trauma* and the possibility of a foreign body, enquiring exactly what has happened and exploring further any feelings of a foreign body.

Finally, depending on the presenting complaints, ask about other factors: type of *discharge* (and what kind of discharge); *itching* or history of atopy (such as sneezing, runny nose, wheezing, and eczema); use of *eye drops* and *cosmetics*; wearing of *contact lenses* and the maintenance of the lenses; presence of predisposing *chronic* or *acute disease* (such as rheumatoid arthritis, cold sores).

Examination of a red eye

Inspection is the most important diagnostic weapon, and again it must be systematic, observing the following features in turn and in particular looking for indicators of damage of the cornea, the iris or deeper structures:

- Pattern of *redness*—into the fornix or pericorneal, vasodilatation or bleeding, superficial or deep, segmental or circular? When the character of the redness is not clear the examiner can try to move the redness with a wet cotton bud—if movable, the cause is superficial.

  Danger signs—redness mainly around cornea or localized involving cornea.

- *Discharge*—watery or purulent?
- *Cornea*—glossy or dull, deformation of the red reflex in the ophthalmoscope, ingrowing vessels, foreign body.

  Danger signs—any corneal abnormality.

- *Anterior eye* chamber—pus (hypopyon), blood (hyphaema), colour of the iris, and size of the *pupil* (compare left and right).

  Danger signs—any abnormality of anterior chamber including difference between pupils.

- *Overall appearance* of prominence.

  Danger sign—protusion of eye (proptosis).

- *Eyelids*—redness, swelling, inside (foreign body), entropion/ectropion, eyelashes.

  If the patient has reported pain, decreased visual acuity, or photophobia on initial questioning, if there is a possibility of trauma to the eye, or if any of the above danger signs are present on inspection, it is necessary to complete the full examination:

- check visual acuity.
- assess pupil size and assess the reaction of the pupils to light.
- look with an opthalmoscope at the cornea, anterior eye chamber, and the vitreous.

Conjunctiva	Cornea	Anterior chamber	Sclera	Eyelid	Orbit
Infection	Foreign body	Iritis	Episcleritis	Chalazion	Cellulitis
Allergy	Abrasion	Acute glaucoma	Scleritis	Blepharitis	Trauma
Injury	Erosion			Herpes zoster	
Dry eye	Keratitis/ulcer				
Subconjunctival haemorrhage					

Fig. 1 Important causes of red eye.

◆ fluorescein stain and inspect the cornea (damaged corneal epithelium will light up green).

◆ assess ocular motility and the position of the eyes in cases of blunt trauma.

If the primary care physician has ophthalmic expertise, it is feasible to assess pain and photophobia with a topical anaesthetic to differentiate between disorders of the cornea and deeper structures. When there is a disorder of the cornea, the patient is free of pain in 10–20 seconds. An increase of pain and photophobia by exposure to light suggests a problem in a deeper structure.

However, in the absence of such specialist expertise it is appropriate to refer patients to an ophthalmologist for this investigation.

Common symptom patterns

On the basis of the history and the examination, it is usually possible to make a firm diagnosis with reasonable certainty. Pain, reduced vision, photophobia, pericorneal redness (and sometimes a defect of the corneal epithelium) occur with *corneal inflammation* and *ulceration* (keratitis). Keratitis is particularly common in relation to use of contact lenses and may complicate infection (e.g. with herpes simplex and zoster); failure to identify a corneal ulcer (Fig. 2) may lead to permanent damage from scarring. Lesions at the edge of the cornea (*marginal keratitis*) often occur in the elderly in association with eyelid disease (as a result of rosacea, entropion, or infective blepharitis) or poor eye closure due to stroke or Bell's palsy (Fig. 3). In all cases, ophthalmic referral is indicated but immediate treatment for any obvious underlying cause should be initiated in primary care (e.g. topical chloramphenicol for staphylococcal blepharitis or acyclovir for herpes zoster).

Pain (not responding to topical anaesthetic), reduced vision, photophobia, and circumcorneal redness are also features of *iritis*. It is associated with inflammation of the ciliary body and consequently iritis may be associated with an abnormal pupil, precipitates in the anterior eye chamber, or even pus in the anterior chamber (hypopyon). Iritis is more common in older patients and is occasionally associated with systemic disease (sarcoid, ankylosing spondylitis) or rarely with infection (syphilis, tuberculosis, herpes zoster). Initiation of treatment for recurrence of iritis with steroids in primary care may be indicated if infective keratitis has been excluded, but only in parallel with re-referral.

Inflammation of the sclera (*scleritis*, Fig. 4) is a possible complication of connective tissue disorders and, like iritis, requires urgent referral. It needs to be distinguished from the more common problem of *episcleritis* (Fig. 5). In both cases, there is localized redness of the sclera associated with dilatation of the episcleral capillaries—but scleritis causes pain rather than discomfort, the redness is often more generalized and more florid, and the involvement of the deeper scleral vessels may give a bluish discoloration to the sclera. The ischaemic process may also lead to blurring of vision.

Severe pain with nausea and vomiting—usually with reduced vision, mid-dilated fixed pupil, pericorneal redness, and steamy cornea—indicates *acute glaucoma* (Fig. 6). It usually (but not invariably) affects elderly patients, and there may be a history of warning haloes or recent use of dilating drops. Onset is rapid and referral should be equally rapid to preserve sight.

Key symptoms and signs which indicate the possibility of these three conditions, and sight threatening problems associated with orbit infection and trauma, are summarized in Fig. 7. If there is any diagnostic doubt, refer to the specialist. In the absence of these warning signs, the diagnosis is likely to be *conjunctivitis, sub-conjunctival haemorrhage* or superficial inflammation (*episcleritis*, a *pterygium*, or a *pingueculum*).

Conjunctivitis (Fig. 8) is often associated with superficial redness, watering, itching, discharge, or feelings of a foreign body. The causes of red eye

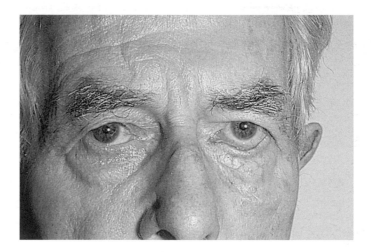

Fig. 3 Ectropion and poor eye closure due to Bell's palsy. (See Plate 13.) [Source: Ellingham and Ellingham in *Oxford Textbook of Ophthalmology* (ed. Easty and Sparrow), Oxford University Press, 1999.]

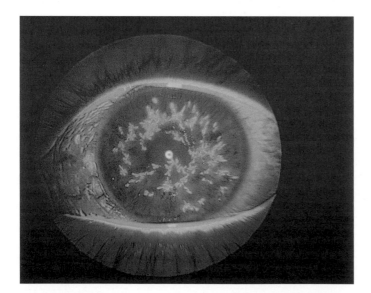

Fig. 2 Corneal damage from dendritic ulcer (stained with fluorescein and viewed with blue light). (See Plate 12.) [Source: Marsh and Easty in *Oxford Textbook of Ophthalmology* (ed. Easty and Sparrow), Oxford University Press, 1999.]

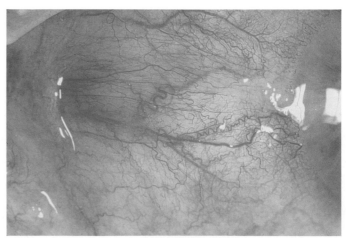

Fig. 4 Scleritis showing dilation of deep vessels and bluish discoloration from scleral thinning. (See Plate 14.) [Source: de la Meza and Foster in *Oxford Textbook of Ophthalmology* (ed. Easty and Sparrow), Oxford University Press, 1999.]

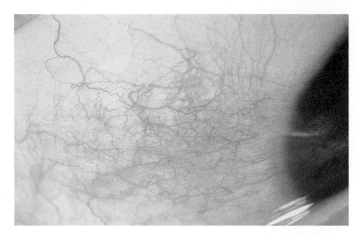

Fig. 5 Episcleritis showing dilatation of superficial vessels only. (See Plate 15.) [Source: de la Meza and Foster in *Oxford Textbook of Ophthalmology* (ed. Easty and Sparrow), Oxford University Press, 1999.]

commonly associated with conjunctivitis are summarized in Fig. 9. When there is no trauma, no evident purulent discharge, and no indications to suggest allergy and disturbances of the tear function think of *viral conjunctivitis*—although some authors think that it is not possible to differentiate between a viral and a bacterial conjunctivitis on the basis of history and examination, and even culture may not provide a definitive diagnosis because of the problem of mixed infections and the limitations of standard microbiology. The diagnosis and management of conjunctivitis is discussed in more detail in Chapter 12.2 by Leung on the 'sticky eye'. The key is to exclude corneal damage from trauma or infection, and corneal

Danger symptoms	Danger signs
Ocular pain	Pericorneal redness
Photophobia	Clouding or staining of
Decreased vision	cornea
	Abnormal pupil
	Proptosis

Fig. 7 Key symptoms and signs suggesting need for urgent referral.

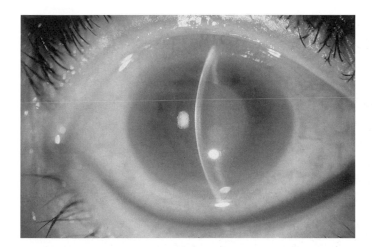

Fig. 6 Acute glaucoma showing red eye, corneal oedema, and fixed oval pupil (white flare from slit lamp reflects shallow anterior chamber). (See Plate 16.) [Source: Kitazawa and Yamamoto in *Oxford Textbook of Ophthalmology* (ed. Easty and Sparrow), Oxford University Press, 1999.]

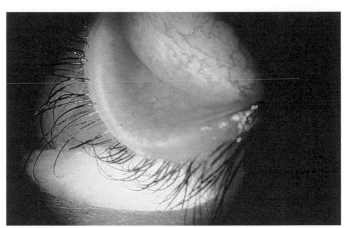

Fig. 8 Acute follicular conjunctivitis caused by adenovirus serotype 8. (See Plate 17.) [Source: Hodge and Smdlin in *Oxford Textbook of Ophthalmology* (ed. Easty and Sparrow), Oxford University Press, 1999.]

Cause	Associations	Discharge	Extra symptoms	Think about
Bacterial infection	Acute or chronic (most bilateral)	Purulent	Sticky eyelashes Oedema of the eyelid	Gonorrhoea in neonates Chlamydia
Viral infection	Acute or chronic (most bilateral)	Watery	Often follicles Oedema of the eyelid Contagious	Herpes Adenovirus Pharyngeal viruses
Allergy	Atopy (Hay fever; asthma) Use of contact lenses	Watery/stringy	Itchy Swollen conjunctiva	Seasonal
Disturbance of tear function	Dry eyes	None or watery	Fluorescein stain	Sicca syndrome
Eyelid problem (blepharitis)	Chronic red lid margins	Often crusts, scales on the eyelid margins	Eczema, seborrhoea	
Eyedrops	Glaucoma drops Dry eyes Allergy	Mostly none	Sometimes itchy Increased by putting drops in the eye	Any drops used Preservatives in artificial tears
Injury	Foreign body Trauma Contact lens	Scant	Visible foreign body Entropion Ectropion	Pay attention for possible penetration!

Fig. 9 Causes of red eye associated with conjunctivitis.

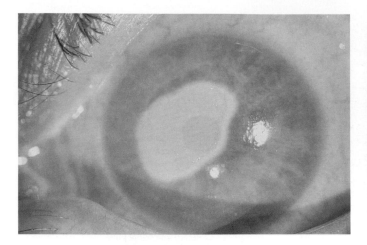

Fig. 10 Corneal abrasion (stained with fluorescein). (See Plate 18.) [Source: Pfister in *Oxford Textbook of Ophthalmology* (ed. Easty and Sparrow), Oxford University Press, 1999.]

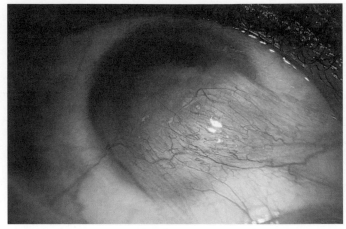

Fig. 12 A pterygium (in this case extending onto cornea and requiring excision). (See Plate 20.) [Source: Larkin in *Oxford Textbook of Ophthalmology* (ed. Easty and Sparrow), Oxford University Press, 1999.]

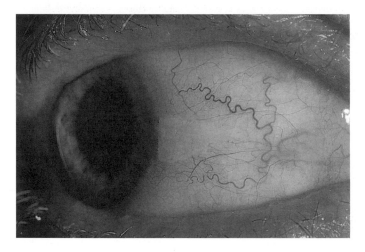

Fig. 11 A pinguecula (an innocent fatty lump on the sclera). (See Plate 19.) [Source: Larkin in *Oxford Textbook of Ophthalmology* (ed. Easty and Sparrow), Oxford University Press, 1999.]

with the development of a *pterygium* and from an inflamed *pingueculum*. Both conditions are associated with past exposure to ultraviolet light. A pinguecula (Fig. 11) is normally seen as a fatty lump on the sclera and is very common in the elderly—but when they become inflamed they cause redness, watering, and soreness. A pterygium is more vascular and wedge shaped in appearance (Fig. 12) but can also flare up to cause similar symptoms of localized redness and soreness. Inflammation may settle spontaneously but referral for confirmation of diagnosis may be appropriate as steroid drops, and rarely excision, may be helpful.

Key points

- Ask about pain, reduced vision, and photophobia.
- Ask about possibility of trauma and foreign bodies.
- Absence of ocular pain, photophobia or decreased vision makes serious pathology of the anterior eye unlikely.
- Redness around cornea, clouding or straining of cornea, abnormal pupils or proptosis merit urgent referral.

Further reading

Blom, G.H., Cleringa, J.P., Louisse, A.C., De Bruin, W., Gooskens, P., and Wiersma, T.J. (1996). NHG standard on red eye. *Huisarts en Wetenschap* **39** (5), 225–38.

Frith, P., Gray, R., MacLennan, S., and Ambler, P. *The Eye in Clinical Practice.* Oxford: Blackwell Scientific Publications, 1994.

Leibowitz, H.M. (2000). The red eye. *New England Journal of Medicine* **343**, 345–51.

staining with fluorescein is mandatory if there is a possibility of corneal ulceration or abrasion (Fig. 10). Although the cornea is sensitive and corneal damage usually presents with pain, this is not invariable and it is better to take the few seconds to use a fluorescein stain than to miss a corneal lesion.

Sub-conjunctival haemorrhage is common and may be spontaneous or associated with trauma. Bleeding gives redness with sharp boundaries without pain or vessel injection. Most resolve spontaneously within 2 weeks, but in case of trauma it is important to exclude serious eye damage of skull fracture. Spontaneous sub-conjunctival haemorrhage due to a coagulation disorder is rare, except in patients on anticoagulants, although it is considered good practice to check blood pressure.

Episcleritis (Fig. 5) is a common cause of localized scleral redness and an uncomfortable eye—which may be painful if you touch it with a cotton bud—but, unlike scleritis, not a painful eye. The cornea on staining, the conjunctivae and vision are all normal. It often resolves spontaneously, or with treatment with anti-inflammatory drugs, and referral is only necessary if the diagnosis is in doubt or if resolution is slow.

As a cause of local vascular redness, episcleritis needs to be distinguished from the more superficial overgrowth of conjunctival blood vessels seen

12.2 **Sticky eye**

Alexander K.C. Leung

Almost everybody has experienced at least one episode of sticky eye in their lifetime. The sticky eye is a common complaint in a primary care setting; it occurs worldwide and affects all ages. The condition commonly results from an exudation of inflammatory cells and a fibrin-rich oedematous fluid from blood vessels in the conjunctiva which combines with denuded epithelial cells and mucus. When the exudate dries, the eyelids may stick together. The most common cause is bacterial conjunctivitis. In most cases, the process is benign and self-limited, but certain unusual causes may pose a threat to vision. The purpose of this chapter is to familiarize primary care physicians with the problem to allow prompt intervention and preclude morbidity.

The most common cause of sticky eye is bacterial conjunctivitis. Other causes include viral, chlamydial, chemical or allergic conjunctivitis, and blepharitis. Parinaud's oculoglandular, Stevens–Johnson and Reiter's syndromes are much less common causes.

Clinical history

The patient's age is often useful in determining a diagnosis. Conjunctivitis in the first 2 days of life may be chemical due to instillation of silver nitrate drops, though these are rarely used nowadays. Ophthalmia neonatorum secondary to *Neisseria gonorrhoeae* typically becomes evident at 2–4 days, *Chlamydia trachomatis* at 5–14 days, herpes simplex virus (HSV) at 6–14 days, and other bacterial infections at 4–30 days after birth.

After the neonatal month, a wide range of organisms can cause conjunctivitis. In general, bacterial conjunctivitis is most common in infants and children; viral conjunctivitis becomes more frequent with increasing age.[1] Infection with *Streptococcus pneumoniae* and *Haemophilus influenzae* is more common in children while *Staphylococcus aureus* is more common in adults.[2] *Streptococcus pneumoniae* affects mainly children in temperate climates during colder months. *Haemophilus influenzae* affects mainly younger children and is more common in warm climates. *Staphylococcus aureus* has no seasonal or climate variation. In sexually active young adults, there may be a possibility of gonococcal and chlamydial conjunctivitis. Bacterial conjunctivitis in the elderly is more commonly associated with a predisposing factor such as blepharitis, keratoconjunctivitis sicca, in-turning lashes, or a blocked nasolacrimal duct.

Viral conjunctivitis is most often caused by *adenovirus*, which may present as follicular conjunctivitis, pharyngoconjunctival fever, or epidemic keratoconjunctivitis.[3] Follicular conjunctivitis, the most common type of ocular adenoviral infection, occurs more commonly in children than in adults.[3] Pharyngoconjunctival fever is usually caused by adenovirus types 3, 4, and 7 and affects mainly children younger than 10 years of age, whereas epidemic keratoconjunctivitis is usually caused by adenovirus types 8, 19, and 37 and occurs mainly in older children, adolescents, and adults. Many of the childhood exanthems such as chickenpox, mumps, rubeola, rubella, and infectious mononucleosis may be accompanied by acute conjunctivitis. Most herpetic ocular infections are caused by HSV-1, though 80 per cent of neonatal cases are caused by HSV-2. Acute haemorrhagic conjunctivitis is usually caused by enterovirus 70 or coxsackievirus A24. Other viruses that cause occasional conjunctivitis include papillomavirus, influenza, molluscum contagiosum, cytomegalovirus, and Newcastle disease.

Ocular infections due to *C. trachomatis*, an obligate intracellular parasite, can occur in two distinct forms: trachoma (associated with serotypes A–C) and inclusion conjunctivitis (associated with serotypes D–K).[2] *Trachoma*, a leading cause of blindness, is endemic in rural areas of developing countries, particularly in Africa, Asia, and the Middle East.[2] Inclusion conjunctivitis is a sexually transmitted disease that occurs in both newborns (ophthalmia neonatorum) and adults (adult inclusion conjunctivitis).

Certain symptoms may suggest a particular diagnosis (Table 1). A purulent discharge strongly suggests a bacterial aetiology, a serous discharge, a viral aetiology, and a mucoid or stringy discharge allergic conjunctivitis.[2] Intense itching, nasal stuffiness, sneezing, and a history of atopy suggest *allergic conjunctivitis*; the most common form is seasonal allergic rhinoconjunctivitis which is an IgE-mediated hypersensitivity reaction precipitated by small airborne allergens and occur in seasons when pollen counts are high.[4] Acute allergic conjunctivitis may otherwise occur in susceptible individuals year-round, being induced by animal dander, dust mites, or some other ever-present antigens. *Gonococcal conjunctivitis* should be suspected when the discharge is copiously purulent.[2]

Patients with *nasolacrimal duct obstruction* usually present with watering and a mucopurulent discharge. This is the most common cause of chronic or recurrent conjunctivitis in infants.

Pain, photophobia, and impaired visual acuity indicate corneal involvement or iritis which may be associated with epidemic keratoconjunctivitis, acute haemorrhagic conjunctivitis, HSV conjunctivitis, and chlamydial conjunctivitis. A history of exposure to other individuals with similar problems, exposure to pool water, or contact with individuals with sexually transmitted diseases suggests infectious conjunctivitis. Contact with pets,

Table 1 Comparison of the clinical manifestations of major causes of conjunctivitis

Clinical manifestation	Bacterial conjunctivitis	Viral conjunctivitis	Allergic conjunctivitis
Discharge	Purulent	Serous	Mucoid
Matting of lids on awakening	Common	Uncommon	Rare
Itching	Mild	Minimal	Marked
Pain	Mild	Mild to moderate without keratitis; severe with keratitis	Absent
Tearing	Moderate	Profuse	Moderate
Photophobia	Mild	Mild to moderate without keratitis; severe with keratitis	Mild
Upper respiratory symptoms	Rare	Not uncommon	Rare
Laterality	Unilateral > bilateral	Bilateral	Bilateral
Conjunctival injection	Yes	Yes	Yes
Palpebral conjunctiva	Papillae	Follicles	Pale and oedematous; papillae may be present
Preauricular adenopathy	Uncommon	Common	None

especially cats, suggests Parinaud's oculoglandular syndrome. An associated upper respiratory tract infection suggests adenoviral infection. A history of use of cosmetics around the eye, contact lens solutions, and especially soft contact lens wear may give a clue to toxic conjunctivitis.

Clinical examination

Conjunctivitis is characterized by dilated capillaries in the conjunctiva that are branching toward the cornea (see Fig. 8 in Chapter 12.1). The presence of papillae suggests allergic or viral, chlamydial and some cases of toxic conjunctivitis. Membranes or *pseudomembranes* may be seen in any severe conjunctivitis, but are typically seen in epidemic, HSV, streptococcal, pneumococcal or diphtheritic conjunctivitis, or Stevens–Johnson syndrome.

In bacterial conjunctivitis, the infection is often unilateral initially but spreads rapidly to the contralateral eye. Viral conjunctivitis is usually bilateral at outset and frequently associated with an upper respiratory tract infection.

Chemosis strongly suggests allergic conjunctivitis. Chemosis may also be seen in HSV and chlamydial conjunctivitis. Petechial haemorrhages may be seen in epidemic keratoconjunctivitis and conjunctivitis secondary to *S. pneumoniae* and *H. influenzae*. More extensive sub-conjunctival haemorrhage is associated with acute haemorrhagic conjunctivitis. Corneal involvement is seen more commonly in gonococcal and viral conjunctivitis. Angular inflammation suggests *Moraxella lacunata* infection.

Marked lid swelling is characteristic of gonococcal conjunctivitis and epidemic keratoconjunctivitis. Greasy scales on the lid margins (cilia collarettes) and ulceration of the lid margins are indicative of blepharitis which may be secondary to staphylococcal infection or seborrhoea. Blepharitis is a common cause of chronic conjunctivitis in older children.

The presence of preauricular lymphadenopathy and pharyngitis is more indicative of viral conjunctivitis. The presence of unilateral granulomatous conjunctivitis and ipsilateral preauricular or submandibular *lymphadenopathy* is suggestive of Parinaud's oculoglandular syndrome. The most common cause of Parinaud's oculoglandular syndrome is cat-scratch disease. Other rare causes include tuberculosis, infectious mononucleosis, tularaemia, syphilis, and sarcoidosis.

Corneal vascularization (pannus), conjunctival follicles, characteristic conjunctival cicatrization, and Herbert's pits are characteristic features of trachoma (Fig. 1). Inclusion conjunctivitis can be differentiated from trachoma as corneal scarring rarely occurs in inclusion conjunctivitis and in trachoma, the upper tarsal conjunctiva is more involved than the lower.

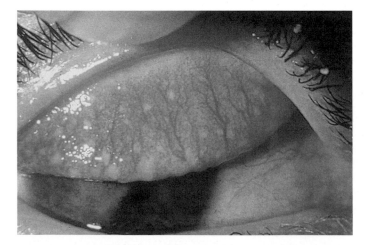

Fig. 1 Trachoma conjunctivitis showing characteristic white-yellow follicles. (See Plate 21.) [Source: Taylor and Vajpayee in *Oxford Textbook of Ophthalmology* (ed. Easty and Sparrow), Oxford University Press, 1999.]

Vesicular lesions on the eyelid, herpes labialis, or corneal lesions are distinguishing features of HSV conjunctivitis. Clinical features of chickenpox, mumps, rubeola, rubella, or infectious mononucleosis suggest the corresponding disease. Lesions of erythema multiforme and involvement of at least two *mucous membranes* suggest Stevens–Johnson syndrome. The presence of arthritis, urethritis or colitis and conjunctivitis together suggests Reiter's syndrome.

Laboratory investigations

Laboratory evaluation is usually not necessary but is essential if conjunctivitis is severe, chronic or recurrent, coexisting with keratitis, or as ophthalmia neonatorum unless due to chemical use.

Conjunctival scrapings for proper stains and culture are the standard laboratory tests. Gram stain provides preliminary information about the presence and relative quantity of bacterial pathogen(s). Gram-negative intracellular diplococci suggest *Neisseria* species. Giemsa stains help to distinguish bacterial infections from other causes of conjunctivitis by revealing the predominant cell type. Neutrophils predominate in bacterial, lymphocytes in viral and eosinophils in allergic conjunctivitis. Multinucleated giant cells and eosinophilic intranuclear inclusions suggest HSV infection whereas intracytoplasmic epithelial inclusions suggest chlamydia. Other tests such as immunofluorescent staining for HSV or chlamydial inclusions should be ordered when indicated.

Management

Topical antibiotics are the mainstay of treatment for bacterial conjunctivitis.[1] Topical chloramphenicol is recommended in the United Kingdom as first line, though it is rarely used in North America because of the risk of aplastic anaemia, although the magnitude of this risk is virtually nil.[5] Topical gentamycin or tobramycin may be used for gram-negative infections and erythromycin, bacitracin, polymyxin B/trimethoprim, or neomycin/polymyxin for gram-positive infections but these agents carry a risk of toxic reaction. Fluoroquinolones (e.g. ciprofloxacin and norfloxacin) are commonly used to treat recalcitrant infections or bacterial keratitis.[2] In general, drops are preferred as ointments may cause blurring of vision. At bedtime, ointments are preferred for their long-lasting effect. Treatment of staphylococcal blepharitis consists of eyelid hygiene.

Infants with gonococcal conjunctivitis are at risk of corneal ulceration and perforation, and so Gonococcal conjunctivitis calls for urgent parenteral therapy with aqueous penicillin G or if resistant strains are possible, cefotaxime or ceftriaxone should be used. In addition, the eyes should be irrigated with saline until the discharge is eliminated.

Infants with chlamydial conjunctivitis are at risk for pneumonia and should be treated with oral erythromycin in addition to topical erythromycin. Adult inclusion conjunctivitis can be treated with oral tetracycline or azithromycin; in pregnant or lactating women, erythromycin is an alternative.

In general, viral conjunctivitis is self-limited and does not require antiviral medication but HSV conjunctivitis, because of the potential for keratitis, calls for treatment with acylovir systemically as well as topically.

Allergic conjunctivitis can be treated with oral antihistamines (e.g. astemizole, loratadine, and terfenadine), topical antihistamines (e.g. levocabastine and antazoline) and topical mast cell stabilizers (e.g. sodium cromoglycate, nedocromil, and lodoxamide).[3]

Ophthalmic referral is required if corneal involvement is possible and for atypical or resistant cases.

Prevention

Because of the low incidence of neonatal conjunctivitis, routine prophylaxis has been abandoned in several industrialized countries. In countries where routine ocular prophylaxis is still practised, erythromycin 0.5 per cent ointment is preferred to silver nitrate drops as it is effective against *C. trachomatis* and does not produce chemical conjunctivitis.

Pregnant women infected with *C. trachomatis* or *N. gonorrhoeae* and their sexual consorts should be treated before delivery. Caesarean section should be planned for mothers who have active HSV infection.

Most pathogens are transmitted by secretions, hand-to-eye contact, and exposure to airborne aerosolized particles. Transmission is a major issue in nurseries, schools, and residential homes. Proper hand-washing and careful handling of secretions may prevent spread of infectious conjunctivitis. Accumulated debris should be removed by wiping from the inner canthus outwards, away from the contralateral eye.

Prognosis

The prognosis depends on the underlying cause. The majority of cases are benign and self-limiting. However, some organisms may cause systemic complications. Otitis media may result from *H. influenzae*, meningococcal meningitis from meningococcal, and pneumonia from chlamydial conjunctivitis. Trachoma, gonococcal, and HSV conjunctivitis may lead to blindness if untreated.

Conclusions

Untreated sticky eyes in less developed countries caused by trachoma and gonococcal infection cause blindness and need effective public health action combining promotion of hygiene with access to treatment. In developed countries, sticky eyes caused by allergy and blepharitis can be a diagnostic and management challenge, but most cases seen by primary care physicians do not threaten sight and are often self-limiting. However, sticky eyes can be associated with concomitant corneal disease and uveitis. Consequently patients with eye pain, photophobia, or impaired vision merit urgent referral for an ophthalmic opinion.

Key points

1. The most common cause of a sticky eye is bacterial conjunctivitis.

2. Chloramphenicol remains the most effective topical antibacterial agent.

3. The conjunctival discharge tends to be purulent in bacterial conjunctivitis, serous in viral conjunctivitis, and mucoid in allergic conjunctivitis.

4. The presence of preauricular lymphadenopathy and pharyngitis suggest viral conjunctivitis.

5. Bacterial conjunctivitis is most common in infants and children; viral conjunctivitis becomes more frequent with increasing age.

6. Eye pain, photophobia, and impaired vision indicate concomitant corneal disease or uveitis and necessitate referral to an ophthalmologist.

7. Proper hand-washing and careful handling of secretions may prevent spread of infectious conjunctivitis.

References

1. Weiss, A., Brinser, J.H., and Nazar-Stewart, V. (1993). Acute conjunctivitis in childhood. *The Journal of Pediatrics* **122**, 10–14.

2. Morrow, G.L. and Abott, R.L. (1998). Conjunctivitis. *American Family Physician* **57**, 735–46.

3. Weber, C.M. and Eichenbaum, J.W. (1997). Acute red eye: differentiating viral conjunctivitis from other, less common causes. *Postgraduate Medicine* **101**, 185–96.

4. Leung, A.K. and Bowen, T.J. (2001). Seasonal allergic rhinitis and food allergy. In *Twenty Common Problems in Pediatrics* (ed. A.B. Bergman), pp. 219–33. New York: McGraw-Hill.

5. Chung, C. and Cohen, E. (2000). Bacterial conjunctivitis. *Clinical Evidence* **4**, 350–5.

Further reading

Weiss, A. (1994). Acute conjunctivitis in childhood. *Current Problems in Pediatrics* **24**, 4–11. (This article provides a comprehensive review of the various causes of acute conjunctivitis in childhood.)

Hirst, L.W. (1991). Conjunctivitis. *Australian Family Physician* **20**, 797–804. (This article provides a practical approach to the management of conjunctivitis.)

12.3 Loss of vision

Denise Mabey

Introduction

Eye consultations account for 1.5 per cent of all general practice consultations in the United Kingdom, with a rate of 50 consultations per 1000 population per year to general practice.[1] Cataract accounts for 5 per cent of all new eye problems, open-angle glaucoma (or suspected glaucoma) for 2 per cent, and macular disease for 1 per cent. In 3 per cent of cases, the general practitioner is unable to make a diagnosis and 14 per cent of all new attendees with eye problems in general practice are referred onward to hospital eye services.[2] Patients may bypass the general practitioner and present directly to an eye casualty department (consultation rate 23 consultations per 1000 population per year in one area of the United Kingdom). Many people with significant visual impairment still do not reach the hospital services.[3]

The cause of loss of vision may be anywhere on the visual pathway from refractive errors of the cornea through to field defects from pathology in the occipital cortex. The initial aim is, from the history, to exclude either sudden, profound, or transient loss and then to seek a pattern in the history and examination to determine the anatomical site and aetiology.

Sudden profound loss of vision

The realization of sudden loss of vision may occur on waking in the morning, by a rapid deterioration during the day, or by inadvertently covering one eye and hence discovering that the other eye cannot see. The latter is not true sudden loss but appears so to the sufferer.

An anterior *ischaemic optic neuropathy* causes a swollen optic disc and may be arteritic (when it is possibly associated with giant cell arteritis) or non-arteritic (when the associations are with hypertension and smoking). *Retinal vein occlusions* with multiple scattered haemorrhages are associated with hypertension, glaucoma, and in people under 50 with systemic vasculitis and hyperviscosity syndromes. Central *retinal artery occlusion* occurs in emboli from the heart or carotid arteries. The retina is pale due

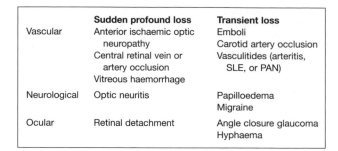

	Sudden profound loss	Transient loss
Vascular	Anterior ischaemic optic neuropathy Central retinal vein or artery occlusion Vitreous haemorrhage	Emboli Carotid artery occlusion Vasculitides (arteritis, SLE, or PAN)
Neurological	Optic neuritis	Papilloedema Migraine
Ocular	Retinal detachment	Angle closure glaucoma Hyphaema

Fig. 1 Causes of sudden profound and transient loss of vision.

to infarction, with a cherry-red spot at the macula. An embolus is visible in 20 per cent of cases.

Optic neuritis, accompanied by pain on eye movements and a relative afferent pupillary defect is found most commonly in young adults. There are usually no abnormal findings on fundoscopy, though the optic disc may be swollen.

Retinal detachments are commonly preceded by floaters and flashes of light and vision is lost if the macula becomes detached. The retina balloons forward into the vitreous.

Transient loss of vision

Visual impairment which is temporary may be in one eye or both and may last from seconds to hours. The range of aetiologies is large and many are treatable. The main causes of transient loss of vision, and of sudden profound loss of vision, are summarized in Fig. 1.

Taking a history

The complaint of loss of vision may mean anything from mild blurring to complete blindness. The three key questions to ask are as follows:

- *Is one eye affected or both?* Ocular and optic nerve disease cause monocular loss, whereas a lesion at or posterior to the chiasm causes binocular loss. Confusion can occur if there is bilateral ocular/optic nerve disease and also because a homonymous hemianopia is often perceived as monocular loss by the patient as they are unaware of the missing field but bump into objects or are unable to read on the affected side.

- *Is the main problem with reading vision, distance vision, or both equally?* Central visual loss is caused typically by macular disease but may occur if the part of the optic nerve which supports the macula is affected, so making reading and recognizing faces the major difficulty, whilst being able to manoeuvre easily around objects. Cataracts, on the other hand, typically cause trouble for distance as they cause myopia, so seeing an approaching bus is more difficult. Age-related macular degeneration, myopic macular degeneration, cilioretinal artery occlusion, central serous retinopathy, and optic neuritis or neuropathy all cause central visual loss.

- *Is the patient at particular risk?* Direct questions should always be asked about diabetes, hypertension, and family history of glaucoma. Diabetes suggests retinopathy or cataract. Hypertension is associated with retinal vein occlusion or an anterior ischaemic optic neuropathy. A family history should be sought for glaucoma or any other eye conditions.

Examination

The various components of visual function that are easily tested in a primary care setting are: acuity, visual field, pupil reactions, and colour vision. They may be affected jointly or separately.

Visual acuity

Acuity is measured with a Snellen chart, usually at 6 m to give acuities written in the form 6/x, or by an ETDRS chart to give a logmar acuity between 0 and 1. Variations for various alphabets and illiterate populations are available. For monocular visual loss, the acuity is proportional to the degree of damage to the central retina or the macular fibres in the optic nerve. If however there is a hemianopic field defect the visual acuities may be normal or only mildly reduced as the remaining half of the field is intact. Re-testing the acuity using a pinhole overcomes refractive errors and gives the best achievable acuity. Reading vision is tested with reading glasses if worn, using a standard chart at a normal reading distance. It is also worthwhile to bring the chart closer, as if that improves the vision then there is some degree of myopia.

Visual field

Visual fields are tested by comparing the observer's field against the patient's, one eye at a time, initially by hand movements and counting fingers in the four quadrants and then defining the areas of loss with a neurological pin. The patterns of loss to search for are: a *homonymous loss* with an occipital/parietal pathology, a *bitemporal loss* with a chiasmal lesion, a *monocular altitudinal loss* with an ischaemic optic neuropathy, a *central scotoma* in optic neuropathy or macular disease, and *gross constriction* in advanced glaucoma.

Relative afferent pupillary defect (RAPD)

This is tested with a bright light swung from eye to eye. The normal is for the pupils to stay constricted as the light moves from one side to the other. A positive RAPD is a pupil that dilates despite the light swing from the other eye, indicating either *optic nerve disease* as in glaucoma or *extensive retinal damage* as in a retinal detachment. Conditions which do *not* cause an RAPD are a dense cataract (although the light is scattered, it still reaches the retina), small lesions at the macula (which can cause profound loss of vision), pathology posterior to the chiasm, and amblyopia.

Colour vision

This can be tested crudely by comparing the brightness of a red object to each eye in turn. The duller red indicates pathology. Various plates exist of which the Ishihara is the most commonly used. To interpret the results, which show red/green colour confusion one should remember that 8 per cent of males and 0.5 per cent of females are colour deficient and also that any pathology which reduces the vision below 6/36 will affect the test. The test is of most use in pinpointing pathology to the optic nerve when colour vision is lost disproportionately to visual acuity.

How to examine the eye

An ophthalmoscope at arm's length is used to determine if there is a red reflex coming back from the retina. An absence means an opacity of the media, most commonly cataract although small pupils may not transmit sufficient light to be easily detected. A naked eye examination will pick up corneal opacities and a dense cataract but little else causing loss of vision. A slit-lamp is used to examine as far as the anterior vitreous and with the addition of a hand-held lens will give a binocular view of the fundus. The ophthalmoscope gives a magnified and monocular view of the back of the eye. The most important fundoscopic abnormalities are shown in Fig. 2.

Principles of management

Sudden profound loss of vision

All cases will require hospital referral—giant cell arteritis and retinal detachment the same day, the others as soon as an appointment can be arranged. In the over-60s, consider *temporal arteritis* and if the history is suggestive and there is a pale swollen optic disc take blood for estimation of

	Haemorrhages throughout retina	Haemorrhages + exudates	Swollen optic disc
Unilateral	Retinal vein occlusion[a]	—	Anterior ischaemic optic neuropathy
Bilateral	Accelerated hypertension	Diabetic retinopathy	Raised intracranial pressure

[a] The addition of cotton wool spots indicates ischaemia and is a bad prognostic sign.

Fig. 2 Important diagnostic abnormalities on fundoscopy.

ESR and CRP then give intravenous hydrocortisone 200 mg and refer urgently for high-dose steroids under surveillance, as side-effects in the elderly should be monitored. Giving a short course of steroids will not affect the positivity of a temporal artery biopsy. If the index of suspicion is low for giant cell arteritis but there is a swollen disc then the likely diagnosis is non-arteritic *ischaemic optic neuropathy*, so advise against smoking and measure blood pressure, urine for protein, ESR, and CRP. If the retina shows multiple haemorrhages suggesting a *retinal vein occlusion* measure blood pressure, full blood count, ESR and CRP, plasma proteins, glucose, lipids, antinuclear antibodies, and in the under-50s, a clotting screen. If the retina is pale and infarcted, showing a *central retinal artery occlusion*, consider retinal embolization. If arteritis is excluded, arrange full blood count, glucose, lipids, autoantibody screen, carotid ultrasound, and echocardiogram.

Transient visual loss

The management depends on the varied underlying causes. Monocular transient total loss of vision (*amaurosis fugax*) may herald retinal artery occlusion. *Intermittent angle closure* is commoner in longsighted people over the age of 50 and causes pain and intermittent coloured haloes around lights. A slit-lamp examination is needed and should be performed by an optometrist the same day.

Screening programmes

Screening programmes run by general practitioners exist for diabetic retinopathy (annual) and may be supplemented by retinal photography. National screening policy varies between countries—some have well-established programmes, particularly for diabetic retinopathy and glaucoma. All countries should have a clear and explicit policy.

Long-term medications

Patients on long-term medication also require careful monitoring which requires the same sort of systematic call–recall as screening. Monitoring must focus not only on the condition but the possibility of complications. For example, patients on glaucoma treatment may suffer breathing difficulties with systemic absorption of topical beta blockers and be unaware of the cause, putting it down to old age.[4]

Implications for quality of life

Loss of visual acuity has major implications for quality of life and general practitioners can help to ameliorate this impact by recognizing the problem and offering appropriate help and advice. In addition, in many countries, the practitioner has statutory obligations in relation to issues such as certifying fitness to drive.

Driving

In the United Kingdom, the requirements for private car use are that the licence holder should be able to read a car number plate at 20.5 m, which equates to an acuity between 6/9 and 6/12. There is also a field of vision requirement of 120° on the horizontal. If the general practitioner knows that a patient does not fulfil these requirements, the patient must be advised to contact the relevant Driver and Vehicle Licensing Authority.

Social services

Of the predicted million people in the United Kingdom eligible, only a quarter have been registered blind or partially sighted and of the remaining three quarters a sizeable proportion are unknown to health and social services.[5] General practitioners must inform themselves of the mechanism to access help from statutory authorities (in the United Kingdom it requires completion of form BD8 by an ophthalmologist).

Getting help and advice

Non-governmental organizations and charities (such as the Royal National Institute for the Blind in the United Kingdom) often provide information and resources for anyone with visual impairment. Again, the general practitioner should provide patients with information about how to access such resources.

Key points

- Giant cell arteritis must always be excluded in over 60-year-olds.
- Safety to drive should be addressed by the general practitioner.
- Many people with impaired vision do not receive the help they need (an estimated 750 000 blind and visually impaired are unknown to statutory services in the United Kingdom).

References

1. Sheldrick, J. et al. (1993). Management of ophthalmic disease in general practice. *British Journal of General Practice* **43**, 459–62.
2. Sheldrick, J. et al. (1992). Demand incidence and episode rates of ophthalmic disease in a defined urban population. *British Medical Journal* **305**, 933–9.
3. Reidy, A. et al. (1998). Prevalence of serious eye disease and visual impairment in a north London population: population based, cross sectional study. *British Medical Journal* **316**, 1643–7.
4. Diggory, P. and Franks, W.A. (1997). Glaucoma therapy may take your breath away. *Age and Ageing* **26** (2), 63–7.
5. Bruce, I., McKennell, A., and Walker, E. *Blind and Partially Sighted Adults in Britain: The RNIB Survey* Vol. 1. The Royal National Institute for the Blind, 1991. (Discusses services available to the visually impaired and their uptake.)

Further reading

Evans, J. Causes of blindness and partial sight in England and Wales 1990–1991. *Studies on Medical and Population Subjects, No. 57.* Office of Population Censuses, 1995. (Gives national data on blindness registration.)

Thylefors, B. et al. (1995). Global data on blindness. *Bulletin of the World Health Organisation* **73**, 115–21. (Provides international data on causes of visual loss.)

12.4 Ptosis and unequal pupils

Peggy Frith

Asymmetry of lid position or of pupil size are not uncommonly noticed, especially by patients who are particularly concerned about their appearance or who delve into medical tomes. They may cause major anxiety, for example, in a professional model or a medical student studying neurology. If the inequality is slight, either alone is unlikely to herald a sinister underlying cause, but if there are other associated clinical features the plot thickens and further investigation may be needed. Sometimes, unequal lid and pupil are noted together, an important observation. The eye with the droopy lid is likely to be the abnormal one, so if the pupil on this side is smaller this could be a Horner's syndrome; if larger, a third nerve lesion. With an acute onset and pronounced inequality, there is more likely to be an important identifiable cause. Immediate action may be necessary.

Simple anatomy

The upper eyelid is maintained by two muscles—the levator supplied by a branch of the third nerve and Muller's muscle supplied by the sympathetic. Drooping may be caused by swelling of the lid, weakness of one of the muscles or a palsy of either nerve, partial or complete.

The iris has a *dual autonomic nerve supply*, parasympathetic to constrict and sympathetic to dilate, so the pupil dilates with a parasympathetic, and constricts with a sympathetic, palsy. The iris itself may be damaged by trauma, ischaemia, or inflammation, or its size altered by systemic or topical drugs.

How significant is the inequality?

Ptosis may be present from birth, in which case it is usually minor and of cosmetic importance, without neurological or functional implications. There may be a family history and old photos taken in babyhood may show that the droop is longer-standing than originally thought. Occasionally, *congenital ptosis* may interfere with the child's vision so that referral to the eye clinic is needed to assess the risk of amblyopia. Note that the upper lid is usually retracted, and not ptosed, in thyroid eye disease, and that facial palsy causes not ptosis, but failure of eye closure.

Slightly unequal pupils are common in otherwise normal people and it may be difficult to be sure if the observation is significant. If there are no other clinical features, and in particular if there is no ptosis, then to wait and watch is reasonable.

Third nerve palsy with a large pupil

A *complete ptosis* is likely to be due to a lesion of the nerve which supplies the levator muscle of the upper lid. This is part of the third cranial (oculomotor) nerve which also supplies other external eye muscles and is associated with parasympathetic fibres running on the outside which constrict the pupil and focus for near vision. With a complete third nerve palsy, once the ptosed lid is lifted the patient will complain that *vision is double* in most directions and a *dilated pupil* may be found. Of course, if the third nerve palsy is partial the ptosis will be incomplete, eye movements may not be affected, and the pupil may be normal. An acute third nerve palsy has several causes, some urgent and possibly compressive, others systemic and involving small blood vessels, with diabetes at the top of the list. Pupil involvement suggests compression.

Alternative rare causes of a complete ptosis include *myasthenia gravis*—in which case the ptosis will be variable, fatiguable, and probably bilateral, though asymmetrical—and iatrogenic after *botulinum toxin* injection. Either of these may cause double vision but myasthenia does not dilate the pupil. There may be other muscles which are weak and fatiguable, for example, affecting eye closure, speech, or proximal limb strength.

Adie's pupil

Adie's pupil is large, usually unilateral—in 80 per cent—and irregular with a characteristic iris reaction. It is typically noticed suddenly in young adults. The diagnosis can be confirmed by a simple pharmacological test and this is important as the finding is almost certain to be innocent, not warranting a scan or CSF sampling. Best to refer to the eye department where the necessary experience, slit-lamp, and dilute pilocarpine are usually available, though not as an emergency.

The patient notices that the pupil is large, especially in bright light which constricts the normally reactive twin, accentuates the inequality and may induce photophobia. There may be difficulty reading with some blurring of near vision and discomfort in the affected eye, though pain is never pronounced and there is no ptosis. Sometimes, there is alarm because a medically trained colleague notices a unilaterally dilated pupil; warning bells ring and the patient is whisked to the nearest casualty department. There are no other neurological features except that some patients have absent lower limb reflexes—the Holmes–Adie syndrome, of unexplained origin. The Adie pupil is thought to be due to pathology in the parasympathetic ciliary ganglion behind the eye within the orbit, and may occasionally follow an attack of herpes zoster ophthalmicus.

The findings are of a pupil which paradoxically reacts better to near effort than to bright light. The pupil is irregular and iris constriction seen by slit-lamp is patchy with spiralling, and 'tonic' as it constricts and redilates slowly. The larger Adie pupil constricts to become smaller within 20 min after one drop of dilute (0.1 per cent) pilocarpine, whereas the normal pupil is unaffected. The patient is impressed to see in the mirror this obvious proof of a positive test and will be relieved to hear that the Adie phenomenon is benign and not associated with stroke, brain tumour, or multiple sclerosis. The difficulty with focus will persist but is rarely disabling and the pupil often becomes smaller over the following months. It is important that the patient understands the name and nature of their unusual pupil, especially to prevent medical bafflement or alarm in the future, for example, after head injury or stroke.

Horner's syndrome with a small pupil

Horner's syndrome associates a small pupil with an incomplete ptosis. It is due to interruption of the sympathetic nerve supply to the eye on the same side, somewhere in a long path from the brain, down the spinal cord, through the autonomic ganglion in the neck, adjacent to the lung apex and back up the carotid arterial tree. The degree of ptosis is usually slight and never complete; usually somewhere above the pupil margin and so not obstructing vision. Loss of sweating on the forehead is possible but rarely found with certainty.

Salient features in the history include trauma to the head or neck sufficient to damage the spinal cord or carotid artery, for instance, a whiplash. Pain or other neurological deficit in the head, neck, upper chest, or arm may indicate the site or suggest a link with migraine. There are many causes, the majority vascular, and a scan of head and neck to include the apex of the lung is usually justified. As a painless and isolated finding, Horner's is unlikely to signal a sinister lesion, except in childhood.

Pupils in an emergency setting

In an emergency setting, pupillary signs are objective, always significant and may be crucial to diagnosis. Key diagnostic pointers are shown in Fig. 1.

Trauma to the eye can dilate the pupil by direct damage to the iris. This may be blunt or penetrating, but either is a sign of significant damage which requires immediate expert assessment in eye casualty. Acute rise in ocular pressure also results in an ischaemic, oval, fixed, enlarged pupil associated with pain and, often also with vomiting. Iritis puts the pupil into spasm so it becomes small and may stick to the lens, looking irregular after dilatation with drops. Argyll Robertson pupils are now very rare; they are small, irregular and react better to near than to light. A lumbar puncture is warranted to test for active CNS syphilis.

Trauma to the head, especially the temple, may rupture the middle meningeal artery so that blood accumulates rapidly as an *extradural haematoma*. This compresses the third nerve so that the ipsilateral pupil dilates progressively as consciousness falls. Heroism with a brace and bit drilled into the temple may save life in this dire emergency—the sort of scenario doctors hope never to meet and certainly never rehearse.

Possibly in the setting of coma, subarachnoid haemorrhage with a dilated pupil suggests rupture of a *posterior communicating aneurysm* which presses on the parasympathetic fibres running on the surface of the third nerve. Raised intracranial pressure alone, especially if lateralized, may cause uncal herniation of the brain with the same result. Either dictates immediate referral to a neurosurgical centre.

Bilaterally dilated pupils in an acute setting may signify fear, muscarinic poisoning as with nightshade or some fungi, or intoxication with tricyclic, amphetamine, ecstasy, or perhaps cannabis. Very occasionally, there is deliberate or inadvertent instillation of atropine-like eyedrops. Bilaterally small pupils suggest opiate use, anticholinesterase poisoning or, if pinpoint sized, pontine haemorrhage.

Equal pupils with an unequal response to light (relative afferent pupil defect) is a very important objective finding. It does not present as inequality of the pupils but as an asymmetrical reaction to direct light shone alternately in one eye then the other. The pupil on the affected side tends to dilate instead of constrict in response. The sign must signify damage on one side to input before the chiasm, and so within the retina or optic nerve on that side. Some causes are central retinal artery occlusion, sometimes retinal vein occlusion; optic nerve compression on one side; unilateral glaucoma; acute optic neuropathy (especially optic neuritis in younger, and ischaemic in older, patients); extensive retinal detachment.

Key points

- Slightly unequal pupils are common and in the absence of ptosis are unlikely to be significant.
- A large irregular pupil in a young person is likely to be due to Adie's syndrome.
- Ptosis is likely to be due to a third nerve palsy or Horner's syndrome.
- Pupillary signs are always significant in an emergency setting.

Further reading

Bacon, A.S. and Collin, J.R.O. (1999). Oculoplastic surgery. In *Oxford Textbook of Ophthalmology* (ed. D. L. Easty and J. M. Sparrow), pp. 1139–42 (including ptosis). Oxford: Oxford University Press.

Brazier, J. and Smith, S.E. (1999). Disorders of the pupil. In *Oxford Textbook of Ophthalmology* (ed. D.L. Easty and J.M. Sparrow), pp. 862–6. Oxford: Oxford University Press. (A two-volume reference book focusing on practical aspects.)

Kardon, R.H. (1998). Anatomy and physiology of the pupil. In: *Walsh & Hoyt's Clinical Neuro-Ophthalmology* 5th edn., Vol. 1 (ed. N.R. Miller), pp. 847–97. Philadelphia PA: Williams and Wilkins. (A five-volume reference tome which covers all possible aspects of common and uncommon dilemmas.)

Important questions	Key answers
Diagnosis?	
Is the inequality of lid or pupil significant?	Marked inequality Recent onset Pain
Which side is abnormal?	Probably the side with droopy lid
Are there associated symptoms or signs?	Lid and pupil both affected
Is this a recognizable pattern?	Third nerve palsy Horner's Adie's
Investigate?	
Should simple tests be done?	Blood sugar Myasthenia antibodies
Refer?	
Refer immediately?	Trauma Reduced consciousness Possible poisoning
Refer for further investigation?	Scan Slit-lamp exam Pilocarpine test

Fig. 1 Key points in assessing and managing pupillary abnormality in primary care.

12.5 Visual disturbances

E. Robert Schwartz

Visual disturbances are often presented urgently to the primary care physician and for the patient or family they are usually quite disturbing symptoms. Unlike many common symptoms, they often present the physician with a diagnostic dilemma.

The history is important in establishing onset, duration, and type of symptom. The key questions to ask are summarized in Fig. 1. Getting the patient to accurately describe the type of visual disturbance that they are experiencing is an important step in establishing the diagnosis. Age and prior medical history will often assist. Illnesses such as diabetes, thyroid, or cardiovascular disease may be important precursors or causes. Trauma, brain tumour, and aneurysm, although rare in primary care practice, may still need to be considered in the differential diagnosis.

Visual disturbances can be classified into five categories:

1. Blurred vision.

2. Sudden loss of vision.

Nature
One or both eyes?
Sudden or gradual?
Migraine, metabolic, vascular history?

Fig. 1 Key questions to ask of a patient with blurred vision.

Monocular blurred vision	Binocular blurred vision
With normal pupils	Improves with pinhole
Macular degeneration	Refractive error
Cataract	Does not improve with pinhole
Retinal vein occlusion	Macular degeneration
Diabetic retinopathy	Cataract
Retinal detachment	Diabetic retinopathy
With abnormal pupils	
Optic neuritis	
Anterior ischaemic optic neuropathy	

Fig. 2 Causes of blurred vision.

3.   Flashes and floaters.

4.   Double vision.

5.   Visual field defects.

This chapter focuses on the causation and management of each.

Blurred vision

The most common complaint is often that of blurred vision. First, it is important to distinguish whether vision is blurred in one eye or both (monocular or binocular). The differential diagnosis of monocular visual loss includes problems with cornea, lens, vitreous, retina or optic nerve, such as cataract, diabetic retinopathy, macular degeneration, or retinal vascular occlusion. The main causes of blurred vision are summarized in Fig. 2.

Refractive error

Blurred vision is most commonly caused by an error of refraction—myopia, hypermetropia, or astigmatism. *Pinhole testing* is the most simple way to confirm whether the patient's visual acuity can be improved by refraction. Glasses and contact lenses traditionally have been the treatment for refractive errors.

Keratitis

Keratitis (corneal inflammation) usually presents with a painful eye and visual acuity is decreased if the lesion is central. On examination, there may be *loss of corneal clarity* and *fluorescein staining* may show epithelium disruption. Corneal oedema and ciliary congestion may also be present. Common causes are dry eye, infections, and trauma (including foreign bodies). Treatment depends upon the underlying cause, but urgent referral to confirm both diagnosis and aetiology is usually indicated. Anti-infective agents are used to manage traumatic or infective keratitis.

Cataract

Cataract describes any lens opacity from the smallest dot to complete opacification. The prevalence of cataract increases with age and 65 per cent of people aged 50–59 have opacities and 100 per cent over 80 years. Depending if the cataract is monocular or binocular, the patient may complain of difficulty in reading, recognizing faces, watching television, seeing in bright light, and driving. Cataracts may be obvious from the opacification of the normally clear lens, best seen against the red reflex, and the retina may appear indistinct on fundoscopy. Although cataract is predominantly a problem of the elderly, congenital cataract presents during childhood and an opaque lens in the newborn merits urgent referral. Other specific causes of cataract in all ages include drugs (particularly steroids), trauma, radiation, diabetes, and hypocalcaemia. Patients experiencing visual difficulty should normally be referred non-urgently for cataract surgery.

Diabetic retinopathy

This is the commonest cause of blindness in the Western world. The longer the duration of diabetes, the more likely the patient is to have retinopathy (about 80 per cent are affected after 20 years). Cataract and chronic open angle glaucoma are more common in diabetics than non-diabetics. Diabetics are also more prone to retinal vein occlusion, and cranial nerve palsies. All adult diabetics should have their pupils dilated and fundi examined yearly by someone with appropriate expertise (e.g. an optician) and the primary care physician has a responsibility to ensure this is done. If retinopathy is identified the frequency of examination may be increased so that in moderate to severe cases it should be performed every 3–4 months.

Two types of diabetic retinopathy may be seen. *Non-proliferative retinopathy* is typified by microaneurysms, dot haemorrhages, and hard yellow exudates with well-defined edges. When they occur in the macular area central vision may be affected. Extensive exudate suggests hyperlipidaemia. *Proliferative retinopathy* is typically characterized by the growth of new vessels on the retina or in the vitreous cavity. These vessels may bleed, causing a sudden decrease in vision due to a vitreous haemorrhage. New vessels also grow on to the iris occluding the drainage angle of the anterior chamber and causing a painful hard eye (rubeotic glaucoma). Laser treatment is normally instigated before there is retinal thickening or vitreous haemorrhage.

Age-related macular degeneration (ARMD)

This common condition of old age is covered in the section on blindness. It seldom occurs in those aged less than 50 years. Exudative ('wet') ARMD may present with distortion of straight lines, rapid onset of visual loss or a blind patch in the central visual field. Symptoms may progress rapidly over a few days or weeks. Non-exudative ('dry') ARMD usually presents with gradual loss of central vision and may be asymptomatic in the early stages.

Effective examination in primary care requires field testing (e.g. Amsler's grid) to detect a central scotoma. Retinal examination may reveal haemorrhages, and screening with pigment. Most primary care physicians will seek an expert opinion to confirm the diagnosis. Patients with sudden onset of visual disturbance or suspicion of wet ARMD should be referred rapidly as laser photocoagulation applied within 72 h can reduce the risk of severe loss of vision in selected cases.

No proven treatment is available for dry ARMD. Oral nutritional supplements may help. Low-vision aids may benefit patients with bilateral macular degeneration. Patients with wet or dry ARMD may be given Amsler's grid as a method of self-monitoring, particularly to detect change in the second eye and ensure early recognition and referral in wet ARMD.

Retinal vein occlusion

This normally presents as a blind area in the visual field. The critical sign is superficial haemorrhages in a sector of the retina along the retinal vein. Other signs are cotton-wool spots, retinal oedema, a dilated and tortuous retinal vein, narrowing and sheathing of the adjacent artery, retinal neovascularization, or vitreous haemorrhage. *Urgent referral is indicated.* Treatment involves retinal laser photocoagulation.

Retinal vein occlusion may be a manifestation of generalized vascular disease, often reflecting underlying diabetes, hypertension, or arteriosclerosis, and should be investigated and managed accordingly by the primary care physician.

Optic neuritis

Optic neuritis causes loss of vision, deteriorating over days. It is almost always unilateral. There is often pain and reduced perception of light intensity. The patient is typically between 18 and 45 years of age. Other focal neurological symptoms may also be present. On examination the critical signs are a *relative afferent pupillary defect* (tested by shining a light into each pupil in turn) and *decreased colour vision*, sometimes associated with a visual-field defects (see Chapter 12.3) typically a central scotoma. Fundoscopy shows a swollen or normal disc with or without haemorrhage. Many cases are idiopathic, but known causes include multiple sclerosis (MS), childhood infections, meningitis, and intraocular inflammation. Patients should be referred to confirm the diagnosis; those with abnormal neurological signs should be referred to a neurologist.

Sudden loss of vision

This topic is covered in more depth in Chapter 12.3 by Mabey. The main ocular causes of sudden visual loss are occlusion of retinal blood vessels, vitreous haemorrhage, optic nerve disorders, trauma, and retinal detachment. A number of causes of visual loss are non-ocular—migraine, syncope, and stroke can all disrupt the visual pathway. The most common ocular cause of sudden visual loss is retinal vascular occlusion or haemorrhage. Transient retinal artery occlusion may cause fleeting blindness for a few minutes—amaurosis fugax (see below). Retinal detachment involving the macula can present as sudden visual loss but the challenge to primary care is to recognize symptoms of detachment at an earlier, treatable, stage. Optic nerve disorders may cause patients to report sudden visual loss, but onset of symptoms is more often gradual. Acute glaucoma leads to rapid visual loss, but usually presents as a severely painful red eye.

Flashes and floaters

The main causes of flashes and floaters are shown in Fig. 3. Migraine is probably the commonest cause of flashing 'scintillating' lights, but as flashing lights and spots can indicate a number of sight-threatening conditions, accurate diagnosis is important. Unless the GP is confident in a diagnosis of migraine or innocent vitreous opacities, urgent referral is indicated. Posterior uveitis and neoplasms are uncommon causes of floaters.

Posterior vitreous detachment (PVD)

The main symptoms are floaters ('cobwebs', 'bugs', or comma-shaped objects which move with eye movement) with flashes of light. The critical sign is *vitreous opacities* which float within the vitreous with eye movement. Other signs include vitreous or retinal haemorrhages, cells in the vitreous, and retinal tears or detachment. The main cause is age related degenerative changes in the vitreous. Patients often refer to the flashes of light as like 'sparks'. Although no treatment is indicated for vitreous detachment alone, if an acute retinal tear is found, laser or cryotherapy is important.

Migraine
Posterior vitreous detachment
Retinal detachment*
Posterior uveitis (uncommon)
Neoplasm (rare)

* Unless the GP is confident in a diagnosis of migraine or innocent vitreous opacities, urgent referral is indicated to exclude this diagnosis.

Fig. 3 Causes of flashes and floaters.

Retinal detachment

Retinal tears and detachment (i.e. separation of the sensory retina from the underlying epithelium) need urgent recognition and referral. The main symptoms are flashes and floaters. Patients may describe a curtain or shadow across the vision. Fundal examination may reveal an area ballooning into the vitreous but patients with suggestive symptoms should be referred urgently for ophthalmic examination whether or not signs of detachment or tear are identified by the GP. Laser therapy, cryotherapy, or scleral-buckling surgery is required within 24–72 h for acute retinal tears.

Double vision

Double vision (diplopia) is caused by the image of an object falling on the fovea of one eye but not of the other. It is often associated with overt squint (strabismus). Concomitant squints (i.e. ones that do not change with the angle of gaze) are most common in childhood, although 'latent squints' leading, for example, to difficulty in maintaining convergence with diplopia on reading or close work, are relatively common in adulthood and merit orthoptic referral. However, the main diagnostic challenge for the GP are paralytic squints caused by palsies of the ocular muscles.

The key diagnostic strategy is to cover each eye in turn. This allows confirmation that the doubling is indeed binocular. With both eyes open the patient is asked to follow an object in the various directions of gaze to discover in which direction separation of the images is greatest. As each eye is covered, the patient is asked to locate the image which is furthest displaced.

Most cases of sudden onset paralytic squint should be referred for an ophthalmic opinion.

Third nerve palsy

Complete palsy gives ptosis, a non-responding pupil, and deviation of the paralysed eye laterally and downwards. However, most oculomotor nerve palsies are incomplete. The most common causes are diabetes, trauma, or stroke. A non-responsive pupil of acute onset suggests an aneurysm at the posterior communicating artery; a reactive pupil suggests the cause may be microvascular disease especially diabetes. Patients with complete palsies require an urgent MRI or CT scan.

Sixth nerve palsy

Weakness of the lateral rectus muscle causes horizontal diplopia worse at distance than near. Diplopia is more pronounced in the direction of the involved lateral rectus muscle. Patients may keep their heads turned to minimize diplopia. Causes include diabetes, multiple sclerosis, compression, stroke, recent lumbar puncture, and myasthenia gravis. Immediate referral for neurologic evaluation is essential if the patient is a young child because of the risk of pontine glioma. Most older patients will have a vascular cause.

Fourth nerve palsy

Weakness of the trochlear nerve causes vertical diplopia, worse when the patient attempts near tasks. Patients complain of difficulty in reading, and again may adopt a compensatory head posture. Causes include trauma, hypertension, diabetes, multiple sclerosis, and myasthenia gravis.

All patients with paralytic diplopia should be advised not to drive. Many elderly patients with paralytic squint will be suffering from a vascular lesion of the central nervous system and should be managed as a minor stroke with appropriate preventive management to minimize the risk of a subsequent major stroke.

Visual field defects

Few practitioners will have access to ophthalmic equipment to test visual fields but all are able to compare a patients peripheral vision with their own and to instruct patients to use an Amsler grid. The simplest distinction is between monocular and binocular defects.

Monocular visual field defects

The most common problems causing monocular visual field defects are glaucoma and the muscular degenerative changes of old age. The presence of an impaired pupillary response to light suggests an optic nerve lesion.

In *glaucoma*, the characteristic visual field losses are arcuate scotomas and nasal defects. Risk of glaucoma is suggested by the presence of factors such as family history of blindness or glaucoma, hypertension, elderly, black race, myopia, previous history of increased intraocular pressure, or chronic steroid use. Fundoscopy may reveal the optic nerve is cupped. Referral is usually necessary for measurement of pressure. Topical glaucoma agents are the first line of defence; surgical treatments may be used in unresponsive cases.

Other causes of monocular field loss include *retinal lesions* such as macular degeneration. Symptoms may include decreased and distorted vision and examination will often reveal decreased visual acuity or colour vision.

Binocular visual field defect

People with bilateral visual loss complain of poor side vision, bumping into objects on one side, or central vision difficulties. The key finding is visual field loss affecting the same field in each eye, of which the commonest cause is stroke. Patients without an explanatory diagnosis need referral to a neurologist for further evaluation.

People with *bitemporal hemianopia* often have vague complaints of peripheral vision loss or other visual problems; women with this condition may have associated changes in their menstrual cycle. The critical sign is bitemporal visual field defect. Visual acuity may or may not be affected. The aetiology is chiasmal lesion due to pituitary tumour. Tilted discs are the only benign cause. Patients should be referred to a neurologist as soon as possible for neurological evaluation and treatment of any underlying condition.

Scotomas

Central scotomas are often bilateral and usually occur in the elderly. They cause reduced visual acuity or a 'patch', leading to not being able to read or recognize faces. They are usually caused by *macular degeneration*.

Conclusions

Consultations for acute visual disturbance are often characterized by anxiety in both the patient and GP. The most important feature of any primary care consultation is the history, and careful questioning is necessary to elicit the key information cited above. In the light of this information, the GP needs to carry out a careful ocular examination to rule out a number of important conditions in which delay can cause irretrievable further loss of vision. These conditions are summarized in Fig. 4. The simple rule is, *if in doubt, refer* for an ophthalmic opinion.

Symptom/sign	Important diagnoses needing referral
Blurred vision	Keratitis—urgent
	Exudative (wet) ARMD
	Retinal vein occlusion
Sudden loss of vision	Retinal vein occlusion
	Retinal detachment—urgent
	Acute glaucoma (but pain predominates)—urgent
Flashes and floaters	Retinal tear or detachment—urgent
Double vision	Cranial nerve palsy
Field defect	Glaucoma suspected
	Unexplained hemianopia

Note: Unless the GP can confidently exclude these diagnoses, referral of patients with these symptoms/signs is mandatory.

Fig. 4 Making a safe diagnosis.

Key points

- ◆ Sudden loss of vision or sudden onset of double vision merits urgent referral.

- ◆ Flashing lights and floaters require urgent referral to exclude retinal detachment unless a firm diagnosis of migraine or vitreous haemorrhage can be made.

- ◆ If in diagnostic doubt, refer.

Further reading

Bezan, D.J. and LaRussa, F.P. *Differential Diagnosis in Primary Eye Care* 1st edn. London: Butterworth-Heinemann, 1999.

Rakel, R.E. *Saunders Manual of Medical Practice* 2nd edn. New York: WB Saunders Company, 2000.

Rhee, D.J., Pyfer, M.F., and Aftab, A. (1999). Office and emergency room diagnosis and treatment of eye diseases. In *The Willis Eye Manual* 3rd edn. (ed. D.J. Rhee and M.F. Pyfer), pp. 1–17. Philadelphia PA: Lippincott Williams & Wilkins.

12.6 Blindness

Suber S. Huang and George E. Kikano

While some eye problems cause immediate symptoms and require attention, it is critical that the primary practitioner be cognizant of the worldwide causes of visual impairment. In the United States, disability from all causes of vision impairment rank third behind cardiovascular disease and arthritis as a major cause of disability in the over 65-year-old population. Inability to see gravely impacts on patient's ability to care for themselves and others. The worldwide cost to society of blindness remains staggering. The World Health Organization (WHO) estimates that there are between 40 and 45 million persons who are so blind that they cannot walk about unaided and 160 million people in the world with disabling visual impairment. The number of blind and visually impaired is expected to double over the next 25 years and the role of primary care physicians in local, national, and international programmes, is crucial in the fight against blindness.[1,2] Blinding disorders can occur in many settings. Acute disease including ocular trauma, external infection, and angle closure glaucoma are often accompanied by acute, painful loss of vision. Acute symptoms of pain and visual loss are easily identified and should be appropriately referred.

Other blinding diseases may be asymptomatic or subtle and require a high index of suspicion for progressive chronic disease. A myriad of ocular complications of systemic disease exists. Blinding complications of endocrine, connective tissue or haematologic disease, hypertension, atherosclerosis, viral infection including HIV, toxic retinopathy, intraocular metastatic tumours, and changes associated with pregnancy all have blinding manifestations which may be undetected until late stages. The main causes of blindness worldwide are shown in Table 1, which is based on a 1997 WHO report.[2] It is important for the primary care physician to be aware that these conditions can be prevented or treated in the majority of cases.

Table 1 Main causes of blindness worldwide

Cataract	43%

Degenerative retinopathy
   Diabetic retinopathy
   Age-related macular degeneration
   Other metabolic degenerative disease
	24%

Glaucoma	15%
Trachoma	11%
Vitamin A deficiency	6%
Onchocerciasis	1%

Cataract

Opacification of the lens is a major health problem and accounts for approximately one-half of all blindness worldwide. In Western countries, this usually occurs later in life, in persons over 50 years of age. It is estimated that 50 per cent of people aged 60 years or more and 100 per cent of people 80 years or older have notable lens opacification. There are an estimated 5 million patients in India, 2 million in China, and at least 3 million cataract-blind in Africa. In India, approximately 3.8 million new persons develop cataract-blindness annually. The number of cataract operations performed annually in India is less than 2 million, and therefore, sight is restored by surgery in only one-half of new cataract-blind. The number of cataract-blind is a universal problem in developing nations worldwide.[3,4]

Cataract is also an important cause of treatable childhood blindness. There are an estimated 200 000 children blind from cataract worldwide, and 20 000–40 000 children with developmental or bilateral cataract are born each year. It is estimated that prevalence of one to four per 10 000 children in industrialized countries and 5–15 per 10 000 children in developing countries develop blindness from cataract.[3–5] Although some risk factors have been identified, no primary preventative treatment is known. Surgical removal of cataracts remains the only proven therapy and can be successful in restoring vision in over 95 per cent of patients without concurrent eye disease. This technology is widely accepted and available in the developing world. In 1993, the World Bank ranked cataract surgery in the most highly cost-effective category—the only surgical intervention to reach that rank.[6] This common cause of visual loss is easily established through visual acuity and screening examinations. Symptoms may include painless progressive loss of vision with diminished ability to see at distance and at near, with glare.

In developing countries, efforts to identify treatable risk factors continue. The role of sunlight, nutrition, diet, dehydration, medication, diabetes, and socio-economic factors in accelerating lens opacification continues to be studied. Worldwide, we must recognize the magnitude of this problem and effect changes in the infrastructure of healthcare delivery, education, and development of screening programmes that will assist in creating regional self-sufficiency and effective allocation of resources.

Age-related macular degeneration (AMD)

An estimated 6 million Americans have visual loss from AMD and another 13–15 million Americans have pre-symptomatic signs. Some form of AMD affects 25 to 30 million people worldwide. It is estimated that costs for medical and long-term care for older Americans who lose their independence each year are $26 billion greater than if they had remained independent that year.[7,8] In an international survey of adults 18 years and older, only 2 per cent of all adults surveyed recognize that AMD is the leading cause of severe sight loss in adults 50 years and older. Only 13 per cent of adults surveyed think that the main purpose of an eye examination is to detect eye diseases at an early stage. In England and Wales, AMD now accounts for approximately 50 per cent of registered blindness.[9]

Two forms of age-related maculopathy exist. 'Dry' AMD is estimated to affect approximately 90 per cent, while 10 per cent develop 'wet' AMD and choroidal neovascularization (CNV) with subsequent bleeding, leakage, or formation of scar tissue. Although less common, wet AMD accounts for 90 per cent of blindness from AMD.

In dry AMD, macular changes are characterized by the deposition of small yellow, discrete, fatty deposits called drusen. Age-related changes may be slow and asymptomatic. Many patients are unaware of AMD and attribute diminished contrast sensitivity and visual acuity to the need for spectacle correction, cataract, or 'getting older'. In wet AMD, abnormal leaking blood vessels due to CNV penetrate the basement membrane of the retina. These vessels lack specialized tight junctions that exist in normal retinal blood vessels. Subsequent bleeding, leakage, exudation, and scar formation often cause acute and rapidly progressive central visual loss. Although age-related changes occur in all races and populations, the prevalence of visual loss is significantly higher in developed countries and especially with a Northern European heritage.

It is estimated that in 1990 choroidal neovascularization had developed in one or both eyes of 150 000–200 000 of the 300 million people in the United States who were 65 years of age or older. Sight-threatening lesions of AMD increase with age from rare at age 50 to 2 per cent prevalence at age 70 and about 6 per cent at age 80. It is estimated that this segment of the population will double in the United States in the next 25 years.[7,8]

Established risk factors for wet AMD include older age, family history, cigarette smoking, low dietary intake or plasma concentrations of anti-oxidant vitamins and zinc, and Caucasian race. Advances in medical care have increased the percentage of the ageing population. Genetic, preventative, and therapeutic interventions continue to be the focus of intense study. Although effective treatment is currently limited, modulation of risk factors and prompt recognition and treatment of exudative disease is critical for vision preservation.

Diabetic retinopathy

Nearly all patients with diabetes of 20 or more years duration will develop some degree of diabetic retinopathy, which parallels the development of diabetic nephropathy and neuropathy. In the United States, an equal number of patients develop blindness from Type 1 and Type 2 diseases. Diabetic retinopathy is the leading cause of blindness in most highly developed countries. Sixteen million Americans have diabetes but only one-half are aware that they have the disease. Diabetes is the leading cause of new cases of legal blindness in working age Americans, the leading cause of chronic renal disease leading to dialysis, and the leading cause of non-traumatic amputation of lower limb.

Retinal damage is characterized by microvascular abnormalities including microaneurysms, intraretinal haemorrhage, and infarctions of the nerve fibre layer of the retina. Abnormal retinal vascular permeability with damage to endothelial cells and pericytes lead to diabetic macular oedema. Macular oedema may produce mild to severe visual loss and may be the first sign to manifest. Advanced retinopathy, including retinal and iris neovascularization, may be asymptomatic. Proliferative diabetic retinopathy (PDR) is characterized by the onset of retinal neovascularization induced by retinal ischaemia. New vessels at the optic nerve and elsewhere in the retina are prone to bleeding, vitreal haemorrhage, fibrosis, and contraction. Fibrovascular proliferation may result in epiretinal membrane formation, vitreoretinal traction, and retinal tears including retinal detachments. Painful neovascular glaucoma results when new blood vessels extend from the iris to plug the trabecular meshwork at the junction of the iris and cornea.

The duration of diabetes is the major risk factor associated with development of diabetic retinopathy. Of patients with Type 1 disease, 25 per cent have retinopathy after 5 years, 60 per cent after 10 years, and 80 per cent after 15 years. PDR is present in approximately 25 per cent of Type 1 patients with 15 years duration of the disease. In Type 2 patients taking insulin, 40 per cent of patients have retinopathy with duration of diabetes less than 5 years and 24 per cent of those not taking insulin at this time. Rates increase to 84 per cent and 53 per cent, respectively, when duration of diabetes is documented up to 19 years.[10–13]

The key alterable risk factor for development and progression of primary and secondary retinopathy remains the control of hyperglycaemia, and this is supported by clinical and epidemiologic studies. Other risk factors include age, type of diabetes, blood pressure, clotting factors, renal disease, use of angiotensin-converting enzyme (ACE) inhibitors, and co-morbid factors associated with cardiovascular disease and mortality. The results of the Diabetes Control and Complications Trial clearly demonstrated that development and progression of retinopathy in patients with Type 1 diabetes could be delayed if glucose concentrations are maintained in the near normal range. The benefits of glucose control were evident both as a primary (patients without retinopathy) and secondary (patients with pre-existing retinopathy) effect.[11] Beyond 3.5 years of follow-up, the risks of progression are five times lower with intensive insulin therapy than with conventional treatment. In the United Kingdom Prospective Diabetes Study (UKPDS), intensive blood glucose control produced a 29 per cent reduction in the need for retinal photocoagulation in the group with intensive glucose therapy as opposed to those with conventional treatment.[12]

The primary care provider is critical for controlling risk factors for micro- and macrovascular disease. One model of cost-effectiveness of intervention in the control of Type 1 diabetic retinopathy predicted that 72 per cent of Type 1 patients will eventually develop PDR requiring panretinal photocoagulation and 42 per cent will develop macular oedema. Prompt referral for at least annual screening and appropriate management of exudative and neovascular complications are crucial to the preservation of vision and prevention of visual loss.[10] Because both macular oedema (the most common cause of visual loss) and neovascularization may be asymptomatic, prevention, and early detection are crucial. Effective laser treatment is available to halt or retard the natural progression of both diabetic macular oedema and neovascularization. However, one epidemiologic study of over 2000 diabetes patients demonstrated that 11 per cent of Type 1 and 7 per cent of Type 2 patients with high-risk PDR had not been seen by an ophthalmologist within 2 years and that 46 per cent of eyes with high-risk PDR had not received recommended laser photocoagulation.[13]

Glaucoma

Glaucoma comprises a variety of conditions that can lead to elevated intraocular pressure which operates in conjunction with vascular, mechanical, and other factors in contributing to optic nerve damage. Chronic open angle glaucoma (COAG) includes both primary open angle glaucoma (POAG) and secondary causes, which may complicate many ocular diseases. POAG is best described as a form of chronic injury to axons of the retinal ganglion cells and optic nerve tissues at the level of the optic disc and lamina cribrosa, usually associated with characteristic visual field defects. Elevated intraocular pressure plays an important, but as yet undetermined, role in optic nerve neurodegeneration. Mechanisms to explain the accelerated and excessive death of the 1 million neurons which comprise the optic nerve include ischaemia, excitotoxicity, apoptosis, autoimmunity, mitochondrial cytopathy, and the role of genetic components.

Glaucoma has been estimated to be the second most common cause of blindness worldwide after cataract. It is estimated that 3 million Americans suffer from glaucoma. The United States National Eye Institute estimates that 120 000 Americans are blinded because of glaucoma and 50 million are at risk. One-half the people with the disease do not know that they have it.[14] Glaucoma is the leading cause of blindness in African-Americans and the second leading cause of blindness in all Americans. Among the 50 million people affected by glaucoma, it is estimated that 7.6 million persons are bilaterally blind from open angle glaucoma (OAG) and angle closure glaucoma (ACG), by the World Health Organization definition of worse than 3/60. The proportion of OAG to ACG varies by race. Chinese have 5 times the amount of ACG as do Europeans and Africans. The ratio of OAG equal that of ACG in people of Chinese descent.[15] In the United States, an

age-adjusted prevalence of 1.55 per cent was noted for POAG. This is similar to a natural history study in African-Americans in West Africa. Demographic risk factors for POAG are African-American descent and older age (>70 years). White people and African-Americans age 70 years or older were 3.5 and 7.4 times respectively, more likely to have glaucoma than race-matched individuals aged 40–50 years. In the Baltimore Eye Survey, first-degree relatives of patients with POAG had a 2.9 times greater odds of having glaucoma than non-relatives.[16,17]

POAG is a particularly insidious disease because of its asymptomatic nature. Significant amounts of peripheral visual fields may be lost in one or both eyes without affecting central vision or activities of daily living. Both the European Glaucoma Society and the American Academy of Ophthalmology recommend a similar approach of screening examinations followed by antiglaucoma treatment to lower intraocular pressure in susceptible individuals. Early intervention by medical, laser, and surgical modalities and the role of neuroprotection of optic nerve function is being increasingly recognized.[18] The prevalence of open angle glaucoma in European, African, and Asian people has been exhaustively studied. Among European-derived people, the best fit of OAG prevalence relates to age as an exponential function which is delayed in comparison to African-derived individuals and comprises greater than 15 per cent of individuals over the age of 90.[17] Because angle closure glaucoma produces rapid pain and visual symptoms, its prevalence tends to be overestimated in series. The true number of patients with asymptomatic POAG worldwide is unknown and contributes to the likelihood that glaucoma will continue to be the second largest cause of bilateral blindness in the world after cataract.

Trachoma

Trachoma is the third most common cause of blindness worldwide after cataract and glaucoma with 150 million people affected in 48 countries. Six million of these people are blind.[19,20] In 1977, the WHO announced an initiative to eliminate trachoma as a cause of blindness by the year 2020. Trachoma is a disease of poverty, initially described in Egypt in 1900 BC, and continues to exist in clusters in the poorest communities. The disease was endemic in Europe and in migrants to the United States in the 1900s. The disease arises from complications associated with *Chlamydia trachomatis*. This obligate intracellular organism has no free-living state and has no animal reservoir for human chlamydial infection. *Chlamydia trachomatis* targets columnar and squamocolumnar epithelial cells and is characteristically an infection of the conjunctiva, genital, respiratory, and intestinal tissues. Repeated episodes of infection throughout childhood and young adulthood are necessary to produce the complications resulting in blindness seen in later life. Repeated infection induces cicatricial changes of entropion, trichiasis, and corneal scarring. A single episode of acute chlamydial infections, as seen in newborns in the United States, is not considered trachoma because of its acute (not chronic) exposure. Active trachoma is a chronic follicular conjunctivitis characterized by invasion of B-lymphocytes (see Fig. 1 in Chapter 12.2). Inflammatory corneal neovascularization and pannus result from chronic disease. Once limbal follicles resolve, depressions remain on the cornea resulting in the key clinical sign of trachoma, 'Herbert's pits'.

Visual loss from trachoma is due to irreversible corneal damage and is worsened by multiple processes including scarring of the Meibomian glands, accessory lacrimal glands, and lacrimal ducts. Insufficiency of tears combined with inturned eyelashes result in progressive corneal opacity.

Although trachoma is not considered a problem in the Western world, it is still prevalent in large regions of Africa, the Middle East, Southwestern Asia, India, Aboriginal communities in Australia, and in small foci of blinding disease in Central and South America. In hyperendemic areas, active disease is most common in pre-school children with prevalence as high as 60–90 per cent.[19,20] Risk factors include poor hygienic conditions, presence of flies that settle on the cornea, cattle (who create an optimal environment for breeding flies), and presence of children with active chlamydial infection. Active disease in adults is almost entirely confined to caretakers of children with trachoma, and adult women are felt to be at much greater risk at developing blinding complications of trachoma than adult men.

Azithromycin taken orally in a single dose was reportedly as effective against ocular chlamydial infections as 6 weeks of topical tetracycline.[21] This has the secondary advantage of eradicating infection and any extra-ocular reservoir, but a control programme must stress multiple strategies for prevention and trachoma control. Disappearance of trachoma in the Western world parallels economic development and improvement in housing, sanitation, and personal hygiene. Visual restoration depends on corneal transplantation. This is rarely available in developing countries and the world availability of suitable corneal donor tissue far exceeds the demand from corneal blinding disorders. Early intervention and tarsal rotation of the eyelids to prevent cicatricial entropion may be effective if instituted early in minor cases of trichiasis. The lack of trained ophthalmic personnel and the overwhelming poverty in which this disease exists make this a most devastating condition.

Onchocerciasis

Onchocercal infection is estimated to produce only 1 per cent of world blindness. However, the WHO estimates that of the 123 million people who live in areas of Africa, Central and South American, Sudan, and Yemen, 17.7 million people are infected with *Onchocerca volvulus*. This results in approximately 270 000 blind individuals and 500 000 who have severe visual impairment.[22] WHO launched the Onchocerciasis Control Programme (OCP) in 1974 but there remain an estimated 15 million infected individuals outside the OCP area. The disease is spread by Simulium black flies, which are the obligate intermediate hosts of *O. volvulus*. Multiple subcutaneous nodules form. Blindness follows invasion of parasites from the skin into either the cornea or the retina and choroid. Retinitis is a post-immune response which results in widespread atrophy of the retinal pigment epithelium and may lead to subretinal fibrosis. An inflammatory response directed against dead and degenerating parasites leads to loss of corneal clarity. In anterior segment and corneal disease, motile worms in the cornea or anterior chamber can be detected by slit-lamp examination after the microfilariae migrate into the ocular tissue. Opacification of the cornea progresses centrally and is accompanied by deep stromal neovascularization. Sclerosing keratitis results in permanent blindness.[23] Because of the immune mediated effects and the presence of posterior segment disease, there is no reliable restorative procedure. In hyperendemic areas, almost every person will be infected and one-half the population will be blinded by onchocerciasis before they die. Once blind, they have a life expectancy of only one-third of the sighted and most die within 10 years.

Control of disease utilizes the strategy of controlling the black fly vector and treating active disease with Ivermectin. It is estimated that in the first 20 years of treatment the prevalence of disease has decreased by 30 million people.[22]

Vitamin A deficiency

A serious and common health problem relates to the clinical manifestations resulting from dietary deficiency of vitamin A. Associated vitamin and protein deficiencies coupled with unsanitary living conditions predispose affected individuals to secondary endogenous and exogenous systemic and ocular infections. Vitamin A deficiency may also arise as a consequence of cystic fibrosis, which is characterized by diminished systemic absorption.[24]

Vitamin A deficiency results in a decrease in conjunctival mucus production. As the bulbar conjunctival vessels become congested, the conjunctival surface dries and becomes irregularly opacified and thickened. Focal white plaques in the interpalpebral area (Bitot's spots) form and may be noted on clinical examination. Xerosis, characterized by severe drying of the conjunctiva and corneal epithelium, results in corneal keratinization and opacity. Secondary inflammatory scarring of the lacrimal gland leads to further drying, severe bilateral visual loss, and blindness. Corneal infections, ectasia, and perforation may occur. Vitamin A retinopathy produces night blindness and eventual degeneration of photoreceptor cells and presumed rhodopsin dysfunction. Retinopathy is characterized by small, irregular, non-discreet, whitish-yellow deposits in the deep retina located in the retinal mid-periphery. Peripheral visual field constriction may occur. Similar symptoms have been reported with hypovitaminosis-A in a patient following colon resection.[25]

Acquired vitamin A deficiency is a problem endemic to the world's poorest regions. A longitudinal prospective study of risk factors contributing to vitamin A deficiency revealed a close, dose–response relationship between the severity of pre-existing vitamin A deficiency and subsequent incidence of respiratory and diarrhoeal infection. Subsequent community-based prophylactic trials of varying designs confirmed that vitamin A supplementation of deficient populations could reduce childhood (1–5 years old) mortality by an average of 35 per cent. Hospital-based trials with vitamin A in children infected with measles revealed consistent reduction in measles-associated mortality in Africa of at least 50 per cent. It is now estimated that improving vitamin A status of all deficient children worldwide would prevent 1–3 million childhood deaths annually.[24–26]

Conclusions

The role of primary care in prevention and treatment of blinding disorders and especially ocular complications of systemic disease cannot be over-emphasized. As the world becomes a more crowded place, it is important to recognize that uncommon presentations of ocular disease may become more prevalent. A high index of suspicion and timely referral for evaluation may prevent or retard the progression of ocular disease and blindness. The role of the primary care physician remains crucial in the prevention, detection, and treatment of blinding disease locally and worldwide. Appropriate intervention preserves the patient's quality of life, the patient's ability to care for themselves, over an increased lifespan, and reduces the chance of morbidity from co-existing disease.

Key points

- ◆ Trachoma still afflicts 150 million people.
- ◆ Onchocerciasis still afflicts 18 million people.
- ◆ Cataract surgery is highly cost-effective.
- ◆ Early recognition of AMD helps preserve vision.

References

1. **Thylefors, B.** et al. (1995). Global data on blindness. *Bulletin of the World Health Organization* 73, 115–21.
2. **WHO prevention of blindness.** (http://www.who.int/pbd/pbl/pbl_home. htm).
3. **Javitt, J.C., Wang, F., and West, S.K.** (1996). Blindness due to cataract: epidemiology and prevention. *Annual Review of Public Health* 17, 159–77.
4. **Livingston, P.M., Carson, C.A., and Taylor, H.R.** (1995). The epidemiology of cataract: a review of the literature. *Ophthalmic Epidemiology* 2 (3), 151–64.
5. **Gieser, S.C. and Schin, O.D.** (1994). Cataract epidemiology and world blindness. *Current Opinion in Ophthalmology* 5 (1), 5–8.
6. **Javitt, J.C.** (1993). Cost-effectiveness of restoring sight. *Archives of Ophthalmology* 111, 1615.
7. **Hawkins, B.S.** et al. (1999). Epidemiology of age-related macular degeneration. *Molecular Vision* 5, 26.
8. **Vingerling, J.R.** et al. (1995). Epidemiology of age-related maculopathy. *Epidemiologic Reviews* 17 (2), 347–60.

9. Evans, J. (1995). Causes of blindness and partial sight in England and Wales 1990–1991. In *Studies on Medical and Population Subjects* No. 57. London: HMSO.

10. Javitt, J.C. and Aiello, L.P. (1996). Cost-effectiveness of detecting and treating diabetic retinopathy. *Annals of Internal Medicine* 124, 164–9.

11. **The Diabetes Control and Complications Trial Research Group** (1995). The effect of intensive diabetes treatment on the progression of diabetic retinopathy in insulin-dependent diabetes mellitus. *Archives of Ophthalmology* 113, 36–49.

12. **UK Prospective Diabetes Study Group** (1991). UK Prospective Diabetes Study (UKPDS). VIII. Study design, progress, and performance. *Diabetologia* 34, 877–90.

13. Klein, R. et al. (1987). The Wisconsin epidemiologic study of diabetic retinopathy. IV. Retinal photocoagulation. *Ophthalmology* 94, 747–54.

14. Coleman, A.L. (1999). Glaucoma. *Lancet* 354, 1803–10.

15. Quigley, H. (2003). http:glaucoma.com/Meetings/3-3/worldwide.htm.

16. Quigley, H.A. and Vitale, S. (1997). Models of open-angle glaucoma prevalence and incidence in the United States. *Investigative Ophthalmology & Visual Science* 38 (1), 83–91.

17. Quigley, H.A. (1996). Number of people with glaucoma worldwide. *British Journal of Ophthalmology* 80, 389–93.

18. Crick, R.P. (1994). Epidemiology and screening of open-angle glaucoma. *Current Opinion in Ophthalmology* 5, 3–9.

19. Mabey, D. and Bailey, R. (1999). Eradication of trachoma worldwide. *British Journal of Ophthalmology* 83, 1261–3.

20. Munoz, B. and West, S. (1997). Trachoma: the forgotten cause of blindness. *Epidemiologic Reviews* 19 (2), 205–17.

21. Schachter, J. et al. (1999). Azithromycin in control of trachoma. *Lancet* 354, 650–5.

22. Pearlman, E. and Hall, L.R. (2000). Immune mechanisms in *Onchocerca volvulus*-mediated corneal disease (river blindness). *Parasite Immunology* 22, 625–31.

23. Hall, L.R. and Pearlman, E. (1999). Pathogenesis of onchocercal keratitis (river blindness). *Clinical Microbiology Reviews* 12 (3), 445–53.

24. Sommer, A. (1993). Vitamin A, infectious disease, and childhood mortality: a 2 solution? *Journal of Infectious Disease* 167 (5), 1003–7.

25. Sommer, A. (1998). Xerophthalmia and vitamin A status. *Progress in Retinal and Eye Research* 17, 9–31.

26. Villamor, E. and Fawzi, W.W. (2000). Vitamin A supplementation: implications for morbidity and mortality in children. *Journal of Infectious Disease* 182 (Suppl. 1), S122–33.

12.7 Eye trauma

Roger Gray

Most eye injuries are minor and self-limiting, and they are also common. It is therefore important to be able to anticipate and recognize the features of more serious damage. This chapter will outline a range of eye injuries, emphasizing some clues in the history and examination which help in the detection of potentially serious damage.

Taking the history

Dust or other wind-blown material getting into the eye is perhaps the commonest and least serious injury, and little additional information is needed from the patient prior to examination. Be careful, however, if the patient or even someone standing close by was using any kind of powered tool at the time, because this greatly increases the risk of a perforating eye injury. Rotary wire brushes can lose their wires, grinders can shower the air with metal or stone fragments, and strimmers/brush-cutters can throw up a great many high-velocity objects. These risks are obviously very much higher if glasses or protective goggles are not worn, and a history of protective eye-wear should be sought in these circumstances. Hammering a chisel is also a classical cause of eye perforation. With prolonged use, a burr develops at the top edge of the chisel, and a fragment can fly off at high speed and puncture the eye. Goggles should always be worn, and the chisel edge kept smooth.

The danger from balls is partly dependent on their size. Footballs, and even tennis and cricket balls, tend to cause more of a problem to the surrounding skin and bone, since the eye is well protected in its bony orbit. On the other hand, shuttlecocks and squash balls can hit the eye very hard because they are too small to be stopped by the orbital rim. Severe injuries can result, including rupture of the eye. Players should wear protective glasses, or even ordinary glasses with plastic lenses.

Chemical injuries can be devastating. The most serious usually involve alkalis, either household cleaning agents, or builders' mortar or plaster mix. The latter can be even more serious because solid pieces can be deposited on the eye and act as an alkali reservoir. Find out how quickly the eye was irrigated after the injury.

Excessive exposure to short wavelength ultraviolet light can temporarily damage the corneal epithelium and cause severe pain. It occurs particularly in welders who have not worn protective eyewear; occasionally someone standing close by can also inadvertently get enough exposure. The condition is known as 'arc eye', and pain does not usually start until some hours after exposure. 'Snow blindness' is very similar.

Symptoms of injury and what they indicate

The *feeling of grit* in the eye (foreign body sensation), is usually caused either by a foreign body or by scratch on the conjunctiva or cornea. Less commonly, the eye is inflamed without being scratched (liquid burns, arc eye). Keeping the eye closed helps the discomfort and sometimes holding the upper lid away from the eye is also helpful. Occasionally, recurrent foreign body discomfort can be a troublesome sequel to a corneal abrasion (recurrent corneal erosion) due to failure of the newly healed corneal epithelium to adhere adequately to its basement membrane, and minimal stress can then dislodge it. Classically, this happens in the early morning when the eyelids are first opened, and the discomfort settles after a few hours.

Aching pain is potentially more serious, because it suggests some irritation to the interior of the eye (iris, or ciliary body) and therefore an injury which is deeper. The ache can be particularly severe in the presence of bright light, due to reactive spasm of the ciliary muscle (photophobia).

Blurred vision can be caused by a variety of injuries, and it is not always a good indicator of serious underlying damage. For instance, a centrally located corneal abrasion can have a major impact on acuity, particularly if the eye is watering as well, yet the prognosis is excellent. On the other hand, a penetrating eye injury from a chisel fragment can present with good vision, but is much more serious. Blood in the eye can cause blurred vision, and this may occur in the anterior chamber (hyphaema), vitreous, retina, or choroid. In the case of vitreous bleeding, floating debris in the visual field may well be a prominent complaint.

Double vision (diplopia) is common after blunt injuries, which can temporarily damage extraocular muscle function without significantly blurring the vision. The diplopia will usually resolve quickly, and without other features of cranial nerve palsy it should not be a cause for alarm. Rarely, the pressure of impact from a blunt injury can fracture bone, usually along the floor of the orbit (blow out fracture of the orbit). Entrapment of fat and sometimes the inferior rectus muscle can then cause vertical diplopia due to restricted eye movements. A good clue to this injury is anaesthesia below the lower lid due to infraorbital nerve damage as it passes along the orbital floor.

Floaters and flashing lights both indicate the possibility of retinal damage, though as already mentioned, a shower of floaters on their own can also indicate vitreous haemorrhage.

Signs of injury, what they mean, and how to deal with them

Sore eyes

A sore eye, with a history suggesting a foreign body or corneal abrasion, is the commonest presentation. In the absence of 'high-risk' injuries such as those involving chisels or powered tools, serious damage is unlikely, but it can be difficult to find the foreign body and/or the corneal abrasion. The vision should be checked, but may not be normal if the central cornea is affected or if the eye is watering profusely. A drop of anaesthetic at this point makes checking the vision easier, and also facilitates examination. Magnification and fluorescein dye should then be used to search for the foreign body (A direct ophthalmoscope with a +10 lens dialled in is a useful light source combined with magnifier.). Small corneal foreign bodies become visible with the magnification, and with the addition of fluorescein and cobalt blue light, any conjunctival or corneal abrasions become easy to see as well (Fig. 1(a)). Sometimes, the abrasions are numerous

and vertically oriented, indicating that the foreign body is lodged under the upper lid (sub-tarsal). Everting the upper eyelid is an important part of any eye exam when a foreign body is suspected, and it is a valuable skill which is easily learnt (Fig. 2).

Black eyes

Another common physical sign is the black eye or peri-orbital haematoma. Due to the vascularity and laxity of these tissues, haematomas can easily close the eye and make examination difficult. Obvious bruising means that some at least of the impact has been absorbed by the skin and bone, so paradoxically the eye may well be undamaged. The edge of the haematoma can be a useful clue to its origin. If the margin is indistinct and well beyond the orbital margin then the orbit is likely to have been spared, but if the margin is well defined and approximates to the orbital margin then be alert to the possibility that the blood originated from the orbital cavity (orbital haematoma). This is much more serious, and raises the possibility of optic nerve compression. This is unlikely; however, unless the eye looks obviously pushed forwards (proptosed) especially if the pupil reactions are normal and extraocular movements are preserved. Another clue to the presence of orbital haemorrhage is the pattern of any sub-conjunctival blood. If the posterior limit of the haemorrhage cannot be seen then it might have started in the orbit. Checking the vision may be difficult, but the lids only

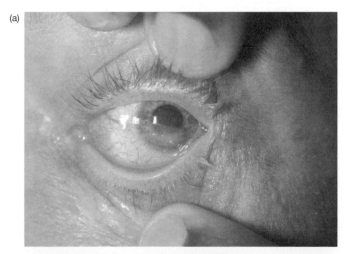

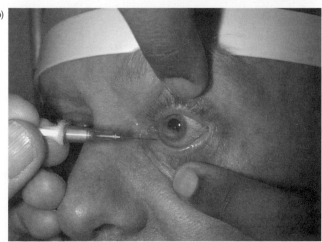

Fig. 1 The use of fluorescein greatly simplifies the task of finding a corneal abrasion or foreign body, as in this case in which a large and inferior corneal abrasion is highlighted (a). A sterile 27-gauge needle mounted on a cotton bud makes an excellent tool for flicking off foreign bodies (b).

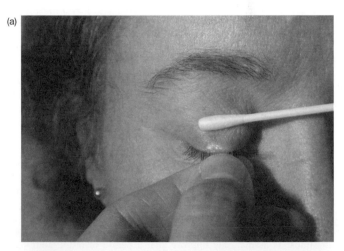

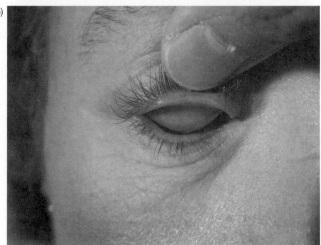

Fig. 2 Lid eversion. Pull down on the upper lashes while pressing backwards at the top of the lid (a). Gentle pressure on the lashes against the skin will keep it everted (b), and releasing pressure coupled with a vigorous blink will return it to normal.

need to open a crack to do this. The narrow aperture may act as a pinhole, which is fortuitous for those who cannot wear their glasses because of bruising or breakage. It is important to have a clearly lit Snellen chart at the right distance. If the lids cannot be held even slightly open *without undue force*, referral of the patient is needed, because rupture of the eye needs to be excluded, and strenuous attempts to force the lids open can squeeze the eye and worsen the injury. A useful test is to press gently on the fellow eye through closed eyelids and feel the natural resistance that the eye should offer. Then compare this with the injured eye. You do not have to press hard, and even with swollen lids it can be surprisingly easy to tell if the eye is soft.

Eye movements should be assessed. Usually, they look intact, in which case it is reasonable to assume that any diplopia is likely to be short lived and not serious.

Carefully examine the pupil reactions. If both react normally to light, this is good evidence that there has been no major damage to the afferent visual system (retina and optic nerve). If one pupil looks larger than the other one and fails to react appropriately to light, it is likely that the sphincter pupillae has been damaged, perhaps permanently (traumatic mydriasis). In addition to the pupil enlargement it is often somewhat irregular as well (magnification may be required to see this). Pupil irregularity is not a feature of third nerve palsy, which is commonly misdiagnosed in this situation even though the eye movements are intact: traumatic third nerve palsies are unlikely to spare everything except the pupil. An irregular pupil can also be due to iris tissue plugging a full thickness corneal laceration, in which case the pupil irregularity will be accompanied by a soft eye and corneal opacification. Any pupil abnormality is an indication for referral.

Blood in the eye

Sub-conjunctival bleeding has already been mentioned in the context of orbital haemorrhage. More often it is due to very minor trauma. Remember though that a small sub-conjunctival haemorrhage can be the only evidence of ocular perforation by something small and very fast like a metal chisel fragment from a hammer blow. Use fluorescein and find out if there has been a tear in the conjunctiva.

Bleeding from the iris can cause hyphaema. This is seen as a layer of blood at the bottom of the eye in front of the iris, with a characteristic horizontal upper border due to gravitational settling. However, this appearance does take time to develop, and if the patient is seen before the blood has settled, then the only signs will be blurring of the iris details and an absent or diminished red reflex. Vision can be dramatically reduced, and can almost as dramatically improve after a period of rest. Traditionally, these patients have often been admitted to hospital for a few days bed rest, though nowadays it is felt that many patients can be managed equally well at home. Vitreous haemorrhage is more difficult to see, and to some extent it has to be assumed if the patient has noticed a sudden shower of floaters, the vision is reduced, and retinal visualization seems obscured in the absence of any obvious cause.

Retinal haemorrhages may be due to shearing injury or valsalva type problems. More rarely they can be markers for an intraocular foreign body. Inflammatory retinal swelling (commotio retinae) can follow a severe blunt injury, and is due to mechanical forces acting through the vitreous jelly to pull or compress the retina.

Haemorrhage anywhere within the eye after trauma is an indication for referral.

Some specific procedures explained

Removing a superficial foreign body

With a needle mounted on a cotton bud, or a fine pair of forceps, and with local anaesthetic eye drops and a good light, it is possible to remove many foreign bodies safely (Fig. 1). Problems arise however when the material is iron based, and particularly if the cornea is involved. Iron rusts very quickly in the warm and wet ophthalmic environment, and a ring of rust is commonly left behind when the iron is flicked off, in which case the patient will need ophthalmic referral. Metallic corneal foreign bodies therefore probably warrant slit-lamp based removal unless they can easily be flicked off. The reason for this is that the cornea is delicate, and scratching it with a needle, etc. can cause unnecessary additional scarring.

Eye irrigation

If a chemical injury is suspected then act quickly. Speed takes priority over the irrigating fluid used. Saline is best, but tap water is perfectly acceptable. Use anaesthetic drops first if available, and ideally find some way in which to squirt water gently over the surface of the eye. A syringe is good, though any pouring vessel will do. Direct the fluid over the cornea, then into the spaces created by pulling the upper and lower lids away from the eye. Finally, evert the upper lid and pour fluid onto the exposed conjunctiva. Throughout, ask the patient to look into all positions of gaze to expose the conjunctiva as much as possible. Five minutes of such treatment should be adequate, though the ideal end point is a normal pH.

Lid eversion

This is an important clinical procedure when an ocular foreign body is suspected. It is easily learnt and entirely painless. Grasp the upper eyelashes and pull the lid gently downward, while at the same time pressing backward at the upper border of the tarsal plate (Fig. 2(a)). A cotton bud is useful, though a paper clip or even a long fingernail will work just as well. Once everted, the lid is kept in place by gently pressing the lashes against the skin (Fig. 2(b)), and when finished, a vigorous blink will return the lid to its normal position.

Padding the eye

This is not always necessary (see Further reading section), because corneal healing times are not speeded up by eye pads. However, the patient will usually be happier with the eye closed, and if a pad is used the most important thing is to ensure that the eye is closed properly underneath it. An eye which opens under the pad is likely to be scratched again, this time iatrogenically. A good technique is to tape the lids together, then apply the eye pad firmly. In some patients with deep-set eyes, it is a good idea to use two eye pads, the one closer to the eye being folded in two and tucked under the brow.

The duration of padding is dependent on the size of the corneal abrasion, and it is not wise to keep the eye padded for more than 24 h without re-examination. For many patients, it is reasonable for the pad to be removed after 24 h, and to come back only if there has not been significant improvement in the discomfort. An antibiotic ointment such as chloromycetin should be used prior to padding, and if photophobia is prominent then a drop of homatropine will help by relieving ciliary spasm. Systemic analgesia may also be helpful, such as regular paracetamol.

Useful eye drops

- Proxymetacaine (minims). An excellent local anaesthetic drop which does not sting.

- Proxymetacaine with fluorescein (minims). Combines two very useful drops.

- Chloramphenicol ointment. Used prior to padding as antibacterial prophylaxis.

- Tropicamide 0.5 per cent (minims). The quickest acting mydriatic to aid fundoscopy.

- Homatropine 2 per cent (minims). Useful to relieve photophobia.

Key points

- Most eye injuries can be accurately diagnosed using a bright light, fluorescein eye drops, and good magnification.

- Everting the upper eyelid is an important procedure during the search for an ocular foreign body.

- Any pupil abnormality is a sign that the eye has been hit hard.

- Irrigate the eye very quickly after chemical spills.

Further reading

Dutton, G. (1995). The GP and eye trauma. *The Practitioner* **239**, 265–71. (There are few articles devoted to eye trauma in a general practice setting. This one is short but well written, it is surprisingly extensive in scope, and has good illustrations accompanying the text.)

Frith, P., Gray, R., MacLennan, S., and Ambler, P. *The Eye in Clinical Practice* 2nd edn. London: Blackwell Scientific Publications, 2001. ISBN 0-632-05895-1. (This book was written specifically for those involved in primary care, and it includes an informative and well-illustrated chapter on eye trauma.)

Kirkpatrick, J.N., Hoh, H.B., and Cook, S.D. (1993). No eye pad for corneal abrasion. *Eye* **7** (3), 468–71. (Patched or not, simple corneal abrasions heal quickly.)

Ragge, N. and Easty, D. *Immediate Eye Care*. Wolfe Publishing Ltd, 1990. ISBN 0-7234-1574-9. (Although written with ophthalmologists particularly in mind, this book does provide a wealth of useful information and excellent photos on the subject of ocular trauma.)

13

Musculoskeletal problems

13 Musculoskeletal problems

13.1 Low back pain and sciatica

*Patrick C.A.J. Vroomen and
Maurits W. van Tulder*

Low back pain has been well documented as a major health problem in industrialized countries. For non-industrialized countries, epidemiological data are largely lacking, yet there is little reason to believe low back pain is not a frequent problem in these countries as well. Lifetime prevalence rate for low back pain in industrialized countries is approximately 75 per cent, indicating that most people suffer an episode of low back pain during their lifetime. Annual incidence is approximately 5 per cent and annual prevalence approximately 25 per cent. The onset of back pain usually occurs between 35 and 55 years of age with no difference between men and women.[1]

Low back pain usually has an acute character with a 90 per cent spontaneous recovery rate within 6 weeks and probably a sizeable number of patients do not consult a GP. In up to one-third of those who do consult their GP, the low back pain may persist beyond 12 months.[2] In 2–7 per cent of cases, the complaints will persist beyond 3 months or patients will have frequent recurrences. Because of the high incidence of low back pain, a fairly large group will end up having chronic low back pain.

For every five patients with pain primarily in the lower back, one patient predominantly has pain radiating into the leg below the buttock, which is referred to as sciatica. Patients with sciatica constitute a different entity because not only does sciatica indicate neurological involvement, but also its diagnosis and management differ from that of low back pain. This problem will therefore be discussed separately.

Though only relatively few people with acute low back pain will seek medical advice, low back pain is still one of the three most frequently presenting complaints in primary care. Primary care physicians will see about two patients with a new episode of low back pain every week.

Risk factors and causes

Risk factors for the development of low back pain are poorly understood. The most frequently reported are heavy physical work, frequent bending, twisting, lifting, pulling and pushing, repetitive work, static postures, and vibrations. Psycho-social risk factors include anxiety, depression, job dissatisfaction, and mental stress at work.[3] Psycho-social risk factors are associated with the risk of developing or perpetuating chronic pain and long-term disability (including work-loss associated with low back pain).

Specific causes for acute low back pain can be identified in only 5–10 per cent of patients. In the other patients, the term non-specific low back pain is often applied because of the weak associations between anatomical abnormality, symptoms, and results of additional diagnostic investigations.

Musculoligamentous injury or degenerative changes are often hypothesized to have caused the pain in the patients with non-specific low back pain.

The specific causes can be divided into two groups: (i) spinal disorders without neurological involvement; and (ii) spinal disorders with neurological involvement. Specific causes of low back pain from spinal disorders without neurological involvement are congenital disorders such as isthmic spondylolisthesis, Scheuermann's disease and spinal stenosis in relation to achondroplasia, spondylolysis, fractures of the vertebral column, infection, inflammation, or segmental instability (defined as more than a 5 mm vertebral shift between flexion and extension). It is important to consider that pain due to abdominal aneurysms and with renal, pancreatic, and uterine disorders can be referred to the back.

Neurological involvement in patients with low back pain originates in the lumbosacral nerve roots. While other neural structures such as the lumbosacral plexus and several nerve disorders may lead to radiating pain in the leg, they are not accompanied by low back pain. In the majority, the nerve root disorder is caused by a lumbosacral disc herniation. The nerve root dysfunction results from both the mechanical pressure on the nerve root and the accompanying aseptic inflammation. Although some of the other causes are rare, the primary care physician needs to consider malignancy, infection, diabetes mellitus, and spinal canal stenosis as causes.

Clinical diagnosis

There are several methods of classifying low back pain, some based on pain distribution, others on pain behaviour, functional disability, clinical signs and symptoms, or anatomical substrate. None of these systems have been critically evaluated. A strategy, both useful, commonly applied and internationally accepted, is to make a triage between:

1. non-specific low back pain;

2. specific low back pain without neurological involvement; and

3. specific low back with nerve root pain.

The diagnosis of non-specific low back pain is based on the exclusion of relevant specific causes. When searching for specific causes, the physician should first focus on features of serious spinal pathology (so-called 'red flags' see Table 1). Such pathology may be suspected primarily on the basis of history and physical examination and can be confirmed by additional diagnostic procedures. Firstly, the patient's age and history should be considered. Secondly, standard history-taking should include considering the distribution and severity of the pain and the relation with time and posture. Thirdly, a standard physical examination should be conducted including inspection of posture, movement and local anatomical derangements, assessment of spinal tenderness on percussion over the spinal processes, or axial pressure, and palpation of the abdomen. In some patients, nerve root disorders may be suspected on the basis of pain distribution and pattern. Then, provocation of pain on coughing, sneezing or straining, weakness, sensory loss, and micturition disturbance (reduction in feeling of urinary passage or incontinence) should be asked for. Also, the diagnostic process should include a neurological examination looking for typical radiating

Table 1 'Red flags': warning signs and symptoms indicating an increased likelihood of serious spinal pathology

Age of onset <20 or >55 years
Violent trauma
Constant progressive, non-mechanical pain (no relief with bed rest)
Thoracic pain
Past medical history of malignant tumour
Prolonged use of corticosteroids
Drug abuse, immunosuppression, HIV
Signs of systemic disease
Unexplained weight loss
Widespread neurology (including cauda equina syndrome)
Structural deformity
Fever

pain in the leg during straight leg raising and bending forward, loss of power (which can be tested by requesting the patient to walk on toes and heels) and loss of reflexes.

Exclusion of specific causes

Specific causes of low back pain may be suspected on the basis of history alone. In 1 per cent of primary care patients with low back pain, a malignancy is the cause.[4] Most frequently, this malignancy is metastatic. Unexplained weight loss also raises suspicion. A history of malignancy in patients with low back pain always necessitates additional investigations. Rheumatological (e.g. Reiter, rheumatoid arthritis, psoriasis, ankylosing spondylitis), metabolic (e.g. osteoporosis, osteochondritis), or infectious diseases (e.g. tuberculosis, septic arthritis) may also cause low back pain. A positive family history, morning stiffness, improvement on exercise, no improvement on lying down, slow onset, an age below 40, and a striking response to non-steroidal anti-inflammatory drugs point to ankylosing spondylitis.[5] When low back pain occurs after potentially traumatic events, spondylolysis, and other fractures may have occurred. Such fractures are more likely and can occur after trivial events in osteoporosis, sometimes in relation to corticosteroid therapy. Compression fractures may explain up to 4 per cent of low back pain cases in primary care.[6] The history may also give clues as to the presence of renal or pancreatic disorders.

Sometimes, inspection reveals structural deformities of the spine. Infectious diseases of the spine should be considered when there is fever, especially when the patient's immune system is compromised or in drug addicts.[6] Palpation of the abdomen may reveal tumours pointing to malignancy or abdominal. If a tumour is detected, auscultation may distinguish cancer from aneurysms. Tenderness on percussion and axial pressure may be painful with vertebral fractures.

Assessment of neurological involvement

The presence of a nerve root disorder is primarily assessed by history-taking and physical examination. The hallmark of neurological involvement in low back pain is a radiating pain into the leg according to a dermatomal distribution, referred to as sciatica.[7] An increase of pain on coughing, sneezing, or straining also increases the likelihood of neurological involvement. Unfortunately, the patient's report of decreased muscle strength and sensory loss is unreliable. In the physical examination decreased muscle strength, sensory loss, reflex disturbance, a positive straight leg raising test, and a provocation of leg pain on bending forwards are associated with nerve root involvement (especially when due to disc herniations). Even when nerve root involvement is already apparent, it is important to specifically check for the presence of paresis or urinary symptoms such as incontinence.

Cauda equina syndrome is likely to be present when patients describe bladder dysfunction (usually urinary retention, occasionally overflow incontinence), sphincter disturbance, saddle anaesthesia, global or progressive weakness in the lower limbs or gait disturbance. This requires urgent referral. The strength of at least iliopsoas, quadriceps, gastrocnemic, and anterior tibial and peroneal muscles should be evaluated. If the investigator can overcome the strength of any of these muscles in a fully cooperative patient, there is a paresis requiring emergency referral. Especially in the first 24 h of such a paresis there is a higher inclination towards surgical treatment. Also, the patient should be asked to walk on heels and toes because this may reveal more subtle weakness of gastrocnemic and anterior tibial/peroneal muscles often undetected on standard muscle testing. As L5 and S1 root disorders constitute 95 per cent of the nerve root disorders disturbed walking on heels and toes are the most frequent signs of weakness.

An important variation on the syndrome described above is the clinical picture of a spinal canal stenosis (also referred to as neurogenic claudication). The pain may be either dermatomal or rather diffuse in the proximal legs. It is often but not always bilateral. Other neurological signs and symptoms may occur. The most important attribute is that the complaints depend on the position of the vertebral column. They are largely restricted to walking and typically do not occur while the patient is seated, rides a bike, or ascends stairs. Even the paresis may wax and wane with walking.

Only one in 100 patients will have a malignancy as the cause of sciatica. An extensive search for malignancy is not warranted in all patients with low back pain and sciatica. Nonetheless, in patients with a history of malignancy, a metastasis should be excluded. Also, in patients with unrelentingly progressive sciatica, or in patients with clear provocation of radicular pain on percussion of the vertebrae a metastatis should be looked for.

Diabetes mellitus may involve lumbosacral nerve roots and may mimic sciatica due to disc herniation. It should be considered as a cause in all diabetics. When more than one nerve root is afflicted, an infection with Borrelia Burgdorferi (Lymes disease) should be considered. Many other causes (e.g. epidural abscess, herpes zoster) exist, but are rare.

Additional investigations

When specific spinal disorders are suspected on the basis of history and physical examination, additional investigations are needed. In cases of sciatica, additional investigations are only required when other causes besides disc herniation are suspected or when disc surgery (see indications for surgery) is seriously considered.

Radiological investigations are the primary additional investigation. Most investigations are sensitive (with the exception of conventional X-rays for some indications), but there is a drawback to this high sensitivity. A number of anatomical derangements can be revealed that have a poor association with complaints and findings. Sometimes these findings may require further management (e.g. with fractures, which are symptomatic in only 10 per cent of patients) but more often the further management of these findings is unclear or unnecessary (e.g. with disc degeneration).

Conventional X-rays are only useful for the identification of spondylolysis and other fractures. For investigation of malignancy, the investigation lacks both sensitivity and specificity. In general, most other abnormalities besides fractures correlate poorly with symptomatology.

Magnetic resonance (MR) imaging is the investigation of first choice when nerve root involvement needs to be demonstrated. It should be underlined that this expensive investigation is only indicated when the clinical picture of sciatica is sufficiently severe and longstanding to consider surgery. MR imaging is also the first-choice option for demonstrating spinal malignancy. A radioisotope scan has a sensitivity similar to MR imaging for showing malignant disease of the spine but it is much less specific. If both are not available, computed tomography (CT) scans are a good second choice.

In general, CT scans have a higher cost-effectiveness when it comes to the demonstration of osseous abnormalities such as fractures. For demonstration of metastatic disease, however, CT scans are inferior to MR scans (but provide a reasonable alternative when MR imaging or radioisotope imaging are not available).

Laboratory investigations may point to cancer, inflammatory or infectious diseases, and diabetes or other metabolic disturbances. Increased calcium and alkaline phophatase levels may hint at malignant disease. Unfortunately, a normal erythrocyte sedimentation rate does not exclude malignancy because approximately 24 per cent of patients with vertebral cancer have a normal sedimentation rate.[8] Needle electromyography may demonstrate nerve root involvement, but because of its lack of sensitivity it should be reserved for cases of sciatica of longer duration where a substantial doubt remains about the presence of nerve root involvement.

Assessing the impact on the patient

History-taking and physical examination serve other important purposes besides establishing a specific cause or the presence of a radicular syndrome. The physician can ask for the severity of pain and the extent of functional disability (interference with daily life). This enables the health care professional to outline a management strategy that matches the magnitude of the problem. Psycho-social risk factors may also be established such as inadequate attitudes and beliefs about back pain (e.g. belief that back pain is harmful or potentially severely disabling or high expectation of passive treatments rather than a belief that active participation will help), inadequate pain behaviour (e.g. fear-avoidance behaviour and reduced activity levels), work-related problems or compensation issues (e.g. poor work satisfaction) or emotional problems (e.g. depression, anxiety, stress, tendency to low mood, and withdrawal from social interaction). Identification of such risk factors should ideally lead to appropriate cognitive and behavioural management. However, in acute low back pain evidence on the effectiveness of psycho-social assessment or intervention is lacking, so evaluation of these psycho-social factors should be reserved for the subacute and chronic stages of disease. Finally, the careful initial examination serves as the basis on which to provide the patient with information regarding diagnosis, management, and prognosis.

Principles of management

The primary care physician has a central role in the management of non-specific low back pain. The initial management of low back pain with sciatica (nerve root involvement) is also the task of the primary care physician. The therapeutic management of specific spinal disorders is generally not the domain of the primary care physician. In the following section, recommendations for the management of non-specific low back pain and low back pain with sciatica are described.

Non-specific low back pain

Various health care providers may be involved in the treatment of acute low back pain in primary care. Although there may be some variations between countries, general practitioners, physiotherapists, manual therapists, chiropractors, exercise therapists, McKenzie therapists, orthopaedic surgeons, rheumatologists, and others, may all be involved. It is important that information and treatment are consistent across professions, and that primary medical care providers closely collaborate with each other and with other primary care practitioners. The management of low back pain depends on the duration of symptoms. In the following, a distinction will be made between acute and chronic low back pain.

Acute low back pain

Treatment of acute low back pain (Box 1) in primary medical care aims at: (i) providing adequate information, reassuring the patient that low back pain is usually not a serious disease and that rapid recovery is expected in most patients; (ii) providing adequate symptom control, if necessary; and (iii) recommending to stay as active as possible and to return to normal activities early, including work.[9] An active approach is the best treatment

Box 1 Recommendations for treatment of acute non-specific low back pain

- Give adequate information and reassure the patient.

- Do not prescribe bed rest as a treatment.

- Advise patients to stay active and continue normal daily activities including work if possible.

- Do not advise specific back exercises, such as strengthening, flexion, and extension exercises.

- Prescribe medication, if necessary for pain relief; preferably to be taken at regular intervals; first choice acetaminophen, second choice NSAIDs.

- Consider a short course of muscle relaxants added to NSAIDs, if acetaminophen or NSAIDs have failed to reduce pain; be aware that benzodiazepines can lead to long-term use and addiction.

- Consider (referral for) spinal manipulation for patients who are failing to return to normal activities.

Box 2 Recommendations for treatment of chronic non-specific low back pain

- The most important objective is to prevent or reduce disability, both physically and mentally, and to improve quality of life and functioning.

- Dependence on medical treatment should be prevented and avoided.

- The emphasis should be on coping with the symptoms together with control of pain.

- Long-term drug treatment should be avoided.

- If necessary, analgesics should only be prescribed in order to facilitate the gradual increase in activities and should be prescribed for a fixed period at fixed times, independent of the presence of pain.

- Refer the patient for exercise therapy to improve daily functioning (there is no evidence to support the recommendation of one specific type of exercises).

- The intensity of the exercises should be increased gradually at fixed times for a fixed period, independent of the presence of pain.

- In case of severe, long-lasting low back pain and disability, or high medical consumption for back pain, refer the patient to a multidisciplinary treatment programme aimed at functional restoration.

option for acute low back pain.[10] Passive treatment modalities (e.g. bed rest and massage) should be avoided as mono-therapy and not be used routinely, because they increase the risk of illness behaviour and chronicity.

Referral to secondary health care is not indicated in the great majority of acute low back pain patients.

Chronic low back pain

The most important objectives of treatment of chronic low back pain (Box 2) in primary medical care are: (i) to prevent or reduce disability, both physically and mentally; and (ii) to limit sick leave.[11] In case of long-lasting chronic low back pain, it is important to identify an increase in disability early, to avoid long-term medical treatment and to help the patient to live with chronic low back pain.[9] Management of chronic low back pain should focus on problems that patients have with activities of daily living, but emotional problems, depression, and other psycho-social factors may play a role. Referral for exercise therapy may be considered if patients need help improving daily functioning. If exercise therapy has failed, if there is serious disability, or if medical consumption is high, patients should be referred for multidisciplinary biopsychosocial rehabilitation.

Referral to secondary health care should be limited to chronic low back pain patients with a suspicion of serious spinal pathology or nerve root pain (see diagnostic triage). There is no evidence that surgery is effective for low back pain unless patients have sciatica/herniated discs, spinal stenosis, or spondylolisthesis.

Low back pain with sciatica

The initial management (Box 3) is aimed at providing adequate information and pain relief. Patients should be instructed that the nerve root is the very likely cause of the pain radiating into the leg and that this nerve root disorder is generally caused by a disc herniation. Such disc herniations occur frequently without giving raise to complaints and fortunately when they do they tend to regress spontaneously in most cases. Approximately 75 per cent of patients will recover spontaneously within 3 months. Patients should be told that the basis of management at first is adequate pain relief (including narcotic analgesics) and hypnotic medication (to induce sleep, not muscle relaxation) if required.

Patients with sciatica are probably more likely to receive inadequate than too much pain medication. A stepwise approach seems reasonable. For instance, a simple analgesic can be prescribed first, adding codeine or substituting naproxen if necessary. Though the benefit of narcotic analgesics has not been specifically demonstrated, they might be prescribed in cases of excruciating pain. The risk of inducing dependence is probably negligible in acute pain syndromes. For pharmacokinetic and psychological purposes, pain medication should be prescribed on a fixed time schedule (time contingent) and not on an 'as needed' basis. There is no added benefit for NSAIDS for sciatica. There is also no evidence that intramuscular steroids or other drugs are superior to placebo. There is as yet no unequivocal evidence that epidural injections with corticosteroids have benefit so referral is not warranted. Prescribing a 2-week regimen of bed rest (only allowing the patient to visit the toilet and shower) does not cure low back pain with

Box 3 Recommendations for the initial management of low back pain with neurological involvement

- Provide adequate information also pointing out the high rate of spontaneous recovery.

- Provide time-contingent pain relief, hypnotic drugs if necessary.

- Avoid strict bed rest.

- Paramedical therapy is not effective in the acute stage, but may guide the patient during recovery.

- Additional investigations are only required when there is suspicion of malignancy or when surgery is indicated; such investigations generally require referral.

- Warning signs and symptoms requiring urgent referral are a history of malignancy, cauda equina syndrome, involvement of multiple nerve roots or onset of paresis.

- An absolute indication for surgery exists for cauda equina only. Paresis is much more controversial as an absolute indication. It may recover with conservative therapy. In patients with pain without cauda equina syndrome or paresis surgery is an elective procedure. The indication depends on severity and duration of pain as well as psycho-social factors. If severe pain has persisted beyond 6–8 weeks, the patient should be referred.

sciatica.[12] Consequently, there is no reason to prohibit the patient to engage in activities of daily life.

There seems to be insufficient evidence supporting the effectiveness of most of the paramedical treatments for nerve root compression.[13] The therapies have been the topic of isolated trials with considerable methodological flaws. Of these, only manipulation had a positive effect in one study. This needs to be confirmed in another study. There is no evidence that traction or exercise therapy are beneficial.

Although surgical therapy for nerve root compression is essentially not a primary care topic, the physician is likely to be confronted with questions concerning this topic. There are great variations between countries concerning the indication for lumbosacral discectomy. This is probably determined to a large extent by cultural differences. Recommendations regarding the indication for surgery are included.

Long-term care

A variety of interventions are employed to prevent (recurrence of) low back pain but most of them lack any evidence of effectiveness. The most frequently reported interventions include back schools and other educational efforts, lumbar supports, and exercises. Ergonomic interventions appear to be frequently employed but have never been properly evaluated. The current evidence suggests that exercises seem to be the only effective preventive intervention. Compliance may be central to the effectiveness of preventive interventions. However, the majority of back pain patients fail to continue recommended exercises. Rather than applying prevention to all low back pain patients, selecting those at risk for developing chronic problems might offer better efficiency.

Social implications

Low back pain is also a major occupational health problem. Collaboration with occupational physicians may be required when back pain occurs in people of working age. Occupational health care for back pain varies considerably among countries depending on the occupational health and social security systems. Back pain is common in all occupations and is a major cause of work absenteeism and disablement. Prevention of work absenteeism and disablement is one of the most important aims of low back pain management in primary medical care. Giving a patient entitlement to absence from work because of non-specific low back pain may be essential in some severe cases, but should be avoided where possible as it is likely to delay rather than hasten recovery. Primary care physicians are recommended to secure consent from the patient for an early discussion with the occupational health practitioner to agree a shared plan for case management.

Low back pain is a major economic burden to society associated with high direct costs of health care utilization and tremendous indirect costs of productivity. However, only few full economic evaluations have been conducted and, consequently, little is known about the cost-effectiveness of the various treatment options for acute and chronic low back pain. Especially, interventions that result in a reduction of work absenteeism and speed up return to work will most likely be very cost-effective. Therefore, future randomized controlled trials are needed that meet the current high methodological standards and include a full economic evaluation.

Key points

- Undertake diagnostic triage on the basis of history and physical examination at the first assessment to exclude relevant specific spinal disorders and radicular syndrome.

- Be aware of psycho-social factors that might influence the prognosis.

- Diagnostic imaging tests (including X-rays, CT, and MRI) are not routinely indicated for non-specific low back pain.

- Do not prescribe bed rest as a treatment.

- Advise patients to stay active and continue normal daily activities including work if possible.

- Refer the patient for exercise therapy to improve daily functioning.

- Reassess patients who are not resolving within a few weeks after the first visit or who are following a worsening course.

- In case of severe, long-lasting low back pain and disability, or high medical consumption for back pain, refer the patient to a multidisciplinary treatment programme.

References

1. Kelsey, J.L. and White A.A. 3rd. (1980). Epidemiology and impact of low-back pain. *Spine* 5, 133–42.

2. Thomas, E., Silman, A.J., Croft, P.R., Papageorgiou, A.C., Jayson, M.I., and Macfarlane, G.J. (1999). Predicting who develops chronic low back pain in primary care: a prospective study. *British Medical Journal* 318, 1662–7.

3. Andersson, G.B.J. (1999). Epidemiological features of chronic low back pain. *Lancet* 354, 581–5.

4. Deyo, R.A. (1988). Measuring the functional status of patients with low back pain. *Archives of Physical Medicine Rehabilitation* 69, 1044–53.

5. Gran, J.T. (1985). An epidemiological survey of the signs and symptoms of ankylosing spondylitis. *Clinical Rheumatology* 4, 161–9.

6. Deyo, R.A., Rainville, J., and Kent, D.L. (1992). What can the history and physical examination tell us about low back pain? *Journal of the American Medical Association* 268, 760–5.

7. Vroomen, P.C.A.J. et al. (1999). Diagnostic value of history and physical examination in patients with sciatica due to disc herniation. *Journal of Neurology* 246, 899–906.

8. Van den Hoogen, J.M.M., Koes, B.W., van Eijk, J.Th.M., and Bouter, L.M. (1995). On the accuracy of history, physical examination and erythrocyte sedimentation rate in diagnosing low back pain in general practice: a criteria based review of the literature. *Spine* 20, 318–27.

9. Van Tulder, M.W., Koes, B.W., and Bouter, L.M. (1997). Conservative treatment of acute and chronic non-specific low back pain: a systematic review of randomized controlled trials of the most common interventions. *Spine* 22, 2128–56.

10. Waddell, G., Feder, G., and Lewis, M. (1997). Systematic reviews of bed rest and advice to stay active for acute low back pain. *British Journal of General Practice* 47, 647–52.

11. Deyo, R.A. and Weinstein, J.N. (2001). Low back pain. *New England Journal of Medicine* 344, 363–70.

12. Vroomen, P.C.A.J. et al. (1999). Lack of effectiveness of bed rest for sciatica. *New England Journal of Medicine* 340, 418–23.

13. Vroomen, P.C., de Krom, M.C., Slofstra, P.D., and Knottnerus, J.A. (2000). Conservative treatment of sciatica: a systematic review. *Journal of Spinal Disorders* 13, 463–9.

Further reading

Waddell, G. *The Back Pain Revolution*. Edinburgh: Churchill Livingstone, 1998.

Nachemson, A.L. and Jonsson, E., ed. *Neck and Back Pain: The Scientific Evidence of Causes, Diagnosis, and Treatment*. Philadelphia PA: Lippincott Williams & Wilkins, 2000.

13.2 Neck pain

Nefyn H. Williams and Jan Lucas Hoving

Epidemiology

Surveys from different countries have shown that neck pain is very common in the community, with prevalence approaching that of low back pain. Lifetime prevalence is 67–71 per cent, 1-year prevalence 12–46 per cent, and point prevalence 13–22 per cent. Chronic neck pain lasting longer than 3–6 months is present in 14–19 per cent of the community. In common with many other musculoskeletal disorders its prevalence is greater in women and in middle age.[1–3] In the Netherlands, 16 GP visits per 1000 people per year are for neck pain.[4] In the United Kingdom, 78 per 1000 registered patients consult their GP over the course of 1 year with 'symptoms involving head and neck', and nine with 'other disorders of cervical region'.[5] This disparity reflects differences in the classification systems used in these studies. Unfortunately, no clear, valid and reproducible classification system has yet been developed.[6]

Neck pain is associated with a history of neck injury, particularly in motor vehicle accidents, and with occupational factors such as repetitive or continuous workload, prolonged sitting, twisting or bending of the trunk, and unfavourable psycho-social working conditions. It is also associated with other musculoskeletal complaints such as back pain, shoulder pain, and headache. This association is stronger with increasing neck pain severity.[1,3,7]

Although most acute neck pain settles within a few weeks of onset, surprisingly little is known about its course in a primary care or community setting. Most studies have investigated chronic pain of more than 6 months duration, in secondary care or occupational settings with a short-term follow-up. In a Dutch study, 50 per cent of the patients with chronic neck pain reported their pain to be less after a follow up of 6 months, with a 30 per cent mean reduction in analgesic consumption and pain.[8]

Studies reporting on prognostic factors have been small with poor methodology, and have suggested that there is a weak association between the presence of pain radiating to the arms, or the presence of neurological signs and a worse outcome. The severity of the pain and a history of previous attacks are also associated with a worse prognosis, but there is no association between the radiological findings of spondylosis and a worse prognosis.[8]

Differential diagnosis

As in low back pain, only a small proportion of patients with neck pain can be diagnosed with definite pathology. There is a wide variation in terminology denoting conditions of the neck. For clinical purposes neck pain can be sub-divided into three groups: possible serious spinal pathology, nerve root pain, and non-specific or mechanical neck pain.

Serious pathological disease

Serious underlying causes are rare and include: fractures, bone metastases, inflammatory arthritides such as rheumatoid disease acute and chronic infection, and less commonly, soft tissue tumours such as meningioma, neurofibroma, and schwannoma. Serious spinal pathology may give rise to neck pain, nerve root pain, or spinal cord compression.

Nerve root pain

Nerve root pain can be defined as pain, motor dysfunction, sensory deficits and/or alteration in reflex activity in the distribution of a specific nerve root, which can extend into any portion of the upper extremity.[9]

The annual incidence of cervical nerve root pain is 0.8 per 1000 population, with peak incidence in those around 50 years of age. The prevalence has been estimated at 3.3 cases per 1000.[10] It can be caused by serious pathology (see above) or foraminal narrowing caused by disc prolapse, spondylosis or spinal stenosis. The relationship between nerve root pain and pathological changes seen on magnetic resonance imaging (MRI) is not straightforward. Nerve root pain may be present in the absence of abnormality, whereas clear pathology may be present in those without symptoms.[11]

Non-specific or mechanical neck pain

This is by far the commonest group of disorders both in the community and presenting in primary care. By the very definition, no pathological cause can be found to explain them. Several underlying mechanisms have been postulated.

Degenerative change and non-specific neck pain

Cervical spondylosis

The combination of disc shrinkage and osteoarthritis of the facet joints is termed *spondylosis*, and is often referred to as *degenerative* change. It is a common radiological finding in patients with non-specific neck pain. The association between these radiological findings and symptoms is weak, so it might be better to describe spondylosis as normal age-related change, similar to grey hair.

Prolapsed intervertebral discs that do not irritate the spinal nerve root may provoke pain in the annulus fibrosus, which is richly innervated with nociceptive fibres. However, it is known from MRI studies that asymptomatic cervical disc protrusions are present in 10–15 per cent of the population.[11]

Trauma and non-specific neck pain

Sprains and strains

Sprained ligaments or strained muscles are frequently cited as reasons for neck pain, but such injuries heal after a few weeks, whereas neck pain often persists for longer.

Whiplash injury

Neck pain and other associated symptoms following a motor vehicle accident are commonly referred to as 'whiplash', although strictly speaking this describes a mechanism of injury rather than a syndrome. The development of acute symptoms of neck pain and headache following such an injury is generally accepted, but the persistence of such symptoms for periods in excess of 6 months following the injury is controversial.[12] The 'whiplash' syndrome exemplifies the need to consider all of the biological, psychological, and social components of an illness.

- *Biological factors.* Placebo-controlled local anaesthetic blocks demonstrate facet joint pain in 60 per cent of subjects with chronic neck pain after a whiplash injury.

- *Psychological factors.* Signs of depression, anxiety, reduced attention, and concentration are common.[13]

- *Social factors.* Although the acute symptoms appear to cross cultural borders, the recovery rate does not. The prevalence of chronic symptoms varies with different cultures, and different systems for payment of health services, and compensations after injuries, but with similar traffic conditions.[13]

Other theories

Other diagnostic labels include facet syndromes, discogenic pain, and somatic dysfunction. However, for any of these, reliable clinical features are either absent or unproven. Further clinical epidemiological studies based in primary care are needed.

Diagnostic approach

Diagnostic triage (see Table 1 and Fig. 1)

The first step is to exclude non-musculoskeletal causes, such as cardiovascular, respiratory, and oesophageal disease, and acute self-limiting infections of the upper respiratory tract and throat. Once it has been established that there is a spinal problem, assessment should distinguish between serious spinal pathology, nerve root pain, and non-specific neck pain. Although the cause of non-specific neck pain remains largely unknown, it can be distinguished from serious spinal pathology and nerve root pain on clinical grounds.

Serious spinal pathology

'Red flag' symptoms

Serious spinal pathology presenting to primary care is rare, but must be excluded in all cases. A number of warning clinical features or *red flags* can be used to raise the suspicion of serious pathology in the neck.

- *Age.* Patients presenting before the age of 20, or with a new or different pain after the age of 55 are more likely to have serious disease.

- *Non-mechanical pain.* Pain that is unrelated to time or physical activity, particularly if it is progressive and unrelenting. Rest or exercise does not relieve it and the patient may not be able to find any position of comfort.

- *Violent trauma.* Severe trauma from a motor vehicle accident or a fall from a height is required to fracture a spine in normal circumstances.

Table 1 Examination routine for neck disorders

Focus	Procedure	Interpretation
General	Posture	Head poked, round shouldered
	Shoulder level	
Soft tissues	Muscle hypertonus	
Gross movements	*Active movement*	
	Forward flexion	Ease of movement and pattern
	Extension	of restriction
	Rotations	
	Side bends	
Shoulder joint	Shoulder elevation	Exclude shoulder pathology
Neurology	*Resisted movements* (always compare left and right)	
	Nerve roots	
	Shoulder	
	Shrugging	C2, 3
	Abduction	C5
	Adduction	C7
	External rotation	C5
	Internal rotation	C6
	Elbow	
	Flexion	C5, 6
	Extension	C7
	Thumb	
	Adduction/abduction	C8
	Finger	
	Abduction/adduction	T1
	Reflexes (if loss of power demonstrated)	
	Biceps	C5, 6
	Brachioradialis	C5, 6
	Triceps	C7
	Plantar	Spinal cord compromise
	Sensory examination (if loss of sensation reported in the history)	
	Passive movements (optional, to localize region of the dysfunction)	

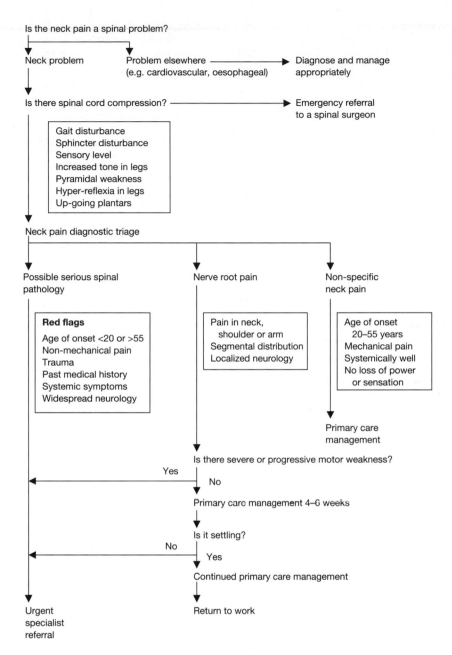

Fig. 1 Diagnostic triage for a patient presenting with neck pain. (Adapted from CSAG back pain guidelines.)

However, minor trauma may fracture osteoporotic bone in post-menopausal women or patients exposed to long-term systemic steroids.

- *Previous medical history.* Many systematic diseases can affect the neck such as rheumatoid disease, tuberculosis, carcinoma, osteoporosis, and HIV infection. Drug abuse and immune suppression may predispose to infection. Systemic steroids and premature menopause are risk factors for osteoporosis.

- *Systemic symptoms.* Alarm symptoms include abnormal weight loss, general malaise, and fever.

- *Widespread neurological symptoms.* Loss of power or sensation involving more than one nerve root. Progressive stiffness in the legs with increasing difficulty walking. Difficulty with micturition or faecal incontinence.

'Red flag' signs

- *Widespread neurological signs.* Weakness involving more than one myotome, and loss of sensation in more than one dermatome. Long tract signs indicating cord compression include spastic gait disturbance, increased muscle tone in the legs, pyramidal pattern of weakness, hyper-reflexia in the legs with clonus and up-going plantar reflexes, loss of position sense in the toes and loss of coordination in the heel–shin test. In the presence of faecal incontinence there may be loss of anal sphincter tone.

The negative predictive value of these 'red flag' clinical findings is high, because if no red flags are present, it is unlikely that any serious spinal pathology has been missed. However, individual positive findings must be interpreted with care as their positive predictive value for diagnosing serious pathology is poor.

Additional diagnostic procedures

When clinical red flags are present initial investigations include a plain radiograph of the cervical spine and erythrocyte sedimentation rate (ESR) measurement. MRI or other imaging is justified in the presence of widespread neurological signs or symptoms. In the absence of red flags, these investigations are unlikely to help, and will lead to a number of false-positive findings. These investigations can help confirm clinical suspicion of severe pathology, but normal results do not exclude it. The decision to refer to secondary care depends upon the severity of the clinical findings and the presence of red flags.

Nerve root pain

Symptoms

This presents as unilateral neck, shoulder and/or arm pain that has a segmental pattern approximating that of a dermatome. It may be associated with altered or absent sensation, or muscle weakness in related muscles. The presence of pain radiating into the arm, or of paraesthesia, is not specific for nerve root pain and may be present in non-specific disorders of the neck.

Signs

- *Observation*. Postural asymmetry may be present with the head held to one side or held flexed, as this position provides the best anatomical decompression of the nerve root. Muscle wasting may be present in long-standing cases.

- *Neck movements*. These are restricted by pain in the neck or sharp pain radiating into the upper extremity, especially during extension, side bending, and rotation towards the affected side.

- *Dural irritation*. The foraminal compression (Spurling) test involves the patient bending their head to one side, whilst the examiner carefully presses down on their vertex. The test is positive if pain radiates to the side to which the head is bent, however, its reliability and predictive value is unknown.

- *Neurological signs*. Nerve root compression may lead to loss of sensation or motor weakness in the affected dermatome or myotome. If weakness is present, the associated deep tendon reflex may also be absent. Nerve root symptoms should arise from a single nerve root. Involvement of more than one nerve root suggests a more widespread neurological disorder.

Non-specific or mechanical neck pain

Patients are usually middle-aged and general health is unaffected.

Symptoms

The essential component of mechanical pain is that it varies with physical activity and with time. Pain may be precipitated by an awkward movement; postural insult, overuse, or they may be no obvious precipitant. The pain may radiate in a non-segmental pattern into the shoulder, down the arm up to the head, or around the scapulae. It will be aggravated by particular movements, postures, and activities and relieved by others. Often activity aggravates the pain and rest relieves it, but sometimes the opposite is true. In any case, the essential component of mechanical pain is that it *varies* with different activities. There may be associated areas of paraesthesia and hyper-aesthesia, but no objective loss of sensation or muscle strength. It may be associated with headache, with pain in other regions of the spine, and with dizziness. Patients may complain of odd sensations that are vague and difficult to describe, such as temperature changes or subjective weakness, but there is no loss of power.

Signs

There are four components to the examination:

- *Positional asymmetry*. There may be asymmetry of posture with the neck pulled to one side as seen in acute torticollis or merely a change in the most comfortable resting position of the neck.

- *Asymmetrical movement restriction*. Neck movement is commonly restricted in an asymmetrical pattern.

- *Soft tissue signs*. These include localized areas of increased muscle tone, palpated as tender bands or nodules.

- *Tenderness*. This can be elicited in many structures including hypertonic muscle and intervertebral joints.

Principles of management (see Fig. 1)

Diagnostic triage categorizes the neck pain into one of three clinical groups.

Serious spinal pathology

Patients with possible serious spinal pathology are referred urgently to the appropriate secondary care specialist. It is better to err on the side of caution and refer patients with equivocal clinical features to avoid missing serious pathology.

Nerve root pain

Nerve root pain of less than 4–6 weeks duration, in the absence of objective neurological signs, should be managed as for non-specific pain. Persistent nerve root pain lasting longer than 6 weeks, or the presence of objective neurological signs, requires secondary care referral. Firstly, to confirm the diagnosis with MRI, and secondly, to consider more invasive procedures such as transforaminal injections or spinal surgery. There is a large overlap in clinical criteria with that of non-specific neck pain, particularly when pain is referred distally and associated with paraesthesia. It is preferable to avoid referral when the diagnosis of nerve root pain is in doubt, to reduce iatrogenic harm from unnecessary orthopaedic surgery. Even so, the percentage of patients with nerve root pain eventually needing surgery is low, and ranges between 8 and 33 per cent.[10] Surgery is usually restricted to patients with persistent or debilitating pain, in combination with loss of power or sensation.

Non-specific neck pain

There is insufficient evidence for the effectiveness of most physical treatments or manual therapies including exercise, mobilization, manipulation, heat or cold, traction, biofeedback, spray and stretch, acupuncture, or laser. Only a small number of studies are available, and the studies are heterogeneous with regard to methodological quality, study populations, interventions, reference treatments, and outcome measures.

A multimodal treatment strategy including exercise plus mobilization or manipulation seems to be the most effective in alleviating pain.[14] There is no evidence that one type of manipulative therapy or exercise is superior to another.[14] The evidence for multidisciplinary biopsychosocial rehabilitation as practised in pain clinics is poor.[15] After an acute whiplash injury, early resumption of normal activity is more effective than immobilization in a cervical collar or rest.[14] In general, activity is good and inactivity is bad, which can be summed up in the aphorism 'rest makes rusty'.

Management strategy

The evidence for some of the treatment approaches for neck pain have been generalized from the larger body of evidence in low back pain research. Most people have neck pain at some stage in their lives. Most episodes resolve within days or weeks, but often recur or become chronic. It should be considered a recurrent fluctuating condition, and any episode of neck pain must be considered in the context of the background of symptoms.

Acute phase (the first 3–4 weeks)

In the early phase, patients need to be reassured that their symptoms are likely to resolve, advised about unfavourable ergonomic and psycho-social working conditions, and encouraged to remain active. Limited courses of simple analgesia or non-steroidal anti-inflammatory drugs (NSAIDs) can be used for pain relief. The use of a cervical collar and prolonged absence from work should be discouraged.

Sub-acute phase (from 3–4 to 12 weeks)

If symptoms persist, referral for a multimodal treatment strategy including exercise plus some form of manual therapy should be considered. Patients should be encouraged to exercise to *move* the painful part; 'rest makes rusty'. Psycho-social factors prolonging the episode should be addressed. Factors to be considered include recognition of fear avoidance beliefs, promotion of positive attitudes to activity and work, tackling associated anxiety and depression, medico-legal proceedings, and family dynamics. Referral to a psychologist or occupational physician may help to address these factors. The hope is that intervention at this stage will prevent progress to chronic symptoms.

Chronic phase (longer than 12 weeks)

Prolonged symptoms become progressively more difficult to treat. If symptoms prevent the patient from engaging in daily activities, low-dose amitriptyline (10–50 mg) can be tried to modify pain and aid sleep. Continuous prescribing of opioid analgesia should be avoided because of the risk of dependency. Psycho-social factors should be re-examined periodically. A course of physiotherapy or spinal manipulation can be given if not tried previously, but should be discontinued if unhelpful. The aim of these treatments should be activation. Passive treatments like massage or electrotherapy are therefore not recommended. Pain clinic referral may now be considered, in particular to a multidisciplinary pain management programme. Referral to an orthopaedic surgeon or rheumatologist is usually unhelpful.

Long-term and continuing care

Nerve root pain

The long-term prognosis for patients with cervical nerve root pain who avoid surgery is good, as 90 per cent are asymptomatic or only mildly incapacitated after 5 years.[10]

Non-specific neck pain

Previous neck pain is an important risk factor for future neck pain. The long-term effects of interventions for neck pain, like most musculoskeletal disorders, has not been convincingly shown. Like low back pain, neck pain is a recurrent condition. Exercise shows promise, particularly when combined with manual therapy. One system of exercise has not been shown to be superior to another. There is insufficient data on neck schools, ergonomic interventions, or modification of biomechanical and psycho-social risk factors.[8,14]

Implications of the problem

Neck pain has a considerable impact on the health and quality of life of individuals and on society as a whole. A population-based study in Canada found that over a 6-month period, 48 per cent had low disability due to varying degrees of neck pain and 5 per cent suffered high disability because of neck pain.[2] In industry, neck disorders account for as many days of lost work as low back pain. In Quebec, 7 per cent of workers' compensation claims are for neck injuries.[12] In the Netherlands, the total cost of neck pain in 1996 was US$ 686 million (522 million Euro), which accounted for 1 per cent of total health care expenditure and 0.1 per cent of the gross domestic product. Indirect costs (absenteeism) accounted for 50 per cent of the total cost.[4]

Modest changes to the prevalence, episode length, and degree of disability would have enormous implications for health, quality of life, and economics. It is thus surprising that so little is known about the natural history and aetiology of this common condition. Future studies should determine which treatment works best for which patient. Better strategies of management in primary care need to be developed, and different primary care interventions tested, in order to prevent patients developing chronic pain and disability. There is a shortage of good high-quality randomized controlled trials with adequate sample size based in primary care. Furthermore, the cost-effectiveness of different neck pain interventions needs to be evaluated.

Key points

- Neck pain patients can be triaged into three groups, those with serious spinal pathology, nerve root pain, and non-specific or mechanical neck pain.

- Mechanical or non-specific pain is by far the commonest group seen in primary care, but its natural history and aetiology remains largely unknown.

- Serious spinal pathology is mainly diagnosed by reference to alarm features ('red flags') in the patient's history and physical examination. Investigations are of lesser importance.

- Principles of management for non-specific pain include avoiding cervical collars, and time off work, using simple analgesia and remaining active, as 'rest makes rusty'.

- Useful interventions include a combination of exercise plus some form of manual therapy.

References

1. Nachemson, A.L. and Jonsson, E., ed. *Neck and Back Pain: The Scientific Evidence of Causes, Diagnosis and Treatment.* Philadelphia PA: Lippincott Williams & Wilkins, 2000. (Evidence-based overview.)
2. Cote, P., Cassidy, J.D., and Carroll, L. (1998). The Saskatchewan health and back pain survey: the prevalence of neck pain and related disability in Saskatchewan adults. *Spine* **23**, 1689–98.
3. Ariëns, G.A.M., Borghouts, J.A.J., and Koes, B.W. (1999). Neck pain. In *The Epidemiology of Pain* (ed. I. Crombie), pp. 235–55. Seattle WA: IASP Press.
4. Borghouts, J.A.J. et al. (1999). Cost of illness of neck pain in the Netherlands in 1996. *Pain* **80**, 629–36.
5. McCormick, A., Fleming, D., and Charlton, J. *Morbidity Statistics from General Practice. Fourth National Study 1991–1992.* London: HMSO, 1995.
6. Buchbinder, R. et al. (1996). Classification systems of soft tissue disorders of the neck and upper limb: do they satisfy methodological guidelines? *Journal of Clinical Epidemiology* **49**, 141–9.
7. Cote, P., Cassidy, J.D., and Carroll, L. (2000). The factors associated with neck pain and its related disability in the Saskatchewan population. *Spine* **25**, 1109–17.
8. Borghouts, J.A.J., Koes, B.W., and Bouter, L.W. (1998). The clinical course and prognostic factors of non-specific neck pain: a systematic review. *Pain* **77**, 1–13.
9. Chesnut, R.M., Abitol, J., and Garfin, S.R. (1992). Surgical management of cervical radiculopathy: indication, techniques and results. *Orthopedic Clinics of North America* **23**, 461–73.
10. Radhakrishnan, K. et al. (1994). Epidemiology of cervical radiculopathy. A population-based study from Rochester, Minnesota, 1976 through 1990. *Brain* **117**, 325–35.
11. Boden, S.D. et al. (1990). Abnormal magnetic resonance scans of the cervical spine in asymptomatic subjects: a prospective investigation. *Journal of Bone and Joint Surgery [American]* **72**, 1178–84.
12. Spitzer, W.O. (1995). Whiplash-associated disorders. *Spine* **20** (Suppl. 8), 1–73.
13. Stovner, L.S. (1996). The nosological status of the whiplash syndrome: a critical review based on a methodological approach. *Spine* **21**, 2735–46.

14. **Gross, A.R.** et al. (1996). Conservative management of mechanical neck disorders: physical medicine modalities for mechanical neck disorders (Cochrane review). In *The Cochrane Library* Issue 1, 2000. Oxford: Update Software.

15. **Karjalainen, K.** et al. (2001). Multidisciplinary biopsychosocial rehabilitation for neck and shoulder pain among working age adults. *Spine* **26**, 196–205.

13.3 Acute joint pain

Jerry G. Ryan and Thomas M. Best

Musculoskeletal pain or dysfunction is the presenting complaint for one of seven patients seen by primary care providers. Although most patients with acute joint pain will have benign, self-limited abnormalities, a small number of patients will require immediate evaluation and treatment. Despite the frequency of these symptoms, surveys of recent graduates of family practice training programmes often indicate a desire for additional training in the diagnosis and treatment of musculoskeletal complaints. A systematic approach to the patient with acute traumatic or atraumatic joint pain will help the primary care provider identify those patients who require immediate intervention as well as devise the most appropriate treatment plan for those patients with less urgent conditions.

Traumatic joint pain

It is beyond the scope of this chapter to provide a detailed listing of all possible traumatic injuries to the peripheral joints. Instead, a general approach to the injured joint will be presented followed by a brief description of common pitfalls encountered in the diagnosis and treatment of injuries to specific joints.

History

The patient is asked to describe the mechanism of injury. The following points in the history will increase the likelihood of a more serious injury.

1. Collision with another individual or structure.

2. Inability to continue with the activity that led to the injury.

3. Effusion of the joint immediately following the injury.

Patients who are able to continue activity, report only minor trauma and do not experience significant pain or effusion of the joint for several hours following the injury are unlikely to require immediate medical or surgical intervention. These patients can be treated conservatively with rest and ice and require more extensive evaluation only if the pain persists for more than 72 h. The importance of an accurate history cannot be overemphasized. For example, a study of 2266 women who underwent arthroscopy revealed that medial meniscus and anterior cruciate ligament (ACL) tears of the knee were correctly diagnosed by history alone in greater than 85 per cent of the patients.

Physical examination of traumatic joint injury

Erythema or warmth of the joint indicates inflammation and requires an immediate evaluation of the synovial fluid. Joint swelling indicates the presence of an effusion. Effusions that arise immediately following an injury are often due to intra-articular bleeding and may indicate ligament rupture or

bony injury. In contrast, effusions that accumulate several hours or days following trauma are most likely due to a gradual accumulation of synovial fluid and rarely require immediate intervention. Supporting ligaments are manually stressed to determine joint stability. A large effusion may distend the joint capsule and prevent adequate assessment of joint stability at the time of injury. If a significant effusion is present, the joint should be protected with a splint or other appropriate methods and reexamined when the effusion has diminished. Severe pain immediately post-injury may also prevent adequate assessment of joint stability. Joint instability indicates rupture or significant injury of supporting ligaments and necessitates orthopaedic referral. Range of motion is documented. Decreased range of motion is often due to disruption of the articular surface, loose bodies within the joint space, or signifcant effusion. Meniscus injuries of the knee can also result in a decreased range of motion. The joint is palpated for the presence of localized pain. Focal pain increases the likelihood of bony injury. Distal pulses, sensation, and muscle strength are carefully evaluated. Patients with evidence of neurovascular compromise on examination require immediate surgical evaluation.

Radiographic evaluation

Although most joint trauma results in ligament or soft tissue injuries, X-rays are frequently obtained to rule out bony injuries. Members of the Division of Emergency Medicine at the University of Ottawa in Ontario, Canada have developed criteria for ordering radiographs of knee and ankle injuries (Table 1). Presence of any of the following necessitates the need for radiographs.

Although the implementation of these guidelines significantly reduced the number of radiographs ordered at the University of Ottawa, similar reductions were not experienced at other institutions after implementation of these rules. In general, the presence of localized bony pain, decreased range of motion, or the inability to continue the activity that led to the injury increases the likelihood of bony injury. Radiographs should be obtained if any of these signs or symptoms are present.

There is disagreement in the literature regarding the value of MRI in the evaluation of joint trauma. A prospective study of 100 patients by Rose and Gold found that MRI and clinical examination have similar accuracy in diagnosing ACL tears and meniscus injury.[1] The authors concluded that MRI added little to the evaluation of a painful knee. Trieshmann and Mosure however found that MRI altered surgical decisions in 27 per cent of the 208 patients studied.[2] MRI was recommended as an effective way to avoid unnecessary surgery. This latter study however excluded patients with effusions, locking of the knee, localized pain, or abnormal radiographic findings. Patients with any of these findings were evaluated with arthroscopy without a prior MRI. A careful history and physical examination will reveal an unstable joint following trauma and referral to an orthopaedist for an urgent orthopaedic evaluation should be based upon the clinical evaluation. Little, if any, additional information is likely to be revealed by a MRI for acute joint trauma.

Table 1 Ottawa rules for ordering X-rays following injury

Ottawa rules for the knee
1. Age 55 or older
2. Isolated tenderness of the patella
3. Tenderness at the head of the fibula
4. Inability to flex to 90°
5. Inability to bear weight immediately or at the time of the exam

Ottawa rules for the ankle
1. Unable to walk more than four steps
2. Bony tenderness on the tip of or along the posterior edge of the distal 6 cm of either malleolus

Treatment

Fracture care is discussed elsewhere in this publication and will not be covered in this chapter. The evaluation and treatment of selected traumatic injuries will be discussed to help the reader when confronted with an injury to these joints.

The RICE (rest, ice, compression, and elevation) approach is frequently mentioned as the initial treatment for soft tissue injuries.

◆ *Rest*—the joint should be placed at rest to protect the joint from further injury or to decrease the level of pain. Prolonged immobilization however may decrease range of motion, decondition supporting muscles, and delay recovery.

◆ *Ice*—decreases joint effusion and joint pain. Allows for early movement of the joint following trauma. Recent interest in alternating heat and cold has not been shown to be superior to simple ice for acute injuries.

◆ *Compression*—helpful to disperse or prevent joint effusion. Elastic compression does not provide structural support to the injured joint.

◆ *Elevation*—due to the difficulty adequately elevating many joints is of limited value. Elevation decreases joint effusion in ankle and knee injuries.

A fifth element, motion, should be added to the care of the injured joint. Passive range of motion exercises immediately following knee, hand, and shoulder surgery has decreased the rehabilitation time for many surgical repairs to these joints. Early motion following ankle sprains has been shown to decrease pain and effusion more rapidly than immobilization of the ankle joint. Early protected motion following selected shoulder injuries improves the active range of motion patients are able to achieve following an injury.

Analgesics

Analgesics may be needed following an acute injury. Non-steroidal anti-inflammatory drugs (NSAIDs) are frequently prescribed for this purpose and will provide adequate analgesia for many acute injuries. A recent literature review regarding the use of NSAIDs for stretch-induced muscle injuries or strains and muscle contusions found little, if any, benefit from these medications beyond their analgesic properties. NSAIDs appear to minimally inhibit the initial post-injury inflammatory reaction but this benefit is offset by later delays in the healing process. For this reason, acetaminophen, and in severe injuries narcotics, are useful analgesic alternatives. Recently, COX-2 inhibitors have been utilized for the treatment of joint injuries but there is no evidence that these agents offer any advantage over traditional and much less costly alternatives.

Evaluating injury to individual joints

The general principles outlined above will, in most instances, identify significant joint injuries. It is useful however to highlight some common injuries and frequently encountered pitfalls while evaluating individual joints.

Shoulder

Acromioclavicular (A-C) ligament

Direct trauma to the anterolateral shoulder will most often result in an injury to the A-C joint, commonly referred to as a shoulder separation. Palpation will reveal focal pain at the A-C joint. Shoulder separations are divided into six categories. A Type 1 injury consists of a strain to the A-C ligament with no evidence of joint space widening on X-ray. A Type 2 injury reveals a widened A-C joint on X-ray but the ligament remains intact. A Type 3 injury results in disruption of the A-C and coracoclavicular ligaments without significant anterior or posterior displacement of the distal clavicle. Patients with Type 3 injuries will usually have a notable bump at the point of the shoulder. All Types 1–3 injuries are initially treated conservatively with initial rest and subsequent physical therapy as soon as symptoms permit. Although surgical repair of Type 2 and 3 injuries is sometimes performed for chronic pain of the A-C joint following injury there is little evidence that outcomes are improved with surgical repair. Resection of the distal clavicle may be performed as an alternative to joint repair. Types 4–6 A-C injuries involve disruption of the A-C and coracoclavicular ligaments and significant anterior or posterior displacement of the distal clavicle. All Types 4–6 injuries require orthopaedic referral for reduction and surgical repair. Fortunately, Types 4–6 injuries are unusual and most A-C injuries can therefore be treated non-operatively.

Rotator cuff

Although most injuries to the rotator cuff are due to chronic overuse, rotator cuff tears may be caused by acute trauma. Elderly patients (>50 years of age) and patients with chronic rotator cuff inflammation are at increased risk for rotator cuff tears. Passive and active range of motion of the humerus should be documented for all shoulder injuries with special attention paid to the patient's ability to abduct the shoulder. Painful abduction of the humerus is the most specific physical finding in patients with rotator cuff injuries. If a patient does not have pain with resisted abduction of the shoulder, an alternative diagnosis should be sought. Most rotator cuff injuries are due to overuse and consist of inflammation but not disruption of the rotator cuff mechanism. Rotator cuff tears are more likely to occur in elderly patients due to falls or young athletes engaged in sports requiring frequent and forceful overhead throwing motions. A careful examination will reveal most rotator cuff injuries but an MRI or an ultrasound of the rotator cuff is indicated if a significant tear is suspected and surgical repair is a reasonable option.

Rotator cuff tendinitis will usually respond to a programme of rest followed by range of motion and strengthening exercises once the initial discomfort has improved. Subacromial corticosteroid injections may be useful in the treatment of rotator cuff tendinitis. Repetitive injections should be avoided due to the increased risk of tendon rupture and compromise of subsequent surgical repair. Surgical intervention is not indicated in the initial treatment of most rotator cuff injuries and should be reserved for patients that have failed an extensive conservative rehabilitation programme. Mantone et al. recently reviewed the available medical literature on treatment of rotator cuff tears.[3] The investigators concluded that early surgical intervention is indicated only in young, active individuals with complete tears of the rotator cuff. Elderly or less active individuals with complete tears and all individuals with partial tears should initially be treated conservatively and surgery performed only in patients who fail conservative measures.

Dislocation of the humeral head

The vast majority of shoulder dislocations are anterior. The most common mechanism of injury is a force applied to the arm in an anterior to posterior direction while the arm is abducted and externally rotated. This force results in the humerus acting as a lever on the shoulder joint disrupting the anterior joint capsule. The humeral head is then dislocated through the disrupted joint capsule and lies anterior to the shoulder joint. Patients with anterior shoulder dislocations are unable to fully adduct and internally rotate the humerus and frequently hold the affected arm in a slightly externally rotated and abducted position. Posterior dislocations account for less than 5 per cent of shoulder dislocations and are almost exclusively due to significant impact to the anterior shoulder such as a motor vehicle accident. It is often possible to relocate the humeral head immediately following the injury before the patient experiences significant muscle spasm. Prior to any attempts to reduce a shoulder dislocation, the neurovascular status of the upper extremity should be carefully evaluated. Compromise of the neurovascular status necessitates an urgent orthopaedic referral to avoid significant injury. Sedation will likely be needed if several hours have passed between the time of injury and the attempt to reduce the dislocation.

Shoulder dislocations are usually apparent on the standard AP X-ray projection. If the diagnosis is still in doubt a Y view of the scapula can be obtained. The humeral head is normally seen overlying the intersection of the scapular spine and the body of the scapula. A dislocation of the humeral head is readily apparent with the Y view. Shoulder dislocations can also result in a depression in the superolateral portion of the humerus termed a Hill–Sachs deformity. The presence of this deformity may be the only indication of a prior shoulder dislocation.

Elbow

Medial and lateral epicondylitis

One of the most frequent causes of elbow pain is inflammation of the muscular insertions at the medial and lateral epicondyles of the distal humerus, commonly referred to as 'golfer's elbow' and 'tennis elbow', respectively. Palpation of the elbow will reveal focal pain overlying the affected epicondyle. Rest, ice, and a strengthening programme are usually sufficient to resolve the inflammation. Infiltration of the muscular insertion with corticosteroids may provide more rapid relief of pain than simple rest but does not effect the overall recovery rate. Prolotherapy has also been evaluated as an alternative treatment of acute epicondylitis and appears to have efficacy equal to corticosteroid injections.

Olecranon bursa

Most effusions of the olecranon bursa are due to an infectious or inflammatory source but trauma to the point of the elbow can also result in an effusion within the olecranon bursa. A traumatic effusion is cool to the touch and non-erythematous. Compression and rest are usually the only treatment necessary for a non-inflammatory effusion. Aspiration of the bursa is indicated if a septic process is suspected or if the size of the effusion compromises range of motion and causes significant pain. Treatment of infectious bursitis is guided by culture of the fluid obtained by aspiration. Antistaphylococcal therapy is appropriate until culture results are known. Non-infectious inflammatory bursitis is treated with rest and NSAIDs. Due to the risk of subsequent infections, corticosteroid injections of the olecranon bursa are reserved for those who have failed conservative therapy.

Wrist

The most common injury to the wrist is a simple sprain followed by contusions and fractures. Pershad et al. prospectively studied the presenting complaints and physical findings paediatric patients presenting to the Emergency Department for wrist injuries to determine if any of these findings can be used to determine the need for radiographs to rule out wrist fractures.[4] Point tenderness over the distal radius and a 20 per cent or greater decrease in grip strength were the only findings that had a significant correlation with the presence of a fracture. Careful attention should be paid to the anatomical snuff-box. Pain in this area can indicate the presence of a scaphoid fracture. Wrist sprains are treated with simple splinting for comfort and analgesics. Treatment of wrist fractures is addressed elsewhere in this publication.

Hand

Finger sprains and fractures are fairly common. Finger fracture will not be addressed here. The most frequently injured joints in the hand are the proximal intraphalangeal (PIP) joints of the fingers and the metatarsal–phalangeal (MP) joint of the thumb. Strains of the IP or MP joints without evidence of dislocation or fracture require only simple rest and buddy taping.

Dislocated joints of the hand can often be reduced at the time of injury by the primary provider. Fractures involving greater than 40 per cent of the articular surface or malalignment following reduction of a dislocated finger require orthopaedic referral and surgical repair.

Treatment of collateral ligament injuries to the thumb (Gamekeeper's thumb) is controversial. There is general agreement that inability to reduce a Gamekeeper's injury and a significant fracture of the base of the phalanx require operative repair. There is less agreement as to the proper approach to a Gamekeeper's injury without these features. A conservative approach is to treat partial tears (<30° of increased laxity at the MP joint) with a thumb spica cast and refer full thickness tears of the collateral ligament (>30° of increased laxity) for surgery.

Knee

The majority of injuries to the knee result in ligament injuries. Effusion of the knee following trauma should always be assumed to be a rupture of the anterior cruciate rupture at the time of initial evaluation. The Ottawa rules are useful for determining the need for radiographs as X-rays are seldom of value in acute knee injuries. The stability of the knee should be carefully assessed and if significant effusion is present the knee should be immobilized and re-examined after the effusion has resolved. Instability of the knee on examination indicates significant ligament disruption and necessitates orthopaedic referral. MRI is not necessary in the initial evaluation of an acute knee injury and decisions regarding initial treatment are based upon a careful history and physical examination. Aspiration of the knee is discouraged unless the effusion significantly impairs mobility. Aspiration adds little to the initial evaluation and carries the risk of introducing an infection. History of a direct fall on the patella necessitates an X-ray to rule out a patellar fracture.

Ankle

As is the case with knee injuries, most injuries to the foot and ankle represent sprains and strains and are the result of an inversion injury. The Ottawa ankle rules are of use in determining the need for X-rays. In the absence of a fracture, essentially all ankle sprains are treated conservatively and do not require surgical intervention. For this reason, radiographs obtained while placing a valgus or varus force on the ankle (stress views) add little to the evaluation of an injured ankle. Persistent ankle pain with normal radiographs should alert the provider to the possibility of a talar dome fracture or an injury to the fibrous syndesmosis between the distal fibula and tibia (high ankle sprain). A CT or MRI may be needed to detect these injuries.

Foot

Fractures of the phalanges and metatarsals due to direct trauma or overuse are common. Most non-displaced fractures will heal with little difficulty and can be treated by the primary care providers. Displaced fractures may require surgical fixation and require orthopaedic referral and will not be reviewed here. Midfoot foot pain may be due to a navicular fracture or fracture-dislocation of the tarsometatarsal articulation (Lisfranc injury). These injuries are often difficult to detect on initial examination and the initial X-rays are often normal. Weight bearing radiographs may improve detection of these injuries. The use of a short-leg walking cast or boot for 2 weeks may be prudent in patient's presenting with midfoot pain and a negative initial evaluation and the patient re-evaluated at the end of this period.

Dislocations of the MP or the IP joints of the feet are unusual, are usually easily reduced by the primary care provider and seldom require surgical repair. Repetitive or forceful hyperextension of the great toe may lead to an inflammatory arthritis of the MP joint referred to as 'Turf toe'. Turf toe will usually resolve with simple taping techniques that prevent extension of the great toe. Metatarsal pain may also be due to overuse inflammation of the MP joint termed metatarsalgia or entrapment of the intermetatarsal digital nerve between the metatarsal heads (Morton's neuroma). Both of these conditions are treated with relative rest and arch orthotics to relieve stress at the metatarsal heads.

Atraumatic joint pain

Atraumatic joint pain can be broadly categorized as inflammatory and non-inflammatory. Each of these categories may be further divided into mono- or oligoarticular (five or fewer joints involved) and polyarticular arthritis. The initial task of the primary care provider is to evaluate the patient for evidence of an inflammatory arthritis. A hot, swollen joint or joints as well as the presence of constitutional symptoms such as fever, weight loss or malaise strongly suggests the presence of infection, sepsis, or systemic rheumatic disease and requires immediate investigation and treatment. A systematic approach to all patients presenting with atraumatic joint pain will help the provider detect those patients requiring urgent intervention.

Initial examination of atraumatic pain

History

Several aspects of the history can be helpful to determine the aetiology of the patient's complaints. Tendonitis, bursitis, and non-inflammatory causes of joint pain tend to have brief periods of early morning stiffness and no constitutional symptoms while rheumatic diseases have prolonged and severe morning stiffness and produce systemic symptoms. Locking or instability of a joint indicates a mechanical defect such as a loose body or other internal derangements. Symmetrical joint involvement can be found in both non-inflammatory joint abnormalities as well as systemic rheumatic disease. Focal tenderness of the joint is typical of trauma or tendinitis but is uncommon for both non-inflammatory and rheumatic disease. As stated previously, the presence of erythema or warmth of a joint always indicates the presence of an inflammatory aetiology and requires further evaluation. The presence of an effusion without evidence of inflammation represents intra-articular damage either due to trauma or non-inflammatory joint disease. Radiographs are of limited value in the evaluation of atraumatic acute joint pain unless there is a history of prior episodes of the same pain.

Evaluation of mono- or oligoarthritis

The patient should always be carefully questioned about a history of trauma or excessive activity prior to the onset of symptoms. If there is no history of trauma, the joint should be evaluated for the presence of an effusion or signs of inflammation. If an effusion is present the joint is aspirated and the fluid sent for the following studies. Effusions of peripheral joints are usually readily apparent from the physical examination. Ultrasound can be used to evaluate less accessible joints such as the hip.

Joint fluid studies

The differential diagnosis is based upon the results of the joint aspirate.

RBC count

The presence of a bloody joint aspirate without an elevated WBC most likely indicates trauma, pseudogout, an underlying coagulopathy, or a tumour. Radiographs are performed to rule out trauma or a bony abnormality. In the absence of an abnormal X-ray a PT, PTT, platelet count, and bleeding time are obtained in the search for a coagulopathy.

WBC count and differential

The presence of more than 2000 WBC/mm^3 of joint fluid or PMNs representing greater than 75 per cent of the WBC's seen on differential represents an inflammatory arthritis. Due to significant variations in the inflammatory response the total WBC is not a reliable means of distinguishing infectious from non-infectious forms of joint pain. Intra-articular crystals, bacterial infection, viral infection, systemic rheumatoid disease, and reactive arthritis are the most common causes of inflammatory joint pain.

Crystals

The presence of crystals in the synovial fluid is highly specific for crystal-induced joint pain. Monosodium urate crystals are found in patients with gout and calcium pyrophospate crystals in patients with pseudogout. The absence of crystals does not rule out a crystal induced arthropathy.

The differentiation of gout from pseudogout is important as pseudogout does not respond to the therapeutic agents used to prevent recurrent episodes of gout.

Culture

If the synovial fluid WBC is greater than 2000/mm^3, the fluid is sent for culture and sensitivity. The diagnosis of septic arthritis is based upon the culture results and not the WBC of the synovial fluid. Cervical, uretheral, pharyngeal, and rectal specimens are obtained for Chlamydia and Gonnococcus cultures if the history indicates an increased risk for sexually transmitted disease. Sterile inflammatory joint fluid necessitates a search for other causes of inflammatory arthritis.

The common causes of sterile inflammatory joint and non-inflammatory fluid and additional studies to evaluate sterile inflammatory joint fluid are shown in Table 2.

Special note should be made regarding the diagnosis and treatment of Lyme disease. Lyme serology should only be obtained if there is a significant exposure to ticks and/or a history of erythema marginatum at the site of the tick bite. Due to the poor sensitivity of Lyme testing the majority of positive results in patients who do not have a high probability of tick exposure represent false positive tests. Routine antibiotic prophylaxis is not recommended for asymptomatic patients in high risk areas with a history of a tick bite.

Diagnosis and treatment

Reactive arthritis is increasingly recognized as the aetiology of several forms of oligoarthritis. Reactive arthritis is defined as a septic arthritis caused by viable bacteria present within the synovial fluid in a non-replicative state. Chlamydia, Yersinia, Salmonella, Shigella, Campylobacter, Clostridium, Ureaplasma, and Streptococcus are potential causes of oligoarthritis. A history of cough, diarrhoea, penile discharge, or cervical discharge requires an evaluation for one or several of these agents by most appropriate method (stool, sputum, urine, or blood cultures).

Polyarthralgia is the manifestation of an underlying systemic disease. Although the differential diagnosis is extensive, several entities should be considered in the initial evaluation. Systemic rheumatic disease must always be considered when a patient presents with acute polyarthralgias. Although the diagnosis of rheumatoid arthritis is based upon the history

Table 2 Common causes and evaluation of sterile inflammatory and non-inflammatory joint fluid

Common causes of sterile inflammatory joint fluid
Rheumatoid arthritis
Juvenile rheumatoid arthritis
Viral infection
Systemic lupus erythematosis
Lyme disease
Sarcoidosis
Spondyloarthopathy

Additional studies to evaluate sterile inflammatory joint fluid
Complete blood count
Sedimentation rate
Rheumatoid factor
ANA
HLA-B27
Lyme serologies
Liver function tests (evaluate for active hepatitis)
Pelvic radiographs (evaluate sacroiliac joints)

Common causes of non-inflammatory joint fluid
Osteoarthritis
Joint injury
Viral infection

and physical exam, the presence of an elevated sedimentation rate, positive rheumatoid factor, and an elevated ANA increase the probability of a systemic rheumatic disease. Joint fluid should be obtained and evaluated as outlined for monoarthritis although the probability of septic or crystal induced arthritis is low if multiple joints are involved simultaneously. If the intial laboratory studies do not suggest systemic rheumatic disease serology for Hepatitis B and C as well as parvovirus should be obtained as these are the most frequently indentified infectious causes of polyarthritis. If no aetiology is determined following this initial evaluation the patient should be referred to a rheumatologist for further evaluation.

Treatment is dictated by the results of the synovial fluid evaluation. Patients at risk for septic arthritis should be placed on intravenous anti-biotics for 72 h until the results of the synovial fluid cutures are complete. *Staphylococcus aureus* remains the most common cause of septic arthritis but broader coverage with either nafcillin and ceftriaxone or vancomycin and ciprofloxin is recommended until the infecting organism is identified and sensitivity studies are available. Patients with gout are started on NSAIDs and/or colchicine for relief of symptoms. Patients with pseudogout will not respond to colchicine therapy and are treated with NSAIDs. The remaining causes of oligoarthralgia represent chronic conditions and rarely require urgent intervention. Treatment is directed at the underlying aetiologies.

Key points

- Taking a careful history of the injury can alone correctly diagnose many cases of traumatic joint pain (85 per cent of meniscal and anterior cruciate ligament tears in knee pain).

- Ottawa rules give useful guidance for the need for X-ray to exclude bony injury.

- A hot swollen joint requires immediate investigation.

References

1. **Rose, N.E. and Gold, S.M.** (1996). A comparison of accuracy between clinical examination and magnetic resonance imaging in the diagnosis of meniscal and anterior cruciate ligament tears. *Arthroscopy: The Journal of Arthroscopy and Related Surgery* **12** (4), 398–405.

2. **Trieshmann, H.W. and Mosure, J.C.** (1996). The impact of magnetic resonance imaging of the knee on surgical decision making. *Arthroscopy: The Journal of Arthroscopy and Related Surgery* **12** (4), 550–5.

3. **Mantone, J.K., Burkhead, W.Z. Jr., and Noonan, J. Jr.** (2000). Nonoperative treatment of rotator cuff tears. *Orthopedic Clinics of North America* **31** (2), 295–311.

4. **Pershad, J., Monroe, K., King, W., Bartle, S., Hardin, E., and Zinkan, L.** (2000). Can clinical parameters predict fractures in acute pediatric wrist injuries? *Academic Emergency Medicine* **7** (10), 1152–5.

Further reading

American College of Rheumatology (1996). Guidelines for the initial evaluation of the adult patient with acute musculoskeletal symptoms. *Arthritis & Rheumatism* **39** (1), 1–8. (An excellent and concise review of the evaluation of the acutely painful joint.)

American Academy of Orthopaedic Surgeons. *Clinical Guidelines for the Evaluation of Joint Pain.* Available through the American Academy of Orthopaedic Surgeons, 6300 North River Rd., Rosemont, IL 60018-4262. (This series of guidelines addresses the available evidence regarding the evaluation and treatment of joint trauma.)

Rose, N.E. and Gold, S.M. (1996). A comparison of accuracy between clinical examination and magnetic resonance imaging in the diagnosis of meniscal and anterior cruciate ligament tears. *Arthroscopy: The Journal of Arthroscopic*

and Related Surgery **12**, 398–405. (A well-done review of the controversy regarding the value of MRI in the evaluation of the acute knee injury.)

Perez, L.C. (1999). Septic arthritis. *Balliere's Clinical Rheumatology* **13** (1), 37–58. (Presents a rationale and simplified approach to joint fluid evaluation.)

Wollenhaupt, J. and Zeidler, H. (1998). Undifferentiated arthritis and reactive arthritis. *Current Opinions in Rheumatology* **10**, 306–13.

Buskila, D. (2000). Hepatitis C-associated arthritis. *Current Opinions in Rheumatology* **12**, 295–9.

Kocher, M.S., Waters, P.M., and Micheli, L.J. (2000). Upper extremity injuries in the paediatric athlete. *Sports Medicine* **30**, 117–35. (Practical review of the most frequent upper extremity injuries in children.)

Clinics in Sports Medicine. W.B. Saunders. (Published four times a year. Each issue devoted to a selected topic. An excellent source of information for the primary care provider as the publication emphasizes the non-surgical treatment of a variety of athletic injuries. Most topics are frequently encountered in the primary care providers' office.)

Woodward, T.W. and Best, T.M. (2000). The painful shoulder. Parts 1 and 2. *American Family Physician* **61**, 3079–88, 3291–300. (A clear review of the examination and treatment of common causes of shoulder pain.)

Mellion, M.B., Walsh, W.M., and Madden, C. *The Team Physician's Handbook.* Lippincott Williams and Wilkins, 2001. (This handbook is written in outline form for ease of information retrieval. The text is written with the non-surgical primary provider in mind. An invaluable resource for health care providers who provide medical services to their local athletes.)

13.4 Chronic joint pain

Wil J.H.M. van den Bosch

This chapter will focus on the two most important causes of chronic joint pain: osteoarthritis and rheumatoid arthritis (RA). Other forms of arthritis like gout (see also Chapter 13.3) are considered more as an acute problem. Joint pain caused by injuries, tumour, and metabolic diseases are discussed in other chapters.

Epidemiology

In the general population 40 per cent of men and 50 per cent of women complain about musculoskeletal problems.[1] Although only a minority of these complaints are considered to be chronic joint complaints, chronic joint pain is common in general practice, in particular among women and in older age. In general practice in the Netherlands the prevalence of osteoarthritis and rheumatoid arthritis together is 6 per cent in men and 10 per cent in women.[2] In patients 75 years and over, the prevalence increases to 37 and 60 per cent, respectively. Figures from secondary care settings are difficult to interpret and extrapolate.

Osteoarthritis

Osteoarthritis is the most common cause of chronic joint pain. It is the single most common cause of disability in older patients, in particular osteoarthritis of the hip or the knee. The MCP joint of the thumb is also involved relatively often. Although all other joints can present chronic pain due to osteoarthritis, this is less common.

During one year, 25 per cent of people over 55 years have a persistent episode of knee pain. Only one in six consult their general practitioner. In 10 per cent, knee pain is caused by osteoarthritis, of which one-quarter are severely disabled.[3] In general practice, musculoskeletal problems accounts for one in 10 of new consultations, 18 per cent of them can be attributed to osteoarthritis.[4] In addition to age and gender, other factors like obesity, joint injuries, and occupational or sport activities are associated with osteoarthritis of the hip and the knee.[5–7] The relationship with obesity and occupational activities means that the prevalence of osteoarthritis is related to social status, with higher prevalence in lower socio-economic groups.

Osteoarthritis has more impact on health-related quality of life than many other chronic diseases. In several studies this impact was only exceeded by depression.[8] For osteoarthritis of the hip it is known that its substantial impact on health status is not strongly related with the degree of damage seen on X-rays.[9] Hip pain is also related to a higher risk on falls.[10]

Rheumatoid arthritis

Rheumatoid arthritis has a prevalence of 0.5–1 per cent of the population. In the Third National Morbidity Study in the United Kingdom, the prevalence was 0.75 per cent in females and 0.35 per cent in males.[11] Another prospective UK study showed an annual incidence rate of 36 per 100 000 for women and 14 per 100 000 for men. RA is rare in men aged less than 45 years. The incidence in men rises steeply with age. The incidence in women increases up to age 45 years, stabilizes to age 75 years, and falls in the very old.[12] Even in countries with universal access to health care, the impact of a well-defined chronic disease like RA seems to be closely linked to the patient's socio-economic situation.[13]

There are no strong risk factors for the development of RA. A multifactorial background is supposed, with a weak genetic component. RA sometimes clusters in certain families. Patients with a family member with RA therefore often think that there is a strong relationship and will fear for having rheumatoid arthritis when they have joint or muscle complaints. There are some hormonal factors. During pregnancy, RA will rarely occur for the first time. Immediately after pregnancy, however, there is a notable increase in the incidence of RA. Oral contraception is supposed to reduce the risk of RA. There are some other factors that are possibly related to RA, like smoking, obesity, and blood transfusions.[14]

Presentation in general practice

Chronic joint pain in the elderly mainly points to osteoarthritis. In most cases, the pain is localized in the joint itself, but sometimes pain is experienced in another area as referred pain. This is particularly true in osteoarthritis of the hip where the pain can be located in the upper leg or in the knee. Pain is usually accompanied by stiffness and diminished function of the joint. In the early stages, this pain starts at the beginning of movement, disappears after some activity, to return after heavy or prolonged activities again. Later, the pain is more continuously present, including in rest and at night. The pain perception and presentation can vary between individuals. There is no strong relationship between the intensity of the pain and the findings on the X-ray. Patients who abstain from using the affected joints with osteoarthritis may experience little pain and may still have serious osteoarthritis.

Chronic joint pain in more joints, especially the small joints of the hand and the feet, point at a polyarthritis. The diagnosis of rheumatoid arthritis is not made very easily. Normally a GP, caring for about 2000 patients, sees one new case of RA about once a year. However, given the chronic nature or the disease, he/she still cares for 10–15 patients with RA in the same population.

Pathophysiological background

Osteoarthritis is characterized by degeneration of articular cartilage followed by the formation of new bone. Inflammation of synovia, so typical for RA, only plays a minor role in osteoarthritis. The process starts with an imbalance between the structure of the cartilage and the stress on the joint. The stress can be negatively influenced by suboptimal position as in dysplasia of the hip, by injuries, by obesity, and by excessive activities during work or sport.[15] The strength of the cartilage decreases in older age. The background of the process of osteoarthritis is not fully understood. Synovial collagenase can penetrate damaged cartilage and its collagen can be further broken down. Superficial erosions of the cartilage arise, leading to hypertrophy and hyperplasia of chondrocytes. Early in this process, there is a chance that the cartilage can repair itself if the circumstances improve. Later on, the process becomes irreversible. Underlying bone will react with remodelling. On the edges of joints hypertrophic spurs appear (osteophytes), followed by osteosclerosis. The joint space narrows. There can also be cyst formation.[16]

In RA, in genetically predisposed persons, a delayed type hypersensitivity reaction to a still not yet identified stimulus starts an immunological process leading to a chronic synovitis and destructive arthritis of joints. The process starts at the microvessels of the synovia. Small vessel lumina get obliterated by thrombi and inflammatory cells, followed by cell infiltration and oedema. The synovia becomes hypertrophic. Later on there will be damage and destruction of cartilage and underlying bone tissue. RA is not only a disease of joints. In the course of the disease up to 50 per cent of all patients show some form of extra-articular disease. There are many other diseases with joint involvement leading to (poly)arthritis, listed in Table 1.

Diagnosis

Osteoarthritis

Osteoarthritis starts as a clinical diagnosis. There is no clinical feature (or a combination of features) that predicts the findings on an X-ray.[17] Early in the development of osteoarthritis of the knee, pain is often only located at either the lateral or the medial joint-line. At a later stage, the knee is enlarged and bony. Crepitation can be heard in motion and there is a reduction in range of movement, especially in flexion. Sometimes a small effusion can be found. X-ray still is the best way to confirm the diagnosis and the seriousness of the disease, when there is a typical clinical picture.

Osteoarthritis of the hip can be suspected when the patient complains about a deep pain in the groin with radiation into the upper leg and when there is a loss of rotation during flexion. In a later stage there can be loss of motion in all directions. X-ray can confirm the diagnosis when necessary. Sonography of the hip can be a way to establish involvement of the synovia. The presence of intra-articular fluid or swelling of the synovia can influence the decision to prescribe NSAIDs or to give intra-articular corticosteroids.

Rheumatoid arthritis

Rheumatoid arthritis is a clinical diagnosis. Making a definite diagnosis in the early stages of the disease is not easy. Time is an important factor. If there is a classical clinical picture with a symmetric polyarthritis of the PIP and MCP joints of both hands with morning stiffness and an elevated ESR for more than 6 weeks, the diagnosis is easy. Unfortunately, complaints often develop more vaguely. Symptoms can start in one joint, can be transient and can initially resemble other diseases, like a subacromial syndrome of the shoulder.

For general practice, the most important investigation is aimed at the establishment of the presence of arthritis. One should be aware of the fact that the detection of arthritis is different for different joints (Table 2).

The clinical investigation is primarily aimed at joints with pain. Arthritis without pain is improbable.[18]

Except for pain at palpation of the joint-line, in most cases there is swelling of the capsule. Red colouring of the joint is typical for a septic arthritis or gout, but not for RA. Morning stiffness can be a sign that helps establish the diagnosis of RA, but it must last for more than 1 h and it should be accompanied by pain, decreased mobility, and swelling of the joints.[19]

An increased ESR supports the existence of an arthritis when the synovia of bigger joints or many joints are involved. A normal ESR, however, cannot rule out RA. ESR is an acceptable method to monitor disease activity in RA. Measuring C-reactive protein has no added value.[20] Additional

Table 1 Differential diagnosis of diseases causing chronic joint pain

	Epidemiology	Male/female	Joints involved	Diagnostics	Therapy
Gout	Incidence 5/1000 patient/year	10:1	Especially MTP big toe	Uric acid crystals in joint fluid	Treatment: colchicine, NSAID Prevention: allopurinol, benzbromaron
Chondrocalcinosis		Female > male	Knee, MCP, wrist, shoulder	Joint fluid: pyrophosphate crystals	NSAID, local steroid joint injection
Reactive arthritis	Incidence 10/1000 patient/year	2:3	Knee, elbow, wrist, ankle	Not specific	NSAID
Septic arthritis	Unknown	1:1	Knee, wrist, shoulder, AC joint	Joint aspiration	Antibiotics, drainage
Ankylosing spondylitis	Prevalence: 0.1–0.2%	3:1	Spine, SI, knee, hip	HLA b27 pos; X-ray sacroileitis; bamboo-spine	Exercise programme, NSAID, sulfasalazine
Mixed connective tissue disease	Unknown		Polyarthritis	Anti RNP pos	Steroids
Polyarteritis nodosa	Unknown	Male >> female	Polyarthritis	Complement < tissue biopsy	Steroids, azathioprine
Acute rheumatic fever	Variable: peak at age 5–15 years	1:3	Hip, knee, ankle, elbow	Increasing level AST	Penicillin; steroids in case of carditis
Reiter's syndrome	Unknown	9:1	Knee, ankle, heels, low back	WBC ↑; HLA b27 pos 65%	NSAID
Behcet's syndrome	Unknown	1.7:1	Knee	Acute phase reactants ↑	NSAID, steroids, cyclophosphamide
Scleroderma	Incidence 0.3:100 000	1:3	PIPs, CPs	Eosinophilia; LE positive 50%; X-ray specific	Steroids, D-penicillamine
Systemic lupus erythematosus	Incidence 40:100 000	1:9		ANA pos	ASA

Table 2 Physical examination of joints to establish arthritis

	Inspection	Palpation	Locomotion
PIP hands	Swelling, atrophy, position	Pain joint line	Flexion more limited than extension
MCP hands	Space between knuckles filled	Tangential pressure pain	Decrease squeeze force
Wrist	Swelling dorsal side	Elevated temperature on painful joint line, especially on the dorsal side	Flexion and extension equally limited
Elbow	Swelling dorsal side, dimples next to olecranon are filled	Painful joint line	Flexion more limited than extension
Shoulder	Atrophy muscles	Not indicated (no added value)	Especially limited exorotation
PIP/MTP feet	Diffuse swelling dorsal side	Pain with tangential pressure	Limited flexion and extension
Ankle	Circular swelling	Painful joint line under both (?) malleoli	Limited plantar flexion
Knee	Swelling next to patella, swelling back of the knee	Painful joint line, hydrops, elevated temperature	Flexion more limited than extension
Hip	Not relevant	Not relevant	Endorotation and flexion more limited than abduction
Generally	Swelling, atrophy, abnormal position	Increased temperature, painful joint line, synovial swelling	Capsular pattern

serological tests are of little use in the establishment of the diagnosis of RA. In general practice, only IgM-RF is important. To demonstrate the presence of IgM-RF, latex-fixation test and Waaler–Rose test are used. The predictive value of the negative RF-test in cases with a strong clinical suspicion of RA and the predictive value of a positive RF-test in presence of doubtful clinical features are both low.[21] Not only the presence, but also the actual RF-level is important.[22] A positive RF-test in the beginning of the disease process indicates a relatively worse prognosis.[23]

For establishing the diagnosis of RA in general practice, X-rays are not the first choice. In a case with serious clinical suspicion, the GP will usually consult a rheumatologist. Erosions in the bone right under the joint surface, especially in the MTP-joints, is quite specific for RA.[24] Ultrasound and MRI are possibly more sensitive than X-rays. The definitive role of these various imaging methods, however, is still not completely clear.[25,26] In many countries, arthritis and even the suspicion of arthritis is reason to refer the patient to a specialist. To lower the threshold for

Table 3 Disease modifying antirheumatic drugs; probable lag time to side-effects

Drug	Lag time (months)	Side-effects
Hydroxychloroquine	2–3	Eyes
Aurothioglucose (IM)	2–3	Skin, kidney, blood
Auranofine (oral)	2–3	Gastrointestinal
Salazopyrine	<2	Gastrointestinal, liver, blood, skin
Cyclosporin	2–3	Kidney, blood pressure
D-penicillamine	>3	Skin, kidney, blood
Azathioprine	>3	Liver, blood
Methotrexate	<2	Gastrointestinal, liver, lung, blood
Leflunomide	<2	Gastrointestinal, liver, blood, blood pressure

referral and to shorten the time between referral and the first visit to the specialist, in some countries special early-arthritis outpatient clinics are created.

If the first symptom of RA is an acute arthritis other diagnoses have to be taken into account (see the chapter concerning acute joint complaints). In the past, GPs themselves tried to treat patients with RA with aspirin and NSAIDs to relieve their pain, to promote mobility, and to increase their functionality. Only in severe cases or in cases where there was insufficient response on treatment, patients were referred to specialist care. However, the recent introduction of disease-modifying drugs have urged a change in this policy. Except for diminishing pain and discomfort, the aim of treatment is now extended to the prevention of joint damage and conservation of joint function in the long term. So now, GPs have reason to refer patients with arthritis and a suspicion of RA to a rheumatologist earlier in the disease process. Treatment of RA with disease-modifying drugs early in the process can postpone joint damage. Although there is consensus that, in general, this is the right approach for most patients, there is still considerable doubt whether in sub-groups of patients these potent drugs may cause more harm than benefit (Table 3). It is also not clear which drug, or which combination of drugs, offers the best effects. It will be a challenge to undertake research to answer these questions.

Principles of management

Osteoarthritis

The treatment of osteoarthritis starts with giving proper information to the patient. Important issues are explanation about the course and information about the causes of this disease. Prevention of extra load to the joints by encouragement to lose weight and refrain from heavy activities at home, during work, and during sport may help. In some cases, a walking stick can be used if the problem is primarily located on one side. The second option is muscle strengthening exercises. Aid from a physiotherapist for this can be useful, but patients have to learn to manage their own disease. Exercises should be aimed at the management of daily activities. In more complicated cases, this support can be given by an occupational therapist, when available in primary (or secondary) care.

Reduction of pain is a better and more realistic treatment goal than trying to reach a complete pain-free state. In mild to moderate cases, paracetamol is a useful option. Paracetamol has an equal effect on pain as an NSAID. In patients with variable pain sensations over the day, giving paracetamol 'on demand' is the best option. In case of more chronic pain, prescription of fixed amounts can offer benefits and generally the total dose will be lower than with on-demand use.

More severe osteoarthritis can be treated by an osteotomy, aimed at a better distribution of the forces on the joint. This may especially be indicated in younger patients, when problems due to congenital anomalies (such as dysplasia of the hip) may be the underlying cause or in cases with asymmetric joint destructions. Many patients benefit from a joint replacement operation.

There are marked socio-economic differences in consultation ratios for osteoarthritis. In the United Kingdom, people in deprived areas consult GPs more often, but are less likely to receive surgery.[27]

Drug treatment for RA

Paracetamol

Painkillers like paracetamol only have a limited effect on the pain. Some patients use them as an additive treatment. In routine use there are few side-effects.

NSAIDs

In many countries, aspirin is still the first choice in drug therapy for RA. It is cheap, but it has considerable side-effects and the half-life is short, so patients need to take tablets every 3–4 h. The biggest problem is gastric–mucosal injury and gastric bleeding due to a combination of direct mucosal injury and platelet inhibition. Efforts to coat tablets of aspirin or to change its structure (non-acetylated salicylates) only partly decreased this problem and increased the price. The next generation of NSAIDs now make it possible to individualize pain medication in patients with chronic joint pain. Looking at the duration of effect, side-effects, and the price, one can make the most appropriate choice. Patients without risk factors such as a history of gastrointestinal disease or recent gastrointestinal complaints, and without hazardous co-medication sometimes can take NSAIDs such as naproxen, ibuprofen, and diclofenac for a longer period without serious side-effects. In patient with risk factors, the newer, but more expensive COX-2 inhibitors can be a better choice. The risk of gastric ulcers and bleeding can also be diminished by adding a proton pump inhibitor or misoprostol to the NSAID. This last medication offers protection of the mucosa of the stomach but does not have much effect on more subjective gastric complaints. Monitoring effect and side-effects of medication in patients with chronic joint pain is an important task for both GP and specialist.

Disease modifying antirheumatic drugs (DMARDs)

There is an increasing list of drugs used for RA. Nowadays, more of these drugs are given early in the disease process and more often also as a combination therapy. One should be careful that the side-effects of treatment do not outweigh the intended benefits.[28] Table 3 shows the lag time and the most important areas where side-effects can be expected.

Corticosteroids

Cortisone was once a wonder drug for RA patients. Then it became clear that cortisone had a lot of side-effects in the long term. It was then thought to be wrong to prescribe cortisone to RA patients. Cortisone was *only* used in a low dose to bridge the time that was needed till the DMARDs that were prescribed had enough effect. Since the risk of osteoporosis can be decreased using biphosphonates, one of the most harmful longer term side-effect of cortisone is now diminished.

Nowadays, there is an increasing amount of evidence that low-dose cortisone not only has a positive effect during treatment, but may also provide benefit for the outcome in the longer term.[29,30]

Cortisone is normally prescribed as tablets. Some patients will benefit from an injection with cortisone when there is a temporary worsening of symptoms or when the patient needs more effective symptom relief, for example, when he or she wants to go on holiday. Cortisone can also be administrated intra-articularly, when there is a single joint that does not respond to systemic treatment.[31]

Tumour necrosis factor (TNF) α-antagonists

One of the most important pro-inflammatory cytokines in chronic polyarthritis like RA is TNF-α. Inhibiting TNF-α has a positive effect on the inflammation process. It is administered intravenously or subcutaneously. It is a very expensive drug and is only used in patients that do not respond to other antirheumatic drugs.

One should always keep in mind that drug treatment is not the only treatment for RA patients. Early in the course of the disease, a patient has to learn to find a balance between rest and avoidance of stress on the one hand, and exercise and increasing physical function on the other hand. Physiotherapists and occupational therapists can offer support.

There are some possibilities for symptomatic therapy to relieve pain. Hydrotherapy, for instance, may have a positive influence on pain in RA and osteoarthritis but the evidence is weak.[32]

Joint replacement therapy is a growing option for patients with disabilities due to imminent deformation of joints or to pain and stiffness that cannot be managed by medication.

Long-term care

For osteoarthritis, after establishing the diagnosis and the severity of the problem, a management plan has to be made. This plan can contain medication to relieve pain, exercise therapy (whether or not by a physiotherapist) and advice about daily activities. Monitoring osteoarthritis is focused on adequate pain relief, maintaining optimal mobility and on controlling progression of the underlying disease process. Apart from pain, specific questions at follow-up consultations about functional status give the best information whether there should be a change in therapy. This implies asking the patient if he or she is able to keep his/her normal social contacts, if he/she can walk to a shop or ride a bicycle. Monitoring in this stage is especially focused on the optimal time to consider a surgical intervention, which has to be thought over carefully. Not only are the patient's pain and mobility an important basis for making this decision, but also his/her general medical condition, the social environment, life expectancy, and capability to participate in a post-surgery rehabilitation programme. The GP can play an important role in preparing the optimal medical and social conditions for such an operation.

Monitoring osteoarthritis is a shared responsibility of the GP and the patient. Clear arrangements have to be made whether the patient will consult the doctor in case of changes in his condition or whether the doctor makes regular appointments with his patient to monitor his condition. One aspect of this monitoring is keeping an eye on medication and on possible side-effects.

Monitoring patients with RA is a shared responsibility of the GP and the rheumatologist. Care that includes both generalists and specialists achieves substantially higher quality than either a generalist or a relevant specialist alone.[33]

In most cases, three different stages in the natural history of RA can be identified. In the first stage, the diagnosis is established and the patient is treated with the drugs that offers him/her the most benefit. In this stage the rheumatologist is the primary caregiver. Many patients with early RA are entered in drug trials. Frequent contact with the specialist is necessary. In this stage, the patient may visit other health such as physiotherapists, occupational therapists, and social workers. Although the GP can also play an important role in this phase in supporting the patient, it is important that there is no disagreement between the advice from the GP and the secondary care team.

In the second stage, the disease in many patients can be stable. A shared-care model with regular care from a GP supported by specialist care in more problematic cases can offer benefits for patients, but the role of primary and secondary care must be very clear to the patient, especially in monitoring side-effects and interactions of medication.

In the third stage, the disease is at an end-stage. There is not much inflammatory activity. The GP takes care of the patient with special attention to the social background. For these patients it can be difficult to travel to a hospital or out-patient clinic. The GP can consult a specialist for support in giving optimal care.

Prognosis

The course of RA is very variable. In some patients, the disease process seems to stop early. These patients have only minor disabilities. The diagnosis of RA is established on fulfilling the ARA criteria. After a couple of years some patients will no longer meet these criteria.[34] In other patients, there is a chronic progressive course with remissions and exacerbations. In about half of all patients with RA, the disease leads to major deformities and disabilities.[35] Nowadays, about 10 per cent of all patients will need a wheelchair sometime in the disease process. Life-expectancy of RA patients is shorter, although there is a shift during the last decade towards a better prognosis.[36]

It is possible to predict functional outcome at 1 year among patients with early inflammatory polyarthritis presenting to primary care using simple clinical variables, like large joint involvement, female sex, and longer disease duration, measured at baseline.[37] The predictions of disability in the long-term can be made more accurately after 1 year follow-up from the onset of symptoms.[38]

Implications

Chronic joint pain has major implications for quality of life. There are physical aspects (not able to do what could be done before and being dependent on others), psychological aspects (depression, loss of autonomy and sexual problems) and social aspects (change of relation with partner, loss of social contacts, work to problems, loss of income, and more costs). For osteoarthritis, surgery and joint replacement can bring a new perspective to life. It is important to ask patients with osteoarthritis about their pain, but also explicitly for functional health status, mobility, possibilities to keep social contacts, and fear or depression. The optimal indication for joint replacement surgery is not solely dependent on the level of pain. For patients with RA, in many cases, the disease has a progressive course that each time changes the patient's perspective. One should carefully give advice about using devices like wheelchairs. Patients should be able to get used to these new aspects of the disease. The introduction of devices like wheelchairs has to be considered in this respect. Professional support by doctors, nurses, and social workers can sometimes be aided by companion patients with the same disease.

Modern medication has increased the importance of managing joint pain well in the early stages. Further research is needed to know if the benefits seen can also be sustained in the longer term.

Key points

- There is no rheumatoid arthritis without arthritis! GPs must extend skills to establish arthritis in different joints.
- A patient with rheumatoid arthritis has a chronic disease with a long-term need for care.
- Chronic joint pain can be best approached by a multidisciplinary team in a shared-care model.

References

1. Miedema, H.S. *Reuma in Nederland; de cijfers* (Rheumatic Complaints in The Netherlands; the Figures). TNO-rapport, Leiden, 1994.
2. Van den Lisdonk, E., van den Bosch, W., Lagro-Janssen, A., and Huygen, F. *Diseases in General Practice* (Ziekten in de huisartspraktijk). Bunge: Elsevier, 1999.

3. Peat, G., McCarney, R., and Croft, P. (2001). Knee pain and osteoarthritis in older adults: a review of community burden and current use of primary care. *Annals of Rheumatic Diseases* **60**, 91–7.

4. Anonymous (1993). Guidelines for the diagnosis, investigation and management of osteoarthritis of the hip and knee. Report of a joint Working Group of the British Society for Rheumatology and the Research Unit of the Royal College of Physicians. *Journal of the Royal College of Physicians London* **27**, 391–6.

5. Lau, E.C. et al. (2000). Factors associated with osteoarthritis of the hip and the knee in Hong Kong Chinese: obesity, joint injury and occupational activities. *American Journal of Epidemiology* **152**, 855–62.

6. Coggon, D., Kellingray, S., and Inskip, H. (1998). Osteoarthritis of the hip and occupational lifting. *American Journal of Epidemiology* **147**, 523–8.

7. Spector, T.D. et al. (1996). Risk of osteoarthritis associated with long term weight bearing sports: a radiological survey of the hips and knees in female ex-athletes and population controls. *Arthritis and Rheumatism* **39**, 988–95.

8. Lam, C.L. and Lauder, I.J. (2000). The impact of chronic diseases on the health-related quality of care of Chinese patients in primary care. *Family Practice* **17**, 159–66.

9. Birrell, F. et al. (2000). The health impact of pain in the hip region with and without radiographic evidence of osteoarthritis: a study of new attenders to primary care. *Annals of Rheumatic Diseases* **59**, 857–63.

10. Nahit, E.S., Silman, A.J., and Macfarlane, G.J. (1998). The occurrence of falls among patients with a new episode of hip pain. *Annals of Rheumatic Diseases* **57**, 166–8.

11. Hochberg, M.C. (1990). Changes in the incidence and prevalence of rheumatoid arthritis in England and Wales, 1970–1982. *Seminars in Arthritis and Rheumatism* **19**, 294–302.

12. Symmonds, D.P. et al. (1994). The incidence of rheumatoid arthritis in the United Kingdom: results from the Norfolk Arthritis Register. *British Journal of Rheumatology* **33**, 735–9.

13. Brekke, M., Hjortdahl, P., Thelle, D.S., and Kvien, T.K. (1999). Disease activity and severity in patients with rheumatoid arthritis: relations to socio-economic inequality. *Social Science & Medicine* **48**, 1743–50.

14. Symmons, D.P. et al. (1997). Blood transfusion, smoking, and obesity as risk factors for the development of rheumatoid arthritis: results from a primary care-based incident case-control study in Norfolk, England. *Arthritis and Rheumatism* **40**, 1955–61.

15. Lequesne, M.G., Dang, N., and Lane, N.E. (1997). Sport practice and osteoarthritis of the limbs. *Osteoarthritis and Cartilage* **5**, 75–86.

16. Hamerman, D. (1989). The biology of osteoarthritis. *New England Journal of Medicine* **320**, 1322–30.

17. Claessens, A.A., Schouten, J.S., van den Ouweland, F.A., and Valkenburg, H.A. (1990). Do clinical findings associate with radiographic osteoarthritis of the knee? *Annals of Rheumatic Diseases* **49**, 771–4.

18. Jones, A., Ledingham, J., Regan, M., and Doherty, M. (1991). A proposed minimal rheumatological screening history and examination. *Journal of the Royal College of Physicians London* **25**, 111–15.

19. Hazes, J.M.W., Hayton, R., and Silman, A.J. (1993). A re-evaluation of the symptom of morning stiffness. *Journal of Rheumatology* **20**, 1138–42.

20. Bull, B.S. et al. (1989). Efficacy of tests used to monitor RA. *Lancet* **ii**, 965–7.

21. Shmerling, R.H. and Delbanco, T.L. (1991). The rheumatoid factor, an analysis of clinical utility. *American Journal of Medicine* **91**, 528–34.

22. Visser, H. et al. (1996). Diagnostic and prognostic characteristics of the enzyme linked immunosorbent rheumatoïd factor assays in RA. *Annals of Rheumatic Diseases* **55**, 157–61.

23. Van der Heyde, D.H.F.M. et al. (1988). Influence of prognostic features on the final outcome in RA: a review of the literature. *Seminars in Arthritis and Rheumatism* **17**, 284–92.

24. Brook, A. and Corbett, M. (1977). Radiographic changes in early rheumatoid disease. *Annals of Rheumatic Diseases* **36**, 71–3.

25. Wakefield, R.J. et al. (2000). The value of sonography in the detection of bone erosions in patients with RA: a comparison with conventional radiography. *Arthritis and Rheumatism* **43**, 2762–70.

26. Boers, M. (2000). Value of magnetic imaging in RA? *Lancet* **356**, 1458–9.

27. Chatervedi, N. and Ben-Shlomo, Y. (1995). From the surgery to the surgeon: does deprivation influence consultation and operation rates? *British Journal of General Practice* **45**, 127–31.

28. Singh, G. et al. (1991). Toxicity profiles of disease modifying anti-rheumatic drugs in rheumatoid arthritis. *Journal of Rheumatology* **18**, 188–94.

29. Götzsche, P.C. et al. (1998). Meta-analysis of short-term low dose prednisolone versus placebo and non-steroidal anti-inflammatory drugs in rheumatoid arthritis. *British Medical Journal* **316**, 811–18.

30. Criswell, L.A. et al. (2000). Moderate-term, low-dose corticosteroids for rheumatoid arthritis (Cochrane Review). In *The Cochrane Library* Issue 2. Oxford: Update Software.

31. Weiss, M.M. (1989). Corticosteroids in rheumatoid arthritis. *Seminars in Arthritis and Rheumatism* **19**, 9–21.

32. Verhagen, A.P. et al. (2000). Balneotherapy for rheumatoid arthritis and osteoarthritis. In *Cochrane Database Systematic Review* Vol. 2. CD000518.

33. MacLean, C.H. et al. (2000). Quality of care for patients with rheumatoid arthritis. *Journal of the American Medical Association* **284**, 984–92.

34. Scott, D.L. and Huskisson, E.C. (1992). The course of RA. *Bailliere's Clinical Rheumatology* **6**, 1–21.

35. Mitchell, J.M., Burkauser, R.V., and Pincus, T. (1988). The importance of age, education and co-morbidity in the substantial earning losses of individuals with symmetric polyarthritis. *Arthritis and Rheumatism* **31**, 348–57.

36. vandenbroucke, J.P., Hazevoet, H.M., and Cats, A. (1984). Survival and cause of death in rheumatoid arthritis: a 25-year prospective follow-up. *Journal of Rheumatology* **11**, 158–61.

37. Harrison, B.J. et al. (1996). Inflammatory polyarthritis in the community is not a benign disease: predicting functional disability one year after presentation. *Journal of Rheumatology* **23**, 1326–31.

38. Wiles, N.J. et al. (2000). One year follow-up variables predict disability 5 years after presentation with inflammatory polyarthritis with greater accuracy than at baseline. *Journal of Rheumatology* **27**, 2360–6.

Further reading

Cush, J.J. et al. *Rheumatology. Diagnosis and Therapeutics*. Philadelphia PA: Lippincott Williams & Wilkins, 1999.

Klippel, J.H., ed. *Primer on the Rheumatic Diseases* 11th edn. Atlanta GA: Arthritis Foundation, 1997.

13.5 Shoulder pain*

*Jan C. Winters and
Danielle A.W.M. van der Windt*

Epidemiology

In general practice, shoulder complaints present as pain at rest and/or when moving the upper arm, that is experienced in (part of) the area from the base of the neck to the elbow. Shoulder complaints due to trauma (fracture or dislocation) will not be discussed in this chapter, but in Chapter 14.2.

Following neck and low back complaints, shoulder complaints take the third position among reasons for consultation with primary care physician for

---

* A substantial part of this chapter has its origin in the recommendations of the Guidelines for Shoulder Complaints of the Dutch College of General Practitioners.

musculoskeletal complaints. About 10 per cent of the population has one or more episodes of shoulder pain during their lifetime. Estimates of the prevalence of shoulder complaints range from 7 to 25 per cent. The annual incidence in general practice of shoulder complaints is estimated between 8 and 25 per 1000 registered patients. For many patients, the complaints tend to be chronic or recurrent. Out of all newly presented episodes of shoulder complaints, 25–50 per cent resolve within 1–3 months, but after 1 year 50–60 per cent of the patients still experience complaints or report a new episode of shoulder pain. Most of these patients (approximately 60 per cent) do not seek further treatment, as the complaints are relatively mild and not disabling.

The following factors may be predictive of a favourable outcome:

◆ rapid onset of severe complaints;

◆ complaints preceded by unusual activities;

◆ complaints due to mild trauma.

Several factors are related to an unfavourable outcome:

◆ previous episodes of shoulder complaints;

◆ long duration of complaints before consultation;

◆ older age;

◆ concomitant neck complaints.

In half of the patients, there are concomitant neck complaints. Neck pain may accompany a painful shoulder, but pain in the shoulder area may also arise from functional limitations in the cervical spine, without a dysfunction of the glenohumeral joint. In one study, 20 per cent of patients with shoulder complaints were shown to have functional limitations of the cervical spine without glenohumeral problems.

Shoulder pain can originate from less common, extrinsic causes, such as cervical disc herniation, rheumatic or neurological conditions, or from referred pain from diseases of the heart, lung, or gallbladder.

Differential diagnosis

Shoulder pain is assumed to originate from overuse and/or degenerative changes of joint capsule and/or rotator cuff, resulting in a mechanical (aseptic) inflammation of these structures. Several classification systems have been described for the classification and diagnosis of shoulder complaints. Most of these systems try to differentiate between different diagnostic entities on the basis of physical examination. However, substantial interobserver variation has been described for the physical examination of the shoulder joint, resulting in only moderate to poor diagnostic agreement.[1,2] Besides that, the findings of physical examination often change in the course of time.[3] Furthermore, in a primary care population the diagnosis at presentation is not a strong predictor of long-term outcome of shoulder complaints.[4]

Finally, a more precise diagnosis often does not lead to a more specific therapy. The available therapeutic possibilities in general practice are limited, and consist mainly of advice, medication, injection, or referral for physiotherapy.

Given the poor reliability of diagnosing shoulder complaints, we will only distinguish shoulder complaints with and without restriction of movement in addition to extrinsic causes, and refrain from using a more specific pathological classification that is based on identification of the source of the lesion. This more simple classification will suffice in a general practice setting.

Thus, based on medical history and physical examination two main groups can be distinguished: (i) patients with restricted passive movement(s) of the glenohumeral joint which can be related to diagnostic entities like capsulitis, frozen shoulder, (peri)-arthritis; (ii) patients without movement restriction, but with a painful abduction.[3] This group can be related to diagnostic entities like (peri)-tendinitis, bursitis, and rotator cuff lesion.

Shoulder complaints without passive restriction of movement

The pain is experienced during and/or at the end of abduction or rotation. The complaints are most frequently experienced during active or passive abduction. These kinds of complaints are presumed to originate from aseptic inflammation or impingement of the subacromial structures. Also the less frequent complaints of the acromioclavicular joint are part of this group, as these are often seen in combination with subacromial shoulder disorders.

Shoulder complaints with passive restriction of movement

Passive mobility is painful and limited in one or more directions of the glenohumeral joint. These findings are presumably caused by an aseptic inflammation of the joint capsule or subacromial structures.

Shoulder complaints originating from extrinsic causes

◆ Pain and functional limitations of the cervicothoracic spine can also be experienced in the shoulder area. Active or passive movement of the cervical spine causes pain in the neck and/or shoulder area.

◆ Cervical disc herniation or carpal tunnel syndrome.

◆ Rheumatic diseases.

◆ Bone metastasis or lung malignancy.

◆ Diseases of heart, lungs, or abdominal problems causing diaphragmatic irritation. Usually, there will be serious accompanying symptoms.

Diagnostic approach

Alarm signals

Although shoulder complaints due to extrinsic causes (except for cervicothoracic function disorders) are rare, the physician should always consider these possibilities when symptoms, or the course of symptoms over time, do not fit the usual picture. One should be cautious with the following:

◆ Severe pain radiating in the arm or hand associated with cervical motion: cervical disc herniation.

◆ Accompanying pain or numbness in the hand, most severe at night: carpal tunnel syndrome.

◆ Combination of shoulder complaints and joint complaints (synovitis) elsewhere: rheumatoid arthritis.

◆ Bilateral shoulder complaints in combination with muscle pain and tiredness: polymyalgia rheumatica.

◆ Persisting shoulder complaints, despite adequate treatment. Malignancy in medical history: malignancy.

Medical history

◆ Location of pain and/or irradiation into the arm.

◆ Restriction of movement of the upper arm.

◆ Co-existing neck pain.

◆ Duration and presumed cause of shoulder complaints.

◆ Severity of complaints; pain at night, not being able to lie on the painful side, limitation of daily activities.

◆ Previous complaints and (success of) treatment.

◆ Relevant co-morbidity, malignancy, fever, other joint complaints.

Physical examination

- Inspection; location of pain as indicated by the patient.
- Active abduction. Pain and/or limitation, comparing painful to healthy side.
- Passive abduction. Pain and/or limitation, comparing painful to healthy side.
- Passive lateral rotation. Pain and/or limitation, comparing painful to healthy side.
- Examination of the cervical spine is carried out when the findings of tests described above are not conclusive or the complaints are suspected to be related to functional limitations of the cervicothoracic spine. (Active and/or passive flexion/extension, lateral flexion left/right and rotation left/right. Pain, limitation and radiation into the arm.)

Other tests for physical examination, such as isometric strength tests, horizontal adduction and passive internal rotation are not necessary. As stated before, these tests will often not contribute to a reliable diagnosis nor have significant consequences for the therapeutic approach.

Diagnostic interpretation

The examiner has to distinguish between

1. Complaints without restriction of movement. Pain is mainly experienced during active or passive abduction.
2. Complaints with restriction of movement of either abduction, external rotation, or a combination of both.

If the examination of the glenohumeral structures is without specific pain or limitations, the possibility of disorders of the cervical spine or one of the more serious extrinsic causes should be considered.

Additional diagnostic procedures

In the majority of cases, additional examination with X-ray, magnetic resonance imaging, computerized tomography, or ultrasonography has no added value, because in primary care it will not influence the therapeutic approach. There is little correlation between radiological findings and shoulder symptoms. Abnormalities are also found in a substantial proportion of persons without shoulder pain.[5] Additional examination should therefore be considered for those cases with a suspicion of serious disorders, who have an aberrant course of symptoms, or do not respond to usual treatment.

Treatment

Essentially, the general practitioner can choose from four therapeutic strategies or combinations thereof:

- Advice, ergonomic instructions, awaiting a spontaneous recovery.
- Analgesics or non-steroidal anti-inflammatory drugs (NSAIDs).
- Injection therapy with a corticosteroid injection with or without lidocaine.
- Referral to a physical therapist.

Advice, ergonomic instructions, awaiting a spontaneous recovery

Although not evidenced based, information regarding the nature and the course of complaints, and advice on how to move the arm without severe pain provocation is an important part of the treatment.

Analgesics or NSAIDs

No studies have been conducted on the effectiveness of analgesics on shoulder complaints, but several studies have evaluated the effectiveness of NSAIDs. Although most of these studies are of relatively poor methodological quality, and have not been conducted in a general practice population, some statements regarding NSAID treatment for shoulder complaints can be made.[6]

- NSAIDs are effective, especially in the first 1–2 weeks.
- There is no specific NSAID to be preferred for shoulder complaints.
- It is unknown if paracetamol (acetaminophen) is equally effective as NSAIDs.
- Few trials have been conducted on the effectiveness of COX-2 antagonists for shoulder complaints. The results seem to indicate a better benefit–risk ratio for nimesulide compared to NSAIDs, due to a lower risk of adverse reactions and at least equal effectiveness. However, further research is needed to confirm these findings and to consider the availability and costs of this type of medication.

Corticosteroid injections

The evidence to support the use of corticosteroid injection therapy is rather weak. Most studies appear to be of relatively poor quality and have been conducted in a specialist setting, mainly involving patients with prolonged symptoms.[7] The results of these studies cannot be extrapolated to patients seen in general practice. Many issues regarding injection therapy still need to be resolved, such as the number of injections given, which steroid to use and in what dose, the additional use of lidocaine, which structure should be injected, and what technique should be used.

Two studies in general practice show favourable short-term results with multiple injections of triamcinolone acetonide.[8,9] In addition, at least four other studies of adequate methodological quality have described favourable short term results of a subacromial injection with triamcinolonacetonide.[7] Research assessing the long-term effectiveness of corticosteroid injections is scarce, but the existing evidence indicates that beneficial effects do not persist after 3–6 months.

Conclusions

- Triamcinolone acetonide is to be preferred, as it is shown to be effective in several randomized controlled trials of adequate methodological quality.
- The adequate dose is 40 mg.
- No statement can be made regarding the additional use of lidocaine, but this is preferred by most physicians.

Injection technique

Several injection techniques are described in the literature. For practical reasons, we describe two techniques, which can easily be learned and applied in primary care: subacromial and intra-articular injection. These two techniques apply to most of the cases in the two symptom groups presented earlier. In case of doubt, one can choose for the subacromial injection because most shoulder pain originates from the structures of the subacromial space or for the combination of the two injections, dividing the dose equally.

Injection into the acromioclavicular joint is not discussed, because shoulder pain due to problems of the acromioclavicular joint are rare and injecting the acromioclavicular joint is difficult.

No exact advice can be given regarding the number of injections given and in which time interval. On pragmatic grounds, we advise a time interval of at least 2 weeks. There is no objection against several injections for one episode of shoulder complaints, but after two injections improvement should be seen, otherwise further treatment with corticosteroid injections is not advisable.

Serious adverse reactions or side-effects are extremely rare. Side-effects are generally limited to facial flushes or some extra pain and discomfort following the injection. Elevated blood glucose levels may occur in insulin dependant diabetes. Incidentally, abnormal menstrual bleeding or postmenopausal bleeding has been reported. With properly applied desinfection and injection technique the risk for a septic arthritis is very low.

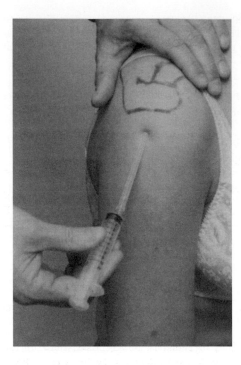

Fig. 1 Execution of a subacromial injection.

Subacromial injection

- *Symptoms:* Pain and/or limitation mostly during abduction.
- *Dose:* 40 mg of triamcinolone acetonide. The addition of 5–10 ml of lidocaine 10 mg/ml can be of used to obtain feedback from the patient on the anaesthetic effect of the injection.
- *Needle:* At least 5 cm long (21G × 2 in. is 0.8 × 50 mm)
- *Execution:* The needle is inserted 2–3 cm on the middle of the lateral side of the acromion under an angle of 50–60° of the upper arm (Fig. 1).

Intra-articular injection

- *Symptoms:* Next to pain and/or limitation in abduction there is also pain and passive limitation of external rotation.
- *Dose:* 40 mg of triamcinolone acetonide. The addition of 5–10 ml of lidocaine 10 mg/ml is optional; the anaesthetic effect is less in intra-articular injections and there is little evidence for the beneficial effect of joint capsule distension.
- *Needle:* At least 5 cm long (21G × 2 in. is 0.8 × 50 mm)
- *Execution:* The needle is inserted 1 cm caudally and 1 cm medially of the dorsolateral angle of the acromion, in a horizontal plane in the direction of the coracoid processus. The needle is inserted totally. This mostly happens without much resistance (Fig. 2).

After an injection there is no need to rest the arm in a sling. The patient can use the arm, and gradually resume activities, but should prevent severe pain provocation.

Physical therapy

Most research concerning the effectiveness of physical therapy for shoulder complaints is of relatively poor methodological quality.[10] Adequate studies show no effect of transcutaneous electrical nerve stimulation (TENS), short wave diathermy, ultrasound therapy, or laser therapy for both acute and chronic shoulder complaints. No valid studies support the use of heat or cryotherapy for acute shoulder complaints. Some evidence exists for a positive effect of exercise therapy or passive mobilizations in chronic shoulder complaints.[11]

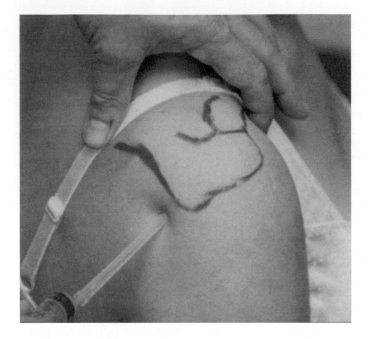

Fig. 2 Execution of an intra-articular injection.

Conclusions

- Physical therapy is not the treatment of first choice in the acute phase of shoulder complaints.
- The use of physical applications is not indicated.
- A referral for exercise therapy or passive mobilizations can be considered if shoulder complaints, interfering with daily activities, persist after the acute phase.

Treatment outline

- Give information regarding the benign nature and course of shoulder complaints:
  - Shoulder pain is troublesome but not dangerous.
  - Most episodes of shoulder pain resolve between 6 and 12 weeks.
  - Move the arm without too much pain provocation, gradually resume activities, be careful with overhand use.
- Analgesic or NSAID, depending on the judgement of the physician, treatment for 2 weeks. If successful this treatment can be continued for 1 or 2 additional weeks.
- If complaints persist, despite analgesics or NSAIDs, a subacromial or an intra-articular injection with a corticosteroid can be given, depending on the findings of the physical examination.
- Consider exercise therapy or mobilizations when pain and disability persists after 6 weeks.

Referral

Most patients with shoulder complaints are treated in general practice. Only 5–10 per cent are referred to a specialist, mostly an orthopaedic surgeon, a rheumatologist, or a specialist in rehabilitation medicine. The appropriateness and indications for surgery are still under discussion. Subacromial decompression or other surgical interventions can be considered, but only after a considerable period of conservative treatment. This means that in most cases a specialist will consider conservative treatment before deciding on surgical intervention.

Implications for daily living

Pain and restriction of mobility due to shoulder problems often cause sleep disturbances and functional disability. Inability to work, loss of productivity, and inability to carry out household activities can be a considerable burden to the patient as well as to society.

Considering the high prevalence of shoulder pain in occupational settings, the economic costs due to loss of productivity (indirect costs) will be much higher than the direct costs of medical care. Little information is available on the economic costs of shoulder pain. Data based on insurance registers, suggest that the percentage of paid sick leave for neck–shoulder pain is approaching that of low back pain.[12]

The reasons for persistence and recurrence of shoulder complaints are less specific and include psycho-social or work-related factors. Occupational research has shown that long-term sickness absence was to a large extent preserved by the work-situation, rather than by individual characteristics. Patients on long-term sick leave perceived their work tasks as monotonous with uncomfortable sitting positions, high demands on precision, higher job constraints, less opportunities for stimulation and development in their jobs, and less possibilities to influence their work.[13]

Further debate

Many issues are still unresolved. Little is known about risk factors for recurrent or persistent complaints, economic implications of shoulder complaints, and the effectiveness of several treatment modalities, including behaviourally oriented interventions, exercise treatment, and manual therapy. Furthermore, criteria need to be developed to guide decisions regarding surgical intervention.

Care for patients with shoulder complaints should be better coordinated between physical therapists, general practitioners, occupational physicians, and specialists. Consensus on diagnostic terminology and classification of shoulder complaints is needed. Multidisciplinary guidelines need to be developed, describing the contribution of each therapist or physician in the management of an episode of shoulder complaints.

Key points

- ◆ The reliability of several aspects of physical examination is poor. The identification of a large number of specific diagnostic entities is not reliable and does not contribute to a rational therapeutic approach. Consequently, a limited and simple examination is sufficient in primary care.

- ◆ Shoulder problems can be classified as
  - complaints without active or passive restriction of movement, but with painful abduction;
  - complaints with passive restriction of movement in one or more directions of the glenohumeral joint;
  - complaints from extrinsic causes.

- ◆ Additional diagnostic procedures have no added value.

- ◆ If advice and/or analgesics are not sufficient NSAIDs are advised; if NSAIDs fail, a corticosteroid injection can be given.

- ◆ The use of physical applications is not recommended; exercises or passive mobilization may be considered for persistent or recurrent shoulder complaints.

References

1. de Winter, A.F., Jans, M.P., Scholten, R.J.P.M., De Wolf, A.N., Van Schaardenburg, D., and Bouter, L.M. (1999). Diagnostic classification of shoulder disorders: inter-observer agreement and determinants for disagreement. *Annals of Rheumatic Diseases* **58**, 272–7.

2. Bamji, A.N., Erhardt, C.C., Price, T.R., and Williams, P.L. (1996). The painful shoulder: can consultants agree? *British Journal of Rheumatology* **35**, 1172–4.

3. Winters, J.C., Groenier, K.H., Sobel, J.S., Arendzen, J.H., and Meybom-de Jong, B. (1997). Classification of shoulder complaints in general practice by means of cluster analysis. *Archives of Physical Medicine and Rehabilitation* **78**, 1369–74.

4. van der Windt, D.A.W.M., Koes, B.W., Boeke, A.J.P. et al. (1996). Shoulder disorders in general practice: prognostic indicators of outcome. *British Journal of General Practice* **46**, 519–23.

5. Liou, J.T., Wilson, A.J., Totty, W.G. et al. (1993). The normal shoulder: common variations that simulate pathologic conditions at MR imaging. *Radiology* **186**, 435–41.

6. van der Windt, D.A.W.M., van der Heijden, G.J.M.G., Scholten, R.J.P.M. et al. (1995). The efficacy of non-steroidal anti-inflammatory drugs (NSAIDs) for shoulder complaints. A systematic review. *Journal of Clinical Epidemiology* **48**, 691–704.

7. van der Heijden, G.J.M.G., van der Windt, D.A.W.M., Kleijen, J. et al. (1996). Steroid injections for shoulder disorders: a systematic review of randomized trials. *British Medical Journal* **46**, 309–16.

8. Winters, J.C., Sobel, J.S., Groenier, K.H., Arendzen, J.H., and Meyboom-de Jong, B. (1997). Comparison of physiotherapy, manipulation, and corticosteroid injection for treating shoulder complaints in general practice: randomised, single blind study. *British Medical Journal* **314**, 1320–32.

9. van der Windt, D.A.W.M., Koes, B.W., Devillé, W. et al. (1998). Effectiveness of corticosteroid injections versus physiotherapy for treatment of painful stiff shoulder in primary care: randomised trial. *British Medical Journal* **317**, 1292–6.

10. van der Heijden, G.J.M.G., van der Windt, D.A.W.M., and de Winter, A.F. (1997). Physiotherapy for patients with soft-tissue shoulder disorders: a systematic review of randomised clinical trials. *British Medical Journal* **315**, 25–30.

11. Ginn, K.A., Herbert, R.D., Khouw, W. et al. (1997). A randomized, controlled clinical trial of treatment for shoulder pain. *Physical Therapy* **77**, 802–11.

12. Nygren, A., Berglund, A., and Von Koch, M. (1995). Neck-and-shoulder pain, an increasing problem. Strategies for using insurance material to follow trends. *Scandinavian Journal of Rehabilitation Medicine Supplement* **32**, 107–12.

13. Ekberg, K. and Wildhagen, I. (1996). Long-term sickness absence due to musculoskeletal disorders: the necessary interventions of work conditions. *Scandinavian Journal of Rehabilitation Medicine* **28**, 39–47.

Further reading

van der Heijden, G.J.M.G. (1999). Shoulder disorders: a state-of-the-art review. *Bailliére's Clinical Rheumatology* **13**, 287–309. (An extensive review discussing all aspects of shoulder complaints in general practice.)

13.6 Hip problems

Samuel B. Adkins

There are several causes of hip problems. These are listed in Table 1. Each of these conditions is found more commonly, or exclusively, within specific age or developmental stages. With the exception of trochanteric bursitis,

Table 1 Hip problems differential diagnosis

Diagnosis	History	Physical findings	Differential diagnosis	Special tests	Treatment	Referral
Developmental dysplasia of the hip	Presence of risk factors, some idiopathic	Positive Barlow/Ortolani testing (only accurate up to 3 months of age), leg skin crease asymmetry	Normal hips	Ultrasound imaging	Abduction splinting, surgery for non-responding patients or those with a late diagnosis	Orthopaedic surgery
Transient synovitis	1–6-year-old children, limp, pain in knee or hip	Afebrile, decreased range of motion	Septic arthritis, Legg–Calve–Perthes disease	CBC < 15 000, erythrocyte sedimentation rate <20	Rest, analgesia, tincture of time (usually resolved within 7 days)	If suspect septic arthritis, for joint aspiration
Septic arthritis	Most <3 years old, may be spread from contiguous osteomyelitis	Toxic appearing, decreased hip range of motion	Transient synovitis, inflammatory arthritis	Joint fluid examination	Surgical decompression of joint, parenteral antibiotics	Urgent orthopaedic surgery
Legg–Calve–Perthes disease	Insidious onset (1–3 months), of limp with hip or knee pain, 4–8-year-old children, males > females	Limited hip abduction, flexion and internal rotation	Inflammatory arthritis, septic arthritis, transient synovitis	Normal CBC and erythrocyte sedimentation rate, plain films positive (early with changes in the epiphysis, later with flattening of the femoral head, or femoral head displacement)	Maintain range of motion, follow position of femoral head in relation to acetabulum radiographically	Orthopaedic surgery if femoral head not well positioned for consideration of splinting or surgery
Slipped capital femoral epiphysis	Acute (<1 month) or chronic (up to 6 months) presentation, pain in groin (referred to knee or anterior thigh), 11–14-year-olds, obese males at increased risk	Leg more comfortable in external rotation, pain and limited internal rotation, chronic presentation may have leg length discrepancy	Muscle strain, avulsion fracture	Plain films widening of epiphysis early, later may see external rotation of femur under proximal epiphysis	Non-weight-bearing, surgical pinning	Urgent orthopaedic surgery for consideration of pinning to prevent further slip
Avulsion fracture	Sudden violent concentric or eccentric muscle contraction, may hear or feel a 'pop'	Pain with passive stretch and active contraction of involved muscle, pain with palpation of involved apophysis	Muscle strain, slipped capital femoral epiphysis	Plain films, if these are negative CT or MRI more sensitive	Five-stage rehabilitation programme of progressive increase in ROM and strengthening (Pappas and Metzmaker)	Orthopaedic surgery if >2 cm displacement, open reduction internal fixation (ORIF), consider physiotherapy
Femoral neck stress fracture	Persistent groin discomfort increasing with activity, increased risk in military recruits and track athletes, female athlete triad (eating disorder, amenorrhoea, osteopenia)	ROM may be painful	Trochanteric bursitis, osteoid osteoma, muscle strain	Plain films may show cortical defects in femoral neck (either superior or inferior surface), bone scan, MRI, CT can also be used if plain radiographs are negative and diagnosis is clinically suspected	Superior surface (compression side)-non-weight-bearing until evidence of healing (usually 2–4 weeks) with gradual return to activities, inferior surface (distraction side) requires ORIF, adequate calcium intake, oestrogen for amenorrhoeic women	Orthopaedic surgery for ORIF
Osteonecrosis	Dull ache or throbbing pain in groin, lateral hip or buttock, history of prolonged steroid use, prior severe trauma (fracture, dislocation), slipped femoral capital epiphysis, congenital dysplastic hip, inflammatory arthritis	Pain with ambulation, abduction, internal and external rotation	Early degenerative joint disease	Plain radiographs, MRI	Protected weight bearing, exercises to maximize soft tissue function (strength and support), total hip replacement	Physiotherapy, orthopaedic surgery

Condition	Symptoms	Signs	Differential diagnosis	Investigations	Treatment	Management
Trochanteric bursitis	Pain over greater trochanter with palpation, pain with walking or running	Pain with palpation of greater trochanter	Ilio-tibial band syndrome, femoral neck stress fracture	Plain films, bone scan, MRI negative for bony involvement	Ice, NSAID, stretching of ilio-tibial band, protect from direct trauma, steroid injection	Physiotherapy
Iliopsoas bursitis	Pain and snapping in medial groin or thigh, worse with standing from seated position	Reproduce symptoms with active and passive flexion/extension of hip	Avulsion fracture	Plain radiographs are negative	Ilio-psoas stretching, steroid injection	Physiotherapy
Ilio-tibial band syndrome	Lateral hip, thigh and/or knee pain, snapping as ilio-tibial band passes over the greater trochanter	Positive Ober's sign	Trochanteric bursitis		Modification of activity, footwear, stretching programme, ice massage, NSAID	Physiotherapy
Meralgia paresthetica	Pain or paraesthesia of anterior or lateral groin and thigh	Abnormality in sensory exam in distribution of lateral femoral cutaneous nerve	Other causes of peripheral neuropathy	NCV testing may be helpful	Stretching of proximal quadriceps, avoid external compression of nerve (clothing, equipment, panus)	Physiotherapy
Hip fracture	Pain in groin or buttock following a fall, most will not be weight bearing	Leg externally rotated abducted and shortened with femoral neck and intertrochanteric fracture (90%), internally rotated, adducted and shortened with sub-trochanteric fracture (10%)	Contusion, sprain	Plain films, nuclear medicine bone scan or MRI if plain films negative	Surgical evaluation, assess risk for future morbidity/mortality	Urgent orthopaedic surgery
Degenerative arthritis	Progressive increased pain and stiffness in thigh and buttocks	Reduced internal rotation early, all motion later, pain with ambulation	Inflammatory arthritis	Plain films help with diagnosis and prognosis	Maximize support and strength of soft tissues, ice, acetaminophen, NSAID, modification of activities, cane to relieve load to joint, total hip replacement	Physiotherapy, orthopaedic surgery

femoral neck and intertrochanteric fractures, and degenerative joint disease, an individual primary care physician rarely sees all the diagnoses that cause hip problems. But all of these diagnoses are seen in primary care. For this reason, and because many of the conditions can lead to long-term or permanent disability at a relatively young age, it is important for all primary care physicians to be familiar with each of the different conditions that can cause hip problems.

Clinical diagnosis

Making the appropriate diagnosis as early as possible is important to reduce the risk of long-term disability and end-stage degenerative joint disease. A carefully performed history and physical examination is the first step in this process. An important point to remember is that patients with hip pathology may present with knee pain. It is therefore important to consider hip pathology in all patients with knee pain.

The physical examination should be systematic and thorough and include examination of the patient while they are standing, walking, transferring from sitting to standing and back to sitting, range of movement, muscle strength, palpation, and special tests such as Ober's when indicated.

Patients may also have referred symptoms into the hip from pathology in the pelvis, abdomen, scrotum, and low back. Clues that will differentiate between hip pathology and referred pain should be sought in the history; an examination of these other areas should be done as appropriate.

Screening in infants

All infants should have a careful examination of their hips to screen for developmental dysplasia of the hip. The risk for this condition is higher if there is a family history, breech presentation, oligohydramnios and for female infants. Screening includes Barlow and Ortolani testing as well as examination of the leg skin creases. These examinations need to be done when the infant is relaxed.

Barlow's test is done with the examiner holding the infant's legs in a flexed position at both the hip and knee. The hip is adducted and posterior pressure is applied to attempt to sublux the hip. Ortolani's test is done with the infant in the same position. The hip is abducted and anterior pressure is applied to the proximal femur in an attempt to relocate the subluxed femoral head. A positive finding for both of these examinations is a distinctive 'clunk' which results from either the subluxation (Barlow) or relocation (Ortolani). Snapping is sometimes confused with this clunk and may cause a false positive result.

Examination of the skin creases is important also, with the affected side more likely to have extra creases, as that limb may be shorter. Skin crease examination is only helpful if the condition is unilateral. Patients who are suspected of having this condition should be evaluated by a physician with special expertise in its management. Early treatment consists of abduction splinting.

Synovitis and septic arthritis

Transient synovitis is a condition of unknown aetiology. This condition may mimic septic arthritis of the hip. Differentiation of these conditions is important, as transient synovitis can be treated with rest and analgesia and usually lasts for less than 7 days. Septic arthritis warrants hospitalization for parenteral antibiotics and consultation with a specialist to surgically decompress the joint.

Patients with toxic synovitis may have had a recent preceding mild viral type illness. Both groups will have pain in the hip, which is exacerbated with motion, especially flexion and extension. They may both appear somewhat toxic, though patients with toxic synovitis are relatively less affected with systemic symptoms. When this diagnosis is suspected a CBC and erythrocyte sedimentation rate should be checked. Of these, the ESR is more accurate, but both have false positive and false negative results. When in doubt, joint aspiration with examination of the fluid is warranted. Septic joints will have elevated WBC counts and organisms present.

Legg–Calve–Perthes disease

Legg–Calve–Perthes disease is a condition that affects the pre-pubescent. It is found in both sexes, but males are more commonly affected. The cause is unknown. These patients present with a limp and complaints of hip pain. Pain may be worse with passive motion, especially internal rotation and abduction. The physical examination may otherwise be normal.

Plain radiographs of the hip should be obtained if this condition is suspected. Treatment for the condition is dependent on whether the patient has normal range of movement or not. If this is normal, and is maintained, further diagnostic evaluation may be performed at the patient and physician's discretion. If the range of motion in the hip is not normal, and plain radiographs are normal, then further diagnostic evaluation should be performed, including consulting a specialist and consideration of MRI scanning of the hip. Patients who are suspected of having this condition should have continued surveillance of their hips, even if their examination and radiographs are normal.

Slipped epiphysis

Slipped capital femoral epiphysis occurs in adolescence. It is more likely to occur around the time of rapid linear growth in late adolescence. It is seen in a 6 : 1 male to female prevalence. Blacks may be at increased risk. Obesity with the appearance of chronic external rotation of the hip (actually retroversion of femoral head and neck) appears to increase the risk of the condition. These patients present with a limp and some degree of hip pain. The degree of pain is dependent on the acuity of the condition. Patients with more chronic slips are less likely to have significant pain.

This is a condition that is especially likely to present with knee pain. *All patients in this age group with a limp and knee pain must have their hips evaluated.*

On physical examination, hip movement is frequently restricted with abduction, internal rotation and flexion most severely affected. Plain radiographs may be diagnostic, with widening or irregularities seen, or a slip at the epiphysis, or they may be normal. If they are diagnostic, referral to a physician with special expertise is essential. The treatment for this condition is still somewhat controversial. Surgical treatment and prolonged bilateral hip spica casting are the two main treatments described in the literature.

Up to 50 per cent of patients will develop bilateral disease. This may be present at the time of presentation, or up to 18 months later. Close monitoring to pick up early disease in the contralateral hip is required.

Avulsion fractures

Avulsion fractures of the apophysis of the attachment of the muscles around the hip joint are not common. They typically occur in active young patients who are involved in strenuous activity. Sites that are more likely include the insertion of the hamstring muscles at the ischial tuberosity ('Hurdler's fracture'), and the insertion of the sartorius muscle at the anterior superior iliac spine ('kicker's fracture'). The patient may report a 'popping' sensation at the time of injury. They will complain of pain with palpation as well as with testing of the inserted muscle's active motion and passive stretch. Treatment for these injuries is dependent on the distance the avulsed fragment is displaced from its insertion site. Surgery to reattach the avulsion is considered for displacements of greater than 2 cm. For this reason, plain radiographs are indicated. With less than 2 cm of displacement, the treatment consists of relative rest with maintenance of range of motion and rehabilitation.

Stress fractures

Stress fractures of the femoral neck are also seen in the young vigorously active patients. This occurs when the bone is chronically fatigued just slightly beyond its capacity. It occurs primarily in two groups: those who have increased their activity level too rapidly and those who have abnormal bone metabolism, usually on the basis of poor dietary practices. Both groups will present with a history of gradual onset of vague pain in the groin, which is aggravated with activity. Further history of an increase in a weight-bearing physical activity or in disordered eating habits should increase suspicion for this diagnosis. Women tend to be more susceptible to the latter cause. A menstrual history should be taken. Women with disordered eating and abnormal bone metabolism will be more likely to have irregular or absent menses.

The physical examination may be normal. When abnormal, pain and limitation in rotation is the most common finding. In advanced stages, pain with walking and a limp may be present. When the diagnosis is suspected, plain radiographs should be obtained. These may be negative in up to 50 per cent of patients initially. Bone scanning or MRI scanning can be helpful when this is the case.

Treatment of this condition must include a reduction in the weight bearing on the affected side. This includes cessation of the activity and the use of crutches for the first several weeks. This is often difficult, as these individuals tend to be strongly motivated to perform their sport or activity. Substitution for the activity with a non-weight-bearing activity (i.e. swimming) may help. If the patient presents with pain at rest, inferior surface fractures, or has continued symptoms despite conservative treatment a surgical referral should be made.

Women who acquire this condition as part of a triad of disordered eating, osteopenia, and menstrual irregularities deserve special consideration as they often have more complex psychological issues contributing to their disease. A multidisciplined approach, which includes psychologist, nutritionist, and physiotherapist along with the physician, may be more successful. All patients with a stress fracture should be counselled on an appropriate diet.

Osteonecrosis

Osteonecrosis is a condition that may be a complication of a prior hip condition. Risk factors are listed in Table 2. Patients present with a limp with or without complaints of pain. The pain is most frequently in the groin. If there is a recent history of trauma it is coincidental. Physical examination may reveal a limp and decreased range of movement. With advanced disease, there may be a leg length discrepancy.

Plain radiographs should be obtained. Early findings may include osteopenia of the femoral head, subchondral sclerosis and cyst formation. As the disease progresses, flattening and collapse of the femoral head occur. Ultimately, the joint is destroyed.

These patients need to modify their activity to preserve the hip joint. This usually requires some modification in weight-bearing activities.

Table 2 Risk factors for osteonecrosis

Hip dislocation
Corticosteroid use
Rheumatoid arthritis
Sickle cell disease
Slipped capital femoral epiphysis
Femoral neck fracture
Alcohol abuse
Systemic lupus erythematosus
Crohn's disease
Legg–Calve–Perthes disease

A physiotherapy consultation, to maintain range of motion should be considered. Surgical referral should happen at the time of diagnosis, as there may be more options available at that time. These patients may eventually require total joint replacement.

Bursitis

Bursitis around the hip is very common with two main sites: trochanteric and iliopsoas. The former is much more common than the latter. Both may present with pain or snapping at the site of the bursa. This is over the greater trochanter for the trochanteric bursitis, and medially over the lesser trochanter for iliopsoas bursitis. Both of these may result from over activity of the muscles that attach near these bursa. Trochanteric bursitis may also result from direct trauma to the lateral proximal thigh.

Trochanteric bursitis is more often symptomatic with erect activities such as walking and running. Iliopsoas bursitis is more likely to be symptomatic when rising from the seated position. The diagnosis needs to be differentiated from avulsion fractures, which are not as likely and usually occur in a more skeletally immature patient. The patient's symptoms are reproduced with palpation of the bursa. Plain radiographs may be needed. Treatment consists of local physiotherapy, application of ice, and stretching exercises. Injection of the trochanteric bursa is effective in up to 90 per cent of patients. Orthotics may be helpful for patients with alignment abnormalities.

Iliotibial band syndrome can cause symptoms similar to trochanteric bursitis. Patients who are at increased risk for this condition include those with a wide pelvis (which explains why it is more common in women) who are involved in activities that require frequent abduction of the hip. Dancers and gymnast, as well as cross-country runners tend to be at higher risk. Its presentation is very similar to a trochanteric bursitis with the exception that there may be more radiation down the lateral side of the thigh, and they will have a positive Ober's test. Lying the patients on their unaffected side and letting the affected knee fall towards the examination table does this test. A positive test is present when the motion is restricted compared to the unaffected side and the patient's symptoms are reproduced. Treatment consists of stretching exercises directed at the lateral thigh, ice and local physiotherapy and if needed modification of activities. Orthotics may be helpful for patients with alignment abnormalities.

Lateral femoral nerve compression

Meralgia paraesthetica is a compression of the lateral femoral cutaneous nerve. This is a pure sensory nerve. Two groups are likely to develop this condition. Very lean active young women, and very obese patients, especially men, who have a panus and wear tight-fitting belts or clothing. The condition results from the compression of the nerve near the superior origin of the inguinal ligament. Patients complain of numbness and pain along the anterior–lateral thigh that may be variable and extend from the inguinal ligament to the knee.

Treatment should include removal of any external compression, modification of activities (limitation of extreme trunk and hip extension), and in rare situations perineural injection. The injection site is found by performing a Tinnel's test along the inguinal ligament. Reproduction of the symptoms with this manoeuvre will direct the location of the injection. This condition may last for a prolonged period of time after therapy is begun. If there has been damage to the axons of the nerve, regeneration may take several months.

Hip fractures in the elderly

Hip fractures are very common. Over 250 000 hip fractures occur annually in the United States. These patients are at significant risk for further morbidity and mortality in the year following the fracture. This means that physicians should take care both in attempts to prevent fracture as well as assessing the patient's risk for a poor outcome following the injury. Risk factors for hip

Table 3 Risk factors for hip fracture

Fair skin females
Tobacco use
Lean body mass
Psychotropic medication use
Dementia
Family history
Caffeine use
Tall stature
Institutional living
Alcohol abuse
Physical inactivity
Previous hip fracture
Impaired vision

Table 4 Risk factors for degenerative joint disease

Family history
Childhood hip disorder
Prior trauma
Obesity
Occupation
Leg length discrepancy
Inflammatory arthropathy

fracture are listed in Table 3. Hip fractures are seen predominately in the elderly, with the risk doubling for every decade over 50 years of age.

There are three types of hip fractures: femoral neck, intertrochanteric, and sub-trochanteric. The first two comprise 90 per cent of hip fractures.

Patients with femoral neck fractures present after a fall and most commonly complain of pain in the groin. Their leg may be externally rotated, abducted, and shortened. In thin patients, there may be swelling in this area. They will probably be unable to bear weight, and plain radiographs should be obtained prior to any attempts at weight bearing. Patients with intertrochanteric fractures present in a similar manner. Patients with sub-trochanteric fractures present with similar histories, but their examination may be somewhat different. They tend to have internal rotation and adduction of the leg instead of external rotation and abduction.

For patients who present with a history of a fall and have complaints of hip pain, especially if they are unable to bear weight, the physician must assume a fracture is present until proven otherwise. After performing a physical examination, plain radiographs should be obtained. If these are negative, nuclear bone scanning, MRI, or surgical consultation should be considered. The rare case when this may not be warranted is for the patient who is already bed bound and severely demented. Decisions for these patients should be made considering their comfort. All patients with hip fractures should be considered for surgical repair, and surgical consultation is indicated.

Degenerative joint disease

Degenerative joint disease (DJD) is a very common chronic disease of the elderly and affects many different joints. Eighty per cent of adults in the United States have DJD in one or more joints. The knees and hips are particularly prone. Younger patients with prior hip problems are at increased risk for early development of this condition. Whites are more commonly affected by DJD of the hip than blacks. European farmers tend to demonstrate some of the highest rates of hip DJD, which may be a result of repetitive activity in their occupation. There are many factors suspected of increasing the risk of hip DJD. These are listed in Table 4.

Patients will present with a history of pain in the hip area, most commonly in the groin or buttocks, which has gradually begun over the coarse of several months or years. The physical examination for these patients should include a systematic general exam, as well as an assessment of their functional capacity. They will usually limp, wanting to limit the stance phase of gait. Strength may be decreased in all of the muscles about the hip. Range of motion will also likely be reduced, with internal rotation and abduction most consistently affected. There may be some crepitance with motion.

Plain radiographs should be obtained. Early findings include narrowing of the joint space (<2.5 mm), subchondral sclerosis, and cysts. Later changes include osteophyte formation, flattening of the femoral head, and further joint space narrowing. Radiographs are helpful in making the diagnosis and following the coarse of disease, but should not be used in making decisions on therapy.

The goal of therapy is to enable the patient to continue to live a productive and pain-free life. Modification of the patient's environment may be necessary. Handrails installed in their homes, to assist in rising from a seated position, elevated seating, including on the commode, and the use of an appropriate cane are all useful aids. Regaining and maintaining range of motion is important and physiotherapy consultation may be helpful. Regular periods of rest during activities that require weight bearing are important in maintaining independence.

Several different medications have been used in treating the pain associated with hip DJD. Non-steroidal anti-inflammatory medications, acetaminophen, and some of the milder narcotics have been used. Because this is a chronic disease, use of these medications can increase the risk for side-effects. Non-medicinal measures should be maximized to limit the need for medication. The newer COX-2 inhibitors have reduced some of the GI risks, but they should still be used cautiously, especially for patients with reduced renal function.

Surgical referral should be made for patients with early onset disease, defined as before age 50, for consideration of an wedge osteotomy which may delay the need for hip replacement. Patients with uncontrolled pain should also be referred for surgical consultation. Hip replacement should be delayed as long as the patient's pain can be controlled. There are several reasons for this, including the complications arising directly from the surgery (infection, thrombophlebitis, etc.) as well as the limited life of the prosthetic. The inability to perform tasks of independent living is also a consideration for joint replacement, but rarely an indication without uncontrolled pain. Another strategy for this condition is prevention. Elderly patients who are at high risk for falling may also benefit from wearing protective hip pads, which are available commercially for the prevention of hip fractures.

Key points

- Diagnoses for hip problems are usually age and development specific.
- Hip fractures, degenerative joint disease, and bursitis are the more common diagnoses.
- Hip problems may present as knee pain.
- Pathology in the pelvis, abdomen, scrotum, and low back may produce hip symptoms.
- Early identification of congenital hip dysplasia through the screening of all infants is necessary to avoid complications.
- Most conditions that present as hip problems are uncommon, but primary care providers must be able to identify the rare aetiology to avoid complications later.

Further reading

Loder, R.T. et al. (2000). Slipped capital femoral epiphysis. *Journal of Bone and Joint Surgery* **82-A** (8), 1170–88.

American Academy of Pediatrics (2000). Clinical practice guideline: early detection of developmental dysplasia of the hip. *Pediatrics* **105** (4), 896–905.

Boyd, K.T., Peirce, N.S., and Batt, M.E. (1997). Common hip injuries in sport. *Sports Medicine* **24**, 273–88.

Zuckerman, J.D. (1996). Current concepts: hip fracture. *The New England Journal of Medicine* **334** (23), 1519–25.

Dieppe, P. (1995). Fortnightly review: management of hip osteoarthritis. *British Medical Journal* **311** (7009), 853–7.

Hoppenfeld, S. *Physical Examination of the Spine and Extremities*. New York: Prentice-Hall, 2000.

13.7 Foot problems

Kees J. Gorter and Richard A. Figler

Epidemiology

Foot complaints are a common health problem. Population surveys have reported a 10–24 per cent point prevalence of self-reported foot complaints in adults, with the highest rates being found in women and in those 65 years of age and older.[1] Three-quarters of the foot complaints have a non-traumatic origin, and more than nine out of 10 of such complaints last over 4 weeks. The main complaints are pain (60 per cent), malpositioning of the toes or toenail problems (20 per cent), numbness or swelling (12 per cent), and skin problems (8 per cent). The forefoot is involved in over 60 per cent of the cases. Being female, having other musculoskeletal disease and other co-morbidity are risk factors for longer-lasting foot complaints. Surprisingly, higher age and obesity are not.

Foot *impairments* are defined as any loss or abnormality of anatomical structure or function (WHO; International Classification of Impairments, Disabilities and Handicaps). The point prevalence of non-traumatic forefoot impairments in people of 45 years and above with forefoot complaints is 65 per cent.[2] Patients on average have more than three forefoot impairments at a time. The majority of these impairments, however, do not contribute to the patients' complaints. Consequently, discerning the difference between a foot impairment and a clinically relevant foot problem is crucial in determining the proper therapeutic approach.

Foot *problems* are defined as different categories of clinically relevant abnormalities to which the foot complaint can mostly likely be attributed. The point prevalence of non-traumatic *forefoot* problems in people of 45 years and above is 21 per cent.[2] It is twice as high in women as in men and increases with age, with the exception of the more than or equal to 75-year age group. The prevalence of musculoskeletal forefoot problems such as hallux valgus and metatarsalgia is 16 per cent, with a gender and age distribution similar to the main group. The prevalence of *non-musculoskeletal* forefoot problems is 5 per cent, irrespective of gender and increases with age. The prevalence of *hindfoot* problems, mainly plantar fasciitis, is 10 per cent.

Presentation in primary care

In general practice, the incidence of presented non-traumatic foot problems is 2–3 per cent and the prevalence is 4 per cent.[3] Just as in the general population, foot problems are present in women twice as often as in men and their number increases with age. In persons of 15 years and above, the incidence of hallux valgus is 0.1 per cent and the prevalence 4 per cent, underlining the chronic nature of this foot problem. Both occurrence rates are in women over seven times as high as in men. There is little detailed information about the occurrence of various other categories of foot problems in general practice.

More than half of persons of 65 years and above seek (para)medical care: 18 per cent paramedical care, mostly podiatrists; 46 per cent the general practitioner (GP), and 36 per cent a medical specialist, mostly orthopaedic surgeons.[4] The others seek other types of care: one of 10 do not seek any type of care; four of 10 use self-care (rest, cold packs, changing shoes, and self-medication); and five of 10 consult a chiropodist for conditions such as nail problems, callosities, and corns.

Aetiology

To understand dysfunction of the foot, clinicians should be familiar with its normal anatomy and development. The foot has 26 bones, two sesamoid bones, and a varying number of accessory ossicles (Fig. 1). Foot problems can be categorized in several ways:

- *According to localization of mechanical dysfunction or structural pathology.* Common local causes of a painful heel are situated at the *hindfoot*, which consists of the calcaneus and the talus (see Box 1 and 'Diagnosis' section). Pain of the middle of the foot is located at the *midfoot*, which is made up of the cuboid bone, the cuneiform 1, 2, and 3 bones, the navicular bone, and the proximal end of the five metatarsals (see Section on 'Diagnosis'). Pain of the distal part of the foot is located at the *forefoot*, which consists of the five metatarsals starting at the midshaft and the phalangeal bones of the toes (see 'Diagnosis' section).

- *According to association with the foot type.* Three main types can be identified: cavus (supinated with high medial longitudinal arch), normal, and planus (pronated with low medial longitudinal arch; flat). Foot problems may be associated with the cavus foot type in which support is present, but shock absorption is lacking, or with the planus foot type in which shock absorption is present, but support is lacking (see 'Diagnosis' section).

- *According to association with other diseases.* Foot problems may be associated with musculoskeletal diseases such as osteoarthritis [subtalar

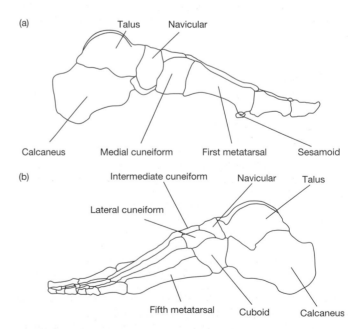

Fig. 1 Bones of the foot: (a) medial aspect; (b) lateral aspect.

Box 1 Common local causes of non-traumatic foot pain

Heel pain

◆ Pain within the heel
  ■ Arthritis/osteoarthritis of the subtalar joint
  ■ Calcaneal apophysitis
◆ Pain beneath the heel
  ■ Tender heelpad
  ■ Plantar fasciitis
◆ Pain medially of the heel
  ■ Tarsal tunnel syndrome
  ■ Tenosynovitis posterior tibial muscle
  ■ Plantar fasciitis
◆ Pain laterally of the heel
  ■ Tenosynovitis peroneal muscles
◆ Pain behind the heel
  ■ Achilles (peri)tendinitis
  ■ Haglund's deformity ('pump bump')
  ■ Retrocalcaneal bursitis (ventrally from Achilles tendon)
  ■ Calcaneal bursitis (dorsally from Achilles tendon)
  ■ Calcaneal apophysitis

Forefoot pain

◆ First metatarsal/first toe
  ■ Hallux valgus (bunion medially from MT-1)
  ■ Hallux rigidus (dorsal callosity)
  ■ Sesamoiditis
  ■ Arthritis/osteoarthritis MTP, PIP, DIP
◆ Toes 2–5
  ■ Abnormal position toes 2–4 (hammer; claw; mallet)
  ■ Abnormal position toe 5 ('curly'; supra-adductus)
  ■ Bunionette (bunion laterally from MT-5)
  ■ Corns (hard digital; soft interdigital)
  ■ Arthritis PIP, DIP
◆ Ball of the foot
  ■ Metatarsalgia
  ■ Morton's neuroma
  ■ Plantar corn [focal intractable plantar keratosis (IPK) Am]
  ■ Localized callus (diffuse IPK, Am)
  ■ Wart
  ■ Arthritis/osteoarthritis MTP
  ■ Metatarsal stress fracture

Arched (cavus) foot

◆ History
  ■ Pain under the foot; laterally
  ■ Complaints increase during walking
  ■ Often tender heelpad; Achilles tenosynovitis
◆ Physical examination

  ■ More rigid foot with little shock absorption; sometimes equinus position; reduced dorsal flexion in the ankle; short posterior tibial muscle; Achilles tenosynovitis due to reduced shock absorption
  ■ High and short medial longitudinal arch and hindfoot inversion (varus position)
  ■ Talar head pointing outwardly
  ■ Consider underlying neurological problems with weakness of peroneal muscles and dorsiflector muscles
  ■ Overloading head of MT-1; steep position of MT-1
  ■ Overloading head of MT-5, basis MT-5, and heel
  ■ Abnormal position toes (claw and hammer; dorsal hard corns)
  ■ In case of a mobile tarsus: tenosynovitis peroneal muscles; overloading lateral hindfoot; prone to ankle inversion
◆ Examination of the shoe
  ■ Lateral side of the sole of the shoe is worn down

Flat (planus) foot

◆ History
  ■ Pain under the foot; medially
  ■ Complaints increase during standing
  ■ Often plantar fasciitis; tenosynovitis posterior tibial muscle
◆ Physical examination
  ■ Sagging of the medial longitudinal arch; forefoot abducted compared to hindfoot; shortening of the lateral longitudinal arch; 'too many toes' sign; hindfoot eversion (valgus position)
  ■ Talar head pointing inwardly; pronation of the tarsus (talo-navicular complex)
  ■ Hypermobile first metatarsal; elevated position of MT-1; insufficient weight bearing
  ■ Varus position first metatarsal; at risk for hallux valgus
  ■ Overloading head of MT-2 and MT-3 with localized callus/plantar corn/metatarsalgia
  ■ Abnormal position toes (hammer; dorsal hard corns)
◆ Examination of the shoe
  ■ Medial side of the sole of the shoe is worn down

joints, first metatarsal–phalangeal joint (MTP-1)], rheumatoid arthritis (arthritis of the foot is an early symptom), psoriasis (inflamed 'sausage' toe), and ankylosing spondylitis (Achilles peritendinitis; bilateral plantar fasciitis). *Metabolic diseases* such as diabetes mellitus (bilateral numbness and increased risk of foot ulcers) and gout (occurs most often in the foot; in 50–70 per cent as an acute, very painful MTP-1 arthritis). Vascular disease (limb ischaemia) and neurological diseases such as polyneuropathy (bilateral numbness) and post-herniated-disc syndrome (one-sided numbness/pain).

Diagnosis

General diagnosis

A diagnosis can frequently be made on the basis of the patient's history, supported by a specific clinical examination. The anatomy of the foot is relatively accessible to palpation and specific testing.

History taking

A history of trauma or overloading suggests a more biomechanical cause of foot complaints. In many of these instances, the foot complaint often decreases after resting and follows a natural course with a spontaneous recovery mostly within 4 weeks. It should be differentiated from systemic rheumatological, vascular, neurological, and metabolic diseases.

Physical examination

Both feet must be examined for comparative purposes. Examination is done in standing and sitting position with the lower legs bared from above the knees to feet.

Gait pattern

When the patient walks, special attention is paid to equal loading of the feet.

Shape and position

The shape of the medial longitudinal arch, the position of the calcaneus in relation to the axis of the lower leg, and the position of the forefoot in relation to the hindfoot are examined in standing position. A non-rigid flatfoot can usually be corrected if, during the Hubscher (or Jack's) test, a tightening of the plantar structures and an increase in the medial arch are seen when the big toe is dorsiflexed with the foot in standing position.

Joints

Besides the range of motion, the pattern of movement, swelling, and localized pain are important when studying joints.

Muscular strength

Tested in the ankle joint (plantar and dorsal flexion), in the subtalar joint (inversion and eversion), and at the level of the toes (plantar and dorsal flexion).

Signs of overloading

If there is an important change in position, especially when combined with limited mobility, there is an increased risk of biomechanical overloading (with an up to seven times increase of local pressure) of the skin and subcutaneous tissues. Patients will usually notice this first because shoes start hurting their feet. Patients with diabetic polyneuropathy, however, may not feel this until after an ulcer has been formed. *Colour of the skin, arterial pulsations, oedema, capillary refill, scars, skin diseases*, and *loss of sensitivity* should also be taken into account as possible clues to explain a patient's foot complaints, especially in older patients and patients with comorbidity.

Assessment of the hindfoot

Tender heel pad

Overloading of the heel due to heavy heel strike or fat pad atrophy in the elderly. In a period of a few months a dull pain is felt beneath the heel. Most serious in the morning. *Physical examination:* tenderness over the heel, which feels distended and sometimes warm.

Plantar fasciitis

Overloading of the foot causes an inflammatory reaction due to traction where the plantar fascia is attached to the calcaneus. Most pain occurs during the first steps after resting and after a period of walking. Pain is most serious in the heel but may radiate towards the forefoot. Almost 90 per cent of the patients improve significantly with conservative care within 6–12 months. *Physical examination:* localized tenderness beneath the medial side of the calcaneus. *Investigations:* X-ray is not recommended since many people without heel pain have a calcaneal spur on the lateral X-ray of the foot. *Referral:* to a rheumatologist should be considered in case of bilateral plantar fasciitis with no improvement within 8–12 weeks to rule out ankylosing spondylitis.

Tarsal tunnel syndrome

Unilateral pain and paraesthesia in the medial part of the hindfoot radiating towards the forefoot, not related to weight-bearing. Often worse at night. Stamping or shaking of the feet sometimes gives relief. Caused by entrapment of the posterior tibial nerve behind the medial malleolus. *Physical examination:* Tinel's sign over the tarsal tunnel (behind medial malleolus towards the heel) can be positive. *Investigation:* as in all entrapment neuropathies laboratory testing for hypothyroidism and diabetes mellitus should be considered. *Referral:* to a neurologist for electrophysiological testing (EMG) should be considered in case of doubt.

Achilles (peri)tendinitis, insertion tendinitis, bursitis, Haglund's deformity

Achilles peritendinitis causes pain and swelling approximately 5 cm proximal from the calcaneus. An insertion tendinitis of the Achilles tendon causes pain immediately where it inserts to the calcaneus. Both may be due to excessive exercises. Retrocalcaneal bursitis lies ventrally from the tendon and calcaneal bursitis dorsally. External pressure due to a tight heel counter in shoes may be the cause. When a prominent calcaneal tuberosity is exposed to excessive pressure or friction due to a rigid shoe counter this causes a swelling just lateral from the insertion of the Achilles tendon (Haglund's deformity). *Physical examination:* tenderness with or without thickening of the tendon proximally from the calcaneus, at the place of insertion, or of the soft tissue anterior or posterior to the tendon. In case of suspected tendon rupture, perform Thompson's test: squeezing of the gastrocnemius-soleus muscles should elicit plantar flexion if the Achilles' tendon is intact. *Referral:* to a rheumatologist should be considered when these problems occur bilaterally and in case of signs of systemic disease (rheumatoid arthritis, ankylosing spondylitis) and to a (orthopaedic) surgeon in case of an Achilles tendon rupture.

Assessment of the forefoot

Hallux valgus

Deformity of the big toe with a valgus position of the proximal phalanx in relation to the first MTP-1 joint. There is a prominent medial first metatarsal head (bunion) and a varus position of the first metatarsal, resulting in a wide foot (splay foot) with plantar hyperkeratosis and sometimes secondary metatarsalgia due to osteoarthritis. People complain of either pain or malalignment and of problems finding properly fitting shoes. *Physical examination:* on visual assessment more than 20° lateral deviation of dig 1 in the MTP joint. *Investigation or referral:* in case of an acute bursitis (bunion) confusion with gout is possible. Aspiration and examination of crystals will confirm the diagnosis gout. This can be done in primary care or by a rheumatologist.

Hallux limitus/rigidus

Osteoarthritis of the MTP-1 joint, sometimes with a dorsal exostosis and callosity. Pain in the great toe when the patient tries to step off on it. To avoid pressing on the big toe, patients roll the foot outwards when walking. *Physical examination:* limited total range of motion less than 75°, definite pain on dorsiflexion. Compare right and left foot. The outer side of the shoe may be unduly worn and the vamp of the dorsum of the shoe has oblique creases instead of the normal transverse.

Abnormal position of toes 2–4

Hammer toe: extension MTP, flexion proximal interphalangeal joint (PIP), neutral or extension distal interphalangeal joint (DIP). *Claw toe:* extension MTP, flexion PIP and DIP. *Mallet toe:* extension MTP and PIP, flexion DIP. These small toe deformities are often painful as a result of secondary hard digital corns. Claw toes are sometimes associated with neurological conditions such as peripheral and hereditary neuropathies and with rheumatoid arthritis.

Abnormal position of toe 5

Varus deformation (curly toe), sometimes overlapping the fourth toe.

Bunionette

Patients complain of pain on the outside of the foot, especially when wearing shoes. The bunionette (tailor's bunion) is a thickening of the bursa over the head of MT-5, with associated excrescence of the bone. Due to excessive pressure or friction of the shoe, the area may be red and swollen.

Metatarsalgia

Primary metatarsalgia is characterized by painful plantar MT-heads and reactive plantar corns or localized callus. This type is most common and originates from the metatarsals, usually due to overloading. Conditions such as Morton's neuroma and metatarsal stress fracture should be absent. Secondary metatarsalgia due to callosities/corns and intra-articular MTP pain can be present in patients with other co-morbidity such as rheumatoid arthritis, gout, and neurological diseases. *Physical examination:* in primary metatarsalgia, there is pain on the plantar aspect of the metatarsal heads 2–5, less at rest and at night, often with localized callus; no dorsal swelling of the forefoot and no pain on tangential pressure. *Investigation:* in case of a suspected stress fracture, a plain X-ray will not be helpful until after 2–3 weeks.

Morton's neuroma

Entrapment neuropathy of the interdigital nerve, usually in between second and third or third and fourth metatarsals. It presents forefoot pain radiating into the toes with often interdigital numbness. *Physical examination:* palpate directly between the metatarsal head to reproduce the patient's pain. This can be combined with tangential pressure (squeeze test); the additional value of a palpable 'click' is in doubt. *Investigation:* in case of doubt diagnostic ultrasound can help.

Arthritis

Forefoot pain also at rest and at night; morning stiffness. *Physical examination:* MTP-arthritis: there may be swelling of the MTP region dorsally; increased space between adjacent toes ('daylight sign'); painful active and passive motion; no radiating pain on tangential pressure. PIP/DIP arthritis: either swelling of several joints often in a symmetrical pattern or swelling of a single toe ('sausage toe'). There may be a relation with oligo- and polyarticular syndromes, such as rheumatoid arthritis, psoriasis, and gout. *Referral:* to a rheumatologist depending on the possibility of systemic rheumatologic disease.

Corns and calluses

Secondary localized callosities due to localized high pressure over a bone. *Physical examination:* hard digital and plantar corns, soft interdigital corns and localized plantar callus are all localized over a bone. In case of doubt, peeling the callosity with a scalpel will show either a homogenous aspect (corn) or a black spotted aspect due to thrombosed end arteries (wart). A more deeply situated foreign body can also cause secondary callosity formation.

Assessing children

The assessment of a child's foot follows the similar format to that of the adult, except that the clinician should appreciate that a number of normal developmental changes exists in the first few years. These variations may differ from adulthood and may concern the parent and even confuse the inexperienced practitioner.

Normal child's foot

The foot structure is flexible, which causes the foot to look flat with a corrigible everted (valgus) heel. To test this flexibility, the child is asked to stand on tiptoe, which normally causes the formation of the medial longitudinal arch. The forefoot is in line with the rear foot. Walking is from heel to toe. By about 8 years of age, the foot adopts the adult morphology.

Abnormal child's foot

It is abnormal when foot structure is inflexible and the everted heel is rigid. Signs of neurological abnormality are a high medial longitudinal arch, tight extensor tendons and difficulty or delay in walking or running, or toe walking. Finally pain, swelling and stiffness of the joints, lesser toe deformities and hallux valgus are abnormal in a child's foot.

Specific

Calcaneal apophysitis (M Sever): usually in boys 8–13 years who complain of a dull ache behind the heel with a gradual onset and exacerbation by jumping. It is not an avascular necrosis but due to a chronic strain from the Achilles tendon at the attachment of the posterior apophysis of the calcaneus. *Physical examination:* tenderness over the lower posterior tuberosity of the calcaneus. *Investigation:* X-rays are normal and are not advised.

Rigid flat feet and *juvenile hallux valgus* are rare findings. It is important to diagnose these abnormalities, however, because of their long-term effects on the foot function.

Principles of management

Foot complaints are often caused by overloading; both rest and patience are, in general, an important advice. Classification of feet into foot types will help to recognize patterns of associated impairments and problems. This is important for treatment, since treatment of forefoot problems may need to start from the hind- or midfoot. Patients with painful forefoot problems and mobility-restricting co-morbidity are at risk of poor physical functioning and poor general well-being (see section titled 'Implications of the problem'). Therefore, besides attention to proper pain medication treatment of co-morbidity should be considered. In all these foot problems, there is (mostly experience-based) knowledge that suitable shoes may often help to improve physical functioning. Knowledge of the anatomy of the shoe is necessary (Fig. 2). Possible lack of shock absorption might be

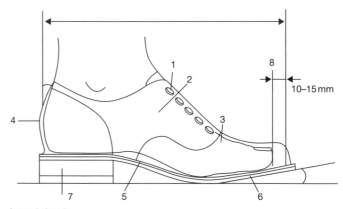

A good shoe has

Points of attention	Good
1. Method of fixation	Laces; buckle and bar; velcro
2. Upper material	Flexible vamp
3. Toecap	Reinforced by toe puff which maintains the shape
4. Stiffener	Strong to prevent medial-lateral sliding of the heel of the foot
5. Distorsion	Shank reinforcement
6. Outsole	Leather/synthetic
7. Heel	Height <3 cm; surface >9 cm^2
8. Length/width/depth	Sufficient (length of the shoe = length of the foot +1 cm)

Fig. 2 Anatomy of the shoe.

important to focus on. Referral to orthotists, podiatrists, and orthopaedic surgeons can be limited to refractory cases.

There is a lack of well-designed randomized clinical trials regarding various forms of specific treatment of foot problems in primary medical care.[5,6] In the following paragraph, therefore, mostly experience-based specific management is described.

Hindfoot

Plantar fasciitis[6]

In the acute stage, non-steroid anti-inflammatory drugs (NSAIDs) can be helpful for 2 weeks to reduce the pain. Possible interactions and side-effects should be taken into account, especially in the elderly. Depending on the foot type, heel cushion (cavus) and medial arch support (planus) can be added. Achilles tendon stretching is advised three times daily 3–5 min. It is advised to incorporate several modalities in combination. If there is no improvement in 6–8 weeks, night splints may be successful in some cases. In case of not sufficiently subsiding serious pain a local corticosteroid injection combined with a local anaesthetic (e.g. 1 ml of 40 mg methylprednisolone with 10 mg lidocaine) can be injected at the point of maximum tenderness. Be sure not to inject through the plantar surface but through the medial part of the heel and parallel to the plantar surface to preserve the integrity of the sole of the foot in order to avoid infection. It is also less painful. This can be repeated two to three times with 3–4-week interval. Be aware of possible risks of local corticosteroid injections as fat pad atrophy and rupture of the fascia.

Tarsal tunnel syndrome

When general measures do not alleviate the problem, referral to an orthopaedic surgeon is advised for a nerve-release operation.

Achilles (peri)tendinitis

In addition to general measures, a heel lift, NSAIDs, heel cord stretching, and if necessary medial arch supports, are helpful. Local corticosteroid injections should be avoided because of risk of tendon rupture.

Heel bursitis and Haglund's deformity

Besides a heel lift, NSAIDs, and a local corticosteroid injection (20 mg methylprednisolone), heel counter adjustment of the shoe is mandatory. Resection of a bony exostosis is seldom necessary.

Forefoot

Hallux valgus[5]

Since there is limited evidence to promote or advise against a certain treatment strategy for symptomatic hallux valgus, there is no need for speedy referral to specialists. The effect of shoe advice (laced shoes, sufficient room at the ball of the foot, restricted heel height, and a sturdy stiffener; possibly stretched shoes), the possible additional effect of foot position improvement by arch supports, and bunion shields can, therefore, be awaited. Surgical intervention may be required to correct the structural deformity. Despite reduction of pain and a (cosmetically) corrected deformity one-quarter to one-third of the patients are not satisfied with these results. It seems advisable that the primary medical care practitioner inquires into the patient's expectations before referring for surgical treatment.

Hallux limitus/rigidus

Non-surgical treatment is directed at limiting the stresses on the MTP-1 joint. Shoes with an extra depth toe box and a stiffened outer sole are helpful. In addition, a metatarsal bar (rocker-bottom sole) added to the shoe will support the hallux in the toe-off phase of gait. Treatment of acute arthritic pain can be started with ice, paracetamol (acetaminophen) three to four times daily 1000 mg or NSAIDs. If necessary an intra-articular injection with corticosteroid (10–20 mg methylprednisolone) will reduce the

pain quickly. When daily function remains impaired surgical intervention is indicated.

Abnormal position toes 2–5

Proper shoes are very important. In painful persistent or progressive contractures, surgical correction is (seldom) advised.

Bunionette

This pain caused by this foot-shoe incompatibility is reduced considerably by wider or stretched shoes. Surgical correction is seldom necessary.

Metatarsalgia

Besides general measures, a variety of methods are employed to disperse weight away from the involved metatarsal(s), including soft shock-absorbing innersoles, moulded shoes with innersoles, and metatarsal bars. Sometimes, especially in deforming rheumatoid arthritis with dorsal dislocation of the MTP joints, surgical intervention is necessary.

Morton's neuroma

Besides wider shoes, a metatarsal bar, and NSAIDs a local methylprednisolone/lidocaine injection (0.5–1 ml of 40 mg methylprednisolone and 10 mg lidocaine solution) can be given in case of much pain. Using a dorsal approach the injection is placed intermetatarsally around the entrapment of the affected interdigital nerve. This can be repeated two to three times with a 3-week interval. If not successful surgical excision is required.

Arthritis

Advice on foot wear is very important; it should provide both support and cushioning. Sport shoes may (temporarily) be a good first choice. NSAIDs are often helpful. If there appears to be a relation with (previously unsuspected) systemic arthritis referral to a rheumatologist for proper medication is advised.

Corns and calluses

Treatment should provide symptomatic relief and also alleviate the underlying mechanical cause. Most lesions can be managed conservatively by use of properly fitting shoes (low heels, soft vamp, and roomy toebox). In addition, several types of orthoses to redistribute local pressure and shear forces may be advised: in case of interdigital corns, a toe spacer is advised. Hard digital corns are a good indication for silicone sleeves. Plantar corn and localized plantar callus are indications for metatarsal pads. Many of these are available without prescription.

Principles of management in children

- *Rigid flat foot* and *juvenile hallux valgus*. These patients should be referred to an orthopaedic surgeon.
- *Calcaneal apophysitis*. This condition usually subsides spontaneously. Sometimes ice and heel lifts will help.

Long-term and continuing care

Opportunities for prevention and health promotion

It is crucial that physicians recognize the complete pathophysiological pattern of a problematic foot. This seems important for treatment and will help when counselling patients with forefoot problems and explaining the reason for the therapeutic advice given, which may concentrate more on the hindfoot or midfoot instead of the forefoot. Especially in bilaterally occurring forefoot impairments, attention should focus on foot type, shoes,[7] and degenerative changes.

Patient education

Patients may believe that their foot complaints are untreatable or are an inescapable phenomenon of ageing.[8] To counteract this, there is need for health promotion to be directed especially towards older people. Written information may complement verbal messages.

Modification of health care seeking behaviour

There are indications that both insoles and shoe adjustments are able to relieve a number of these complaints.[9] Interventions of this nature usually carry only a small risk of iatrogenic damage which is of great importance especially in the older age group. Many of these patients might be helped in primary care and specialist care is less often necessary.

Health issues

In patients with mobility-restricting morbidity such as osteoarthritis, rheumatoid arthritis, serious cardiovascular or lung disease, and co-occurring foot problems, treatment of foot problems may improve their mobility. Patients with diabetes mellitus and both polyneuropathy and signs of overloading of the feet (corns and calluses) are at high risk for a diabetic foot ulcer. Besides regular examination the patient and the primary medical care practitioner, shoe advise and insoles are strongly recommended.

Implications of the problem

Foot problems are associated with an increased risk of falls, limitation of mobility, decreased levels of physical functioning,[10] disability, and possibly, also loss of productivity.[11] Foot pain is independently associated with poor general health perception in people with foot problems.[2] The influence of foot problems on health care use and costs is, however, not clear. The natural course of most common foot problems is not known in primary medical care. Prognostic studies are needed to assess who is at risk for a poor outcome. Treatment is mostly experience based. Effectiveness studies can assess medication and non-invasive treatment (shoe adjustments or insoles) in people with foot problems.

Key points

- Foot problems can be categorized according to the localization of the pain. Knowledge of the anatomy of the foot is important to understand dysfunction.

- Classification of feet into foot types will help to recognize patterns of associated problems. Adequate treatment is available for foot problems presented in primary medical care, but it is mostly experience based.

- Shoes should be adjusted to the feet instead of the other way around. Knowledge of the anatomy of the shoe is important.

References

1. Gorter, K.J., Kuyvenhoven, M.M., and de Melker, R.A. (2000). Nontraumatic foot complaints in older people: a population-based survey of risk factors, mobility, and well-being. *Journal of the American Podiatric Medical Association* **90**, 397–402.

2. Gorter, K.J., Kuyvenhoven, M.M., and de Melker, R.A. (2000). Nontraumatic forefoot problems and foot function in people of 45 years and above. *Arthritis and Rheumatism* **43**, S129.

3. Lamberts, H., Brouwer, H., and Mohrs, J. *Reason for Encounter-, Episode- and Process-Oriented Standard Output from the Transition Project* (2 Vols).

Amsterdam: University of Amsterdam, Department of General Practice/Family Medicine, 1991.

4. Gorter, K.J., Kuyvenhoven, M.M., and de Melker, R.A. (2001). Health care utilisation by older people with non-traumatic foot complaints: what makes the difference? *Scandinavian Journal of Primary Health Care* **19**, 191–3.

5. Ferrari, J., Higgins, J.P.T., and Willimas, R.L. (2000). Interventions for treating hallux valgus (abducto-valgus) and bunions. In *The Cochrane Library* Issue 1. Oxford: Update Software.

6. Crawford, F., Atkins, D., and Edwards, J. (2000). Interventions for treating plantar heel pain. In *The Cochrane Library* Issue 3. Oxford: Update Software.

7. Frey, C. et al. (1993). American Orthopaedic Foot and Ankle Society women's shoe survey. *Foot and Ankle* **14**, 78–81.

8. White, E.G. and Mulley, G.P. (1989). Footcare for the very elderly people. A community survey. *Age and Ageing* **18**, 275–8.

9. Postema, K. et al. (1998). Primary metatarsalgia: the influence of a custom moulded insole and a rockerbar on plantar pressure. *Prosthetics and Orthotics International* **22**, 35–44.

10. Bowling, A. and Grundy, E. (1997). Activities of daily living: changes in functional ability in three samples of elderly and very elderly people. *Age and Ageing* **26**, 107–14.

11. Gorecki, G.A. (1973). Preliminary investigation of lower extremity impairments among men in heavy industry. *Journal of the American Podiatric Association* **63**, 47–56.

Further reading

Jahss, M.H. *Disorders of the Foot and Ankle*. Philadelphia PA: W.B. Saunders Company, 1991. (An excellent and comprehensive textbook of orthopaedics (2 Vols). It covers a great variety of subjects ranging from anatomy and biomechanics to treatment of common and of more specific foot problems. Several chapters can be very useful both as a manual and a reference for primary care physicians.)

Coughlin, M.J. (2000). Common causes of pain in the forefoot in adults. *Journal of Bone and Joint Surgery. British. Volume* **B**, 781–90. (Very practical approach of the cause and the mostly outpatient treatment of painful common forefoot problems as seen by an orthopaedic surgeon. The vast majority of these are useful in primary care as well.)

Pyasta, R.T. and Panush, R.S. (1999). Common painful foot syndromes. *Bulletin of Rheumatic Diseases* **48**, 1–4. (The authors use patient vignettes to show clearly that evaluation of the painful foot requires obtaining a pertinent history and performing a systematic examination directed by the patients' complaints.)

West, S.G. and Woodburn, J. (1995). Pain in the foot. *British Medical Journal* **310**, 860–4. (In the ABC series of the BMJ, this article contains a lot of condensed information on foot pain caused both by common and more seldom occurring diseases. Special emphasis on rheumatologic foot problems.)

13.8 Tennis elbow

Willem J.J. Assendelft and Sally Green

Introduction

'Tennis elbow' has many analogous terms, including 'lateral elbow pain', 'lateral epicondylitis', 'rowing elbow', 'tendonitis of the common extensor origin', and 'peritendonitis of the elbow'.

Tennis elbow is characterized by pain over the lateral epicondyle of the humerus and pain on resisted dorsiflexion of the wrist.

Tennis elbow is common with a population prevalence of 1–3 per cent.[1] Peak incidence is between 40 and 50 years of age, and for women between 42 and 46 years of age the incidence increases to 10 per cent.[2,3] The incidence of lateral elbow pain in general practice is four to seven per 1000 patients per year.[3,4]

Tennis elbow is considered to be an overload injury, typically following minor and often unrecognized trauma of the extensor muscles of the forearm.[5] Large-scale high-quality studies on risk factors and prognosis are lacking. Many risk fisk factors have been suggested, but in fact none is empirically confirmed. Despite the title tennis elbow, even tennis is a direct cause in only 5 per cent of those with epicondylitis. Tennis elbow is generally self-limiting. In a general practice trial, 80 per cent of the patients with elbow pain of already greater than 4 weeks duration, following an expectantly awaiting policy were recovered after 1 year.[6] Only a very small percentage of those with tennis elbow progress to needing surgical intervention.

Diagnosis

When a patient presents with pain in or around the epicondyle the general practitioner takes a history including:

◆ location of the pain and radiation when present;

◆ provoking activities;

◆ duration and fluctuation of complaints;

◆ aetiology according to the patient;

◆ previous episodes, course, and treatment.

Differential diagnosis

Two-thirds of elbow pain in primary care is caused by lateral epicondylitis, 5 per cent by medial epicondylitis, and 9 per cent by an olecranon bursitis. In general epicondylitis, being an insertion tendinopathy, can be easily distinguished from intra-articular causes or bursitis by examination of aggravating activity, localization of the pain, and resisted muscle tests.

Physical examination

The general practitioner has the patient dorsiflex the wrist against resistance, with the wrist in a neutral position and the elbow fully stretched. In addition, the general practitioner palpates the elbow on the locus of maximum pressure pain. Additional examinations do not add to the diagnosis. The various other resistance and palpation tests for tennis elbow do not have added value. Radiographs will not help to confirm diagnosis either, since the 5–25 per cent calcifications that are seen do not confirm the diagnosis or have a prognostic meaning. Only when an intra-articular cause is suspected the sedimentation rate may be used to exclude an inflammation and a radiograph to investigate the possibility of a loose body, osteochondritis dissecans, or a bone tumour. There are no valid studies known about the prognostic or confirmative abilities of value of ultrasonic diagnosis.

Evaluation

The diagnosis of tennis elbow or lateral epicondylitis can be made with pain on or near the lateral epicondyle (eventually with radiation in the underarm) that is provoked or increases with:

◆ movements of the wrist;

◆ pain on dorsal flexion of the wrist against resistance;

◆ pressure pain on or around the lateral epicondyle.

Absence of pressure pain makes the diagnosis epicondylitis very unlikely.

With atypical findings on examination or when the pain seems to originate from a different locus, additional examination of the elbow is indicated. When concomitant neck pain or dermatomal sensory changes exist the cervical spine is examined, including an arm stretch test for detection of nerve irritation or cervical hernia.

Treatment

Advice and patient education

The general practitioner explains that the ailment is caused by an overload of the extensor muscles of the wrist. The amount of disability is partially dependent on the force exerted by these muscles. The force increases when squeezing hard, dorsiflexion of the wrist, or turning of the lower arm. The duration of complaints cannot be predicted. However, the average duration is about half a year.[7] No treatment has a proven effect on the duration of the episode. The general practitioner advises to await spontaneous recovery. The impact on daily activities can be discussed and practical solutions sought. Absolute rest is not necessary. The ability to use the arm is determined by the amount of disability various activities provoke. If pain increases the level of activities should be decreased.

There is evidence from meta-analysis of three trials that topical NSAIDs are significantly more effective than placebo with respect to pain.[8] No trial has directly compared oral and topical NSAID and so no conclusions can be drawn on the best route of administering NSAID in tennis elbow.

Injections

Corticosteroid injections have been compared in randomized controlled trials to placebo injections, local anaesthetic, or other conservative treatment (elbow support, NSAID, physiotherapy).[9] Almost all studies showed favourable short-term follow-up results for pain relief. After 6 weeks or longer, no differences in favour of corticosteroid injections could be detected. Two high-quality trials show that injection therapy has a far lower cure-rate at 6 months and longer than NSAIDs and expectantly awaiting, respectively.[10,11]

An injection is therefore only indicated for relieving pain in the short-term (Box 1, Fig. 1). Different suspensions are used. Relatively little corticosteroid suspension in a low dosage is needed. From research, no recommendations for a certain corticosteroid can be made. An anaesthetic can be added. Anaesthesia after injection provides feedback on the injection technique and may prevent post-injection pain. However, injection without addition of an anaesthetic is also possible. Some potential adverse effects of injection have been reported. However, in trials, post-injection pain

Box 1 Injection technique

Triamcinolone acetate 10 mg/ml can be used, optionally mixed with lidocaine 2% in a 1 : 1 mixture. No more than 1 ml should be injected, to prevent volume effects, possibly causing more post-injection pain. A thin needle is required. The length of it is irrelevant, since the skin at the epicondyle is relatively thin.

The needle is inserted vertically at the site of the insertion of extensors, this is the place where the vertical aspect of the epicondylus becomes horizontal. With the needle the most painful spots are identified and on each spot a drop of 0.1 ml is injected. In general, 3–6 drops are sufficient. When an anaesthetic is added dorsiflexion against resistance can be applied with the needle still in its place. If this is still painful further drops are still needed.

The patient is instructed to prevent any activities that normally provoke the pain. Absolute rest or a sling is not necessary.

The duration of effect differs individually. A period of at least 2 weeks before the next injection is advised. Normally, a series of maximally three injections is given.

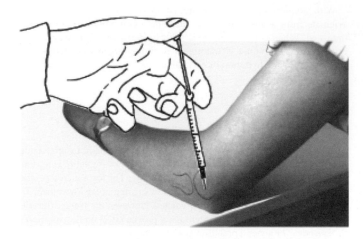

Fig. 1 Injection technique. Photo: Department of Continuous Professional Development, Dutch College of General Practitioners.

(11–58 per cent) and local skin atrophy (17–40 per cent) were equally reported in corticosteroid injection and control groups, therefore more likely to be due to observer bias than to true effects of the injected corticosteroids.

Other treatments

The effectiveness or preventive abilities of braces, tapes, stretching exercises, ice application has not been proven. In addition, the effectiveness of various physiotherapeutic interventions, shock wave therapy and acupuncture remains unclear.[6,12–14]

Surgery has not been studied in controlled trials. Three-quarters of the follow-up studies report success of 80 per cent and over. Generally, operation is not recommended if complaints exist less than 1 year.

Current debate

Because of the lack of methodologically sound studies supporting or refuting most of the treatment interventions used in the treatment of tennis elbow, many aspects of the approach (patient education, NSAIDs, timing of referral for operation) is based on common sense, although there is some evidence for the use of topical NSAID. No clear and consistent psycho-social or physical risk factors have been derived from research yet. Many treatment options are insufficiently studied. In addition, some clinicians and researchers tend to regard epicondylitis as a part of the repetitive injury syndrome.

Key points

- When untreated the prognosis of tennis elbow is favourable— 80 per cent recover completely within a year.
- Corticosteroid injections are only indicated for severe pain or functional limitation.
- X-ray examination is unnecessary.

Acknowledgements

We thank R. Buchbinder, P.A.A. Struijs, and N. Smidt for their contributions to the reviews underlying the recommendations in this chapter.

References

1. **Allander, E.** (1974). Prevalence, incidence and remission rates of some common rheumatic diseases and syndromes. *Scandinavian Journal of Rheumatology* **3**, 145–53.
2. **Card, M.D. and Hazleman, B.L.** (1989). Tennis elbow—a reappraisal. *British Journal of Rheumatology* **28**, 186–90.
3. **Verhaar, J.** (1994). Tennis elbow: anatomical, epidemiological and therapeutic aspects. *International Orthopedics* **18**, 263–7.
4. **Hamilton, P.G.** (1986). The prevalence of humeral epicondylitis: a survey in general practice. *Journal of the Royal College of General Practitioners* **36**, 464–5.
5. **Murtagh, J.E.** (1988). Tennis elbow. *Australian Family Physician* **17**, 90, 91, 94–5.
6. **Smidt, N. et al.** (2001). Physiotherapy for lateral epicondylitis: a systematic review. In *Conservative Treatments for Tennis Elbow in Primary Care* [thesis] (ed. N. Smidt), pp. 13–45. Amsterdam: EMGO Institute.
7. **Hudak, P., Cole, D., and Haines, T.** (1996). Understanding prognosis to improve rehabilitation: the example of lateral elbow pain. *Archives of Physical Medicine and Rehabilitation* **77**, 568–93.
8. **Green, S. et al.** (2001). Non steroidal anti-inflammatory drugs (NSAIDs) for lateral elbow pain. In *Cochrane Library* Issue 4. Oxford: Update Software.
9. **Smidt, N., Assendelft, W.J.J., Van der Windt, D.A.W.M., Hay, E.M., Buchbinder, R., and Bouter, L.M.** (2002). Corticosteroid injections for lateral epicondylitis: a systematic review. *Pain* **96**, 23–40.
10. **Smidt, N., Van der Windt, D.A.W.M., Assendelft, W.J.J., Devillé, W., Korthals-de Bos, I., and Bouter, L.M.** (2002). Corticosteroid injections for lateral epicondylitis are superior to physiotherapy and a wait and see policy at short-term follow-up, but inferior at long-term follow-up: results from a randomised controlled trial. *Lancet* **359**, 657–62.
11. **Hay, E. et al.** (1999). Pragmatic randomised controlled trial of local corticosteroid injection and naproxen for the treatment of lateral epicondylitis of the elbow in primary care. *British Medical Journal* **319**, 964–8.
12. **Buchbinder, R. et al.** (2002). Shock wave therapy for lateral elbow pain (Cochrane review). In *Cochrane Library* Issue 1. Oxford: Update Software.
13. **Green, S. et al.** (2001). Acupuncture for lateral elbow pain. In *Cochrane Library* Issue 4. Oxford: Update Software.
14. **Struijs, P.A.A. et al.** (2001). Orthotic devices for tennis elbow (Cochrane Review). In *The Cochrane Library*. Oxford: Update Software.

13.9 Hand and forearm problems

Dennis Y. Wen

Introduction

Problems involving the upper extremity and specifically the hand, wrist, and forearm, are a common presenting complaint to primary care physicians. In our modern industrialized society, proper functioning of the fingers, hands, and wrists becomes essential not only for occupational pursuits, but also for activities of daily living as well as recreational and sporting endeavours. This chapter will discuss the recognition, diagnoses, and management of common hand, wrist, and forearm entities likely to be encountered by the primary care physician. Many of these conditions can be considered repetitive strain injuries. Acute traumatic conditions will not be discussed, as they are covered in other chapters. The proper examination

Table 1 Clinical syndromes of hand and forearm

Condition	Symptoms/location	Mechanism	Physical examination
Carpal tunnel	Paraesthesiae palmar thumb, index, middle, and ring fingers; often worse at night	Repetitive strain; median nerve entrapment by transverse carpal ligament	Tinel's; Phalen's; thenar atrophy if severe
Ulnar nerve entrapment	Paraesthesiae ring and small fingers; worse with elbow flexed and at night	Usually ulnar nerve entrapment in cubital tunnel at elbow	Tinel's at cubital tunnel; symptom reproduction with elbow flexed; intrinsic atrophy and weakness if severe
DeQuervain's	Radial wrist pain, worse with movement	Repetitive strain	Tender EPB, APL tendons at radial styloid; Finkelstein's
ECU tendonopathy	Dorsal ulnar pain, worse with movement	Repetitive strain	Tender ECU tendon at distal ulna; pain with resisted wrist extension and ulnar deviation
TFCC injury	Ulnar wrist pain; can be dorsal, volar, or both; worse with movement	Repetitive strain, or acute trauma	Tender TFCC, dorsal, volar, or both
Kienbock's	Mid-dorsal wrist pain, swelling; painful flexion and extension	Unknown; ?repetitive strain or acute trauma	Tender swelling over dorsal lunate bone; decreased ROM; plain radiographs with lunate sclerosis
Trigger finger	Snapping, locking of finger or thumb with flexion and/or extension; may be painful or painless	?Repetitive strain	Snapping, locking with DIP or PIP joint movement; tender thickening at A-1 pulley at metacarpal head
Dupuytren's contracture	Painless palmar contractures, most commonly small and ring fingers	Unknown; genetic	Palmar cords and nodules; finger and palm contractures
Ganglion cysts	Usually dorsal, radial nodules; can be painful with wrist extension; may be occult or asymptomatic	Unknown; ?repetitive strain	Nodular swelling at dorsal scapholunate junction

EPB, extensor pollicis brevis; APL, abductor pollicis longus; ECU, extensor carpi ulnaris; TFCC, triangular fibrocartilage complex; ROM, range-of-motion; DIP, distal interphalangeal; PIP, proximal interphalangeal.

and management of these conditions can help decrease symptoms and restore essential functioning of the upper extremity (Table 1).

Clinical syndromes

Carpal tunnel syndrome

One of the most commonly encountered repetitive overuse entities in the upper extremity is carpal tunnel syndrome, which is an entrapment neuropathy of the median nerve as it crosses the carpal tunnel at the level of the wrist. Population prevalence estimates in adults range from 0.5 to 7 per cent.[1,2] Blue-collar workers have higher prevalence rates than white-collar workers and those unemployed.[3] Pregnancy, hypothyroidism, amyloidosis, rheumatoid arthritis, as well as other metabolic conditions are often associated with carpal tunnel syndrome.[1] The roof of the tunnel is formed by the transverse carpal ligament, which extends from the radial-sided carpal bones to the ulnar-sided carpal bones. The tunnel contains nine of the finger flexor tendons along with the median nerve. The median nerve can become mechanically compressed within the tunnel due to increased pressure, usually from tenosynovitis of the flexor tendons.

Symptoms include pain, paraesthesiae, and dysaesthesias in the median nerve sensory distribution, which includes the volar surface of the thumb, index, middle, and radial half of the ring fingers. The sensory innervation of the radial portion of the palm usually does not pass through the tunnel. However, patients have often not paid close attention to the exact distribution of symptoms, and will describe it as 'all over' or 'the whole hand'. Symptoms often occur during sleep or with activity. More severe cases can have constant symptoms. Patients often describe being awoken by the paraesthesiae and having to flick their wrist back and forth in a radial-ulnar direction to reduce symptoms. Symptoms may also include non-specific descriptions of weakness, awkwardness, or incoordination of the hand and fingers.

Generally, the dorsal hand is not involved, nor is the wrist itself. If symptoms definitely involve the dorsum of the hand, it is unlikely to be

from carpal tunnel syndrome and more likely could be from radial nerve entrapment syndromes or radiculopathy from the cervical spine. Wrist and forearm symptoms usually do not occur directly from carpal tunnel syndrome, but the hand symptoms from carpal tunnel syndrome can radiate into the wrist and forearm. The concurrent flexor tenosynovitis can also cause some volar wrist and forearm symptoms. Definite neurologic symptoms occurring proximal to the wrist suggests more proximal compression of the median nerve or radicular conditions from the cervical spine.

Physical examination begins with visual inspection of the hands and wrists for any obvious deformities or swelling. Attention should be paid to the prominence of the thenar eminence at the palmar base of the thumb, whose musculature is innervated by the recurrent median nerve. Any noted atrophy compared with the opposite hand suggests long-standing severe carpal tunnel syndrome. Provocative testing includes eliciting a Tinel sign or a Phalen sign. A positive *Tinel sign* occurs when the examiner percusses the median nerve at the level of the wrist with a finger, and paraesthesiae in the median nerve distribution are reproduced. A positive *Phalen sign* occurs when median nerve distribution paraesthesiae are reproduced by passively holding the patient's wrist in a hyperflexed position for 30–60 s. The sensitivity, specificity, and reproducibility of the Tinel and Phalen signs are unclear,[2–4] but if exact reproduction of the patient's symptoms occur with these tests, the diagnosis is supported. Strength testing of the thenar musculature can be checked by resisted opposition of the thumb, which can be deficient in more severe long-standing cases.

Additional testing such as plain radiographs are usually not necessary, except to rule out other suspected conditions. Electromyelography and nerve conduction studies can corroborate the diagnosis in unclear cases, but are not routinely necessary. It must be kept in mind that severity of electrodiagnostic findings often do not correlate well with severity of symptoms, and both false negatives and false positives are common.[2,3] Thus, electrodiagnostic testing has a limited role in making the diagnosis of carpal tunnel syndrome when the diagnosis is clear from the history or examination. Advanced imaging such as CT scan or MRI scan are not generally helpful, except to rule out other entities.

Management involves measures to decrease the pressure on the median nerve at the carpal tunnel. Relative rest of the involved hand and wrist can be helpful. Splinting the hand in near neutral flexion-extension has been shown to decrease carpal tunnel pressures.[1] Removable splints can be used during sleep, or can also be used during daily activities. Anti-inflammatory medications, local icing, and physical therapy to work the finger flexor muscle–tendon units are of questionable benefit, but can be tried along with splinting.

If a trial of splinting is not successful in reducing symptoms, a local corticosteroid injection can be tried. The role of local injections is somewhat controversial. Most studies indicate relief of symptoms with injection, but recurrences occur.[1] The injection is generally performed with a mixture of local anaesthetic such as lidocaine or bupivacaine or both, along with a corticosteroid. The needle is placed into the volar wrist at the level of the proximal wrist crease just ulnar to the palmaris longus tendon. Avoidance of the ulnar artery is essential. If the patient experiences marked paraesthesiae, pain, or dysaesthesias during the injection, re-direction of the needle is indicated to avoid possible direct nerve injection.

Referral for consideration of surgical intervention is appropriate for continuation of symptoms despite conservative treatment, especially if motor weakness or thenar atrophy appears. For long-standing cases, or late presenting cases, with significant motor weakness or atrophy, early referral may be indicated before neurologic changes become irreversible. Surgical carpal tunnel release can be performed open or arthroscopically and the relative merits of each technique are often debated.

Ulnar nerve entrapment (cubital tunnel syndrome)

Entrapment neuropathy of the ulnar nerve is much less common than carpal tunnel syndrome. The most common site of entrapment is at the cubital tunnel as the nerve wraps around the postero-medial elbow. Symptoms involve paraesthesiae in the fourth and fifth digits, often worse at night or with bent-elbow activities. A Tinel's sign can be elicited by percussing the ulnar nerve just posterior to the elbow, although the sensitivity and specificity of this test has not been documented. Atrophy or weakness of the intrinsic hand muscles (dorsal and palmar interossii, including the adductor pollicis) suggests severe or long-standing entrapment. Atrophy is best noted on the dorsum of the hand. Weakness can be tested by resisted finger abduction and adduction. Reproduction of symptoms by holding the elbow in an extreme flexed position for 30–60 s can also aide in diagnosis.

Electrodiagnostic studies can help with the diagnosis, but as with carpal tunnel syndrome, false positives and false negatives occur. Limited data exist on treatment, but conservative measures with rest from aggravating bent-elbow activities are usually tried first. Elbow splints that limit flexion can help and may need to be worn at night. For recalcitrant long-standing cases, or those with muscle weakness, surgical intervention with ulnar nerve transposition may be necessary.

DeQuervain's syndrome

The most common overuse tendinopathy of the wrist is DeQuervain's syndrome, which involves the abductor pollicis longus (APL) and extensor pollicis brevis (EPB) tendons as their sheaths course over the distal radial styloid. This is quite commonly seen in primary care, although actual prevalence figures are lacking.[5] Limited data suggest that repetitive motions of the wrist and ulnar deviation motions of the thumb can contribute to this condition.[5] An association with the postpartum state has been noted.[6] Patients present with diffuse radial-sided wrist pain without antecedent trauma. Crepitus and local swelling may be present in more severe cases.

On inspection, swelling of the tendon sheath along the radial styloid and extending proximally may be noted in severe cases, but is not a consistent

or usual finding. Patients are often quite tender to palpation, localized to the APL and EPB tendon sheaths at the distal radial styloid and slightly beyond. The rest of the wrist and thumb are usually unremarkable. Range of motion testing is sometimes difficult due to patient discomfort, but can be normal except in wrist ulnar deviation. *Finkelstein's test* is performed by flexing the thumb into the palm and passively ulnar deviating the entire wrist and thumb, causing maximal stretch of the APL and EPB tendons. Sharp pain, worse than the opposite asymptomatic wrist, elicited with this manoeuvre corroborates the diagnosis. Strength testing by resisted thumb extension often provokes pain and weakness. Radiographs and more advanced imaging is usually not necessary except to rule out other conditions.

The differential diagnosis includes other entities producing radial-sided wrist pain. Scaphoid fractures involving the middle or proximal thirds will have local tenderness in the anatomic snuff box just dorsal to the APL and EPB tendons. Usually, a history of significant direct trauma is also present. Similarly, a distal radius fracture can be suspected after trauma. Plain radiographs can be obtained if fracture is suspected. Osteoarthritis involving the base of the thumb at the carpo-metacarpal joint is a common alternative diagnosis, but usually the tenderness is localized to the carpo-metacarpal joint that is more distal to the area involved with DeQuervain's. Plain films may demonstrate the thumb base arthritis. An occult ganglion cyst should also be considered.

Local icing, anti-inflammatory medications, and splinting can be tried as initial treatment, despite the lack of controlled treatment trials. Splints must immobilize both the wrist and the thumb metacarpo-phalangeal (MCP) joint, and are commercially available. A simple wrist splint that does not include the thumb MCP joint will not be effective. Although some cases will respond to splinting and anti-inflammatory medications, more severe and long-standing cases often do not. Therefore, injection of corticosteroid into the tendon sheath is often recommended initially, along with splinting. Alternatively, local injection can be tried after failing a trial of splinting. Injection is performed with a mixture of local anaesthetic and corticosteroid. A small bore needle (27 or 30 gauge) is placed into the APL and EPB tendon sheath at the level of the radial styloid, but not into the tendons themselves. Often, finding this small space is difficult, but if successful, Finkelstein's test and resisted thumb extension should become less painful. Both of these manoeuvres can be attempted prior to withdrawing the needle in order to confirm correct placement of the mixture.

The role of physical therapy with stretching and strengthening exercises for the wrist and thumb extensors is unclear. Very little data support exercises, but can still be tried. When conservative approaches fail, or if injections are needed too frequently, surgical referral is indicated. The sheath containing the APL and EPB tendons is divided longitudinally, followed by post-operative splinting.

Extensor carpi ulnaris tendinopathy

The second most common overuse tendinopathy in the wrist and hand involves the extensor carpi ulnaris (ECU) tendon at the level of the wrist and distal ulna. This is seen much less commonly than DeQuervain's. Repetitive wrist motion including pronation and supination, and ulnar deviation, are thought to contribute to the development of this condition. Patients present with insidious onset dorsal-ulnar wrist pain related to use and movement. The ECU tendon runs within a sheath attaching it to the ulnar side of the distal ulna bone. Traumatic rupture of the sheath is possible although somewhat rare, and will result in painful snapping at the distal ulna with pronation and supination movements.

Localized swelling may or may not be present around the ECU tendon at the distal ulna. Tenderness can usually be localized to the tendon. Resisted wrist extension and resisted ulnar deviation can reproduce symptoms. The main differential diagnosis along with ECU tendinopathy for ulnar-sided wrist pain is an injury to the triangular fibrocartilage complex (TFCC). This complex structure of ligamentous and cartilaginous components lies between the distal ulna and the ulnar carpal bones, specifically the triquetrum and lunate. The tenderness in TFCC injuries is more diffuse than for ECU tendinopathy and can be ulnar-sided and volar-sided, instead of just dorsal-sided as for ECU tendon problems. Further complicating matters, the ECU tendon has a connection to the TFCC and it is possible for both conditions to co-exist. Distal ulna and ulnar styloid fractures also present with ulnar-sided wrist pain, but usually a history of direct trauma is present.

Plain radiographs are generally normal, but can be used to rule other entities such as distal ulnar fractures. Occasionally, MRI is useful if the diagnosis is unclear, or if TFCC pathology needs to be evaluated.

Treatment involves resting the wrist, often with the aid of a splint, although no data exist from controlled studies. Local ice and anti-inflammatory medication may help with symptoms. A wrist splint can usually prevent wrist flexion and extension, as well as wrist radial and ulnar deviation, but cannot prevent wrist pronation and supination unless the elbow is simultaneously immobilized. Therefore, a below-elbow splint can help prevent some of the offending motion, but not all. An above-elbow splint or cast limits all motion at the wrist and ECU tendon, but is extremely inconvenient for the patient. Furthermore, the risk of elbow contractures increases with prolongation of elbow immobilization, especially in elderly individuals. Thus, usually a below-elbow removable wrist splint is tried first, and above-elbow immobilization can be considered a later option. A local injection with a mixture of local anaesthetic and corticosteroid can often be helpful, and can be tried upon failure of below-elbow splinting, and before above-elbow immobilization. Similar to the situation with DeQuervain's, physical therapy with stretching and strengthening exercises is of questionable benefit, but can still be tried.

Failure of these treatments along with protracted symptoms warrants surgical consideration, which involves decompression of the tendon sheath. A subluxed ECU tendon along with a ruptured sheath is also an indication for surgical intervention, although prolonged casting can be attempted prior to surgery with knowledge that successful healing of the torn sheath is unpredictable without surgery.

Trigger finger

Trigger finger is commonly seen in primary care and presents with snapping or locking of the fingers or thumb with flexion and/or extension, sometimes worse upon first awakening or after prolonged use. This may be painful or painless. Force may be needed to either flex or extend the finger in order to overcome the snapping and locking. Degeneration and thickening of the tendon pulley sheath, specifically the A-1 pulley located in the palm at the level of the metacarpal head, causes the stenosing effect. Repetitive overuse is thought to contribute, although not proven.[7] This condition can involve any of the fingers including the thumb.

Physical examination reveals no abnormalities in the finger distal interphalangeal (DIP) or proximal interphalangeal (PIP) joints themselves. A tender nodule can be noted at the pulley sheath located in the palm at the metacarpal head. Often, a snapping sensation can be felt with the palpating finger over the pulley sheath as the PIP and DIP joints are flexed and extended. Radiographs are generally normal and not necessary.

Local ice, anti-inflammatory medications, splinting, and rest from any offending activities can be tried initially, but are often unpredictable. Therefore, local corticosteroid injections may be attempted early on in the treatment course since the success rate in controlled trials is much higher.[8,9] A mixture of local anaesthetic and corticosteroid is injected near the nodule at the tendon pulley sheath with a small bore needle (25 or 27 gauge). Relief of pain may be immediate, but the triggering or locking may take several days or longer to recede. Although initial relief of symptoms is often obtained with local injections, the recurrence rate is high. Repeat injections can be performed for recurrences, although should be limited to a total of three or four. If injections are either unsuccessful, or recurrences persist, surgical release of the pulley sheath is indicated.

Triangular fibrocartilage complex injuries

As aforementioned in the ECU tendinopathy section, the TFCC is a complex structure of ligamentous and cartilaginous components between the distal ulna and the triquetrum and lunate carpal bones, and is an important cause of ulnar-sided wrist pain. Injury to components of the TFCC can occur from trauma, such as a fall onto the wrist or traction or torsion of the wrist, or can occur from repetitive overuse. Prevalence rates are lacking, but are somewhat common in primary care. Patients present with ulnar-sided wrist pain, often diffuse and vaguely localized. Crepitation and popping can also be present. Swelling usually is not a prominent feature.

Local tenderness over the TFCC is usually found on physical examination. The tenderness can be along the dorsal side, along the ulnar side just palmer to the ECU tendon, or along the volar side, or usually all three areas. Axial loading of the ulnar wrist with passive pronation and supination can reproduce pain and crepitus. Plain radiographs are generally normal. Arthrography and MRI can show the abnormalities of the injured TFCC, but are not extremely reliable, and their accuracy can vary from institution to institution.

The differential diagnosis includes ECU tendinopathy, distal ulnar fracture, luno-triquetral ligament injury (which can be considered part of the TFCC), or distal radio-ulnar joint injury (which can also be considered part of the TFCC). Distinguishing TFCC proper pathology from luno-triquetral ligament or distal radio-ulnar ligament injuries can be difficult, but initial treatment may be similar.

Treatment can initially involve local ice, anti-inflammatory medications, rest, and splinting, but is often unsuccessful in significant cases. No data exist from controlled treatment trials. Similar to the situation for ECU tendinopathy, above-elbow immobilization to avoid wrist pronation and supination can be more efficacious than below-elbow splinting, but also more complicated and inconvenient. For cases recalcitrant to below-elbow splinting, local injection into the TFCC can be tried. A mixture of local anaesthetic and corticosteroid is injected from the dorsal side. This can often relieve symptoms either temporarily or permanently. For cases with unsuccessful injections or recurrences, repeat injections or above-elbow casting may be attempted. Failures with these treatment modalities require surgical referral. Arthroscopic or open techniques of diagnosis along with debridement and repair may be indicated.

Kienbock's disease

Kienbock's disease refers to an avascular necrosis of the lunate bone for which the aetiology and pathophysiology is unknown. The condition is relatively rare, but can be seen in primary care. Kienbock's generally occurs in young adults and purported aetiologies include a single traumatic event, or repetitive microtrauma. An ulna bone slightly shorter than the radius (ulnar minus variance) is thought to be a predisposing factor. Patients present with pain usually dorsal-sided, around the lunate bone located in the middle (radial-ulnar) of the proximal carpal row. Swelling and limitation of range of motion is often quite prominent.

Dorsal swelling around the lunate can be noted on physical examination. Localized tenderness over the dorsal lunate is found. Limitation of range of motion, especially wrist extension, along with pain can be demonstrated. Plain radiographs can reveal sclerosis of the lunate bone and even collapse of the bone in more advanced cases. There are some less advanced cases of Kienbock's that have normal plain films; therefore, an MRI scan is indicated if still suspected.

Differential diagnosis includes dorsal wrist capsule impingement or impaction, or an occult ganglion cyst, both rather benign conditions. Other, more serious conditions may include scaphoid fracture, scapholunate ligament disruption, lunate fracture or dislocation, and luno-triquetral ligament tear, all of which are generally of traumatic aetiology. Radiographic features, perhaps with advanced imaging such as MRI, can help distinguish these conditions.

Treatment options are somewhat limited for Kienbock's disease, and are mostly surgical. Hence, early referral is indicated once diagnosis is made. Ice, anti-inflammatory medications, and casting may relieve symptoms, although no well-controlled trials exist, but these measures probably do little to alter the course of the disease. Untreated cases have potential for arthritic changes and chronic pain. The surgical goal is to unload the lunate, either by shortening the radius or by lengthening the ulna. Surgical results are often unpredictable and treatment trials are lacking. More advanced cases and surgical failures may require one of several fusion procedures.

Ganglion cysts

Ganglion cysts are commonly seen soft tissue tumours of the wrist. The majority are located dorsally and arise from the scapholunate ligament. Volar-sided wrist ganglions are less common and arise from either the radiocarpal or scaphotrapezial joints and are intimately involved with branches of the radial artery. Their aetiology is unclear although some seem to be associated with trauma or chronic stress. Some are asymptomatic, but others can cause chronic pain with extremes of wrist flexion and extension.

A large cyst or several interconnected cysts can be found on physical examination. They are usually firm and sometimes tender. Dorsal ganglions are found at the joint line and become more prominent with wrist flexion. Occult dorsal ganglions exist that are often difficult to detect as they are hidden within the dorsal wrist joint. Sometimes, only palpable tenderness without a mass is present. Volar ganglions are usually found on the radial wrist just proximal to the wrist joint line and may be pulsatile due to their connection with the radial artery. Plain radiographs are mainly used to rule out other conditions. Ultrasound and MRI can detect ganglions, but are not routinely necessary.

Asymptomatic or minimally symptomatic ganglions may not need treatment and can just be observed. Wrist splinting for reduction of symptoms can be tried. Attempted aspiration or corticosteroid injection of ganglions is often done, but failure and recurrence rates are high. Surgical intervention is indicated for symptomatic cysts failing conservative management. Excision of the cyst can be performed open or arthroscopically.

Dupuytren's contracture

Dupuytren's contracture is characterized by thickening and contracture of the palmar fascia resulting in gradual flexion contracture of the fourth and fifth fingers. No actual flexor tendon involvement occurs, distinguishing it from trigger finger. Bilateral involvement can occur. The aetiology remains unknown, but familial occurrences suggest a genetic predisposition. The condition is uncommon, with population prevalence estimates varying widely by race, ancestry, and age.[10] The greatest concentration is in those of northern European descent. The prevalence is higher in alcoholics and diabetics, and increases with increasing age. There is no known association with repetitive strain. Pain is not usually present. However, functional deficits can occur with advancement of the contracture and cosmetic appearance may become a concern.

Management is operative when functional limitations become intolerable and consists of fascial dissection and contracture release. Surgical results are generally satisfactory, but recurrences can occur. Controlled treatment trials are lacking and multiple surgical techniques have been proposed. A trial of splinting in order to slow the progression of contracture can be tried prior to surgery, but is of unproven benefit.

Key points

- If symptoms involve the dorsum of the hand, carpal tunnel syndrome is unlikely.
- Injections of steroid is the most effective treatment for trigger finger.
- Splinting often helps overuse tendinopathies.
- The main indication for surgical referral of Dupuytren's contracture is intolerable functional deficit.

References

1. **Marshall, S.** (2001). Carpal tunnel syndrome. In *Clinical Evidence* Issue 5 (ed. S. Barton), pp. 717–28. London: British Medical Journal Publishing Group.

2. **D'Arcy, C. and McGee, S.** (2000). Does this patient have carpal tunnel syndrome? *Journal of the American Medical Association* **283**, 3110–17.

3. **Atroshi, I. et al.** (1999). Prevalence of carpal tunnel syndrome in a general population. *Journal of the American Medical Association* **282**, 153–8.

4. **Massy-Westropp, N., Grimmer, K., and Bain, G.** (2000). A systematic review of the clinical diagnostic tests for carpal tunnel syndrome. *The Journal of Hand Surgery* **25A**, 120–7.

5. **Moore, J.S.** (1997). DeQuervain's tenosynovitis: stenosing tenosynovitis of the first dorsal compartment. *Journal of Occupational and Environmental Medicine* **39**, 990–1002.

6. **Skoff, H.D.** (2001). 'Postpartum/newborn' deQuervain's tenosynovitis of the wrist. *American Journal of Orthopedics* **30**, 428–30.

7. **Moore, J.S.** (2000). Flexor tendon entrapment of the digits (trigger finger and trigger thumb). *Journal of Occupational and Environmental Medicine* **42**, 526–45.

8. **Saldana, M.J.** (2001). Trigger finger: diagnosis and treatment. *Journal of the American Academy of Orthopedic Surgeons* **9**, 246–52.

9. **Speed, C.A.** (2001). Corticosteroid injections in tendon lesions. *British Medical Journal* **323**, 382–6.

10. **Ross, D.C.** (1999). Epidemiology of Dupuytren's disease. *Hand Clinics* **15** (1), 53–62.

Further reading

Saar, J.D. and Grothaus, P.C. (2000). Dupuytren's disease: an overview. *Plastic and Reconstructive Surgery* **106**, 125–34. [Overview of epidemiology, possible mechanisms, clinical presentation, and treatment (conservative and surgical) options.]

Allan, C.H., Joshi, A., and Lichtman, D.M. (2001). Kienbock's disease: diagnosis and treatment. *Journal of the American Academy of Orthopedic Surgeons* **9**, 128–36. (Overview of aetiology, diagnosis, staging, and treatment options.)

14

Common emergencies and trauma

14 Common emergencies and trauma

14.1 Out-of-hospital cardiac arrest

Andrew K. Marsden

Introduction and overview

Cardiac arrest is the ultimate emergency. At one time, the management of cardiac arrest was believed to be the prerogative of hospital practice and, even then, merely a gesture made in an attempt to avert the process of dying. However, effective community programmes the world over have demonstrated that successful resuscitation is achievable and primary care practitioners should now be skilled in cardiopulmonary resuscitation (CPR) and prepared to make determined attempts at resuscitation where appropriate.

The culture change came with the realization that two-thirds of deaths from coronary heart disease occurred before hospital admission and that most resulted from ventricular fibrillation (VF), a potentially treatable condition. Pantridge in Belfast pioneered the concept of the mobile coronary care unit, bringing the defibrillator and advanced life support skills from the cardiac ward to the patient's home. In the 1970s, Cobb in Seattle trained paramedics to provide defibrillation and bystanders to provide basic life support. Chamberlain in Brighton introduced 'cardiac ambulances' to the United Kingdom with paramedics trained to recognize and treat life-threatening cardiac dysrhythmias. Automated, semi-automatic advisory defibrillators (AEDs) are now readily available and are relatively inexpensive. They are in frequent use by trained first-aiders, and primary care physicians undertaking emergency work should know how to access and use this equipment. Increasingly sites of public gatherings such as sports stadia and shopping malls have AEDs on site, and physicians who are there on a social basis should be prepared to use them.

Sudden death and heart disease

In 1993, approximately 1.25 million Americans suffered a myocardial infarction, of whom about 500 000 died. These deaths were heavily concentrated in the first hour after the onset of symptoms, with approximately one-half of the mortalities occurring less than 1 h after the onset of symptoms, and the great majority of these prior to the patient's arrival in hospital.

In the United Kingdom, approximately 300 000 people suffer an acute myocardial infarction (AMI) each year and, of these, about 140 000 die. The 28-day mortality is nearly 50 per cent, making AMI the biggest killer disease in the Western world; 50 per cent of the deaths from heart attack occur in the first 75 min after the onset of symptoms and 75 per cent of deaths will have occurred in 3 h. On occasions, AMI may occur without pre-existing symptoms, sudden death being the first evidence of the condition. Ventricular fibrillation is the immediate antecedent cause in over 50 per cent of these deaths.

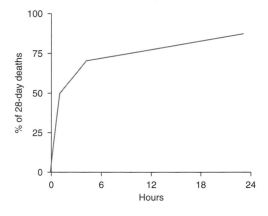

Fig. 1 Mortality curve for coronary heart disease. [Recommendations of a Task Force of the European Society of Cardiology and the European Resuscitation Council. *European Heart Journal* **19**, 1140–64 (1998).]

Figure 1 shows the 28-day mortality curve for coronary heart disease and emphasizes the narrow time-window of opportunity if such mortality is to be addressed. Good rates of survival from VF are feasible, and increase significantly in episodes of VF which occur in cardiac-monitored patients or when skilled professionals are present at the time VF occurs.

Cardiac arrest and the primary care physician

Most patients who experience chest pain, especially those in rural communities, will still call their general practitioner (GP) or primary care physician in preference to calling the emergency services, so that the GP is often in the best position to provide emergency treatment. Myocardial infarction is the commonest cause of cardiac arrest managed by GPs, and a small minority of patients will have a cardiac arrest in the presence of their primary care physician, further emphasizing the importance of maintaining skills in CPR and of ensuring that basic resuscitative equipment is available in the primary care setting.

A management strategy—the chain of survival

The concept of the 'chain of survival' (Fig. 2) was developed by Cummins, a Seattle emergency physician, who identified the links contributing to successful resuscitation out-of-hospital.[1] The chain is only as good as its weakest link. Each of the links forms a component of evidence-based guidelines for CPR, guidelines which have been agreed the world over through the International Liaison Committee on Resuscitation (ILCOR) and presented in Europe through the European Resuscitation Council (ERC) and the

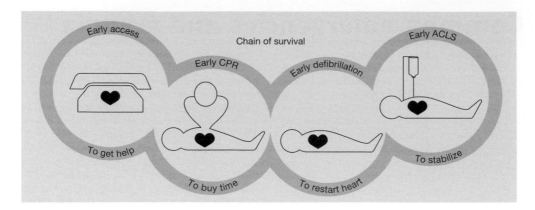

Fig. 2 The 'chain of survival'.

Resuscitation Council (United Kingdom). A complete set of guidelines together with explanatory notes can be downloaded from the Resuscitation Council's website (www.resus.org.uk).

Early awareness

This precedes the formal links in the chain. It is clearly important, through public education campaigns, for patients to be aware of the significance of chest pain as a dangerous warning signal prompting immediate action.

Early access

A telephone call to the emergency services is often the first action required. Most countries have dedicated emergency numbers for this purpose. The ambulance, fire service, or paramedic control centre is likely to have a system of prioritizing calls, so that life-threatening chest pain or cardiac arrest calls will result in an emergency response. Response times are critical, and emergency care providers use a range of technologies to ensure that response times are kept to a minimum. First aid and CPR instructions can be provided by telephone to the caller. In the United Kingdom, the British Heart Foundation has published good practice guidance which recommends a 'dual response' by the GP and the ambulance service.

Early CPR

CPR 'buys time' until a defibrillator can be deployed. Left untreated, the mortality from VF increases at 20 per cent per minute of fibrillation so that early defibrillation is the primary determinant of survival. CPR extends the window of opportunity for successful defibrillation. There has been much emphasis in recent years on education of the general public in basic life support (BLS) with the British Heart Foundation 'Heartstart UK' emergency life support training schemes supplemented by national campaigns such as 'Save a Life' and the '999 Lifesaver' Roadshows. The Heart and Stroke Foundation sponsors both public awareness campaigns and BLS and advanced cardiac life support (ACLS) education for health care professionals throughout the United States and Canada.

The components of CPR follow the ABC approach. The airway must be opened [using head tilt-chin lift (or jaw thrust when a neck injury may be present)] and the breathing checked. If absent, ventilation in BLS is provided by expired air resuscitation using the mouth-to-mouth method, although the importance of this has been de-emphasized recently, adding at least in part to the general unwillingness of the public to engage in mouth-to-mouth resuscitation. If initial ventilations do not result in the signs of a circulation being present, then chest compressions should be delivered. The combination of expired air resuscitation and chest compression (100 per minute) in a ratio of 2 : 15 is known as CPR. The algorithm for BLS is shown in Fig. 3.

Health care professionals will use adjuncts to facilitate BLS. The pocket mask with supplemental oxygen is easier to use than the bag-valve-mask,

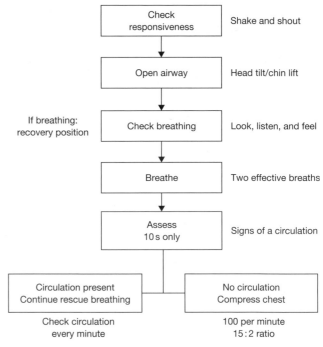

Fig. 3 Algorithm for basic life support. (With kind permission of The Resuscitation Council, UK.)

which requires a two-person technique for effective use. Airway adjuncts may include oropharyngeal or nasopharyngeal tube airways. Ventilation can be improved when the bag-valve device with oxygen reservoir is connected to a laryngeal mask airway, which is safe, effective and easy to use.

As BLS is a practical subject routinely taught on emergency life support courses, the procedural details will not be described here. However, practitioners should ensure that they remain competent in applying the BLS algorithm and the techniques of assessment of unresponsiveness, opening the airway, expired air resuscitation, the use of a pocket mask, chest compressions, the recovery position, and the management of choking.

Early defibrillation

VF is the disordered electrical storm accompanying myocardial ischaemia or conduction defect. It is the cause of over 70 per cent of cardiac arrests. Although it can, occasionally, be terminated by a precordial thump

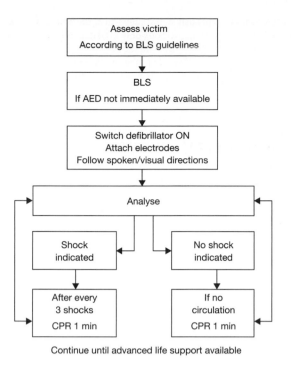

Fig. 4 Algorithm for advisory defibrillation. (With kind permission of The Resuscitation Council, UK.)

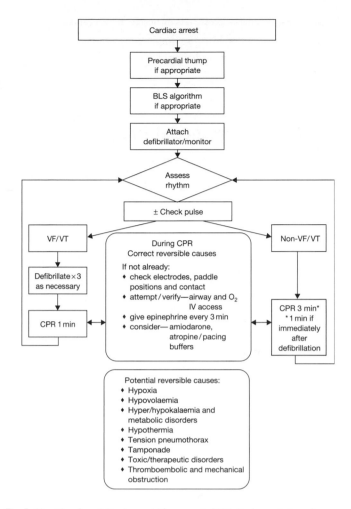

Fig. 5 Algorithm for adult advanced life support. (With kind permission of The Resuscitation Council, UK.)

(indicated in witnessed or monitored arrests when the defibrillator is not immediately at hand), its definitive management is by the delivery of a direct current electrical shock across the heart. The biggest predictor of survival in cardiac resuscitation is the speed of delivery of the first defibrillating shock. Over the years, extensive research has been undertaken on the best way of delivering the shock—published defibrillation guidelines (Fig. 4) reflect the current view. Effective defibrillation requires good contact of the electrodes with the chest wall, which is best achieved by the use of adhesive electrode pads. At present, the sequence of shocks for the adult (200 J, 200 J, 360 J in the first stack with subsequent stacks of three shocks each at 360 J) is based on a monophasic waveform. However, the latest generation of defibrillators employ the more efficient biphasic waveform with the delivered energy adjusted accordingly: the latest devices are able to accurately predict the patient's impedance (resistance) to defibrillation and adjust the amplitude and duration of the waveform accordingly. This technology has enabled small, lighter defibrillators to be developed. The diagnostic routines and treatment algorithms are software driven, so that the machines can operate semi-automatically with the operator having only to press a button to deliver the shock when indicated. Manual over-ride is also provided.

Early advanced life support

Because of the way that AEDs operate it is now customary to divide the rhythm abnormalities associated with cardiac arrest into *shockable* (VF or pulseless ventricular tachycardia) or *non-shockable* [asystole or pulseless electrical activity, PEA (formally known as electromechanical dissociation)] rhythms. The treatment algorithms are adjusted accordingly, but with the emphasis being placed on the early recognition and correction of a shockable rhythm (Fig. 5).

When treating *shockable* rhythms, the defibrillating shocks are given in stacks of three with no pause for pulse check or CPR between the shocks in each stack. Between the stacks, emphasis is placed on CPR and interventions aimed at improving coronary and cerebral perfusion or addressing the underlying cause (see below).

The management of *non-shockable* rhythms is supportive (mainly CPR) whilst the underlying cause is being addressed. Supportive therapy includes definitive airway care, including bag and mask ventilation through a laryngeal mask airway or a cuffed tracheal tube, chest compressions, and vascular access to allow the administration of cardioactive drugs. Adrenaline (epinephrine) administered as 1 mg i.v. (10 ml of 1 : 10 000) every 3 min of arrest is employed for its alpha-adrenergic actions which cause vasoconstriction and increase myocardial and cerebral perfusion pressure. Some evidence suggests that vasopressin should be used as the drug of first choice, and it is currently the recommended choice for this role in ACLS guidelines.

The role of most other drugs in cardiac resuscitation remains controversial. However, atropine in incremental doses up to a total of 3 mg may be given in asystole to provide total vagal blockade and the antiarrhythmic amiodarone in a dose of 300 mg is now considered the drug of choice for refractory VF.

Other than enhancing CPR, the extra provision of advanced life support is aimed at determining and treating, where possible, the underlying causes. These have been listed as the four *H*s and the four *T*s:

Hypoxia—ensure adequate oxygenation and ventilation

Hypovolaemia—consider a fluid challenge of repeated aliquots of crystalloids until return of a circulation

Hyper/hypokalaemia and metabolic disorders

Hypothermia (see below)

Tension pneumothorax—decompress by needle thoracocentesis

Tamponade—decompress by pericardiocentesis

Toxic/therapeutic disorders—administer an antidote (e.g. naloxone) if appropriate

Thromboembolic and mechanical obstruction.

Resuscitation in special circumstances

Children

The emphasis in resuscitation in children should be on the management of hypoxia and hypovolaemia. An infant with a heart rate below 60 bpm should be considered in cardiac arrest and given chest compressions. The algorithm for paediatric advanced life support is shown in Fig. 6.

Trauma

Major trauma presenting in cardiopulmonary arrest carries a dismal prognosis. The emphasis should be on rapid transfer to hospital, with attention to the airway, with cervical spine control predominating. A fluid challenge to return a circulation can be attempted whilst en-route to hospital but this must not be allowed to delay the delivery of the patient to an institution where surgical attention can be given to internal haemorrhage and organ derangement.

Immersion and hypothermia

In hypothermia (whether complicating near-drowning or from another cause), core body temperatures below 30°C are likely to induce VF. This may correct spontaneously if, but only when, the body is warmed—ideally through core rewarming methods only available in hospital. There is little point attempting to give more than the first three shocks at the scene whilst the body remains in VF from hypothermia. Resuscitation attempts should be abandoned only after the patient is warmed to 32–34°C, or when active warming attempts are unable to raise core temperature at a rate greater than 1C°/h.

Post-resuscitation care

The return of spontaneous circulation following resuscitation of cardiac arrest out-of-hospital is most gratifying but without vigorous after-care a successful outcome is not assured. Definitive airway care with 100 per cent oxygen (controlled by blood gas monitoring) should be provided for unconscious patients or those unable to maintain their own airways, otherwise oxygen is given at lower concentration by mask. About one-third of post-arrest patients will require a short period of ventilatory support. In some, correction of acid–base and metabolic abnormalities following the period of organ ischaemia will be required. In others, cardiac or other end-organ failure needs to be addressed. There is a high incidence of re-arrest, especially from re-fibrillation, so that constant cardiac monitoring is essential. A 12-lead diagnostic ECG should be performed. Unless the resuscitation was unduly prolonged or involved traumatic procedures, myocardial infarction patients who have survived a VF arrest should be considered for coronary re-perfusion with thrombolytic agents.

Results of resuscitation out-of-hospital

In recent years, there has been an encouraging increase in the success of resuscitation from out-of-hospital cardiac arrest with about 8 per cent of survivors being discharged from hospital and remaining alive at 1 year.[2] Survival from resuscitated shockable rhythms ranges from a median 12 per cent across most emergency medical service systems to 50 per cent or more when the moment of VF was witnessed by a practitioner with immediate access to a defibrillator. The survival from asystole—about 2 per cent—is poor, but much asystole recorded in the existing outcome databases results from untreated VF and it is expected that the incidence of this 'secondary asystole' will diminish with improved response times to heart attacks in the community and the wider availability of AEDs. The responsibility of primary care physicians should extend beyond their ability to respond to cardiac arrest out-of-hospital. By contributing to community awareness and involvement, particularly by providing patients with excellent advice as to how to seek care when they develop chest pain (either for those patients with a history of ischaemic heart disease, or those at risk) and by encouraging patients to participate in BLS training programmes, primary care physicians can make meaningful contributions to the health of their patient populations.

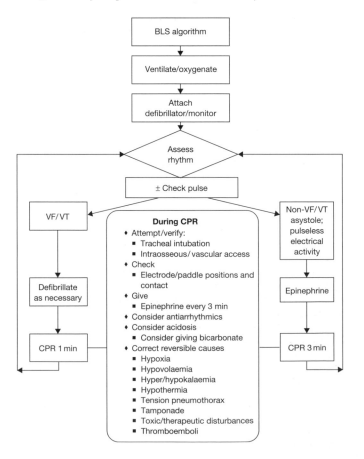

Fig. 6 Algorithm for paediatric advanced life support. (With kind permission of The Resuscitation Council, UK.)

Key points

- Out-of-hospital cardiac arrest can be expected relatively frequently in general practice.
- Ventricular fibrillation complicating myocardial infarction is the commonest precipitant.
- Management follows the principles in the 'chain of survival'.
- Automated external defibrillators provide an easy means of treating VF.
- Good survival rates are possible.
- The primary care physician has a role in community awareness, and treatment of out-of-hospital cardiac arrest.

References

1. Cummins, R.O. et al. (1991). Improving survival from sudden cardiac arrest: the 'chain of survival' concept. *Circulation* **83**, 1832–47.
2. Cobbe, S.M. et al. (1996). Survival of 1476 patients initially resuscitated from out of hospital cardiac arrest. *British Medical Journal* **312** (7047), 1633–7.

Further reading

Bossaert, L., Handley, A., Marsden, A., Arntz, R., Chamberlain, D., Ekstrom, L., Evans, T., Monsieurs, Y., Robertson, C., and Steen, P. (1998). European Resuscitation Council Guidelines for use of automated external defibrillators for EMS providers and first responders. *Resuscitation* **37**, 91–4.

Bossaert, L., ed., for the European Resuscitation Council. *European Resuscitation Council Guidelines for Resuscitation.* Amsterdam: Elsevier, 1998. (The definitive current evidence base for the practice of resuscitation in Europe.)

Colquhoun, M.C. (1998). The use of defibrillators by general practitioners. *British Medical Journal* **297**, 336. (A useful practical review article.)

Colquhoun, M.C., Handley, A.J., and Evans, T.R. *ABC of Resuscitation* 4th edn. London: BMJ Publications, 2002. (From the BMJ's 'ABC' series, this book contains 20 articles covering different aspects of resuscitation in practice.)

Department of Health. *National Service Framework for Coronary Heart Disease.* March 2000. www.doh.gov.uk/nsf/coronary.htm. (The standards of practice for the delivery of early coronary care.)

Pai, E.R., Haites, N.E., and Rawles, J.M. (1987). One thousand heart attacks in the Grampian: the place of cardiopulmonary resuscitation in general practice. *British Medical Journal* **294**, 352–4.

Rawlings, D.C. (1981). Study of the management of suspected infarction by British immediate care doctors. *British Medical Journal* **282**, 1677–9.

Resuscitation Council, UK. *Resuscitation Council Guidelines*, 2000. www.resus.org.uk. (An excellent website containing all the Resuscitation Council's publications, including its guidelines, policy statements, frequently asked questions, and details of practical training courses.)

Weston, C.F.M., Penny, W.J., and Julian, D.G. on behalf of the British Heart Foundation Working Group (1994). Guidelines for the early management of patients with myocardial information. *British Medical Journal* **308**, 767–71. (The extant guidelines for the management of myocardial infarction out-of-hospital.)

14.2 Fractures and limb trauma

Arun Sayal

Introduction

The spectrum of illness seen in orthopaedic injuries ranges from trivial to limb and life threatening. Musculoskeletal injuries account for 3–5 per cent of all primary care office visits. The majority tends to be less severe, treated non-operatively, and can be well managed by the primary care physician. However, some cases require specialist referral. Prompt recognition of the need for and urgency of referral optimizes patient care and makes efficient use of specialists.

General principles

The mechanism of injury and subsequent symptoms are essential aids in diagnosis. Falls (especially in the elderly) can be due to any of a number of precipitating medical conditions such as arrhythmia, ischaemia, seizure, stroke, infection, medication side-effects, etc. The possibility of non-accidental trauma should be considered in all patients, especially if the history is vague, inconsistent with the injury or if there has been unreasonable delay in seeking treatment. Asking about previous problems with either the injured joint or the opposite one enables the clinician to better determine the extent of acute injury. The patient's vocational and recreational demands help determine the goals for recovery and the need for a rehabilitation programme.

The injured limb must be examined down to the skin prior to X-ray to ensure that an open fracture ('compound' in out-dated terminology) does not exist. Open fractures require emergent referral to hospital. Neurovascular integrity must be confirmed, and any compromise should be referred immediately. Examine the joint above and below the suspected site of injury to rule out the possibility of a second injury or of referred pain (e.g. hip injuries presenting with knee pain). Particularly with children, palpate the likely source of pain last. Once the child feels discomfort, fear may cause the rest of the exam to appear falsely painful and difficult to conduct.

Radiology

In acute limb trauma, when indicated, plain radiography is almost always the initial investigation of choice. Children fall often, usually without any significant consequence. They rarely complain persistently unless there is an abnormality. Also, in children the growth plates tend to be weaker than the ligaments. Therefore, children are more likely to suffer fractures than sprains. Fractures are also more common in the elderly due to weaker bones; a lower threshold to order X-rays should be the rule in dealing with the young and old. The correct views must be ordered to accurately diagnose fractures (e.g. for a distal radius injury, X-ray the 'wrist' and not 'forearm'). Two views at right angles to each other are the minimum requirement. In some cases, special views are indicated (e.g. scaphoid).

Specialist referral

If there is *any doubt* about whether a fracture requires operative treatment (either open or closed reduction), then referral is indicated. Closed injuries that are neurovascularly intact can wait a few days from time of injury until reduction. Any delay in consultation of more than a few days should only be undertaken with prior approval of the surgeon.

The more likely an injury is to be complicated, the more likely the case should be referred to a specialist. Intra-articular fractures require anatomic reduction and are at significant risk for osteoarthritis. The majority should be referred early. All pathologic fractures should be referred.

While X-rays are very good at diagnosing fractures, they are not perfect (especially if a 'stress' or 'fatigue' fracture is suspected). If there is a high clinical suspicion of a fracture but the initial X-rays are normal, the injured limb should be appropriately protected and further investigations or follow-up arranged. Conversely, if an X-ray suggests a fracture, but the area is not tender, then the diagnosis of an acute fracture is suspect.

The concept that 'sprains' are minor injuries requiring little medical attention is misleading. While the majority of sprains heal without long-term consequences, some result in chronic joint instability and require operative repair. It is important to recognize that small avulsion fractures, though seemingly trivial, often represent significant ligamentous injuries.

Analgesia

Inadequate treatment of acute musculoskeletal pain occurs with unintended frequency. Short courses of prescription analgesics should be considered when dealing with acutely painful injuries. NSAIDs should be prescribed if significant inflammation is present.

A well-known mnemonic for the treatment of acute soft tissue injuries is 'RICE'—rest, ice, compression, and elevation. Patients are better served by replacing the word 'rest' with 'restricted activity', thus encouraging patients to carefully make use of the injured limb as the pain allows. This decreases the stiffness, atrophy, and proprioceptive loss that often occur with unnecessary immobilization.

Terminology

Comfort with the orthopaedic *nomenclature* is necessary to appropriately manage cases. A *fracture* simply refers to a loss of continuity of the bone cortex. Terms such as 'hair-line', 'crack', and 'break' do not, strictly speaking, imply escalating degrees of injury.

A *dislocation* refers to a complete loss of continuity between two articular surfaces. *Subluxation* (also called an 'incomplete dislocation') is a partial loss of continuity between two articular surfaces. *Displacement* is present if the bony ends of the fracture have moved relative to each other. Dislocation, subluxation, and displacement are always described with the position of the distal anatomy relative to the proximal. *Angulation* refers to the amount of 'tilt' (measured in degrees) a fracture deviates from the anatomic position. Classically, angulation has been described by the direction of the point of the angle formed at the fracture site (see Fig. 1). The phrase 'the distal fragment is angulated in' the direction in which it has tilted from the anatomic position is increasingly accepted.

Shoulder injuries

Many acute shoulder injuries will present to a primary care practice. The usual mechanism is a fall on the shoulder tip. Common to all is the potential for disabling stiffness (particularly in the elderly) if immobilized longer than necessary. Ensuring the restoration of shoulder range of motion after any upper extremity injury is essential.

Clavicle fractures

The clavicle is one of the most commonly fractured bones in the body. The most frequent site of fracture (~80 per cent) is the middle third of the clavicle. The usual mechanism is a fall on the shoulder tip. Patients present with pain with shoulder movement, localized tenderness, often a step

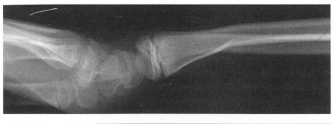

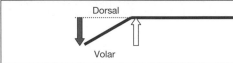

Fig. 1 X-ray of a Smith's fracture in a child. The white arrow shows the older classic method of determining angulation (in the direction of the point of the angle formed at the fracture site, i.e. *dorsal* angulation). The black arrow represents the newer terminology. It describes the direction in which the distal fragment has tilted from the anatomic position. In this case, 'the distal fragment is angulated *volarly*'.

deformity and angulation. X-rays will usually confirm the diagnosis. Some authors recommend a 'figure-of-eight' bandage. However, treatment with a simple sling heals equally well, offers the same or better patient comfort and is not associated with axillary vein thrombosis (a potential complication with the 'figure-of-eight'). Management consists of a sling as required (usually 2–4 weeks) and protected activities for 2–4 weeks after that. Referral is only required if the fracture fails to heal by 6 weeks.

Fractures of the distal third of the clavicle are less common (~15 per cent) but more problematic. Clinically, they will usually have local swelling and tenderness. Distal clavicle fractures are better appreciated on X-rays of the shoulder as opposed to clavicle views. These fractures often have associated tears of the coracoclavicular ligaments and are at greater risk for delayed or non-union. Fractures of the distal third of the clavicle should be referred early to orthopaedic surgeons.

Acromio-clavicular joint injuries

These are more commonly referred to as 'shoulder separations' and are usually caused by falling on the shoulder tip with the arm adducted. In a grade I injury there is a stretch of the acromio-clavicular (A-C) ligaments with tenderness of the A-C joint on examination. Grade II is a tear of the A-C ligaments with tenderness and a mild step-off deformity of the joint. Grade III injuries tear the A-C and coracoclavicular ligaments with the distal clavicle prominently 'floating'. Higher-degree injuries (grades IV–VI) will rarely be seen in a primary care practice. Clinical examination will often reveal the degree of injury. X-rays of the A-C joints (taken standing both with and without weights) can confirm the diagnosis. Grade I injuries are treated with a sling for 7–10 days, with no heavy lifting or contact sports until the site is non-tender and a full range of motion has returned (usually about 2 weeks). Grade II injuries require about 10–14 days in a sling and restricted activities for about 6 weeks. The treatment for grade III injuries is controversial. For some patients, consideration should be given to primary operative repair but most can be managed conservatively. Grade III injuries of the A-C joint should be referred for orthopaedic opinion.

Shoulder dislocations

Gleno-humeral dislocations that present to a primary care office should be referred to an emergency department for prompt reduction and appropriate follow-up.

Proximal humerus fractures

Fractures of the proximal humerus are frequently seen in the elderly after falls. Approximately 85 per cent of fractures of the proximal humerus are undisplaced or minimally displaced (<1 cm). These can be treated with a sling for 1–2 weeks and early mobilization. The major complication is loss of range of motion, so careful follow-up and exercises are required. If the fracture is displaced more than 1 cm, angulated more than 45°, or associated with a dislocation, then prompt referral is indicated for closed or open reduction.

Elbow injuries

Elbow injuries commonly result from falls either on the outstretched hand or directly on the point of the elbow. Careful palpation of the areas most commonly fractured (supracondylar, radial head, and olecranon) often suggests the injury clinically. The presence of an elbow effusion on the lateral X-ray is a very important finding. A normal X-ray demonstrates a small anterior fat pad and no posterior fat pad. On the lateral elbow X-ray, (see Fig. 2) billowing out of the anterior fat pad (the 'sail sign') and/or the presence of a posterior fat pad are evidence of an intra-articular effusion, most commonly from a fracture. If no fracture is seen, treatment depends on the patient's age. For an adult, the diagnosis is most likely to be a very subtle radial head fracture (even if not seen on X-ray) and the patient can be

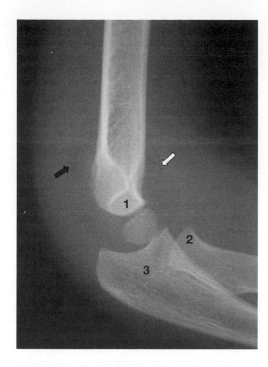

Fig. 2 X-ray of a child's elbow showing an effusion but no definite fracture. The anterior 'sail' sign (white arrow) and/or the posterior fat pad (black arrow) are evidence of an elbow effusion. (1) humerus; (2) radius; and (3) ulna.

treated with analgesia, a sling and follow-up weekly until the symptoms resolve. For a child, a supracondylar fracture through the growth plate must be presumed. This requires urgent referral for a posterior slab and follow-up.

Fracture of the radial head

This is the most common adult fracture about the elbow. The mechanism is a fall on the outstretched hand and presents with elbow pain, maximal over the radial head and exacerbated by pronation/supination. Undisplaced radial head fractures are treated with a sling, analgesia, and early mobilization. Brief plaster immobilization is reserved for those with severe pain. If the radial head is displaced or comminuted, then referral to an orthopaedic surgeon is indicated.

Supracondylar fractures and olecranon fractures

These require urgent referral for assessment for possible surgery.

Fractures of the coronoid process

These fractures (anterior lip of the ulna at the elbow) can be seen after hyperextension injuries to the elbow. These are often more significant than they appear. They often represent a spontaneously reduced elbow subluxation (or less commonly dislocation) and suggest a significant ligamentous injury. They should be referred for plaster immobilization and early orthopaedic follow-up.

Pulled elbow

Patients with a pulled elbow (radial head subluxation) are commonly seen in primary care offices. This generally affects children between 6 months and 5 years of age. Laxity of the annular ligament around the radial head allows the bone to sublux when longitudinally pulled and/or twisted. The child's arm has usually been pulled (not fallen on), often in play, and after a brief cry, the child is hesitant to move the arm. The child with a pulled elbow is usually fairly comfortable at rest. Clinically, there should be no

evidence of an elbow effusion. The arm should be examined from the clavicle to the fingers to rule out other injuries. If the history and examination are consistent with a pulled elbow, then attempting reduction without ordering X-rays is recommended. However, if there is reasonable clinical suspicion of a fracture, then X-ray the elbow first. Normal X-rays (no evidence of fracture *or* effusion) are consistent with a pulled elbow and attempting reduction is acceptable.

The reduction is attempted by putting one thumb on the radial head and the other hand holding the wrist. Gentle forearm supination is followed by elbow flexion, with the thumb feeling for the reassuring 'click' of reduction. This movement is often uncomfortable for the child. The child should be moving the arm spontaneously within a few minutes. This must be seen before discharging the patient. If the manoeuvre was unsuccessful, then reduction can be attempted by fully pronating the arm and then elbow flexion. If still the patient does not move the arm normally, then X-rays should be taken (if not already done) to rule out any occult fracture. If the X-rays are normal and there is no other area of clinical concern, the arm should be placed in a sling and the patient re-examined the next day. Should the reduction be unsuccessful the following day, then referral is indicated.

Wrist and hand injuries

The commonest mechanism for injuring the wrist is a fall on an outstretched hand. The most common fracture seen in adults is a fracture of the distal radius. A Colles' fracture is a dorsally displaced, impacted fracture of the distal radius with the distal fragment angulated dorsally. Much less common is a Smith's fracture (often called a 'reverse Colles'). It results from a fall on the dorsum of the hand, with the distal fragment angulated volarly. These fractures require plaster immobilization as a minimum, and often reduction and as such should be referred to an emergency department for further treatment.

Children who complain of persistent wrist pain after a fall are much more likely to have a fracture than a sprain. Tenderness and swelling are present. The buckle (or torus) fracture is best seen on the lateral X-ray. If there is tenderness over the growth plate and the X-ray shows soft tissue swelling but no fracture, then a Salter I growth plate fracture has occurred. Treatment for Salter I fractures and anatomically aligned buckle fractures is forearm plaster immobilization for about 3 weeks. Fractures that are angulated less than 15° will often remodel over time. The decision to reduce is based on many factors and patients should be referred to an ED for further assessment. Fractures angulated more than 15° require urgent referral to an orthopaedic surgeon for reduction.

Scaphoid

Every patient with an acute 'wrist injury' should be carefully examined for a fracture of the scaphoid (also known as the navicular bone). Tenderness in the anatomic snuff-box after a fall on the outstretched hand is suspicious for a scaphoid fracture. It is helpful to deviate the wrist ulnarly when palpating the snuff-box to better reveal the scaphoid. Comparison palpation of the opposite snuff-box should be performed since many people are tender in the absence of injury. Other clinical signs may include palmar scaphoid tenderness (palpation at the base of the thenar eminence), pain with axial loading of the first metacarpal (pushing in on the thumb), and pain with gripping. Particular attention is paid to scaphoid injuries because of the risk of non-union and avascular necrosis, which can lead to severe, chronic wrist pain and requires operative treatment. When ordering X-rays, scaphoid views should be specifically requested. If the X-rays reveal a fracture, immobilization and referral to an orthopaedic surgeon are indicated. The patient with a significant clinical suspicion of a fracture and normal X-rays (~10 per cent of scaphoid fractures) should be immobilized in a thumb-spica cast for 10–14 days and then re-examined. Alternatives for the patient with a clinically fractured scaphoid and normal X-rays include a CT scan or bone scan.

Boxer's

Fractures of the fourth or fifth metacarpal neck often follow a closed fist punch. These fractures require referral for cast immobilization and possible reduction.

Phalanx fractures

Phalanx fractures will commonly present to a primary care office. Rotation of any degree is an indication for reduction but is rarely appreciated radiographically. It must be detected clinically by gently flexing the fingers and noting that: (a) the fingers point toward the scaphoid bone without scissoring; (b) the nailbeds are parallel; and (c) the flexed injured hand resembles the flexed uninjured hand. Treatment depends on fracture stability. If the fracture pattern is transverse *and* there is no requirement for reduction, the fracture is stable and can be buddy-taped for about 3 weeks. If the fracture pattern is oblique or if the fracture requires reduction (because of angulation, rotation, or displacement), then it is unstable. Unstable phalanx fractures should be referred for reduction (if needed), plaster immobilization, and follow-up with a hand specialist.

Isolated distal tuft fractures do not require any specific treatment. If they co-exist with an associated nail avulsion, then referral is indicated for an intricate nail bed repair.

Mallet fingers

These occur due to sudden hyperflexion injuries to the distal interphalangeal (DIP) joint. The result is either a tear of the extensor tendon or an avulsion fracture of the distal phalanx dorsally. In either case, the distal phalanx is noted to droop and the DIP cannot be actively extended. X-rays will differentiate the fracture from the extensor tendon injury. If the avulsed fragment involves more than a third of the joint space, then referral is indicated for possible open reduction and internal fixation. For smaller bone fragments and for all extensor tendon injuries, treatment requires splinting the DIP in slight extension for 6 weeks without any allowance of flexion.

Hip injuries

Acute hip injuries are common in the elderly. Unfortunately, they often result in debilitating hip fractures. Diagnostically, they are relatively uncommon in a primary care office given the immobility that results. Of note, it is not always the fall that causes the hip fracture. Many patients with a hip fracture will state that they heard a crack while twisting on the leg, and the pain caused them to fall. Almost always, patients with acute hip fractures will be non-ambulatory. The pain is often felt laterally about the hip. Pain felt medially about the groin after a fall may represent a pelvic ramus fracture. Physical examination should include compression of the iliac wings and palpation of the pubic symphysis looking for signs of a pelvic fracture. An active or passive straight leg raise will be extremely painful (if possible at all) for the patient with a fractured hip. Gentle log rolling of the femur will cause significant pain. Often, the affected leg is shortened and externally rotated. X-rays of the hip will most often reveal the anatomic site of the fracture—femoral neck, intertrochanteric, or much less commonly, sub-trochanteric. If there is a high clinical suspicion of fracture and the X-rays do not confirm the diagnosis, then an urgent CT scan or bone scan should be arranged. Patients with fractured hips should be referred urgently for open reduction, internal fixation or hemiarthroplasty. Acute pelvic fractures should be referred urgently for orthopaedic opinion. The majority of isolated pelvic rami fractures are treated conservatively with bed rest and analgesia.

Knee injuries

The majority of acute knee injuries involve soft tissue damage as opposed to a fracture, a disproportionate number of which will require operative treatment. The primary care physician must be comfortable diagnosing knee injuries in order to separate out those that require referral from those that do not. The history and physical examination of the injured knee is more challenging in the first few days after injury. Due to the pain and decreased mobility, the patient usually does not yet know if there is pain with squatting, swelling with activity, giving way, locking, etc. Many clues are available on history-taking. Determining the mechanism of injury is essential. A twisting injury suggests a meniscal tear; a valgus strain (a force directing the knee medially) often injures the medial collateral ligament (MCL); a sudden deceleration injury can damage the anterior cruciate ligament (ACL). Swelling that occurs within an hour or two of injury represents blood in the joint. An acute haemarthrosis is most often due to either a fracture (of the patella, femur, or tibia) or an ACL tear. Swelling that takes hours to develop represents inflammatory fluid and is more typical of meniscal tears.

On physical examination, observe the patient both walking and squatting. Perform the examination with the patient lying on a bed and not sitting in a chair. Effusions are detected by the fluid bulge sign (for small effusions) and patellar ballotment (for larger effusions). The patient should perform a straight leg raise. This ensures that the knee extensor mechanism is intact and rules out a complete tear of either the quadriceps or patellar tendon. The knee should be palpated completely. Tenderness isolated to the joint line suggests meniscal pathology. Tenderness along the medial side above and below the joint line is usually an MCL injury with or without meniscal damage.

The 'patellar apprehension' test is useful to detect patellar instability. The test is performed by gently directing the patella laterally and noting pain or quadriceps tightening. A valgus strain will stress the MCL and a varus strain tests the less commonly injured lateral collateral ligament (LCL). Testing of the ACL requires an anteriorly directed force behind the proximal tibia while stabilizing the distal femur.

The anterior drawer test requires the knee to be flexed at 90°, which is usually very painful in the acute setting. Pain causes muscle spasm, which renders the test far less reliable.

The Lachman test, performed with the knee at 20–30° of flexion, is often more useful acutely. However, it too can give false reassurance of ACL integrity if there is significant pain and muscle spasm.

Ligament injuries can be graded clinically, based on the physical examination. Grade I injuries represent a stretch of the ligament, with no laxity noted. Grade II injuries are incomplete tears that open slightly with stress, but with a definite endpoint. Grade III tears are complete disruptions with sometimes less pain but laxity and no definite endpoint.

Radiographs of the acutely injured knee reveal a fracture in less than 7 per cent of patients who present to an emergency department. This figure is probably less for patients presenting to a primary care practice. The Ottawa Knee Rules were devised, validated, and subsequently shown to decrease the use of knee X-rays by 21 per cent without missing fractures. Suggested criteria include any of the following:

1. age 55 years or older;

2. isolated tenderness of the patella;

3. tenderness at the head of the fibula;

4. inability to flex to 90°; or

5. inability to weight bear both immediately and in the emergency department (defined as unable to transfer weight twice onto each lower limb regardless of limping).

All fractures about the knee require urgent orthopaedic referral and should be kept non-weight-bearing. Early referral is indicated for grades II and III ACL tears and grade III MCL tears. Other ligamentous injuries and suspected meniscal injuries should be treated with weight bearing as tolerated, removal from sporting activities and knee flexion–extension exercises to maintain range of motion and strength. The routine use of immobilization splints for acute meniscal or ligamentous injuries should be discouraged because of the atrophy and stiffness that results. Follow-up on a weekly or biweekly basis is required to ensure that symptoms improve and that more significant pathology is not subsequently revealed. Failure to steadily progress to the pre-injured state or delayed diagnosis of a more serious ligament injury requires referral.

Ankle and foot injuries

The vast majority of ankle injuries presenting to a primary care office is sprains. The mechanism is most often inversion. This results in damage to the lateral ligament complex of the ankle. Pain and swelling around the lateral malleolus is very common after inversion injury. Pain on the medial side of the ankle is less often present. In examining ankles after inversion injuries, particular attention must also be paid to lateral aspect of the foot. Sudden inversion can cause an avulsion fracture at the base of the fifth metatarsal due to contraction of the peroneus brevis tendon.

Much less commonly, external rotation forces can be directed at the ankle and result in fractures of both the medial malleolus and the proximal fibula. Therefore, it is important to remember that 'the ankle examination starts at the knee' and carefully palpate distally from there when examining ankle injuries.

The Ottawa Ankle Rules (Fig. 3) have been validated and shown to reduce the need for ankle X-rays without missing significant fractures.

Sprained ankles should be treated with restricted activity, ice, compression bandage, and elevation as a minimum. NSAIDs may be beneficial. Exercises and often referral to a physiotherapist are needed to maintain range of motion and strengthen the supporting muscles and tendons. Removable ankle braces that allow plantar and dorsiflexion but prevent inversion are useful acutely and serve as protection when the patient returns to sport. The use of plaster immobilization for sprained ankles should be discouraged.

Small avulsion fractures of the lateral malleolus represent ligamentous injuries and should be treated like sprains.

Isolated fractures of the lateral malleolus without significant pain around the medial malleolus are stable and can be treated in an 'air-inflated' ankle brace for 3–4 weeks. Isolated fractures with significant pain on the medial side are potentially more serious. Significant pain around the medial malleolus often represents at least a moderate injury to the deltoid ligament. Lateral malleolus fractures with a significant deltoid injury are potentially unstable and should be referred, immobilized, and followed by orthopaedic surgeons.

A fracture of both the medial malleolus and anywhere along the fibula (from fibular head to lateral malleolus) is unstable by definition and requires urgent orthopaedic referral for probable open reduction and internal fixation.

Fractures of the base of the fifth metatarsal must be differentiated from proximal shaft fractures of the same bone. Avulsion fractures of the base are due to inversion injuries, and occur proximal to the joint between the fourth and fifth metatarsal bases. They can be treated symptomatically with weight bearing as tolerated, analgesics and brief plaster immobilization if the pain is severe. Even if significant displacement is present, the vast majority of these fractures heal without problem. However, one type of fracture of the proximal shaft of the fifth metatarsal (distal to the intermetatarsal joint) is far more significant. The history is one of gradually increasing pain with athletic training. The result is a type of 'acute on chronic' stress fracture at the proximal shaft of the fifth metatarsal known as a Jones' fracture. This fracture is notoriously prone to non-union and requires urgent referral for either prolonged plaster immobilization (6–8 weeks) or primary open reduction and internal fixation.

Ruptured Achilles tendon

Acute tears of the Achilles tendon may be missed if not specifically sought. The history is usually a sudden snap at the back of the heel. Testing for resisted plantar flexion is *not* sufficient to rule out the diagnosis. Patients should lie prone (or kneel on a chair) with their feet over the edge. Palpate along the Achilles tendon feeling for a gap. Also, squeeze the mid-calf and note if the foot plantar flexes (Thompson's test). Failure of the foot to plantar flex suggests a tear of the Achilles tendon. Any suspicion of an Achilles tendon rupture requires prompt orthopaedic referral.

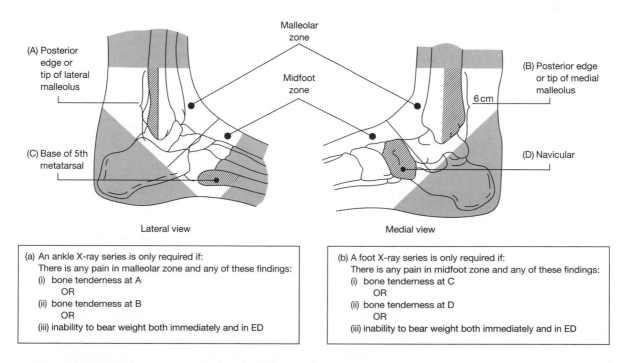

Fig. 3 The Ottawa Ankle Rules. Indications for X-rays in adults after acute ankle injury. (Reprinted with the permission of Dr Ian Stiell.)

Further reading

Andersen, K., Jensen, P.O., and Lauritzen, J. (1987). Treatment of clavicular fractures: figure-of-eight bandage versus a simple sling. *Acta Orthopaedica Scandinavica* **57**, 71–4.

Stiell, I. et al. (1997). Implementation of the Ottawa Knee Rule for the use of radiography in acute knee injuries. *Journal of the American Medical Association* **278**, 2075–9.

Stiell, I. et al. (1994). Implementation of the Ottawa Ankle Rules. *Journal of the American Medical Association* **271**, 827–32.

McRae, R. *Practical Fracture Treatment* 3rd edn. Edinburgh: Churchill Livingstone, 1994. (Concise, thorough, relatively inexpensive, excellent illustrations/X-rays; if a primary care physician wants one acute fracture textbook, this is the one.)

Tintinalli, J.E., Kelen, G.D., and Stapczynski, J.S., ed. *Emergency Medicine— A Comprehensive Study Guide* 5th edn., Chapters 259–63, 266–9. New York: McGraw-Hill, 2000. [Good acute orthopaedic sections; since it is an emergency text, limited in that deals mostly with initial (and not long-term) management.]

Rockwood, C.A., Green, D.P., Bucholz, R.W., and Heckman, J.D., ed. *Rockwood and Green's Fractures in Adults* 4th edn. Philadelphia PA: Lippincott-Raven, 1996. (Comprehensive orthopaedic reference textbook.)

Barkin, R.M. and Rosen, P., ed. *Emergency Pediatrics: A Guide to Ambulatory Care* 4th edn., Chapters 66–8. St Louis MO: Mosby-YearBook, 1994. (Practical for acute pediatric problems seen in a primary care office.)

14.3 Control of haemorrhage

Gary Ward

Introduction

Haemorrhage is defined as the loss of circulating blood volume from the cardiovascular system. This can lead to the physiological changes associated with shock, which is a clinical syndrome associated with inadequate tissue perfusion. The single most important aspect of managing this syndrome is its early recognition. Without such recognition, the victim develops progressive physical signs which, if not treated early, may become irreversible, leading to organ damage and eventually death. It is imperative that the clinician is able to recognize not only the clinical symptoms of shock but also be able to predict such clinical progression and to treat it appropriately and aggressively, thus reducing not only mortality but also morbidity. Whilst recognizing that haemorrhage is the principal cause of shock, the clinician must also be able to recognize other causes of this syndrome and to treat them appropriately.

This chapter is concerned with recognizing haemorrhage and shock and also with the initial measures which can be employed to support the patient until definitive care can be provided.

Pathophysiology of shock and haemorrhage

Loss of circulating blood volume leads to the clinical syndrome of shock, in which there is tissue hypoxia secondary to inadequate tissue perfusion. In the short term, this may produce reversible changes of extra and intracellular acidosis, but if the shock continues for a prolonged period of time, irreversible changes occur to intracellular structures which eventually lead to cellular dysfunction and death.

As inadequate tissue perfusion and hypoxia develop, cells convert from aerobic to anaerobic metabolism. The speed with which shock develops can have a profound effect upon the ability of tissues to survive this insult. If blood loss occurs over several hours then the tissues can undergo some degree of adaptation to the relative under-perfusion. However, if rapid loss of circulating blood volume occurs then the body has little time to adapt and the symptoms and signs of shock develop.

The susceptibility of different tissues to inadequate tissue perfusion is very variable. The brain is the most susceptible organ with a warm ischaemic time of only 3–5 min, compared with 20 min for renal tissue and several hours for skin. Some organs can still recover after such periods of ischaemia.

Types of shock

Haemorrhagic shock is only one form of shock which can affect the body. Any insult which results in inadequate tissue perfusion can lead to the clinical syndrome of shock. Shock can be divided into several different types. In absolute hypovolaemia there is a true reduction in the circulating whole blood volume. Haemorrhage, burns, and salt and water depletion can all lead to this process. Other conditions cause a relative hypovolaemia in which the normal circulating blood or plasma volume is present but the vascular bed through which it circulates has been increased, causing cardiovascular changes aimed at maintaining normal tissue perfusion. An example of this is anaphylaxis, where massive vasodilatation leads to a significant drop in blood pressure. Cardiogenic shock is due to an inadequate pumping ability of the heart. This can be primarily due to myocardial dysfunction occurring in the setting of ischaemia or an arrhythmia or secondarily due to medication, hypoxia or an acute rise in after load. Obstructive shock is due to a reduction in either venous return or outflow from the heart, such as in pulmonary embolism or cardiac tamponade.

Staging of hypovolaemic shock

Hypovolaemic shock can be divided into a series of simple stages or classes from I to IV (Table 1), although in reality the process of development of shock is a continuous process and the physiological parameters measured at any point in time represent only a snapshot of the processes which are occurring within the body. It should also be remembered that not all of these parameters need to be measured in order to determine that the patient is in shock. The individual response to hypovolaemia is highly variable and will depend upon factors such as age, degree of fitness, pre-morbid disease, and medication.

Table 1 Classification of hypovolaemic shock

	Class I	Class II	Class III	Class IV
Blood loss				
Percentage	<15	15–30	30–40	>40
Volume (ml)	750	750–1500	1500–2000	>2000
Blood pressure				
Systolic	Unchanged	Unchanged	Reduced	Very low
Diastolic	Unchanged	Raised	Reduced	Very low
Pulse pressure	Unchanged	Narrowed	Widened	Unrecordable
Pulse (beats/min)	Slight tachycardia	100–120	120–130	>130
Capillary refill	Normal	>2	>2	Undetectable
Respiratory rate	Normal	Normal	15–20	>20
Extremities	Normal	Pale and sweaty	Pale and sweaty	Pale and cold
Complexion	Normal	Pale	Pale	Ashen
Mental state	Alert	Anxious	Anxious and confused	Drowsy and confused
Urine flow rate (ml/h)	>30	20–30	10–20	0–10

The anatomy of haemorrhage

Haemorrhage can occur internally or externally. External haemorrhage is almost invariably traumatic, and major external haemorrhage is usually from the large vessels of the limbs. Spontaneous, and occasionally life-threatening, haemorrhage can be the result of relatively minor trauma to a varicose vein of the leg. Arterial blood is lost from a high pressure system and generally results in blood spurting from a wound; because arterial blood is oxygenated, it is usually bright red. Venous haemorrhage comes from a low pressure system; the blood is relatively unoxygenated and is dark red or purple in colour. Internal haemorrhage may be due to trauma or to disease processes affecting the vascular system (e.g. aortic aneurysm) or viscera (e.g. haemorrhage from oesophageal varices or peptic ulceration). If a major arterial vessel is breached, loss of circulating volume can be rapid and catastrophic. If, however, blood loss is due to blunt trauma to an internal organ, blood loss may be principally from the venous system and the development of shock can be slow and insidious. Because of the significant volumes present within the visceral cavities, large volumes of blood can be lost without any external evidence of blood loss, apart from changes in physiologic parameters. The notable exception is a penetrating wound to the pericardium which can result in the syndrome known as cardiac tamponade. Only small volumes of blood within the pericardial sac are required to produce this syndrome which may lead to a catastrophic loss of cardiac output, resulting in pulseless electrical activity (PEA) in which there is a normal electrical rhythm, but no associated cardiac output. This syndrome can be recognized by the findings of shock, raised jugular venous pressure, and muffled heart sounds.

While haemorrahge may result in easily detectable signs, such as abdominal distention with guarding and rebound, it is prudent to remember that massive collections of blood can collect in the retroperitoneal space with alteration of vital signs, but no signs of distention or peritoneal irritation. Exsanguinating haemorrhage can also accompany a major pelvic fracture, and even a fracture of the femur may result in losses of up to 1 l of blood (Fig. 1).

Management of haemorrhage

Patients with significant haemorrhage due to trauma are likely to require transfer to a facility where definitive treatment can be provided, but the primary care physician may be required to attempt to control haemorrhage at the scene of an accident. This must be undertaken with due regard to the general condition of the patient, and before approaching the patient the clinician should first ensure that it is safe to enter the area the patient is in.

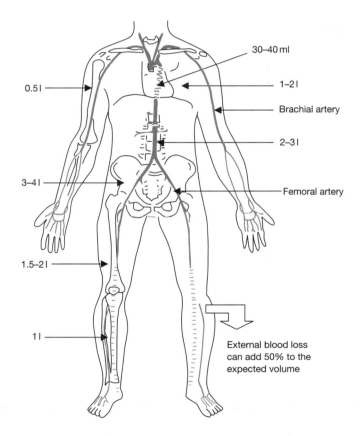

Fig. 1 Potential blood loss resulting from fractures and vascular injury.

Adequate control of the airway and breathing are essential in injured patients; the first action is to determine the patient's level of consciousness and the patency of the airway, together with an assessment of the possibility of spinal injury and the need for immobilization (Box 1). In the severely injured patient oxygen, if available, should be given. If necessary, help should be summoned at an early stage and, when these initial procedures have been performed, attention can be turned to the control of haemorrhage and the treatment of shock.

The patient should be carefully examined for signs of external haemorrhage and, if these are present, measures should be taken to control the

Box 1 Summary of actions

- Ensure safety, assess conscious level, airway, and cervical spine. Apply direct pressure to site of external haemorrhage, with limb elevation and tourniquet if required.
- Gain vascular access and provide fluid replacement.
- Check for limb ischaemia.

blood loss. Patients should be presumed shocked unless proven otherwise. The only necessary acute intervention is to apply direct pressure on the wound with a gloved hand. The use of tourniquets and/or attempts at clamping or ligating vessels at this stage are more likely to cause harm than result in benefit. Simple measures will control the majority of external haemorrhage, which is likely to be principally venous in origin. If this does not succeed and the haemorrhage is from a limb, the limb should be elevated and direct pressure applied. In the case of arterial haemorrhage, direct pressure should be applied to the major artery supplying the area from which the bleeding has occurred. If this is unsuccessful, a tourniquet may be required. A useful method of controlling haemorrhage is the application of a blood pressure cuff proximal to the bleeding point. This should be inflated above the systolic blood pressure to prevent further bleeding, whilst a firm dressing is applied. The cuff can be deflated to allow return of the blood supply to the affected limb.

If partial or complete amputation of a limb has occurred, the arterial vessels often contract due to spasm, markedly reducing initial blood loss. For this reason, dressings should be checked regularly, to ensure that further blood loss does not occur when spasm resolves. The blood supply to the remainder of the limb should be assessed to ensure that ischaemia either due to the vascular damage or a constriction device is not evident.

If there is no sign of external haemorrhage but the patient has signs of shock, it must be presumed that the source of bleeding is in one of the body cavities. There is little that can be done to control haemorrhage of this kind, and the patient requires urgent transfer to hospital.

Following these initial procedures to control haemorrhage, the next step is to gain venous access. This should be done using two large bore (ideally 16-guage) venous cannulae, if available, using the largest visible and accessible vein. The ante-cubital fossae are preferred, but if this is not possible other sites, such as neck, groin, or foot veins should be used. Intravenous fluid replacement should commence as soon as possible.

Summary

- Haemorrhage is only one cause of the clinical syndrome of shock.
- Early recognition of shock is the most important part of management.
- The clinician must never forget that assessment of the airway and breathing should come before the circulation.
- External haemorrhage can usually be controlled by simple manoeuvres.
- Internal haemorrhage is unlikely to be controlled in the out-of-hospital setting.

Further reading

Skinner, D., Swain, A., Peyton, R., and Robertson, C. *Cambridge Textbook of Accident and Emergency Medicine*, 116–39. Cambridge: Cambridge University Press, 1997.

Resuscitation Council (UK). *Advanced Life Support Course* 4th edn.

American College of Surgeons Committee on Trauma. *Advanced Trauma Life Support for Doctors* 6th edn., 1997.

14.4 Head and neck injuries

Matthew W. Cooke

Head and neck injuries are both extremely common. The primary care practitioner may encounter these when called to an incident or when they are the subject of an office visit. In the latter case they are usually not so severe, but it is still important to exclude serious injury. Any person with a significant head injury may also have a neck injury.

Acute head injury

Every year in the United Kingdom, 10–15 people in every 100 000 suffer a severe head injury, 15–20 people a moderate head injury, and 250–300 people suffer a mild head injury. One hundred and fifty thousand people will suffer a loss of consciousness of over 15 min. People aged 15–29 are the group most likely to suffer a head injury and males are five times more likely to sustain head injuries than females.

Approximately half of head injuries are caused by road accidents and these are often the more severe injuries. Cycling accounts for approximately 20 per cent of all head injuries in children, and an 85 per cent reduction in risk of head injury can be achieved by the use of cycle helmets. Domestic and industrial accidents account for 20–30 per cent, sports and recreational injuries for 10–15 per cent, and assaults for 10 per cent.

Management of the head injured patient who is not fully conscious

The seriously injured brain must be protected from the secondary injuries caused by hypoxia, hypercarbia, and poor perfusion. The assessment and treatment of these patients is undertaken in the order of potential threat to life.

Firstly, assess whether the scene is safe for you and the casualty. Do not move the casualty unless you or they are in danger.

Then follow the ABCD approach in assessing the casualty's urgent needs. *Airway* should be cleared whilst the neck is immobilized (see later). If oxygen is available this should be given as at high a concentration as available. The adequacy of *breathing* should be assessed; if ventilation is inadequate then it should be assisted with a bag-valve-mask device if available. *Circulation* should be assessed and external haemorrhage controlled using direct pressure. As long as the systolic blood pressure is over 90 mmHg, no immediate action is required. If the blood pressure is below this level, then an infusion of crystalloid fluids can be commenced and 2 litres given rapidly.

When this assessment and treatment has been undertaken, then D (for *disability* or neurological *disorder*) can be assessed. The most important aspect of this examination is the rapid assessment of the level of consciousness. The simplest assessment is the AVPU score determining whether the person is *a*lert, responding to *v*ocal stimuli, to *p*ainful stimuli, or is *u*nconscious. The pupils are also checked at this stage to determine if they are reacting to light and are equal in size. As time permits then a full assessment of the level of consciousness can be undertaken using the Glasgow Coma Scale (Table 1).

Any patient with a Glasgow Coma Score (GCS) of less than 15 should be assessed in hospital for their injuries. Coma is defined as a GCS of 8 or below; these patients are at severe risk because of the severity of injury but also because of the inability to control their own airway (see Chapter 11.7).

Management of the fully conscious head injury (GCS = 15)

Assessment of the fully conscious patient after head injury should include a history relating to the mechanism of injury, paying particular attention to the forces that may have been involved. Loss of consciousness and amnesia

Table 1 The Glasgow Coma Scale

Eye opening	
Spontaneously	4
To speech	3
To pain	2
No eye opening	1
Best motor response in upper limbs	
Obeys commands	6
Localizes to pain	5
Withdraws to pain	4
Abnormal flexion to pain	3
Extension to pain	2
No motor response	1
Best verbal response	
Normal speech	5
Confused	4
Inappropriate words	3
Inappropriate sounds	2
No verbal response	1

are common symptoms from head injuries. Other neurological symptoms should also be sought. Examination should include an assessment of the level of consciousness and examination of the eyes, including pupillary changes and fundoscopy. The cranial nerves and peripheral nervous system should be examined. Isolated neurological loss is uncommon but can be an important indicator of serious intracranial pathology.

A head-injured person should be referred to hospital if any of the following are present:

* Impaired level of consciousness at any time since the incident.

* Amnesia for the incident or subsequent events.

* Neurological symptoms, for example, severe persistent headaches, frequent nausea and vomiting, altered behaviour, and seizures.

* Clinical evidence of a skull fracture, such as a cerebrospinal fluid (CSF) leak from ears or nose, periorbital haematoma, boggy swelling on scalp.

* Co-existing major extracranial injury.

* High-risk mechanism of injury, for example, possible penetrating injury, high-energy incident (e.g. golf ball blow), potential non-accidental injury.

* High-risk co-morbidity, for example, anticoagulant treatment.

* Adverse social factors, for example, supervision inadequate for observation at home.

* Inability to accurately assess, for example, child, intoxicated.

Skull X-ray should be undertaken in a person with a history of loss of consciousness, amnesia, a scalp laceration/bruise/swelling of more than 5 cm or down to bone, persistent headache or vomiting, a violent mechanism or mechanism with high local energy (e.g. a golf ball blow) and associated severe maxillofacial injury. In a child, skull X-ray should also be undertaken if the child has fallen greater than twice its height, on to a hard surface or in suspected non-accidental injury.

If the X-ray is normal, those who have a GCS of less than 15, are difficult to assess (e.g. drunk, pre-existing neurological disorders), persisting neurological signs or symptoms (including headache and vomiting), bleeding diathesis, co-existing disease, or lack of appropriate supervision at home, should have a period of observation.

CT scan is the definitive investigation of acute head injury. Patients who have continuing coma after resuscitation, a fracture, or other abnormality on skull X-ray, deteriorating conscious level or developing neurological signs should have an urgent scan. Those who are observed should be scanned if they have continuing confusion, headache, or vomiting.

Indications for scanning are becoming wider as scanning facilities become more acessible and so it is important to know local protocols.

If there is no indication for X-ray, then the person can be given appropriate advice and discharged home, provided there is a responsible adult who can supervise them. The advice should include making medical contact if any of the following occur: worsening or persistent headaches, despite taking paracetamol, frequent vomiting, seizures, double vision, problems with balance, increasing drowsiness. The patient should also be advised to rest for 24 h and not to take alcohol, hypnotics, or tranquillizers.

It is important that relatives and employers are warned about the possible effects of a minor head injury, and for plans to be made accordingly. These might include not rushing to return to work, keeping stress to a minimum in the short term, and abstaining from alcohol. Studies have shown variable rates for return to work after minor head injury from less than half at 2 weeks[1] to 95 per cent by 3 months.[2] Difficulties are made worse if the person has a mentally demanding job where there is a narrow margin for error. The general conclusion is that the majority of people who experience a minor head injury make a full recovery, usually after 3–4 months. However, there is a very small sub-group whose recovery is incomplete.

Although rates and patterns of recovery may differ between individuals, many people experience headaches, dizziness, nausea, vomiting, confusion, disorientation, lethargy, impaired concentration, memory problems, intolerance to light and noise which can lead to anxiety and depression immediately after their injury. Usually, the events immediately before the incident, and those for some time afterwards, may not be remembered, even though the person may have been conscious for the majority of that time. All these symptoms are common after a minor head injury. Usually these symptoms of post concussion syndrome will gradually disappear, although the recovery period may vary from a few days to as long as a few months. If symptoms are severe or worsening then the patient should be referred for investigation, including CT scanning. Abnormalities are unusual if the person is fully conscious. However, previously unrecognized co-existing conditions may be detected. After exclusion of other pathologies, treatment consists of analgesics and antiemetics. More severe cases may require specialized care including cognitive rehabilitation, psychotherapy, stress management, vocational counselling, and pain management.[3]

Acute neck injury

Patients with an acute neck injury may present in the primary care physician's office or may be encountered when passing a road traffic incident. Accidents involving speeds of greater than 30 miles/h (48 km/h), a fall of greater than 10 ft (3 m), and significant injury above the clavicles should all act as warnings of potential cervical spine injuries. Horse riding and diving are particularly high-risk activities. As mentioned earlier, all patients with a head injury should be suspected of having an acute neck injury.

When approaching the person with a possible neck injury, it must be presumed that there is a serious injury until proved otherwise. The person should be told not to move their head. Calling to a person from the side will automatically get them to turn towards you, therefore try to approach from in front and give instructions not to move. As soon as possible try to immobilize the neck. This is most simply undertaken by holding the person's head just above the ears. If possible support your forearms on the person's chest or shoulders so as to brace the neck region. When an ambulance arrives, formal immobilization using a rigid collar, side supports, and tape can be used instead of the manual immobilization. Immobilization with a rigid collar only is inadequate.

If the mechanism of injury suggests the possibility of a cervical spine injury and there are no other life-threatening injuries, the neck can then be assessed in three stages. Firstly, by determining that the patient is fully conscious, not intoxicated and able to cooperate with a clinical examination. Secondly, there should be no central neck pain, bony cervical spine tenderness, or any peripheral sensory or motor neurological signs. Thirdly, the patient's ability to actively move the neck through a full range of pain-free movement is assessed.

If these criteria are not satisfied then further investigation to exclude spinal injury is required. Initially, plain radiography should be undertaken of the whole of the cervical spine ensuring that the films demonstrate the base of the skull through to the top of the first thoracic vertebra. Those with neurological loss that persists for more than a few minutes need to have a specialist assessment to determine if MR scanning is required. An ambulance should be requested and spinal immobilization continued until it can be replaced by a hard collar and full support. The person should not be moved from their location unless they are in imminent danger. If the patient is moved, spinal immobilization must be maintained.

A common pitfall is the older person who has fallen down stairs and complains of upper neck pain. This must be presumed to be an odontoid peg fracture until excluded by X-ray. Many such patients walk in to the surgery or hospital because they think it cannot be serious.

Acute neck sprain

Acute neck sprain is a common condition seen routinely in primary care and emergency departments. It is usually the result of injury. It appears to affect females more than males. It also affects adults more than children, which may be a reflection of the relative time spent in cars and of the protection provided to children by their head being against the seat and, often, being in a specific child seat with added protection to the head and neck. The incidence of acute neck sprain appears to be increasing. In America, there are over 1 million neck sprain injuries per year.

Mechanisms

This injury is traditionally said to involve damage to the ligaments, joint capsules, and muscles of the cervical spine without disruption of bone or neurological impairment. Recent research has shown that the explanation of the continuing symptoms may be related to causes other than the musculoskeletal structures of the neck, including subchondral fractures, facet joint disruption and the effects of the injuring force on other structures including the brain. Referred to as 'whiplash injury', it commonly occurs in motor vehicle accidents as a result of an acceleration–deceleration injury to the neck. The patient is often the driver or a front seat passenger in a car that has been struck from the rear, although other mechanisms are not uncommon. If a head restraint is improperly adjusted or absent, the neck may extend until the occiput impacts upon the posterior chest wall. However, neck sprain may result from other types of trauma.

Clinical picture

Resultant pain and disability may be immediate in the more severe injury and at this end of the spectrum radiographic examination is often required to exclude bony damage. More frequently, the patient will give a history of minimal symptoms during the first hour or two followed by a progressive increase in pain and limitation of movement and function over the next few hours. It is not uncommon for patients to present after the condition has worsened overnight and symptoms typically peak at 48 h. Three to five per cent of those exposed to a rear shunt road traffic incident will develop symptoms with 0–3 days. Eighty per cent of these patients have pain and/or stiffness of their neck. Pain is usually confined to the neck though may also be experienced over the occiput and between the scapulae. Extension into the latter two areas is associated with a worse prognosis with an increased likelihood of long-term neck problems. Limitation of movement varies considerably but may be so severe as to preclude normal daily activity for a prolonged period. Other associated symptoms include headaches, light-headedness, dizziness, impairment of concentration, psychological complaints, and vertigo. Some symptoms are related to injury to other structures, including cranial nerve injury, sympathetic chain injury, and brain stem dysfunction. Subjective parasthesiae in the upper limb in the presence of a normal neurological examination may have a similar aetiology but arouse suspicion of possible cord injury. Temporo-mandibular

dysfunction is associated with acute neck sprain and probably results from a co-existing acceleration–deceleration injury to the joint capsule and ligaments. Brain injury, with no other symptoms, may cause attention deficit, headaches and memory disturbance. Worsening of migraine is also documented to occur after neck injury. Symptoms of ophthalmic dysfunction are not uncommon. Dizziness is due to inner ear dysfunction related to the acceleration–deceleration forces.

Examination

Examination should take into account the patient's posture and range of neck movement. Gentle palpation often elicits greater tenderness over the musculature (resulting from spasm); midline tenderness should be regarded with suspicion, particularly if severe, although this may be due to posterior interspinous ligament damage. Marked midline tenderness or the presence of a palpable step mandates urgent referral (with cervical spine immobilization) to an emergency department for further investigation, likewise any clinical suspicion of neurological deficit. Any indication for X-ray (see earlier) is also an indication for spinal immobilization pending the investigation.

No cause and effect relationship has been established between the severity of the injury and the specific symptoms.

Management

The principle of management is to encourage an early return to normal movement and function. Reduction of pain and swelling are key to facilitating this process. A triad of analgesia, local heat, and gentle exercises forms the basis of treatment. Perhaps the most important investment by the physician is the time that it takes to explain the reason for the discomfort and loss of movement. A brief description of the downward spiral of pain and reflex spasm helps the patient to understand that in this instance the degree of pain does not equate to injury severity, and helps encourage early mobilization. The most important advice is that early movement can often prevent long-term problems.

Analgesia in the form of a non-steroidal anti-inflammatory analgesic is important. If this does not fully relieve the pain then paracetamol (acetaminophen) can be added to the regime. It is important for the person to realize that painkillers should be used early to enable mobilization. Ice can also be applied to the back of the neck for its analgesic and anti-inflammatory action. If pain is not relieved by these means then the use of a muscle relaxant, for a short period, may be advantageous.

Exercise (Box 1) should be started as early as possible. If exercises are not undertaken in the first 2 weeks, then they have been shown to have no

---

Box 1   A sample exercise regime

- Be sure you are sitting upright in a good position before commencing the exercises. Use smooth slow movements.

- Draw yourself up straight with your shoulders back, tuck in your chin to make a double chin, then relax.

- Turn your head round to look over right shoulder, hold your head in that position for a few seconds, now turn to the left and hold it there. Repeat this 10 times slowly.

- Looking straight ahead try to touch your ear down to your right shoulder, hold that position for a few seconds and repeat to the left; do this 10 times.

- Bend your head forwards and backwards slowly, stopping at the extremes each time, do this 10 times.

- Try and do these exercise every 2 h, until you can move your neck normally.

advantage. Exercises should be undertaken soon after ice and about 30 min after pain relief has been taken to maximize their benefit. One visit to a physiotherapist for full instruction on exercises has been shown to be advantageous.[4] Further physiotherapy should be given to those with severe symptoms, poor prognostic signs and those with pre-existing neck problems. Physiotherapy should be instituted early to prevent stiffness rather than waiting to refer only those who develop it. Pulsing electromagnetic field therapy gives good pain relief in the early stages. There is no evidence supporting the use of neck traction or other physical therapies.

Soft collars have been used commonly in the past. Evidence suggests that they are of no benefit and, because they prevent early movement, they may make stiffness worse, which will delay recovery. They do offer good pain relief in the early stages and it is therefore important to explain to the patient that the disadvantages of the collar outweigh the short-term pain relief. Use of a pillow or rolled-up towel to support the concavity of the neck at night and for short periods during the day will provide pain relief without the prolonged immobilization of a collar.

Advice on continuing care of the neck is important. This will help to speed up recovery and prevent future aching in the neck. Posture is important and the simple action of pulling the chin back and sitting up straight is often sufficient to improve posture. The patient should examine their work environment to ensure that their seat is correctly positioned and allows them to maintain a good posture throughout the day. Long periods leaning over a desk or staring at a computer screen will inevitably cause some neck stiffness. Advice should be given on moving the neck or changing activities every 20 min.

Follow-up

Finally, review is not always necessary but patients should be encouraged to return if they experience persistent or different symptoms. Referral for physiotherapy or for further investigation may be required. A lower threshold for referral should be adopted in the very young, the elderly and those difficult to assess.

Most people with an acute neck sprain will only have pain and stiffness for a few days. There is no good evidence that mild to moderate neck sprains lead directly to chronic neck problems. This is partly because both the injury and chronic neck pain are common conditions in the general population. Ten per cent of those with acute neck sprain will develop some chronic complaints that will impact on their level of functioning. Indicators for the development of a chronic problem are unclear but may include rapid onset of symptoms, intensity of the initial pain, pain between shoulder blades, reversal of the normal neck curvature, severity and duration of stiffness, and pre-existing neck symptoms or upper limb pain. However, some investigators have failed to identify any reliable prognostic factors. One study showed that long-term severe symptoms were unrelated to treatment.

There is no evidence that delayed symptoms are causally related to previous injury. They are more likely to be due to coincidental neck problems.

Conclusions

Head and neck problems can both present because of an acute injury or because of continuing problems. In the acute severe head injury, careful assessment is needed to determine who needs immediate first-aid measures followed by hospital treatment. In the less severe head injury, thorough assessment is needed to determine those who can be reassured and allowed home with appropriate supervision and advice. Patients should all be warned of the long-term effects of minor head injuries and encouraged to return if they persist. Patients with neck pain who do not require X-ray can be managed in primary care with careful explanation and encouragement to mobilize the neck. There is great debate over the role of neck injury in chronic neck symptoms, but early resolution of symptoms is the best way of reducing any risk of continuing symptoms.

Key points

1. Head injuries require careful assessment to select those requiring further investigation.

2. Head injuries not requiring investigation should be discharged to the care of a responsible adult with appropriate advice.

3. Any person with an acute neck injury should have the neck immobilized until injury can be excluded.

4. Soft tissue injuries of the neck need early mobilization, facilitated by pain relief and reassurance and not obstructed by the use of a soft collar.

References

1. Haboubi, N.H., Long, J., Koshy, M., and Ward, A.B. (2001). Short-term sequelae of minor head injury (6 years experience of minor head injury clinic). *Disability & Rehabilitation* 23 (14), 635–8.
2. Powell, T.J., Collin, C., and Sutton, K. (1996). A follow-up study of patients hospitalized after minor head injury. *Disability & Rehabilitation* 18 (5), 231–7.
3. Legome, E. Post concussive syndrome. eMedicine, http://www.emedicine.com/emerg/topic865.htm.
4. McKinney, L.A., Dornan, J.O., and Ryan, M. (1989). The role of physiotherapy in the management of acute neck sprains following road-traffic accidents. *Archives of Emergency Medicine* 6 (1), 27–33.

Further reading

American College of Surgeons Committee on Trauma. *Advanced Trauma Life Support Course for Physicians*. Philadelphia PA: American College of Surgeons, 1997.

The Society of British Neurological Surgeons (1998). Guidelines for the initial management of head injuries: recommendations from the Society of British Neurological Surgeons. *British Journal of Neurosurgery* 12 (4), 340–52.

Rø, M., Borchgrevink, G., Dæhli, B., Finset, A., Lilleås, F., Laake, K., Nyland, H., and Loeb, M. SMM-report 5/2000: Whiplash injury—diagnosis and evaluation. Health technology assessment and a systematic review. The Norwegian Centre for Health Technology Assessment (SMM), 2000.

On behalf of Joint Royal Colleges Ambulance Liaison Committee and Faculty of Pre-Hospital Care (1998). Position statement on spinal immobilisation. *Pre-hospital Immediate Care* 2, 169–72.

Johnson, G. (1996). Hyperextension soft tissue injuries of the cervical spine—a review. *Journal of Accident & Emergency Medicine* 13, 3–8.

14.5 Non-accidental injuries

Brian Schwartz and Roberta Schwartz

Introduction

Non-accidental injury is a term that encompasses all sorts of trauma resulting from levels of violence ranging from trivial to lethal. Injuries may be related to a single event or repeated trauma.

This chapter will address patterns of non-accidental injury seen most often in primary care, namely, presentations of physically abused individuals. The management of the multiple traumatized patient who presents to an emergency department is beyond the scope of this textbook. Moreover, the treatment of injuries that have occurred as a result of deliberate injury perpetrated by an individual unknown to the patient will not be addressed specifically here.

There are three distinct populations in which non-accidental injury is described: children, the elderly, and other adults. We shall arbitrarily define a child as a person age 16 or under and dependent on a parent or guardian, and an elder as a person 65 years or over and often dependent on a child or caregiver.

Physical abuse usually occurs in the context of at least one of other forms of abuse, including sexual, emotional, psychological, and financial abuse. The practitioner should recognize these components of power and control in the abusive relationship (see also Chapter 9.11).

Epidemiology

The prevalence of abuse in various communities has been estimated through public surveys to be relatively constant. For example, the proportion of women, who have ever been subjected to physical violence in various countries is as follows: United States 25 per cent, Canada 29 per cent, Australia 23 per cent, Finland 22 per cent, Chile 26 per cent, Korea 37 per cent, England and Wales 23 per cent, and Holland 20 per cent.[1] These estimates depend on the definition used (some cultures will not define some forms of physical violence as abusive) and the population studied. About one in seven women in a primary care setting admits to being abused in the past year.[2]

The prevalence of child abuse in communities may be related to economic and social conditions. In Canada, the estimated incidence of physical abuse of children is about 1200 cases per 1 million population per year. The prevalence of abuse in street youth and teenage runaways is much higher. Children witness over 70 per cent of abuse occurring in the home, with attendant morbidity.

Due to under-reporting, the prevalence of elder abuse is likely to be even higher than the 3.2 per cent figure quoted in one study.[3]

The natural history of the 'disease' of abuse is that of escalation, sometimes leading to mortality in the form of homicide or suicide. For example, between 30 and 40 per cent of female homicides are caused by an intimate male partner (compared to about 4 per cent of male homicides). Child abuse leading to death is less common, although more publicized in Western societies and under-reported in others. Deliberate injury to children and adults is condoned and even encouraged in many cultures.

Subsequent to identification of deliberate injury as the cause of the trauma, a victim may be further battered if interventions are not accomplished. Furthermore, an adult victim (usually female) who has left the home and/or relationship is at significantly higher risk of further injury or homicide if stalked by the perpetrator.

Presentations in primary care

Few data document the true frequency of abused individuals in primary care, due to the fact that only a small percentage of injured patients are appropriately identified as victims. Neither the patient nor the perpetrator will disclose the true cause of injury. The patient will not disclose due to her (95 per cent of adult abuse victims are females) fear of further harm. In the case of child abuse, the patient may be non-verbal and physically dependent on the abuser. In elder abuse, financial control is another element. Since abuse is common in immigrant populations, there may be language barriers to obtaining a true history of the events, and fear of deportation may inhibit disclosure.

Only about 10 per cent of abused victims are identified as such upon presentation. Moreover, non-accidental injury accounts for up to a third of all female trauma patients presenting to emergency departments.[2] The incidence of detection increases when universal screening questions are used.

Frequently, a victim is assaulted many times before presenting to a health care professional. Over 50 per cent of patients presenting to health care providers with non-accidental injuries have been assaulted more than 10 times by the same partner. Children or elders who are assaulted may not present for medical care due to their dependence on the perpetrator. A delayed presentation is often accompanied by a false history.

Causes

The underlying determinants of violence against children, partners, and elders are complex. Definitions include the components of *power* and *control* as aetiologic factors in the abusive relationship. The perpetrator uses deliberate injury, along with other forms of abuse such as name-calling, psychological harassment, and financial manipulation to exert control over the victim.

Co-morbid factors in physical abuse include drug or alcohol use, mental illness, a history of abusive or violent behaviour, and the witnessing of abuse as a child. There is no evidence supporting the notion that socio-economic status, religion, ethnicity, age, sexual orientation, or levels of education are determinants of physical abuse. Indeed, deliberate injury is found in all segments of society. However, the extent of reporting varies in many cultural groups because of the stigma and isolation resulting from disclosure.

How to make a diagnosis

The essential aspect of diagnosing non-accidental injury is to *recognize the presentations!* Injury patterns have been described, primarily by paediatricians, which may alert the practitioner to the fact that a patient's injuries were deliberately inflicted. There are two cardinal rules:

1. if the physical findings are not explained by the history, suspect abuse;

2. injuries at different stages of healing suggest repeated abuse (Table 1).

Table 1 Specific examples of injury patterns that are predictive of abuse

Childhood injuries	Adult (partner) injuries	Elderly injuries
Shaken baby syndrome	Facial and orbital injuries	Signs of being restrained (wrists, ankles)
Burns to hands, buttocks	Penetrating injury	Broken eyeglasses
Multiple unusual lesions	Upper arm injuries	Abdominal trauma
Multiple or unusual fractures (see Table 2)	Symmetrical injuries	Genital trauma/infection
Upper arm injuries	Abdominal/genital injuries	Fractured ribs

Table 2 Fractures in children that suggest abuse

Any fracture in a child less than 12 months
Multiple fractures
Fractures at different stages of healing
Spiral fractures of long bones (femur, humerus)
Metaphyseal fractures
Rib fractures (especially posterior)
Avulsion fractures of lateral clavicle or acromion

Table 1 outlines specific examples of injury patterns, which are highly predictive of abuse.

The *shaken baby syndrome* is a description of neurological injury caused by intracranial haemorrhage resulting from vigorous shaking or a rapid deceleration injury (hitting a wall or bed) of an infant by a parent or caregiver. The presentation is that of decreased mental status, behaviour change, or failure to thrive, without external evidence of injury. While retinal haemorrhages may be seen on fundoscopic examination, diagnosis is made with non-contrast computer axial tomography. It is useful to remember that significant head injuries and long bone fractures are *not* caused by falls from a bed or change table. Table 2 lists types of fractures in children that should lead the physician to consider non-accidental injury.

Children (and sometimes adults) may be subject to unusual forms of physical punishment, which include bites (multiple contusions in the shape and size of human dentition), cigarette burns (small punctate lesions), and oral lacerations from forced feeding.

Clinical examination and radiography may reveal multiple fractures at different stages of healing. This is almost always accompanied by a false history of a one-time event. Delays in presentation to health care professionals are common. A skeletal survey or bone scan may reveal unsuspected new or old fractures.

The most common injuries to non-elder adults are facial contusions and fractures.[4] For example, a blowout fracture to the orbit is caused by an object the size of a fist striking the face, not by a fall down a flight of stairs.

Female adults are particularly prone to victimization during pregnancy. Injury to the abdomen, thorax, and genitalia occurs with high frequency.

Upper arm injuries in children and adults are the result of grabbing and squeezing by the assailant, and findings are often symmetrical. Fending off of the attacker may cause fractures and contusions of the forearm.

The abused elder may present with injuries accompanied by signs of neglect in addition to the delays and inconsistencies described above. Changes in behaviour, altered mental status, and paranoid ideation may be indistinguishable from presentations due to other causes. In the case of abuse, the patient may be fearful of the caregiver and other clues such as the injuries noted in the chart should be sought.

Patients who suffer deliberately inflicted injury by a loved one may present as detached or evasive. Caregivers may appear indifferent, angry, or overly friendly.

If the practitioner suspects, even remotely, that an injury has been caused by a deliberate act, he/she must have a method that will establish a diagnosis, effectively treat the injuries and initiate secondary prevention. Prevention of further injury in the abusive relationship is the most important element in the reduction in morbidity and mortality from non-accidental injury. The 'ABCs' is a practical way to remember the following methodology (Box 1) in treating patients with injuries caused by physical abuse.

Asking and behaviour

First, the physician must *Ask* about deliberate injury. While this may seem intuitively obvious, there are issues surrounding this simple part of the

Box 1 The ABCs of non-accidental injury

- Asking
- Behaviour
- Clinical care
- Documentation
- Education
- Follow-up

history. What if the patient is non-verbal or demented? Are there dangers if the patient discloses? How do cultural, ethnic, and language differences affect the patient's response?

Asking requires that a patient who can verbally communicate be questioned alone and in confidence. The practitioner should explain that it is his or her practice that all patients must be interviewed alone. If the partner or caregiver is reluctant to leave the interview, the possibility of abuse is more likely.

The question should be direct, but formed in a way that is non-judgemental and non-threatening. For example: 'We know that your injuries can be caused by another person. Has this happened to you?'

In primary or emergency care, a number of short screening tools have been developed. Here is one example:

1. 'Have you ever been hit, kicked, punched or otherwise hurt by someone recently? (in the past year? ever?) If so, by whom?'
2. 'Do you feel safe in your current relationship?'
3. 'Is there a partner from a previous relationship who is making you feel unsafe now?'[5]

For patients who are not able to communicate, you must look for corroborating evidence of deliberate injury. Observe the patient's *behaviour*. If a child or elder is withdrawn, evasive, or does not interact normally with their parent or caregiver, this may be a clue to the possibility of deliberate injury. In the case of an abused adult, the patient may be withdrawn, with the partner providing the history. Observe the parent/caregiver's behaviour. It may be controlling over the patient, or overly solicitous to the health care staff. Historical details may be filled in even if the patient is capable of providing some description of the event. Recognize your own intuition: if the history and physical findings do not match, and the patient's behaviour is not appropriate for the presentation, suspect deliberate injury.

Principles of management—clinical care, documentation, and education

The keys to appropriate management are to provide appropriate *clinical care*, to ensure complete *documentation*, and provide *education* to the patient.

The practitioner must render clinical care after the diagnosis of non-accidental injury is made or suspected. If there is threat to life or limb, care must be given in the first instance appropriate to the circumstances. Airway management, oxygenation, and maintenance of perfusion are paramount. The patient with chest, abdominal, neurological, or orthopaedic injuries should be referred for surgical management. This does not preclude, however, communicating your suspicions to the attending surgeon to ensure follow-up. The victim of deliberate injury is not served well if discharged to the care of the perpetrator.

Documentation of all injuries and information surrounding the events is necessary for many reasons. First, it documents your clinical impression on the record for communication with consultants and other health care professionals. Second, it provides the best evidence for legal action against the assailant if and when it is needed. Third, it is an aid for you if you are called

Table 3 Normal ageing of bruises

Age (days)	0–2	2–5	5–7	7–10
Description	Purple, tender	Red/blue	Green/yellow	Yellow/brown

as a witness in any legal proceedings. In many countries, the legal process may drag on for years, and an accurate written description, accompanied by photos or sketches, will form the truest account of the events and findings at the time of injury.

When documenting the patient's history, use quotes if possible. Rather that write 'patient's husband pushed her down the stairs', or 'patient was pushed down the stairs', note that, 'patient states: "my husband pushed me down the stairs"'. This avoids any assumptions on the part of the physician, and accurately reflects the substance of the interview. Describe all injuries in detail, noting size and apparent age of bruises (see Table 3), deformities, and neurovascular status. Many physicians use body diagrams to depict areas of suspected fracture, contusion, and abrasion.

Patient education must be undertaken in the initial stages of treatment of non-accidental injury. Upon disclosure, the practitioner should assess the patient's risk of further injury by asking the following questions:

1. Has the perpetrator threatened to kill her or threatened suicide?

2. Has anyone else (children, relatives) been threatened with injury or death?

3. Is there access to weapons in the home, and has the perpetrator ever used them?

Establish a safety plan. For a child, the local child protection agency should be notified. Most democratic countries have a legal requirement to do so. For an adult, some societies have deemed it a legal obligation for a health care provider to report suspected abuse, but this is not universal. In urban areas, there are often shelters available for the victim, or she may be able to stay with friends or relatives for protection. Unfortunately, there are still many geographic areas (often rural) and cultures where a protected environment is impossible to find, or is unacceptable to the patient due to the risk of being found, the shame of leaving the home, or financial hardship. In such cases, a discussion about safety and referral for ongoing supportive individual counselling is indicated, if available. If admission to the hospital is not indicated for treatment of injuries, it may be indicated for protection of the patient, particularly in the abused elder.

It is essential during the education process to assure the patient that the abuse is not her fault, and *not* related to a problem in the marriage or relationship. The emotional and psychological control exhibited by the perpetrator includes the notion that the victim 'deserves' his or her punishment. In the case of children, many societies still condone forms of hitting or spanking, but demonstrable injury due to corporal punishment is never appropriate. Similarly, any injury inflicted on an adult by a partner, child, or caregiver is the result of psychopathology and control issues in the abuser. A failed or problem relationship is not the cause of physical violence, and marital therapy is not indicated until the abuse stops. Indeed, couple therapy may lead to exacerbation of abusive behaviour if it has not previously been identified and addressed. The practitioner should communicate these facts to the patient and appropriate protective and legal agencies notified when required.

Continuing care

Appropriate *follow-up* and referral are essential in the secondary prevention of injury and emotional/psychiatric sequelae from domestic violence. Abused children generally must be reported to and assessed by the local child protection agency. Physicians must be familiar with the legal requirements in their countries. Adults may be encouraged to report assault to the local law enforcement. Many jurisdictions have legal requirements to report injured adults. Moreover, some countries and states have educational secondary prevention programmes for perpetrators who have been identified and charged with assault. Therefore, if the victim chooses to leave, a safety plan backed up by law enforcement is recommended.

If the patient has chosen not to disclose, or upon disclosure has decided not to notify law enforcement (in jurisdictions where it is not mandatory), her autonomy must be respected. It is incumbent on the physician to understand that she may be willing to allow the situation to continue due to financial, emotional, or cultural factors. Furthermore, the risk of further harm is higher after the victim has left the assaulter's domain.

The follow-up and protection of abused elderly patients is most difficult as institutionalization and resources, which may be scarce, are often necessary.

While it is self-evident that the treatment of injuries requires appropriate medical or surgical referral and follow-up, the patient will also need psychological treatment and support. Post-traumatic stress disorder is a common component of traumatic injuries of any kind, in particular those suffered at the hand of a loved parent, partner, or child.

The most important and beneficial long-term strategy for morbidity reduction is primary prevention. So-called 'zero tolerance' of the infliction of physical injury as a disciplinary tool is essential in all societies, and physicians have a responsibility to speak out against violence. Public awareness programmes are crucial, as are educational programmes specific to those groups whose cultures condone physical punishment to family members. Prominent citizens, clergy, or other influential members of a society may be helpful in spreading the message of non-violence.

Implications of non-accidental injury

Non-accidental injury is a systemic public health problem, similar in scope and severity to smoking, substance abuse, and poverty as a social issue with profound medical consequences. In fact, many of these factors co-exist and may be causally related.

Children who are abused exhibit psycho-social behaviour problems, and later on are at increased risk of abusing their children. Children who witness assault at home are at risk of becoming victims or perpetrators in adulthood. It is unknown whether psychological interventions are effective in halting this generational cycle of domestic violence.

The post-traumatic stress disorder related to deliberate physical injury often leads to substance use and economic depravity. This has direct and indirect costs in terms of productivity, job loss, and morbidity/mortality in the form of self-harm and suicide. Without primary and secondary prevention the problem persists through generations and cultures.

Children and adults who are abused are at risk of presenting with other medical conditions. Patients with so-called functional abdominal pain, headache, or pelvic pain have an increased incidence of abuse in their background. Patients who present repeatedly with these complaints should arouse the practitioner's suspicion of pre-existing or ongoing abuse. When this suspicion is present, the question should be asked.

Pregnant women who are assaulted are at higher risk of complications of pregnancy and childbirth.

Primary care practitioners who care for assaulted individuals must work together with law enforcement, the legal system, and social agencies to reduce the incidence of non-accidental injury inflicted in the home.

While it is clear that mandatory reporting of child abuse results in improved outcomes, it remains controversial whether or not mandatory reporting of adult abuse to law enforcement reduces the incidence of further injury. Although initial studies from the United States indicated positive results, these have not been replicated. Long-term studies are required to clarify the role of mandatory reporting.

The economic implications of child and elder abuse relate to the costs of guardian care in hospitals, institutions or, in the case of children, foster care. Direct health care costs are related not only to the treatment of injuries, but also to the morbidity of the medical complaints, substance use, and psychiatric sequelae in these patients. Moreover, the costs to society in terms of job and productivity loss are enormous. A Dutch study reported that domestic violence cost the state more than 150 million Euros a year in health care and lost working time.[6] In the United States, the cost approaches $2 billion per year.

The key areas for primary care research include the extent to which early identification and intervention reduce morbidity and mortality, and what interventions are most effective in the prevention of non-accidental injury. The challenge for primary care practitioners is to work with social agencies, law enforcement, and cultural groups in their communities to implement identification and intervention schemes, which can be critically evaluated.

Key points

1. Suspect physical abuse when the history and physical do not match.

2. Look for injuries at different stages of healing.

3. Remember the ABCs:

   (i) Ask—alone if possible;

   (ii) Behaviour—the patient's and partner/caregiver's;

   (iii) Clinical care—treat injuries;

   (iv) Documentation—accurately and with quotes;

   (v) Education—safety plan and resources;

   (vi) Follow-up—referral to appropriate agencies, admission for treatment/protection.

4. Children require protection; competent adults require autonomy.

References

1. **Statistics Canada**. *Family Violence in Canada: A Statistical Profile*. Catalogue no. 85-24-XIE, Ottawa, 1999, p. 20.

2. **Eisenstat, S.A. and Bancroft, B.A.** (1999). Domestic violence. *New England Journal of Medicine* **341** (12), 886–92.

3. **Pillemer, K. and Finkelhor, D.** (1988). The prevalence of elder abuse: a random sample survey. *Gerontologist* **28**, 51–7.

4. **Muelleman, R.L., Lenaghan, P.A., and Pakieser, R.A.** (1996). Battered women: injury locations and types. *Annals of Emergency Medicine* **28** (5), 486–92.

5. **Feldhaus, K.M.** et al. (1997). Accuracy of 3 brief screening questions for detecting partner violence in the emergency department. *Journal of the American Medical Association* **277**, 1357–61.

6. **Diamantopoulou, A.** Violence against women: zero tolerance. Closing address of the International Conference, Lisbon, May 6, 2000.

Further reading

Reese, R.M., ed. *Child Abuse: Medical Diagnosis and Management*. Philadelphia PA: Lea and Febiger, 1994. (This book is an excellent reference on child abuse.)

Tintinalli, J., ed. *Emergency Medicine: A Comprehensive Study Guide* 5th edn. American College of Emergency Physicians. New York: McGraw Hill, 2000, pp. 1949–62. (The chapters on Child Abuse, Domestic Violence, and Elder Abuse are a concise review of the issues dealing with acute presentations of abused individuals.)

Jacobson, N. and Gottman, J. *When Men Batter Women; New Insights into Ending Abusive Relationships*. New York: Simon and Schuster, 1998. (This is for primary care practitioners who wish to delve into the dynamics of abusive relationships.)

Cramer, K.E. (1996). Orthopaedic aspects of child abuse. *Pediatric Clinics of North America* **43** (5), 1035–46. (An excellent review of injury patterns in child abuse.)

14.6 Burns

Gillian Smith and Keith P. Allison

Epidemiology

Burns are a common form of trauma worldwide. In 1991, the United States reported 5053 burn-related deaths, and 2 million patients seeking treatment for burns.[1] In the United Kingdom, burns account for approximately 250 000 injuries per year affecting 0.5 per cent of the population and leading to 175 000 accident and emergency attendances, 15 000 admissions to hospital, and 1000 deaths.[2]

Initial care for this huge group of patients tends to be provided by family, friends, ambulance personnel, voluntary organizations, and family medical practitioners. Rapid and professional initial assessment, appropriate first aid, treatment, and transfer of patients can profoundly influence subsequent management and outcome.

Burns can happen in isolation but care should be taken not to overlook other injuries. Most burns occur within the home, in the kitchen, or bathroom. There is a strong link with low socio-economic status, family tensions, overcrowding, and poor housing. The young, the elderly, and anyone without direct control of their environment (e.g. alcoholics, epileptics, multiple sclerosis patients, and diabetics) are particularly at risk. In the developing world, flame burns are more common, due to the use of open fires, kerosene lamps and poorly maintained heating devices, and the lack of legislation, which is key in accident prevention.

Accidents can occur, through carelessness or unsafe working practices, in those who use heat, chemicals, and electricity (e.g. the electroplating industry and use of acids). Burns are also sustained, mainly in young men, in conflicts, parasuicide, suicide, and homicide attempts. Increasingly, complex weaponry is leading to an increase in the incidence of burns. In World War II, burns comprised 1.5 per cent of British casualties, whilst in The Falkland Islands War, this rose to 14 per cent and in The Yom Kippur War, up to 70 per cent of tank battle casualties sustained burns.[3]

Aetiology

Burns may be classified in several ways. Describing a burn by the causative agent is found by some authors to provide more useful information, which determines the need for additional care or surgery.

Classification of burns

Burns are traditionally classified as being either superficial, partial thickness, or full thickness. Superficial (first degree) burns involve injury to the outer epidermal layer of the skin, and are characterized by red, inflamed, painful skin, usually without blister formation. Partial thickness (second degree) burns involve injury deeper into the skin, involving both epidermis and dermis, and are characterized by blister formation and are usually painful. In full thickness (third degree) burns, the full depth of the skin may be damaged, producing a charred or leathery appearance. There is no blood flow in the area and therefore no capillary refilling. The burn is insensate due to destruction of nerve endings. Patients with full thickness burns may have areas of superficial burns at the edges, and may still have severe pain.

A more meaningful approach is to classify burns according to the causative agent, as follows:

1. Flame burns, which occur when the patient or their clothing has caught fire. These are usually full thickness injuries.

2. Scalds, due to immersion, spill, or hot fluids. These are often from hot drinks or baths, producing mixed depth injuries with deeper elements underlying the initial point of contact. Hot fat or cooking oils tend to

produce deeper burns as the temperature and heat retention of oil are greater than those of water.

3. Electrical burns:

(i) Low voltage (<1000 V) injuries tend to produce small, full thickness burns at the point of contact. The skin injury may require minimal care but there is a risk of cardiac injury and patients should be transferred to hospital for examination, including an electrocardiograph (ECG). ECG changes, related symptoms, or persistent tachycardia are indications for hospital admission for observation.

(ii) High voltage (>1000 V) injuries are often extensive, involving widespread tissue damage which may not be apparent on initial assessment. Muscle damage can release myoglobin, which can lead to renal failure. There is also a risk of cardiac arrhythmia or arrest due to myocardial damage. The morbidity and mortality of this kind of injury is very high.

(iii) Lightning strike (massive DC shock) may produce cardiac arrest, but prolonged resuscitation may also be successful. Associated fractures and dislocations are likely.

4. Chemical burns are usually due to acids, alkalis, petrol, and other industrial compounds. They occur most often in the workplace. Their severity depends on the concentration of the causative agent and the duration and area of contact. The mainstay of treatment is irrigation with water or saline. Neutralizing agents should generally be avoided, as a local chemical reaction can be generated which itself produces further heat.

5. Radiation burns, generally sunburn and flash burns, occur when the patient or the clothing has not caught fire. The severity of injury depends on the intensity of the heat, the distance from the source of heat and the duration of exposure.

Differential diagnoses

Burns need to be distinguished from cold injury, including frostnip and frostbite, and also from toxic epidermal necrolysis, also known as scalded skin syndrome, a condition in which desquamation occurs, resembling a superficial burn. Causes of toxic epidermal necrolysis include drug reactions, cutaneous staphyloccocal infection, and graft-versus-host disease.

Diagnosis

History

It is always important to find out as much information about the patient, the event and the source of injury as possible.

- When, where, and how did the burn occur? Was the patient in an enclosed space (increased chances of an inhalational injury)? What temperatures were involved (e.g. tea, baths, and molten metals)? Is any information available about chemicals or antidotes?

- What was the patient wearing?

- Has any first aid been administered already?

- Has the patient had to jump or fall from a window to escape the fire? Consider other injuries.

- What was the pre-morbid condition of the patient?

Special considerations

Airway

The principal initial threat to life following a burn is damage to the upper airway. Oedema caused by direct thermal damage can develop rapidly. Signs of burnt hair or soot in the nostrils or mouth or facial and neck involvement

of any type must alert the rescuer or casualty staff to the possibility of early airway obstruction. Occasionally, a patient may need elective endotracheal intubation; if this is delayed, a surgical airway may well need to be created, and this procedure can be difficult because of soft tissue swelling.

Cervical spine immobilization may be required when there is co-existent trauma or when the circumstances surrounding the event are unclear.

Respiration

Burns sustained within an enclosed environment carry a risk of smoke or chemical inhalation injury. This is the commonest cause of death in house fires. Key signs, which must not be missed, are increased respiratory rate, hoarseness, wheeze, stridor, carbonaceous sputum, intercostal muscle recession, and use of accessory muscles of respiration. All patients with suspected airway or chest injury must receive 100 per cent oxygen.

The upper airway filters heat well, so thermal damage to the lower airways is unusual. Superheated steam may, however, reach as far as the alveoli. The constituents of smoke are varied and depend on the materials burning and the temperatures reached (polyvinyl chloride can yield 75 different products including hydrochloric acid, phosgene, and cyanide). These create local tissue reaction and damage in the airways and lung parenchyma. Smoke inhalation is the commonest cause of death in the first hour after burns.

Inhaled carbon monoxide binds preferentially to haemoglobin leading to hypoxia. Patients experience headache, nausea, and an altered level of consciousness. Pulse oximetry can be misleading, because the oximeter cannot differentiate between carboxyhaemoglobin and oxyhaemoglobin. The patient may be hypoxaemic despite an apparently satisfactory pulse oximetry reading.

The signs and symptoms of inhalational injury may not be immediately apparent, particularly if there is no upper airway damage. Symptoms may develop up to 48 h following the fire.

Burn severity

Burn severity has tended to involve assessment of total body surface area (TBSA) of burn and depth of injury, although assessment is often inaccurate and has a limited bearing on initial management of the patient.

Aides memoire for calculation of burn size include Wallace's rule of nines (which is not applicable to children under the age of 14 years), use of patient's hand (= 1 per cent TBSA) and Lund and Browder pictorial charts.

A simpler and more rapid method of assessment to convey the size of injury is to calculate if half of the patient's body is burnt. If it is not, then is the area burnt less than or more than half of this, and so on (100→50→25→12.5 per cent, etc.).

Escharotomy

Full thickness, circumferential burns of the chest or limbs can cause respiratory embarrassment and compartment syndromes, respectively. In children, who rely on abdominal respiration, full thickness burns of the abdomen can cause respiratory compromise. The effect of the burnt tissue is to produce constriction as burn oedema develops. This tourniquet effect may be released by means of longitudinal incisions through the burnt tissue along the full extent of the burn. When incised, the wounds gape allowing restoration of movement and circulation. This procedure requires hygiene, coagulation diathermy, and frequently, blood transfusion.

Non-accidental injury

A high index of suspicion for the possibility of non-accidental injury should be present in burnt children and in the elderly. The pre-hospital care of the burn remains unchanged but the initial history and examination are very important, as the involvement of other health care agencies may be required. Hospital referral to a specialist should be considered. Meticulous records must be kept and clothing should be brought in with the patient.

Burns in children

Most burns occur in children between 18 months and 3 years of age. In developed countries, the majority are scalds. Non-accidental injury should always be considered. The mortality rate in children is lower than in adults but there are specific differences in the pathophysiology:

- The head takes up a greater proportion of the surface area.
- Smaller airways mean that airway problems may develop with less swelling.
- The larger surface area to volume ratio makes them prone to hypothermia.
- Venous access may be challenging and intraosseous infusion should be considered.
- Children compensate well for hypovolaemia and signs are subtle until advanced. A urine output of 1–2 ml/kg/h should be the minimum acceptable. Fluid overload can lead to hyponatraemia and cerebral oedema.
- Young children are prone to hypoglycaemia, due to their lack of glycogen stores.
- Toxic shock syndrome occurs mainly in toddlers with small burns.
- Long-term problems include growth inhibition for several years after the burn, with no compensatory catch-up phase, limitation in respiratory reserve after inhalational injury, joint contractures, and impaired breast development.

Primary care management of patients with burn injury

Always use a SAFE approach

- Shout/call for help;
- Assess the scene;
- Free from danger—remove the casualty from danger and avoid danger yourself;
- Evaluate the casualty.

Stop the burning process and remove the burning source

- Remove all burnt/burning clothing (unless adherent to the patient), and jewellery, and bring bagged clothing to hospital for examination.
- Chemical burns require a prolonged period of irrigation. Specific information for dealing with the chemical concerned should be obtained and brought with the patient to hospital. The burn should be irrigated thoroughly until pain or burning has subsided. Clingfilm covering is likely to worsen the effects of chemical burns, and wet dressings are preferred. Powder injuries may be worsened by contact with water, so that powder should be brushed off before irrigation.

Actively cool

Actively cool the burn wound for 10 min (in developed countries where ambulance services have a priority dispatch system, the dispatcher gives this information prior to staff arrival).

- Water should not be ice cold.
- Be aware of the risk of hypothermia, especially in children.
- Cool pads should not be applied to large trunk burns in children.

Cover

Cover the burnt area, if possible using a cellophane or plastic film such as clingfilm or cleanfilm.

- Be aware of constricting effect of wrapping!

- Keep the patient warm (wrap the patient up in blankets or duvet).
- For small burns, continue to cool the burn for analgesia, using a wet towel on top of the clingfilm.
- Be mindful of iatrogenic hypothermia.
- There are numerous dressings available for pre-hospital burn care. Clingfilm fulfils all criteria for a wound covering as it is cheap, clean, conforms and seals in nerve endings, is easily stored and one size suits all.
- Clingfilm may theoretically worsen the effect of a chemical burn and so wet dressings only should be used in these instances.
- Water-jel™ type products have their merits for small area burns, facial burns, or in environments where water for cooling is not readily available.

Assessment of airway with cervical spine stabilization, breathing, circulation

Oxygen, when required, should be given at a high flow rate via a non-rebreathing mask. Oxygen is not required if the burnt area is small and there is no suspected inhalation injury.

Assessment of burn severity

- In order to estimate the size of burned area, use the half burnt/half not approach (serial halves: 100→50→25→12.5 per cent).
- Do not use rule of nines in children but remember other aides memoire.
- Mechanism of injury—the type of burn is very important (flame, scald, electrical, chemical, cold), as is the duration of injury.

Vascular access

- Attempt cannulation for burns greater than 25 per cent TBSA.
- Start fluid replacement once cannulated.
- Cannulation may also be required to allow administration of analgesia.
- Limit the number of attempts to two.
- Cannulation through burnt skin is not ideal but is acceptable. Consider the intraosseus route in young children.
- Do not allow cannulation procedures to unnecessarily extend the on-scene time.
- Fluid replacement must be started if time to hospital is more than 1 h from time of injury (1000 ml for adult, 500 ml for child 10–15 years, 250 ml for 5–10 years, no fluids for under 5 s).
- Where transfer time is prolonged, burn size assessment must be more accurate and fluid replacement for resuscitation should be guided by the Parkland formula, giving 4 ml/kg per per cent burn with half of this volume given in the first 8 h after the burn.
- Crystalloid (normal saline or Ringers lactate) is the fluid of choice.
- Intravenous fluid should be warmed.

Analgesia

- Use intravenous opiate titrated to effect. In adults, include an antiemetic.
- Other options for analgesic which may be considered in children include intranasal diamorphine and nasal fentanyl.

Transport

- Information back to the emergency department/base hospital should be provided, regarding the age, gender, details of the incident, resuscitation problems, relevant treatment given, and the estimated time of arrival.

◆ Alert the emergency department/base hospital for:

 ■ more than 25 per cent (1/4) total body surface area burn;

 ■ airway concern (singed nasal hair, peri-oral charcoal);

 ■ high voltage (>1000 V) electrocution;

 ■ carbon monoxide poisoning (confined space);

 ■ associated serious injuries (e.g. decreased level of consciousness).

◆ All treatment should be carried out with the aim of reducing on-scene times and delivering the patient to the appropriate treatment centre.

◆ Initial transport should be to the nearest appropriate emergency department or base hospital, unless local protocols allow direct transfer to a burns facility. The patient should be transferred to a specialist burns care unit, when required, as soon as possible, ideally within 4 h of injury.

Specialist referral

Criteria for burns unit referral vary in different countries, and may relate to the facilities available. If in doubt, discussion with a specialist unit is advisable.

In general, the following should be referred:

◆ burns requiring fluid resuscitation (adult >15 per cent, child >10 per cent TBSA);

◆ full thickness burns;

◆ electrical burns;

◆ chemical burns;

◆ non-accidental injury;

◆ burns with other associated trauma;

◆ respiratory burns;

◆ burns in patients with complex medical problems;

◆ burns affecting specialized areas such as the hands, genitals, and face.

Multiple casualties

If multiple casualties are present, some or all who have burns, it may be necessary to invoke a local disaster plan. A triage system, in which agreed criteria determine treatment priorities, is likely to be used.

Long-term care

Facilities available for burns rehabilitation show even greater disparity between countries than those for treatment. In the United States, there is a move towards ambulatory service and home care, in addition to greater use of burns rehabilitation centres. Regular integrated physiotherapy and occupational therapy are essential. Burns camps, to improve self-esteem and teach coping strategies, are becoming popular although there is not yet any objective evidence of their benefit.

Scar management

Burns taking longer than 2 weeks to heal have a high risk of forming hypertrophic scars, especially if they span a flexor surface. Scar management techniques include time-consuming regular washing and moisturizing of all scars, use of silicone gels and custom-made pressure garments. Itching may remain a problem despite antihistamines and regular moisturizing. Scars require protection from the sun with a high factor suncream. Patients' self-consciousness is related not to the severity of scarring, but to their own perception of it. Some may request cosmetic camouflage. Others require scar revision surgery for either functional or aesthetic reasons.

Scar revision

Scar revision, ideally after a minimum interval of 12 months, may include one or a combination of the following: excisional techniques, dermabrasion, z-plasties, laser resurfacing, split skin grafting, tissue expansion techniques, the application of cultured keratinocytes, artificial dermal substitutes, or local/distant flap reconstruction. Scar contracture over flexor surfaces is a frequent problem, but the techniques of tissue expansion, microsurgical free tissue transfer and artificial dermal substitutes may provide the capability to reconstitute these areas with good quality tissue. Children, in particular, may expect a series of scar revisions for contracture as they grow. Joints require regular passive and active stretching exercises and are at risk of heterotopic ossification.

Implications

Psychological implications

Psycho-social support is essential in all major burns, facial burns, and a surprising number of small burns. Family relationships can be strained with the hospitalization of one of the family members. Inability to work, undertake child care, or perform other roles can have a significant effect. The prevalence of post-traumatic stress disorder varies in studies from 8 to 45 per cent. There is a higher risk in those with pre-burn affective disorder, delerium, or severe pain during treatment and less social support. Counselling and marital therapy may be required. Patient support groups can be helpful as self-consciousness, poor self-esteem, and anxiety are common.

Health economic implications

Return to previous employment will depend on the individual's degree of physical and psychological disability. The patient's disability may have implications for family health or in extreme situations their survival. The length of time off work, burn size, and pre-injury employment are all predictors of eventual return to work. The patient is likely to need re-training, encouragement, and support provided by an integrated team to embark on a new career. Regular hospital attendance has economic implications for obtaining and retaining employment.

Uncertainty and controversy

The long-standing controversy on the use of colloid or crystalloid for resuscitation fluid was complicated by a heavily criticized metanalysis in 1998 from the Cochrane injuries group, which suggested a higher rate of death in the albumin-treated group.[4]

Growth hormone given to burns patients may reduce their weight loss, improve their wound healing, and shorten hospital stay.

Increasing survival of patients with large body surface area burns due to technical advances in care is placing an increased emphasis on rehabilitation, outreach, and funding for this kind of care.

Prevention

The consequences of burn injuries can be devastating and far-reaching. Recognition of the causative factors involved in burns and subsequent data collection, will provide the evidence to produce legislation and help prevent particular types of incident, particularly those involving domestic furniture and clothing. Continuing public education, including the encouragement of the use of smoke detectors, is of great importance in preventing burn injuries.

Key points

- Burn injuries are common and may be associated with other traumatic injuries.

- The initial care of any burn injury involves basic first aid, dressing, analgesia, and transport to a secondary care facility.

- Primary care includes family care, child protection, psychological welfare, and long-term rehabilitation.

References

1. Kao, C.C. and Garner, W.L. (2000). Acute burns. *Plastic and Reconstructive Surgery* **101** (7), 2482–92.

2. National Burn Care Review Committee Report. *Standards and Strategy for Burn Care; A Review of Burn Care in the British Isles.* http://www.baps.co.uk/documents/nbcr.pdf.

3. Sparkes, B.G. (1997). Treating mass burns in warfare, disaster or terrorist strikes. *Burns* **23** (3), 238–47.

4. Cochrane Injuries Group Albumin Reviewers (1998). Human albumin administration in critically ill patients: a systematic review of randomised control trials. *British Medical Journal* **317**, 235–40.

Further reading

Cole, R.P. (1999). The UK albumin debate. *Burns* **25**, 565–8. (Critical review of Cochrane Injuries Group metanalysis.)

Settle, J.A.D., ed. *Principles and Practice of Burns Management.* London: Churchill Livingstone, 1996. (Definitive textbook on UK burn care.)

Herndon, D., ed. *Total Burn Care.* Saunders, 1996. (Definitive textbook on US burn care.)

American Burn Association, http://www.ameriburn.org.

International Society for Burn Injuries, http://www.worldburn.org. (Updated website on international burns care.)

Burn Survivor Resource Centre, http://www.burnsurvivor.com. (Medical and legal links with discussion forum for burns victims.)

14.7 Poisoning

John Henry

Epidemiology

Acute and chronic poisoning by drugs, chemicals, traditional remedies, plants, and animal venoms is a world-wide problem, numerically greater in developing countries where there is low awareness of the hazards, more toxic plants and venomous snakes, and little control of industrial use. The family physician or general practitioner may be confronted by isolated cases of exposure in patients of any age, ranging from neonates to the elderly. However, there are two main age peaks in the incidence of poisoning, due to accidental ingestion by small children and suicidal gestures in younger adults. Poisoning can also affect all the members of a household, workplace, or community due to multiple exposures from a common source. This may be by ingestion from contaminated food or water supply, or by inhalation of toxic gases or sprays.

Poisoning in primary care

Although poisoning is one of the less common problems occurring in primary care, it is the primary care practitioner who is the first person to see and diagnose the patient in most cases of poisoning. The practitioner may need to intervene urgently to save life, or may have to act as triage point, diagnostician, detective, or counsellor. A common-sense approach is therefore needed, and the poisonings that are most likely to occur in the locality need to be well known. Very little extra equipment is required, though a small number of antidotes should be included in the doctor's bag. Information on the toxicity of a drug, chemical substance, animal or plant, together with advice on management, is now readily available from poison centres in most countries.

Possible causes

The most fundamental cause of poisoning is the underlying reason behind the poisoning rather than the substance taken. Accidental poisoning is the term given to childhood exposure, because although the child has initiated the action through natural exploratory curiosity, it lacked knowledge about the consequences. This type of poisoning occurs from the ages of 6 months to 5 years with a peak at 18 months to 2 years. Frequently, this type of ingestion is of minimal toxicity, but the incident gives rise to great concern by the parents. The other types of poisoning which may occur in small children are iatrogenic and non-accidental. Iatrogenic poisoning occurs especially in premature infants and neonates, where a small error in dose can cause life-threatening toxicity (especially with drugs such as chloramphenicol, theophylline, and digoxin). Non-accidental poisoning may range from a carer's attempt to sedate a child in order to quieten it to Munchhausen's syndrome by proxy. These are summarized in Table 1.

In teenage children, deliberate self-harm and substance misuse are the commonest causes of poisoning. In early adult life, deliberate self-harm in the form of parasuicidal gestures is common, while all through adult life poisoning can occur in industrial settings. Serious suicidal attempts become more common and are more likely to be successful especially in males over the age of 45 years. There may be underlying factors such as mental or physical illness, alcohol or substance misuse, unemployment, and marital separation.

Diagnosis of poisoning

In every case, the history should include an assessment of the patient, the toxin involved, the route of exposure, and the aetiology (Table 2). Physical assessment of the patient should document vital signs, level of consciousness, pupil size, and any other abnormalities found so that deterioration or recovery can be objectively measured.

The diagnosis of poisoning is most often apparent from the history and circumstances, but the physician may need to suspect poisoning when the patient presents with unexplained symptoms or collapse or coma without any apparent cause. Intentional poisoning of a child or an adult by another person may present with a misleading history and clinical findings which do not fit with a medical illness. Suspicion of poisoning and further advice

Table 1 Causes of childhood poisoning and the ages at which they commonly occur

Iatrogenic (neonate to 6 months)
Accidental (6 months to 5 years, peak age 18 months)
Non-accidental (up to 2 years)
Substance abuse (over 10 years)
Deliberate self-harm (usually over 12 years)

Table 2 Key features of the clinical history and examination in poisoning

Patient: vital signs, age, weight, medical conditions, current medications
Poison(s): number, identity, quantity, toxicity, manufacturer
History: time of exposure, symptoms, time of exposure, first aid given
Route of exposure: ingestion, injection, inhalation, eye/skin exposure
Aetiology: accidental, suicidal, intentional

Table 3 Plan of action in acute poisoning

Ensure your own safety
Stabilization of patient: ABC—CPR
Assess severity
Take as full a history as possible from patient, relatives, and bystanders
Perform a brief clinical examination
Decide management strategy
Consider measures to reduce absorption: activated charcoal
Consider specific antidotes, e.g. naloxone, atropine
Psychiatric assessment; follow-up

is required in these rare cases. The patient who claims he has been poisoned must be listened to carefully to decide whether the suspicions are justified and the symptoms are consistent with poisoning. A minority of these have actually been poisoned, while most are suffering from a paranoid delusion of poisoning. In these cases, the alleged source of the poisoning is vague and the symptoms are ill-defined.

It is common practice to measure salicylate and paracetamol (acetaminophen) levels when it is known or suspected that these drugs have been ingested. It is especially important with paracetamol (acetaminophen) since there may be no symptoms even in a potentially fatal overdose.

Principles of management

The first step in management (after ensuring that there is no danger to oneself, especially from fumes or smoke in cases of poisoning by inhalation) is to decide whether the poisoning presents an immediate threat to life, and whether an urgent intervention such as cardiopulmonary resuscitation is required (Table 3). In extreme cases, external chest compression and mouth-to-mouth resuscitation may be needed. This is not contra-indicated by infections such as AIDS or hepatitis C, and exhaled poisons such as cyanide or carbon monoxide are not poisonous to the medical attendant even if giving mouth-to-mouth resuscitation. The most dangerous circumstance is the risk of swallowing regurgitated poison such as cyanide or organophosphates. It is always preferable to use a non-return airway. When cardiopulmonary resuscitation is required, it should be continued for as long as the patient's condition requires it, or until further help becomes available.

When the eyes and/or skin have been contaminated by corrosives or pesticides, the eyes must be attended to first and washed out continuously with clean water for 20–30 min. The skin should be washed vigorously with water, paying particular attention to thinner areas of the skin (axillae, groins, and face).

Ingested corrosives, acids, or alkalis should be treated by immediately giving the patient a few cups of water to drink in order to dilute and so prevent damage to the tissues. However, after 10–20 min this action may well be too late and the patient may be unable to swallow, with saliva evident in the mouth.

In the case of ingested solid or liquid poisons, the question arises as to whether the gut should be decontaminated. Although mothers may make their child vomit by tickling the back of its throat, there is no evidence that inducing emesis by tickling the throat or giving syrup of ipecacuanha has any effect on the course of the poisoning. Emptying the stomach by gastric lavage rarely has a place in the hospital setting, but has no place in primary care; the practice has now been abandoned in North America. If the ingestion was less than 1 h ago, activated charcoal may be given as a suspension in water. This is specially prepared charcoal with a large surface area giving it a high adsorbent capacity, which adsorbs most drugs and poisons in a ratio of about one part poison to 10 parts charcoal. The dose is 25–50 g for an adult and 1 g/kg body weight in a child. Exceptions include iron, lithium, alcohol, methanol, ethylene glycol, corrosives, acids and alkalis, and where oral antidotes or medication need to be given. One other method of decontaminating the intestine is by whole bowel lavage. This involves giving isotonic fluid, using solutions normally used for preparation of the bowel for X-ray procedures. The adult dose is 500 ml to 2 l per hour, given until the effluent is clear. It can be used to clear the gut of sustained release preparations, iron, lithium, heavy metals, and illicit drug packets.

Substances involved in poisoning

Alcohol

Alcoholic drinks cause the typical signs of intoxication (slurred speech, ataxia, confusion, and aggression). Larger amounts can cause vomiting, coma, and hypoventilation, with the risk of aspiration of vomit. If the patient is unconscious, management is as for the comatose patient. Remember that a single bottle of spirits could be fatal for a non-drinker. However, provided the airway is protected, the patient will usually metabolize the alcohol and recover. Activated charcoal has no place in management.

Paracetamol (acetaminophen)

Paracetamol (acetaminophen) is the most widely available analgesic worldwide, and is safe in therapeutic use, but overdose of over 300 mg/kg can cause liver failure and sometimes kidney failure. It is important to note that during the first 48 hours the patient remains conscious and there may be few or no initial symptoms apart from malaise, nausea, and vomiting. Treatment is usually given if the patient has taken more than 150 mg/kg. Fatal liver damage can be prevented by giving an antidote (e.g. N-acetylcysteine) within 10–12 h of ingestion, so that every case needs to be carefully assessed and where possible referred urgently to hospital for measurement of blood levels and treatment. Some patients are at increased risk of liver damage; those taking enzyme inducing agents (e.g. phenytoin, rifampicin, heavy alcohol users); and those who are malnourished or who have been fasting recently.

If the patient presents within 1 h of ingesting a potentially toxic amount, give activated charcoal (Table 4) and arrange hospital transfer. If this is impossible or the patient refuses transfer, methionine or acetylcysteine or any protein-containing food can be given, as these will help to protect the liver from damage.

Salicylates

Common features of acute toxicity from aspirin and other salicylates include vomiting, dehydration, tinnitus, deafness, sweating, warm extremities, and hyperventilation. Severe poisoning is likely to cause coma, convulsions, pulmonary oedema, and cardiovascular collapse. If any of these occur, the outcome is likely to be fatal. However, the patient is likely to remain conscious and alert for many hours even after a large overdose. Out-of-hospital management includes giving activated charcoal (Table 4) and fluids to drink if tolerated. Hospital assessment is essential for any symptomatic patient, and repeated levels of drug need to be measured, as drug levels can rise for many hours after a large ingestion.

Table 4 Key points about activated charcoal

Extremely large surface area (1000 m²/g)
Most substances bound; weak binding by van der Vaals forces
Not effective for alcohols, lithium, iron, corrosives, petroleum distillates, cyanide
Recommended 10 : 1 charcoal to drug ratio for effectiveness
Dose: adults, 25–50 g; children, 1 g/kg
Most effective when given soon after ingestion (<1 h)

Patients with chronic salicylate poisoning generally do not present with gastrointestinal symptoms, although they may be dehydrated. The commonest presentation is one of intellectual change, including lethargy, disorientation, or hallucinations. Patients with chronic salicylate poisoning will have more serious toxicity at a given serum salicylate concentration than an acutely poisoned patient. An elevated INR or prothrombin is frequently present. It is a notoriously covert presentation, and must be considered in any patient presenting with unexplained central nervous system dysfunction, particularly in the presence of a mixed acid base disturbance. In these patients, it is important to remember to treat the patient and not the salicylate level, as otherwise patients will be significantly under-treated.

Tricyclic antidepressants

Symptoms of overdose include tachycardia, dilated pupils, cardiac arrhythmias and hypotension, hot dry skin, and dry mouth. Convulsions, respiratory depression, and coma can occur. If the patient presents within 1 h of ingesting a potentially toxic amount, give activated charcoal (Table 4) whilst awaiting transfer to hospital.

Selective serotonin re-uptake inhibitors (SSRIs)

These may cause few or no symptoms even after large overdoses. However, many patients experience gastrointestinal upset and drowsiness, while some develop tachycardia, muscle stiffness, and hypertension. Convulsions may occur. If the patient presents within 1 h of ingesting a potentially toxic amount, give activated charcoal (Table 4) whilst awaiting transfer to hospital.

Benzodiazepines

These are relatively safe when taken in overdose, although they can cause life-threatening problems particularly in older people and patients with severe chronic obstructive airways disease. Symptoms of overdose range from drowsiness, ataxia and nystagmus to hypotension, respiratory depression, and coma, particularly if benzodiazepines have been taken with alcohol or other CNS depressants. The effects of benzodiazepines can be reversed with flumazenil which should only be given in hospital and even in that setting, patients are generally treated conservatively only.

Opioids

Features of opioid poisoning include a progressive depression of the CNS leading to drowsiness, coma, respiratory depression, and ultimately, respiratory arrest. The patient will usually have pinpoint pupils and a slowed respiratory rate. There may also be hypotension, tachycardia, and hallucinations. Initial management depends on the patient's level of consciousness:

- If the patient is conscious and presents within 1 h of ingesting a potentially toxic amount of an opiate give activated charcoal.

- If respiration appears inadequate, assess closely, clear the airway, and give mouth-to-mouth ventilation.

- If the patient has respiratory depression or impaired consciousness give naloxone 0.4–2.0 intravenously (IV) and repeat every 2–3 min up to a maximum 10 mg (this can be given by intramuscular (IM) or subcutaneous injection if the IV route is not feasible).

The duration of action of some opioids (e.g. dihydrocodeine, dextropropoxyphene, and methadone) can outlast that of an IV or IM dose of naloxone and deterioration may later occur despite initial reversal. Repeated doses, or an infusion, of naloxone may be required. Naloxone may not reverse the effects of buprenorphine, so improvement may be delayed.

Iron tablets

Early symptoms of iron overdose include nausea, vomiting, abdominal pain, and diarrhoea. The patient's vomit and stools may be grey or black. Haematemesis and rectal bleeding may occur and in severe cases coma and shock. Most patients, especially children, will need measurement of serum iron, possibly gastric lavage and deferoxamine treatment, even if their symptoms have resolved within a few hours.

Caustic chemicals

Ingestion of caustic chemicals may cause severe burns and oedema of the mouth, pharynx, upper airway, and upper gastrointestinal tract. If the patient is conscious and able to swallow, give water or milk (three cupfuls) immediately to dilute the acid or alkali. Do not give neutralizing chemicals as the heat released can cause further injury. If vomiting occurs, the oesophagus may be damaged. Patients suspected of ingestion of caustic chemicals should be referred to hospital.

Carbon monoxide

Carbon monoxide is produced when carbon-containing fuels burn in air, and poisoning occurs when insufficient oxygen reaches the fire and when products of combustion accumulate. Motor exhaust fumes are an important cause of poisoning. Immediate features of exposure include headache, weakness, tachypnoea, dizziness, nausea, and agitation. Vomiting, impaired consciousness, respiratory failure, myocardial infarction, and cerebral oedema may occur in severe cases. If several people experience symptoms such as headache and vomiting, it is important to consider carbon monoxide poisoning as a possible cause. Give oxygen at a high concentration while awaiting transfer to hospital.

Organophosphates and carbamates

Organophosphorus and carbamate insecticides are used to control insects in homes and gardens. They are also very widely used agriculturally in tropical countries. They can cause serious poisoning which may be fatal through inhalation, skin contact, or ingestion. The amount which causes toxicity varies between chemicals, and some products contain petroleum distillate which can cause pulmonary oedema if aspirated.

The onset of symptoms may be delayed for up to 12 h. Symptoms include confusion, exhaustion, nausea, vomiting, diarrhoea, wheezing, sweating, salivation, and fasciculation of the muscles. The patient may have miosis, bradycardia, incontinence, and seizures. Pulmonary oedema and loss of consciousness are serious signs. After clearing the airway of secretions, the most important treatment is to give atropine in large doses (2 mg at a time) until the mouth is dry. Diazepam can be given to relieve anxiety and control seizures. Hospital care is essential in all but the mildest cases.

Drug misuse

Illicit drugs are an increasing problem in every society. Many different substances can be misused, from glue or petrol sniffing, to cannabis to 'hard' drugs. The popularity of a substance varies with age and social scene. Heroin causes the largest problem, and poisoning can occur due to an excessive dose in a naive user as well as to a 'regular' dose in a person who has become tolerant. It is important to remember that 10 mg of heroin intravenously could be fatal for a non-user, but the average user who presents to an addiction centre for help is taking 750 mg daily. Tolerance starts to be lost after a couple of days of abstinence, and toxicity can then occur from the user's normal dose. Management of toxicity is described above (opioids). Abscesses and infectious illnesses are a further problem apart from toxicity.

Cocaine causes massive surges in blood pressure due to widespread constriction of blood vessels, and chest pain is the commonest complication requiring medical attention. It usually resolves within a few hours without causing any apparent long-term damage. Every patient with symptoms following cocaine use should be given diazepam intravenously in relatively large doses, and those with chest pain should be given aspirin as for any patient with acute cardiac chest pain. Beta-blockers are contra-indicated. Hallucinations, aggression and convulsions, and cerebrovascular accidents may also follow cocaine use. Long-term users can develop accelerated atheroma.

Hallucinogens (LSD, some types of mushrooms, some plants) can lead to a sought after hallucinatory experience in which visual images are distorted and pleasant. However, the experience may be disturbing or frightening and physical restraint may be necessary. If possible, try to 'talk down' the patient one to one in a quiet dimly lit place. If this fails, intravenous diazepam is the best drug to calm the patient.

Ecstasy (MDMA) is now popular as a 'dance drug'. Some people may develop hyperthermic collapse due to dancing for too long without replacing fluid, and the urgent treatment is intravenous fluid, which should bring down the pulse rate and enable normal temperature regulation. Rarely, some people drink too much fluid and become confused or develop convulsions, because this drug causes a surge in levels of antidiuretic hormone. Most patients will recover naturally provided no more fluid is given.

Flunitrazepam (Rohypnol)

A benzodiazepine commonly used in European practice but less commonly used in North America, has often been cited as a 'date rape' drug. It is, in its original formulation, both clear and odourless as well as tasteless, but now has a blue dye added. It has frequently been used in social settings such as drinking establishments to cause altered levels of consciousness in female patrons so that they may be subjected to sexual abuse. Rohypnol has the properties of many benzodiazepines, including being a potent sedative, as well as inducing retrograde amnesia. While it has no long-term deleterious effects, patients who have been poisoned with it will frequently present to primary care practitioners or emergency departments with a vague sensation of having been anaesthetized and subsequently sexually assaulted. Patients will metabolize the drug spontaneously, and have no need of medical management other than the appropriate psychological and legal supports for any abuse which they have experienced.

Gamma hydroxybutyrate (GHB)

This drug, used in European practice as a procedural sedative, although not used medically in North America, has extremely potent, but short-term and spontaneously reversing side-effects. The classic presentation is one of the sudden onset of unresponsiveness, associated with hypotension and bradycardia and sometimes muscle twitching. Patients are generally rapidly transported to an emergency department, where a variety of sinister underlying causes such as an intracranial haemorrhage may be considered. The drug is generally metabolized spontaneously and quickly, and within a period of 30–60 min patients may recover rapidly, with normal vital signs. The drug may be detected by testing for it in a toxicology laboratory. There are, for all intents and purposes, no long-term side-effects from the drug, but it is often administered to unwary patrons as a 'date rape' drug. Conducting confirmatory testing may be important for pursuit of police proceedings. The only necessary intervention is support of vital functions.

Cardiac glycosides

Apart from chronic therapeutic toxicity with the drugs digoxin or digitoxin, digitalis (foxglove; *Digitalis purpurea* or *Digitalis lamata*), or oleander plants (*Nerium oleander* or yellow oleander; *Thevetia peruviana*) may be involved in self-poisoning.

Nausea, vomiting, cardiac arrhythmias, hypotension, and death may result. The patient should be given activated charcoal if able to swallow and immediately transferred to medical care supporting cardiac output by external chest compression if necessary. A plasma potassium concentration over 5.3 mmol/l is an indication of severe poisoning. If available, digoxin-specific Fab antibodies should have sufficient cross-reactivity to bind with all the cardiac glycosides.

Lead

In children, lead poisoning most commonly results from pica due to ingestion of lead paint from old buildings. Surma (black eye cosmetic made from lead sulfide) is another cause. In adults, lead poisoning may arise from contaminated water supplies or from occupational causes—painting or manufacturing.

Children usually present with anaemia and failure to thrive. Adults present with abdominal pain, constipation, muscle weakness (wrist or foot drop) and in the most severe cases, encephalopathy, with convulsions. The diagnosis may be suspected by finding punctate basophilia on a blood film and confirmed by measuring blood lead concentrations.

Prognosis and long-term care

The long-term outlook following acute poisoning is generally good. The great majority of poisonings leave no permanent damage. The main limitation is when the poisoning has been due to deliberate self-harm, and the patient may be suffering from depression or schizophrenia, with alcoholism as another complicating factor. In these cases, there is a risk of further episodes of self-poisoning or of suicide by another method, and long-term antidepressant or antipsychotic medication may be indicated.

Where a patient has been poisoned in the course of their occupation, one needs to decide whether the exposure has been intentional, whether carelessness has been involved, and whether the safety practices are deficient or absent. The practitioner can then advise the patient and the employers appropriately.

Poisoning due to substance misuse carries the risks associated with the substance and the mode of use (e.g. IV injection, which may lead to bacterial or viral infections), and long-term contact with an addiction centre or agency may help to minimize the dangers and improve prognosis.

In a small number of poisonings, there may be long-term morbidity. Carbon monoxide and organophosphates are important examples. Lead poisoning in children may lead to developmental delay and permanent mental impairment, whereas in adults eventual full recovery is the rule even after severe poisoning.

An important role of the primary care physician whose patient has suffered a poisoning is to decide on the aetiology of the event. For those in whom it is felt that this was a purposeful gesture, it is imperative that the family physician decide on the degree and depth of depression, and either initiate treatment or make an appropriate referral. For those where accidental poisoning has occurred, the family physician must ensure that the household and/or work site are equipped with adequate safety measures. For those cases in which criminal intent is suspected, the authorities must be notified.

Key points

- ◆ Childhood poisoning is usually accidental and very rarely fatal.

- ◆ In adults, the most serious poisonings occur from intentional overdose of drugs or in developing countries from pesticide ingestion.

- ◆ Swallowed poisons require gastric lavage or activated charcoal within 1 h.

- ◆ Antidotes are required in few cases; the most important are acetylcysteine for paracetamol (acetaminophen), naloxone for opioids, and atropine for organophosphates.

- ◆ Most poisoned patients recover with supportive care alone.

Perhaps the single most important role for the primary care physician is to counsel new parents on appropriate safety measures for the home in order to prevent unnecessary tragedy.

Further reading

Henry, J.A. and Wiseman, H., ed. *Management of Poisoning. Handbook for Healthcare Workers.* Geneva: World Health Organization, 1997, pp. 315.

American Academy of Clinical Toxicology, European Association of Poisons Centres and Clinical Toxicologists (1997). Position statements. *Clinical Toxicology* **35**, 699–762.

14.8 Drowning and inhalations

D. Anna Jarvis

The World Health Organization (WHO) in 1999 named drowning as the fifth commonest cause of accidental death worldwide. The extent of the problem is unrecognized because 50 per cent of victims die at the scene, and under-reporting of submersion injuries is common. The male/female ratio, sites of drowning, and associated problems (child maltreatment and neglect, head and neck trauma, alcohol and drug ingestion) vary across age groups and from country to country.

Definitions

Drowning is defined as death within 24 h of suffocation by submersion in a liquid medium. *Near-drowning* is survival for at least 24 h after suffocation by submersion in a liquid medium. These definitions are unsatisfactory. Young children drown in shallow bodies of water, without full submersion, because they lack the necessary motor skills to extricate themselves. Drowning victims die after more than 24 h of intensive care from conditions directly related to drowning events such as post-hypoxic cerebral oedema and adult respiratory distress syndrome. Orlowski and Szpilman[1] propose that drowning be defined as 'suffocation by immersion or submersion in any liquid medium caused by the entrance of liquid into the airways, that partially or fully compromises ventilation or oxygen exchange'.

Epidemiology

Drowning incidents peak in the pre-school and adolescent/young adult age groups. Marked male predominance is related to increased risk-taking behaviour, use of drugs and alcohol, and exposure to aquatic sports and occupations. In North America, the male : female ratio increases from 3 : 1 in young children to 6 : 1 in adolescents. In Brazil, no sex differential is noted under 1 year of age, males drown five times as frequently across all ages with a 8.7 : 1 ratio between ages 20 and 29 years.

National statistics may not identify high-risk populations. Mackie[2] reports that Australian indigenous people have a higher than average drowning incidence in both the under 5 years and the 25–34-year-age groups. Overseas tourists account for 25 per cent of all scuba-related drownings and a disproportionate percentage of non-boating and ocean drownings. In the United States, drowning is the third commonest cause of unintentional injury across all ages. In some states (California, Florida), drowning is the leading cause of death among pre-schoolers. Drowning is the leading cause of death in native Alaskans at all ages. Studies have reported positive blood alcohol levels in 10–50 per cent of US adolescent drownings.

Under 1 year of age, bath tubs, buckets, and other household water catchments are common drowning sites. Child maltreatment and neglect must always be considered. In the United States, Australia, and South Africa, 70–90 per cent of deaths from drowning occur in residential swimming pools. In non-industrialized nations, natural bodies of water (rivers, lakes, dams, oceans) are more common sites. Countries with life-saving associations report significant numbers of near-drowning rescues annually. On Rio de Janeiro beaches, there were approximately 290 rescues for each death, and on US beaches (1996), 62 747 rescues with eight cases of near-drowning for each death.

Pathophysiology

Aspiration

The primary mechanism of injury in drowning is hypoxia with secondary metabolic and respiratory acidosis. Initial aspiration of water causes breath-holding or laryngospasm with active and passive swallowing. As hypoxia worsens, aspiration of fluid into the lungs occurs, so-called 'wet drowning'. In 10–20 per cent of drownings, asystole occurs before termination of laryngospasm or breath-holding, so-called 'dry drowning'. Swimmers who hyperventilate to prolong submersion time may lose consciousness or develop non-perfusing cardiac rhythms before critical hypoxia is appreciated.[3–5]

Aspiration of either fresh or salt water results in interruption of surfactant production, alveolitis, pulmonary oedema, obstructed alveolar-capillary gas exchange, shunting, and profound hypoxia. The exact volume of aspirated fluid needed to cause critical hypoxia is unknown. Aspiration of 1–3 ml/kg of water in humans has been shown to produce marked decreases in PaO_2 and in pulmonary compliance. Aspiration of chemicals, sand, vegetation, sewage, and other particulate matter may further complicate matters, though mechanical lung damage, hypoxia, and inflammatory responses. The theoretical electrolyte disturbances in salt water drowing are rarely encountered. Only case reports from Dead Sea drownings and submersion events in chemical liquids have documented marked electrolyte abnormalities.

Cold-shock response

Tipton and others[3] have described the *cold-shock response* to sudden immersion in cold water, probably the cause of the majority of drowning incidents and deaths in open waters in the United Kingdom. The response is seen at water temperatures below 25°C with maximum response recorded at 10°C, and its incidence is inversely proportional to water temperature. The initial response is a gasp, followed by uncontrolled hyperventilation for 2–3 min. During hyperventilation, victims may panic due to a sensation of dyspnoea and aspirate and ingest cold water. In the United Kingdom, 60 per cent of drownings occur within 3 m of safety, and two-thirds of the victims were considered 'good swimmers'.

Hypothermia

Hypothermia is defined as a core body temperature less than 35°C. The rate of body cooling depends on:

- water temperature and ambient weather conditions;
- victim's age, body surface area to mass ratio, insulation;
- underlying metabolic and cardiovascular status;
- concomitant injuries or ingestants.

Young children are more prone to hypothermia because of their relatively large head size, large body surface area to mass ratio, reduced subcutaneous fat content, and ineffective shivering. Consciousness is gradually impaired as core temperature falls. At body temperatures less than 34°C, most victims aspirate water (unless wearing a personal flotation device with a 'spray hood') and lose neuromuscular control. Swimming and actions to secure safety become increasingly impaired. Most victims are non-responsive at 30°C.

Stone reported a 6–7 per cent decrease in cerebral blood flow with each 1°C fall in body temperature. All cerebral activity ceases at 22°C. Ventricular fibrillation may occur at 28°C and asystole at 24–26°C. Cardiovascular responses to cold immersion include peripheral vasoconstriction, a 42–49 per cent increase in heart rate and a 59–100 per cent increase in cardiac output. Increased myocardial workload along with simultaneous maximal catecholamine response may result in cardiac dysrhythmias. Patients with underlying cardiovascular disorders are particularly prone to adverse outcomes. This is the proposed mechanism for sudden cessation of struggling/swimming described by eyewitnesses of drowning events.[6]

Diving response

The diving response is a mammalian reflex of apnoea, marked peripheral vasoconstriction and bradycardia initiated by sudden immersion of the face in cold water. This reflex is mediated through the ophthalmic division of the trigeminal nerve. Slowed cerebral metabolism and shunting of available blood to the brain prior to massive aspiration of water may explain full neurological recovery of some children after prolonged submersion in cold water. Rapid cerebral cooling secondary to swallowed and aspirated water (after loss of consciousness) are also significant factors. The diving reflex persists in about 15 per cent of adults. The interactions of cold-shock and diving responses may result in fatal cardiac arrhythmias after the breath-holding phase of cold water exposure.

Management

Rescue

A panicky victim may injure the rescuer. The conscious victim is best approached with a flotation device positioned between victim and rescuer. The apnoeic victim should have mouth-to-mouth respirations initiated in the water. Effective cardiac compressions cannot be applied in water, therefore the victim should be retrieved before attempting cardiac massage. When possible, victims wearing life jackets who have a clear airway should be recovered in the horizontal position. The possibility of cervical spine trauma must be considered if the victim is in shallow water.

Out-of-hospital management

The principles of out-of-hospital management are:

- timely relief of hypoxia;
- restoration of cardiovascular stability;
- prevention of further heat loss;
- speedy transfer to hospital.

If no spontaneous respirations are observed, mouth-to-mouth ventilation should continue until personnel and equipment are available for endotracheal intubation. If spontaneous respirations are present, the victim may be positioned on the right side (if there is no suspicion of a spine injury) with the head slightly dependent, to decrease the possibility of aspiration. The Heimlich manoeuvre is not indicated as it may induce vomiting, aggravate spinal and visceral injuries, and delay intubation. When oxygen is available, it should be administered to victims who have any respiratory symptoms. Significant hypoxia may be present with few clinical signs. It is difficult to detect pulses in hypothermic victims. The unresponsive, apnoeic victim should receive cardiac massage until advanced life support providers and equipment are available. Heat loss should be limited by removal of wet clothes and wrapping the victim in dry

blankets/sheets. Surface heating should be delayed until cardiac output has been normalized.

En route to hospital, advanced life support providers should maintain optimal oxygenation. Electrocardiographic monitoring may indicate the need for application of cardiopulmonary resuscitation algorithms. Hypothermic victims with *ventricular fibrillation* or *asystole* may not respond to *defibrillation*, *epinephrine* or *vasopressin* (see Chapter 14.1). Effective ventilation and cardiac compressions must be maintained, and intravenous/intraosseous access secured for administration of fluids and drugs. Glucose-containing solutions are only administered in cases of documented hypoglycaemia.

Emergency department management

A rapid, accurate initial assessment of victims is important (Fig. 1). It is equally important to review the drowning incident and subsequent management with the transport team and find out about the victims' previous health.

Patients in cardiopulmonary arrest need full resuscitative efforts until they are rewarmed to 33°C. Intubation is essential in anticipation of the development of pulmonary oedema. Continuous positive airway pressure (CPAP) starting at 5–10 cm H_2O should be applied with ventilation rates above normal for age. The aim is to maintain oxygen saturations greater than 90 per cent with inspired oxygen concentration (FiO_2) less than 0.5 and acceptable blood pressures. It may be necessary to increase CPAP or positive end-expiratory pressure (PEEP) to 10–15 cm H_2O. High pressures may reduce blood pressure and damage lung tissue. Intermittent endotracheal suctioning may be necessary to clear oedema fluid and aspirated debris. It is preferable not to administer diuretics because most drowning victims have decreased intravascular volumes and benefit from saline in 20 ml/kg boluses.

Cardiac compressions should be maintained until adequate cardiac output is established or the patient is warmed to 33°C. Cardiopulmonary bypass is the fastest method of rewarming, although not widely available. Rewarming may be achieved with inhaled oxygen and intravenous fluids

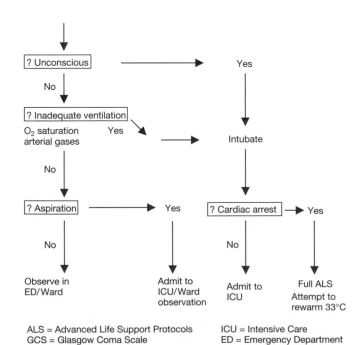

ALS = Advanced Life Support Protocols
GCS = Glasgow Coma Scale

ICU = Intensive Care
ED = Emergency Department

Fig. 1 Initial assessment of victims. [*Adapted from:* Golden, F.St.C., Tipton, M.J., and Scott, R.C. (1997). Immersion, near-drowning and drowning. *British Journal of Anaesthesia* **79**, 214–25.]

warmed to 40°C in conjunction with body cavity irrigation (bladder, stomach, colon, peritoneum, and pleural cavity). Further heat loss should be prevented by covering the patient, including the scalp with, dry, warm blankets. Surface warming should be delayed until the core temperature is 32°C to avoid skin burns. Between 28 and 30°C, the myocardium may respond to drugs and electricity. *Ventricular fibrillation* and *Torsades de Pointe* are commonly encountered rhythms during rewarming from profound hypothermia. There are reports of successful recovery after 4.5 and 5.5 h of effective cardiac massage in profoundly hypothermic patients. Once sinus rhythm is established, epinephrine or dopamine infusions may be necessary to maintain adequate rates and cardiac output.

Patients with ventilatory failure and/or hypothermia should be intubated and ventilation supported as outlined above. Patients with evidence of aspiration and adequate ventilation should receive oxygen and close monitoring for signs of respiratory distress or poor perfusion. These patients may benefit from CPAP or BiPAP administered by mask. They need admission to an intensive care or high dependency unit. Patients with no evidence of aspiration, respiratory compromise, or significant injury need close observation for 6–24 h. Oxygen saturations and/or serial arterial blood gases are indicated as late onset pulmonary and cerebral oedema may develop rapidly. These patients may be observed in emergency, a short stay or inpatient unit depending on the severity of the near-drowning episode and hospital facilities.[4,5]

All drowning victims require:

- rectal temperature measurements 15 cm from the anal verge;
- blood tests—arterial gases, glucose, electrolytes, haematology, renal function, coagulation studies, and drug screen (adolescents and adults);
- chest X-rays (further imaging may be indicated);
- electrocardiogram;
- urinalysis.

It is unusual to document abnormal electrolytes. Rhabdomyolysis has been described in cold water drowning. Severe metabolic acidosis (pH < 7.1) is associated with a poor outcome and should be treated with ventilation and sodium bicarbonate infusions of 1–2 mmol/kg.

Treatment in intensive care

Patients who need ventilatory support, ongoing central warming techniques, invasive monitoring, and management of significant other injuries are candidates for intensive care. Delayed effects of profound hypoxia include cerebral oedema, acute respiratory distress syndrome, coagulopathy, renal tubular necrosis, and multisystem failure. It is preferable to withhold antibiotics and screen endotracheal secretions daily for signs of infection. Patients known to have been submerged in sewage may be started on antibiotics at the time of admission.

Prognosis

A variety of scales have been devised to try to identify patients who benefit from prolonged resuscitative efforts. In Canadian, USA, UK, and Australian experience, the majority of patients who present to hospital in cardiac arrest or coma will either die or survive with severe neurological compromise (see Chapter 14.1). No system is 100 per cent predictive. Anecdotal stories of miraculous recoveries abound, particular involving younger children submerged in frigid water. Factors associated with poor outcomes include:

- age less than 3 years;
- submersion greater than 5 min;
- water temperature greater than 10°C;
- post-rescue resuscitation delay greater than 10 min;
- initial pH less than 7.1;

- blood glucose greater than 11 mmol/l;
- arrival at hospital in cardiac arrest, GCS less than 6, fixed dilated pupils.

The outcome for near-drowning victims tends to be bimodal, death or good survival. Death occurs in 30–50 per cent of victims. Approximately 11 per cent overall survive with severe neurological sequelae of anoxic cerebral encephalopathy. In victims with cardiopulmonary arrest and core temperatures of 34°C or higher, resuscitative efforts in the hospital should not be continued beyond 25 min.[1,4,7–10]

Prevention

No discussion of drowning is complete without consideration of preventive measures. There has been no decrease in pre-school age drownings in countries with intensive water safety campaigns. An American Academy of Pediatrics survey found that few paediatricians routinely advise families about water/swimming safety. Quan[4] reported that 8 per cent of near-drowning patients admitted to a tertiary care paediatric centre may have been victims of child maltreatment or neglect. Drowning deaths in residential pools are significantly decreased when four-sided isolation fencing is legislated (compared to three-sided fences with the house providing the fourth side).[2,4,11] All pool owners should know basic life support techniques.

Nearly 40 per cent of all drownings result from boating accidents. Many indigenous peoples who work on water never learn to swim, and alcohol is detected in two-thirds of victims of boating-related drownings. Positive blood alcohol levels have been reported in 10–50 per cent of drowned adolescents. Youths and young adults infrequently wear personal flotation devices (PFDs). In Canada, there are laws against drinking and operating aquatic vehicles, but the laws are poorly enforced. Concerted efforts to enact and enforce drinking laws and routine use of PFDs (like seat belts in cars) should reduce the number of drownings in the boating/aquatic sector.

In Australia, better education of tourists in technical aspects of diving, and ocean safety has been proposed to decrease drowning among visitors. Worldwide, both general public and health providers underestimate the impact of drowning on society. Most victims are previously healthy individuals with normal life expectancy. The loss of human potential is immeasurable.[2]

Key points

- Drowning is the fifth commonest cause of death.
- The incidence of drowning shows a bimodal age pattern— preschool children and adolescents/young adults.
- Fifty per cent of victims die at the scene.
- Eleven per cent survivors are neurologically impaired.
- Seventy to 90% of drowning in industrialized nations occurs in residential pools.
- Alcohol contributes to 10–50% of drowning deaths in adolescents.
- Victims who arrive at hospital with vital signs absent rarely survive neurologically intact.

References

1. **Orlowski, J.P. and Szpilman, D.** (2001). Drowning—rescue, resuscitation, and reanimation. *The Pediatric Clinics of North America* **48** (3), 627–46.
2. **Mackie, I.J.** (1999). Patterns of drowning in Australia, 1992–1997. *Medical Journal of Australia* **171**, 587–90.
3. **Golden, F.St.C., Tipton, M.J., and Scott, R.C.** (1997). Immersion, near-drowning and drowning. *British Journal of Anaesthesia* **79**, 214–25.

4. Quan, L. (1999). Near-drowning. *Pediatrics in Review* **29** (8), 255–9.

5. Weinstein, M.D. and Krieger, B.P. (1996). Near drowning: epidemiology, pathophysiology, and initial treatment. *The Journal of Emergency Medicine* **14** (4), 461–7.

6. Stone, H.H., Donnelly, C., and Frosbese, A.S. (1956). The effect of lowered body temperature on cerebral hemodynamics and metabolism of man. *Surgery, Gynecology and Obstetrics* **103**, 313–17.

7. Conn, A.W., Montes, J.E., Barker, G.A., and Edmonds, J.F. (1980). Cerebral salvage in near-drowning following neurological classification by triage. *The Canadian Anaesthetists' Society Journal* **27** (3), 201–10.

8. Graf, W.D., Cummings, P., Quan, L., and Brutocao, D. (1995). Predicting outcome in pediatric submersion victims. *Annals of Emergency Medicine* **26**, 312–19.

9. Szpilman, D. (1997). Near-drowning and drowning classification: A proposal to stratify mortality ADD: based on the analysis of 1831 cases. *Chest* **112**, 660–5.

10. Zuckerman, G.B., Gregory, P.M., and Santos-Damani, S.M. (1998). Predictors of death and neurologic impairment in pediatric submersion injuries. The Pediatric Risk of Mortality Score. *Archives of Pediatric and Adolescent Medicine* **152**, 134–40.

11. Thompson, D.C. and Rivara, F.P. (2000). Pool fencing for preventing drowning in children. In *Cochrane Database Systematic Review* Issue 2, CD001047.

14.9 Electrical injuries

D. Anna Jarvis

Electrical injuries, including lightning strikes, are traditionally recorded with 'burns'. They account for 3–4 per cent of burn centre admissions in Kentucky (United States) and 5.6 per cent in Birmingham (United Kingdom). The incidence of electrical injuries is unknown due to underreporting of domestic, recreational, and industrial events. Approximately 1000 deaths per year are caused by electrical injuries in the United States, of which 100 are due to lightning.[1–3]

Epidemiology

Paediatric electrical injuries have a bimodal distribution, affecting children less than 6 years, and older children and adolescents. Low-voltage injuries predominate in younger children, and high-voltage injuries in older children, adolescents, and adults. Deaths from electrical injuries are mostly preventable. Lightning injuries occur mainly in males 15–44 years of age engaged in work or recreational activities.[2,3]

Pathophysiology

Tissue damage from electric energy increases with the energy applied and the duration of contact:

$$\text{Energy} = (V^2/R) \times T$$

where, V is the voltage applied, R the resistance to current flow, and T the duration of current flow.

Tissue damage is determined by:

- tissue resistance;
- path of electrical current;
- type of current, frequency, and duration.

Tissue resistance

Body tissues vary greatly in their resistance to electrical flow, and graded from least to greatest are: nerves, blood vessels, muscles, skin, tendon, fat, and bone. Skin resistance increases with age and thickness and markedly decreases with high water content or surface moisture. The foetus is particularly susceptible to electrical injury and death.[1,2,4]

Path of electrical current

Electrical currents tend to flow towards the ground from the point of contact. The path taken through the body indicates potential internal injuries. The hand to hand pathway has a mortality of greater than 60 per cent due to spinal cord transection at the level of C4 to C8. The hand to foot pathway has a mortality of greater than 20 per cent due to cardiac dysrhythmias. The foot to foot pathway has a mortality of less than 5 per cent. Pregnant victims of household or lightning shocks with minimal or no injury may experience foetal deaths due to a hand to foot pathway of the current.

Lightning may affect a victim through *direct strike, side flash, stride potential,* or *flashover*. The direct strike is potentially most serious as the current flows through the longitudinal axis of the victim. A side flash is deflected current from another victim (or object such as a tree). Stride potential describes lightning that first hits the ground then enters one leg of the victim and exits through the other leg. Mortality rates of 30 per cent are reported in stride potential victims with leg burns. In the flashover phenomenon, lightning flows outside the body, and may 'blow off' the clothes, leaving pathognomonic feather-like dermal burns.[2,5]

Type of current, frequency, and duration

In alternating current (AC), the electron flow changes with a certain frequency/second. One hertz (Hz) = 1 cycle/second. Household AC, usually 50–60 Hz, stimulates muscle tetany. Victims may be unable to let go of the power source, resulting in prolonged exposure to current, greater heat production, and thermal injury. Low-voltage AC is more likely to produce ventricular fibrillation. Direct current (DC) is greater in energy and causes a single massive muscle contraction. Victims are usually thrown clear of the DC source. Significant thermal burns are infrequent. Examples of DC current include lightning strikes, defibrillation, and artificial pacemakers. DC and high-tension AC are more likely to cause asystole.

The potential for injury increases with the voltage. Low voltage is defined as less than 1000 volts (V). Household electrical lines in Europe distribute 220 V, and in North America 110 V. Flash burns and charring are more common with higher voltages. High-tension wires may transmit 10 000–1 000 000 V. Lightning may exceed 10^7 V.[1,3,5–7]

Management

Rescue

Rescuers must ensure that all electrical current is shut off before a victim is approached. Rescuers should be insulated and equipped with wooden-handled or insulated wire cutters. Damaged electrical wires must be secured as they may whip about when current is restored. Lightning can hit a site more than once. Victims should be removed to a safe place if stormy weather persists. Victims of electrical injury who experience prolonged apnoea or cardiac arrest have better outcomes than other categories of trauma victims. They should receive aggressive treatment with full ACLS and ATLS protocols en route to hospital. The cervical spine must be immobilized until spinal trauma has been ruled out. Data collection should start at the scene including: voltage and type of current, evidence of additional trauma (fall, explosion, or fire), duration of electrical injury, apnoea, and cardiopulmonary arrest.

Emergency department management

It is important to rapidly identify any need for ongoing cardiopulmonary resuscitation. Oxygenation and ventilation should be maximized while vital signs are obtained and two large bore intravenous lines are established. In the presence of shock or extensive tissue damage, a normal saline or Ringer's lactate 20 cm³/kg bolus should be administered. Electrical injuries are deceptive, in that there may be few external signs of extensive internal tissue damage. Fluid therapy must be based on urine output of 2 ml/kg/h in infants and toddlers and 1–1.5 ml/kg/h in older children and adults.

Once initial stabilization has been accomplished, a meticulous head to toe secondary survey is needed. A 12-lead cardiogram, urinalysis and base-line blood count, electrolytes, blood gas, and renal function may indicate significant internal injuries. In conscious patients, further investigations and admission to hospital are based on: history of the event, estimated electrical injury, examination, initial investigations, or the patient's pre-morbid medical status. Fatovich and others have pointed out that asymptomatic patients with low-voltage electrical events do not need investigation or admission to hospital.

Patients with altered level of consciousness require admission to an intensive care unit and urgent radiological investigations to rule out spinal, intracranial, chest, or skeletal injuries. Patients with extensive burns or soft tissue injuries should be referred to an appropriate plastic surgeon/burn unit.

Central venous pressure monitoring may be necessary to optimize fluid therapy in patients with intracranial injuries and extensive soft tissue damage and/or renal impairment. Superficial burns should be cleaned, debrided, and dressed with silver sulfadiazine or mafenide acetate. Tetanus prophylaxis is essential. Fasciotomies may be indicated. The role of parenteral antibiotics is controversial. Many burn specialists withhold antibiotics until there is evidence of infection.

Complications

Electrical exposures may result in significant occult injuries. Repeated clinical examinations and ongoing vital sign monitoring are essential for early detection of injuries and complications. Myocardial damage may occur without elevated cardiac enzymes. Minimal skin burns may overlie coagulated, necrotic muscles and deeper tissues. Damaged muscles can lead to myoglobinuria, hyperkalaemia, and renal failure. Compression fractures of the vertebral bodies, long limb fractures, head, spinal, or internal organ injuries may result from massive muscle contractions or as a result of impact with the ground or other solid objects.[5,8]

In the first 24 h after significant electrical injuries, victims may develop compartment syndromes, adult respiratory distress syndrome, third space pooling, and neurological syndromes. Loss of consciousness, amnesia, and confusion are common after high-voltage injuries. Full recovery can be anticipated if neurological findings are due to the electrical injury and not hypoxia, trauma, or haemorrhage. Spinal cord injuries which present immediately also have a good prognosis. Internal organ damage is rare. Stress ulcers and paralytic ileus are the commonest gastrointestinal complications. Ileus that persists more than a few days may indicate more serious occult visceral injury.

Over subsequent days to weeks, delayed thrombosis and blood vessel rupture may lead to bleeding. Victims of electrical burn may experience exsanguinating haemorrhage when eschar seperates. Patients and their families must know the signs of impending haemorrhage and emergency management. Delayed onset neurological syndromes include peripheral nerve injuries, reflex sympathetic dystrophy, motor neuropathies, spinal cord lesions, impotence, bladder dysfunction, cognitive impairment, depression, anxiety, and post-traumatic stress disorder.

More than 50 per cent of patients with lightning injuries experience tympanic membrane rupture. Hearing loss is both conductive and sensori-neural at high frequencies. Eye injuries may present early, for example,

hyphaema, or up to years later with cataracts. All victims must be informed of the need for appropriate monitoring for delayed complications.[7–9]

Prevention

Parents must be instructed to 'child proof' their home to prevent younger children chewing on electrical wires or live plugs. Children need to be taught electrical safety and the dangers of climbing trees or flying kites near electrical wires. All age groups need to know that they should seek shelter and avoid metal objects, trees, bodies of water, and high ground during lightning storms. The safest action if caught outdoors is to find the lowest ground and lie curled up. Knowledge of bystander CPR and how to activate emergency medical services also saves lives.

Enforcement of appropriate industrial standards for protective clothing and equipment, along with safe working practices, would greatly reduce electrical injuries and deaths among young adults.

Key points

- ◆ Approximately one in five electrical deaths is caused by lightning.

- ◆ Body tissues vary in resistance to electrical flow (nerves and blood vessels are least and fat and bone most resistant).

- ◆ Skin resistance increases with age and thickness, and decreases with moisture.

- ◆ Low-voltage alternating current usually induces ventricular fibrillation.

- ◆ High-voltage alternating current and direct current usually induce asystole.

- ◆ Extensive deep tissue injuries and foetal death may occur with minimal or no external injuries.

- ◆ Complications may present immediately or up to years later.

References

1. Smith, M.L. (2000). Pediatric burns: management of thermal, electrical, and chemical burns and burn-like dermatologic conditions. *Pediatric Annals* 29 (6), 367–78.

2. Jain, S. and Bandi, V. (1999). Electrical and lightning injuries. *Critical Care Clinics* 15 (2), 319–31.

3. Lee, R.C. (1997). Injury by electrical forces: pathophysiology, manifestations, and therapy. *Current Problems in Surgery* 34 (9), 677–765.

4. Fish, R.M. (2000). Electric injury. Part III: Cardiac monitoring indications, the pregnant patient, and lightning. *The Journal of Emergency Medicine* 18 (2), 181–7.

5. Fish, R.M. (1999). Electrical injury. Part I: Treatment priorities, subtle diagnostic factors, and burns. *The Journal of Emergency Medicine* 17 (6), 977–83.

6. Fatovich, D.M. and Lee, K.Y. (1991). Household electrical shocks: who should be monitored? *Medical Journal of Australia* 155, 301–3.

7. Baily, B. et al. (1995). Cardiac monitoring of children with household electrical injuries. *Annals of Emergency Medicine* 25 (5), 612–17.

8. Fish, R.M. (2000). Electric injury. Part II: Specific injuries. *The Journal of Emergency Medicine* 18 (1), 27–34.

9. Thomas, S.S. (1996). Electrical burns of the mouth: still searching for an answer. *Burns* 22 (2), 137–40.

15

Skin and soft tissue problems

15 Skin and soft tissue problems

15.1 Hair-related problems

B.C. Gee and Jennifer Powell

Hair is not essential for health and survival in humans but abnormalities in its growth density and pattern, or alterations in its colour and texture often lead to great distress. The psychological burden of hair problems impacts upon social and sexual interaction and may lead to social isolation. Management therefore requires not only treatment of possible underlying systemic disease, but also psychological help and support. Often, a single consultation will not suffice, especially if the patient falls into a poor prognosis group. Public health aspects such as ensuring that close contacts with head lice are treated also fall into the primary care remit. Provision of resources will need to be planned accordingly.

Most consultations relate to alopecia (hair loss), but scalp infections and infestations, inflammatory conditions, excess hair, and hair shaft abnormalities are all common problems that may lead to consultation.

In primary care, the new episode rate for hair disorders is 2.2/100/year, with a peak of 3.5/year in the 15–24 age group. There is very little difference between men and women. A general practitioner (GP) can therefore expect to see approximately five new cases a year. This is certainly an underestimate as patients frequently mention their hair concern as a 'by the way', others consult their hairdresser or non-medical 'hair specialists'. Consultations for head lice, a perennial problem, are not included in these data.

Approaching a patient with hair loss

Patients consult a doctor regarding hair loss for many reasons. They may have noticed themselves that their hair is thinning or that there is increased shedding, or the hairdresser has pointed out a bald spot that has not been apparent before. It is important to approach the patient sympathetically and allow time for them to voice their anxieties.

History

A good history will cover the following areas: duration, speed of onset, previous episodes, hair care, response to treatment, anybody else affected, current and past systemic problems, present medications, and family history.

Examination

The approach should be systematic. Note the pattern of hair loss, the scalp surface, and the hair shaft (Fig. 1).

A gentle pull of approximately 50 hairs from the scalp surface distally (trichogram), will indicate the amount of shedding and suggest the presence of weathering. Telogen hairs are club hairs, and should be no more than five of 50 pulled hairs—(normal anagen : catagen 90 : 10). If this is

Pattern—diffuse, patchy, marginal, localized.

Scalp surface—looking for signs of inflammation, e.g., scaling, erythema (perifollicular or diffuse). The presence of scarring may be difficult to determine but is manifest by partial or complete loss of follicular orifices.

Hair shaft—signs of trauma: broken ends, irregular length hairs may indicate trichotillamania. The presence of an 'exclamation mark' hair is pathognomonic of alopecia areata. If lice themselves are not identified, eggs may be seen dotted along the hair shaft.

Fig. 1 Clinical examination of hair related problems—what to look for.

significantly increased then telogen effluvium is present. If the hair shafts break on a gentle pull then it suggests a hair shaft abnormality.

Hairs can be mounted and viewed under light microscopy. To obtain the best result, at least 50 hairs preferentially plucked rather than cut should be sent in a folded card with a clear history to a dermatologist who specializes in hair. If a scalp biopsy is required, referral to a dermatologist is advisable—although not difficult technically to perform, biopsies may be difficult to interpret. If the biopsies need to be done in the community, send two 4-mm punch biopsies requesting both vertical and horizontal sections.

Historically, the differential diagnoses for hair loss is divided into scarring and non-scarring alopecia. The most common non-scarring alopecia to present is alopecia areata (AA).

Alopecia areata

This condition relates to patchy hair loss on any hair-bearing surface. Alopecia totalis refers to complete loss of scalp hair and alopecia universalis to complete loss of body hair.

Examination reveals patches of non-scarring alopecia (Fig. 2). Inflammation is often subclinical and therefore erythema and scaling may be absent. 'Exclamation mark' hairs are pathognomonic of alopecia areata (AA)(Fig. 3) but may not be present.

If patches are small and few, the patient can be advised that regrowth is likely to occur spontaneously between 6 and 12 months. Factors that predict a poor prognosis for regrowth are: pre-pubertal presentation, a pattern of loss at the scalp margins (ophiasis), multiple lesions especially those away from the scalp, and rapid onset of extensive disease. Interestingly, not only does the initial hair regrowth appear unpigmented but AA tends to spare white hair, which explains reports of stress causing the sufferer to go 'white overnight'!

Nothing more than discussion of the natural history is warranted in limited disease. First-line treatments consist of topical immunosuppression in the form of topical steroid application. Response should be seen in 3 months, and if not, the treatment should be stopped.

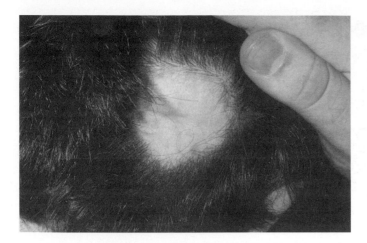

Fig. 2 Patches of non-scarring alopecia. (See Plate 22.)

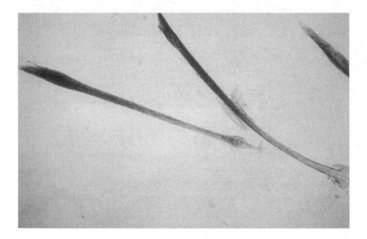

Fig. 3 'Exclamation mark' hairs in alopecia areata. (See Plate 23.)

Intralesional and oral steroids are probably best left to dermatologists to prescribe, because although regrowth is common whilst the patient is using steroids, hair loss may be resumed on cessation of treatment. If hair growth persists then spontaneous resolution would have occurred anyway. Other treatments offered by the hospital include:

- dithranol which works as an irritant;
- topical sensitizers such as diphencyprone (DCP);
- immunosuppressants such as cyclosporin, PUVA, and methotrexate have also been used with some benefit.

A referral to a dermatologist is justified to confirm the diagnosis, discuss certain therapies and, in the United Kingdom, for provision of a wig.

Common baldness (androgenetic alopecia)

Patients regularly consult the GP for help with common baldness (androgenetic alopecia), and also commonly bring it up as a secondary issue.

This form of alopecia is inherited and androgen-dependent. There are no accurate prevalence rates but some authorities consider that it approaches 100 per cent in Caucasian males, and 60 per cent in females. The main clinical feature of common baldness is the progressive miniaturization of terminal hairs into short and unpigmented vellus hairs. This accompanies shortening of the anagen phase and increased shedding in telogen. The *hair shedding* often leads the patient to seek advice.

The diagnosis in men is generally made without difficulty, but if women present with other androgenetic manifestations such as acne and hirsutism (coarse terminal hair in male body hair distribution) then an underlying endocrine pathology should be sought.

Minoxidil and finasteride are the most efficacious treatments. Minoxidil (a hypertensive agent) by serendipity was found to cause hypertrichosis (excess hair—non-androgen dependent). It is thought to work by increasing the anagen phase duration thereby increasing shaft diameter. The effect is hard to evaluate but studies have shown 15 per cent of patients have regrowth, 50 per cent have no progression of loss, and 35 per cent continue to lose hair. The 5 per cent preparation causes distant hypertrichosis in women and is not recommended.

Finasteride, a selective inhibitor of 5-alpha reductase isoenzyme type 2, has been shown to show an improvement in patients with mild to moderate vertex scalp hair loss. Regrowth is more impressive than minoxidil and unlike the latter will not cause shedding if stopped.

Hormone replacement therapy (HRT) in post-menopausal women may improve androgenetic alopecia as will antiandrogens such as cyproterone acetate and spirononolactone.

Diffuse alopecia

Diffuse alopecia has many causes: a detailed medical history and systemic examination is required.

Drugs including cytotoxics, wafarin, heparin, antithyroid agents, and vitamin A derivatives (retinoids) are frequent causes.

Telogen effluvium occurs when a significant number of follicles prematurely enter catagen, quickly followed by telogen. The precipitating event such as childbirth, febrile illness, surgery, haemorrhage, 'stress', and ingestion of certain drugs can then be dated as hairs take approximately 2–3 months to be shed. If the cause is not readily identifiable, then iron deficiency and hypo- and hyperthyroidism should be considered. Patients will often expect a blood test and are therefore happy to acquiesce.

Nutritional hair loss is seen mainly, but not exclusively, in Third World countries. Protein-calorie malnutrition results in various hair changes. Diffuse alopecia is caused by the increased number of deluge hairs and anagen follicles becoming dystrophic. There is also partial loss of pigment (black hair looks reddish). Axillary hair is often sparse. *Zinc deficiency* either as a result of dietary deficiency or an inherited disorder such as acrodermatitis enteropathica causes sparse brittle hair. This is unlikely to occur alone without systemic features. Zinc supplements in healthy patients are not indicated.

Trichotillomania presents with patchy hair loss which may be unilateral. The hairs are broken and are of different lengths. Onychophagia (biting of nails) may result in dystrophic nails but pitting is not a feature as in AA. Another useful sign to differentiate between AA and trichotillomania is the presence of lower-lid eyelashes—if absent, the diagnosis is likely to be AA as they are too short to be plucked.

Chronic traction alopecia may be more diffuse and occur along hairlines and partings. It is common in Afro-Carribean women due to the methods used to style their hair.

Scarring alopecia

Generally, if scarring is present then a dermatogist's opinion should be sought. A useful classification is folliculocentric scarring alopecia (pustular and lymphocyte mediated) and secondary scarring alopecia.

Folliculocentric pustular alopecia

Alopecia characterized by pustules centred on the hair follicles has four common causes:

- *Dissecting cellulitis of the scalp*—akin to hidradenitis suppurativa (HA) in the scalp.
- *Acne keloidalis nuche*—keloidal plaques in young Afro-Caribbean males.
- *Follicultis decalvans*—primarily affects the scalp of both sexes but can involve the beard, axillary, pubic, and inner thigh hair.
- *Tinea capitis*—see later.

Mild cases may respond to protracted courses of antibiotics (e.g. tetracycline 500 mg bd for 6 months) and topical antiseptics (e.g. chlorhexidine washes). However, most cases will need more aggressive treatments such as oral retinoids, complex antibiotic regimens, or surgery that can only be provided by secondary care.

Lymphocyte-mediated scarring alopecia

There are two common forms of lymphocyte mediated scarring alopecia—discoid lupus erythematosus (DLE) and lichen planopilaris. Typically, 5 per cent of patients with DLE will progress to systemic lupus erythematosus (SLE). Topical and intralesional steroids with sun avoidance are the mainstays of treatment. If the condition is widespread antimalarial drugs such as hydroxychloroquine are helpful.

Lichen planopilaris (lichen planus of hair follicles) presents as hyperkeratotic papules with perifollicular erythema. Body hair may also be involved. Other clues such as typical lichen planus affecting skin, nails, and buccal mucosa may be present. Potent topical steroids and oral steroids may be helpful, but the alopecia is permanent and disfiguring.

Secondary scarring alopecia

This describes alopecia that is cicatricial and not centred on follicles. Common causes of secondary alopecias include morphea (en coup de sabre), lichen sclerosus and atrophicus, burns (thermal and chemical), radiation, and neoplasia.

Infections and infestations

Tinea capitis is common in children all over the world. Uncomplicated infection will not cause scarring, but, there are two types of infection namely kerion and favus that do. Kerions are well circumscribed, crusted, boggy areas (Fig. 4). Cervical lymphadenopathy is usually present. The most common cause worldwide is *Microsporum canis*, although *Trichophyton tonsurans* predominates in North America. Favus is seen in rural areas and is associated with poor hygiene and poor nutrition. Clinically, cup-shaped yellow crusts are seen. The aetiological agent is *T. schoenleinii. M. canis* and *T. schoenleinii* fluoresce green under Wood's light. When sending specimens for culture the yield is higher if plucked hairs as well as scalp scrapings are sent to the laboratory. Griseofulvin is prescribed at a dose of 10 mg/kg for 6–8 weeks for children. It is the only oral antifungal licensed for children in the United Kingdom but in adults terbinafine and itraconazol are routinely used.

Pediculosis capitis (infestation with head lice) is seen worldwide. Nits (oval eggs fixed on the hair shaft) make the diagnosis (Fig. 5) and can be more readily identified under Wood's light. Treatment to all close contacts is required simultaneously. Permethrin, malathion, and synergized pyrethin have all been shown to be effective. Applications should be left on for 12 h, and then washed off. This should be repeated for 7–10 days. A good adjunctive treatment is 'bug busting' which involves combing wet hair for 30 min every third day with a fine-toothed comb over a 2-week period. This practice alone is not sufficient.

Secondary syphilis can present as the classical 'moth-eaten scalp'. However, syphilis may also present as acute diffuse alopecia. Serological tests are advised.

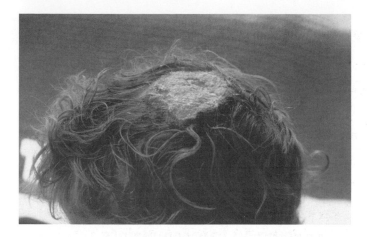

Fig. 4 Kerions in *Tinea capitis* infection. (See Plate 24.)

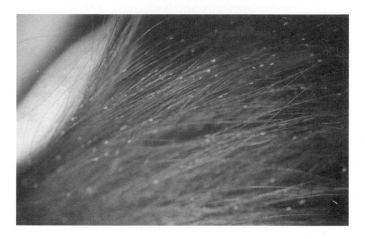

Fig. 5 Nits in *Pediculosis capitis* infestation. (See Plate 25.)

Hirsutism

Hirsutism is defined as growth of terminal hairs under the influence of androgens in women, in areas where secondary sexual hair grows in men at puberty. It is often subjective. Racial differences should be taken into account before launching into superfluous investigations (hypertrichosis is excessive growth of hair for a particular site and age of patient—e.g. maybe associated with naevi or drug administration).

Investigation

If the hirsutism is mild, the menstrual cycle is regular, and there are no features of virilism no further investigation is required. Women with moderate hirsutism with or without menstrual irregularities should be screened for polycystic ovarian syndrome by ultrasonography. Severe hirsutism with a short history or very severe with a long history should be investigated for an androgen-secreting tumour and will need a referral to an endocrinologist.

Treatment

Bleaching, waxing, sugaring, and depilatory creams are useful cosmetic treatments. There is no evidence to support the notion that shaving stimulates hair growth. Lasers are effective if not permanent treatment.

Electrolysis is permanent but painful. Antiandrogen tablets such as Dianette® (35 µg ethinyloestradiol and 2 mg cyproterone acetate) taken for 21 days out of 28, and spironolactone 50–200 mg daily are usually beneficial.

Hair shaft abnormality

If hair loss occurs in childhood, it may be as a result of a hair shaft abnormality. Children who have abnormal hair and other systemic signs should have hair sent for microscopic analysis. Characteristic signs such as pili torti (twisting through the longitudinal axis) may be seen and can be used as a diagnostic aid. There are many congenital and acquired syndromes in which characteristic hair abnormalities provide the easiest form of diagnosis.

Other common hair complaints

Patients will also complain of greasy hair. Uncomplicated grease and scales are likely to be due to seborrhoeic dermatitis. This inflammatory condition is thought to be worsened by the yeast, *Pityrosporum ovale*. Antifungals such as ketoconazole shampoo and tar-based shampoos are effective.

Scalp eczema manifested by scaling erythema and a tender itching scalp is usually responsive to topical steroids in lotion or mousse form, and tar shampoos.

Scalp psoriasis with silvery scaling plaques, may in addition to steroid and tar preparations need salicylic acid to descale the affected areas prior to treatment.

Patients may also seek advice about chemical and physical hair damage from shampoos, dyes and bleaches, hair waving/straightening, backcombing and hot drying, etc. The hair may be excessively weathered or matted and tangled. Stopping the trauma to the hair, using conditioner, and seeking the help of an understanding hairdresser are all helpful.

Conclusions

If the diagnosis is not clear, referral to a dermatologist is advised. Biopsies are always difficult to interpret and therefore should be done in the hospital setting. Many hair problems are chronic and these patients need moral support as well as medical input.

Key points

1. Hair problems are common and immediately obvious. They cause considerable distress.

2. Psychological support is an important aspect of treatment.

3. The diagnosis is usually clear from the history and pattern of the abnormality.

4. Referral to a dermatologist is advised if the patient requires investigation (including hair microscopy or scalp biopsy) or second-line treatment.

Further reading

Dawber, R.P.R. *Diseases of the Hair and Scalp* 3rd edn. Oxford: Blackwell Science, 1997. (Comprehensive textbook.)

Sinclair, R. (1998). Male pattern androgenetic alopecia. *British Medical Journal* **317**, 865–9. (Clinical review by a leading authority on hair disorders.)

Sperling, L.C., Solomon, A.R., and Whiting, D.A. (2000). A new look at scarring alopecia. *Archives of Dermatology* **136**, 235–42.

Burgess, I. (2001). Head lice. *Clinical Evidence* **5**, 1165–8. (Systematic review.)

Website

www.Oxfordhair.org. (Site of international hair federation, also supplies links.)

15.2 Nail disorders

Patricia Sunaert and Eric van Hecke

The nail apparatus develops in the embryo as an epidermal protrusion. The nail plate in humans is a protective covering for the fingertip and toetip. The nail plate of the fingers plays an important role in many subtle finger functions.

The nail plate consists of the keratinized flattened cells of the nail matrix that have lost their nuclei and form a compact horny layer. It is formed by the nail matrix, situated beneath the nail fold and is attached to the nail bed. The matrix is almost completely covered by the proximal nail fold. The part of the matrix visible under the nail plate is the lunula. The space between the nail fold and nail plate is covered by the cuticle. The nail plate shows fine longitudinal, parallel ridges that become more apparent with age.

Fingernails grow faster than toenails. Speed of growth diminishes with age. Complete outgrowth of a fingernail takes 6 months, of a toenail 12–18 months.

Table 1 summarizes the common nail disorders seen in general practice. The diagnosis and management of each condition is set out below.

Nail trauma

Brittle nails

Brittle finger nails are common in women and due to frequent contact with water and detergents. Logical therapeutic advice is the avoidance of water and detergents. Intake of vitamins or minerals is useless.

Ingrowing toenail

Most ingrowing nails are located at the big toe. Predisposing factors are morphological anomalies of the toe, ill-fitting footwear, and excessive trimming of the lateral edges of the nail. The nail plate pushes into the lateral nail fold and causes a painful inflammatory reaction and secundary bacterial infection. Granulation tissue develops. Therapy in the first instance is conservative: correct footwear, correct nail cutting, insertion of

Table 1 Nail disorders seen in primary care

Trauma	Infection	General skin problems	Tumours
Brittle nails	Acute paronychia	Psoriasis	Warts
Ingrowing toenail	Chronic paronychia	Lichen planus	Mucoid cysts
Onychogryphosis	Onychomycosis	Alopecia areata	Fibromas
Subungeal haematoma			Exostoses
Onycholysis			Glomus tumours
Luconychia			Naevi
Melanonychia			Melanomas

cotton wool under the free edge of the nail plate, application of silver nitrate, of antibiotic and steroid creams. In case of relapses, surgical intervention consists of simple nail avulsion combined with use of phenol.

Onychogryphosis

Onychogryphosis of the big toe is mostly seen in the elderly. The nail plate thickens, discolours, and grows in a spiral. Neglect and ill-fitting footwear are possibly contributing factors. In case of major nuisance, extraction and even destruction of the nail and matrix is a therapeutic option.

Subungeal haematoma

Subungeal haematoma is usually traumatic in origin. Therapy consists of drilling an opening through the nail plate with a needle. Subsequently, onycholysis can develop, depending on the impact of the trauma.

Onycholysis

Onycholysis is the separation of the nail plate from the nail bed. It can be traumatically induced, as well by an acute as by a chronic repititive trauma.

Leuconychia striata

Leuconychia, white spots of the nails, are often due to trauma at the cuticula or matrix. It is the most common nail disturbance in children. Parents ascribe it, often wrongfully, to dietary shortages. Therapeutic advice consists of avoidance of repetitive trauma as nail biting.

Melanonychia

Melanonychia are brown to black longitudinal bands from the nail fold to the distal edge of the nail. They are common in dark races but rare in white people.

Nail infections

Acute paronychia

Acute paronychia (whitlow) is a bacterial infection, usually due to *Staphylococcus aureus* although mixed infection of aerobic and anaerobic bacteria are found. Acute trauma, nail biting, and aggressive manicure can cause a portal of entry at the proximal nail fold. Inflammation of the nail fold follows and the nail fold becomes red, swollen, and extremely painful. Eventually pus is discharged. Therapy will consist of warm compresses in the initial phase. In case of abscess formation, drainage will lead to resolution. It may not be mistaken for herpetic whitlow (herpes simplex infection of the finger).

Chronic paronychia

Chronic paronychia is secondary to separation of the nail fold from the nail plate. The cuticula is absent. Inflammation of the nail fold results, which becomes secondarily infected, often with *Candida albicans*, other yeasts, and bacteria. Finally, the nail plate will be involved. The initial pathologic event is an irritative contact dermatitis, due to constant contact with water and detergents, often seen in housewives, dish washers, and bar keepers. Clinically, the nail fold is red, swollen, and slightly painful. Occasionally, there is discharge of a white purulent material. The nail plate shows transverse ridging and green-black discoloration at the lateral edge, probably due to Pseudomonas super-infection. Often, several fingers are involved though not all. Therapy will consist primarily in avoiding contact with water (cotton and vinyl gloves, barrier creams, use of household machinery). Since bacterial and yeast infections are common and can co-exist, use of antibiotics and/or antimycotics seems justified under guidance of cultures. Topical steroid and antimicrobial creams (antibiotic, antifungal-azole, nystatin) and even a course of oral antibiotics (penicillinase resistant broad spectrum) or an antimycotic (azole) can be given. A chronic paronychia of one finger not answering therapy should arouse suspicion of malignancy.

Onychomycosis

Onychomycosis is any fungal infection of the nail (Fig. 1). Tinea unguium is an infection of the nail by dermatophytes. Most fungal infections of the toenails are caused by dermatophytes (over 90 per cent). Yeasts and moulds account for less than 10 per cent and the existence of mould onychomycosis is debatable. Finger onychomycosis is usually a concurrent phenomenon with chronic paronychia. Onychomycosis of the toenails is very common and increases with age. It is rare in children (<1 per cent), is common in adults (2–5 per cent), and reaches prevalences of 20 per cent in those of age over 60.

Tinea unguium is mostly found in people having tinea pedis for a long time. Heat and high humidity (result of wearing shoes) are predisposing factors. The big toenail is usually the first to be affected. In most cases, the fungus starts to invade the nail bed and the ventral nail plate from the distal margin. In rare cases, the infection occurs through the dorsal nail plate or even the proximal nail fold, mainly in immunocompromised patients. Clinically, a subungeal hyperkeratosis develops which can be seen through the nail plate as a white or yellow spot, sharply demarcated, and slowly progressing over months and years from distal to proximal (DLSO or disto-lateral subungeal onychomycosis). Superficial white onychomycosis (SWO) with white discoloration of the surface of the nail plate and proximal subungeal onychomycosis (PSO) with subungeal hyperkeratosis, spreading from the proximal nail fold are rare clinical pictures. All these types of onychomycosis can finally result in a total destruction of the nail plate: total dystrophic onychomycosis (TDO). It is sometimes difficult to distinguish an onychomycosis from a nail psoriasis or a traumatic dystrophy of the nail. Laboratory confirmation of a fungus infection is advisable. Direct microscopic examination and culture is best done with the crumbling material scraped from under the nail plate. Most cultures yield *Trichophyton rubrum* as the causative fungus (90 per cent).

Before taking a decision whether to treat or not, one has to consider the following: the complaint is often purely cosmetic and since many patients are old and on multiple drug therapy for unrelated conditions, antifungal therapy will expose them to serious drug reactions as a result of drug interaction. Finally, antifungal therapy is long and costly. Consequent mechanical complaints can be adjusted with podologic techniques. Local treatment with antifungals is disappointing with the possible exception of amorolfin in a nail lacquer for SWO. The most effective treatment is terbinafine 250 mg daily for 3 to 4 months. The nail is left in place and will gradually grow to full length in 9–12 months. An alternative is itraconazole in three or four 'pulses' (400 mg daily for 1 week with 3-week interval).

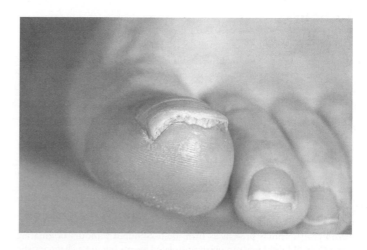

Fig. 1 Onychomycosis (fungal infection) of the nail. (See Plate 26.)

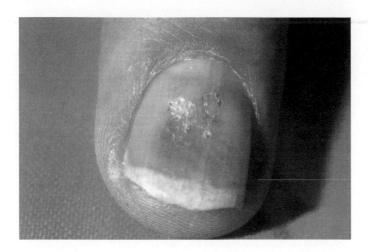

Fig. 2 Nail showing psoriasis. (See Plate 27.)

Nail anomalies in skin disease

Nails are involved in many skin diseases but sometimes the nail changes are the only sign of the skin disease. Diagnosis and treatment are often difficult and require the expertise of a dermatologist.

Psoriasis

Psoriasis frequently involves the nails (Fig. 2). The 'oil spot' is a yellow-brownish discoloration of the nail plate due to a psoriasis plaque under the nail plate. Pitting of the nail plate is very common. Less common are linear transverse red-blue lines, subungeal haemorrhages known as 'nail splinters'. Subungeal keratosis and deformation of the nail plate are seen in serious forms of psoriasis. Nail psoriasis is often taken for onychomycosis.

Lichen planus

Nails are involved in up to 10 per cent of patients, usually mildly. In severe cases, lichen planus leads to atrophy of the nail plate which can disappear totally. Pterygium unguis is sometimes seen.

Alopecia areata

Nail changes are common in alopecia areata, mainly pitting of the nail plate. They point to an unfavourable prognosis.

Tumours

Periungeal warts

Warts can develop at the nail fold (periungeal wart) or under the free edge of the nail plate. Treatments are multiple (salicylic acid plaster, liquid nitrogen, cautery, CO_2 laser vaporization). X-ray and bleomycin treatment have to be rejected.

Mucoid cysts

Mucoid cysts are common and occur mainly at the dorsal aspect of the distal phalanx but can be peri- or subungeally located. They present as soft, flesh-coloured compressable nodules. Puncture of the cyst is usually sufficient treatment. Excision is indicated if there is a connection with the joint.

Periungeal fibroma

Periungeal fibromas present as firm, flesh-coloured tumours originating from the nail fold. They can occur as isolated events but are a characteristic sign of tuberous sclerosis (Koenen tumours).

Subungeal exostosis

Subungeal exostosis is a localized outgrowth of bone under the nail plate. It causes pain by lifting the nail plate. The diagnosis is made by an X-ray. Treatment is surgical.

Glomus tumour

Glomus tumours are benign proliferations of glomus bodies. The tumour presents as a painful blue coloration under the nail plate. Treatment is surgical.

Pigmented lesions

A naevus in the nail matrix may cause a longitudinal pigmented stripe in the nail plate. Melanoma of the nail apparatus is rare. It presents in different ways. A chronic swelling of the proximal nail fold, resembling chronic paronychia, not responsive to classic treatment, raises suspicion of melanoma. The appearance of a blue-black pigmentation on the neighbouring skin (Hutchinson's sign) is very suspicious. Another presentation is a fast growing wart-like, non-pigmented thickening of the nail bed. Formation of a pigmented band in the nail plate may also indicate a melanoma. A melanoma can develop out of an existing naevus. Any suspicion should incite referral.

Nail disorders in non-dermatological disease

Some nail anomalies are associated with non-dermatological disease but their predictive value is limited. Beau's lines develop a few weeks after an acute infection. They are transverse depressions of the surface of all the nails. Clubbing accompanies chronic lung and heart disease.

Key points

- ◆ Trauma and infection of the nail are the most common problems in general practice.

- ◆ Frequent contact with water and detergents is an important cause of nail disorders like chronic paronychia and brittle nails. Appropriate advice should be given.

- ◆ To the unexperienced, abnormal nails are generally considered 'fungal', leading to long, ineffective, and costly treatments. Confirmation of the diagnosis of onychomycosis should be undertaken before starting therapy. Not all onychomycosis has to be treated with oral antifungals.

- ◆ Subungeal melanoma is rare but one should be suspicious when a nail problem does not respond to conventional treatment.

Further reading

Dawber, R.P.R., Baran, R., and de Berker, D. (1998). Disorders of nails. In *Rook/Wilkinson/Ebling Textbook of Dermatology* (ed. R.H. Champion, J.L. Burton, D.A. Burns, and S.M. Breathnach), pp. 2815–68. Oxford: Blackwell Scientific Publications.

Rounding, C. and Hulm, S. (2001). Surgical treatments for ingrowing toenails (Cochrane Review). In *The Cochrane Library* Issue 2. Oxford: Update Software.

Crawford, F., Hart, R., Bell-Syer, S., Torgerson, D., Young, P., and Russell, I. (2001). Topical treatments for fungal infections of the skin of the foot (Cochrane Review). In *The Cochrane Library* Issue 2. Oxford: Update Software.

Evans, E.G.V. and Sigurgeirsson, B. (1999). Double blind, randomized study of continuous terbinafine compared with intermittent itraconazole in the treatment of toenail onychomycosis. *British Medical Journal* **318**, 1031–5.

Bull, M.J.V. and Gardiner, P. *Surgical Procedures in Primary Care*. Oxford: Oxford University Press, 1995. (For surgical procedures.)

Buxton, P.K. *ABC of Dermatology*. London: BMJ Publishing Group, 1998.

15.3 Pruritus

Walter A. Forred

Pruritus occurs in all communities. There are age-related clusters in the young, atopic patient under the age of 10 years, and in the elderly patient, afflicted with xerosis. The symptom of itching is so common, with a myriad of aetiologies, that one cannot reliably estimate prevalence or incidence in the community. The natural history is likewise variable. A number of patients are treated and cured or their symptoms spontaneously disappear. Other patients are treated with multiple therapies to little or no avail.

Itching can be produced by numerous physical and chemical stimuli experimentally (Table 1). Within the skin there are no specialized itch receptors. Rather, polymodal nociceptor nerves at the epidermal–dermal junction modulate the itch sensation. These nociceptors, non-myelinated nerve C-fibres and A-delta fibres, are located in the dermal–epidermal junction. The impulses are then conducted by the non-myelinated C-fibres to the central nervous system. Within the central nervous system, in the substantia gelatinosa, the C-fibres interact with spinal interneurones and A-fibres. When scratching stimulates the A-fibres, they inhibit the C-fibres, thus reducing the itch sensation.[1] This reduction of itch may be effected by the release of endorphins by the A-delta fibres. Curiously, though, endorphins may in turn produce itching.

Pruritus, or itching, is probably the most common dermatological reason for patients to present to the physician. It is difficult to treat itching. For centuries, many treatments have been tried, some with limited success and others without. There is no one simple answer to the question of what causes pruritus and with what to treat it.

Aetiology

The aetiologies of pruritus are myriad. For simplicity, they are categorized as localized or cutaneous causes, generalized or systemic causes, and psychogenic or neurotic causes. They are summarized in Table 2.

Table 1 Chemical mediators of pruritus

Amines	Histamine, serotonin, dopamine, adrenalin, melatonin
Proteases	Tryptases, chymases, carboxypeptidases, papain, kallikrein
Opioids	Morphine, endorphin
Eicosanoids	Prostaglandin-E_2, prostaglandin-H_2
Cytokines	IL-1 to IL-11, TNF-α and TNF-β
Neuropeptides	Substance P (SP), neurotensin, calcitonin gene-related peptide, neurokinin A

Cutaneous causes

Common irritants

Irritants producing local inflammation and pruritus may cause contact dermatitis. Common aetiologies of contact dermatitis include plants (e.g. poison ivy) rubber, wool, nickel, or topically applied 'caine' anaesthetics.

Infestations and bites

Scabies can cause moderate to severe itching. Sea bather's eruption (due to jellyfish larvae) and other insect bites frequently trigger itching.

Xerosis

Xerosis, or dry skin, is the most common instigator of pruritus. Moderate to severe itching characterizes xerosis. Bathing too often, old age, and high temperatures with low humidity may be contributing factors. The elderly are particularly afflicted with xerosis.

Dermatoses

Atopic dermatitis affects one in 20 pre-school children. The most distressing symptom of atopic dermatitis is pruritus. Atopic dermatitis results in lichen simplex chronicus which is a localized disorder of the skin. Repeated scratching produces lichenification of the skin. These pruritic patches lead to more scratching and thus more lichenification in a vicious cycle. Pruritic vesicles followed by scaling, fissures, and lichenification characterize dyshidrotic eczema. The hands and feet are most often affected.

Other cutaneous causes

Anogenital pruritus is a difficult condition to treat. Infestations, psoriasis, and dermatophytosis should be excluded as causes. Other aetiologies include neurodermatitis, oral antibiotics, atopic dermatitis, beer drinking, haemorrhoids, soiling, and colorectal cancer. Very frequently, the patient has self-treated to excess, exacerbating the problem.

Systemic causes

Drugs

Drugs most often produce pruritus by a cholestatic mechanism. These include anabolic steroids, cephalosporins, chlorpropamide, cimetidine, erythromycin estolate, gold, non-steroidal anti-inflammatory drugs (NSAIDs), nicotinic acid, oral contraceptives, penicillin, phenothiazines, phenytoin, progestins, and tolbutamide. Many other drugs can also produce pruritus. Other pharmacological agents act on the C-polymodal nociceptors to produce the itch sensation. These include alcohol, cocaine, chloroquine, heroin, morphine, and meperidine.

Endocrine

Hyper- and hypothyroidism can bring about pruritus. This may be secondary to the associated xerosis with these ailments. Carcinoid syndrome frequently manifests as pruritus when there are high levels of circulating serotonin and/or histamine.

Table 2 Causes of pruritus

Cutaneous	Systemic	Psychogenic
Irritants	Drugs	Delusions of parasitosis
Infestations and bites	Liver disorders	Psychogenic pruritus
Dry skin	Thyroid disease	Neurotic excoriation
Anogenital disorders[a]	Renal failure	
	Pregnancy	
	Infection	
	Malignancy	
	Iron deficiency	
	Aquagenic[a]	

[a] See text.

Hepatic

Cholestasis, whether intrahepatic or extrahepatic can cause pruritus. Intrahepatic aetiologies include primary biliary cirrhosis, drug use, hepatitis, and sclerosing cholangitis. Extrahepatic causes are due to obstruction of the biliary tree from calculi, scarring, or malignancy.

Malignancy

Many types of malignancy can cause pruritus. Included in the list are visceral cancers, mycosis fungoides, multiple myeloma, central nervous system tumours, lymphoma, leukaemia, and occult tumours.

Renal failure

Renal failure probably causes pruritus through secondary hyperparathyroidism that is associated with the disorder. The majority of patients receiving haemodialysis have pruritus.

Infection

The classic infective aetiologies of pruritus include varicella and rubella. HIV, *Giardia lamblia*, and systemic parasitosis may also be infective aetiologies.

Pregnancy

Pruritus gravidarum is a common problem. It consists of intense, generalized pruritus in the absence of skin lesions. The onset is late in pregnancy and disappears with delivery. It is due to cholestasis and increased circulating bile salts. The second pregnancy-related cause of itching is pruritic urticarial plaques of pregnancy (PUPP). There are urticarial plaques on the trunk and proximal extremities. It occurs in the third trimester, usually in primigravida women.

Other systemic causes

Many other causes of pruritus exist. Iron deficiency is a reversible cause of pruritus. Perhaps one of the most frustrating is aquagenic pruritus wherein pruritus is induced by contact of the skin with water. It may occur with polycythemia vera, Hodgkin's disease, or mastocytosis. In pure aquagenic pruritus, the sexes are affected equally and the population is young to middle aged. A family history of aquagenic pruritus exists in two-thirds of patients. The itching begins when the skin is in contact with water and lasts for 1–2 h. A separate form of aquagenic pruritus affects elderly women without a family history of the malady. It occurs in the winter and the symptoms last for 10–20 min.

Psychogenic causes

Delusions of parasitosis

Psychotic patients with schizophrenia may have delusions of parasites or insects crawling on their skin (formication). These delusions are also observed in ethanol withdrawal syndrome.

Psychogenic pruritus

Pruritus may occur at the mere mention of insects crawling on the skin. Frequently, the clinic staff will scratch after a patient with scabies has been to the clinic. Likewise, the weak stimulation of clothing lightly rubbing on the skin has caused pruritus in some patients (remember the itchy wool clothing from childhood).

Neurotic excoriation

Neurodermatitis is most frequently seen on the dorsum of the foot and the medial aspect of the ankle. The itch–scratch cycle is continual, even occurring at night. Chronic lichenification and dermal pigmentary changes are often noted in the affected areas.

Making a diagnosis

The most important aspect of the diagnosis of pruritus is a thorough history and physical examination. Failure to take the time to obtain a detailed history will lead the examiner astray. Important historical points include localization and extent of the itch. Elicit the quality of the sensation and its severity. What was the time of occurrence, the duration of the symptom and its periodicity? Have there been any provocative factors, ingestions of new or different food or medications, occupational exposure, or travel exposure? Has the home environment changed (new pets or hobbies) and do other household members itch? Has there been emotional stress or a history of a previous skin disorder or allergy?

A complete physical examination is necessary to exclude internal diseases. A meticulous examination of the skin is crucial to identify such occult signs as a small cluster of vesicles or a single scabetic burrow. The examiner should make note of changes in the skin, hair, or mucous membranes. Exact descriptions of palpability, colour, size, margins, configuration, location, and extent of the lesions aid in differentiation of localized versus generalized pruritus. Recording these dermal findings with accurate drawings or photographs may be of help when reviewing the case.

In cases of localized pruritus, simple laboratory tools are necessary. These include a potassium hydroxide (KOH) fungal preparation of skin scrapings or a plain skin scraping to identify scabies. Frequently dermal biopsy is useful in the definitive diagnosis of a dermal lesion.

In generalized pruritus, a broad approach to significant internal diseases is warranted. This includes obtaining a complete blood cell count with manual differential, thyroid function tests, hepatic profile, blood chemistries (complete and basic metabolic profiles), HIV, chest X-ray, urinalysis, and stool for ova, parasites, and blood. Other more specialized studies such as computerized tomography (CT) of the chest, abdomen, and pelvis or mammography may be indicated by history and physical examination in some instances.

Management

Optimal therapy for generalized pruritus is treatment of the underlying cause or avoidance of the insulting agent. If, however, there is no treatment or no underlying aetiology defined, non-specific palliative therapies may be applied. Precipitating factors should be avoided.

Topical treatment

Topical treatment is commonly the first step in the management of itching. The most important of these treatments is hydration of the skin. The cooling effect of menthol or zinc oxide and the anaesthetic effects of phenol (in calamine lotion), camphor, or one of the 'caine' drugs is usually attempted initially. A cream formulated with camphor, menthol, and eucalyptus has been used for nearly a century for the treatment of the itch of sunburn. These topical agents are effective in the management of sunburn and have usually been tried by the patient before seeking consultation with the physician. Grandmother has usually prescribed baking soda baths, which supply hydration of the skin, helping with the itch. Topical low-potency corticosteroids may be of benefit for short-term treatment but are to be avoided chronically. They are effective only if there is inflammation in the skin. These topical corticosteroids may also temporarily relieve the itch of atopic dermatitis or eczema. Pramoxine hydrochloride can be applied topically for the treatment of mild to moderate itching. The emollients will aid in the relief of the itching in xerosis because they aid in rehydration of the skin. The discomfort of pruritus from post-herpetic neuralgia is often relieved with capsaicin cream topically. Doxepin cream 5 per cent can be used for the treatment of itch without the side-effects observed in orally administered tricyclic antidepressant compounds or diphenhydramine cream.

Ultraviolet B (UVB) phototherapy has been utilized for the treatment of pruritus associated with chronic haemodialysis, psoriasis, and AIDS-associated eosinophilic pustular folliculitis. The light source generates UVB in the 290–320 nm wavelength. Only those experienced in light therapy should use this treatment. The mechanism of action is inhibition of the release of histamine.[2]

Table 3 Sedative effect of antihistamines used to treat pruritus (non-sedating = 1, highly sedating = 4)

Class	Generic name	Sedative effect
Phenothiazine	Promethazine HCl	4
	Trimeprazine	3
Piperazine	Hydroxyzine	3
	Cetirizine	2
Ethanolamine	Diphenhydramine HCl	4
	Clemastine fumarate	3
Ethylenediamine	Tripelennamine HCl	3
	Pyrilamine maleate	2
Alkylamine	Chlorpheniramine maleate	2
	Bromopheniramine maleate	2
Piperidine	Cyproheptadine	2
	Terfenadine[a]	1
	Astemizole[a]	1
	Loratadine[a]	1
	Ketotifen fumarate[a]	1
	Fexofenadine[a]	1

[a] Non-sedating.

Systemic treatment

Systemic treatment is usually undertaken because topical measures have provided no relief. The most common agents used are the oral antihistamines. They block the chemical sensitivity of nociceptors, which facilitate the itch sensation. Either sedating or non-sedating antihistamines may be used (Table 3). Antihistamines are not effective in all cases of pruritus. Tricyclic antidepressants have also been used to treat the itch of chronic urticaria. These agents are potent antagonists at the histamine-receptor sites. Of this class of agents, doxepin has a greater affinity for both H_1 and H_2 receptors than other agents or the sedating antihistamines.[3]

Cholestyramine has been used to treat pruritus of chronic renal failure and pruritus gravidarum. It is administered orally as 5 g twice a day. Other agents found to be effective in the treatment of renal failure associated pruritus are activated charcoal, heparin, and UVB light therapy. Cirrhosis associated pruritus has been successfully treated with naloxone hydrochloride and naltrexone. Naltrexone is an oral opiate receptor antagonist that can be administered on a daily basis.[4] Rifampicin has been reported in the successful treatment of primary biliary cirrhosis.

Transcutaneous electrical nerve stimulation (TENS) is successful in the short-term management of pruritus. The long-term efficacy of TENS treatment has not been studied.[5] In severe nocturnal pruritus, the use of sedating drugs such as phenobarbital or the benzodiazepines are useful. Systemic corticosteroids, particularly prednisone, are frequently used to treat pruritus. These agents treat the inflammatory process in the skin, clearing the pruritus.[6]

Pruritic popular eruption (PPE) of HIV is severe, unremitting and unresponsive to traditional antipruritic therapy. Because pentoxifylline inhibits the production or action of TNF-α, pentoxifylline is effective in the treatment of PPE.

Long-term and continuing management

Many of the underlying causes of pruritus are self-limiting while others are chronic in nature. The more chronic conditions include atopic dermatitis and eczema, xerosis, neurodermatitis, lichen simplex chronicus, and pruritus secondary to malignancy, chronic renal failure, and hepatic failure. The treatment of these chronic conditions can be frustrating for the clinician as well as the patient. In all of these conditions, it is extremely important to provide appropriate hydration of the skin. Although there are no specific treatments that are successful in all patients, an organized trial of

previously proven therapies can be administered. It is important to understand that the pruritus may not be cured but rather controlled.

Pruritus is a symptom of a multitude of underlying problems. It primarily affects quality of life by its continual annoyance. The ability to concentrate and sleep is interrupted by pruritus. Many patients are anxious and depressed by the chronic nature of the pruritus. Patients often have a sense of guilt because of the time and money spent on treating their 'illness'. This impacts their professional, social, and personal activities, disrupting their life.

Key points

- Pruritus has multiple aetiologies.
- Diagnosis is based primarily on history and physical examination.
- Optimal therapy is treatment of the underlying cause.
- Cessation of itching is the principal goal for the patient.
- Skin hydration and topical agents are the first line of therapy.
- Systemic agents are usually antihistamines and/or corticosteroids.
- Pruritus may be chronic and incurable.

References

1. Teofoli, P. et al. (1996). Itch and pain. *International Journal of Dermatology* **35**, 159–66.
2. Phillips, W.G. (1992). Pruritus. *Postgraduate Medicine* **92**, 34–46.
3. Millikan, L.E. (1996). Treating pruritus. *Postgraduate Medicine* **99**, 173–84.
4. Metze, D. et al. (1999). Efficacy and safety of naltrexone, an oral opiate receptor antagonist, in the treatment of pruritus in internal and dermatological diseases. *Journal American Academy of Dermatology* **41**, 533–9.
5. Tang, W.Y.K. et al. (1999). Evaluation on the antipruritic role of transcutaneous electrical nerve stimulation in the treatment of pruritic dermatoses. *Dermatology* **199**, 237–41.
6. Millikan, L.E. (2000). Pruritus: unapproved treatments or indications. *Clinics in Dermatology* **18**, 149–52.

Further reading

Fleischer, A.B. (1995). Pruritus in the elderly. *Advances in Dermatology* **10**, 41–59. (A review of itching in the geriatric population.)

Hägermark, Ö. and Wahlgren, C. (1995). Treatment of itch. *Seminars in Dermatology* **14**, 320–5. (A review of the treatment options for pruritus.)

Krajnik, M. and Zbigniew, Z. (2001). Pruritus in advanced internal diseases. Pathogenesis and treatment. *The Netherlands Journal of Medicine* **58**, 27–40. (An analysis of the systemic illnesses that can contribute to pruritus.)

Leung, A.K.C. (1998). Pruritus in children. *Journal of the Royal Society of Health* **118**, 280–6. (A synopsis of the etiologies and management of pruritus in children.)

Lowitt, M.H. and Bernhard, J.D. (1992). Pruritus. *Seminars in Neurology* **12**, 374–84. (A discussion of the pathophysiology of pruritus. A description of pathways and central processing is included.)

15.4 Pigmented skin lesions

Ashfaq A. Marghoob, Allan C. Halpern, and Carlos A. Charles

Pigmented skin lesions encompass both melanocytic and non-melanocytic neoplasms. Non-melanocytic pigmented lesions include seborrohoeic keratosis, pigmented basal cell carcinoma, and pigmented actinic keratosis just to mention a few. Melanocytic neoplasms of the skin include lesions such as common naevi, atypical moles (dysplastic naevi), congenital melanocytic naevi, blue naevi, Spitz naevi, lentigines, and melanoma. This chapter will concentrate on three common benign melanocytic neoplasms encountered in clinical practice—common acquired naevi, atypical or dysplastic naevi, and congenital melanocytic naevi. All three of these lesions have been identified as risk factors for melanoma (Table 1). In addition, some of these lesions may also be precursors to melanoma. However, while melanomas may arise in association with any one of these potential precursor naevi, the overwhelming majority of these melanocytic naevi never progress to melanoma. The last part of this chapter will discuss some important aspects about melanoma.

Common melanocytic naevi

The most frequently encountered melanocytic neoplasm is the common acquired melanocytic naevus. Common naevi begin appearing at approximately 6 months of age and their numbers continue to increase until the third decade of life. The number of common naevi an individual develops is due in part to two factors: their genetic predisposition and the amount of sun (ultraviolet) exposure received.[1] On average, Caucasian individuals in their third decade of life will acquire approximately 30 melanocytic naevi. It is unusual to develop new naevi after the age of 40, therefore, new naevi developing in older individuals should be viewed with suspicion. Common naevi are usually symmetric, with a homogeneous light to dark brown colour. Their borders are fairly sharp and they rarely attain a diameter larger than 5 mm. The topography of common naevi can be flat, dome-shaped, sessile, or pedunculated. Histologically, common naevi are composed of nests of naevo-melanocytes. The primary location of these nests within the dermis and/or epidermis defines a naevus as junctional, compound, or interdermal.

The presence of many (≥50) common melanocytic naevi is a powerful risk marker for melanoma and their presence can be used to identify persons that may benefit from periodic skin cancer screening examinations (Table 1).[2–4] Furthermore, numerous studies have shown that as the number of melanocytic naevi increases so does the relative risk for melanoma (Fig. 2(a)).[3,4] The ultimate aim of screening is to identify melanoma in its early and thus curable stages. Most of the melanomas that develop in these individuals arise de novo, however, in some cases they can develop in association with a common melanocytic naevus.[5]

Aside from the removal of naevi for cosmetic reasons, common melanocytic naevi do not require treatment unless they develop suspicious changes or become symptomatic (i.e. itching, pain).[6] Obviously, any naevus that begins to bleed needs to be evaluated closely. Individuals who have hundreds of common naevi may benefit from having their cutaneous surface photographed.[7] These photographs can serve as a baseline to which future skin examinations can be compared. The aim of photographically assisted follow-up is to help the examiner detect new and/or changing lesions within a background of many naevi. The physician can thus focus their attention on those lesions at greatest risk for being early melanomas. If the changes were deemed suspicious for melanoma, then an excisional biopsy of the lesion would be most desirable.

Atypical moles (dysplastic naevi)

Examination of individuals in familial melanoma kindreds led to the identification of a particular naevus—the dysplastic naevus (atypical mole). This naevus was observed to occur more frequently in individuals that developed melanoma. Since the description of dysplastic naevi in the setting of familial melanoma, numerous studies have shown that these naevi can also occur sporadically. Approximately 7 per cent of Caucasians have atypical (dysplastic) naevi. These atypical or dysplastic naevi are benign acquired melanocytic naevi that clinically resemble melanoma in that they frequently manifest some degree of asymmetry with indistinct borders, have colour variegation, and often have a diameter greater than 6 mm (Fig. 1).[8] They frequently will have a macular (flat) component, and on histology will have some degree of architectural disorder and cytologic atypia.[9] Like common acquired melanocytic naevi, atypical moles may first begin to appear during early childhood; however, most will not become fully clinically manifest until puberty.[3] Unlike individuals with common naevi, it is not unusual for persons with atypical naevi to continue to develop new lesions throughout life.[3] Both genetics and ultraviolet light

Table 1 Risk factors for malignant melanoma

Naevus type	Risk of malignant melanoma
Common melanocytic naevi	
Many (≥50)	↑
Atypical moles/dysplastic naevi	
Few (1–4)	↑
Many (≥5)	↑ ↑
Atypical mole syndrome/dysplastic naevus syndrome	
No personal or family history of melanoma	↑
Personal but no family history of melanoma	↑ ↑
One family member with melanoma	↑ ↑ ↑
Two or more family members with melanoma	↑ ↑ ↑ ↑
Congenital melanocytic naevi	
Small	↑?
Medium	↑
Large	↑ ↑

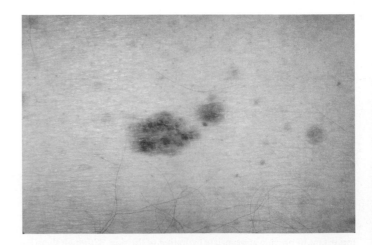

Fig. 1 Atypical mole (dysplastic naevus). (See Plate 28.)

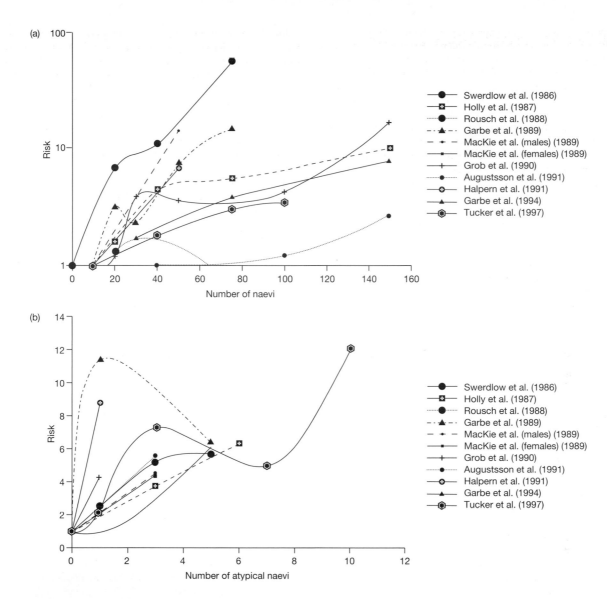

Fig. 2 Multiple studies have shown that (a) the relative risk of melanoma increases as the number of common melanocytic naevi increase and (b) the relative risk of melanoma increases as the number of atypical moles increase.

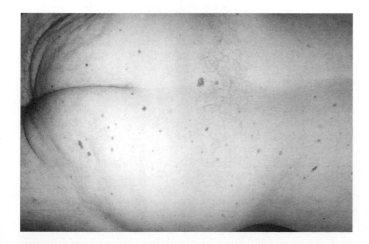

Fig. 3 Atypical mole syndrome. Notice the presence of multiple naevi on the relatively sun protected area of the buttocks. (See Plate 29.)

exposure may be involved in the phenotypic expression of atypical moles. However, though most acquired naevi develop on skin that receives intermittent sun exposure (i.e. back), it is not uncommon for atypical moles to also develop in relatively sun-protected areas such as the scalp and groin.[10] The presence of atypical moles, independent of the total number of common naevi, places an individual at high risk for developing melanoma (Fig. 2(b)).[3,4]

Patients with multiple atypical moles and common naevi have what has come to be known as the atypical mole syndrome or dysplastic naevus syndrome (Fig. 3).[3] Atypical mole syndrome can occur sporadically; however, in many individuals it appears to be an inherited disorder in which the affected individuals begin to develop atypical (dysplastic) naevi during childhood and continue to develop multiple dysplastic naevi over their lifetime. These individuals are at high risk of developing melanoma (Table 1), and these melanomas tend to develop at a younger age as compared to melanomas occurring in non-affected individuals.[3] The 10-year life-table risk for developing melanoma in a patient with the atypical mole syndrome is estimated to be approximately 12 per cent.[8] In addition, these individuals are also at increased risk of developing multiple melanomas. In fact, after the diagnosis of a melanoma, approximately 35 per cent of patients with the atypical mole syndrome will develop a subsequent unrelated primary melanoma.[8] Not all patients with this syndrome are at equal risk for developing melanoma. The magnitude of the risk depends on factors such as the number of naevi, personal or family history of melanoma, and family history of dysplastic naevi (Table 1).[3] Individuals with dysplastic naevi who have at least two blood-related family members with melanoma have a greater than 80 per cent lifetime risk for developing melanoma.[3]

All patients with atypical moles and the atypical mole syndrome should be instructed on the importance of sun avoidance and sun protection. They need to be under life-long skin cancer surveillance, ideally conducted by a health care provider experienced in the evaluation of pigmented lesions. To complement the periodic physician-based skin examinations and to increase the probability of detecting early melanoma it is recommended that these patients perform monthly self-skin examinations.[8] The use of baseline total body photographs may prove to help not only the physician but also aid the patient at efficiently examining their own skin.[7]

The prophylactic removal of all atypical moles is not justified since the risk of any given dysplastic naevus developing into a melanoma is small. In addition, most melanomas develop de novo and not in association with a dysplastic naevus. Thus, the removal of all dysplastic naevi will not eliminate the risk for developing melanoma. The alternative to prophylactic excision is periodic skin examinations with the aim of finding new or changing pigmented lesions that may represent early melanomas. These lesions can be evaluated carefully and biopsied if warranted. Baseline total body photography can greatly assist in the follow-up examination of these patients.

Congenital melanocytic naevi

Congenital melanocytic naevi are melanocytic naevi that are present at birth or become apparent shortly after birth. Approximately 1 per cent of infants have a congenital melanocytic naevus. They usually present as brown, multishaded pigmented lesions with sharply demarcated borders, often with a mammillated surface and hypertrichosis (Fig. 4). Congenital melanocytic naevi generally grow in proportion to the growth of the child. They are typically classified according to the size they attain, or are predicted to attain, in adulthood. Congenital melanocytic naevi that are less than 1.5 cm in greatest diameter are classified as small, medium congenital naevi measure between 1.5 and 19.9 cm, and large congenital melanocytic naevi measure at least 20 cm in greatest diameter.[11] The very large congenital naevi are also known as giant naevi.

Melanoma can develop within any congenital melanocytic naevus, but the risk of developing melanoma appears to correlate, at least to some degree, with the size of the naevus.[11] Individuals at greatest risk are those with large congenital melanocytic naevi. The estimated lifetime risk of developing melanoma in patients with large naevi is between 4.5 and 10 per cent, and the relative risk is between 101 and 1046.[11] Individuals with large congenital naevi can develop melanoma at any age, however, 70 per cent of the melanomas are diagnosed in children under the age of 10. These primary melanomas can occur within the large naevus or within the central nervous system. In 23 per cent of patients who present with metastatic disease, the primary site of the melanoma cannot be found. It is possible that in these patients the focus of the primary melanoma is 'hidden' somewhere within their large congenital melanocytic naevus.

Individuals with large congenital melanocytic naevi are also at risk of neurocutaneous melanocytosis, an entity in which the leptomeninges contain excessive amounts of melanocytes and melanin.[12] Malignant degeneration of these melanocytes results in development of primary central nervous system melanomas. However, benign proliferation of melanocytes within the leptomeninges can also result in serious complications and even death. The 5-year cumulative risk for developing melanoma and/or neurocutaneous melanocytosis in individuals with large congenital melanocytic naevi is reported to be between 2.3 and 3.3 per cent.[12] Patients with large congenital naevi that are at greatest risk for developing melanoma and/or neurocutaneous melanocytosis are those that have multiple satellite congenital naevi, and those in whom the large congenital naevus is located on the back, head, or neck area (Fig. 5).[11]

Congenital melanocytic naevi that are less than 20 cm in diameter have a reported lifetime risk for developing melanoma of between 0 and 6.3 per cent.[11] Some recent studies evaluating medium-sized congenital naevi did not reveal an increased risk for melanoma developing in naevi of this size.[11] However, there are many case reports and series of cases that clearly show that melanomas can and do develop in congenital naevi that are less than 20 cm in diameter and therefore these lesions do need monitoring.[13] In contrast to large congenital melanocytic naevi, melanomas developing in smaller congenital naevi tend to develop at or after puberty.

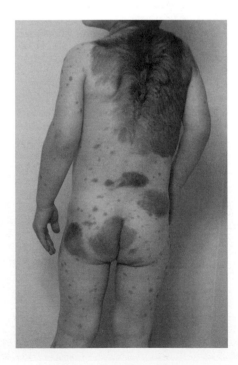

Fig. 5 This patient with a large congenital naevus on the back and with multiple satellite naevi is at high risk for developing neurocutaneous melanocytosis. (See Plate 31.)

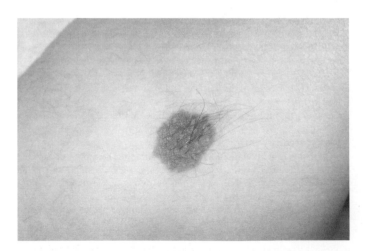

Fig. 4 Medium-sized congenital melanocytic naevus. (See Plate 30.)

For congenital naevi less than 1.5 cm in diameter, the risk of developing melanoma is considered to be low enough that prophylactic removal of these lesions is not warranted.[14] However, if a small congenital naevus develops suspicious changes, becomes symptomatic, or is irregular, then an excisional biopsy may be justified.

The management of patients with congenital melanocytic naevi needs to be tailored for each patient and naevus. Surgical removal of congenital naevi, especially large or clinically atypical congenital naevi, may lower the risk for developing melanoma. However, excision cannot eliminate the risk since it is sometimes impossible and often impractical to remove every naevus cell and melanomas have developed from remnant naevus cells. Furthermore, surgical excision does not eliminate the risk of developing extracutaneous melanomas as can occur in patients with neurocutaneous melanocytosis. If surgical excision is selected as the treatment of choice, it should ideally address the risk of malignant transformation, achieve satisfactory cosmetic results, and maintain adequate function. An alternative to prophylactic excision; especially for those naevi that are uniform, light coloured, even textured, and without nodules; is close clinical surveillance. Any changes suspicious for melanoma should be biopsied and appropriately treated. Baseline photographs of the naevus can be utilized for comparison during subsequent skin examinations to help detect subtle changes within these naevi. For those patients at increased risk for neurocutaneous melanocytosis, obtaining a screening MRI scan of the brain should be considered.

Melanoma

Melanoma, a malignancy derived from the pigment producing cells of the skin known as the melanocytes, is the deadliest form of skin cancer. The incidence of melanoma continues to rise and despite advances made in chemotherapy and immunotherapy, the prognosis for advanced disease remains poor. The key to survival is early detection and surgical excision of localized cutaneous melanoma.

Both genetics and the environment play important roles in the pathogenesis of melanoma. In addition to common melanocytic naevi, dysplastic naevi and congenital melanocytic naevi, other factors associated with a heightened risk for developing melanoma include fair skin, freckles, red hair, blond hair, light coloured eyes, a tendency to sunburn, an inability to tan, and a family history of melanoma. Intermittent bursts of intense ultraviolet radiation exposure appear to be the most important environmental risk factor for melanoma.

Any new, changing, or symptomatic pigmented lesion should be examined closely.[6] The clinical signs of early melanoma can be remembered by the 'ABCDE' rule. Melanomas will frequently manifest some or all of the following features: *a*symmetry, *b*order irregularity, *c*olour variegation,

changing *d*iameter, and *e*nlargement (Fig. 6). However, some melanomas may lack these features. If after careful inspection of the suspect pigmented lesion a diagnosis of melanoma cannot be ruled out then a biopsy should be performed. The preferred method of biopsy is a total excision biopsy. The pathologist should be requested to step-section the specimen. Step-sectioning may help detect a focus of melanoma occurring within an otherwise benign naevus (i.e. dysplastic naevus). Furthermore, by minimizing sampling error, step-sectioning helps to determine the maximum tumour thickness (i.e. Breslow thickness). The Breslow thickness is one of the most important predictors of survival and the depth of the tumour also dictates the extent of surgery that may be required. The current recommendation is that melanomas less than 1 mm in thickness be excised with a 1 cm margin of normal skin, and tumours greater than 1 mm should be excised with a 2–3 cm margin. In addition, patients with melanomas greater than 1 mm in Breslow thickness may be candidates for sentinel lymph-node biopsy. Patients with documented lymph-node metastasis may undergo therapeutic lymph-node dissection. Subsequently, these patients may be eligible for adjuvant therapy with interferon and/or experimental melanoma vaccine. Patients with distant metastasis (i.e. liver, lung, brain, soft tissue, etc.) may benefit from chemotherapy.

Patients with a history of melanoma are at increased risk for developing new primary skin cancers. Thus they should have skin cancer surveillance examinations performed at regular intervals throughout their life so as to detect early, localized metastatic disease and to help detect new primary melanoma and non-melanoma skin cancers at an early stage.

Conclusions

Common melanocytic naevi, dysplastic (atypical) naevi, and congenital melanocytic naevi are relatively prevalent lesions that are likely to be encountered by all general practitioners. It is imperative that the examining physician be aware of the significance of these benign pigmented melanocytic naevi. Persons with these melanocytic naevi are at increased risk for developing melanoma. Once these persons are identified, skin cancer screening and primary prevention (i.e. avoidance and protection from excessive ultraviolet exposure) efforts can be directed towards them. It is hoped that these efforts will help detect early and thus curable melanomas and lead to a decrease in the melanoma mortality rate.

Key points

- ◆ People with melanocytic naevi are at increased risk of developing malignant melanoma and should be offered advice on sun exposure and self-examination.

- ◆ The clinical signs of melanoma can be remembered by the ABCDE rule: *a*symmetry, *b*order irregularity, *c*olour variegation, changing *d*iameter and *e*nlargement.

- ◆ Some melanomas lack ABCDE features—if in doubt undertake excision biopsy or refer.

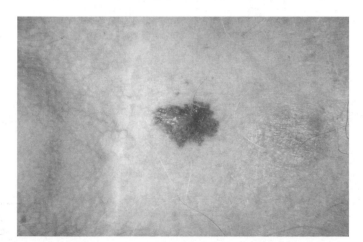

Fig. 6 Malignant melanoma demonstrating some of the 'ABCD' features of melanoma. (See Plate 32.)

References

1. **Kelly, J.W.** et al. (1994). Sunlight: a major factor associated with the development of melanocytic naevi in Australian school children. *Journal of the American Academy of Dermatology* **30**, 40–8.
2. **Holly, E.** et al. (1987). Number of melanocytic naevi as a major risk factor for malignant melanoma. *Journal of the American Academy of Dermatology* **17**, 459–68.
3. **Slade, J.** et al. (1995). Atypical mole syndrome: risk factor for cutaneous malignant melanoma and implications for management. *Journal of the American Academy of Dermatology* **32**, 479–94.

4. Tucker, M.A. et al. (1997). Clinically recognized dysplastic naevi. A central risk factor for cutaneous melanoma. *Journal of the American Medical Association* 277, 1439–44.

5. Marks, R., Dorevitch, A.P., and Mason, G. (1990). Do all melanomas come from 'moles?' A study of the histological association between melanocytic naevi and melanoma. *Australasian Journal of Dermatology* 31, 77.

6. Rigel, D.S. and Carucci, J.A. (2000). Malignant melanoma: prevention, early detection, and treatment in the 21st century. *CA: A Cancer Journal for Clinicians* 50, 215–36.

7. Halpern, A.C. (2000). The use of whole body photography in a pigmented lesion clinic. *Dermatologic Surgery* 26, 175–80.

8. Marghoob, A.A. (1999). The dangers of the atypical mole (dysplastic naevus) syndrome. Teaching at-risk patients to protect themselves from melanoma. *Postgraduate Medicine* 105, 147–8, 151–2, 154.

9. Consensus Development Panel on Early Melanoma (1992). Diagnosis and treatment of early melanoma. *Journal of the American Medical Association* 268, 1314–19.

10. Abadir, M.C. et al. (1995). Case-control study of melanocytic naevi on the buttocks in atypical mole syndrome: role of solar radiation in the pathogenesis of atypical moles. *Journal of the American Academy of Dermatology* 33, 31–6.

11. Marghoob, A., Kopf, A., and Bittencourt, F. (1999). Moles present at birth: their significance. *Skin Cancer Foundation Journal* 17, 36–98.

12. Bittencourt, F.V. et al. (2000). Large congenital melanocytic naevi and the risk for development of malignant melanoma and neurocutaneous melanocytosis. *Pediatrics* 106, 736–41.

13. Illig, C. et al. (1985). Congenital naevi less than or equal to 10 cm as precursors to melanoma: 52 cases, a review, and a new conception. *Archives of Dermatology* 121, 1274–81.

14. Bono, A. et al. (1994). Let's stop worrying about pigmented skin lesions in children. *European Journal of Cancer* 30A, 417.

15.5 Acute skin rashes

Lyn Clearihan

The skin, as the largest organ of the body, is prone to insult both from within and without. Its variety of responses are, however, limited, making a clear clinical differentiation difficult between the more than 60 conditions producing an acute skin rash. Good clinical acumen, experience, and a basic knowledge of how the skin responds to insult, aids a speedy diagnosis and provides a basis for managing for best outcomes.

Epidemiology and prevalence

All age groups and ethnic groups are prone to acute skin rashes, although some conditions have a greater predilection for:

- Specific *age groups*—for example, viral exanthems such as erythema infectiosum and roseola infantum are conditions of childhood, while pemphigus vulgaris appears in older people.

- *Gender*—for example acute cutaneous lupus and erythema nodosum are much more frequent in women, whereas granuloma annulare and Sweet's syndrome have more than twice the prevalence in men.

- *Geographic locality*—for example, polymorphous light eruption is more common in those from Northern climes whereas cutaneous larva migrans is quite common in Asia, Africa, and central America.

- *Race*—for example pseudofolliculitis barbae is more prevalent in African-Americans.

Disorders of the skin are among the commonest reasons for seeking a medical consultation. They can result in both physical and emotional problems. In America alone, a skin condition was named as limiting social relationships in 6.8 million people. Acute rashes due to drug reactions add to the costs of care. Although on a community level the problem is small compared to the large number of drugs ingested, on a hospital level the escalating nature of the problem has prompted some to call this 'an epidemic of modern civilization'. Contact or allergic eczema contributes a substantial morbidity to occupational health in Western countries, with an estimated cost to the American economy in billions of dollars annually.

Seeking medical care

The impetus for seeking medical care may relate to whether the patient feels ill or the rash is symptomatic. The sudden appearance (i.e. over hours to days) of a rash may cause concern that the patient has 'caught' something or is contagious, putting friends or family at risk. A 'label' may not always be easy to provide, even though it often eases patient anxiety. By grouping the problem into broad categories, the practitioner can often develop an effective management plan and provide suitable public health advice. Categories may relate to either the most common problems (Table 1), the appearance of the rash or its symptoms.

Making the diagnosis

A holistic approach

Although the rash is the immediate focus of attention, it is important not to lose sight of the whole patient. What does this rash mean to the patient? What are their concerns and why have they presented today with this problem? Knowledge of the patient's background or other medical problems may provide insight to questions such as: does the patient suffer with other known illnesses or are they on any prescribed medications (remembering that a rash can appear after months to years of continual usage); are there any emotional issues that the patient has been dealing with? Establishing whether the patient is ill or not will also affect the likely diagnostic options.

Physical examination

Avoid confining the examination to just the presenting lesion. Asking the patient to undress and examining their entire skin may reveal other lesions or related problems. Mucous membranes and nails may reveal diagnostic clues (e.g. Wickham's striae in lichen planus or Koplik spots in measles). A thorough examination also needs a good light, preferably natural, although the use of some diagnostic aids are best used in subdued lighting (such as a Wood's light).

Three attributes of specific lesions should be considered:

- Pattern recognition and the distribution of the eruption.

- Characteristic appearances and the morphology of the primary lesions (if treatment has been given, the lesion may be a response to treatment rather than the primary problem).

- Associated symptoms or signs.

Table 1 Common conditions which produce an acute skin rash

Eczema
Contact dermatitis
Urticaria
Viral exanthems
Drug reactions

Palpation, as well as inspection, is often useful. Induration or thickening are important diagnostic signs, implying the involvement of structures deeper than the epidermis.

The distribution

The symmetry of lesions may suggest either an exogenous or endogenous cause. For example, contact dermatitis rarely produces a symmetrical rash whereas acute eczema will often involve both flexures.

The involvement of specific body areas may provide further clues. A generalized rash that also involves the palms and soles of the feet or the mucous membranes has a limited number of causes. The great masqueraders, secondary syphilis and HIV, should always be considered. An erythematous, annular rash appearing in the same site within a few hours of consuming a particular drug may be due to a fixed drug eruption (the tongue and glans penis are common sites). In many countries, phenolphthalein contained in a number of over-the-counter medications is the offending substance.

Other conditions have specific predilections for certain parts of the body, for example, lichen planus often appears around the wrists and ankles. A papular, itchy rash on the penis is a common manifestation of scabies. A maculopapular rash starting on the head and progressing rapidly (within 24–36 hours) to the trunk is likely to be rubella.

Characteristics and morphology

The morphology of the rash helps differentiate the likely structures involved. For example, the presence of scale always indicates epidermal involvement, whereas the presence of a papule or nodule means dermal involvement. Some understanding of morphological terms is useful for establishing broad categories of conditions and may be useful for the pathologist (Table 2). While a large number of conditions will result in a maculopapular presentation, there are a smaller number that will produce vesicles, bullae or a vasculitic rash (Tables 3 and 4).

Signs which demonstrate particular lesion characteristics may be helpful. For example:

- Nikolsky's sign in vesicular lesions demonstrates the dislodgement of the epidermis by lateral finger pressure or the lateral extension of a bullae.
- Koebner phenomenon involves changes, such as vitiligo, psoriasis or warts in regions which have been previously exposed to trauma.

Drug eruptions can appear in any guise but the most frequent is a symmetrical exanthem like eruption. A full discussion of the commonly implicated drugs are available in the references at the end of this chapter. In most cases, the rash improves on stopping the drug with a few notable exceptions—erythema multiforme major, toxic epidermal necrolysis, and exfoliative dermatitis. These conditions may result in mortality and will require hospital care.

The behavioural characteristics of certain rashes may also provide clues to their diagnosis. For example:

- The herald patch of Pityriasis rosea (this is sometimes mistaken as tinea). In addition, lesions often have a distinct collarette of scale and may be arranged in a Christmas tree (fir tree) pattern.
- The papules and plaques of lichen planus present as violaceous, flat topped lesions.
- The dome-shaped lesions of molluscum contagiosum tend to appear in groups and may be mistaken for warts in the genital area.
- The vesicular lesions of herpes zoster are usually unilateral, following a specific dermatome.

Associated symptoms

Many rashes can produce itch, but only five main conditions cause extreme itch:

- acute eczema/contact dermatitis;
- scabies;
- urticaria;
- insect bites; and
- drug reaction.

Table 2 Dermatological descriptive terms for specific lesions

Flat lesions

Macule—a flat lesion. Not palpable. Less than 2 cm in diameter

Patch—also flat and not palpable. It is greater than 2 cm in diameter

Raised lesions

Papule—this is an elevated lesion that can be palpated above normal skin. It is less than 1 cm in diameter

Nodule—these are usually 1–5 cm in diameter and are raised above the surrounding skin

Plaque—this is also elevated. It has a flat top and edges are either distinct or blend into surrounding skin. They are larger than 1 cm in diameter

Cystic lesions

Vesicles—raised, fluid-filled lesions, less than 1 cm in diameter

Pustules—a vesicle with a cloudy appearance due to the presence of leucocytes. May indicate infection but not always

Bulla—a raised fluid filled lesion which is greater than 1 cm in diameter

Table 3 Infectious causes to consider in the differential diagnosis of an acute skin rash

Maculopapular[a] (including plaques and nodules)	Vesicular[a] (including pustules and bullae)	Purpuric or generalized erythema
Candida	Folliculitis	Cellulitis
Epstein–Barr virus	Furuncles/carbuncles	Erysipelas
Enteroviruses—viral exanthems in children	Hand, foot, and mouth disease	Gonococcaemia
Erythema infectiosum—5th disease	Herpes simplex	Meningococcaemia
Gianotti–Crosti syndrome	Herpes zoster	Rocky mountain spotted fever
Measles	Impetigo	Scalded staphylococcal syndrome
HIV	Molluscum contagiosum	Septicaemia
Rickettsial infections	Neonatal congenital syphilis	
Roseola infantum—6th disease		
Rubella		
Scarlet fever		
Secondary syphilis		
Tinea		
Tinea versicolour		

[a] These forms may occur either with or without erythema.

Table 4 Other conditions to consider in the differential diagnosis of an acute skin rash (drug reactions may present in any morphological form)

Maculopapular (including plaques and nodules)	Vesicular (including pustules and bullae)	Purpuric or generalized erythema
Acute cutaneous lupus erythematous	Acute eczema	Erythema nodosum
Acute cutaneous paraneoplastic syndrome	Acute cutaneous paraneoplastic syndrome	Henoch–Schonlein purpura
Erythema multiforme	Contact dermatitis	Hypersensitivity vasculitis
Erythema (polyarteritis) nodosum	Eczema herpeticum	Pemphigoid
Guttate psoriasis	Erythema multiforme	Stevens–Johnson syndrome
Kawasaki syndrome	PLEVA	Toxic epidermal necrolysis
Insect bites	Polymorphous light eruption	Toxic shock syndrome
Lichen planus	Pomphylox	
Lyme disease	Porphyria cutanea tarda	
Pediculosis		
Pityriasis rosea		
Polymorphous light eruption		
Scabies		
Sweet's syndrome		
Urticaria		

Fever or systemic symptoms are also important. Not all causes of rash and fever (e.g. toxic epidermal necrolysis and Stevens–Johnson syndrome) are due to infective causes but they will be high on the list of diagnostic possibilities. In managing fever in young children, the use of aspirin should be avoided due to its relationship to Reye's syndrome.

History

A dermatological complaint is unique among medical problems in that the physical examination often precedes an in-depth history, however integrating the history with the examination is often practical and time saving. This can be supplemented by a more detailed history once a differential diagnosis is in mind. The following 10 questions will cover the core areas of interest:

1. Is the rash itchy?
2. How long has it been present/when did it develop?
3. Has this happened before? If so, how long did it last?
4. What were you doing at the time it started?
5. Have you been unwell recently/do you feel sick now?
6. Does anyone else you know have anything similar?
7. Have you treated it or has it changed in character or distribution since it started?
8. Are you taking any medications, or been on any in the last month?
9. Have you been travelling recently or had unprotected sex?
10. What type of work do you do?

If the diagnosis is still unclear, there are a small number of specific investigations which may help. Unfortunately, the only definitive way of confirming that a rash is due to a drug reaction is by withdrawing the drug and demonstrating an improvement in the rash.

Useful office tools and investigations

A hand-held magnifying lens—this simple instrument is invaluable for identifying lesion characteristics.

A Wood's light—this is a hand-held ultraviolet light. Certain conditions fluoresce different colours (e.g. tinea capitis appears green). However, a negative result does not exclude the condition and it is not helpful on dark skins.

Diascopy—this involves pressing a glass slide against a lesion to distinguish whether it will blanch. Extravasated blood such as purpura, will not but erythema will.

Skin biopsies—may be either shave, punch, or excision and are the most useful diagnostic procedure in dermatology. These are office procedures but need to be performed under sterile conditions. An active lesion needs to be biopsied and if this has an expanding edge a segment of this needs to be captured.

Skin scrapings for microscopy and culture—may be useful for detecting fungi. A Tzanck preparation from scraping the base of a vesicle may be diagnostic in conditions such as herpes zoster, herpes simplex, varicella, and pemphigus.

Patch testing—may help identify the causative agent in contact allergic dermatitis. It is not useful for food allergies and is operator dependent for a useful result.

Serology—may be helpful in certain conditions but needs to be directed toward a specific diagnosis.

Management

The broad spectrum of conditions and the self-limited nature of many, often warrants a wait and see approach, although delay in instituting therapy in a small number of conditions may be life threatening (e.g. meningococcaemia).

General issues

◆ Explanation and reassurance are very important for easing patient anxiety. Patient education with handouts is often helpful especially in situations where school exclusion periods may apply, or there are issues of infectivity particularly in relation to pregnant patients.

◆ Symptomatic advice, again supported by patient handouts may be helpful. Simple suggestions such as avoiding hot showers or the benefits of frequent tepid baths to relieve the itch of a pruritic rash are useful. Products containing menthol and phenol will often be valuable for their soothing properties. In acute dermatoses, using a soap substitute and a wet dressing (either as a soak or a lotion) can be of immediate benefit. Identifying the causative agent and removing the patient from further contact are essential for effective management in contact dermatitis. This, plus the use of an oral antihistamine, help symptoms in acute urticarias.

◆ Empirical therapy with topical steroids may be used even without a clear diagnosis. This can cause problems such as tinea incognito or may alter the appearance of the original rash making a clinical diagnosis difficult. For these reasons, this practice should be avoided.

Specific issues

◆ Topical corticosteroids have transformed the management of acute inflammatory dermatoses. There are numerous preparations available. These are categorized into groups depending on increasing strength and potency. In terms of acute rashes, it is better to be aggressive but remember to avoid using high potency steroids on the face, flexures, and on infants. Also avoid ointments on weeping areas. Giving an explanation of the reasons for use and the need for short-term treatment is more likely to increase compliance. As the rash improves, concurrent use of emollients may reduce the need, or frequency of use, of topical steroids.

◆ How much cream? A 30 g tube will cover the entire body. In advising patients on the amount to apply, use of the finger tip unit (FTU) may be helpful. This is the amount of cream that will cover a fingertip to the distal interphalangeal joint and is roughly 0.5 g. The face and neck will need 2.5 FTU whereas the leg requires 6 and an arm (excluding the hand) requires 3 FTU. Match the vehicle (i.e. lotion, gel, cream, or ointment) to the lesion, skin type, and area of the body involved.

◆ The development of antiviral agents (acyclovir, 800 mg five times per day, famciclovir, 250 mg t.d.s and valaciclovir, 1000 mg t.d.s) have provided real benefits in terms of shortening the duration of disease and its infectivity for both herpes zoster and genital herpes simplex. Accurate diagnosis is essential as their maximum benefit is achieved in the first 72 hours. These agents are also useful in specific cases of varicella but again have to be used early.

◆ Acute urticaria. Identifying the causative agent allowing avoidance is the most effective management but as 50 per cent of causes are unidentifiable this may be difficult. Symptomatic treatment of the itch, plus H1 antihistamines will usually suffice. In a small number of cases a short course of oral prednisolone may be needed.

◆ Prevention is the key issue for many infective conditions. Global immunization programmes are attempting to reduce the incidence and prevalence of common infections such as measles and rubella. The development of new vaccines such as those against varicella and meningococci offer hope of reduced morbidity and complications from these conditions.

Conclusions

Due to the diversity of conditions that can produce acute rashes, they are likely to be an ongoing problem for the primary care practitioner in the twenty-first century. For many conditions, prevention holds the key to effective management but as the number of drugs available in the community increases and the range of potential environmental toxins and allergens does likewise, drug reactions and the prevalence of contact dermatitis are likely to be a continuing problem. Atopic dermatitis still offers mystery as to its cause. Urticaria can be distressing and in the majority of cases a cause is difficult to elucidate. The development of a number of new vaccines may see the eradication of a number of infections but effective global immunization campaigns are still needed.

Future aids in refining the diagnosis and better preventive strategies are likely to be the ongoing thrusts of care for this ubiquitous group of problems.

Key points

1. Acute skin rashes are common problems in the community and primary care.

2. Using broad categories and remembering that common things occur commonly is helpful in establishing the diagnosis.

3. Drug reactions are ubiquitous—virtually any type of rash may be due to a drug.

4. Have a high index of suspicion for the great chameleons, secondary syphilis and HIV.

5. Skin biopsy is one of the most useful tools in establishing the diagnosis.

6. Always have a diagnosis in mind before starting treatment.

Further reading

Bigby, M. (2001). Rates of cutaneous reactions to drugs. *Archives of Dermatology* **6**, 765–70.

Buxton, P.K. *ABC of Dermatology. Hot Climates Edition*. London: BMJ Books, 1999.

Fitzpatrick, T.B. et al. *Color Atlas and Synopsis of Clinical Dermatology*. New York: McGraw-Hill, 2001.

Friedman, P.S. (1998). Allergy and the skin. 11—contact and atopic eczema. *British Medical Journal* **316**, 1226–9.

Habif, T.P. et al. *Skin Disease. Diagnosis and Treatment*. St Louis MO: Mosby, 2001.

Lawley, T.J. and Yancey, K.B. (2000). Alterations in the skin. In *Harrison's Principles of Internal Medicine* 15th edn. (ed. E. Braunwald et al.), pp. 305–9. New York: McGraw Hill.

Murtagh, J. *General Practice*. Sydney: McGraw-Hill, 1998.

Resnick, S.D. (1997). New aspects of exanthematous diseases in childhood. *Dermatology Clinics* **2**, 257–66.

Ryan, T.J. (1996). Diseases of the skin. In *Oxford Textbook of Medicine* 3rd edn. (ed. D.J. Weatherall, G.G. Ledingham, and D.A. Warrell), pp. 3703–33. Oxford: Oxford Medical Publications.

Shah, M., Lewis, F.M., and Gawkrodger, D.J. (1997). Patch testing in children and adolescents: five years' experience and follow up. *Journal of the American Academy of Dermatology* **37**, 964–8.

15.6 Chronic skin rashes

Richard Anstett

This chapter deals with four common and extremely important conditions in primary care—lichen simplex, rosacea, lichen planus, and seborrhoeic dermatitis. Each condition causes chronic skin lesions that can impact substantially on quality of life. It is therefore important that they are recognized and managed appropriately by the general practitioner.

Lichen simplex chronicus

Lichen simplex chronicus, previously referred to as neurodermatitis, is an eczematous rash that occurs from repeated scratching in a localized area of the body (Fig. 1). The areas involved include those easily reached such as wrists and ankles, the upper back, the genital and perianal area, and the back of the ear.

The condition is primarily a problem of adults but may be seen in children who have eczema and may contribute to bacterial overgrowth in

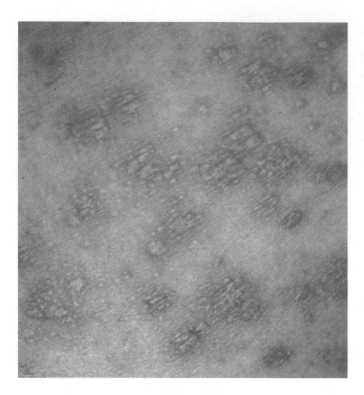

Fig. 1 An eczematous rash or lichen planus. (See Plate 33.)

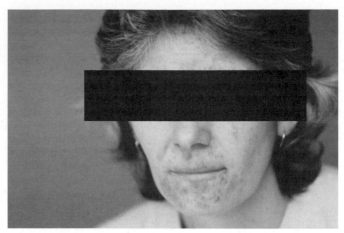

Fig. 2 Rosacea characterized by papules and papulopustules on the face. (See Plate 34.)

children due to chronic irritation. Since the condition is initiated by the itch–scratch cycle, there is no particular predilection for the condition on the basis of gender, race, or living circumstance.

The most plausible explanation for the condition is that an individual finds a particular part of his/her body itchy. Scratching the itch is pleasurable so the behaviour continues until a localized patch of dermatitis develops. A differential diagnosis should include any systemic cause of pruritus such as advanced liver disease, as well as dermatologic conditions including nummular eczema, contact dermatitis, and in particular in tropical settings, a variety of fungal infections.

History is critical, although some patients may be reticent about admitting to a 'self-inflicted lesion'. Since the lesions have the appearance of any chronic dermatitis with scaling leading to lichenification, the typical locations become important in the differential diagnosis. Biopsy and histologic evaluation should rarely be necessary.

The condition fits into the category of 'nuisance' relative to the severity of other dermatologic conditions. Dermatologic referral should only be considered if the diagnosis is in doubt or if simple management has failed. Evaluation for internal problems may be indicated if there is a generalized pruritus of unexplained origin and psychological consultation may be indicated if anxiety plays a major role in the aetiology. Patients need to be informed that the cycle will not stop until they cease the itching. Mid-range steroid ointments may be used for 2–3 weeks, although weaker preparations should be considered for the anal–genital areas and for the axilla. Oral antihistamines such as doxepin may be used especially at bedtime to control itching while the patient is asleep.

Health education which focuses on the patient's awareness of the nature of the problem is critical. The use of over-the-counter topical steroid ointments and oral antihistamines may avoid unnecessary doctor visits.

Rosacea

This condition is characterized by papules and papulopustules that appear primarily over the central region of the face on a striking erythematous base (Fig. 2). The stages of rosacea include periods of blushing that eventually become persistent erythema. Eventually, there is the development of the papules and papulopustules, usually around the fourth and fifth decades. In some individuals, a permanent and disfiguring sebaceous gland hypertrophy occurs, particularly on the nose (rhinophyma).

The condition is common in fair-skinned individuals of Northern European background and is rare in dark-skinned individuals. Milder cases of rosacea more frequently occur in women but the disfiguring sebaceous hypertrophy is more likely to occur in men.[1] Rosacea is commonly seen in temperate climates with Caucasian populations and much less frequently in the tropics and in dark-skinned individuals.

A number of co-morbidities are associated with rosacea, none of which have been shown to be causative. These include gastric problems including acid reflux disease, infestation with *Helicobacter pylori*, hypertension and migraine headaches.[2] It is widely recognized that what rosacea patients do have in common is a predisposition to facial flushing. Conditions to consider in the differential diagnosis include acne, perioral dermatitis, folliculitis, lupus erythematosus in a malar distribution. In developing countries, or where individuals may suffer from severe malnutrition, B-complex deficiencies may present with symmetric facial lesions.

The history of blushing and flushing of the face for years prior to the development of papulopustules in a central facial distribution is highly suggestive of rosacea. Acne can generally be eliminated by the absence of comedones in rosacea. The predominantly central rather than perioral distribution favours rosacea over perioral dermatitis. Lesions of lupus erythematosis are not typically papulopustular. The lesions associated with excessive use of topical steroids on the face may look very much like rosacea but can be differentiated by a history of such use. Specialist referral should be limited to cases in which the diagnosis is in doubt or appropriate treatment has been less than successful. Further laboratory or histologic examination is rarely indicated. Only resistant cases need to be managed by a dermatologist. Metronidazol is highly effective as a topical treatment and is available as a cream, gel, or lotion. Clindamycin is also available as gel solution and lotion. Topical therapy should continue for 1–2 months before it is considered unsuccessful. At that time an individual may switch to a different topical or add systemic antibiotics such as tetracycline 500 mg b.i.d. for 1 month, with gradual reductions to a dose of 250 mg daily for another 1–2 months. If potential significant sun exposure is a problem, the clinician may prefer erythromycin. Rosacea aggravated by the use of topical steroids may call for 3–6 months of oral antibiotic therapy before success is achieved. The flushing component of rosacea may be treated more effectively with the avoidance of hot foods and beverages, alcohol, and other substances that produce facial flushing.

For patients with severe or continued recurrences, a very low-dose oral antibiotic such as tetracycline or erythromycin 250 mg q.d. may be sufficient to suppress the condition. Patients should be advised to seek help as early as possible in order to start treatment early in the clinical course of the condition.

Chronic or recurrent facial dermatologic conditions have potential significant impact on the emotional, social, and occupational lives of individuals. Psychological counselling may be important in this regard, as well as public education about the nature and cause of the condition.

Lichen planus

This condition is characterized by violaceous flat-topped papules, usually seen on the wrists and legs and in acute form may cover the entire body. Mucous membrane lesions on the lips or in the oral cavity have a white appearance. Small crossing white lines called Wickham's striae may be noticed and are pathognomonic for the diagnosis. They have a lacy appearance on mucous membranes. They are occasionally seen on the penis and may become generalized. They first appear as pink and as they mature they take on a more purple colour. The development of the lesions tends to be rather sudden and may last 6–12 months, or occasionally, for years. Pruritus may be mild or severe. Lesions may occur at sites of previous injury (Koebner phenomenon).

Worldwide prevalence tends to be slightly less than 1 per cent of the population and no racial predilection has ever been noticed. While men tend to be affected by the condition in midlife, it occurs later in women.

The cause of lichen planus is unknown. A classification scheme has been proposed, identifying three types of lichen planus: (i) idiopathic; (ii) drug associated; and (iii) associated with other diseases. In all cases, cell-mediated immunity plays a major role in triggering the disease. Recently, association of lichen planus with a variety of infectious diseases has been noted including herpes simplex, syphilis, HIV, and amoebiasis.[3] Hepatitis C virus has been implicated in the initiation of lichen planus lesions.[4]

Papular lichen planus may take the form of discoid lupus psoriasis, pityriasis rosea, and Bowen's disease. Hypertrophic lichen planus can appear similar to psoriasis and lichen simplex chronicus, and Kaposi's sarcoma. Oral lichen planus may appear as leucoplakia candidiasis, secondary syphilis, or pemphigus. The diagnosis can be confirmed with histopathologic and immunofluorescent evaluation, both of which are usually unnecessary in the primary care setting and unrealistic throughout most of the world. The appearance of the typical papule of lichen planus in the common distribution of wrists, legs, genitalia, and oral cavity is sufficient to make the diagnosis.

Consultation is indicated if the diagnosis is in question or the lesions have failed to respond to appropriate therapy. Antihistamines are used for severe itching, and relatively high potency steroids are used topically for localized disease. Intralesional triamcinolone may be used for hypertrophic lesions. For generalized lichen planus, prednisone is used usually for 3–4 weeks at a gradual taper. Corticosteroids in an adhesive base such as Orabase may be used for oral lesions.

Since lichen planus may be drug induced, identification and avoidance of the causative drugs and chemicals is important. Identification of life stressors which may have initiated the disease, and appropriate psychological counselling may nullify future episodes. Long-term medical and psychological consequences of prolonged oral steroid therapy may have to be addressed.

Simple lichen planus falls into the category of an 'itchy nuisance' to most patients. However, the sudden onset of a generalized episode of lichen planus may be traumatic and terrifying to a patient and may call for significant psychological intervention. The patient's overall quality of life and occupational capacity may be temporarily affected, not only by a generalized episode of lichen planus, but by the consequences of chronic steroid therapy.

Seborrhoeic dermatitis

In infants, the condition takes on the appearance of yellow, greasy scales commonly seen on the scalp (cradle cap). Similar lesions may be

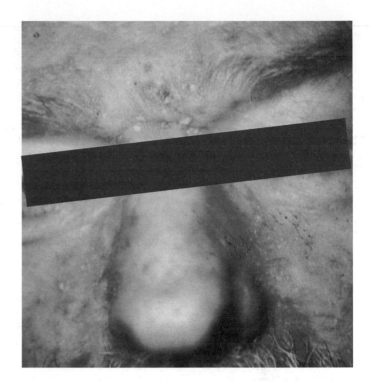

Fig. 3 Seborrhoeic dermatitis present as greasy scales. (See Plate 35.)

seen in the diaper area and axilla. In adults, present are greasy scales and yellow-red macular patches and papules on the scalp and its margins, the eyebrows, the eyelashes, the nasolabial fold, the ear canals, and on the chest (Fig. 3).

Extremely common in infancy, particularly the first 6 months of life, the lesions are occasionally seen in adolescents, more commonly in adulthood, and in geriatric populations. The condition is known worldwide with no particular predilection for gender, race, location, or skin tone. The condition is extremely common in primary care and has been recently recognized as a co-morbidity with HIV infection.[5]

The cause of seborrhoeic dermatitis' unknown, the disease is associated with increased sebum production in infants, but this association has not been found in adults. Areas of the body in which sebaceous follicles are present tend to be the sites of predilection, including the face, ears, scalp, and trunk. The yeast *Pityrosporum ovale* has been implicated in the condition, although no specific causative pathway has been explained.[6] Drugs associated with seborrhoeic dermatitis include arsenic, gold, and cimetidine.

Typical cases are not difficult to diagnose because of the classic distribution and lesion appearance as described above. Classic seborrhoeic dermatitis tends to form diffuse scaling areas while psoriasis produces sharply demarcated plaques. Seborrhoeic dermatitis may appear more like psoriasis in intrigineous areas. The lesions may present as diaper dermatitis in infancy and be confused with Candida. The condition in a perioral distribution may be confused with perioral dermatitis in adults. Essential atopic eczema in infants could be confused with seborrhoeic dermatitis. Extensive or recalcitrant disease should make the clinician think of immunodeficiency and, in particular, HIV disease.

In infancy, parents should be encouraged not to over-treat and limit therapy to mild antifungal or keratolytic shampoos, reserving topical steroids for the most severe cases. In adults, patients need to realize that the condition is chronic and recurrent. For the mildest form of seborrhoeic dermatitis, 'dandruff', using a mild keratolytic such as 2.5 per cent selenium sulphide is usually effective. In more severe cases, topical corticosteroids or ketoconazole as a shampoo may be added two to three times a week. On the ears and scalp borders, a steroid ointment used daily usually produces effective control. This is not to be applied to the face. On the face, 2 per cent ketoconazole applied daily and/or a hydrocortisone cream is usually sufficient. On the eyelids, warm soaks may be sufficient to remove the lesions adherent to the lids. If not, a low-dose hydrocortisone in an ophthalmic preparation is usually adequate.

Patients should be instructed on the possibility of secondary infection and the need for prompt treatment. Since many of the treatments for seborrhoeic dermatitis are available over the counter, careful patient education will assist in the proper use of these treatments and will reduce unnecessary clinic visits.

Chronic facial lesions may have emotional implications related to self-esteem and social success.

References

1. **Jansen, T. and Plewig, G.** (1997). Rosacea: classification and treatment. *Proceedings of the Royal Society of Netherlands* **90**, 144.
2. **Rebora, A.** et al. (1995). May *Helicobacter pylori* be important for dermatologists? *Dermatology* **191**, 6.
3. **Boyd, A.S. and Melder, K.H.** (1991). Lichen planus. *Journal of the American Academy of Dermatology* **25**, 59.
4. **Daoud, M.S.** et al. (1995). Chronic hepatitis C in skin diseases: a review. *Mayo Clinic Proceedings* **70**, 559.
5. **Schechtman, R.C.** et al. (1995). HIV disease and Malassezia yeasts: a quantitative study or patients presenting with seborrheic dermatitis. *British Journal of Dermatology* **133**, 694.
6. **Bergbrant, I.N.** (1995). Seborrheic dermatitis and Pityrosporum yeasts. *Current Topics in Medical Mycology* **6**, 95.

Further reading

Freedberg, I.N., Eisen, A.Z., Wolff, K., Austen, K.F., Goldsmith, L.A., Katz, S.I., and Fitzpatrick, T.B., ed. *Fitzpatrick's Dermatology in General Medicine* 5th edn. New York: McGraw Hill, 1999.
Epstein, E. *Common Skin Disorders* 5th edn. Philadelphia PA: W.B. Saunders, 2001.
Habif, T.P., Campbell, J.L., Quitadamo, N.J., and Zug, K.A. *Skin Disease, Diagnosis and Treatment*. St Louis Mo: Mosby, 2001.
Fitzpatrick, T.B., Johnson, R.A., Wolff, K., Palano, N.K., and Suurmond, D., ed. *Color Atlas and Synopsis of Clinical Dermatology* 3rd edn. New York: McGraw Hill, 1997.

15.7 Acne

Lyn Clearihan

The skin is our window on the world. The way we see ourselves and how others see us, affects how we think and feel. It is hardly surprising then that dermatological problems are one of the commonest medical complaints, and with an estimated 90 per cent of boys and 80 per cent of girls in the 16–17 year age bracket affected, acne vulgaris is amongst the most frequent of these in Western countries.

Although acne is basically a self-limited condition leaving the 'spotty teenager' to just endure a right of passage can have potentially serious long-term physical and psychological sequelae, warranting a very proactive approach to the problem. Although a cure is still not possible, containing

the disease early can result in cosmetic improvement with a reduction of depression and social isolation.

Incidence and prevalence

Although a peak incidence occurs during the teenage years, acne vulgaris is not just a problem of youth. In a significant number of people (especially women), acne may continue well beyond their 20s and in a small number of cases, appears in their 30s and 40s. The latter is linked to the use of the contraceptive pill, cosmetics, or antibiotics.

Girls have an earlier peak incidence (14–16 years of age) than boys (15–17 years), but boys have a higher overall prevalence (although this gender trend is reversed in later years) and tend to suffer more severe forms of the disease. Although acne is found in all ethnic groups, it does appear to have a lower prevalence in non-Western populations.

Natural history

The natural history of acne vulgaris is variable. It can remit and then worsen without obvious cause and in some countries a flare may be noticed during winter. Some individuals experience a few lesions while others experience more severe, disfiguring disease. In general, the longer it persists untreated, the more severe it tends to be, having been noted to result in scarring after only 3 years. There are a number of myths involving acne (see Table 1), the perpetuation of which only adds to the misery of the sufferer.

Costs of care and use of services

It has been estimated that in America alone, 17–28 million people suffer with some degree of acne and that the cost of care for this problem may run into billions of dollars. In many cases, care is sought from family, friends, the media, or other sources rather than a medical advisor. As there are many over-the-counter preparations sold for this condition, easy access and embarrassment may result in many trying self-prescribed products prior to prescription items, adding further to the costs of therapy. Unfortunately, many products only have surface exfoliating benefits and fail to act on the blocked follicle itself making them of doubtful efficacy.

In most countries, medical care for this problem can be accessed from specialists (dermatologists), family doctors, or outpatient clinics. Services, however, are not universally accessible and cost for both care and medication may be a limiting factor. In the post-teenage years, the main users of medical services for this problem are women.

What causes acne?

The actual cause of acne is still shrouded in mystery. The fact that it often runs in families suggests a genetic basis but the pattern of inheritance is not

Table 1 Myths about acne

1. That you will outgrow acne
2. That it is a normal part of adolescence
3. That it is a mild condition without serious consequences
4. That it is caused by diet
5. That it is due to inner toxins that need to be purged
6. That it is due to poor hygiene
7. That sunlight will cure acne
8. That some cosmetics are specifically designed to improve acne
9. That squeezing or picking at pustules or 'pimples' will make them go away

clear. A number of factors are known to contribute to, or be associated with, its development (see Table 2).

Androgens, however, are known to play a central role and their increase in production during the pre-pubertal period is intimately connected to the subsequent development of acne. They contribute to both an increase in size of the sebaceous glands and an increase in production of sebum. The pathogenesis has been studied extensively and the development of acne is thought to be related to the interplay of four pathogenic factors:

- increased sebum production;
- an altered pattern of follicular keratinization resulting in hyperkeratinization;
- microbial colonization of the pilosebaceous unit with *Propionibacterium acnes*;
- release of inflammatory mediators into the follicle and surrounding dermis.

Increased sebum production

Sebum is a mixture of triglycerides, fatty acids, wax esters, and sterols and is essential for the health and hygiene of the skin. Acne severity and sebum production appear to be directly related. The excess sebum causes swelling of the follicle and possibly contributes to hyperkeratinization via a reduction in linoleic acid, which seems important for normal keratinization function.

Hyperkeratinization

Hyperkeratinization results from an altered pattern of keratin production. The combination of increased keratinous material and sebum results in swelling and blockage of the follicle with early comedone formation.

The role of *Propionibacterium acnes*

Propionibacterium acnes is an anaerobic pleomorphic diphtheroid which colonizes the follicle. It is an important part of the inflammatory reaction. It is the main source of follicular lipases. These are released from the bacteria and hydrolyze triglycerides into free fatty acids, which cause inflammation both within the follicle and the dermis when they are extruded after follicle rupture. *P. acnes* also produces hyaluronidases, proteases, and chemotactic factors, all of which may be important in the inflammatory process. Resistance of this bacteria to antibiotic therapy has noticeably increased over recent years due to the more widespread use of both topical and systemic antibiotics.

Table 2 Factors contributing to or associated with acne

Drugs including hormones (glucocorticosteroids—topical and systemic, corticotrophins (ACTH), oral contraceptives, anabolic steroids), halogens (bromides, iodides/iodine), and other (phenytoin sodium, isoniazid/rifampicin, lithium, haloperidol, dantrolene, quinine, vitamin B12)

Occupational exposure to certain products such as *oils, coal tar, chlorinated phenols*

Some *cosmetics* are comedogenic and can induce acne when used over many years

Natural *sunlight* may improve mild acne but can make inflammatory acne worse. Care is needed when prescribing medications that can cause a photosensitivity reaction

Occlusion and pressure on skin (e.g. from a chin strap or resting chin on hand) can be a cause of acne. Sometimes termed acne mechanica

Many women experience a *pre-menstrual flare*

Acne may be worse in individuals who *sweat* a lot

Making the diagnosis

Acne vulgaris is very much a clinical diagnosis. The primary lesion is the microcomedone, the precursor of the comedone (see Fig. 1). Although it is not pathognomonic for acne, it is the essential pathological unit. The following four types of lesions may be found in varying degrees:

- non-inflammatory
    - *comedones* either closed (whiteheads) or open (blackheads);
- inflammatory
    - *papules,*
    - *pustules,*
    - *nodules* (also known as nodulocystic).

Comedones have an intact follicular wall. When this ruptures the contents extrude into the surrounding dermis provoking a foreign body reaction. The resultant lesions depend on the extent of the inflammatory response (see Fig. 2). As acne is a pleiomorphic condition, a mixture of

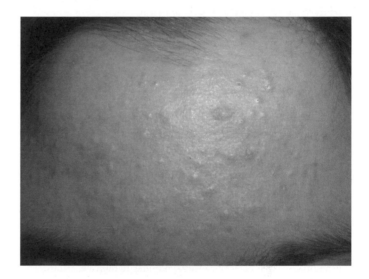

Fig. 1 Mild acne, demonstrating both closed and open comedones. This photograph was supplied by Dr Chris Baker. (See Plate 36.)

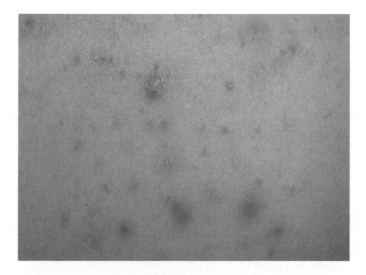

Fig. 2 Severe acne showing papules, pustules, and cysts. This photograph was supplied by Dr Chris Baker. (See Plate 37.)

lesions often co-exist, along with the characteristic scar of acne, the punched out pit. Both the type and number of lesions predominating will determine the classification of mild, moderate, or severe. In inflammatory acne, the condition is regarded as mild if only a few papules/pustules are present and no nodules; moderate if a few nodules are accompanied by an increased number of papules/pustules; and severe if all three types of lesions are present in increased numbers. Nodulocystic is the most severe form.

Acne vulgaris invariably affects the face. The shoulders, chest, and upper back may also be involved, especially in more severe acne (particularly in males).

Distress, embarrassment, and some irritation or discomfort are common accompaniments of acne. The presence of severe pain, however, warrants a specialist referral.

Variant presentations

Acne vulgaris rarely causes a diagnostic dilemma although there are a number of conditions which may cause confusion (see Table 3). It may also present in one of a number of variant forms:

- *Acne conglobata*—a particularly severe form affecting the face, trunk, and arms. It is more prevalent in boys.

- *Acne fulminans*—severe acne coupled with a systemic response with fever, malaise, and joint pains. A hypersensitivity response to *P. acnes*, is thought to be the cause.

- *Neonatal and infantile acne*—this occurs either during the neonatal period or early childhood. Generally, it clears spontaneously but in rare cases may last upto 5 years of age.

- *Pyoderma faciale*—affects mainly adult women and produces large erythematous, necrotic lesions.

- *'Mallorca acne' or acne aestivalis*—although not true acne, as there are no comedones, this papular/pustular rash appears after sun exposure in women in their 20s or 30s. Its distribution is mainly on the shoulders and trunk.

Laboratory investigations are not appropriate for this condition. A notable exception is with a woman in her 30s or 40s with features of hyperandrogenism or polycystic ovary syndrome. In this case, an hormonal workup with free testosterone, FSH, LH, and DHEA-S measurement would be appropriate.

Managing for best outcomes

Instituting treatment as early as possible is associated with avoiding or reducing scarring, limiting disease duration, and reducing psycho-social distress. Treatment protocols are a balance between maximizing outcomes while minimizing side-effects.

Rational therapy dictates directing treatment to the underlying pathological processes. Unfortunately, only isotretinoin, a potent oral retinoid, acts on all four of these. It is highly effective for severe acne but it has a number of problems (see Table 4) and is very expensive.

There are a number of topical medications available in the therapeutic armamentarium for acne (Table 5). There are, however, a number of problems which beset effective management.

- Most of the topical preparations can cause a local reaction with scaling, erythema, burning on application, or itch (especially the retinoids). Reactions will often settle if they can be tolerated for a few weeks.

- Most medications have to be used for prolonged periods of time (4–6 weeks in general) before any improvements are seen and maintenance therapy is needed to suppress acne activity. Poor compliance is one of the major reasons for treatment failure making patient education an essential component of effective management.

Table 3 Differential diagnosis and distinguishing features from acne

Condition	Distinguishing features
Acne rosacea	There are no comedones with this condition and its distribution is centrally on the face
Perioral dermatitis	Tends to affect women. Its distribution is mainly around the mouth and chin but may be paranasally. Lesions are papulovesicular. There are no comedones
Gram negative folliculitis	
Staphylococcus aureus	This involves infected hair follicles and may be anywhere on the body
Pityrosporum	Tends to occur on the trunk
Pseudomonas	Is often related to hot tub use
Pseudofolliculitis barbae	Affects males. Is distributed on the face and tends to be related to shaving
Steroid-induced folliculitis	All lesions are at the same stage of development
Keratosis pilaris	These are follicular-based papules and pustules. Tend to occur on the face, the posterolateral aspects of the upper arm and the trunk
Senile comedones	Also known as Favre–Racouchot syndrome. Comedones are present

Table 4 Oral medications used for the management of acne

Antibiotics	Tetracyclines. These are usually first choice with a starting dose of 500 mg b.i.d, with a slow reduction after a satisfactory response. GI tract disturbances are main side-effects
	Doxycyclines 50–100 mg daily are sometimes preferred to the tetracyclines
	Erythromycin, either 500 mg b.i.d or 333 mg b.i.d, depending on the ester chosen. GI side-effects are common
	Trimethoprim/sulfamethoxazole DS is sometimes tried if above is unsuccessful
	Minocycline. This has the least recorded bacterial resistance but has quite a high side-effect profile (pneumonitis, hepatitis, and in rare cases, pseudotumour cerebri)
Oral isotretinoin	The most potent acne medication available
	Potent teratogen. Female patients must have a negative pregnancy test and be using contraception
	Numerous side-effects. Commonest are dry and cracked lips, dermatitis, and nose bleeds
	Usual starting dose is 1 mg/kg/day
	Course length is about 20 weeks. A second course may be needed if relapse occurs
	Its use may be limited by cost and restricted prescribing
Oral contraceptive pill	Very effective for mild to moderate acne
	Choose an antiandrogenic progesterone
	A specific pill combining cyproterone and ethinyloestradiol has been developed specifically for women to treat acne. It is an effective contraceptive
Spironolactone	This is effective in selected patients, especially if they are hirsute and have features suggestive of hyperandrogenism

Table 5 Topical medications used for the management of acne

Benzoyl peroxide (BPO)	Antimicrobial plus keratolytic May bleach clothing Strengths of 2.5, 5, and 10% plus a variety of vehicles
Azelaic acid	Antimicrobial and keratolytic Useful if patient cannot tolerate BPO Use with caution in darker skinned patients as can cause bleaching of the skin
Isotretinoin and tretinoin	Most potent comedogenic agents First generation retinoids Apply at night 30 min after washing and drying affected area Initial flare on starting therapy is common Additive photosensitivity reactions may occur New formulations are under development to reduce side-effects
Adapalene	Synthetic retinoid Similar clinical efficacy to tretinoin but possibly reduced side-effect profile
Tazarotene	Another synthetic retinoid Seems to have less of a problem with photosensitivity than other retinoids but not available in all countries
Topical antibiotics	Erythromycin 2% gel Clindamycin 1% lotion Meclocycline cream (not available in every country) Sodium sulfacetamide 10% and sulfur 5% (new preparations are looking at subtracting the sulfur component)
Intralesional corticosteroids	These may be useful in severe acne if cystic lesions are present

◆ *P. acnes* resistance to antibiotics is a growing problem and is now seen as an important cause of treatment failure. Antibiotic resistance was not noted until the late 1970s. Resistant strains have now been reported to all the clinically useful antibiotics for acne except minocycline, although recently resistant strains have been noted in the United States. Newer preparations combining a topical antibiotic with either a retinoid or benzoyl peroxide have not demonstrated the same resistance problems to date and seem generally better tolerated.

Possible treatment regimens are outlined below according to the severity of the condition and the degree of inflammation at presentation.

Mild non-inflammatory

1. A salicylic acid wash may be useful although simply washing the affected area with water and non-perfumed soap is sufficient prior to applying topical medications.
2. Topical retinoids are the most effective anticomedonal agents and should be first-line therapy. Start with the lowest concentration and slowly increase if necessary. Topical benzoyl peroxide (BPO) may also be considered as initial therapy or combined with a topical retinoid after 4–6 weeks if necessary.

Mild inflammatory

1. Initiating therapy nightly with a topical retinoid (isotretinoin/tretinoin) is often effective.
2. If this treatment is ineffective after 4–6 weeks, consider adding BPO in the mornings (plus or minus a drying agent such as sulfacetamide/sulfur) or a topical antibiotic (new formulations are evolving which

combine products in the one vehicle). Azelaic acid is a useful option for patients unable to use either BPO or a retinoid.
3. If after a further 6 weeks, the response is still inadequate consider the use of an oral antibiotic (see below).

Moderate non-inflammatory

1. A trial of topical therapy with either retinoids alone or in combination with BPO or topical antibiotics may be sufficient to improve the condition.
2. If improvement is not sufficient, combine a topical therapy with an oral antibiotic, remembering to start with a sufficiently effective dose and maintain therapy for at least 6 months.
3. In a young woman, consider an oral contraceptive with weak androgenic properties.
4. Other medications, such as spironolactone may be useful in selected patients.

Moderate inflammatory

1. Topical therapy using a retinoid in the evening and BPO in the mornings should be initiated.
2. Depending on the degree of inflammation and the number of papules/pustules or nodules, oral antibiotics may be commenced initially or after first assessing the response to topical therapy.
3. For continuing papules, consider injecting them with intralesional steroid (triamcinolone acetonide).
4. In suitable patients, consider using oral contraceptives, cyproterone, spironolactone, or low-dose oral corticosteroids.

Severe acne

1. Topical therapy combined with oral antibiotics can be tried, but the possibility of scarring can be a real risk in this group.
2. Oral isotretinoin is the mainstay of therapy in this group and should be used early to prevent scarring.
3. Intralesional corticosteroid injections may be considered for large cystic lesions.
4. Comedone removal was a common treatment method in the past but is used less frequently today as it may cause scarring and does not prevent new comedones. It is sometimes used to reduce the potential for inflammatory lesions.

What of the future?

Although the overall prevalence of acne seems to have dropped over the last two decades, it is still the source of much misery and distress, being associated with depression, social isolation, and unemployment.

The search for better understanding and more effective treatments are predicated on the fact that successful management of acne is associated with improvements in quality of life. Areas of interest include, developing more targeted therapies through a better understanding of how androgens exert their effect on the pilosebaceous unit; developing a greater understanding of why some individuals are more affected than others; developing better tolerated therapies which require shorter durations of therapy and finding ways to overcome increasing bacterial resistance by an ongoing search for other antimicrobial therapies.

New developments in laser and cosmetic surgery are also offering new hope to those afflicted with acne scarring, although the mainstay of therapy will remain prevention. The human interpretation of this condition is an ongoing source of interest and underpins the search for a better understanding of the social issues which influence its morbidity. Perhaps, more light will be shed on this ubiquitous problem as part of the unravelling of the secrets of the human genome, bringing with it relief from the considerable morbidity associated with it.

Key points

1. Acne cannot be cured but it can be improved and contained.

2. Acne is not an insignificant condition with the potential for serious physical and psychological sequelae.

3. It must be managed in partnership with the patient to ensure compliance with prolonged treatment.

5. Modern treatments are effective, especially oral tretinoin which offers ongoing disease suppression. Its use, however, is limited due to teratogenicity, side-effects, and cost.

6. Each patient will need an individual treatment plan, where the benefits and efficacy are balanced against the possible side-effects.

Further reading

Atkan, S., Ozmen, E., and Sanli, B. (2000). Anxiety, depression and the nature of acne vulgaris in adolescents. *International Journal of Dermatology* **39**, 354–7.

Cooper, A.J. (1998). Systematic review of *Propionibacterium acnes* resistance to systemic antibiotics. *Medical Journal of Australia* **169**, 259–61.

Cunliffe, W.J. and Gould, D.J. (1979). Prevalence of facial acne vulgaris in late adolescence and in adults. *British Medical Journal* **1**, 1109–10.

Glass, B. et al. (1999). A placebo controlled clinical trial to compare a gel containing a combination of isotretinoin (0.05%) with gels containing isotretinoin (0.05%) or erythromycin (2%) alone in the topical treatment of acne vulgaris. *Dermatology* **199**, 2442–7. (This RCT demonstrates the benefit of combination therapy over single therapy in sustained efficacy with some diminishing of adverse events.)

Goodman, G. (1999). Acne and acne scarring: why should we treat? *Medical Journal of Australia* **171**, 62–3.

Goulden, V., Stables, G.I., and Cunliffe, W.J. (1999). Prevalence of facial acne in adults. *Journal of the American Academy of Dermatology* **41**, 577–80. (The importance of this study is the fact that it is community based, giving some idea of prevalence in an adult population.)

Landow, K. (1997). Dispelling myths about acne. *Postgraduate Medicine* **102**, 94–112.

Ross, J.I. et al. (2001). Phenotypic and genotypic characterisation of antibiotic-resistant *Propionibacterium acnes* isolated from acne patients attending dermatology clinics in Europe, the USA, Japan and Australia. *British Journal of Dermatology* **144**, 339–46.

Stathakis, V., Kilkeeny, M., and Marks, R. (1997). Descriptive epidemiology of acne vulgaris in the community. *Australasian Journal of Dermatology* **38**, 115–23.

Stern, R.S. (2000). Medication and medical service utilisation for acne 1995–1998. *Journal of the American Academy of Dermatology* **43**, 1042–8.

Strauss, J.S. and Thiboutot, D.M. (1999). Diseases of the sebaceous glands. In *Fitzpatrick's Dermatology in General Medicine* 5th edn. (ed. I.M. Freedberg et al.), pp. 769–84. New York: McGraw Hill. (This chapter provides an indepth discussion of the pathophysiology of acne and our current understanding plus an overview of management.)

Thiboutot, D. (2000). New treatments and therapeutic strategies for acne. *Archives of Family Medicine* **9**, 179–87.

White, G. (1998). Recent findings in the epidemiologic evidence, classification and subtypes of acne vulgaris. *Journal of the American Academy of Dermatology* **39**, S34–7.

15.8 Psoriasis

Steven R. Feldman

Psoriasis is characterized by thick scaly plaques on a red base in characteristic locations. There is rapid growth of epidermal cells caused by inflammation. The diagnosis is normally made purely on the clinical appearance and distribution of the lesions. The lesions may be itchy, painful or bleeding, and may be associated with arthritis. The skin lesions impact on patients' psycho-social functioning. Most treatments work by reducing the inflammation in the lesions.

Epidemiology

Psoriasis affects about 2 per cent of the population in Europe and the United States.[1] It is somewhat less common in Asians. It may be less common in Blacks, though this may be due to under-reporting. Psoriasis is more common at higher latitudes. It is worse in winter months and is improved with sun exposure.

Psoriasis occurs equally in men and women and can affect individuals of any age. There are two peaks of incidence, one in the late teens and early 20s, the other in the 50s and 60s.[2] Earlier onset is generally associated with more severe disease.

Both genetics and environment influence the expression of psoriasis. The strongest evidence for the genetic component is the higher concordance for psoriasis in monozygotic versus dizygotic twins. About 90 per cent of patients report a positive family history of psoriasis. There are at least four genetic regions containing genes involved in psoriasis, including genes in the HLA group.

Frequency in primary care

The care of psoriasis patients often falls to dermatologists in the United States, much less so in the United Kingdom. While psoriasis is the seventh most common skin condition seen by dermatologists in the United States, it is not among the 20 most common skin conditions seen by US family physicians.[3]

Possible causes

The underlying cause of psoriasis is very poorly understood. This often frustrates patients. Flares and remissions are common, though some lesions are usually present even during the remissions.

Psoriasis may be exacerbated by streptococcal infection and by drugs (including lithium and beta-blockers). Psoriasis lesions may also occur in areas of trauma. This is called the 'Koebner phenomenon'. Excessive alcohol intake, smoking, and obesity may also be risk factors. Psoriasis is also seen in some patients with human immunodeficiency virus infection.

How to make a diagnosis

History

The history in psoriasis is usually of limited value in determining the diagnosis. Useful information for planning treatment includes past treatments and their efficacy, presence of arthritis, and history of alcohol use or other causes of hepatic disease. A history of recent streptococcal infection may indicate the need for antibiotic treatment.

Examination

The clinical examination is essential for diagnosis and determination of the type of treatment. Psoriasis lesions are usually thick and scaly on a red base

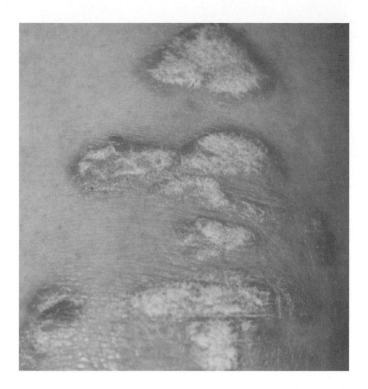

Fig. 1 Psoriasis plaques are thick, red, and scaly. The borders of the lesions are usually very sharp. (See Plate 38.)

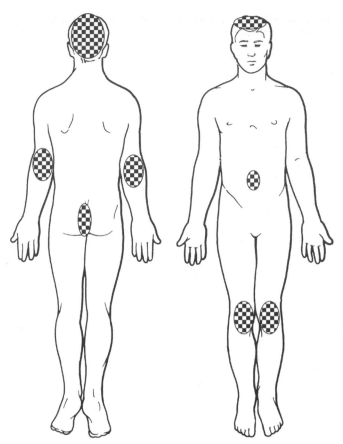

Fig. 2 Psoriasis may affect any area of the skin, but there are some areas that are characteristically involved. The elbows and knees are the most commonly affected sites. The head, umbilicus, and gluteal cleft are also commonly affected. Nail dystrophy may also occur. Palm and sole involvement is not uncommon, can be incapacitating and may be difficult to control.

(Fig. 1). They have a sharp, well-defined border. They tend to occur in characteristic locations including the scalp, elbows, knees, umbilicus, and gluteal cleft (Fig. 2). Psoriasis may also cause pitting of the nails and separation of the nail from the nail bed. When red and scaly plaques are identified in other areas, identification of involvement of the characteristic areas will often confirm the diagnosis.

Psoriasis is usually easily differentiated from atopic dermatitis (eczema). Psoriasis involves the extensor aspects of the knees and elbows, while atopic dermatitis involves the flexor surfaces. Psoriasis lesions are thicker, redder, and more sharply demarcated than atopic dermatitis lesions.

Guttate psoriasis consists of small drop-shaped psoriasis lesions. It usually occurs suddenly, precipitated by streptococcal upper respiratory infection. It must be differentiated from pityriasis rosea. Unlike the irregularly shaped psoriasis lesions, pityriasis rosea lesions are oval and follow the skin lines. Often, the presence of preexisting psoriasis lesions of the scalp, elbows, or knees will help in differentiating these conditions.

Investigation

Laboratory tests are not needed for the diagnosis of psoriasis. Biopsy is only rarely required in atypical cases.

Specialist referral

A referral to a specialist is indicated when the diagnosis is uncertain or to help plan a treatment regimen when first line therapies have not been sufficiently effective.

Referral to a specialist is also indicated for the treatment of pustular or erythrodermic psoriasis. In pustular psoriasis, small sometimes coalescing pustules are scattered over the psoriasis plaques. Erythrodermic psoriasis refers to psoriasis that involves the entire integument. These may be life threatening when severe.

Principles of management

General principles

Many different treatments are available for psoriasis. Patients can be treated with topical therapy alone if they feel they can reasonably apply topical medications to all their lesions. Phototherapy or systemic therapy is used when the psoriasis is too extensive for topical therapy alone.[4]

The psycho-social impact of psoriasis must be addressed for all patients. Realistic expectations should be set. The goal will be to bring the lesions under control. Complete clearing of all lesions is rarely accomplished. Attempting to do so by using aggressive treatments to clear the last few lesions may result in side-effects worse than the disease.

It is usually helpful to combine two or more treatments.[5] The stronger medications are used initially to get the disease under control. Safer medications are then used to maintain long-term control of the psoriasis.

Patients with psoriasis are often frustrated by the chronicity of their disease and limited efficacy of treatments. Non-compliance is a frequent result, further limiting treatment efficacy. Encouraging patient participation in the development of the treatment plan may help encourage greater compliance.

Topical steroids

Topical corticosteroids are the usual initial treatment for localized psoriasis in the United States. Psoriasis is much less responsive to topical corticosteroids than is atopic dermatitis. High (fluocinonide) or super-high (clobetasol propionate, betamethasone dipropionate) potency corticosteroids are used, usually twice daily. For sensitive skin areas such as the face or intertriginous areas, low (hydrocortisone) or medium (triamcinolone) potency topical corticosteroids are used. Ointment vehicles are generally used in psoriasis to help moisturize the dry, scaly plaques.

Other topical treatment

Frequent use of moisturizers can also help improve psoriasis. Tar preparations, especially when used in conjunction with phototherapy, may be helpful. Topical anthralin preparations, rarely used in the United States because of their staining and irritancy, are effective. Topical vitamin D analogues (calcipotriol, calcipotriene) are also very useful. These work slowly and may be associated with irritation. By using topical corticosteroids initially to complement the vitamin D analogue, the speed of clearing is increased while the potential for irritation is vastly decreased. Once a good response is achieved, patients may taper off the topical corticosteroid in order to prevent local atrophy or systemic corticosteroid side-effects. There is the potential for hypercalcaemia when vitamin D analogues are used in large quantity (over 120 g per week of topical calcipotriol 0.005 per cent).

Phototherapy

An effective and very safe treatment for patients with more generalized psoriasis is phototherapy. This can be in the form of sunlight or office-based ultraviolet B (UVB) light treatments. Use of an ultraviolet A (UVA) tanning bed may also provide some benefit when office-based UVB light treatments are inaccessible. Topical treatment to the thickest lesions will help speed clearing.

PUVA, a combination of psoralen (a photosensitizer) and UVA light, is more effective than UVB light treatments. It causes a high risk of cutaneous malignancy, however. It must be done in carefully controlled environments as the combination of psoralen and excessive UVA exposure will result in severe burns, sometimes fatal.

Systemic treatment

Oral retinoids (acitretin) have limited benefit for psoriasis by themselves. They are more useful when used in a low dose in combination with phototherapy.[6]

Some patients with severe disease require systemic medications such as methotrexate or cyclosporine. They are generally used in low doses with the goal of getting the lesions down to a bearable level. Methotrexate requires frequent monitoring for effects on haematologic and hepatic function. Liver biopsy is also recommended at intervals to monitor for chronic hepatotoxicity not detected by serum liver function tests.[7] The use of cyclosporine is generally reserved for short-term use of the treatment of severe flares. Long-term use of cyclosporine results in nephrotoxicity. Etanercept (Enbrel) is effective for psoriatic arthritis, and early data suggest that TNF inhibitors are also effective therapy for patients with psoriasis.

Long-term and continuing care

Once the lesions of psoriasis have been controlled, the frequency of therapy may be reduced. Patients with localized disease may find that the use of moisturizers alone or intermittent use of topical corticosteroids or topical vitamin D analogues are sufficient to maintain control of the disease. Patients with more extensive disease may benefit from sun exposure or a home UVB phototherapy device to maintain control of the disease.

Quality of life issues

Psoriasis impacts on every dimension of health-related quality of life. The magnitude of this impact is as great as that of other medical conditions such as diabetes, myocardial infarction, and depression. Patient may spend over an hour a day taking care of their psoriasis. They may use multiple medications, frequently availing themselves of alternative medicines. About 25 per cent of patients report having wished they were dead because of their psoriasis.

The most bothersome aspects of psoriasis are itching, appearance, scaling, and patients' inability to control the psoriasis. The odours, costs, side-effects, messiness, and time-consuming nature of psoriasis treatments are also problematic and frequently result in poor compliance. Patients often are bothered by their doctor's dismissive, 'you have to learn to live with it', attitude. If one is aware of the specific aspects that are of concern to patients with psoriasis and ask patients about these specific areas of concern, an improved outcome can be expected.

Self-help organizations

Joining an organization of other patients with psoriasis is helpful for many patients where such organizations are accessible. These organizations help reduce the sense of isolation that accompanies the disease. In the United States, the National Psoriasis Foundation (NPF) helps educate members about the disease, helping to reduce the sense of frustration and increasing patients' sense of empowerment. Useful information from the NPF is accessible worldwide (in English and Spanish) through their website, www.psoriasis.org.

Treatment summary

Treating limited areas of psoriasis

Low-cost approach:

1. Start with moisturizers twice daily (BID) and tar ointment every 4 hours (qhs).
2. If not sufficiently effective, add high-potency topical corticosteroid ointment BID.
3. If not sufficiently effective, add dithranol qd or vitamin D analogue BID.

High-efficacy approach (sequential therapy):

1. Start with vitamin D analogue plus superpotent topical corticosteroid BID
   (i) after 2 weeks (or after clearing) reduce use of superpotent topical corticosteroid to weekend use;
   (ii) if the condition remains clear, taper off the corticosteroid;
   (iii) if good control is maintained, taper off the vitamin D analogue.
2. Alternative approaches include superpotent topical corticosteroid every morning (qAM) and topical dithranol or tazarotene qhs.

Treating extensive areas of psoriasis

1. Initial therapy with UVB (or sun exposure or tanning bed lamps if UVB not available). Use in conjunction with tar or vitamin D analogue ointment for greatest efficacy. If there is severe pruritus, add 0.1 per cent triamcinolone ointment to worst areas.
2. Second-line therapies include psoralen plus UVA light, addition of oral retinoid therapy or low-dose methotrexate therapy (generally these are prescribed by dermatology specialists).

When to refer

The primary indication for referral is if the diagnosis of psoriasis is uncertain. Referral should be considered if the psoriasis has not responded to initial measures described above.

Key points

* The diagnosis of psoriasis is made on the characteristic appearance and location of the lesions.

* Twenty per cent of patients also have arthritis.

* Psycho-social impact is large and needs to be addressed.

* Two major types of psoriasis (for treatment purposes) are localized disease and generalized disease.

* Localized disease may be managed with topical agents (corticosteroids, vitamin D analogues, retinoids, tar, anthralin).

* Generalized disease may be managed with phototherapy (including sun exposure) or systemic agents.

* Patients can be directed to www.psoriasis.org for information about psoriasis.

References

1. **Koo, J.** (1996). Population-based epidemiologic study of psoriasis with emphasis on quality of life assessment. *Dermatologic Clinics* **14**, 485–96.

2. **Elder, J.T., Henseler, T., Christophers, E., Voorhees, J.J., and Nair, R.P.** (1994). Of genes and antigens: the inheritance of psoriasis. *The Journal of Investigative Dermatology* **103**, 150S–3S.

3. **Fleischer, A.B. Jr., Feldman, S.R., and McConnell, R.C.** (1997). The most common dermatologic problems identified by family physicians, 1990–1994. *Family Medicine* **29**, 648–52.

4. **Pardasani, A.G., Feldman, S.R., and Clark, A.R.** (2000). Treatment of psoriasis: an algorithm-based approach for primary care physicians. *American Family Physician* **61**, 725–33, 736.

5. **Lebwohl, M.** (1997). Topical application of calcipotriene and corticosteroids: combination regimens. *Journal of the American Academy of Dermatology* **37**, S55–8.

6. **Spuls, P.I., Witkamp, L., Bossuyt, P.M., and Bos, J.D.** (1997). A systematic review of five systemic treatments for severe psoriasis. *British Journal of Dermatology* **137**, 943–9. (See comments.)

7. **Roenigk, H.H. Jr., Auerbach, R., Maibach, H., Weinstein, G., and Lebwohl, M.** (1998). Methotrexate in psoriasis: consensus conference. *Journal of the American Academy of Dermatology* **38**, 478–85.

Further reading

Griffiths, C.E. et al. (2000). A systematic review of treatments for severe psoriasis. *Health Technology Assessment* **4**, 1–125. (This article provides a systematic review of treatments for severe psoriasis. It provides comprehensive coverage of the topic and references to original evidence.)

Rapp, S.R. et al. (1997). The physical, psychological and social impact of psoriasis. *Journal of Health Psychology* **2**, 525–37. (This article provides a detailed description of the broad impact of psoriasis on patients' lives. It includes information on the specific aspects of the disease that affect patients' well-being.)

Lebwohl, M. et al. (1995). Topical therapy for psoriasis. *International Journal of Dermatology* **34**, 673–84. (This review provides a more detailed discussion of topical therapy with references to the original evidence.)

Feldman, S.R. (2001). Advances in psoriasis treatment. *Dermatology Online Journal* **6**, 1. (This review provides more detail on the many treatments available for psoriasis. It describes both the general approach and the specific treatments, including tables relating key points.)

15.9 Eczema and dermatitis

Richard A. Nicholas

Dermatitis is defined in the Oxford English Dictionary as 'an acute, or chronic, non-contagious, simple inflammation of the skin, characterized by the presence of itching papules and vesicles which discharge a serous fluid, or dry up'. Dermatitis and eczema are terms that are often used interchangeably to describe a group of non-infectious, inflammatory skin conditions. They can present in a variety of ways, but commonalities include the presence of erythema, dryness, and itching, often with the presence of vesicles and papules with predominantly unclear borders.

The acute stage of an eczematous condition presents as intensely red itching skin, often with the presence of vesicles or blisters. As the condition progresses, the itching may moderate and transform to a burning or stinging pain associated with a fissuring, erythematous, dry appearance. If present long enough, the condition progresses to lichenification, with thickened skin, chronic excoriations, and fissuring.

Dermatitis is the most common skin diagnosis (16.4 per cent) made by family physicians in the United States.[1] Inflammation, primarily in the epidermis, may extend into the dermis. Scratching or fissuring may interrupt the epidermis, evidenced by excoriations, weeping, oozing, or crusts.

There are several types of dermatitis with varied patterns from multiple causes, generally with distinctive clinical findings. These are summarized in Table 1. The more common entities include atopic dermatitis, contact dermatitis, seborrhoeic dermatitis, nummular eczema, stasis dermatitis, and hand dermatitis.

Atopic dermatitis

The most common dermatitis in childhood, this disease occurs in up to 12–14 per cent of children, and most (80–90 per cent) develop the disease before age 7.[2–4] Mild childhood disease persists into adulthood only about 10 per cent of the time; with severe disease in childhood, as many as 80 per cent continue with persistent problems.[5,6] Research into the pathogenesis of atopic dermatitis suggests a complex inflammatory process involving mast cells, lymphocytes, and infiltrating leucocytes, associated with abnormal regulation of IgE production.[7] However, there does not appear to be any systemic immunosuppression. Structural abnormalities of the skin, including

Table 1 Common types of eczema and dermatitis

Atopic eczema

Contact eczema: a localized reaction that includes redness, itching, and burning where the skin has come into contact with an allergen (an allergy-causing substance) or with an irritant such as an acid, a cleaning agent, or other chemical. Contact dermatitis refers to any dermatitis arising from direct skin exposure to a substance

Seborrhoeic eczema: yellowish, oily, scaly patches of skin on the scalp, face, and occasionally, other parts of the body

Nummular eczema: coin-shaped patches of irritated skin—most common on the arms, back, buttocks, and lower legs—that may be crusted, scaling, and extremely itchy

Neurodermatitis: scaly patches of skin on the head, lower legs, wrists, or forearms caused by a localized itch (such as an insect bite) that becomes intensely irritated when scratched

Stasis dermatitis: a skin irritation on the lower legs, generally related to circulatory problems

Pompholyx (dyshidrotic eczema): irritation of the skin on the palms of hands and soles of the feet characterized by clear, deep blisters that itch and burn alteration of the lipid composition of the stratum corneum reduce the capacity of the skin to bind water thereby compromising the barrier function of the skin making it vulnerable to external irritants.

Diagnosis

A detailed set of criteria for diagnosing atopic dermatitis developed by Henifin and Rajka in 1980 is available.[8] Primary care providers will find diagnostic guidelines developed by Williams et al.[9] most valuable (Table 2).

There are acute, sub-acute, and chronic forms of atopic dermatitis. In the acute phase, the disease presents as an intensely pruritic red papular eruption that may be vesicular with weeping, exudation, and crusting (Fig. 1). There are usually excoriations and the skin may be secondarily infected. The sub-acute form is less vicious. Itching, though present, is less severe, and there continue to be numerous excoriations. The chronic form exhibits thickening (lichenification), increased skin markings and hyperpigmentation. *Staphylococcus aureus* colonizes the skin in 95 per cent of people with atopic dermatitis.[10] All three skin reaction patterns can co-exist in the same individual.

Distribution of lesions differ somewhat depending on the age of the individual and is helpful in arriving at a diagnosis. In children, lesions usually start during the first 2 or 3 months of age on the cheeks, around the ears, scalp, and on the extensor surfaces of the extremities.

As the disease progresses to about age 2, the area affected migrates to include the antecubital and popliteal fossae. By age 5, the face is less involved but the thighs and buttocks, chest and back become inflamed.

Table 2 Diagnosis of atopic eczema in children

Must have: an itchy skin condition (or parental report of scratching or rubbing in a child)

Plus at least three of the following:
1. History of involvement of the skin creases such as folds of the elbows, behind the knees, fronts of ankles, or around the neck (including cheeks in children less than 10 years old)
2. A personal history of asthma or hay fever (or history of atopic disease in a first-degree relative in children less than 4 years of age)
3. A history of general dry skin in the past year
4. Visible flexural eczema (or eczema involving cheeks/forehead and outer limbs in children less than 4 years old)
5. Onset before age 2 (not used if child is less than 4)

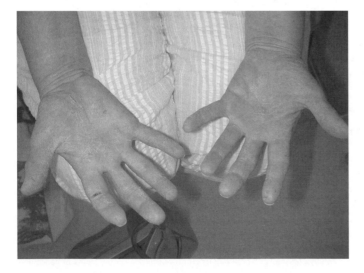

Fig. 1 Acute form of atopic dermatitis. (See Plate 39.)

In older children and adults, lesions are usually in the flexural areas, neck, wrists, ankles and extensor surfaces, although acute exacerbations can involve the entire body.

Associated conditions

Many patients with atopic dermatitis have allergic disease such as asthma or hay fever (allergic rhinitis). The allergic phenomenon occurs in either the patient or the patient's family. The allergy may be IGE mediated, and while not diagnostic, IGE levels may be elevated. Skin hypersensitivity often can be demonstrated by patch tests, but this has little clinical significance and does not indicate that particular agent precipitates atopic dermatitis.

Other skin changes may be associated with atopic dermatitis. One of the most common is xerosis (dry skin). Atopic dermatitis is often referred to as the 'dry skin' disease. Most with atopic dermatitis have dry skin.[11] Close examination reveals the skin to be rough, with fine scales and perifollicular accentuation. Keratosis pilaris, secondary icthyosis vulgaris, and hyperlinear palms and soles often accompany atopic dermatitis.

Some other common findings are eyelid dermatitis, Denny–Morgan folds (extra infraorbital folds), cataracts, and orbital darkening. Eyelid dermatitis can be quite severe leading to excessive rubbing and scratching and subsequent thinning of the cornea and development of keratoconus. Cataracts, either anterior or posterior subcapsular do occur. Orbital darkening is due to lichenification, hyperpigmentation, and/or oedema secondary to inflammation.

Principles of treatment

The goals of treatment are to control the disease by restoring hydration, decreasing itching and inflammation, and identifying and eliminating external factors that may initiate or exacerbate the disease. The patient and/or parents should know it is unlikely that the disease will be cured but very likely that it can be adequately controlled. The evidence base for treatment of atopic dermatitis is limited. Reasonable randomized controlled trials exist for the use of oral cyclosporine, topical corticosteroids, psychological approaches, and UV-light therapy. Insufficient evidence exists for the use of other therapies, even those that have been long-standing mainstays of treatment.[12]

Hydration

Hydration of the skin can be accomplished easily and inexpensively by body temperature water soaks for 15–20 min once or twice daily followed by application of a greasy preparation or moisturizer to prevent water loss due to evaporation. An indication that adequate soaking has occurred is observation of wrinkling of the skin over the pads of fingers and toes. Vegetable fat (Crisco in the United States) application after patting off excess moisture is inexpensive and effective, but any good moisturizer will do. Ointments are most effective because they are the most occlusive, but they are also the messiest to use. Strong soaps and long hot showers and baths should be stopped. Use soaps with a neutral pH and minimal defatting activity.

Table 3 Topical corticosteroid potencies (From British National Formulary, 2001)

Potency	Example
Mild	Hydrocortisone 1%
Moderate	Clobetasone butyrate 0.05%
Potent	Betamethasone valerate 0.1%
Very potent	Clobetasol proprionate 0.05%

The preparation containing the least potent drug at the lowest strength which is effective should be the one of choice.

Topical corticosteroids

These preparations are effective in reducing redness and inflammation. They should be used with care and are most effective when applied within a few minutes of soaking or bathing. These agents have been classified into groups according to potency as determined by their activity on a vasoconstrictor assay (Table 3). The lowest potency that is effective should be used (group one is the most potent). This may be a 1 per cent hydrocortisone in aquaphor or other moisturizing preparation (especially in children) or 0.025–0.1 per cent concentration of triamcinolone. Use of topical steroids should be carefully monitored; stronger preparations should not be used on the face or intertriginous areas that might become occluded, that is, armpits, groin, etc.

Tacrolimus, may prove to be an effective topical alternative to corticosteroids. The 0.1 per cent concentration of tacrolimus ointment is used for adults, while the lower 0.03 per cent concentration is for both children (ages 2 and above) and adults for short-term and intermittent long-term therapy. This agent lacks the significant systemic side-effects of cyclosporine and the cutaneous side-effects of topical corticosteroids.

Systemic corticosteroids

The occasional flare of the disease requires aggressive treatment. Unfortunately, dramatic improvement with systemic steroids may be accompanied by an equally dramatic reoccurrence once the systemic steroid is discontinued. Systemic preparations should be avoided except for short-term management.

Tar compounds

Tars are excellent anti-inflammatories that are inexpensive with few side-effects. When marked inflammation has decreased, corticosteroids can be discontinued and replaced with topical tar preparations. Two to 5 per cent Liqour Carbonis Detergens in a moisturizing base is effective. Marketed products such as Psorigel and Pragmatar work well also.

Antibiotics

Some acute flares are triggered by infections. Because of the high carrier state of *S. aureus* in atopic dermatitis, it is difficult to evaluate whether the patient has an acute infection. However, many flares are due to *S. aureus* and may respond to antibiotic treatment. Sensitivity studies should be done before initiating antibiotic therapy since resistant organisms are not uncommon.

Antipruritic agents

Itching is an exasperating symptom that is difficult to manage. Although antihistamines are used extensively, there is some doubt about their effectiveness. Sedating antihistamines are certainly of value, especially in children. Therapy with an H_1 and H_2 blocking agent such as Doxepin may be effective in adults. Do not use topical antihistamine or anaesthetics.

Referral

Severe episodes of atopic dermatitis that are refractory to treatment should be referred to a dermatology consultant for treatment with other more complicated methods such as allergy therapy, phototherapy, PUVA, cyclosporine, gamma interferon, and thymopentin.

Contact dermatitis

Contact dermatitis is skin inflammation resulting from contact with either an irritant or allergen with resultant itching, redness, swelling, oozing, and scaling. Initially contact dermatitis manifests as red, swollen, and blistered areas. Later stages may be crusted or scaly. Chronic inflammation may cause the skin to appear lichenified and thickened.

Identification and avoidance of the offending substance may be difficult, but the location and pattern of skin inflammation can provide clues to the aetiology. Patch testing with the suspected offending agent to the surface of the skin can confirm the clinician's suspicions.

Avoiding the substance is usually curative. Symptomatic treatment involves hydrating the skin, topical corticosteroids and emollients, and avoiding other sensitizing or drying agents.

Nummular (discoid) dermatitis

People with atopic dermatitis, allergic, and irritant contact dermatitis, psoriasis, and tinea corporis often present with coin-shaped ('nummular' or 'discoid') lesions. Nummular dermatitis itself is an idiopathic eruption that appears most frequently on the extremities and trunk. The cause is unknown, but there may be a personal or family history of asthma, allergies or atopic dermatitis or similar disorder. It is characterized by coin-shaped lesions that develop gradually with no apparent cause or precipitating factor and no specific distribution. More common in the winter, the lesions start as moist, red, papules and/or vesicles that develop crust and slowly enlarge to dry, scaling, well-demarcated, itching plaques (Fig. 2). There is often considerable lichenification because of lesions that itch incessantly so the afflicted person rubs and scratches them over time.

The characteristic shape, absence of other skin disease, and no identifiable cause are clues to the diagnosis. Differential diagnosis includes the above-mentioned diseases plus xerosis, xerotic eczema, and the 'oid, oid' disease predominant in Jewish males described by Sulzberger and Gerbe,[13] that probably is a variant nummular eczema.

The course of this disease varies from person to person. It may regress with treatment, but may recur at intervals for years. The main principles and stages of treatment are shown in Table 4.

Pompholyx

This hand dermatitis is also known as dyshidrosis or dyshidrotic eczema. Pompholyx is an idiopathic, pruritic, symmetric eruption of the hands and/or feet that starts as tense vesicles on the palm and soles with little

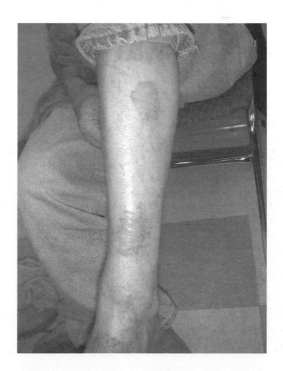

Fig. 2 Coin-shaped ('nummular' or 'discoid') lesions on the leg. (See Plate 40.)

Table 4 Treatment of nummular (discoid) eczema

1. Maintain skin hydration—warm water tub soaks
2. Maintain uniform environment not hot or cold
3. Moderate to low humidity
4. Mild skin cleansers and moisturizers
5. Mid-potency topical corticosteroids twice daily, under occlusion with plastic wrap or suit if severe
6. Topical coal tar preparations locally
7. Aggressive treatment of secondary infections
8. Ultraviolet treatment or natural sunlight
9. Occasional intermittent oral corticosteroids for severe flares

Table 5 Treatment of pompholyx

1. During the acute onset phase intermittent cold compresses using water or soothing solution as Burow's solution two or three times a day
2. Soaks or compresses using weak solutions of potassium permanganate, aluminium acetate, or vinegar in water, may be applied for 15 min four times a day. This will dry up blisters
3. Then apply a medium to strong potency corticosteroid
4. Use of occlusion with a wet glove or plastic wrap is effective
5. For severe cases, short-term courses of oral corticosteroids are prescribed for 2 or 3 weeks and occasional long-term use is necessary for maintenance
6. Tar preparations are effective for treatment and maintenance
7. Products like Psorigel, Balnatar, 10% Liquor Carbonis in Nivea Oil are useful

If none of these methods give relief, referral to a specialist who has experience with psoralen and UVA is indicated.

inflammation. Typically, the lateral aspects of the fingers are involved. The vesicles usually subside in 3–4 weeks and are followed by erythema, scaling, and later, lichenification, although recurrent waves of vesiculation can recur.

The cause of pompholyx is unknown although it frequently occurs in people who are atopic with a propensity or family history of hay fever, asthma, or atopic eczema. Occasionally, a pompholyx-like syndrome is caused by allergy to metals such as nickel. In susceptible individuals, stress can induce pompholyx. The main principles and stages of treatment are shown in Table 5.

Stasis dermatitis

Stasis dermatitis is an eruption that follows venous stasis and oedema. The skin rash is not the first indication of disease. It is associated with varicose and dilated veins. There is frequently a history of deep venous thrombosis or surgery or injury to the extremity. The patient's first symptoms will usually have been swollen legs, indentation due to stockings, aching, and heavy feeling at the end of the day and often pruritus. Later, the skin may be dry, with red papular, indiscreet, itching eruptions. There may be thickened brown haemosiderin hyperpigmentation distributed throughout the lesions. There is often a blotchy appearance to the skin, and erosions or ulcers may be infected in long-standing cases.

Control of oedema is essential. Lower leg compression is accomplished with fitted support stockings. If the oedema is severe or there are erosions or ulcers, compression with Unna Boots is most effective. Before compression dressings are applied, vascular studies can differentiate between arterial or venous aetiologies. Management of stasis dermatitis is summarized in Table 6.

Table 6 Management of stasis dermatitis

For dermatitis:
1. Cool intermittent compresses with water or Burow's solution until acute inflammation and/or exudation has subsided
2. Mild to moderate topical corticosteroid application every 3 or 4 h
3. Topical and/or oral antibiotic if infection is suspected

For oedema and venous congestion:
1. Elevation of involved legs
2. Fitted support stockings
3. Superficial vein stripping

For erosions or ulcers:
1. Antibiotics if infected
2. Daily to weekly whirlpool followed by application of a lytic enzyme
3. Application of Silvadene as an anti-inflammatory and to stimulate replication of keratinocytes
4. Weekly debridement followed by application of mild topical corticosteroid and Unna Boot

Key points

- Dermatitis and eczema are terms that are often used interchangeably.
- Maintaining skin hydration is an important element of treatment.
- The corticosteroid of choice is the least potent at the lowest strength that is effective.
- Control of oedema is essential in managing stasis dermatitis.

References

1. Fleischer, A.B. Jr., Feldman, S.R., and McConnell, R.C. (1997). The most common dermatologic problems identified by family physicians, 1990–1994. *Family Medicine* **29**, 648–52.

2. Herd, R.M., Tidman, M.J., Prescott, R.J., and Hunter, J.A.A. (1996). Prevalence of atopic eczema in the community: the Lothian atopic dermatitis study. *British Journal of Dermatology* **135**, 18–19.

3. Kay, J., Gawkrodber, D.J., Mortimer, M.J., and Jaron, A.G. (1994). The prevalence of childhood atopic eczema in a general population. *Journal of the American Academy of Dermatology* **30**, 35–9.

4. Bleiker, T. et al. (2000). The prevalence and incidence of atopic dermatitis in a birth cohort: the importance of a family history of atopy. *Archives of Dermatology* **136** (2), 274.

5. Rystedt., I. (1985). Prognostic factors in atopic dermatitis. *Acta Dermato-Venerologica* **65**, 206–13.

6. Roth, K. (1964). The natural history of atopic dermatitis. *Archives of Dermatology* **89**, 206–13.

7. Bos, J.D., Kapsenberg, M.L., and Smitt, J.H. (1994). Pathogenesis of atopic eczema. *Lancet* **343** (8909), 1338–41.

8. Henifin, Rajka. (1980). Diagnostic features of atopic dermatitis. *Acta Dermato-Venerologica Supplement* (*Stock H*) **92**, 44–7.

9. Williams, H.C., Burney, P.G., Pembroke, A.C., and Hay, R.J. (1994). The UK Working Party's diagnostic criteria of atopic dermatitis. II. Observer variation of clinical diagnosis and signs of atopic dermatitis. *British Journal of Dermatology* **131**, 397–405.

10. Leyden, J.J., Marples, R.R., and Kligman, A.M. (1974). *Staphylococcus aureus* in the lesions of atopic dermatitis. *British Journal of Dermatology* **90**, 525–30.

11. Linde, Y.W. (1992). Dry skin in atopic dermatitis. *Acta Dermato-Venerologica Supplement* **177**, 9–13.

12. Hoare, C. et al. (2000). Systematic review of treatments for atopic eczema. *Health Technology Assessment* **4** (37), 1–191.

13. Sulzberger and Gerbe. (1937). Nine cases of distinctive discord and lichenoid chronic dermatitis. *Archives of Dermatology* **36**, 247–72.

15.10 Skin infections

Gary W. McEwen

This chapter deals with the main skin infections seen in general practice—impetigo, folliculitis and furunculosis (boils), cellulitis, erysipelas, dermatophyte and yeast infection, warts, herpes, and molluscum. It also, for completeness, deals briefly with infestations.

Impetigo

This occurs frequently in children and adults as a primary or secondary process. It presents clinically in several forms; bullous or non-bullous (crusted).

Impetigo contagiosa is the non-bullous form characterized by tiny vesiculo-pustules leading to the typical findings of yellow exudation and crusts that appear on the exposed areas. The crust can be removed easily leaving behind a red moist surface that soon produces fresh exudate (Fig. 1). The lesions spread by autoinnoculation centrifugally, leading to large circular areas and as the name implies is very contagious. Children under 6 years old are most often affected. Both *Streptococcus pyogenes* and *Staphylococcus aureus* are the primary pathogens alone or together. The lesions may occur primarily in normal skin or secondarily from arthropod bites, varicella, and dermatitis. Acute glomerulonephritis is an unusual but well-documented complication that may result from the streptococcal organism; rarely, cellulitis or rheumatic fever may also result.

Treatment includes gentle skin cleansing to remove the crusts and a short course of an antibiotic. In many countries, resistance to penicillin is high and a penicillinase-resistant antibiotic is recommended for staphylococcal infections. Mupirocin ointment or cream is an effective topical therapy for impetigo that is localized in healthy children. The nares are a reservoir for *S. aureus* and should be treated with oral or topical treatment if repeated episodes of impetigo develop.

Bullous impetigo is a staphylococcal toxin mediated process that is found in both adults and children. Neonates may develop this during the first or second week of life and aggressive treatment is indicated due to a high risk of pneumonia and septicaemia. Adults present with large non-inflammatory

bullae that rupture, leaving circinate crusty lesions. The lesions are usually localized and may resemble bullous pemphigoid or bullous arthropod bites. A culture is normally negative for bacterial growth as a staphylococcal phage toxin mediates the blisters. The treatment is systemic with penicillinase resistant antibiotics such as dicloxacillin. Complications include development of staphylococcal scalded skin syndrome and local invasion leading to lymphadenopathy, cellulitis, and scarring.

Folliculitis and furunculosis

Folliculitis manifests in a number of ways depending on the aetiology. Infection with bacteria, fungi, yeast, and viruses may result in folliculitis. There are some non-infectious processes such as eosinophilic folliculitis, acne keloidalis nuchae, and irritant folliculitis that manifest as folliculitis also.

Staphylococcus aureus accounts for the greatest proportion of the bacterial causes of folliculitis. The tiny folliculocentric pustules are commonly seen in the beard and perinasal areas but may occur in other places such as the groin and buttocks. A gram stain and culture will help to confirm the pathogenesis, but treatment should be initiated with oral antibiotics. Patients with repeated infections should have the nares treated with mupirocin ointment daily as nasal carriers are not uncommon.

Pityrosporum folliculitis is caused by overgrowth of the yeast *Pityrosporum ovale* (*Malassezia furfur*). Its appearance is characterized by mildly pruritic monomorphous pustules on the upper back and chest. Adolescent and adult populations are primarily affected and the disorder is often misdiagnosed as acne vulgaris. Some cases may result from yeast overgrowth after corticosteroid therapy. Treatment with topical zinc, selenium sulfide, or ketoconazole shampoos are effective. Systemic treatment with the azoles may be necessary, but griseofulvin is ineffective.

Herpes simplex virus is a rare cause of folliculitis and should be considered in a patient with a difficult vesicular folliculitis.

Furuncles, or boils, are deep-seated inflammatory nodules that begin around a hair follicle, but often develop into abscesses. Carbuncles are less follicule oriented and more extensive, deep, and painful. They have multiple interconnected tracts under the skin with several to many surface pustules. They are more painful and serious than furuncles. Furuncles arise in hair-bearing sites and seem to favour areas prone to friction and heavy perspiration such as the buttock, axillae, neck, and face. Both carbuncles and furuncles may arise primarily, or resulting from another primary skin disorder such as eczema or abrasions where bacteria gain access from a compromised skin barrier. Both carbuncles and furuncles may lead to abscess formation and cellulitis and bacteraemia in some cases. Systemic symptoms and leucocytosis are seen more commonly with carbuncles. Lesions on the face around the nose and lips are exceptionally dangerous as spread may occur to the brain through the facial and angular veins and the cavernous sinus. A culture will usually yield *S. aureus* and treatment involves local application of moist heat, and oral antibiotics. Patients with fever or cellulitis require intravenous antibiotics. Lesions with fluctuance should be incised and drained with continuation of antibiotics.

Cellulitis and erysipelas

Cellulitis is infection of the subcutaneous and dermal tissues caused primarily by *S. aureus* and *S. pyogenes*. Usually, there is a wound or portal of entry for the bacteria. The result is a spreading erythema of the involved area, which is normally tender and slightly infiltrated. Streaking from the area, lymphatic involvement may be found. Fever, chills, and sepsis may result. Cellulitis of the legs in patients with chronic lymphoedema and venous stasis should prompt evaluation for tinea infections of the nails and feet that may provide a portal of entry for pyogenic bacteria. These patients are also more likely to have repeated episodes and may require suppressive antibiotics. Healthy patients with uncomplicated disease may be treated with oral antibiotics. Patients with streaking from lymphatic involvement, or constitutional symptoms, or underlying illness or conditions such as

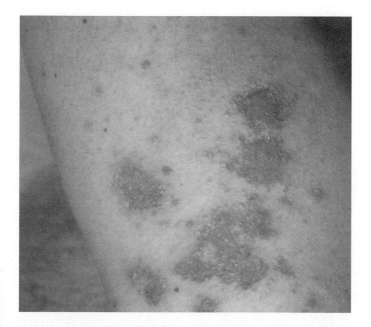

Fig. 1 Non-bullous form of impetigo characterized by crusts. (See Plate 41.)

diabetes, stasis, and lymphoedema should receive parenteral antibiotics and close monitoring for bacteraemia.

Erysipelas is an acute form of cellulitis caused primarily by beta-haemolytic group A streptococcus. The striking clinical findings are a rapidly progressing erythema and brawny oedema with an advancing peripheral edge. The face and legs are the sites most often affected. Bacteraemia or deep cellulitis may result. Like cellulitis, there is often a portal of entry for the bacteria, such as a scratch or fissure. Recognition is not difficult, but an acute contact allergic dermatitis can cause some confusion because of the localized pattern of inflammation in each condition. Treatment with oral antibiotics in uncomplicated cases is usually successful. Parenteral antibiotics should be administered to high-risk populations such as infants, elderly, diabetics or immunocompromised patients, or patients who do not respond to oral therapy.

Dermatophyte and yeast infections

Fungal infections on the skin can be categorized as superficial and deep. The superficial skin, hair, and nail infections commonly referred to as ringworm or tinea are primarily caused by dermatophytes. The different clinical manifestations may be classified based on the particular site of infection (see Table 1). The treatment is based on the location of the infection.

Most dermatophyte infections of the skin can be treated with topical antifungal medications. The scalp and nails usually require systemic medication for the best chances of mycological and clinical cure. Other concurrent medications should be noted as significant drug interactions may occur.

Tinea capitis, scalp ringworm, is a very contagious infection seen most commonly in children. It may be transmitted throughout the family and school via fomites. The scales laden with organisms may be transmitted readily by close contact with an often-asymptomatic carrier. In the United States, *Tinea tonsurans* is the most common pathogen causing an endothrix and inflammatory changes of the skin and breakage of the hair shaft with a characteristic 'black dot' pattern. *T. tonsurans* infection is acquired from humans. Other causative fungi include *Microsporum audouinii* which spreads from human to human and *Microsporum canis* which spreads from animals such as cats and dogs and causes a fluorescent ectothrix.

Diagnosis and treatment of scalp ringworm is discussed in Chapter 15.1. Some common complications of tinea capitis include the formation of a kerion, a dermatophytid skin reaction, and secondary impetigo. Permanent scarring alopecia may ensue unless adequate therapy is provided.

Onychomycosis is a very common infection of the nail plate. The infection is classified based on the location of the infection. Most infections occur distally and under the nail, but infections of the proximal nail fold and on top of the nail plate are seen. Both dermatophytes and candidal yeast species may be pathogenic. The proximal subungual white onychomycosis caused by *T. tonsurans* is found almost exclusively in the setting of systemic infection with human immunodeficiency virus (AIDS). The distal subungual infection leads to the characteristic changes of yellow discoloration and lifting of the nail plate (onycholysis). The infection spreads proximally leading to yellow brittle thickened and eroded nail plate changes. Diagnosis and treatment are discussed in Chapter 15.2. The differential diagnosis of dystrophic yellow nails includes psoriasis, lichen planus, and a number of other skin diseases.

Athlete's foot (tinea pedis) is a particularly common condition present in about 15 per cent of the general population. Swimming pool users, athletes, and industrial workers are at particular risk. Infection can be persistent and can spread to other parts of the body and to other people. Most people can be treated effectively with topical allyamines and azoles. Creams are usually preferred to dusting powders that may exacerbate skin irritation.

Pityriasis vesicolor is a common fungal skin condition caused by the Pityrosporum yeast, which causes spreading discrete brown scaly patches in light-skinned individuals or decolorized patches in dark-skinned individuals on the back or trunk. It is traditionally managed with selenium sulfide shampoo. Topical azole antifungals are also effective but need to be prescribed in large quantities. Administration of oral ketoconazole 400 mg followed by rigorous exercise to sweat is effective. Relapse is common, particularly in the context of immune suppression.

Candidal skin infections may be treated with topical azoles or nystatin. Failure to respond to topical treatment is an indication for systemic treatment.

Warts and molluscum

Human papillomavirus (HPV) is the cause of warts and is by far the most common viral infection of the skin. This DNA virus has many different types, but typing is rarely useful in clinical practice. Certain types are known to induce cervical dysplasia leading to carcinoma. Wart types on the hands and feet are normally not found in the genitalia. Warts are easily recognized, but not so easily treated.

Common warts

Verrucae vulgaris, common warts, are normally seen in young adults and children on the hands and feet. Clinically, they are non-inflammatory, hyperkeratotic papules that contain the tiny black punctate dots that are thrombosed and dilated capillaries. Warts differ from callosities, in that they break up the dermatoglyphics of the skin. Sub-clinical lesions are often present. Patients who bite their nails seem to be affected more severely in the periungual areas. Treatment for the common wart in healthy patients must be tempered by the fact that spontaneous resolution is the rule.

Most warts resolve within 3 years and rarely is it necessary to excise a wart unless the diagnosis is in question. Treatment with destruction and immunotherapy is the rule. Topical salicylic acid preparations are widely available and very effective when combined with salt-water soaks, occlusion with tape, and gentle paring of the keratinous debris of the wart with a fingernail file. Cryotherapy with liquid nitrogen is very useful, but great care must be used to avoid scarring, nerve damage, and hypopigmentation. The delivery of liquid nitrogen cryotherapy by spray or cotton-tip applicator to the wart should last 15–20 s or so to achieve a thaw time of 30–45 s. This leads to a blister and separation of the skin under the wart with desquamation.

Cantharone, a blistering agent from the blister beetle, immunotherapy with topical compound DCP, simple tape occlusion, and injection of candidal antigen have all been used. Surgical ablation with carbon dioxide laser and electrodessication devices are commonly used, but like all other treatment modalities does not guarantee a cure. Even hypnosis and the power of suggestion have their proponents.

Flat warts

Flat warts, verruca plana, are characterized clinically by the smooth, 1–3 mm flat-topped, well-defined slightly tan or hypopigmented papules located on the face and hands of children and young adults. Generally, they occur in groups and spread easily with autoinnoculation. This feature can aid in the

Table 1 Classification of dermatophyte infection by site

Onychomycosis	Fingernail or toenail
Tinea capitus	Hair of scalp
Tinea barbae	Beard
Tinea faciei	Face
Tinea corporis	Body in general
Tinea manus	Hands
Tinea pedis	Feet
Tinea cruris	Groin

diagnosis of this lesion. Treatment of several lesions with cryotherapy is usual, but should be avoided for multiple lesions for cosmetic reasons, especially when located on the back of the hands or face. Flat warts undergo more frequent spontaneous remission than common warts. Topical medications that may be useful include topical tretinoin, imiquimod cream, 5-fluorouracil cream, and cantharone.

Plantar warts

Plantar warts are the most difficult wart to treat leading to frustration on the part of the physician and patient. Salicylic acid in higher concentrations in combination with paring and tape occlusion are useful. Destructive methods including cryotherapy and electrodessication may prove to be too painful. Immunotherapy with DCP or candidal antigen injections may help. Laser or traditional surgery should be the very last result as the scars may be painful and recurrent wart within the scar may prove difficult to clear. Intralesional bleomycin is an excellent treatment, but costly and may induce necrosis and distal sclerosis.

Genital warts

Genital warts, also known as condyloma acuminata, are the most common sexually transmitted disease and are discussed in Chapter 15.14. Infection is frequently sub-clinical and unknown to the patient leading to asymptomatic shedding of the virus. Genital wart infections with certain HPV types are closely associated with cancers of the cervix, glans penis, anus, vulvovaginal area, and periungual skin. Condyloma acuminata are characterized clinically by the 1–5 mm lobulated papules that may form large cauliflower-like masses in moist intertriginous areas. A careful history and physical is necessary to exclude other sexually transmitted diseases. The differential diagnosis of these masses in the intertriginous areas should include secondary syphilis, also known as condyloma lata. Evaluation of genital warts should also include a Pap smear of the cervix in women or the anus of men or women engaged in anal intercourse. Treatment with topical medication and destructive therapy is the rule. Cryotherapy and electrodessication are effective, but may leave hypopigmentation and scarring. Topical medications including imiquimod cream, 5-fluorouracil cream, and podophylotoxin are useful. Trichloroacetic acid and podophyllin are chemicals that may be used in the office. Partners of these patients should be referred for evaluation as well.

Molluscum contagiosum

Molluscum is caused by a poxvirus and spread by skin-to-skin contact. As the name implies, it is readily spread in several patient groups; children, adults (sexually), and the immunosupressed. The lesions are characterized by dome-shaped papules with a small umbilicated central core. Lesions may be quite large and resemble skin tags, pustules, and furuncles. The infectious virus particles are discharged by rubbing and autoinnoculation is common. Treatment is determined by the clinical setting, but should be tempered by the self-limited nature of the condition, usually less than 2 years. Cryotherapy with liquid nitrogen is a simple and effective nonsurgical treatment. There are many other topical treatments; tape stripping, potassium hydroxide application, cantharone, 5-fluorouracil, cidofovir, imiquimod cream, trichloracetic acid, and podophylotoxin gel. Surgical curettment and shave removal is effective, but may leave scarring. Treatment of molluscum in the setting of immunosuppression and atopic dermatitis can be difficult.

Other common viral infections

Herpes simplex virus was mentioned above as a rare cause of folliculitis. A more common manifestation of skin infection with herpes simplex virus in

general practice is the cold sore (herpes labialis). Limited evidence from randomized controlled trials (RCTs) suggests that pain and duration of symptoms from this recurrent problem can be reduced with early application of topical antiviral agents (e.g. acyclovir). Oral systemic treatment has been shown to reduce the duration of lesions when initiated at the onset of the typical prodromal symptoms of burning and tingling. It can also reduce the number of outbreaks in individuals with recurrent lesions (more than 6 per year). However, it may not block the spread of infection as a number of patients continue to shed virus asymptomatically despite treatment with topical or oral agents. There is little good evidence of the effectiveness of other agents (including topical acyclovir) as prophylaxis, although ultraviolet sunscreen may be effective. Systemic treatment may be necessary for persistent labial lesions and for buccal and vaginal lesions. Herpes simplex also causes genital infection (see Chapter 6.5).

Herpes zoster, which presents clinically either as chickenpox or shingles, is discussed elsewhere in this book. Fig. 2 shows a typical case of shingles affecting the T2 dermatome on the left side with clear midline demarcation. Oral treatment with antiviral agents (acyclovir, famiclovir, and valacyclovir) reduce the relative risk of post-herpetic pain in shingles by about 50 per cent. Antidepressants may also be effective. Evidence for the benefit of adding a steroid to antiviral treatment is conflicting.

Orf is caused by a DNA pox virus transmitted from farm animals. It is most commonly seen in farm workers but may also be seen in those returning from farm vacations. It presents as a solitary lesion, usually on the hand, with an incubation period of up to 4 weeks. It usually resolves

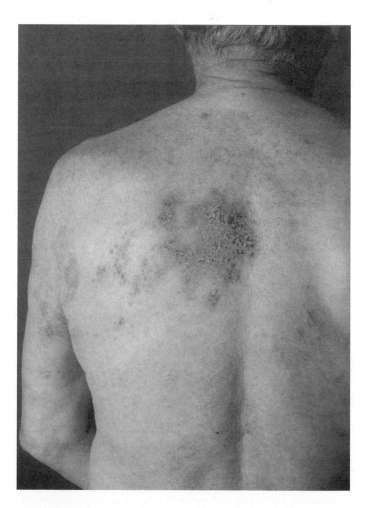

Fig. 2 Typical case of shingles affecting the T2 dermatome on the left side. (See Plate 42.)

Table 2 Tropical skin infections

Condition	Distribution	Cause	Clinical features
Leprosy	Worldwide	*Mycobacterium leprae*	Macular, papular or nodular, anaesthetic skin lesions; neuropathy associated ulceration and tissue loss
Leishmaniasis	Worldwide	Protozoa transmitted by sandflies	Slowly growing ulcerating skin lesion with granulating base; erosive sore at junction of nose and mouth
Onchocerciasis	Africa, South America	Filaria transmitted by blackflies	Intensely itchy papules; spotty depigmentation of shins and abdomen (leopard skin); keratitis and iritis
Loasis	West Africa	Filaria (loa)	Continuously migrating lesions (with egg-size Calabar swellings)—worms migrate at about 1 cm/h
Larva migrans	Worldwide	Hookworms	Intensely itchy subdermal, aimlessly wandering, track from hookworm larvae migrating from site of egg

spontaneously within a further 6 weeks. The only indication for therapy is secondary bacterial infection.

Common infestations

The most common infestations seen in general practice in the developed world are lice and scabies. The diagnosis of head lice (pediculosis capitis) is discussed in Chapter 15.1. The infection is essentially harmless although sensitization may result in local irritation and erythema. Secondary infection may occur through scratching. The most commonly used chemical treatments for elimination of lice are malathion and permethrin. They should be applied as an aqueous lotion to dried hair, left on the hair overnight, and then washed off. Both chemicals are more effective than shampooing alone but the effect achieved may depend on local resistance. Adverse reactions are uncommon. Combing is probably less effective than chemical treatment but in combination with chemical treatment has no additional adverse effects except minor discomfort. All members of a family or other social group should be treated.

Body lice (pediculosis corporis) are seen most commonly in people living in deprived or insanitary conditions. Secondary bacterial infection is common through excoriation. They can be treated effectively with carbaryl, malathion, or permethrin but the provision of clean clothing and bathing facilities is essential for cure.

Infection of coarse body hair with lice (*Pthirus pubis* or 'crabs') is by direct body contact, usually sexual intercourse. Lice are about 2 mm in length and difficult to see; as with scalp hair eggs (nits) can sometimes be identified adherent to the hair shaft. Single application of malathion or carbaryl is usually effective.

Scabies is common—and a particularly important and sometimes difficult diagnosis in primary care. It is caused by a mite which lives on the skin and burrows to feed and mate. It causes intense itching, although this is caused by sensitization and does not occur until 3–4 weeks after infestation. Diagnosis depend on finding adult mite burrows and associated papular eruptions; mites can sometimes be retrieved from the head of the burrow. Treatment is with malathion or permethrin applied all over the body at night without bathing (paying particular attention to finger and toe webs and under fingernails). A bath should be taken after 24 h. All household or body contacts should be treated. Antihistamines and calamine may help itching, which takes time to subside.

Tropical skin infections

The most important skin infections seen in tropical climes (and increasingly imported to temperate climes through air travel) are leprosy, leishmaniasis, onchocerciasis, loasis, and cutaneous larva migrans. Detailed consideration of these conditions are beyond the scope of this book but the main clinical features are summarized in Table 2. Confirmation of diagnosis and treatment is best left to someone with experience of the condition.

Further reading

Odom, R., James, W., and Berger, T. *Andrews' Diseases of the Skin* 9th edn., London: Saunders, 2000.

Freedburg, I.M. *Fitzpatrick's Dermatology in General Medicine* 5th edn., New York: McGraw Hill, 1999.

Schachner, L. and Hansen, R. *Pediatric Dermatology* 2nd edn., 1995.

BMJ Clinical Evidence, 2002. (Updated 6 monthly—this summarizes current clinical evidence on treatment effectiveness and has a section on skin disorders.)

15.11 **Bruising and purpura**

R. Stephen Griffith

On examination of the vertex of the scalp of a newborn infant, the first bruise of life is often evident. Many more will follow. Bruising occurs whenever a provocative event, such as trauma, infection, or failure of the haemostatic mechanisms, allows enough erythrocytes to escape the microvascular system into the epidermis or dermis to be visible. Bruising is such a common event, it may be considered normal, especially in toddlers and the elderly—in the former due to repeated traumas associated with exploration of their environment, and in the latter due to the loss of stromal support which results in extravasation of blood due to minor, unrecognized trauma. However, bruising in the absence of trauma may be an indication of underlying conditions ranging in severity from cosmetic to fatal. When unexplained bruising is present, the health care provider must evaluate the patient to determine who needs reassurance and who needs further evaluation or referral.

Everyone understands the term 'bruise' and it is the term most frequently used. However, it is non-specific, encompassing haematomas, petechiae, ecchymoses, and purpura. The more specific terms will be used in this chapter. A haematoma, or contusion, is a palpable mass of extravasated blood that develops between tissue planes, frequently associated with oedema and usually secondary to a significant trauma. If a haematoma is associated with a pathologic condition, there will usually be associated purpura in other areas; thus, haematoma formation will not be discussed separately. 'Purpura' is used to describe extravasation of formed elements of blood into the dermis or epidermis. Purpura does not blanch on external pressure. 'Petechiae' is a more specific term, referring to purpuric lesions less than 3 mm in diameter. When less than 1–2 days old they are a brilliant red, but after a few days they fade to brown as the erythrocytes break down. In time, there remains only a rusty brown stain of remaining haemosiderin pigment. 'Ecchymoses' refer to purpuric lesions greater than 3 mm in diameter. They are often confluent and irregular in shape. In evaluating a patient, it is important to distinguish the above lesions from erythema, which is a reddened area of skin, and telangiectasias, which are 1–3 mm masses of dilated capillaries. Since the blood in both of these conditions is intravascular, they readily blanch with external pressure. It is also important to distinguish between purpuric lesions that are palpable and those that are macular, since the causes may be different.

Purpura is often a reflection of what is occurring throughout the body. The skin is a window into what is happening systemically, and the health care provider must keep in perspective that visible lesions may be just the 'tip of the iceberg'.

Purpuric bleeding occurs at the level of the microcirculation—the terminal arterioles, the capillaries, and post-capillary venules. Microvascular physiology is a complex interplay of active endothelial cells, connective tissue support and protection, and haemostatic mechanisms that prevent the egress of erythrocytes while allowing the passage of nutrients and by-products of cell metabolism. Disturbance of any component of the microvascular structure or function can result in purpura.

There are innumerable causes of purpura. Table 1 lists the most common causes of purpura. The following discussion will emphasize the more common causes of purpura and those less common conditions which should be considered by the primary care provider due to the serious nature of the affliction.

Causes of purpura

Abnormalities of haemostasis

Abnormalities of platelets

Platelet-related purpura is generally petechial and superficial on skin and mucous membranes. This may be due to a decrease in the number of platelets or a result of poorly functioning platelets. Thrombocytopaenia can come from a variety of causes involving decreased production (bone marrow replacement, aplastic anaemia, etc.) or increased destruction (idiopathic thrombocytopaenic purpura, hypersplenism, drug-dependent immune mechanisms, sepsis, disseminated intravascular coagulation). Platelet dysfunction is most commonly caused by medication administration, especially aspirin, but may be due to underlying conditions, such as uraemia, or, rarely, inherited disorders. With inadequate platelet activity, microscopic breeches in the endothelium do not get 'plugged', and purpura results.

Diagnosis of thrombocytopaenia can easily be accomplished by a platelet count, while a bleeding time is required to establish platelet dysfunction. Treatment is directed at the underlying cause. Platelet transfusion can be given for life-threatening haemorrhage.

Plasma coagulation abnormalities

Coagulation abnormalities usually present as ecchymoses and larger haematomas instead of the petechial bleeding more characteristic of the platelet disorders. Hereditary deficiencies of clotting factors are the prototypical causes, classically Factor VIII (haemophilia), Factor IX (Christmas disease), or von Willebrand's disease (which also is associated with an abnormality of platelet aggregation). Hepatic dysfunction may result in inadequate production of coagulation factors. Iatrogenic causes include treatment with heparinoids or coumarin compounds. Diagnosis is established with prolongation of the prothrombin time or the partial thromboplastin time, and treatment can be directed accordingly: replacing clotting factors with fresh frozen plasma or cryoprecipitate for critical bleeding, vitamin K for coumarin excess or hepatic dysfunction, or protamine for heparin excess.

Disseminated intravascular coagulation (DIC) is a consumptive coagulopathy that is usually caused by sepsis. Because of ongoing clot formation, the platelets and the coagulation factors can be depleted, resulting, paradoxically, in bleeding. This is a life-threatening event that can lead to purpura fulminans—extensive bleeding into large areas of the skin indicating severe clotting abnormality. Treatment is aimed at the underlying cause and support with appropriate transfusions of platelets and clotting factors.

Haemorrhagic disease of the newborn deserves special consideration. At birth, the level of vitamin K dependent coagulation factors is normal, but the level of vitamin K in the newborn is low since it does not readily cross the placenta. The major source of vitamin K is as a by-product of bacterial colonization of the intestine, which takes a few days to develop. Breast milk contains low levels of vitamin K. As a result, the coagulation factors are rapidly depleted, and bleeding can result. It usually occurs on day 2 or 3 of life, and manifests as purpura and gastrointestinal bleeding. Bleeding from the nose and umbilicus can also occur, or even intracranial bleeding. Treatment with vitamin K should be given immediately, with the use of fresh frozen plasma reserved for critical bleeding. Administering vitamin K prophylactically at birth to all newborns is very effective in preventing this condition.

Table 1 Causes of purpura

Infection (See text)

Small vessel vasculitis
  Hypersensitivity vasculitis
  Henoch–Schönlein purpura
  Serum sickness
  Mixed cryoglobulinaemia
  Urticarial vasculitis
  Associated with connective tissue disease:
    SLE; rheumatoid arthritis; Sjögren's syndrome
  Dermatomyositis/polymyositis
  Inflammatory bowel disease
  Goodpasture's syndrome
  Relapsing polychondritis
  Behçet's disease

Decreased mechanical strength of the microcirculation
  Solar purpura (senile purpura)
  Scurvy
  Hypercortisolism
  Heritable disorders of connective tissue
  Amyloidosis

Abnormalities of haemostasis
  Platelet abnormalities
  Plasma coagulation abnormalities

Larger vessel vasculitis
  Polyarteritis nodosa
  Wegener's granulomatosis
  Allergic angiitis and granulomatosis (Churg–Strauss syndrome)
  Lymphomatoid granulomatosis
  Temporal arteritis
  Takayasu's arteritis

Other causes
  Mechanical purpura
  Purpura simplex
  Progressive pigmenting purpura
  Factitial purpura
  Psychogenic purpura
  Associated with malignancy
  Toxins and venoms
  Embolic phenomena
  Assault and abuse
  Drugs

Vasculitis

This broad spectrum of disorders is characterized by purpura and histologic findings on skin biopsy of vessel-directed inflammation. These disorders can be divided into small vessel vasculitis and larger vessel vasculitis.

Small vessel vasculitis

These disorders are termed leucocytoclastic vasculitis (Fig. 1). They are caused by an immune mechanism wherein immune complexes leak between endothelial cells resulting in complement activation, chemotaxis, and subsequent neutrophil infiltration. Catabolic enzymes are released from the lysed neutrophils (leucocytoclasis) causing disruption of the endothelium and leakage of erythrocytes resulting in purpura. Since there is surrounding inflammation, these lesions are palpable purpura. The antigen leading to the immune complex formation is rarely identified; an exception would be the Hepatitis B surface antigen. Drugs, chemicals, and micro-organisms can all serve as the stimulus for a vasculitis. These lesions have a predilection for the dependent areas such as legs and feet. As the lesions age, ulceration or bullae formation may occur, particularly in the larger lesions. A comprehensive review of the causes of the vasculitis is beyond the scope of this chapter, but the major types can be reviewed in Table 1.

A leucocytoclastic vasculitis that merits discussion is Henoch–Schonlein purpura (HSP). This disorder is characterized by palpable purpura, renal disease, joint pain, and abdominal pain. It occurs most frequently in children between 2 and 11, but may occur at any age. It is mediated by an IgA antibody with unknown antigen. The most common presentation is petechiae and ecchymoses symmetrically on the legs and buttocks, with associated joint or abdominal pain. The disease is usually self-limited with a good prognosis, but it can lead to severe glomerulonephritis and renal failure. Treatment is symptomatic with close monitoring of renal function.

Large vessel vasculitis

These disorders, listed in Table 1, are characterized by inflammation of small, medium, and large vessels. The most common such disorder is polyarteritis nodosa. Some conditions, such as connective tissue diseases, infections, and drug-related vasculitis may cause both large and small vessel vasculitis. The skin findings usually are not the predominate symptoms of these disorders, but may be the initial symptom.

Treatment of the vasculitis disorder is determined by the underlying cause. It may involve removal of the offending antigen, if known (discontinue drug, treat infection), supportive care, corticosteroids, or even immunosuppressive agents.

Infections

Infections may cause purpura by several mechanisms, including direct vessel wall invasion, direct effect of a toxin released by the infecting organism on the vessel wall, thrombocytopaenia, DIC, immunologically mediated vasculitis, and septic emboli. Many bacteria, viruses, fungi, and protozoal infections have been associated with purpura, but the presentations are not specific enough to allow discrimination based on the skin findings. Some of the infections cause a clinical picture that is highly specific, and will be discussed in more detail.

Rocky Mountain spotted fever is caused by *Rickettsia rickettsii*. The organism is transmitted by tick bite, and the fever begins after an incubation period of 3–12 days. The rash typically appears within 1 week of the onset of fever, beginning on the hands, wrists, feet, and ankles, then spreading centrally to the trunk. The lesions begin as red macules and rapidly progress to petechiae. In fulminant cases, the rash can progress to large ecchymoses and purpura fulminans with areas of necrosis. Treatment with antibiotics as early in the course of the disease as possible is of paramount importance.

Another *Rickettsia* infection, epidemic typhus caused by *R. prowazekki*, has been responsible for severe epidemics in the past but is less common today. The vector is the body louse. The rash of epidemic typhus begins as red macules in the axillae and on the trunk, progressing to purpuric lesions and spreading to the extremities, usually sparing the hands and feet. Early antibiotic treatment is the mainstay of treatment.

Neisseria species also commonly cause purpuric skin lesions. Skin lesions are the presenting symptom in meningococcaemia in the majority of cases. The lesions are characteristically small, stellate, purplish-grey, palpable purpura that are quite tender. They may rapidly progress to purpura fulminans. While most common on the lower extremities, the rash can appear anywhere. Prompt recognition and management with antibiotics and supportive care are necessary to prevent progression and death. Disseminated gonococcaemia, caused by *N. gonorrhoeae*, also presents with palpable purpura, some with pustular centres. The lesions tend to be few and widely distributed. Arthralgias and fever are usually associated with the rash, and antibiotics are necessary for the treatment.

Purpura fulminans refers to rapidly progressive haemorrhagic necrosis of the skin, with haematologic features of DIC. It is most commonly related to severe bacterial infections with sepsis, but can also be idiopathic, following a 'preparatory' infection, such as varicella or streptococcus. Rarely, it is seen in newborns associated with protein S or C deficiency. Treatment is supportive, antibiotics as appropriate for the underlying infection, replacement of coagulation factors and platelets as indicated, and heparin to stop DIC.

Decreased mechanical support of the microcirculation

Minor trauma usually does not result in bruising. However, if the connective tissue that supports and protects the microcirculation is inadequate, then minor—often unnoticed—trauma can result in bleeding.

Solar purpura

This is also called purpura of ageing or 'senile' purpura. This condition is frequently seen in the ageing population. It is most commonly present on the extensor surfaces of the forearms and can be extensive. It is thought to be caused by sunlight-induced collagen degradation. Because of the resultant decreased support, the skin is fragile to shear forces. This fits with the patient's history that even the slightest force results in purpura or even a laceration. Reassurance and protection are indicated.

Scurvy

Scurvy is a disease of collagen metabolism caused by a deficiency of vitamin C, which prevents cross-linking of collagen fibres, thus decreasing its strength and support to the microcirculation. Purpura develops after about 90 days of vitamin C deprivation. An associated skin finding is corkscrew hair.

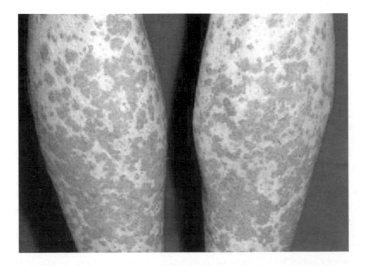

Fig. 1 Leucocytoclastic vasculitis of posterior legs. (See Plate 43.)

The treatment is vitamin C replacement. It takes only 10 mg per day to prevent scurvy.

Hypercortisolism

Purpura is frequently seen in patients with corticosteroid excess, whether primary Cushing's syndrome or from exogenous corticosteroids. Cortisol inhibits collagen synthesis, leading to decreased connective tissue and easy bruising. Clinically, the purpura looks much like solar purpura, but in the setting of a Cushingoid patient. Prolonged use of potent topical steroids can also lead to localized areas of skin atrophy then purpura.

Heritable disorders of connective tissue

The classic disorders of this group are the Ehler–Danlos syndromes ('elastic man syndrome'), but also in this group are osteogenesis imperfecta, pseudoxanthoma elasticum, and Marfan's syndrome. Purpura often develops with slight trauma, lacerations are frequent, and healing is abnormal, resulting in re-injury.

Amyloidosis

In this condition, amyloid infiltrates the space between the endothelium and the basement membrane of the vessels, resulting in decreased flexibility and strength of the vessels. Extravasation of blood can occur, and purpura may be the presenting symptom in some patients. The distribution of purpuric lesions in amyloidosis is typically on the face, an unusual distribution that may help in the diagnosis of this unusual condition.

Other causes

Mechanical purpura

The haemostatic integrity of the microvascular system can be overcome by significant changes in pressure. Excessive valsalva forces, such as with lifting heavy weights or pushing in labour, or protracted vomiting or coughing episodes can result in purpura. Likewise, tourniquets or other restrictive bands can cause purpura.

Purpura simplex

One common reason for visits to ambulatory clinics, particularly in young, otherwise healthy women, is easy bruisability, without the predisposing fragile skin as seen in solar purpura. The lesions are usually solitary, but they may recur. They are sometimes called 'Devil's pinches'. The patient complains of a stinging sensation, usually on the legs, followed by the development of a bruise. Though bothersome, the condition is benign and not commonly associated with more serious pathologies.

Progressive pigmented purpuras

This group of disorders has as a common pathway of pathogenesis—dilatation of dermal capillaries with occasional endothelial proliferation. The vessels are fragile and break with minor trauma, resulting in purpura, most commonly on the anterior lower leg. These are chronic or subacute in nature. Histologically, there is extravasation of erythrocytes with lymphocytic infiltration but no granulocytic infiltration. Clinically, it appears as orange-red or 'cayenne pepper' macules, with lesions eventually fading only to be replaced by new lesions. The aetiology of the disorders is unknown. They rarely cause symptoms except mild itching and the cosmetic appearance. Therapy is not necessary or effective. Schamberg's disease is the most common disorder of this group.

Factitial purpura

This is most frequently caused by self-inflicted wounds, such as placing a drinking glass around the mouth and sucking the air out to induce perioral mechanical purpura. Occasionally, patients will surreptitiously take heparin or coumarins to cause bleeding. Underlying psychopathology may not be obvious, and these patients can be a great challenge.

Psychogenic purpura

This condition, also termed Gardner–Diamond syndrome, may or may not be a subset of factitial purpura. Purpuric lesions occur most commonly on the extremities following trauma or emotional upset. The lesions begin as nodule and develop into ecchymoses; pruritus and pain may occur. Some authors have suggested the condition is due to autosensitization to extravasated erythrocytes, leading to a dermal inflammation. The lesions may take months to years to resolve. The condition occurs most commonly in women, and they frequently go from physician to physician seeking answers.

Associated with malignancy

Neoplastic diseases of the endothelium can result in purpura and haemorrhagic lesions. Chief among these is Kaposi's sarcoma. Other less common tumours of the vascular system can also lead to purpuric lesions. A direct endothelial cell defect is the cause of these lesions.

Lymphomas and leukaemias have also been associated with purpuric lesions, and the skin findings may be the first sign of the illness. The proposed mechanism is a hypersensitivity reaction to tumour antigens.

Toxins and venoms

Bites by arthropod and venomous snakes can cause purpura by local anticoagulant effects, direct destructive effects on the microvasculature, or systemically by inducing DIC. This diagnosis should be considered if localized, non-symmetric purpura develop.

Embolic phenomena

Fat embolism occurs some hours after a fracture of a long bone. Clinical signs include hypoxia, dyspnoea, and sometimes mental status change. Frequently, non-palpable petechial lesions will develop over the trunk and face. Cholesterol embolism occurs most often after disturbance of atherosclerotic vasculature by the use of catheters or after surgery. Non-palpable purpura will be observed 'downstream' for the disturbed plaque.

Assault and abuse

It is self-evident that after an assault, bruising will occur. The health care provider must always keep in mind the possibility of abuse, especially in children and the elderly. Unusual configuration or location of bruises or a history that is not compatible with the pattern of injury should suggest the possibility of abuse, and should be addressed accordingly.

Drugs

Pharmaceuticals can cause purpura by inducing thrombocytopaenia or by hypersensitivity vasculitis, as mentioned earlier in the chapter. Most classes of drugs have been associated with purpura and a drug side-effect should be considered in anyone taking medications.

Differential diagnosis of purpura

With the vast number of diagnoses to consider in a patient who presents with purpura and the considerable overlap in symptoms, the approach to an undifferentiated patient with purpura can be quite challenging. Figure 2 shows a flow chart that may be of help for the initial evaluation. A careful history and physical will often be all that is required to reach a diagnosis, but limited laboratory evaluation may be helpful. A complete blood count including platelet count, prothrombin time, and partial thromboplastin time are the most commonly ordered tests, with more specialized test occasionally to confirm a specific diagnosis, for example, an ANA test. A skin biopsy may be helpful, especially in the evaluation of palpable purpura.

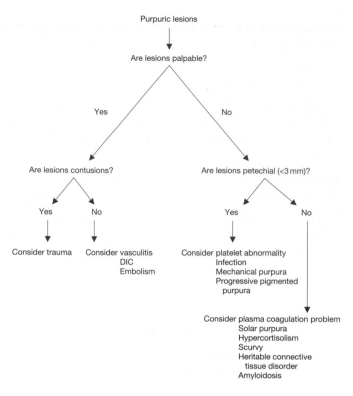

Fig. 2 Flow chart for evaluation of purpura.

Summary

Purpura should be approached as a symptom that provides clues to the underlying condition, the severity of which may range from the simple and benign to the devastating and rapidly fatal. The clinician must take into consideration the distribution and appearance of lesions, the presence of associated symptoms (e.g. fever, pain), the age and overall health of the patient, the timing (sudden onset or not), and exposures to medications or toxins. Although history and physical examination will point toward the correct diagnosis in most cases, laboratory evaluation and skin biopsy may be necessary. An organized approach can help discover the correct diagnosis and lead to appropriate treatment.

Key points

- Purpura should be approached as a symptom that provides clues to the underlying condition.

- Prophylactic vitamin K at birth is very effective at preventing haemorrhagic disease of the newborn.

- Henoch–Schönlein purpura is usually a self-limited disease but close monitoring of renal function is essential.

- Meningococcal bacteraemia often presents with purpuric skin lesions—prompt recognition and management is necessary to prevent death.

Further reading

Baselga, E., Drolet, B., and Esterly, N. (1997). Purpura in infants and children. *Journal of the American Academy of Dermatology* **37**, 673–705.

Jaffe, F. (1994). Petechial hemorrhages: a review of pathogenesis. *The American Journal of Forensic Medicine and Pathology* **15** (3), 203–7.

Kitchens, C. (1984). The purpuric disorders. *Seminars in Thrombosis and Hemostasis* **10** (3), 173–89.

Piette, W. (1994). The differential diagnosis of purpura from a morphologic perspective. *Advances in Dermatology* **9**, 3–23.

Schreiner, D. (1989). Purpura. *Dermatology Clinics* **7** (3), 481–90.

Stevens, G., Adelman, H., and Wallach, P. (1995). Palpable purpura: an algorithmic approach. *American Family Physician* **52** (5), 55–62.

Vora, A. and Makris, M. (2001). An approach to investigation of easy bruising. *Archives of Diseases in Childhood* **84**, 488–91.

Fitzpatrick, T. et al., ed. *Dermatology in Clinical Medicine.* New York: McGraw-Hill, 1993.

Habif, T. *Clinical Dermatology.* St Louis MO: The C.V. Mosby Company, 1990.

15.12 Lumps in and under the skin

Richard P. Usatine and Gunjan Sharma

Lumps in and under the skin come in all shapes, sizes, colours, and textures. These lumps are most often benign growths but occasionally can be pre-malignant or malignant. While virtually all skin lesions other than flat macules and superficial scaly lesions may be considered lumps, we will focus on a set of common skin growths that are often seen in the offices of primary care physicians. We are purposely leaving out naevi, melanomas, acne, and various infections of the skin which are covered in other chapters. The lumps we will be covering can be divided into the three categories shown in Table 1.

It is essential to be able to distinguish between benign and malignant growths in order to detect skin cancers at the earliest stage. Skin cancers that go undetected can result in cosmetic deformities, functional disturbances, or loss of life.

Patients are often concerned about new skin growths because they fear skin cancer, are disturbed by the appearance of the growth, have symptoms such as pain or itching, are worried by bleeding from the growth, or find the growth gets in the way of normal life activities. For these reasons, primary care physicians need to be able to diagnose and treat most types of skin growths whether they are benign or malignant. It is also appropriate to make timely referrals to other skin specialists when the diagnosis and or treatment are beyond the limitations of your knowledge and skills.

Table 1 Types of skin lumps seen in general practice

Benign growths—cherry angiomas, epidermal and pilar cysts, dermatofibroma, lipoma, neurofibroma, pyogenic granulomas, seborrhoeic keratosis, sebaceous hyperplasia, skin tags (acrochordon)
Pre-malignant growths—keratoacanthoma
Malignant lesions—basal cell carcinoma, squamous cell carcinoma

Epidemiology

As we age, we continue to develop new skin growths over time. The skin growths can be part of the normal ageing process such as the acquisition of seborrhoeic keratoses. Sun exposure is the greatest preventable risk factor for the development of malignant growths. Seborrhoeic keratoses are the most common benign neoplasm and develop on the back, face, and extremities of many older persons. Sebaceous hyperplasia is a common skin condition that occurs particularly on the face of adults and the incidence increases with ageing. Keratoacanthomas usually are seen in male patients, most commonly age 50–70 and are distributed over sun-exposed areas. Basal cell carcinoma (BCC) occurs most commonly in Caucasians between the ages of 40 and 80. Squamous cell carcinoma (SCC) occurs more commonly in white men older than 55.

The relative frequencies of skin malignancies are:

- BCC 80 per cent;
- SCC 16 per cent;
- melanoma 4 per cent.

All skin growths are more common with ageing. In particular, seborrhoeic keratoses and cherry angiomas are very common in middle aged and elderly persons. Over 25 per cent of adults have acrochordons (skin tags) and these are found more commonly in patients that are overweight in areas where there is skin friction. Neurofibromas and pyogenic granulomas are the least common of all the benign growths discussed in this chapter.

The majority of lumps in and under the skin are idiopathic. Some lumps that have identified causes are shown in Table 2.

Diagnosis

Most skin lumps can be diagnosed on the basis of their appearance and how they feel. Our clinical acumen improves as we learn to recognize the common and uncommon patterns in which these growths appear. Pattern recognition involves recognizing:

- the shape, size, colour, and distribution of the growths;
- whether the growths are soft, hard, or blanch;
- their depth within or under the skin.

Diagnostic features for skin growths which often cause confusion are shown in Table 3. A fuller descriptions of each lesion is given below.

Cherry angiomas are often dome shaped and 0.1–0.4 cm in diameter. These superficial vascular spots look like cherries, are soft and blanch with pressure.

Epidermal cysts often have a central punctum or pore that may drain foul-smelling white or clear keratinaceous material. These cysts may be superficial in areas of thin skin around the face and ears and deeper below the thicker skin of the back and neck. These cysts may become inflamed and tender. Pilar cysts are a type of epidermal cyst found on the scalp.

Dermatofibromas are discrete, firm nodules, 0.3–1.0 cm in diameter that are non-tender and often have a hyperpigmented halo. They are most commonly found on the legs of adults and may show a central umbilication with pinching.

Lipomas are subcutaneous and are soft, rounded, or lobulated. They are usually movable under the overlying skin.

Seborrhoeic keratoses (SKs) are stuck-on, warty, well-circumscribed, scaly hyperpigmented lesions. They often may be diagnosed on the basis of their clinical appearance only. Close inspection with magnification often will demonstrate the presence of horn cysts or dark keratin plugs. They occur on back, trunk, face, abdomen, and extremities. SKs can show many of the features of a malignant melanoma, including an irregular border and variable pigmentation. The key differential diagnostic features are the surface characteristics. Melanomas have a smooth surface that varies in elevation, colour density and shade. SKs preserve a uniform appearance over their entire surface. If there is a significant suspicion of melanoma, full thickness biopsy should be performed. A shave biopsy can be performed when suspicion of melanoma is very low but the diagnosis is slightly uncertain.

Sebaceous hyperplasia has the appearance of a yellowish papule with umbilication without ulceration on the face of an adult. It is important to differentiate sebaceous hyperplasia from nodular BCC—squeeze to look for sebum. A shave biopsy should be performed if not certain. If many lesions are present, shave the most suspicious one.

BCCs appear as nodular, superficial and sclerosing lesions, in that order of prevalence. Nodular BCCs begin as small, firm, dome-shaped papules, with a smooth surface reflecting a loss of the normal pore pattern. The surface has a pearly white, translucent appearance. As these lesions enlarge, they may ulcerate centrally or peripherally, leaving a small bloody crust or a scar at the site of ulceration. Superficial BCCs and SCC in situ appear as red or pink scaling plaques, occasionally with shallow erosions or crusts (Fig. 1). Differentiation between these two similar lesions requires biopsy. Sclerosing BCCs are colourless, flat, macular tumours, with an atrophic surface and a hard, indurated consistency. They may resemble scars and are easily overlooked.

Table 2 Skin lumps with known cause

Dermatofibromas can be caused by trauma, a viral infection, or an insect bite
Pyogenic granulomas often occur at a site of minor trauma and are more common in pregnancy
Keratoacanthomas may be associated with tar exposure; an increased incidence is seen in immunocompromised patients
Predisposing factors to the development of basal cell carcinoma are chronic ultraviolet sunlight exposure, arsenic, and ionizing radiation
Causes of squamous cell carcinoma include ultraviolet radiation, old burn scars, chronic inflammation, PUVA therapy, radiation therapy, arsenic, tar, immunosuppression, smoking, xeroderma pigmentosum

Table 3 Making a differential diagnosis

Simple lumps	Pigmented lesions	Bleed easily	Dome shaped
Epidermal cyst—contains keratinous material, may have central punctum	Melanoma—smooth surface, even if variation colour and elevation	Squamous cell carcinoma—slow growing scaly red lesion	Nodular basal cell carcinoma—slow growing, central ulceration later
Dermatofibroma—discrete, firm, may have pigmented halo	Seborrhoeic keratosis—stuck on appearance, irregular surface with keratin plugs/horns	Pyogenic granuloma—fast-growing red papule	Keratoacanthoma—rapid growth, keratin core
Lipoma—soft, rounded, may be movable under skin			

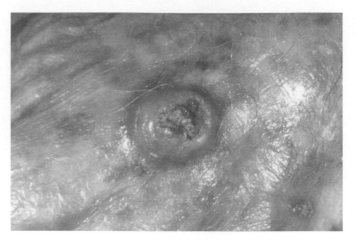

Fig. 3 Keratoacanthoma is a dome-shaped nodule with a central keratotic core. (See Plate 46.)

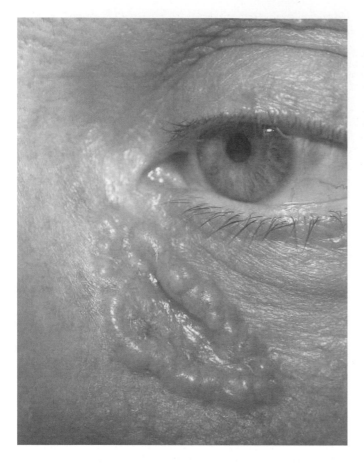

Fig. 1 Nodular basal cell carcinoma showing a raised border, a smooth pearly surface, and telangiectasias. (See Plate 44.)

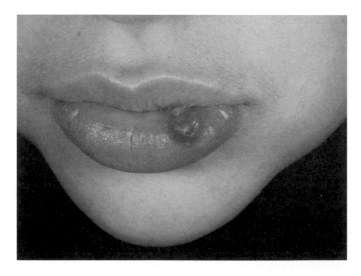

Fig. 2 Erythematous friable papule indicating diagnosis of pyogenic granulomas. (See Plate 45.)

SCCs of the skin may present as slowly growing scaly red lesions particularly on the face and scalp. They are frequently hyperkeratotic and can be friable and bleed easily.

The diagnosis of BCC and SCC is confirmed by histologic examination after biopsy. A shave biopsy or a 2–4 mm punch biopsy usually provides

sufficient tissue for diagnosis. Lesions that are above the skin or are thick may be biopsied by a shave biopsy. A punch biopsy is suggested for flat lesions such as sclerosing BCC. Diagram the area on the chart from which the biopsy is taken, because healing of small lesions may make the site difficult to discern if further treatment is necessary.

Pyogenic granulomas are diagnosed based on the clinical history of an erythematous papule that bleeds easily and has developed over a few days to weeks (Fig. 2). The classic distribution is head, neck, extremities, and gingiva. They are seen more commonly in pregnancy. Because an amelanotic melanoma can resemble a pyogenic granuloma, it is wise to send the removed lesion for histologic examination.

Keratoacanthomas appear with the sudden onset of a solitary, rapidly growing dome-shaped nodule with a central keratotic core (Fig. 3). A history of such a lesion which is rapidly growing should alert the clinician to the diagnosis. Excisional biopsy is a good method for diagnosis and to differentiate keratoacanthoma from SCC.

Skin tags (acrochordons) are pedunculated lesions on narrow stalks occurring around axilla, neck, groin, and under the breasts.

Principles of management

Biopsy options include the shave biopsy, punch biopsy, and the fusiform or elliptical biopsy. The following material will give specific recommendations for treatment of the growths covered in this chapter. These are only recommendations based on the literature, the authors experience and the interpretation of common standards of practice. Primary care physicians should consider availability of equipment, the standards of practice in his or her community, and patient preference to determine the treatment of any specific growth seen in his or her practice (Table 4).

Cherry angiomas

Small cherry angiomas can be electrodesiccated with low current with or without anaesthesia. Settings of about 1.5–2 W are suggested when using the Hyfrecator electrosurgical instrument. This can be done without anaesthesia for small lesions. For larger lesions—use lidocaine with epinephrine for anaesthesia and shave the angioma off with a #15 scalpel. Use electrodessication for the base. Chemical haemostasis is an alternative to electrocoagulation if the angioma was removed completely by the shave procedure.

Table 4 Management options for skin lumps

Reassuring the patient and doing nothing
Reassuring the patient and monitoring the growth over time
Biopsy the growth if it is suspected to be malignant
Excising the growth for cosmetic or functional reasons
Using cryotherapy to destroy the lesion
Using electrosurgery (with or without curettage) to destroy the lesion
Using a topical medication

Dermatofibromas

It is best to convince patients to leave their dermatofibromas alone because surgical removal can result in a scar that is more painful and unsightly than the original dermatofibroma. Cryotherapy is one alternative, but is not very effective. Surgical punch excision may be used to remove small dermatofibromas. Larger lesions may require a fusiform excision.

Epidermal cysts

Most epidermal cysts can be left alone and not excised. If excision is planned, one should remove the entire cyst wall and the irritating contents. After local anaesthesia, the skin above the cyst can be opened with a linear incision, a fusiform incision, or a 4 mm punch biopsy. Using the first two methods, the surgeon may attempt to remove the cyst intact. If the cyst opens, one should remove all the cyst wall and its contents to prevent post-surgical inflammation and re-growth of the cyst. When using a small punch biopsy hole that is smaller than the actual cyst, the punch is cut into the cyst itself and the contents of the cyst are expelled with external pressure. Then the cyst wall is removed through the open hole. In some cases, the cyst is inflamed or infected. Then an incision and drainage should be done and the cyst wall removed after the inflammation resolves.

Neurofibromas

Appropriate methods to remove a neurofibroma include excision with a shave, a punch biopsy if it is small, or an elliptical excision if the lesion is large.

Pyogenic granuloma

A pyogenic granuloma is best treated by shave excision, curettage of the base and then electrosurgery. Because these are very vascular lesions, it is good to let the lidocaine and epinephrine work for at least 10 min to get the maximal haemostatic effect from the epinephrine. Sometimes a small tourniquet can be used for a few minutes during the initial shave excision. The curette is used to scrape out any remaining vascular tissue and electrodessication can destroy any remaining tissue to prevent re-growth.

Seborrhoeic keratoses

Destructive methods to treat SKs can be used if the diagnosis is certain. Cryotherapy with a 1 mm halo is fast and easy. One must be careful to not overfreeze and cause permanent hypopigmentation of the skin. Electrodessication and curettage is another safe and easy method. The tissue after electrodessication is so soft that even a moistened gauze pad can be used to do the curettage.

Sebaceous hyperplasia

Sebaceous hyperplasia is purely of cosmetic concern unless the lesion resembles a BCC. If the diagnosis is uncertain the shave biopsy can be used for diagnostic and therapeutic purposes. Some methods for the treatment of sebaceous hyperplasia are: cryotherapy, shave excision, electrodessication, and pulse dye laser. Accutane could be prescribed if it is severe.

Skin tags

Snip excision with sharp iris scissors is a reliable method for removing skin tags. Ethyl chloride can be used for topical refrigerant anaesthesia. Haemostasis with aluminium chloride is sufficient. Electrosurgery is good method for the removal of multiple small skin tags. Cryotherapy works variably depending upon the size, smaller is better. If a skin tag has a large base, use lidocaine and epinephrine and then shave off with #15 scalpel. If the skin tags are classic and have a benign appearance, they often do not need to be sent to pathology. If you are uncertain, you may send the most suspicious ones.

Keratoacanthoma

A superficial shave biopsy is not an adequate technique when dealing with a keratoacanthoma because these lesions are invariably much deeper and will recur if treated only with a superficial shave biopsy. After the deep shave, performing a superficial curettage and desiccation to prevent recurrence is recommended. Consider referral to a dermatologic surgeon, especially for multiple lesions. Oral retinoids or intralesional chemotherapy may be options in such cases.

Basal cell carcinoma

There are many treatments available for BCCs. While a shave biopsy is a common diagnostic technique, it is not the definitive treatment for any type of BCC. After a diagnosis with a shave biopsy, there are number of options to remove the remaining BCC. Curettage and electrodessication is an excellent method of treatment for small nodular and superficial BCCs. This cycle is repeated three times. The fusiform (elliptical) excision can be used for diagnostic and therapeutic purposes. Cryosurgery is one treatment option for small superficial BCCs because it is quick and gives good cosmetic results. Mohs surgery gives meticulous margin control and low recurrence rates. It is particularly useful in sclerosing BCCs, recurrent BCCs, and BCCs in cosmetic and functional areas. Radiation is the treatment of choice for patients who are not operative candidates. Refer any SCCs to a dermatologic surgeon unless you have significant experience treating non-melanoma skin cancers.

Patient education

Patient education is an important part of the treatment of skin growths. Also, patients should be given informed consent before performing surgery. Risks such as pain, scar formation, bleeding, infection, and recurrence should be explained regardless of whether you are removing a benign or malignant lesion. Specific suggestions about how to discuss various skin growths with patients follow.

Can be left alone

Cherry angiomas—Reassure patients that these are benign and are best left alone. Large ones may bleed if they become traumatized, but the bleeding can be stopped with pressure.

Lipomas—Most lipomas can remain untreated. The resulting scar over an excised lipoma can be more noticeable and look worse than the lipoma itself. A lipoma may be excised with a fusiform excision when patients insist on removal. Large and deep lipomas may need to be removed in the operating room.

Skin tags or acrochordons—May be left but can get caught in clothing and necklaces and bleed or get inflamed. Multiple lesions may develop and there are no ways to prevent development of new lesions except for weight loss if the patient is overweight.

Risk of recurrence

Epidermal cysts—Let patients know that epidermal cysts can recur even after surgery.

Dermatofibromas—Patients should be advised that lesions may recur and that the hyperpigmentation may persist despite treatment.

Neurofibromas—Before treating neurofibromas, you should tell patients that these lesions can recur or the area of the excision can become indented.

BCC and SCC—There is a risk of recurrence which varies based on the type and location of the lesion along with the treatment type used.

Discuss cancer risk

Seborrhoeic keratoses(SK)—because melanoma can look like an SK, patients should be educated about the signs and symptoms of melanoma (ABCDEs of melanoma). If the patient feels that the SK is developing features that are suggestive of melanoma, he or she must return for evaluation and possible excision. Unfortunately, there are no ways to prevent development of new SKs.

Keratoacanthomas are not invasive but can become quite large and involute and cause severe scarring. If the scarring occurs on structures such as the ears or nose, disfigurement may result.

BCC or SCC patients should be educated about the direct relationship of these cancers to cumulative sun exposure. Discuss sun-protection measures (e.g. wearing hats and long sleeves, avoiding midday sun, and using sunscreens). Teach skin self-examination with attention to any new lesions that do not resolve within 6–8 weeks. Educate patients to watch for changes in scar sites (e.g. elevation, ulceration, induration). Emphasize the importance of follow-up, because new lesions will develop in 40–50 per cent of patients.

Conclusions

While patients have many reasons to seek medical care for skin growths, the primary care physician needs to understand the diagnosis and natural history of the skin growths in order to appropriately educate the patient about the management options available. Treatment options include reassurance, observation, biopsy, surgical removal, or destruction by cryotherapy, curettage, or electrosurgery. It is appropriate to make timely referrals to other skin specialists when the diagnosis and or treatment are beyond the limitations of your knowledge and skills.

Key points

1. It is essential to be able to distinguish between benign and malignant growths in order to detect skin cancers at the earliest stage.

2. While patients have many reasons to seek medical care for skin growths, the primary care physician needs to understand the diagnosis and natural history of the skin growths in order to appropriately educate the patient about the management options available.

3. Pattern recognition is an effective method for diagnosis. Biopsy is usually only needed when malignancy is suspected.

4. Biopsy options include the shave biopsy, punch biopsy, and the fusiform (elliptical) biopsy.

5. Not all skin growths need to be treated or removed. Reassurance is often the best treatment for benign growths such as cherry angiomas, sebaceous hyperplasia, seborrhoeic keratoses, and skin tags.

6. It is appropriate to make timely referrals to other skin specialists when the diagnosis and or treatment are beyond the limitations of your knowledge and skills.

Further reading

Goldstein, B.G. and Goldstein, A.O. *Practical Dermatology* 2nd edn. St Louis MO: Mosby-Year Book, Inc., 1997.

Habif, T. *Clinical Dermatology: A Color Guide to Diagnosis and Therapy* 3rd edn. St Louis MO: Mosby, 1996.

Usatine, R., Moy, R., Tobinick, E., and Siegel, D. *Skin Surgery: A Practical Guide.* St Louis MO: Mosby-Year Book, Inc., 1998.

15.13 Photosensitivity

Sandra Marchese Johnson

Photosensitivity disorders are fairly common. They are most frequently managed by primary care providers. The most common, polymorphous light eruption (PLE), occurs in about 14 per cent of the light-skinned population in America and as high as 24 per cent in Scandinavia.

A photosensitive reaction should always be considered when a patient seeks care for a rash that is confined to areas of the skin that are exposed to light. These reactions are abnormal cutaneous responses to ordinary light exposure. The person afflicted may complain of allergy to the sun because of itching or burning after exposure. Frequently, a patient with a light-sensitive reaction will present with a rash on exposed skin surfaces that cannot be explained, or with reported skin symptoms after sun exposure that resolved before the visit.

Clinical history

A diagnosis can often be made solely on the basis of history.[1] But there are times when the history is insufficient for diagnosis and laboratory studies and/or a biopsy is required. There are more complicated photosensitive disorders that require phototesting in order to achieve an accurate diagnosis. The testing requires sophisticated and expensive apparatus. These diseases require referral to a consultant dermatologist.

The common photosensitive disorders can be differentiated by determining historical events surrounding the onset of symptoms. The age of the patient when symptoms were first noted is especially important. Some good questions to ask are listed in Table 1.

Knowing about medicinal and cosmeceutical exposure including prescription drugs, over-the-counter medications, herbal remedies, plants,

Table 1 Questions to ask about photosensitivity

1.	How long does it take for the skin reaction to develop and how long does it last?
2.	Have you ever had a similar reaction?
3.	How old were you when you first experienced this condition?
4.	What do you put on your skin?
5.	What is your occupation?
6.	What medications do you take?
7.	Do you have other symptoms?
8.	Are other organ systems involved?
9.	Does light coming through a window glass cause symptoms?
10.	Does anyone else in your family have similar problems?

and perfumes are essential because all can be sources of photosensitization. A family history of photosensivity may lead to identification of a genodermatosis. Learning about other organ system involvement may provide information about a systemic disease with skin manifestations. The interval between sun exposure and skin reaction will help delineate between solar urticaria (minutes) and PLE (hours to days). The occupation and recreation of the patient will provide information about exposure to photosensitizing agents. Artificial light sources such as welding arcs and computer terminals may exacerbate symptoms. The duration of individual lesions will help to distinguish between solar urticaria (resolves quickly) and porphyrias (may persist for months). Seasonal variation will differentiate between PLE (worse in spring and early summer) and actinic prurigo (persists all year). UVB light is filtered by window glass, but UVA light is not. If the degree of photosensitivity is affected by glass filtering then one has a clue to the wavelengths responsible for photosensitivity. Associated systemic and cutaneous symptoms may also provide clues such as pruritus with photoallergy or burning with porphyrias. Involvement of other organ systems may also prompt one to consider diseases such as dermatomyositis and porphyrias.[2]

Knowing the time between exposure to light and the onset of the skin disorder will help to differentiate between the various diseases. Some are acute starting within a few minutes or hours after exposure and may resolve in hours or a few days. These include drug-related photosensivity and solar urticaria. Others are chronic, with slower onset and are persistent. These include porphyria cutanea tarda (PCT), lupus erythematoses, and hydroa vacciniforme. The most common of the photosensitive diseases, PLE, is between the acute and chronic for it has features of both.

Clinical examination

Most photosensitive patients have sharply demarcated eruptions, small papules coalescing to plaques and small vesicles, limited to exposed skin (Fig. 1). Areas commonly spared include the upper eyelids, submental area, post-auricular area, upper lip, and skin creases. The face may be relatively spared due to hardening or chronic exposure.[2] Photocontact dermatoses will usually be limited to the site of application. Sometimes the primary skin lesions will provide clues to the diagnosis. Patients with PCT present with blisters and milia whereas people with solar urticaria will present with urticarial papules and plaques.

Some patients present without appreciable skin pathology at the time of the physical examination. This is especially true for people with solar urticaria and PLE. Patients with a chronic or persistent photodermatosis may not have skin lesions to observe at the time of presentation. These include PCT, and chronic actinic dermatosis (CAD).

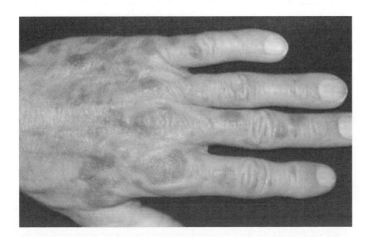

Fig. 1 A photosensitive patient having sharply demarcated eruptions, small papules coalescing to plaques, and small vesicles. (See Plate 47.)

Laboratory evaluation

A skin biopsy with immunofluorescence may provide information to determine the cause and to rule out other possibilities in the differential diagnosis. Systemic lupus erythematosus (SLE), dermatomyositis, porphyrias, hydroa vacciniforme, photoallergy, and phototoxicity can often be differentiated histologically. A biopsy should also rule out a light-aggravated dermatosis.

Laboratory tests that may be helpful to determine the type of photosensitive disorder include circulating antinuclear antibody (ANA) and extractable nuclear antigens, anti-SSA (Ro), and anti-SSB (La). Further laboratory workup for porphyrias include plasma, stool, and urine porphyrins. Anti-Jo-1 or other anti-tRNA synthetases will be positive with dermatomyositis.[3]

Differential diagnosis

A photodermatosis can occur at any age but differentiation by age of onset is effective for diagnosing the common diseases. Table 2 lists the age that many of the conditions first occur.

Photodermatoses beginning at a young age

Juvenile spring eruption (JSE) is a variant of PLE that occurs in spring. It probably occurs much more frequently than reported because when it starts it is usually mild and with natural skin hardening it ceases. It is more common in boys but can occur in either sex. The early typical case will present as a mild minute papular rash occurring on the ears and malar eminences of the face. The rash occurs after the first prolonged exposure to the sun. Usually the lesions last only a few days, so that a physician does not always see the clinical manifestations. JSE can be more severe with larger papules, blisters, and crusts and for this the primary care provider is consulted. Treatment may be limited to reassurance of the parents, avoidance of sun exposure, and/or application of a mild corticosteroid cream such as 0.025 per cent Triamcinolone, twice daily until clear. Usually the rash will clear in about 4 days. Relapses will often occur yearly for several years and then disappear because the skin hardens, however some develop PLE later.

Actinic prurigo usually presents with pruritic excoriated papules on the bridge of the nose. The chest and upper back, other areas of the face, arms, and legs can also be involved. It may be difficult to distinguish from PLE. Some of the differentiating features are that the patients affected are younger, have a positive family history, and have perennial involvement. Exposed skin is involved and the lesions may persist in winter in contrast to juvenile spring eruption that does not. Scarring is uncommon but may occur. Young girls are usually affected. The condition may remit in adolescence.[4,5] There has been an association with HLA-DR4 in British patients.[6]

People with erythropoietic protoporphyria complain of burning pain almost immediately after exposure to the sun. There may be no visible skin lesion with the symptoms. The burning pain is often worse when the weather is windy. After recurrent episodes there may be small scars around the mouth and face. Diagnosis is confirmed by laboratory finding of increased protoporphyrin concentrations in the red blood cells.

Table 2 Photodermatoses starting at different ages

In childhood	At maturity	In advanced age
Polymorphous light eruption	Polymorphous light eruption	Chronic actinic dermatitis
Juvenile spring eruption	Solar urticaria	Drug-induced photosensitivity
Actinic prurigo	Drug-induced photosensitivity	Dermatomyositis
Erythropoietic protoporphyria	Porphyria cutanea tarda	Cutaneous T-cell lymphoma
Hydroa vacciniforme	Lupus erythematosis	

Hydroa vacciniforme is very rare and presents with vesicles that scar. The children resemble those affected with varicella zoster virus but are otherwise healthy. Hydroa vacciniforme is important to differentiate from the other conditions because of its high propensity of scar formation. It may remit in adolescence.[4] Strict ultraviolet avoidance is strongly encouraged for people with hydroa vacciniforme.

Photodermatoses starting at maturity

Polymorphous light eruption occurs most frequently in young adult women. It is a relatively common idiopathic photosensitive disorder. There does not appear to be a familial tendency or relationship to skin type. Pruritic vesicles and papules affect the neck and arms and peak at 72 h after exposure.[4] The face may be involved in children. Solar simulation may confirm the diagnosis. ANA, anti-SSA, and anti-SSB are normal.

Solar urticaria is less common than PLE. The condition can appear abruptly and at any age. The primary lesion is an urticarial papule or plaque that arises within 10 min of exposure and resolves within a couple of hours.[1] Associated symptoms can include itching and burning.[4]

There are cutaneous manifestations of SLE, which are photosensitive lesions. There is a variant of LE, sub-acute cutaneous lupus erythematosus, in which the skin is usually the only affected organ. The clinical manifestations of LE are protean. The lesions may mimic PLE or they may be bullous or exanthematous. The lesions of LE usually persist longer than those of PLE.[1] LE may also be differentiated from PLE by positive delayed (up to 3 weeks) phototesting, positive direct immunofluorescence at the dermal–epidermal junction on a skin biopsy with immunoglobulins and complement, a positive anti-SSA (Ro) and/or positive.

Porphyria cutanea tarda and pseudoporphyria cutanea tarda (pseudoPCT) usually presents with skin fragility, blisters, milia and sclerodermoid changes on photoexposed skin. Uroporphyrins I, II, and III are positive in PCT and help to make the diagnosis.

Drug-induced photodermatoses can be divided into phototoxic, photoallergic, and photocontact. A phototoxic drug eruption will occur in every person if given enough of the agent and enough light. It is often considered an aggravated sunburn and will resolve when the drug is withdrawn. The most common culprits are tetracycline antibiotics, psoralen, phenothiazines, non-steroidal anti-inflammatory drugs, thiazide diuretics, and sulfonylureas. Most drugs are phototoxic but some can cause phototoxic and photoallergic reactions. Antihistamines and compounds containing sulfa or sulfur derivatives are common culprits.[5]

Photodermatoses starting at advanced age

Chronic actinic dermatitis presents as erythematous eczematous skin on chronically exposed skin. The areas usually involved include the dorsal hands, face, and neck. Non-exposed skin may become involved in severe cases. Endogenous eczema or contact dermatitis may co-exist and confuse the clinical picture. The clinical manifestations often persist into the winter when the patient has limited exposure. Occasionally, the diagnosis of cutaneous T-cell lymphoma will need to be ruled out.[3] Cutaneous T-cell lymphoma may be indistinguishable from clinically chronic actinic dermatitis. It is diagnosed by CD8 and CD4 studies that show a predominance of CD4 cells.

Patients with dermatomyositis may present with photosensitivity and violaceous telangiectatic patches on the neck, dorsal hands, and in a periocular distribution on the face.

Phytophotodermatitis

This is a relatively common photochemical sensitivity that can occur at any age. The eruption is eczematous, confined to areas exposed to the sun that have been contact with an inciting agent. Inciting agents are often plant materials such as limes, celery, figs, or parsnips. Oil of Bergamot often found in fragrances is another common agent. The affected area frequently has a bizarre distribution. It becomes brown or tan in a few days. Though it may cause much concern to the patient and family, it is innocuous and usually requires no treatment other than reassurance.

Treatment

Wavelengths that reach the earth include ultraviolet, visible light, and infrared rays. UVC is less than 280 nm and is absorbed by the ozone layer. UVB rays are from 280 to 320 nm. UVA rays are from 320 to 400 nm.[1] Because UVA makes up such a greater percentage of the solar spectrum that we are exposed to, it makes sense that most photodermatoses are due to wavelengths that fall in the UVA range. Thus all patients, with or without suspected photosensitivity, should wear broad-spectrum sunscreens that cover wavelengths in both UVB and UVA ranges. Most patients with photosensitivity respond to use of sun-blocking agents and avoidance of sun exposure.

The current recommendations for photoprotection include: (i) liberal application of sunscreen at least 30 min before going outdoors on children 6 months of age and older; (ii) the higher the sun protection factor (SPF) the better; (iii) re-apply sunscreen every 2 h or more especially when partaking in swimming or outdoor activities; (iv) wear sunglasses, a hat, and tightly woven fabric; and (v) avoid outdoor activities between 10:00 a.m. and 4:00 p.m. standard time.[7]

If this is not practical, hardening of the skin may be accomplished with progressive exposure. Hardening will not alleviate all photodermatoses but frequently helps with PLE and JSE.[8]

Polymorphous light eruption

There is a wide range of severity of JSE and PLE. Mild PLE are usually controlled by avoidance and protection against sunlight. Application of a mild Group IV–VII topical corticosteroid preparations will enhance the treatment. Severe chronic PLE requires more aggressive treatment such as oral corticosteroids and/or photodesensitization with UVB or UVA light.

Drug-induced photosensitivity

Drug induced photosensitive disorders include photoallergic reactions, phototoxic reactions, and phytophotodermatitis. Careful history will identify drug, plant, and other chemical allergens which can cause photosensivity. Treatment consists of eliminating contact with or ingestions of these allergens. During the period of time after elimination of the offending agents local treatment with mild topical steroid is indicated.

Actinic prurigo

In addition to avoidance of sunlight and broad-spectrum skin barrier protection, sedative antihistamines and mild topical steroid application will help reduce this condition. Patients who have recalcitrant disease should be referred to a consultant for potential UVB desensitization or PUVA treatment.

Chronic actinic dermatitis

This highly debilitating disease may respond to topical emollient and corticosteroid (Groups IV–VI) therapy. Ingestion of synthetic beta-carotene 180 mg/day prior to exposure has been reported to be effective in preventing severe reactions.[9] If these are not effective PUVA combined with oral prednisone may provide relief.

Porphyria cutanea tarda

Oral low-dose chloroquin and serial phlebotomy to remove excess hepatic iron stores are effective. Weekly removal of 500 cm³ of blood until the serum ferritin level reaches the lower limit of normal is the goal. Then, levels of circulating and excreted porphyrins continue to decline and cutaneous lesions improve. If low-dose chloroquin is administered, liver function studies must accompany administration.

Key points

1. Determine time course of reaction.
2. Take a careful history (see Table 1).
3. Observe any clinical findings: if possible have patient return when the rash is present.
4. Perform initial laboratory investigation and/or biopsy if indicated.
5. Remove any potential sensitizing agents.
6. Refer to specialist when indicated.

References

1. Roelandts, R. (2000). The diagnosis of photosensitivity. *Archives of Dermatology* **136**, 1152–7.
2. Kim, J.J. and Lim, H.W. (1999). Evaluation of the photosensitive patient. *Seminars in Cutaneous Medicine and Surgery* **18** (4), 253–6.
3. Champion, R.H., Burton, J.L., Burns, D.A., and Breathnach, S.M., ed. Cutaneous photobiology. In *Rook/Wilkinson/Ebling Textbook of Dermatology* Chapter 25, pp. 982–93, 1998. Oxford: Blackwell Science.
4. Ferguson, J. and Ibbotson, S. (1999). The idiopathic photodermatoses. *Seminars in Cutaneous Medicine and Surgery* **18** (4), 257–73.
5. Epstein, J.H. (1999). Phototoxicity and photoallergy. *Seminars in Cutaneous Medicine and Surgery* **18** (4), 274–84.
6. Menage, H.P. et al. (1996). HLA-DR4 may determine expression of actinic prurigo in British patients. *Journal of Investigative Dermatology* **106**, 362–7.
7. Pao, C. et al. (1994). Polymorphic light eruption: prevalence in Australia and England. *British Journal of Dermatology* **130**, 62–4.
8. Anderson, D., Wallace, H.J., and Howes, E.I.B. (1989). Juvenile spring eruption of the ears. *Clinical and Experimental Dermatology* **14**, 462–3.
9. Arndt, K., LeBoit, P., Robinson, J., and Weintroub, B.U. *Cutaneous Medicine and Surgery, An Integrated Program in Dermatology* Vol. 1. Philadelphia PA: W.B. Saunders, 1996, pp. 768–71.
10. Lim, H. and Cooper, K. (1998). The health impact of solar radiation and prevention strategies. Report of Environmental Council, American Academy of Dermatology. *Journal of the American Academy of Dermatology* **41** (1), 81–101.
11. Rosen, C.F. (1999). Photoprotection. *Seminars in Cutaneous Medicine and Surgery* **18** (4), 307–14.
12. Kawada, A. (2000). Risk and preventive factors for skin phototype. *Journal of Dermatological Science* **23**, S27–9.

15.14 Genital disorders

Alena Salim and Jennifer Powell

Introduction

Skin diseases affecting the female and male genitalia are a significant and important group of dermatological conditions that may be associated with considerable morbidity, discomfort, and embarrassment. The disorder may be confined to the genitalia or may be part of a generalized dermatosis. Sometimes it is difficult to determine the exact aetiology and it is therefore important to examine the rest of the skin and mucous membranes for other clues to the diagnosis. It should also be remembered that the appearances of common dermatoses affecting the genitalia may be altered since the area is moist and characteristic scaling may be lost. In addition, a 4 mm punch biopsy of skin is a useful diagnostic tool and is easy to perform under local anaesthetic in the outpatient clinic.

In general, presenting symptoms may be divided into three main groups:

1. itching, with or without soreness, and possibly with a rash;
2. pain or 'burning' confined to the genital area;
3. erosions, lumps, and non-healing lesions.

To allow comparison, the presentation in male and female patients of four important dermatoses (lichen sclerosus, lichen planus, intraepithelial neoplasia, and genital psoriasis) is juxtaposed in Figs 1–4. However, for simplicity, the text below deals with men and women separately.

The female genitalia

Rashes

Eczema

The term eczema is used synonymously with dermatitis and for practical purposes eczemas are sub-divided into two main groups, *endogenous* and *exogenous*. Endogenous eczema, such as atopic and seborrhoeic dermatitis, arises as a result of a genetic predisposition, and exogenous eczema, for example, irritant and allergic contact dermatitis results from contact with external substances. Common irritants include vaginal discharge, urine, faeces, soap and other toiletries. Common allergens affecting the vulva include the active constituents of medicaments, for example, neomycin and corticosteroids, other constituents of medicaments such as preservatives (e.g. ethylenediamine in Tri-Adcortyl® cream) and biocides, local anaesthetics, perfumes, spermicides, and rubber chemicals found in condoms.

Vulval eczema commonly presents with pruritus, dryness, soreness, and dyspareunia. On examination, there may be erythema mild scaling and excoriations of the vulva in the acute phase and thickening (lichenification) in the chronic phase.

Secondary infection is common and may exacerbate the symptoms. Therefore, swabs should be taken to exclude infection with Candida or pathogenic bacteria (e.g. staphylococcus and streptococcus).

Treatment involves giving advice on general vulval care such as avoiding all irritants, allergens, and fragranced toiletries, washing with a bland emollient soap substitute, and wearing loose non-restrictive, non-occlusive clothes. Moderately potent (e.g. clobetasone butyrate 0.05 per cent) to potent topical steroids (e.g. beclomethasone dipropionate 0.025 per cent) may be used to bring the inflammation under control and the potency reduced as the condition improves. Sometimes, a topical steroid cream combined with an antifungal is needed and any symptomatic bacterial infection should be treated with oral antibiotics.

Lichen simplex

Any pruritic dermatosis of the vulva can lead to scratching and chronic rubbing. Typically, the vulval skin appears lichenified (thickened with accentuated skin markings, dry, and rugose), scaly and hypo- or hyper-pigmented. The problem then becomes a self-perpetuating one as an itch–scratch cycle is established.

The aim of treatment is to break the itch–scratch cycle. Reassurance and explanation are the key to successful treatment. Patients should be advised about general vulval care and a potent topical steroid (e.g. beclomethasone dipropionate 0.025 per cent) may be needed for short periods in the early stages to bring the condition under control, but this should be gradually tapered as things improve. If scratching at night is a problem, the use of a sedating antihistamine is often very helpful.

Psoriasis

Psoriasis affects 2 per cent of the population and tends to run a chronic course. Typical psoriatic erythematous scaly plaques may appear on the

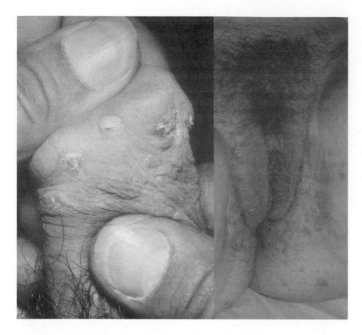

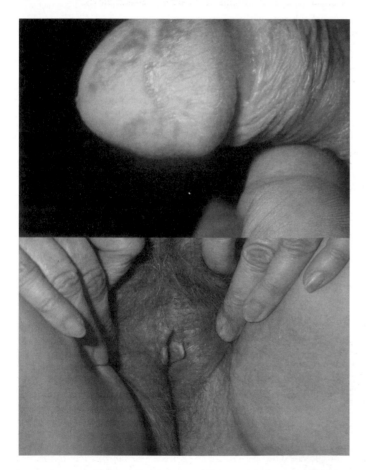

Fig. 1 Genital psoriasis. (See Plate 51.)

Fig. 3 Lichen sclerosus. (See Plate 48.)

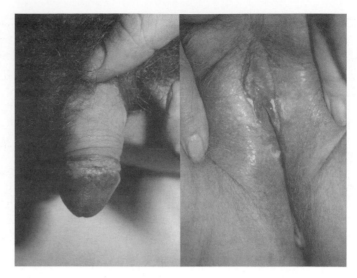

Fig. 2 Lichen planus. (See Plate 49.)

Conventional treatments (such as coal tar) for psoriasis are usually too irritant to apply to the vulva and therefore mild–moderate potency topical steroids are commonly used in combination with topical antibiotics/antifungals (e.g. clobetasone butyrate 0.05 per cent alone or with oxytetracycline and nystatin) if secondary infection is suspected.

Lichen planus

Lichen planus is an inflammatory dermatosis, which has a female preponderance and a peak incidence between 30 and 60 years. The exact aetiology is unknown although it is thought to be immune mediated and certain drugs (e.g. quinine and β-blockers) and infections (such as hepatitis C) may induce a lichen planus-like eruption.

Lichen planus can affect the vulva in two ways. The first is with the typical violaceous flat-topped papules and plaques with white streaks on the surface which affect other body sites simultaneously. The second is an uncommon type of erosive lichen planus, which may affect the vulva, vagina, and gingiva (Fig. 2). The latter patients complain of severe vulval symptoms with pain, burning, dyspareunia, and post-coital bleeding. On examination, the inner labia minora and vestibule are usually affected and the vulval epithelium appears bright red with erosions. Scarring and destruction of the normal vulval architecture may occur.

Referral to a dermatologist is needed to confirm the diagnosis by skin biopsy. The differential diagnoses include lichen sclerosus, immunobullous disorders, infection (herpes simplex virus) and plasma cell vulvitis (Zoon's vulvitis).

Erosive lichen planus tends to run a chronic course that is resistant to treatment. Patients need to be given advice about general care of the vulva. Very potent (e.g. clobetasol propionate) and potent topical (e.g. beclomethasone dipropionate) steroids are helpful in some patients and steroid foam or suppositories may be needed for those with vaginal involvement.

Patients need long-term follow-up since there is the small risk of transformation to squamous cell carcinoma.

Lichen sclerosus

Lichen sclerosus (formerly known as lichen sclerosus et atrophicus) is a chronic inflammatory skin disease that causes significant discomfort and morbidity. It affects women more than men (ratio of 10:1) and although it can occur in all age groups it usually affects post-menopausal women in the fifth and sixth decades. It can also occur in children where the manifestations may be easily mistaken for sexual abuse.

mons pubis and labia majora (Fig. 1). More commonly, the characteristic silvery scale tends to be absent in flexural psoriasis and the areas of erythema on the vulva tend to be well demarcated and this provides a diagnostic clue. The labia minora are not involved.

Although the exact aetiology of lichen sclerosus is unknown it is thought to be autoimmune mediated and is associated with autoantibodies and a number of autoimmune disorders (e.g. vitiligo, alopecia, pernicious anaemia, and thyroid disorders). Immunogenetic studies have also shown an association with HLA class II DQ7.

Lichen sclerosus most commonly affects the anogenital area although extragenital sites may also be involved. The most common presenting symptoms in women are of pruritus, soreness, dysuria, dyspareunia, and pain on defaecation. The classical clinical appearance of lichen sclerosus is ivory white pallor of the vulva, which may extend posteriorly to affect the perianal area in a figure of eight pattern (Fig. 3). There is often associated atrophy and there may be telangiectasia, purpura, erosions, fissures, and hyperkeratosis. As the disease progresses, the architecture of the vulva may become distorted with resorption and fusion of the labia minora and narrowing of the introitus.

The differential diagnosis of lichen sclerosus includes vitiligo (which may co-exist), erosive lichen planus, scarring mucous membrane pemphigoid, and lichen simplex. Patients need to be referred for a diagnostic skin biopsy and should be assessed for associated autoimmunity by means of a full blood count, glucose, thyroid function, serum B12 and autoantibodies [antinuclear antibodies (ANA), thyroid autoantibodies, smooth muscle antibodies, mitochondrial antibodies, and gastric parietal cell antibodies].

Patients with lichen sclerosus require detailed explanation and information regarding the nature of the disease, its natural history, treatment, possible association with malignancy, and reassurance that it is not contagious. Self-help groups such as the lichen sclerosus society may be helpful in this respect.

Advice about general care of the vulva is important. A very potent topical steroid (such as clobetasol propionate) is used initially to bring the disease under control, applying the ointment twice a day for approximately 3 months. The use can then be decreased to 'as and when required'. Patients need to be advised that only the affected areas should be treated and a mirror is helpful in this respect.

There is a small risk, approximately 5 per cent, of malignant transformation to squamous cell carcinoma in areas of lichen sclerosus and patients therefore need long-term follow up often by means of specialist departments sharing care with the primary care team. Patients need to be examined for non-healing erosive or warty lesions that may signify development of malignancy.

Blisters, erosions, and ulcers

Erythema multiforme

A severe variant of erythema multiforme associated with mucosal involvement (oral, ocular, and genital) is called Stevens–Johnson syndrome. Attacks may be recurrent and are commonly precipitated by infection, especially herpes simplex, and drugs although some cases are idiopathic. On examination, blisters and painful shallow ulcers are seen on the labia. Treatment includes withdrawal of any precipitating medication, treatment of the underlying infection and symptomatic relief with local applications. Systemic steroids may be needed in severe cases.

Autoimmune bullous diseases

Autoimmune blistering diseases may affect the skin and mucous membranes, including the vulvovaginal region. In these diseases, antibodies are directed at normal components of the epidermis and basement membrane zone.

The autoimmune bullous disorders may present with intact blisters (e.g. bullous pemphigoid), erosions and ulcers (pemphigus vulgaris), and scarring (mucous membrane pemphigoid).

Referral to a dermatologist is needed to confirm the diagnosis by means of histology, direct and indirect immunofluorescence. Differential diagnoses include erosive lichen planus, lichen sclerosus, herpes simplex infection, and Stevens–Johnson syndrome.

Treatment is with very potent (e.g. clobetasol propionate) and potent topical steroids (e.g. beclomethosone dipropionate) and general care measures previously mentioned are also important.

Behçet's syndrome

Behçet's syndrome is a multisystem disease of unknown aetiology. It commonly affects men more than women in the third and fourth decade. In women, the vulvar lesions typically affect the labia minora and are usually deep, painful, persistent ulcers that vary in size. The ulcers may lead to destruction of the vulvar tissue and scarring is common.

Associated manifestations may include oral ulceration, ocular lesions, pathergy (pustulation after venepuncture), other skin lesions (non-specific macules, papules, nodules, and pustules and vasculitis), arthritis, neurologic manifestations, and thrombotic disease.

Recurrent aphthosis

Patients with recurrent aphthosis present with recurrent oral and genital ulcers. These tend to be more frequent and more superficial than those of Behçet's syndrome and no features of Behçet's are identified. The cause is unknown. Treatment of early lesions with potent topical steroid can be very effective.

Fixed drug eruption

Fixed drug eruptions tend to occur more frequently on the penis than the vulva and are discussed under the male genital dermatoses.

Pre-malignant conditions

Vulval intraepithelial neoplasia (VIN)

The term vulval intraepithelial neoplasia (Fig. 4) includes all the lesions formerly called Bowen's disease, bowenoid papulosis, and carcinoma in situ. The classification is graded I–IV depending on the depth and degree of dysplasia. VIN I is not always a precursor to VIN II and III and may resolve spontaneously. VIN II and III are precursors of cancer and are becoming more common. This is thought to be secondary to the increasing prevalence of dysplastic types of human papillomavirus (HPV), for example, type 16.

Patients complain of pruritus and soreness and may present with non-healing lesions, eroded, crusty erythematous areas or warty, pale, pigmented lesions. The lesions may be multiple or single.

Referral to a gynaecologist or dermatologist initially is appropriate since the diagnosis needs to be confirmed on biopsy. Treatment options include surgical excision and laser therapy.

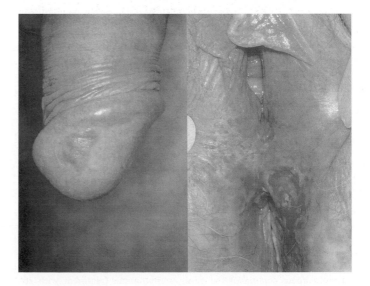

Fig. 4 Intraepithelial neoplasia. (See Plate 50.)

Vulval pain syndromes

The vulval pain syndrome refers to conditions of vulval pain in association with a normal vulva. It primarily describes two conditions, vulvar vestibulitis and dysaesthetic or essential vulvodynia. Patients with vulval pain syndrome have usually been extensively investigated and often treated ineffectively for infectious and/or dermatologic disease. It is thought that the condition is part of the wider group of neuropathic pain syndromes, which include glossodynia, scrotodynia, the chronic perianal pain syndrome and post-herpetic neuralgia.

Vulvar vestibulitis tends to affect young women and patients complain of pain on touch or attempted vaginal penetration (superficial dyspareunia and discomfort on insertion of a tampon). On examination, there is tenderness in the area of the vestibule and possibly some erythema.

Essential or dysaesthetic vulvodynia tends to affect older women and is characterized by symptoms of chronic vulval pain, burning, stinging, discomfort, irritation, and rawness. Pruritus does not tend to be a feature and on examination the vulva usually looks normal.

Assessment of these patients involves a thorough history and careful examination to exclude any potentially treatable conditions. A detailed explanation of the condition and reassurance is needed. Information about patient support groups is also very helpful.

General vulval care measures should be introduced. Topical local anaesthetic and lubricants may be beneficial before sexual intercourse in those with vulvar vestibulitis. Tricyclic drugs, as used for other chronic pain syndromes such as amitriptyline, are useful in dysaesthetic vulvodynia. The dose needs to be started low (10 mg nocte) and gradually increased. Doses of 50–75 mg are usually sufficient for symptomatic relief but doses of up to 150 mg may be required. Patients who have recalcitrant symptoms may benefit from referral to the local pain clinic and psycho-sexual counselling is also of benefit in some.

The male genitalia

Male genital dermatology encompasses a wide variety of skin lesions and rashes. These may affect the genitalia only or form part of a generalized dermatosis.

Rashes

Eczema

The penis may be affected by an irritant or allergic contact dermatitis. Typical irritants include soap, disinfectants and antiseptics, urine, faeces, and smegma. Patients may complain of pruritus and present with ill-defined erythematous scaly patches. Typical contact allergens affecting the penis include rubber additives and latex in condoms, spermicides, lubricants, and topical local anaesthetics. Patients may present with swelling of the penis, erythema, and scaling.

It is important to obtain a detailed history of all topical products used and if an allergic contact dermatitis is suspected referral to a dermatologist for patch testing is indicated.

The scrotal skin is frequently involved in eczema. *Lichen simplex* is the most frequent type seen and this is associated with lichenification. Pruritus is persistent and rubbing is often sustained by rubbing through trouser pockets. An itch–scratch cycle is established and this needs to be broken as in women.

For all eczemas, simple measures such as avoiding tight occlusive clothes, soaps and perfumed products, and keeping cool should be employed. Washing with a bland emollient soap substitute such as aqueous cream or emulsifying ointment is also helpful. Mild topical steroids (e.g. hydrocortisone) may occasionally be needed for short periods of time but this should be used cautiously and sparingly, especially on the scrotum since the absorption of topical preparations is greatly enhanced through the scrotal skin. In acute eczema of the penis, symptomatic treatment with cold compresses is helpful.

Psoriasis

Psoriasis may occur solely on the glans or shaft presenting with thin, pale, erythematous well-defined plaques or may be part of a generalized dermatosis. Psoriasis is sometimes confined to the inguinal folds, scrotum, and penis and as in women it tends to present with bright red well-defined erythematous plaques. The differential diagnosis includes tinea cruris but the plaques or homogeneous with no central clearing to suggest tinea.

Low-potency topical steroids often mixed with antibacterial/anticandidal creams (e.g. clobetasone butyrate 0.05 per cent alone or with oxytetracycline and nystatin) are useful to treat these areas.

Lichen planus

Lichen planus may involve the glans or the shaft of the penis with typical violaceous flat-topped papules with a white streaky pattern on the surface. Other body sites are usually simultaneously affected. Treatment is with mild topical steroids and the condition tends to resolve in 1–2 years.

Zoon's balanitis

Zoon's balanitis (plasma cell balanitis) is an inflammatory condition of the penis of unknown aetiology, which tends to affect uncircumcised middle-aged or elderly men. This characteristically affects the glans penis and prepuce and presents as an indolent, reddish brown circumscribed plaque with a shiny, smooth surface. The surface may also be stippled with tiny red specks.

The differential diagnosis includes penile intraepithelial carcinoma and referral to a dermatology or urology department is needed for diagnostic skin biopsy. This shows the characteristic features of a subdermal infiltrate of plasma cells.

Circumcision is usually curative for Zoon's balanitis, however, other treatment options include the carbon dioxide laser and photodynamic therapy.

Lichen sclerosus

Lichen sclerosus (formerly called balanitis xerotica obliterans) occurs in middle-aged men (although it may also occur in childhood and adolescence) and affects the glans penis and prepuce. Interestingly, compared to women perianal involvement is uncommon and the association with autoimmune diseases and autoantibodies is also less common in men.

Lichen sclerosus presents with ivory white atrophic macules or plaques on the glans penis and may be associated with bullae, erosions, telangiectasia, and petechia. Scarring also develops in men and the prepuce may become adherent to the glans, the coronal sulcus obliterated and the external meatus narrowed and scarred. Patients may complain of pruritus, phimosis, dysuria, and painful erections.

Potent topical steroids (e.g. clobetasol propionate 0.05 per cent) are indicated especially if there is meatal involvement. These are safe to use under supervision and for short periods of time. Circumcision is advisable if there is a phimosis.

Ideally, long-term follow-up of these patients is needed since there is a risk of squamous cell carcinoma developing at affected sites. This is often difficult, so it is important to counsel the patient at the time of diagnosis, so he is aware of future risks.

Infections

Candida is commonest cause of infective balanitis. It most commonly occurs after intercourse with an infected partner and predisposing factors include diabetes and a recent course of antibiotics. Symptoms may include mild burning and pruritus and on examination the glans has a typical glazed appearance and there may be surrounding eroded satellite pustules, which extend on to the groins. Swabs need to be taken to confirm the diagnosis, ideally from both the patient and his sexual partner and diabetes should also be excluded. Treatment is with topical anticandidal cream and in severe cases oral therapy may be indicated. It is important that both the patient and his partner are treated at the same time.

Other causes of balanitis include bacterial, commonly streptococcus, trichomonal, and chlamydial infections.

Pigmentary disorders

Vitiligo

Vitiligo may affect the penis and scrotum in the same way as the rest of the body presenting with asymptomatic hypopigmented macules. The condition can be distinguished from lichen sclerosus since the lesions are asymptomatic and show no atrophy, scarring, telangiectasia, purpura or textural change. The rest of the body needs to be examined especially the hands and face for other commonly involved sites in vitiligo.

Lentigines

Lentigines are acquired hyperpigmented macules which may occur on the glans or shaft of the penis. These lesions are not uncommon and are usually asymptomatic and benign. The lesions tend to be small, uniform in colour, size, outline, and pigmentation, hence easily distinguished from a melanoma.

Blisters, erosions, and ulcers

Infections

The commonest infective causes of genital ulceration are herpes simplex and syphilis. Clinically herpes presents as an intact or ruptured vesicle or an area of chronic ulceration. In the primary infection, symptoms include pain, burning, pruritus, and urethritis and constitutional symptoms occur in 50 per cent of patients.

The diagnosis of herpes simplex is confirmed by taking swabs for viral culture and these need to be placed in a special viral transport medium. Patients should be treated with oral antiviral drugs (e.g. acyclovir, famciclovir, or valacyclovir) at the start of an attack and should be referred to the genito-urinary medicine clinic to exclude other sexually transmitted disease.

Erythema multiforme

Erythema multiforme may involve mucous membrane sites such as the eyes, oral mucosa, penis, and vulva. This spectrum of disease is called Stevens–Johnson syndrome and is usually precipitated by infections (e.g. herpes simplex) and drugs (e.g. sulfonamides). Treatment involves stopping the offending drug, treating any underlying infection, and symptomatic treatment with bland emollients, analgesia, and good hygiene and nursing care.

Autoimmune blistering disorders

The autoimmune blistering disorders such as pemphigus vulgaris, bullous pemphigoid, and mucous membrane pemphigoid may all affect the penis and occur infrequently. Patients with a suspected diagnosis should be referred to a dermatologist for confirmation of the diagnosis.

Fixed drug eruptions

Fixed drug eruptions may present as well-defined erythematous patches, plaques, or bullae that resolve with hyperpigmentation. A detailed history is needed to obtain the classic history of the rash recurring after each exposure to the offending drug. The commonest drugs causing this are sulfonamides, penicillins, tetracylines, phenolphthaleins, and non-steroidal anti-inflammatory drugs.

Papules and nodules

Condyloma acuminata

Condyloma acuminata (viral warts) present as soft velvety, hyperplastic, or sessile lesions commonly on the coronal sulcus, preputial border, and urethral orifice. These are acquired by sexual contact and patients need to be referred to the genito-urinary clinic for treatment and to exclude the co-existence of other sexually transmitted diseases. Sexual partners of the patient should also be examined thoroughly. Treatment options include podophyllin, imiquimod, cryotherapy, electrocautery, and laser therapy.

Molluscum contagiousum

Molluscum contagiousum is a viral infection, which commonly affects infants and young adults. Lesions may occur at any body site and also genital and paragenital areas. The lesions are skin-coloured papules which have a central umbilication and are usually asymptomatic. No treatment is needed since the lesions resolve spontaneously over a period of 3–18 months. Before involution, the lesions often become pruritic and inflamed. Sexual transmission is the usual cause in adults, however in infants, although sexual abuse remains a possibility, most cases arise from autoinoculation.

Scabies

The genitalia of males suspected of suffering with scabies should always be examined especially when there are no obvious burrows at other sites. The penis and scrotum are often involved displaying erythematous papules, nodules, and burrows. The patient and all household contacts should be treated at the same time with an appropriate antiscabies preparation.

Seborrhoeic keratosis

Seborrhoeic keratosis present as warty lesions with a stuck on appearance and vary in colour from yellow through brown to black. These are benign lesions and differentiated from melanocytic naevi and melanomas by the presence of keratin cysts on their surface.

Epidermoid cysts

Epidermoid cysts may present as papules or nodules on the scrotum and although asymptomatic can cause significant embarrassment to patients. There is often a central punctum and if the lesions discharge the contents are cheesy and smell offensive. The lesions can be easily excised.

Angiokeratomas

Angiokeratomas may affect the scrotum and present as punctate angiomas often have a rough surface. Other body sites may also be affected. These lesions are benign and no treatment is needed other than reassurance.

Pre-malignant conditions

Penile intraepithelial neoplasia

Penile intraepithelial neoplasia (PIN) is an increasingly encountered umbrella term that encompasses erythroplasia of Queyrat, Bowen's disease, and bowenoid papulosis, but as yet there is no formal consensus on the clinico-pathological classification of this entity. PIN may present quite non-specifically and it is important to consider this diagnosis in any patient with a presumed inflammatory or infective balanitis that has not responded to treatment. Patients should be referred to a urologist or dermatologist for diagnostic skin biopsy. Treatment options include topical 5 per cent fluorouracil cream, circumcision, excision, photodynamic therapy, laser therapy, and radiotherapy.

Key points

1. Some genital problems cause considerable morbidity and distress, but may present late because of patients' anxiety or embarrassment. Others may be asymptomatic, yet still lead to problems later, so it is important to recognize abnormal signs.

2. Prompt referral to specialist units usually leads to an early diagnosis, often with the help of a biopsy—a quick, simple procedure performed in clinic under local anaesthetic.

3. Many genital disorders respond well to treatment, both in control of symptoms and limitation of progression of disease.

4. Some genital disorders are associated with development of malignancy. Follow-up and/or information given to patients must be planned accordingly.

Further reading

Ball, S. and Wojnarowska, F. (1998). Vulvar dermatoses: lichen sclerosus, lichen planus and vulval dermatitis/lichen simplex chronicus. *Seminars in Cutaneous Medicine and Surgery* 17, 182–8.

Bunker, C.B. (2001). Topics in penile dermatology. *Clinical and Experimental Dermatology* 26, 469–79.

Edwards, A. and Wojnarowska, F. (1998). The vulval pain syndromes. *International Journal of STD & AIDS* 9, 74–9.

English, J.C., Laws, R.A., and Keough, G.C. (1997). Dermatoses of the glans penis and prepuce. *Journal of the American Academy of Dermatology* 37, 1–24.

Powell, J. and Wojnarowska, F. (1999). Lichen sclerosus. *Lancet* 353, 1777–83.

16

Old age

16 Old age

16.1 Falls in the elderly

Alicia Curtin

Falls are the leading cause of accidental death among persons 75 years of age and older. Falls account for significant mortality and morbidity among older persons, costing the United States, 6 billion dollars per year.[1]

Although there is a temptation to view falls as a single, significant event, the fact is falls are multifactorial in nature. A fall is 'an event which results in a person coming to rest inadvertently on the ground and other than a consequence of the following: loss of consciousness, sudden onset of paralysis as in a stroke, or epileptic seizures'.[2] Many falls are the result of cumulative effects of impaired gait and balance, medical illnesses, and environmental factors. This fact has prompted the classification of potential risk factors and aetiologies of falls. Frequently, older persons are not aware of the risk factors and do not report falling unless an injury has occurred. Identifying and targeting the population at greatest risk with multifactorial interventions is essential to the prevention and reduction in the incidence of falls and fall-related injuries in older persons.

Epidemiology

In the United States, accidents are the sixth leading cause of death in persons over the age of 65 and falls account for two-thirds of these deaths.[3] The annual incidence of falls ranges from 30 per cent in persons over the age of 65 to 50 per cent in persons over 80 years of age.[4] Rates of fall-related deaths for older persons increase sharply with advancing age and are consistently higher among men than women. This trend may be related to the higher prevalence of co-morbid illness among men than women of similar age.[5]

Falls in the older person are also a strong predictor of placement in a nursing home facility. Compared with older persons who have not had a fall, older persons who have fallen have a greater than threefold rate of requiring placement in a nursing home facility.[6] Given the loss of independence and privacy and the financial costs associated with institutionalization, the identification of preventable risk factors is a priority in reducing the incidence of falls.[6]

Similar trends are seen in other countries. In a cross-national analysis, falls are the leading specified mechanism of injury death in all countries except Australia, Israel, and France (see Fig. 1). More than 85 per cent of deaths due to falls in all the countries except Israel are classified as unintentional. In the over-74 age group, there is considerable cross-national variation by sex, with rates peaking in France and West Germany. In France, West Germany, and the United Kingdom, fall rates for females are 50 per cent higher than for male. Japan has by far the lowest national death rate related to falls. The interpretation of these comparative analyses studies is limited due to the inconsistencies in reporting and recording the causes of death.[7]

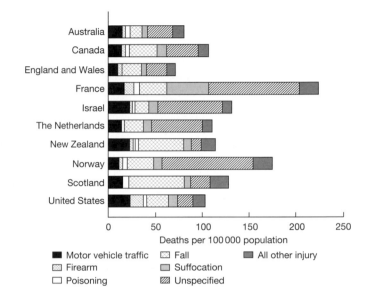

Fig. 1 Average annual injury death rates by mechanism among persons 65 years of age and over: Injury International Collaborative Effort (ICE) countries, selected recent years.[3]

Although significant mortality is associated with falls, a majority of falls do not result in serious injuries. In the United States, 30–50 per cent of falls result in minor soft tissue injuries, such as abrasions, bruises, and lacerations.[8] Approximately 1 per cent of these falls result in hip fracture, 3–5 per cent in other types of fractures, and an additional 5 per cent result in severe soft tissue injury, such as haemarthroses, joint dislocations, sprains, and haematomas.[9]

Hospitalization rates for hip fracture differ by age and are higher for Caucasian women than for other groups. Rates increase with advancing age for both sexes but are consistently higher for women in all age categories. This gender difference may be related to the prevalence of osteoporosis in older Caucasian woman. Compared with Caucasian women aged 65 years and older, African-Americans of comparable ages have greater bone mass and are less likely to sustain a fall-related hip fracture.[5]

The nursing home population is generally older, sicker, more cognitively impaired, and more functionally dependent than their community-dwelling counterpart. In nursing homes, 30–40 per cent of the residents fall each year. Incidence rates of falls for nursing home residents are approximately three times the rate for community-dwelling older persons. In fact, nursing home residents have a disproportionately high incidence of hip fracture and higher mortality rates associated with hip fracture compared to community-dwelling older persons.[10]

Almost half of ambulatory nursing home residents will fall each year and more than 40 per cent have more than one fall. About 4 per cent (range 1–10 per cent) result in fractures and 11 per cent (range 1–36 per cent) result in other serious injuries, such as head trauma, soft tissue injuries, and lacerations.[10]

Falls are also an important marker of frailty. Of older persons who are hospitalized for a fall, only about one half are alive 1 year after. This indicates the seriousness of underlying disease and the need to ameliorate the symptoms of chronic illness to prevent further risks of falling.

Aetiology

The complexity of reducing the incidence of falls is due to their multifactorial aetiology. Three groups of risk factors have been identified in the literature, intrinsic, extrinsic, and the situation or activity a person is engaged in when the fall occurs. Intrinsic factors are inherent in the older person who falls. Extrinsic factors are circumstantial to the older person who falls. These factors are most often associated with ambulatory older persons than among those who are frail and ill. Most situational falls occur when older persons are engaging in activities (see Table 1).

Intrinsic factors include chronic diseases such as cardiovascular disease, neurological disorders, dementia, depression, visual problems, and the use of certain drugs such as sedatives, tranquillizers, antidepressants, antihypertensives, and diuretics. Certain cardiovascular diseases such as cardiac arrhythmias (heart block, sick sinus syndrome, and bradycardia), postural hypotension related to decreased baroreceptor sensitivity and hypertension increase the older person's risk for falls.

Neurological disorders such as Parkinson's disease greatly affect the older person's postural stability and gait. Cerebrovascular events and seizures also put the older person at risk of falling. Lower extremity neuropathies related to spinal stenosis or diabetes may also alter the older person's gait and stability. Vertebrobasilar syndrome produces episodic symptoms of dizziness and ataxia provoked by hyperextension of the neck. Transient ischaemic attacks caused by carotid atherosclerosis also increase the older person's risk of falls. Older persons with dementia are at an increased risk of falling because of lack of judgement and insight, decreased attention span, and agitation. Depression also interferes with attention and motivation and may contribute to falls risk.

Osteoporosis is not considered a risk factor, but it does predispose older persons to fractures of the hip, vertebrae, distal forearms, and pelvis, especially in older Caucasian women. The risk of falling, bone strength, and the force of the impact will ultimately determine the risk of osteoporotic fractures in the older person and may contribute to the higher falls-related mortality rates seen in older women than men.

Visual acuity, adequate depth perception, and distant-edge-contrast sensitivity are important for maintaining balance, proprioception, and detecting and avoiding hazards in the environment. Ocular diseases such as macular degeneration, cataracts, and glaucoma can impair vision and increase the older person's fall risk.

Table 1 Risk factors for falls in older persons

Intrinsic factors	Extrinsic factors	Situational/activity-related factors
Age	Environmental hazards	Climbing
Cognitive impairment	Inadequate lighting	Walking on uneven
Muscle weakness	Slippery or icy surfaces	surfaces
Foot problems	Loose rugs	Rising from a chair
Polypharmacy	Low soft chairs	Turning around
Sensory impairment	Low toilet seats	Reaching
Gait and balance	High steps	
impairments	Ill-repaired stair treads	
Postural hypotension	Ill-fitting shoes	
Depression		
Chronic illnesses		
Acute illnesses		

Polypharmacy can lead to confusion, cardiac arrhythmias, and poor coordination. Centrally acting medications such as sedative hypnotics, neuroleptics, and antidepressants have been associated with an increased risk of falls.[11] Other classes of medications such as narcotic analgesics, antihypertensives, anticonvulsants, and antiarrhythmics may impair the older person's sensorium and gait stability. In addition, the total number of medications and recent changes in medication dosages have also been implicated. The use of alcohol may affect cognition, gait, and balance and increase the older person's risk of falls.

Foot problems such as callouses, bunions, or anatomical deformities may also alter the older person's gait pattern and provide incorrect proprioceptive information. This will cause gait instability and increase the risk of falls.

Age-related changes in the older person's gait and balance increase the risk of falls. This includes age-related decline in vestibular function, which contributes to increase body sway. This becomes worse in the dark because of the older person's reliance on visual and sensory input. Changes in the proprioceptive system including peripheral nerves, cervical articular mechanoreceptors, and posterior column, may cause instability with position changes or when walking on uneven surfaces. Age-related changes in gait pattern and decreased muscle strength are intrinsic factors that predispose the older person to falls.

Acute illnesses such as exacerbation of congestive heart failure, pneumonia, urinary tract infections, and other infectious processes may precipitate falls by temporarily impairing cognition and function. Metabolic disturbances, such as hypoglycaemia, hyperglycaemia, anaemia, electrolyte imbalances, and hypoxaemia may acutely affect the older person's cognition and thereby increasing the risk of falling.

A small proportion of falls are the result of a single overwhelming intrinsic event such as a stroke, or a single disease process such as Parkinson's disease. However, most falls are a result of the cumulative effects of intrinsic, extrinsic, and activity-related behaviour in the older person. A careful and focused assessment and interventions aimed at ameliorating chronic disease symptoms and identifying modifiable risk factors will reduce the risk of falls in certain populations of older persons at risk.[2]

Assessment

A detailed multidimensional function-oriented assessment is essential to identify causes and potentially modifiable risk factors for the older person who has fallen or who is at risk of falling. As part of any history, the older person should be asked if he or she has had a fall in the past year (see Fig. 2).

Depending on the target population, the type of assessment warranted will vary. A brief assessment should be performed as part of a routine assessment for low-risk older persons. For high-risk older persons, such as those who fall repeatedly, live in a nursing home or present to the physician after a fall, a detailed comprehensive assessment is necessary. This assessment should include a detailed history about the circumstances of the fall, the older person's risk factors for falls, a review of the medications, co-morbid illnesses, and alcohol use, a review of systems for acute medical symptoms, current cognitive and functional status, and an assessment of environmental hazards (see Fig. 2).[11]

Physical examination should focus on the identified risk factors obtained in the history. This examination should include an assessment of basic neurologic function including mental status, muscle strength and tone, lower extremity peripheral nerves, proprioception, deep tendon reflexes, cerebellar function, and tests of cortical extrapyramidal function.

A cardiovascular examination should include heart rate and rhythm, postural pulse and blood pressure (lying and standing with a 5-min interval between each reading). Visual screening and an examination of the lower extremities, especially the feet, for deformities, ulcerations, or other structural or painful processes, are important.[11]

In addition, a careful examination of the older person's functional performance is necessary. Balance and gait are affected by the cumulative effects of disease and age-related changes and impairments in neurologic,

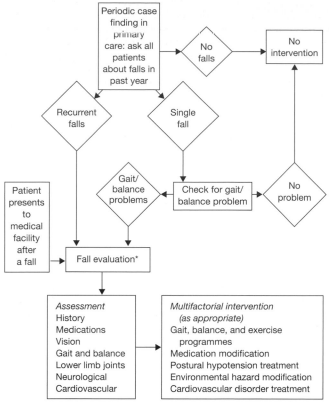

Fig. 2 Algorithm summarizing the assessment and management of falls. (*Reproduced from*: American Geriatrics Society, British Geriatrics Society, and American Academy of Orthopaedic Surgeons Panel on Falls Prevention (2001). Guideline for the prevention of falls in older persons. *Journal of the American Geriatrics Society* **49**, 664–72, with permission.)

sensory, and muscular functioning.[4] It is also important to remember that gait abnormalities may also represent a compensatory manoeuvre to increase gait stability by the older person. For example, a stooped posture or broad base stance with small steps may indicate an adaptive gait pattern by the older person to compensate for decreased muscle strength, kyphosis, and mild osteoarthritis of the knees and hips.

Observations of gait initiation, step height and length, step continuity, symmetry, path deviation, trunk sway, walking stance, and turning while walking are important in assessing for gait abnormalities. The 'get up and go test' and the performance-oriented assessment of mobility are two simple screening tests that can be administered in the clinical setting. The older person is asked to rise from the chair, to stand momentarily with eyes opened and closed, then nudged on the sternum, to walk 10 ft, and to return and sit in the chair.[12]

A normal gait pattern of an older person includes a slightly widened base of support between the feet and minimal vertical or lateral movement of the pelvis. The stance and swing phase of the older person's gait pattern alternates with each leg. The stance phase starts with heel strike with the foot in full contact with the floor to toe push. There should be no breaks or stops in the stride and step lengths should be at least the length of the foot and equal over most cycles. The swing phase is after the toe push off the floor and the foot is advanced to the next position. The swing foot should completely clear the floor, but by no more than 1–2 in. There should be minimal trunk motion and the step path should be straight. When turning, steps should be smooth and continuous.[12]

In the analysis of gait and balance, abnormal findings may indicate specific disease processes or problems. For example, if the older person has difficulty rising from a chair, this may indicate proximal muscle weakness,

deconditioning, or arthritis, (especially of the hips or knees). Instability when first standing may indicate postural hypotension, multisensory deficits, or lower extremity weakness. Decreased step height and length may indicate compensation for decreased vision or proprioception, fear of falling, or Parkinson's disease.[12]

Other screening manoeuvres, such as neck turning while standing, back extension by reaching up, bending over, and standing on one leg unsupported for 5 s, all simulate movements used in daily activity. As the person performs these manoeuvres, movements, or gestures that suggest instability, such as staggering or grabbing objects for support, are noted. The use of these simple manoeuvres assists in detecting obvious functional problems and identifies potential areas for improvement. If an older person uses an assistive walking aid, such as a cane or walker, proper use of the device must also be assessed.

Depending on the history and physical examination, further laboratory and diagnostic tests may be warranted. It may be useful to obtain a complete blood count, chemistries, thyroid function tests, and drug levels if the history and physical examination indicate a potential problem in these areas. Electrocardiogram and holter monitor may be considered if a cardiac arrhythmia is suspected. Neuroimaging may be helpful for older persons with neurological deficits and gait abnormalities, but these tests should not be used indiscriminately. Referral to specialists such as a neurologist, cardiologist, ophthalmologist, or podiatrist, may be indicated if the older person needs further evaluation for specific problems identified on the assessment.

Management

The goal of management is to minimize the risk of falling without compromising mobility, functional activities, personal independence, and an acceptable quality of life.[4] The appropriate interventions will depend on the history, physical examination, and if the older person reports a previous fall, the circumstances of that fall.

For example, the goal for healthy older persons who have not experienced a fall, is to maintain or improve balance, gait, flexibility and endurance, and to maintain mobility and functional independence.[4] For older persons who have experienced a fall, treatment is focused on reducing subsequent falls and their associated morbidity by eliminating or modifying as many contributing risk factors as possible. Initial treatment of acute or reversible deficits such as urinary tract infections, pneumonia, congestive heart failure, metabolic disturbances, or medication side-effects may result in major improvements in the older person's gait and balance. However, falls tend to be associated with several contributing risk factors that are chronic processes and impairments. These processes and impairments are modifiable, but not curable, and they therefore require multiple treatment strategies.

Specific recommendations developed by the American Geriatrics Society Panel on Falls in Older Persons target specific populations depending on place of residence. Recommendations for a community-dwelling population should include: gait training and advice on the appropriate use of assistive devices, review and modification of medications, especially psychotropic medications, exercise programmes, with balance training as one of the components, treatment of postural hypotension, modification of environmental hazards, and treatment of cardiovascular disorders including cardiac arrhythmias.[11]

Specific recommendations for nursing home and the assisted living populations include staff education programmes, gait training, advice on the appropriate use of assistive devices, and review and modification of medications, especially psychotropic medications.[11]

Exercise programmes should focus on strength and balance training. Tai Chi, an oriental martial arts form, may increase stability and balance and reduce the incidence of falls.[11] A referral to physical therapy for gait and balance training and an evaluation of the need for an assistive device is helpful in increasing gait stability. Appropriate exercise prescription along with good supervision, continuity, and persistence are elements of a successful exercise programme. The physical therapist may also be effective by teaching the older person strategies for getting up from the floor or by encouraging the older person's confidence in performing the activities of daily living.

Reviewing medication and reducing or stopping the use of certain medications may reduce the risk of falls. Older persons taking four or more medications or taking psychotropic medications, such as sedative-hypnotics, neuroleptics, and antidepressants, should be targeted. Reduction of medications is an important component of any effective fall-reducing intervention.

Assistive devices such as canes and walkers and other fall prevention equipment including bed alarms, motion monitors, low beds, and hip protectors are an important part of the multifaceted approach to reducing falls in the older person. The use of hip protectors in high-risk groups may not reduce the incidence of falls, but may reduce the incidence of hip fractures associated with falling.[11] Providing protective padding for the hips of an older person at risk for falls may be a promising approach if the padding is comfortable and non-restrictive. The use of restraints, such as a vest posey or wrist restraints, has not been proven to prevent falls. Restraints have actually lead to immobility, pressure ulcers, and serious injuries. In fact, reduction of restraints in nursing homes does not increase the incidence of injurious falls.[11]

Staff education and behavioural training programmes may be helpful in reducing falls in the older person. In-service training to staff to teach them to reorient confused older persons, to maintain routine toileting schedules for older persons with incontinence, and to supervise ambulation and transfers may assist in the prevention of falls. Assisting older persons to be active and increasing their awareness of the potential risk factors in the environment may also assist in the reduction of falls.

A home safety assessment may be useful in discovering potential hazards in the older person's environment, which may contribute to or cause a fall. Common environmental hazards in the home include loose throw rugs, slippery wet floors, cords and wires on the floor, cluttered hallways and rooms, low toilet seats and chairs, and high steps and worn stair treads. Footwear can also be hazardous. Ill-fitting shoes, slippers without soles, and high-heeled shoes are unsafe. Repairing loose rugs, providing adequate lighting especially in stairways, railings, and safety equipment in the bathroom and proper fitting shoes, are an important part of a multifaceted plan to reduce the extrinsic risk factors in the older person's home environment.

The treatment of chronic diseases, such as cardiovascular disease (i.e. syncope, orthostatic hypotension, bradycardia), osteoporosis, and neurological disorders, is essential in the overall plan of care for the older person who has fallen.

Long-term and continuing care

Falls are an important marker of frailty and nursing home admission. Falls can have serious consequences for physical mobility and quality of life. Loss of mobility can result both from fracture-related disability and self-restricted activity caused by fear of falling and lack of confidence. Families may also impose restrictions on the mobility and independence of the older adult after a fall. This leads to further functional decline, social isolation, and feelings of helplessness.[10]

Prevention strategies must balance the need to reduce risks and the need to maintain the older person's mobility and personal autonomy. Older persons need to be screened regularly for risk factors. Despite our progress in understanding the aetiology of falls, there still remains a lack of knowledge of the most effective strategies to reduce the incidence of falls. Public health education programmes for older persons should focus on surveillance of the problem, prevention and health promotion activities such as exercise and nutrition, and regular physician visits. Reducing the incidence of falls may subsequently reduce disability in this population and consequently the need for nursing home admission.

Implications

With increased public awareness and education, older persons have become more active and more conscious of the role of diet and nutrition in reducing age-related decline in physical health. In addition, the popularity of life care communities and congregated living among older persons may play an important role in maintaining social networks and mobility levels. Many of these communities provide group activities, including a variety of exercise programmes such as Tai Chi, yoga, strengthening training, golf, dancing, swimming, and aerobics. These factors may help delay the onset of fall events that can threaten independence and quality of life.

The effects of falls extend beyond the obvious physical trauma. The psychological effects can have lasting and damaging consequences for older persons. Fear of falling may contribute to reduced mobility, self-limited activity, and social isolation. Families may also become overprotective and restrict the independence of the older person after a fall. These restrictions lead to further decline in function and increase risk of subsequent falls.[8,13] Further research needs to focus on this cohort of older persons in developing strategies to decrease their fear of falling and increase their confidence in performing their activities of daily living.

Understanding the many risk factors associated with falls and the most appropriate, cost-effective strategies to modify these risks and the morbidity related to falling, requires a multidisciplinary approach. This approach will lead to the further refinement and development of effective strategies in fall prevention for older persons.

Further research is also necessary to evaluate the cost-effectiveness of intervention strategies and the effectiveness of targeting high-risk persons. In addition, the necessary type, intensity, duration, and frequency of an exercise programme needs to be determined in order to prescribe the most effective and efficient plan of care.

Key points

1. Falls are the leading cause of accidental deaths in persons 75 years and older.
2. The aetiology of falls is multifactorial, requiring a comprehensive assessment and the identification of modifiable risk factors.
3. The comprehensive assessment of falls should include history of falls, fall risk factors, review of medications and co-morbid illnesses, current cognitive and functional status, and environmental hazards.
4. The physical examination should include an assessment of basic neurological function, cardiovascular and musculoskeletal examination, vision and hearing screening, and gait and balance assessment.
5. Management of falls requires a multifaceted approach including exercise training, medication reduction, the diagnosis and treatment of specific chronic/acute illnesses, optimizing sensory input, and home safety evaluation.

References

1. Barclay, A. (1988). Falls in the elderly: is prevention possible? *Postgraduate Medicine* 83, 241–4.
2. Kellogg International Work Group Preventing Falls by Elderly (1987). The prevention of falls in later life. *Danish Medical Bulletin* 34, 1–24.
3. Fingerhut, L.A., Cox, C.S., and Warner, M. et al. (1998). International comparative analysis of injury mortality: findings from the ICE on injury statistics. *Advance Data from Vital and Health Statistics* No. 303, pp. 1–20. Hyattsville MD: National Center for Health Statistics.

4. Tinetti, M. (1996). Falls. In *Geriatric Medicine* 3rd edn. (ed. C. Cassel, H. Cohen, E. Larson, D. Meirer, N. Resnick, L. Rubenstein, and L. Sorensen), pp. 528–34. New York: Springer-Verlag.

5. Stevens, J.A. et al. (1999). Surveillance for injuries and violence among older adults. *Morbidity Mortality Weekly Reports. CDC Surveillance Summary* **48** (8), 27–50.

6. Tinetti, M. and Williams, C. (1997). Falls, injuries due to falls and the risk of admission to a nursing home. *New England Journal of Medicine* **337**, 1279–84.

7. Rockett, I.R. and Smith, G.S. (1989). Homicide, suicide, motor vehicle crash and fall mortality: United States' experience in comparative perspective. *American Journal of Public Health* **79**, 1396–400.

8. Nevitt, M., Cummings, S., Kidd, S., and Black, D. (1989). Risk factors for recurrent nonsyncopal falls: a prospective study. *Journal of American Medical Association* **261**, 2663–8.

9. Sattin, R. (1992). Falls among older persons: a public health perspective. *Annual Review of Public Health* **13**, 489–508.

10. Rubenstein, L., Josephson, K., and Robbins, A. (1994). Falls in the nursing home. *Annals of Internal Medicine* **121**, 442–51.

11. American Geriatrics Society, British Geriatrics Society, and American Academy of Orthopaedic Surgeons Panel on Falls Prevention (2001). Guideline for the prevention of falls in older persons. *Journal of the American Geriatrics Society* **49**, 664–72.

12. Tinetti, M. (1986). Performance-oriented assessment of mobility problems in elderly patients. *Journal of the American Geriatrics Society* **34** (2), 119–26.

13. King, M. and Tinetti, M. (1995). Falls in community-dwelling older persons. *Journal of the American Geriatrics Society* **43**, 1146–54.

Further reading

American Geriatrics Society, British Geriatrics Society, and American Academy of Orthopaedic Surgeons Panel on Falls Prevention (2001). Guideline for the prevention of falls in older persons. *Journal of the American Geriatrics Society* **49**, 664–72. (Consensus of evidence-based guidelines for the prevention of falls in older persons.)

Rubenstein, L., Josephson, K., and Robbins, A. (1994). Falls in the nursing home. *Annals of Internal Medicine* **121**, 442–51. (Review article.)

Sattin, R. (1992). Falls among older persons: a public health perspective. *Annual Review of Public Health* **13**, 489–508. (Review article.)

Tinetti, M. et al. (1994). A multifactorial intervention to reduce the risk of falling among elderly people living in the community. *The New England Journal of Medicine* **331** (13), 821–7. (Primary research examining specific strategies in reducing the risk of falling for older persons in the community.)

16.2 Gait and movement disorders

Alexander H. Rajput and Ali H. Rajput

Introduction

Normal ageing processes lead to changes in all the organs and physical function capacity declines in old age—a 75-year-old man cannot run as fast as at age 25 years. The evolution of walking on two feet occurs subsequent to the infant learning to crawl on four limbs. This newly evolved faculty therefore suffers early with age.

Normal balance and ambulation require integration of position sense, the visual system, vestibular organs, motor strength, and motor function coordination. Optimally functioning systems allow for well-controlled physical activity including gait and balance. Decline in the function of these organs leads to general motor slowing and decreased ability to compensate for any error. Missing a step, which would not be hazardous at young age, could significantly increase the risk of fall in old age.

Movement disorders are common illnesses and some are concentrated in old age. Physical slowing is also a feature of some well-known movement disorders. Distinguishing normal age-related motor slowing from pathological causes is essential.

Chronology and biology run parallel courses. Age-related motor decline is symmetrical. Any significant difference from others of the same age is a strong indication of disease.

Gait disorders

Epidemiology

Balance and gait difficulties are common in the elderly population. Approximately 15 per cent of the general population aged 60 years and older have some degree of gait abnormality. The frequency increases with advancing age.

Several systems noted below are critical for normal gait and balance. Dysfunction of any one or a combination of these factors may be the basis of gait abnormality. In nearly half of the elderly with gait abnormality, there is one identifiable cause and in another 30 per cent there is more than one cause. Even after extensive investigations, the cause cannot be identified in nearly 20 per cent.

Presentation to primary care

Patients may present as feeling unsteady, veering to one side or the other, shuffling feet, postural changes, or falls. Because of the multifactorial nature of gait and balance, all appropriate systems must be considered.

1. Vestibular—A history of vertigo with or without alteration in hearing localizes to the vestibular apparatus. The patient may not report spinning but may have a sensation of 'waves'. Often, these patients will have transient dizzy feelings on rising from a lying position or with turning the head quickly. These patients may show short duration nystagmus coinciding with the subjective dizzy feeling.

2. Visual—Gait changes associated with visual dysfunction may be due to change in visual acuity such as cataracts and macular degeneration, or visual field loss. Occasionally, patients are unaware of a visual field deficit until detected by the examiner.

3. Motor—Stroke, myopathy, or peripheral neuropathy all cause muscle weakness affecting gait. The hemiparetic gait seen in stroke consists typically of the arm held in adduction and internal rotation with flexion at the elbow and wrist, and extension of the leg with foot drop. The weak leg circumducts (goes around in a semicircle to take the next step) so that the toe will not catch on the floor. Proximal lower extremity weakness seen in myopathy results in inability to stand from a seated position without pushing off with the hands, and inability to rise from a squatting position without assistance. If there is weakness of the hip musculature (especially the hip abductors), the gait will appear 'waddling' like a duck. Foot drop is typically due to a root or peripheral nerve disorder. So the foot does not catch on the ground, there is exaggerated hip flexion and elevation of the leg. The front of the foot strikes the ground before the heel. This characteristic gait is called 'steppage' gait.

4. Sensory impairment—Loss of position sense also results in gait difficulty, especially in the dark, as the visual system is not able to compensate for impaired proprioception. The loss of vibration sense in the lower limbs is part of normal ageing; position sense, however, remains intact

in normal old age. Therefore, examination of position sense at the toes is a critical part of the assessment in patients with gait difficulty.

5. Mechanical involvement—Arthritis is common in the elderly and contributes to gait difficulty by affecting the axial skeleton lower limb musculature.

With advancing age, arthritis of the hip and knee joints becomes a common problem. Arthritis will produce painful interference in walking. Hip joint arthritis will produce inguinal or buttock pain which is made worse when standing and walking. There is also a reduced range of hip joint movements due to pain. Often in these patients there is tenderness over the mid inguinal ligament area. Arthritis at the knee joints will similarly produce limitation of some movements at the knee and there may be tender points around the knee joint.

When the cause of gait difficulty is not identifiable in the above major categories, referral to a specialist is indicated. Neurologists are often asked to evaluate patients with gait disturbance, as there are a number of neurological conditions affecting various levels of the nervous system that may impair gait, including the movement disorders.

Gait disorders in movement disorders

The gait difficulty in movement disorders is not attributable to visual, sensory, motor weakness, or vestibular dysfunction. In movement disorders, the gait difficulty is due to one or a combination of the following:

◆ focal or generalized change in posture;

◆ difficulty regaining balance after postural displacement;

◆ major change in tone;

◆ inability to initiate movement;

◆ reduced or altered speed of movement;

◆ presence of involuntary movements which interfere with gait;

◆ lack of proper coordination of movements;

◆ inability to stop intended movements; or

◆ impaired central mechanisms for gait integration.

Patients with dementia may also have gait difficulty. Advanced Alzheimer's disease patients fall frequently.

Gait apraxia is an example of central sensorimotor integration dysfunction causing gait abnormality. Gait apraxia is characterized by an inability to use the lower limbs when attempting to walk. Leg function is normal when tested lying down with no weakness, sensory loss, or incoordination. These patients have a broad-based gait and walk as if the feet are 'glued' to the floor. Visual cues such as a line on the floor do not improve the gait. The triad of gait apraxia, dementia, and urinary incontinence is seen in normal pressure hydrocephalus (NPH).

Diagnosis of gait abnormality

History

The onset in most cases is insidious but depending on the cause, for example, stroke, it may be sudden. In most cases (except stroke), the disability is progressive if untreated. Patients may present with any number of the complaints listed below.

The history should be obtained in an attempt to identify the cause of the gait difficulty. For the purpose, the following leading questions should be asked. Are you having pain which prevents you from walking normally? Are your legs so weak that they may give out when you walk? Do you have a feeling that objects are going around or moving when you walk? Is the difficulty in walking present regardless if you walk in the light or in the dark?

Pain in the hip, knee, or foot which makes walking difficult may be due to bursitis or arthritis. When gait difficulty is present only in the dark but the gait is normal in the light, it indicates loss of position sense in the lower limbs. Gait difficulty due to vestibular and cerebellar function abnormalities

is present in the light as well as in the dark. In the case of vestibular dysfunction, patients frequently experience dizziness when turning in bed, sitting up quickly, or on sudden turning of the head to one side or the other.

Physical examination

Examination begins when the patient walks into the room. Observe whether the patient walks unassisted, holds onto a person or object to steady himself, or is brought in a wheelchair. Normal elderly people have a slightly flexed posture and shorter stride length with a slightly wider base compared to younger persons. Flexed posture greater than expected by age is seen in Parkinson's syndrome (PS) and thoracic kyphosis.

Ask the patient to arise from a chair with arms folded in front. Difficulty arising without assistance is seen with proximal leg weakness and advanced parkinsonism.

Gait initiation failure results in inability to start walking upon standing and is seen in PS and gait apraxia. Visual cues (asking the patient to step over a line or stick) improve the gait in PS but not in gait apraxia.

Parkinsonian gait is characterized by a narrow base, reduced armswing (often asymmetric), and exaggerated flexion at the waist and neck. The gait is 'shuffling' because of reduced stride length and problems picking the feet off the ground. Turning difficulties, and less commonly, propulsion and retropulsion are seen in PS and are discussed under the heading 'Parkinson syndrome'. Postural instability is seen in moderate to advanced disease, and will be discussed below.

Postural instability is tested by facing the patient, asking him/her to place his/her feet shoulder width apart and giving him/her a modest pull towards the examiner. The patient is prepared for the next part, when the examiner stands behind the patient and pulls the patient towards the examiner. *More than two steps on gentle pull is abnormal.* Uncontrolled propulsion or retropulsion and the inability to move the feet represent more advanced impairment. By age 70 years, approximately 70 per cent of the general population have postural instability. Hence, impaired postural reflexes in the elderly are not diagnostic of neurological disease.

If a patient cannot walk without assistance or spontaneously falls during gait testing, the posture is obviously unstable. If the posture is unstable with a forward pull, it will nearly always be unstable with a backward pull. The degree of force used should be modest, as even young healthy persons can be displaced by a strong pull.

Cerebellar disorders and *gait apraxia* each has a wide base. Gait apraxia has already been discussed earlier. Cerebellar gait is unsteady and 'lurching'. Features supportive of a cerebellar disorder include limb ataxia, dysarthria, and nystagmus.

Tandem gait is tested by asking the patient to walk with one foot in front of the other—heel touching toe. It is easier for the patient to do with arms outstretched to the sides. Difficulty or inability to do tandem gait is a major feature of *cerebellar disorders*. However, anything which significantly interferes with gait would make tandem walking difficult. Some impairment may be seen in normal elderly people.

Romberg testing is performed by asking the patient to stand with eyes closed and feet together. A positive test requires that the patient break his/her stance; swaying back and forth only does not constitute a positive test. Positive Romberg is a sign of *impaired position sense.*

Investigations

History and clinical assessment dictate the investigation of a gait disorder. For example, a patient with vestibular dysfunction needs an otologic assessment. Imaging studies to rule out normal pressure hydrocephalus (NPH), cerebellar masses or atrophy, or vascular causes for gait difficulty (i.e. ischaemic lesions in the basal ganglia or cerebellum) are appropriate. Subdural haematoma can result from falls and requires investigation in the setting of head trauma.

Referral

Referral will be discussed under movement disorders.

Principles of management in gait disorder

The two main arms of management are: (i) treat the underlying cause(s); and (ii) supportive care. Supportive care includes walking aids such as a cane or walker, and making the home environment safer, that is, moving to a one-storey house without stairs. If available, a referral to physiotherapy for formal gait assessment, including risk of falls, and recommendations regarding assistive devices is valuable.

NPH is treated with ventriculoperitoneal shunting.

Long-term and continuing care in gait disorder

The goal is to keep the patient ambulatory as long as possible. Once a person is no longer safe to walk alone despite assistive devices (i.e. cane or walker), he/she is likely better off in a wheelchair.

Continuing care includes ensuring that all medical disorders and contributing conditions are treated or accounted for, especially the sequelae of immobility. Risks of immobility include deep vein thrombosis with possible subsequent pulmonary embolus, atelectasis, pneumonia, and skin ulcerations that may become secondarily infected. Despite limited mobility, patients should change positions and do some physical activity and stretching exercises to avoid deconditioning and contractures.

Implications of gait disorder

Falls are the major risk in patients with gait disorders. Falls may result in minor or major problems, for example, hip fracture, subdural haematoma, etc. If a patient sustains serious injury, he/she may be subsequently unable to resume walking independently for physical/psychological reasons. Falls should be prevented whenever possible.

Home environments often have to be modified (i.e. elimination of stairs in the house, elevators available in apartment, etc.) or changed completely by having the patient move in with family or into a nursing home. The effect on the spouse and/or caregiver cannot be ignored, as the patient cannot be left unattended if there is significant fall risk. Some activities may be eliminated if the risk of falling is too great. Functional independence is at stake, depending on the cause of the gait disorder and the success of treatment.

With an ageing population and increasing prevalence of neurological conditions, gait disorders will become more frequent and physicians and health care systems need to be prepared for this. Improved medical therapy for these conditions as well as appropriate supportive care will enable persons to remain independent longer and also reduce the burden of the caregiver.

Movement disorders

Movement disorders can be divided into two groups based on age at onset age. Some movement disorders begin at younger age but do not reduce life expectancy, for example, essential tremor (ET). The second group is those disorders with onset in old age, for example, PS. We will discuss these two disorders below.

Parkinson's syndrome

Epidemiology

Onset of PS before the age of 30 years is extremely rare and only 7 per cent of PS patients develop their symptoms before the age of 40 years. The prevalence of PS is 1.5 per cent in those 65 and older. The prevalence rate of PS is seven times greater in those over age 75 compared to the population between age 40 and 60 years. Mean onset age of PS is approximately 62 years.

The most common PS variant is idiopathic Parkinson's disease (IPD), the cause of more than three-quarters of all PS cases. Pathologically, IPD is characterized by Lewy bodies and neuronal loss in the substantia nigra part of the midbrain. The second most common cause of PS is drug-induced, usually secondary to neuroleptic medication. Other less common variants include progressive supranuclear palsy (PSP), and multiple system atrophy (MSA). We no longer see new cases of post-encephalitic parkinsonism.

Presentation to primary care

The most common presentation mode is upper limb tremor, which is often first noted by the spouse or a family member. Reduction in size of handwriting (micrographia) and softer voice (hypophonia) are also common complaints. Approximately 15 per cent of PS present as gait problems or generalized slowing without tremor. The diagnosis in such cases is frequently delayed.

Differential diagnosis

The patients with tremor onset should be distinguished from the other common cause of tremor, ET. In typical PS cases, there is additional bradykinesia and rigidity, which are not part of ET. Those who have onset of generalized slowing/gait difficulty need to be distinguished from normal age-related slowing. Age-related slowing is symmetrical while PS is asymmetrical in most cases. In the event the family physician cannot make the diagnosis, the patient may be tried empirically on levodopa/carbidopa 100/25 mg three times daily for 4–6 weeks. With improvement, the diagnosis of PS is confirmed. Alternatively, the patient may be referred to a specialist if the diagnosis or response to levodopa/carbidopa is in question.

Other uncommon variants of PS include the following:

1. Progressive supranuclear palsy (PSP)—These patients have vertical gaze palsy in addition to parkinsonian features. They typically present with early falls, and have minimal tremor.

2. Multiple system atrophy (MSA)—These patients have parkinsonian features as well as autonomic dysfunction, for example, postural hypotension, impotence, and bladder incontinence.

3. Diffuse Lewy body disease (DLBD)—Parkinsonism and dementia characterize this condition. Early onset dementia, diurnal fluctuations in cognition and early unexplained falls are common in DLBD and are not seen in typical Parkinson's disease.

These disorders respond poorly to treatment and suspected patients should be referred to a neurologist.

Diagnosis

PS is a clinical diagnosis. Two of the three are required to make the diagnosis of PS: resting tremor, bradykinesia, and rigidity.

Resting tremor is tested by asking the patient to lie supine with all four limbs fully supported against gravity. This is important when there is resting tremor of the upper extremity with ipsilateral lower extremity resting tremor in the seated position, as the tremor in the lower limb may simply be transmitted from the upper extremity resting upon it. Asking the patient to close his/her eyes, squeeze your finger and count backwards out loud will bring out subtle tremor not otherwise seen.

Bradykinesia should be tested by asking the patient to perform repetitive movements, for example, both arms simultaneously pronating/supinating rapidly, or rapidly tapping the index finger against the thumb. The involved side will show a decline in amplitude, slowing or even arrest of the movement.

Rigidity means constant increase in tone with passive movement. The increase in tone is independent of direction and velocity, in contrast to spasticity. Rigidity is best tested at the wrist by slow circular passive movement while holding the forearm fixed with the other hand.

Reinforcement brings out rigidity and is done by asking the patient to tap the opposite foot on the floor while you are moving the wrist. Tell the patient 'please do not help me or resist the movements'. Patients who do not comprehend the command or are unable to cooperate due to cognitive decline may carry out the movements that the examiner is passively performing, and may provide excessive resistance, or may help at one and oppose at the next assessment. This is called 'gegenhalten'.

Other supportive features on examination are diminished facial expression and soft (hypophonic) and rapid (tachyphemic) speech.

Distinction between IPD and other PS variants is not critical in primary care practice although a history of neuroleptic or metoclopramide (a gastrointestinal medication) use is very important as drug-induced parkinsonism resolves by merely discontinuing the offending agent.

Gait difficulty and gait testing

A shuffling gait with stooped posture and diminished armswing, often asymmetric, is seen in PS. Interestingly, the tremor of PS is often worse when walking. Gait initiation failure characterized by an inability to take the first step is a common late-stage feature of PS. That would be most evident when there is a doorway or border to cross, or on attempts to change direction.

Turning is impaired in PS. Instead of a pivot and change in direction, the patient may take several small steps to turn. This is called 'en bloc' turning as the entire body turns as a single unit.

The patient may exhibit propulsion and/or retropulsion when walking, which refers to uncontrollable forward and backward steps, respectively. Postural stability testing is discussed under gait disorders.

Investigations

In typical PD, no imaging studies or blood tests are required. In atypical PS, imaging or autonomic function testing may assist in making the diagnosis, but such patients are best referred to a neurologist.

Management

The mainstay of PS therapy is levodopa. Adverse effects of levodopa include nausea and emesis, hallucinations, orthostasis, and confusion. Other medications used in PS include dopamine agonists, anticholinergics, monoamine oxidase inhibitors, and amantadine. Some patients with early PS may not require medical therapy but should be followed regularly. Once there is postural instability (more than two steps with backward pull), treatment must be initiated. Further details are provided in Chapter 11.3.

Essential tremor

ET is the most common pathological tremor in the elderly. The next most common cause of tremor and the most disabling disorder is PS, which was discussed above. Onset of ET may be at any age and typically presents with a history of hand tremor interfering with activities such as eating soup with a spoon, writing, or threading a needle. There is often a positive family history of tremor.

Tremor in PS is present at rest and may be minimal or absent in some patients. In contrast, the tremor of ET is a postural and kinetic (action) tremor. There is no bradykinesia or rigidity in ET, though severe tremor may give the feeling of cogwheel rigidity. The remainder of the neurological examination is normal, though a minority of ET may also have head or voice tremor. Unlike PS, gait is not affected in ET.

Improvement of tremor following alcohol ingestion is non-specific as tremor due to other conditions may also improve. The most effective medications for ET are beta-blockers, primidone, or clonazepam.

Please refer to Chapter 11.3 for further details on tremor.

Referral

Referral to a specialist is appropriate if the diagnosis is uncertain, if there is a poor response to medical therapy, or if investigations are not available to the primary care physician (i.e. imaging studies). In Western countries, referrals are often patient driven.

Long-term and continuing care of movement disorders

ET does not impact gait or life expectancy. However, all parkinsonian syndromes do impact gait and life expectancy. Long-term management is similar to that described under gait disorders with the addition of medication additions and adjustments as warranted.

Implications of movement disorders

Tremor causes embarrassment for many and can have a tremendous impact on social functioning. Some may avoid social activities altogether because of the tremor. The bradykinesia and rigidity are more disabling than the resting tremor in PS. Patients may have to give up their occupation, as they can no longer keep up with the daily rigours of work. When patients get too slow and stiff or there is postural instability, patients should consider stopping driving. As gait is impaired in PS, the implications are similar to those outlined under the section titled 'Implications of gait disorders'.

Key points

- Gait disorders are often multifactorial in the elderly.
- Gait disorders impact functional independence.
- Tremor is the most common movement disorder symptom.
- Essential tremor is the most common pathological cause of tremor.
- Parkinson syndrome is the most disabling condition associated with tremor, and the most common movement disorder affecting gait.
- The prevalence of both gait disorders and movement disorders will increase as the population ages.

Further reading

Thompson, P.D. and Marsden, C.D. (2000). Walking disorders. In *Neurology in Clinical Practice* (ed. W.G. Bradley, R.B. Daroff, G.M. Fenichel, and C.D. Marsden), pp. 341–54. Boston MA: Butterworth-Heinemann.

Nutt, J.G. and Horak, F.B. (1997). Gait and balance disorders. In *Movement Disorders: Neurologic Principles and Practice* (ed. R.L. Watts and W.C. Koller), pp. 649–60. New York: McGraw-Hill.

Rajput, A.H. (1997). Movement disorders and aging. In *Movement Disorders: Neurologic Principles and Practice* (ed. R.L. Watts and W.C. Koller), pp. 673–86. New York: McGraw-Hill.

Rajput, A.H. (1993). Parkinsonism, aging and gait apraxia. In *Parkinsonian Syndromes* (ed. M.B. Stern and W.C. Koller), pp. 511–32. New York: Marcel Dekker.

Van Allen, M.W. and Rodnitzky, R.L. *Pictorial Manual of Neurologic Tests* 2nd edn. Chicago IL: Year Book Medical Publishers, 1981.

16.3 Infections

Suzanne F. Bradley

Epidemiology

Prevention of deaths due to infectious diseases during the twentieth century has contributed substantially to increased life expectancy. However, despite improvements in health care, infectious diseases remain a significant cause of morbidity and mortality in older people. The prevalence of infectious syndromes and their aetiologic agents is dependent upon the setting in which the infection is acquired. Among community-dwelling elderly and residents of chronic care facilities, respiratory and urinary tract infection are most common followed by infections of soft tissue and the gastro-intestinal tract. Among hospitalized elderly, urinary tract infection occurs most often followed by pneumonia, surgical wound infections, and bloodstream infections.

Diagnosis of infection in the older adult

Recognition of infection can be difficult. Abnormal physical findings or complaints may be erroneously ascribed to pre-existing medical conditions or an effect of 'normal old-age'. The febrile response may be absent or blunted in infected older adults. Normal baseline temperatures of elderly patients are often lower and maximal febrile responses may be sluggish or delayed. Anti-inflammatory medications can alter signs of inflammation further delaying diagnosis and treatment.

An attenuated inflammatory response leads to the absence of classical clinical signs and symptoms of infection. One-third of elderly patients do not have an elevated white blood cell count and many will not have localizing symptoms or focal findings on physical examination. Other non-specific symptoms and signs such as acute change in mental status, functional status, appetite, and respiratory rate have been associated with infection in the elderly. The diagnosis of infection should be considered in any older patient who has an acute change in function even if they lack fever or leucocytosis.

Implications

The atypical presentation of infection may lead to misdiagnosis and delay in treatment. The diagnoses of cholecystitis, appendicitis, diverticulitis, meningitis, endocarditis, and miliary tuberculosis are frequently missed in older adults. Mortality from these infectious syndromes is two- to 20-fold higher in the elderly when compared with death rates in young adults.

Prevention

Ageing alone, increased presence of co-morbid illnesses, or more frequent medical interventions and their complications have been suggested as possible factors that contribute to increased morbidity and mortality from infection in the elderly. Age-related factors that independently increase risk of infection include alterations in the immune system, normal flora, anatomy, and nutrition with increasing age. Efforts at prevention of infection in older adults should target those risk factors that are potentially reversible. Examples of prevention strategies will be discussed under the various clinical syndromes discussed below.

Urinary tract infection (UTI)

Epidemiology

Overall, UTI is the most common cause of infection in the elderly. The incidence of bacteriuria increases as a function of age and debility. Bacteriuria increases with the increased prevalence of prostatic hypertrophy in older men and decreased oestrogen levels in older women. With declining oestrogen levels, vaginal pH increases and normal colonizing flora are replaced with pathogenic gram negative bacilli. Other diseases that increase with age such as nephrolithiasis and neoplasms can result in urinary obstruction, urinary stasis, and the development of infection. Cerebrovascular accidents, diabetic neuropathy, cystocoeles, rectocoeles, and bladder diverticuli also impair bladder emptying. Use of urinary catheters increases the risk of UTI and associated bloodstream infections substantially.

Diagnosis

UTI, while common, can be overdiagnosed in older adults because significant pyuria ($\geq$10 WBC per low power field) is common; it is found in 30 per cent of elderly without symptoms of UTI. In addition, a high proportion of ambulatory women and men aged 65 years and older will have significant bacteriuria without symptoms. Asymptomatic bacteriuria may be present in almost 50 per cent of debilitated nursing home residents. Therefore, the diagnosis of UTI in the elderly cannot be made by the presence of bacteriuria ($\geq$ 105 CFU bacteria per millilitre) or pyuria alone.

The diagnosis is dependent upon symptoms referable to the urinary tract such as new onset on frequency, urgency, dysuria, or flank pain. Chronic symptoms or odiferous urine does not correlate with the presence of UTI. Treatment invariably results when cognitively impaired patients cannot describe their symptoms. It should be recognized that treatment for possible UTI might suppress other infections seen in older adults. Abdominal symptoms and pyuria can be found with nephrolithiasis, diverticulitis, inflammatory bowel disease, or intra-abdominal abscess in proximity to the genito-urinary tract.

In the older adult with symptomatic bacteriuria and pyuria, the most likely pathogen depends upon gender and whether the organism was acquired in the community or health care setting. In the absence of genito-urinary abnormalities, most UTIs in healthy elderly women are due to susceptible *Escherichia coli*. In healthy men, *E. coli*, *Proteus mirabilis*, and enterococci are the most common causes of UTI. In nursing home residents, *E. coli* and *Proteus* species are prevalent, but more resistant gram negative bacilli begin to emerge. In elderly patients with hospital-acquired infection, *E. coli* is still the predominant pathogen, but *Proteus aeruginosa* occurs with increasing frequency, followed by *Candida albicans* and other gram negative bacilli. Many elderly institutionalized patients will have infection due to multiple organisms even without an indwelling catheter.

Management

In a setting where antibiotic resistance is likely, treatment choices should be based on gram stain, most likely organism, and local resistance patterns until urine and blood culture results are known. Since many elderly people are persistently bacteriuric, success of therapy should be guided by relief of symptoms rather than by negative urine cultures. Treatment of asymptomatic bacteriuria in older adults does not prevent UTI, renal failure, or reduce mortality.

The optimum duration of therapy in ambulatory elderly women with uncomplicated UTI is not defined; 7 days of therapy has been recommended for cystitis, as relapse is common with 3 days of therapy. In institutionalized elderly women, 14 days of therapy has been recommended because pyelonephritis is common and cannot be readily distinguished from cystitis. Since infections in men are almost always complicated by the presence of structural or functional abnormalities, duration of treatment for UTI should be 2 weeks. If symptoms recur after that time, a longer course of antibiotics may be prescribed to treat a presumptive chronic bacterial prostatic focus. Use of antimicrobial agents which penetrate into prostatic tissue (quinolones, trimethoprim–sulfamethoxazole) is required for 6–12 weeks. Treatment of bacteriuria related to urinary devices should be considered only when symptoms occur, for example, fever for which no other cause is evident.

If fever, bacteraemia, and bacteriuria fail to improve rapidly despite isolation of an organism susceptible to therapy, early investigation to look for obstruction or abscess by ultrasound or computerized tomography (CT) should be considered.

Prevention

In patients with recurrent UTI ($\geq$three episodes per year), reversible causes of obstruction and urinary stasis should be sought and treated. In older women with recurrent UTI and normal anatomy, single doses of antibiotics such as trimethoprim–sulfamethoxazole, nitrofurantoin, or a quinolone can be tried post-coitally or daily. Topical treatment with intravaginal oestriol normalizes vaginal flora and decreases the incidence of infection in elderly women. Daily ingestion of cranberry juice may reduce pyuria and bacteriuria in elderly women.

Reasons for the use of chronic indwelling urethral catheters should be identified and the underlying condition treated by alternative means if possible. It is not clear that intermittent urethral catheterization is associated with fewer infections. Routine catheter changes or irrigation with antibacterials are not effective in preventing infection. Prophylactic use of antibiotics reduces infection rates, but resistance is common.

Respiratory tract infection

Epidemiology

Pneumonia remains one of the most common causes of admission to hospital and one of the top 10 causes of death in older adults. Asymptomatic oropharyngeal colonization with pathogenic gram negative bacilli increases with increasing age and debility; rates of colonization vary from ~10 per cent in healthy community-dwelling older adults to more than half of elderly hospital patients. Gram negative bacilli thrive with reduced salivary flow or xerostomia. Changes in salivary gland function occur with normal ageing, autoimmune disease, radiation therapy, and the use of drugs with anticholinergic side-effects. Older adults are also exposed to pathogens that cause respiratory disease as a consequence of medical care. Pathogens are transmitted by the hands of health care personnel or by exposure to other patients.

Mechanisms to prevent aspiration of oropharyngeal secretions are also impaired. Immobility, cognitive decline, and impaired gag reflex due to co-morbid diseases or the use of sedatives contribute to aspiration. Age-related decline in lung elasticity, respiratory musculature, and the development of kyphosis can contribute to decreased cough, airway collapse, and reduced mucociliary clearance. Obstructive airway disease, emphysema, neoplasm, or bronchiectasis can also reduce mucociliary clearance. Achlorhydria is common in older adults as a consequence of ageing itself or the use of acid blocking agents. Increased gastric pH allows proliferation of pathogens otherwise destroyed by stomach acid.

Diagnosis

The prevalence of some pathogens is increased in older adults. In community-dwelling elderly, potential pathogens include *Streptococcus pneumoniae*, *Haemophilus influenzae*, and less commonly gram negative bacilli. In nursing home and hospital patients, gram negative bacilli and *Staphylococcus aureus* are more likely causes of pneumonia.

Streptococcus pneumoniae is the most common cause of bacterial pneumonia in the elderly and follows aspiration of normal oropharyngeal flora. *H. influenzae* and *Moxarella catarrhalis* also colonize the respiratory tract of smokers or patients with underlying pulmonary disease. *S. aureus*, pneumococci, and group A beta-haemolytic streptococci may cause superinfection following influenza infection in the elderly.

Legionella pneumophila, other *Legionella* species, *Chlamydia pneumoniae*, and *Mycoplasma pneumoniae* may cause atypical pneumonitis in the elderly. *Legionella* occurs predominantly in older persons with underlying illness. Influenza, parainfluenza, respiratory syncytial virus, and adenovirus have also been associated with atypical pneumonia in elderly persons.

Common underlying diseases with similar presentations may obscure the diagnosis of pneumonia in older adults especially if fever and leucocytosis is absent. Sputum gram stain, cultures of sputum and blood can be useful in establishing the diagnosis of typical bacteria pneumonia and optimizing treatment. Identification of atypical causes of pneumonia is more difficult and may require special culture media, rapid diagnostic testing, or use of serology. Collection of clinical specimens from older patients who are unable to cough or cooperate is difficult.

Management

Empiric initial therapy which treats both typical and atypical pathogens have been recommended for community-acquired or nursing home acquired pneumonia. Choice of therapy should be based on local resistance patterns and guidelines. For debilitated elderly, guidelines have recommended intravenous beta lactam–beta lactamase inhibitor combinations (piperacillin–tazobactam) or third-generation cephalosporins (ceftriaxone) in combination with a macrolide (azithromycin) or quinolone (ciprofloxacin). For healthy community-dwelling elderly, therapy with oral agents may be appropriate. For nosocomially acquired pneumonia, therapy should target resistant gram negative bacilli, *S. aureus*, and *Legionella*. Lack of clinical response or the setting of an outbreak should prompt consultation with a microbiologist or infectious diseases physician.

Prevention

Despite the predilection for respiratory infection in older adults, some preventative measures may be effective. Vaccines have been shown to be efficacious for influenza and the prevention of invasive pneumococcal disease (see Chapter 16.9). Other measures to prevent respiratory illness include the avoidance of sedating drugs, feeding tubes, and unnecessary use of gastric acid-reducing medications. Infection control education of health care personnel may reduce the transmission of potential pathogens.

Tuberculosis (TB)

Epidemiology

In the developed world, approximately one-quarter of all cases of active TB and more than one-half of the deaths due to this disease occur in persons over the age of 65. While most cases of TB occur in community-dwelling elderly persons, cases also occur in nursing home residents. Many persons with latent TB now survive into old age with conditions that lead to waning cell-mediated immunity and reactivation, that is, renal failure, malignancy, diabetes mellitus, malnutrition, and corticosteroid use (see also Chapter 2.2).

Diagnosis and management

The onset of TB in the aged is usually described as insidious, but acute presentations may occur. Because cardiopulmonary disease is common in the aged, chest roentenographic findings suggestive of TB are frequently misinterpreted. Findings may be atypical, such as lower lobe infiltrates, adenopathy, and pleural effusions, but the upper lobe involvement is noted most commonly. Pulmonary TB is the most frequent presentation in the elderly, but extrapulmonary TB is more common than in younger persons.

Smears and culture of body fluids and tissues should be directed by abnormalities noted on routine clinical or laboratory examination. istopathology may demonstrate caseating granulomas. The tuberculin test may be unrevealing as anergy is a common finding in 25 per cent of older patients with active infection. In the elderly person with positive smears or a clinically compatible illness, empiric therapy (isoniazid, rifampin, ethambutol ± streptomycin) must continue until culture results are known. Treatment choice should be based on likelihood that the patient has a resistant organisms, risk of toxicity, and potential for drug interactions.

Prevention

Prevention of TB involves identification, isolation, and treatment of active cases and their contacts. In countries where the prevalence of tuberculous infection is low, skin testing with purified protein derivative has been used to identify elderly persons with latent infection. Elderly persons without evidence of active TB who have had documented conversion of their skin test from negative to positive that cannot be explained by prior exposure should be offered treatment for latent infection for 9 months. In the United States, most native elderly patients with latent infection harbour susceptible organisms acquired in their youth. Choice of therapy for latent infection should be based on similar factors considered for treatment of active infection.

Skin, soft tissue, and osteoarticular infection

Age-related changes in skin integrity, co-morbid illness, waning immunity, and increased exposure to pathogens contribute to the increased frequency of soft tissue infections seen in the elderly.

Herpes zoster

As cell-mediated immunity wanes with increasing age, the prevalence of herpes zoster increases. Painful blisters on erythematous bases in dermatomal distribution are the hallmark of herpes zoster infection. Clinical suspicion, Tzanck smear for giant cells, and less commonly by demonstration of the virus by culture or rapid tests make the diagnosis. Treatment with antivirals (acyclovir) is recommended for persons with ophthalmic zoster, or disseminated disease, and those who are immunocompromised. Persons aged 50 years and older should also receive therapy to reduce the risk of post-herpetic neuralgia.

Scabies

Elderly residents of nursing homes may be exposed to scabies, an ecoparasite that is easily transmitted from person to person or by fomites. In older persons, scabies may induce little inflammatory response. As a result, the rash in the elderly patient with scabies may be atypical, pruritus uncommon, and infestation heavy as the infection remains undetected for prolonged periods of time. Diagnosis is generally made when staff present with more typical manifestations and the organism is detected on skin scraping. Isolation of infected persons, disinfection of linen and clothing, and prolonged treatment of heavily infested patients with permethrin or ivermectin may be necessary to eradicate the infection. All nursing home patients with unexplained rashes should be examined for the presence of scabies particularly before topical steroids are given.

Skin ulceration

The skin is a major barrier to microbial invasion. In the aged, alterations in skin integrity may occur as a result of dermal atrophy, decreased mobility with resulting pressure and shearing injury, incontinence with maceration, malnutrition, vascular disease, oedema, and increased prevalence of diabetes mellitus. Greater than 50 per cent of diabetics are of age 60 years and older. Breaks in skin barriers can lead to superficial infection and spread to deep tissue and bone.

The choice and duration of antibiotic therapy for soft tissue infections is dependent on the depth and anatomic location of the ulceration, presence of co-morbid disease, community or nosocomial acquisition, and local resistance patterns. Blood cultures should be obtained in patients with cellulitis or deeper infections; cultures of purulent wounds may be useful in guiding therapy. In addition to antibiotics, identification of reversible underlying causes for ulceration may be necessary to establish a treatment plan and prevent future infections.

Preservation of skin integrity is the major goal in prevention of skin infections. Rapid, early mobilization of the patient can prevent pressure ulcers. Avoiding shearing forces when moving a patient is essential. Treatment of incontinence, avoidance of maceration and oedema, and improvement in nutrition may help maintain skin integrity. Identification of peripheral artery disease amenable to by-pass surgery can reduce ischaemia and promote healing. Neuropathic extremities must be identified early and protected by daily foot inspection and use of appropriate footwear.

Diarrhoea and gastroenteritis

Epidemiology

Diarrhoeal illness or gastroenteritis is common among older adults, particularly the disabled. It is estimated that one-third of nursing home residents will get diarrhoea each year. In the United States, most deaths due to diarrhoea occur in persons aged 75 years and older. Reduced stomach acid and intestinal motility may allow the proliferation and slow the egress of pathogens from the gastrointestinal tract. Medications and underlying diseases seen with increasing age alter intestinal motility.

Diagnosis

Gastrointestinal symptoms due to infection are mediated primarily by direct invasion by the organism or by the elaboration of toxins. Invasive or toxin-mediated inflammatory colitis in older adults is characterized by tissue destruction, abdominal pain, bloody stool, and the presence of faecal leucocytes.

Food-borne outbreaks of non-typhoidal *Salmonella* gastroenteritis have been a significant problem in nursing homes, with fatality rates as high as 10 per cent. Complications of enteric fever such as perforation and death are greatest in persons aged 50 years and older. The toxigenic bacteria enterohaemorrhagic *E. coli* (EHEC) and *Clostridium difficile* also are reported commonly among older adults, particularly in the long-term care setting. Food-borne infection with *E. coli* 0157:H7 has been associated with bloody diarrhoea and haemolytic uraemic syndrome. Mortality rates as high as 30 per cent have been reported with this infection.

Clostridium difficile infection ranges from a mild self-limited antibiotic-associated diarrhoea to toxic megacolon. Increased frequency of carriage and infection in the elderly has been associated with increased antibiotic use, decline in phagocytosis of the organism by neutrophils, inability of serum to neutralize toxins, and increased exposure in nursing homes. Most elderly persons who carry a toxin producing *C. difficile* strain will not develop manifestations of disease, and underlying disease and debility may be important co-factors for development of symptoms.

Non-inflammatory diarrhoea is characterized by watery stool without blood, mucous, or tissue destruction. Enterotoxin-producing strains of *Bacillus cereus*, *C. perfringens*, and *S. aureus* have been implicated in outbreaks of food-borne disease in nursing homes. Water-borne outbreaks of *Giardia lamblia* in nursing homes have been described with rare cases related to food contamination and a child-care programme. Wintertime outbreaks of watery diarrhoea associated with vomiting, respiratory symptoms, fever, or headaches have been associated with Norwalk-like agents, enteroviruses, or rotavirus infections.

Diagnosis of bacteria gastroenteritis is made primarily by culture of stool for bacteria or assays of stool for toxins. The pseudomembranes of *C. difficile* can be demonstrated by sigmoidoscopy. Identification of giardia in stool by smear or antigen detection may be difficult and high clinical suspicion should lead to empiric treatment with metronidazole. Serologic diagnosis or stool antigen detection for non-inflammatory diarrhoea is rarely practical in individual patients and should be reserved for outbreaks.

Management

Early identification and treatment of dehydration is important for treatment of all gastrointestinal infections. Antibiotics are generally not recommended for self-limited gastroenteritis in healthy persons, but quinolones (ciprofloxacin) may be indicated in frail elderly patients. For mild symptoms of *C. difficile*, antibiotics should be discontinued. For more severe disease, oral metronidazole or vancomycin may be given. Relapses after therapy are frequent, but most patients respond to a second course of the same therapy.

Prevention

At home or in institutions, faecal–oral transmission of gastrointestinal pathogens is preventable by careful attention to water sanitation, food preparation, and disinfection of hands and environmental surfaces. Use of disposable thermometers and sporicidal disinfectants have been useful in the control of *C. difficile*.

Bloodstream infection

Primary bloodstream infection

Primary bloodstream infections can occur in older adults as a consequence of waning cell-mediated immunity, achlorhydria, and other host factors. Increased frequencies of bloodstream infections due to tuberculosis, *Listeria monocytogenes*, and non-typhoidal salmonellosis have been noted in older adults. Bacteraemia and meningitis due to *L. monocytogenes* has been found commonly in older adults, particularly those with co-morbid illness. This organism is widespread in nature and has become an increasingly important cause of food-borne disease. Extraintestinal salmonellosis predominates at the extremes of age and is associated with antecedent vascular disease, gallstones, malignancy, and cirrhosis.

Secondary bloodstream infection

Gram negative bacteraemia following UTI or pneumonia is most common in the community and nursing home setting, reflecting the relative frequency of these infectious syndromes. *E. coli* and *Klebsiella* species account for the majority of bloodstream infections in those settings. In hospitals, gram positive cocci account for almost half of bloodstream infections; many of these nosocomial infections are associated with devices or procedures.

The source of secondary bacteraemia is important prognostically in older adults; survival rates are greatest following intravascular catheter-related, genito-urinary tract, and gastrointestinal tract infections. The poorest survival occurs in elderly patients with bacteraemia following pneumonia. A poor outcome following bacteraemia is particularly likely in elderly persons who are afebrile, receive delayed or inappropriate treatment, or who present with end-organ damage (sepsis syndrome).

In elderly patients with suspected bacteraemia, empiric therapy should be based on whether the organism was community or nosocomially acquired and the most likely source. Foreign bodies associated with the infection should be removed if possible. Definitive therapy should be based on results of blood cultures and antimicrobial susceptibilities.

Methicillin-resistant *S. aureus*

Epidemiology

Staphylococcus aureus infection is commonly found in older adults, causing soft tissue and bone infection, bacteraemia, pneumonia, and endocarditis. The risk of *S. aureus* infection increases when there is underlying disease, such as diabetes mellitus or need for dialysis, and functional dependency rather than ageing alone. The prevalence of *S. aureus* infection has been described most often in hospitalized patients, most of which are elderly. How often *S. aureus* infection occurs among healthy community-dwelling elderly and residents of nursing homes is essentially unknown.

Greater attention has been paid to the epidemiology of methicillin-resistant strains of *S. aureus* (MRSA) infection in hospitals and chronic care facilities. In some hospitals, almost one-third of blood stream *S. aureus* infections are due to methicillin-resistant isolates. Risk of infection with MRSA seems to correlate with the underlying severity of patient illness. In chronic care facilities and in the community, infection due to MRSA appears to be less common than in hospital.

It is clear that patients who have been in hospital or in nursing homes can become asymptomatically and chronically colonized with MRSA for months to years. MRSA colonization seems to occur most commonly among patients most dependent on others for their care. The presence of wounds, intravenous catheters, and enteral feeding tubes are just a few of the factors that may predispose the patient to become colonized with MRSA. MRSA colonization itself may be a marker of severe debility and increased mortality.

Diagnosis

A positive culture for MRSA is not a sufficient reason to begin treatment. It is important to differentiate MRSA infection from asymptomatic colonization. Signs and symptoms of clinical syndromes compatible with *S. aureus* infection (soft tissue infection, pneumonia, bacteraemia, endocarditis) should be sought. In the absence of clinical findings, asymptomatic colonization with MRSA should be assumed.

Management

In patients with MRSA infection, antimicrobial susceptibilities should be obtained as resistance to many antibiotic classes is common. Depending upon the clinical diagnosis and antimicrobial susceptibilities, oral (trimethoprim–sulfamethoxazole) or intravenous therapy (vancomycin) should be initiated. Systemic antibiotics should not be used to try to eradicate colonization with MRSA. Recolonization and resistance commonly follow antibiotic treatment for MRSA carriage.

Prevention

The spread of MRSA infection and colonization can be prevented or reduced by careful adherence to local infection control guidelines. Geographic areas with a low prevalence of MRSA may have more stringent policies to prevent introduction of the organism into the health care system. The most stringent policies should be considered in patient populations where infection risk is greatest, for example, acute care hospitals.

For the individual MRSA carrier, risk of infection may be increased following surgical procedures. Reduction in the number of MRSA shed in the perioperative period may reduce the risk of surgical wound infection. A brief course of intranasal mupirocin prior to surgery will transiently decolonize the patient of MRSA.

Key points

- Symptoms and signs of infection in older adults may be blunted or absent.
- Abnormal findings on history, physical, or laboratory examination should not be ascribed to 'normal ageing'.
- Delay in diagnosis and treatment of infections may account for poor outcomes in older adults.
- The predominant infectious syndromes and pathogens seen in older adults vary as a function of debility and acquisition in the community, nursing home, or hospital.
- Some risk factors can be reversed or modified to prevent infection in older adults.

Further reading

Reviews

Yoshikawa, T.T. and Norman, D.C., ed. *Infectious Disease in the Aging*. Totowa NJ: Humana Press, 2001.

Crossley, K. and Peterson, P. (1996). Infections in the elderly. *Clinical Infectious Diseases* **22**, 209–15.

Nicolle, L. et al. (1996). Infections and antibiotic resistance in nursing homes. *Clinical Microbiology Reviews* **9**, 1–17.

Sen, P. et al. (1994). Host defense abnormalities and infections in older persons. *Infections in Medicine* **11**, 34–7.

Davies, P. (1996). Tuberculosis in the elderly. Epidemiology and optimal management. *Drugs & Aging* **8**, 436–44.

Lorber, B. (1997). Listeriosis. *Clinical Infectious Diseases* **24**, 1–11.

Shimoni, Z. et al. (1999). Nontyphoid *Salmonella* bacteraemia: age-related differences in clinical presentation, bacteriology, and outcome. *Clinical Infectious Diseases* **28**, 822–7.

Ravdin, J. and Guerrant, R. (1983). Infectious diarrhea in the elderly. *Geriatrics* **38**, 95–101.

Bradley, S.F. (2002). *Staphylococcus aureus* infections and antibiotic resistance in older adults. *Clinical Infectious Diseases* **34**, 211–16.

Selected observational studies

Emori, T. et al. (1991). Nosocomial infections in elderly patients in the United States, 1986–1990. *American Journal of Medicine* **91** (3B), 289S–93S.

Wasserman, M. et al. (1989). Utility of fever, white blood cells, and differential count in predicting bacterial infections in the elderly. *Journal of the American Geriatrics Society* **37**, 537–43.

Meyers, B. et al. (1989). Bloodstream infections in the elderly. *American Journal of Medicine* **86**, 379–84.

Table 1 Common non-specific symptoms of illness in the elderly

Confusion
Apathy
Weakness
Lethargy
Fatigue
Anorexia
Weight loss
Dyspnoea
Immobility
'Stuck in a chair'
'Take to bed'
Drowsiness
Poor concentration

16.4 Non-specific presentations of illness

Tzvi Dwolatzky, A. Mark Clarfield, and Howard Bergman

Introduction

The clinical presentation of illness in the frail elderly is frequently non-specific and/or atypical. The absence of typical signs and symptoms was emphasized by Osler in his description of the presentation of lung infection: 'Pneumonia in the aged may be latent and set in without a chill; the cough and expectoration are slight, the physical signs ill-defined and changeable, and the constitutional symptoms out of all proportion to the extent of the local lesion'.

Nascher's classic 1914 text[1] also dealt with this phenomenon. 'Another frequent source of error in diagnosis is due to obscure symptoms which may be unnoticed or uninterpretable ... another source of error ... is in the interpretation of symptom complexes. We often find in maturity a number of symptoms which taken collectively are diagnostic of a certain disease. In senility every symptom must be traced to its source before we determine its relation to the disease which we suspect.'

This phenomenon may lead to a significant delay in the diagnosis of disease and consequently to an increase in morbidity and mortality among older patients. For example in one study, the presentation of lower respiratory tract infection with non-specific symptoms such as confusion, lethargy, and poor eating was associated with a significant increase in 30-day mortality.[2] Thus, the primary care physician is often faced with a diagnostic challenge and significant professional responsibility in caring for the frail elderly.

Common non-specific presentations of illness

Functional loss is the final common pathway for most clinical problems in older persons. Unlike younger patients who often exhibit a single, specific symptom or sign, older patients frequently present with non-specific problems that are in fact expressed as functional deficits. A high index of suspicion for a new medical problem in any older patient who presents with an acute change in function is advisable.

The importance of recognizing that illness may present with a change in functional status as opposed to more classical symptoms and signs was emphasized by Bernard Isaacs who coined the term 'Geriatric Giants' to describe the common syndromes of immobility, instability, incontinence, and intellectual impairment.[3] Many diseases involving various organ systems may present with these symptoms leading to both diagnostic difficulties and therapeutic confusion.

Table 1 lists some common non-specific symptoms of illness in the elderly.

The mechanism of atypical presentation of illness

The exact mechanism that results in this atypical presentation is not well understood. It is known that age has a profound effect on all physiological functions, especially the immune system and host defense mechanisms. Also, many factors such as nutrition, environmental chemicals, ultraviolet radiation, genetics, illnesses, and drugs may affect immune function over the years. The combination of immunosenescence, age-related loss of thermal control of the central nervous system, decreased vasoconstriction, and the loss of muscle mass and shivering control may often lead to a blunted fever response.[4,5] Age-related changes of the cardiovascular system as well as physical deconditioning may affect the haemodynamic response to stress and cause orthostatic changes with a decrease in cerebrovascular perfusion. Neurological changes associated with ageing may predispose the older patient to confusion and to changes in the level of consciousness.

Factors affecting disease presentation

Non-specific presentation may occur as a result of numerous factors in addition to the loss of physiological reserve. The physician frequently encounters difficulties in obtaining an adequate history from the older patient. Visual impairment, hearing loss, language difficulties as well as confusion and aphasia may limit the patient's ability to communicate. Paranoid behaviour will prevent the patient from describing symptoms accurately. The depressed may minimize symptoms, whereas the 'heart-sink' or the anxious patient may exaggerate them. The physical examination can mislead. For example, normal ageing changes of the skin can be confused with conditions such as hypothyroidism.

An additional problem involves the presence of multiple pathology. The older patient often suffers from many diseases and as a result may present with a symptom that may well be caused by any one or a combination of these pathologies. For example, ischaemic heart disease, chronic lung disease, and reflux oesophagitis can all present with dyspnoea. Medications are an important cause of symptoms such as confusion, fatigue, incontinence, gastrointestinal complaints, and falls. Polypharmacy, a common problem in the elderly, often leads to both adverse drug reactions and interactions and may limit a patient's response to illness.

The non-specific presentation of common conditions

Infections and the fever response

Although older people can present classically, the clinical features of infection in the elderly are often non-specific, atypical, or even absent. In the frail elder there is often a blunted fever response and the patient with significant infection may be afebrile or even hypothermic. This response has been attributed to both central and peripheral changes that occur due both to ageing and the effect of chronic disease on various organ systems.[4] Not surprisingly, the absence of fever may delay diagnosis and treatment and lead to higher morbidity and even mortality. The above notwithstanding, it should be noted that the presence of a raised temperature in elderly patients is more frequently associated with a bacterial infection,[6] the most common involving the urinary tract, the respiratory system, skin or soft tissue, and the gastrointestinal tract.

Infections in the elderly can present with a decline in functional status alone, with non-specific symptoms and signs. When infection is suspected, rapid clinical evaluation should be initiated. This includes a focused history and physical examination. Careful attention should be directed towards the following: oropharynx, conjunctiva, skin (specifically looking for pressure sores), chest, heart, abdomen, perineum and perirectal area, central nervous system, and mental status.[7] A recent change in functional status should be carefully noted. Temperature should be measured and monitored every few hours, as a change from baseline may be significant. It is preferable to measure rectal temperature, since impaired peripheral vasoconstriction may lead to a greater and variable difference between skin and core temperature.

Laboratory investigations should include a white blood cell (WBC) and differential count. Even if no other tests are available, as a diagnostic tool that is simple and inexpensive, the WBC and differential are quite useful for predicting bacterial infection in elderly patients.[6] Whenever possible, relevant cultures should be taken.

Dehydration commonly accompanies fever and infection in elderly patients, and many of the non-specific presentations of infection, such as weakness, fatigue, drowsiness, and confusion may indeed be related to dehydration. Fluid replacement often results in a rapid improvement in symptoms even without specific antimicrobial therapy.

Urinary tract infections (UTI)

Younger patients with infections of the upper urinary tract are frequently symptomatic, with symptoms and signs including fever, rigours, dysuria, frequency, urgency, nocturia, incontinence, and renal angle tenderness. However, the older patient may present with non-specific symptoms, such as confusion, anorexia and functional decline or with recent onset of incontinence. In complicated UTI, there may be signs of septic shock with hypotension and poor peripheral perfusion indicating that immediate therapeutic intervention is indicated.

It should be kept in mind that most older persons with bacteriuria are asymptomatic[7] and it has been observed that untreated asymptomatic bacteriuria is not associated with increased morbidity and mortality. To add to the confusion, the association of non-specific symptoms with bacteriuria does not necessarily indicate the presence of symptomatic infection, as these symptoms may well be due to other causes. Unless UTI is

clearly present, the patient should therefore also be evaluated for other illnesses prior to commencing antibiotic therapy.

Pneumonia

The clinical diagnosis of pneumonia in the older patient can be exceedingly difficult to make, as the classical symptoms are frequently absent, especially in the very frail. Dyspnoea and cough may be absent. However, tachypnoea is often seen, with a respiratory rate of greater than 25 breaths per minute associated with impending respiratory failure, an emergent situation where if available, oxygen saturation should be monitored via pulse oximetry. Where pneumonia is suspected, a chest radiograph (CXR) should be performed. An abnormal CXR demonstrating a new infiltrate compatible with pneumonia is the most reliable diagnostic method, but it should be kept in mind that in the early stages the CXR may be read as normal. Only with time, rehydration, and progression of the infectious process will the pneumonia become visible on film.

Cardiovascular disorders

Coronary artery disease

In more than 80 per cent of older patients with clinical coronary heart disease, angina pectoris is the presenting symptom.[5] The clinical presentation of angina pectoris in older persons is often classical. However, it may also present as pain in the back or the shoulders, and this may easily be misinterpreted as degenerative joint disease. Pain with a burning nature in the epigastrium is also often misdiagnosed as peptic ulcer disease or as reflux oesophagitis as these conditions are also common in older patients. Occasionally, dyspnoea rather than pain may be the major complaint. Other symptoms include syncope with exertion, coughing, palpitations, and episodes of confusion.

As in the younger diabetic, myocardial infarction in the elderly may be unrecognized or even silent. In the Framingham Study, acute infarction was unrecognized in approximately 25 per cent of patients, with 52 per cent of these presenting atypically.

Congestive heart failure (CHF)

While older patients with CHF may present with the usual symptoms of dyspnoea on exertion, paroxysmal nocturnal dyspnoea, orthopnoea, oedema, and fatigue, they often exhibit non-specific symptoms.[8] These may include weakness and fatigue, cough, drowsiness, and confusion. The patient may also complain of nausea and anorexia with abdominal discomfort. Insomnia is common due to orthopnoea and nocturia and sometimes the presenting complaint may be inability to sleep except when seated.

With CHF, any of the patient's symptoms may be attributed to other conditions. For example, dyspnoea may be attributed to respiratory disease or to anaemia, weakness and fatigue to anaemia or deconditioning, and oedema to venous insufficiency. For this reason, heart failure is often underdiagnosed in elderly patients and the primary care physician should maintain a high index of suspicion for this condition. When available, CXR and especially cardiac ultrasound can be of great help in confirming the diagnosis.

Neurological disease

Cerebrovascular disease

Stroke is a leading cause of morbidity and mortality among elderly patients and the incidence and prevalence rates increase with age and should be suspected in the presence of focal neurologic signs or symptoms of sudden onset. However, especially in the older, frail patient, stroke may present with non-specific and non-focal symptoms or signs (Table 2). A recent change in function should alert the physician to the possibility of an acute cerebral

Table 2 Non-specific presentations of stroke

Dizziness
Syncope
Vertigo
Ataxia
Seizures
Confusion
Delirium

insult. Focal seizures may mimic stroke and should be considered in any older person who develops focal motor or sensory disturbances of short duration. Seizures are often the sequelae of a cerebral infarct, and may even manifest as the presenting symptom. While cerebrovascular disease is the most common cause of seizures in the elderly,[5] other causes should also be considered, such as primary or secondary tumours, degenerative diseases, metabolic conditions, and trauma, among others.

Confusion is a frequent presenting symptom in the older patient with a stroke, varying from mild confusion to a florid delirium, with restlessness, agitation, aggressive behaviour, hallucinations, and fluctuations in mental status. It is important to note that an acute confusional state is frequently unrecognized, and failure to recognize delirium may have serious consequences.

Subdural haematoma

Subdural haematoma (SDH) presents the primary care physician with a major diagnostic dilemma. The older person often has some degree of atrophy of the brain, with the intracranial veins stretched and more fragile than in youth. To add to the diagnostic difficulties, a haematoma in the subdural space may initially be tolerated reasonably well. The clinical presentation is often sub-acute and non-specific, with manifestations including seizure, ataxia and gait disturbance. The patient may frequently present with confusion or delirium. This may be particularly difficult to diagnose in the demented where worsening confusion and behavioural disturbances can develop.

In any older patient with these symptoms or with a decline in previous functional ability, SDH should be considered. This is particularly true if there is a history of recent head trauma—even minor, headache, change in the level of consciousness, or other neurological abnormalities. The clinical suspicion of SDH warrants further evaluation, whenever possible by CT scan.

Endocrine disorders

Thyroid disease

The higher prevalence of thyroid disease in the older patient, as well as the paucity of specific clinical signs and symptoms necessitates that thyroid disorders be considered in the differential diagnosis. However, thyroid function tests may be affected by other associated conditions as well as by some medications, and this may lead to misinterpretations of the results and to misdiagnosis.

Hypothyroidism often develops insidiously and in many cases the patient's condition is understandably attributed to ageing. The classic signs such as cold intolerance, weight gain, oedema of the face and eyelids, paresthesia and muscle cramps, were shown in one study to actually be less frequent in older patients. Also, when these symptoms were present, they were often incorrectly attributed to other conditions.

The older patient with hypothyroidism may present with decreased appetite and weight loss. Dry skin and hair loss is common. Carpal tunnel syndrome, especially bilateral, is an important form of peripheral neuropathy that is found in these patients. The patient may be apathetic with poor concentration and cognitive impairment. While hypothyroidism is often considered as one of the 'reversible' causes of dementia, a relatively small number of these patients have been shown to improve on hormone replacement. The severely hypothyroid patient may develop behavioural problems, such as paranoia and delusions, and hallucinations and psychosis may occur. The apathetic patient with anorexia and weight loss may well be diagnosed as suffering from depression.

Hypothyroidism is an important cause of sleep apnoea, and this problem has been shown to improve with therapy. The myopathy associated with hypothyroidism may lead to proximal muscle pain and stiffness, and this presentation may be misdiagnosed, for example, as polymyalgia rheumatica. Patients may present with joint pain and stiffness as well as joint effusions. The most frequent effects of hypothyroidism on the cardiovascular system in the older patient include bradycardia, pericardial effusion in up to 50 per cent of patients with overt hypothyroidism, and diastolic hypertension. Other common findings include anaemia and hypercholesterolaemia.

Hyperthyroidism most commonly results as in the younger patient from Grave's disease (diffuse toxic goitre), and toxic multinodular goitre is also common in the elderly, especially in regions of relative iodine deficiency. The absence of typical findings of hyperthyroidism in the elderly was first described in 1931 by Lahey as 'apathetic hyperthyroidism'. Apathy and anorexia are found more often in the older than the younger patient, and may be mistakenly attributed to depression or to malignancy.

Confusion is an important presenting symptom of hyperthyroidism in the elderly. The older patient may present with supraventricular tachycardia, particularly atrial fibrillation. Weight loss is often significant and the patient may complain of constipation. Muscle weakness involving the proximal muscles may cause a significant limitation in function. Unlike younger patients, a palpable goitre is absent in at least half of the older patients. The classic eye findings of hyperthyroidism occur less frequently in the elderly. Tremor, nervousness, and sweating are also less common.

Diabetes mellitus

Diabetes mellitus is a common condition affecting older patients. However, a lack of consensus as to what constitutes diabetes in the elderly, as well as atypical presentation, has led frequently to its underdiagnosis in the elderly. The diagnostic criteria of the American Diabetes Association requires that the patient present with 'classic diabetes symptoms plus a random glucose level of >200 mg/dL'. However, these symptoms are frequently absent in the elderly or they may be incorrectly attributed to other conditions. For example, polyuria may be considered to be a symptom of either an enlarged prostate or of heart failure or the use of diuretics. Polydypsia is often absent, and when present is often a harbinger of a hyperosmolar state.

Non-specific symptoms of hyperglycaemia include visual changes, anorexia and weight loss, urinary incontinence, gait disturbances, confusion, and mental changes or even coma. The patient may present with recurrent infections and poor wound healing. A significant delay in diagnosis may result in an initial presentation related to one of the long-term sequelae of the disease, such as renal failure, diabetic foot, or blindness. The physician should thus be alert to the possibility of diabetes developing in the older patient and should initiate adequate treatment as soon as the diagnosis has been confirmed.

Other common conditions

Depression

Depression in older persons is very common and may present in many ways. The usual classic symptoms as defined in the DSM-IV may be present, but the diagnosis of depression in the elderly is frequently not easy. The patient often presents with a change in his functional ability, and this may well occur in particular after suffering a loss, such as the death of a spouse. Social activity may be significantly curtailed, and the desire to perform usual tasks may be limited. There may be a lack of motivation and drive. The patient's physical appearance may indicate a lack of interest and self-esteem.

Cognitive symptoms are frequent. This may vary from a loss of concentration and memory impairment to dementia (pseudodementia) but it should be noted that pseudodementia is not common, and that when assessing such patients the physician should rather consider the diagnosis of Alzheimer's disease with an associated depression. The depressed patient may present with delusions or psychotic symptoms. The older patient who expresses suicidal intentions should be referred for psychiatric assessment, as there is an especially increased risk of suicide with advancing age, especially in men.

Many depressed older patients will present with non-specific somatic symptoms and as a result will often undergo unnecessary investigations in an attempt to rule out physical disease.

Polymyalgia rheumatica and giant cell arteritis

Polymyalgia rheumatica (PMR) and giant cell arteritis (GCA) are closely related conditions that are almost always seen in patients over the age of 50. The mean age of onset for both conditions is 70 years, with an increasing incidence with age. Both conditions are not uncommon in the elderly, with a reported prevalence of PMR of 550 per 100 000 and of GCA of 234 per 100 000. The diagnosis of these conditions is often difficult as they frequently present with non-specific symptoms rather than the classic symptoms of these disorders.[9]

The classic presentation of PMR includes morning stiffness and pain and tenderness of the proximal girdle muscles and neck. The pain may be severe and limit activity and may be aggravated by joint movement. The symptoms are usually symmetrical. The onset is often insidious but may be abrupt.

GCA commonly presents with headache that may be severe. Visual loss may occur in up to 20 per cent of patients. Other visual symptoms such as diplopia or ptosis may occur. Rarely, visual hallucinations may precede visual loss. The patient may frequently complain of scalp tenderness or of claudication of the jaw or the tongue. There are non-classic manifestations of organ involvement in about 10 per cent of patients. This includes involvement of the vascular system, with angina pectoris or myocardial infarction, or even aortic dissection. The patient may suffer transient ischaemic events or even stroke. Dementia as a result of GCA has been described. Respiratory involvement may manifest as a cough or sore throat, as hoarseness or as lung infiltrates. Sensorineural hearing loss may occur. Renal involvement may lead to proteinuria or haematuria.

Non-specific constitutional symptoms (Table 3) occur in about one-half of those affected with these conditions. These may be the only presenting symptoms and this often leads to misdiagnosis. Early recognition, especially of GCA, is essential in preventing possible catastrophic consequences such as blindness and stroke. A high index of clinical suspicion and the appropriate laboratory investigations will lead to early effective treatment with corticosteroid therapy.

Surgical conditions

Many surgical conditions present atypically in the older person. It is thus essential to maintain a high index of suspicion in treating this age group. A few examples will have to suffice.

Table 3 Non-specific constitutional symptoms of PMR and GCA

Low-grade fever
Night sweats
Anorexia
Weight loss
Malaise
Fatigue
Depression

In a study that assessed the clinical presentation of acute appendicitis in the elderly, only 20 per cent of patients presented with all the classical manifestations of fever, anorexia, right lower quadrant pain, and leukocytosis. Their lack caused a significant delay in diagnosis and 72 per cent already had perforation at the time of surgery. Nausea and vomiting was common. The lack of more specific clinical signs was particularly prominent in confused or demented patients. Hip fracture can present as isolated pain in the knee. Also, asymptomatic hip fracture (usually impacted) without a definite history of trauma is well described.

Conclusions

The frail older patient can suffer from multiple pathology, polypharmacy, a lack of physiological reserve and often presents with non-specific symptoms and signs of disease. This phenomenon frequently leads to a delay in diagnosis and may be associated with an increase in morbidity and mortality. A recent change in the functional status of the patient demands a careful assessment. The primary care physician should be aware of the atypical presentations of common disorders in the elderly and maintain a high index of suspicion of the underlying aetiologies. Although atypical presentation offers the family doctor a clinical and intellectual challenge, careful history taking, a guided physical examination, and standard laboratory tests will usually suffice to allow the clinician to make at least a provisional diagnosis and provide appropriate treatment.

Key points

- Atypical presentation is common, especially in the frail elderly.
- Anything can cause almost any symptom, but there are some typical geriatric syndromes.
- A recent change in function demands careful assessment.
- A careful history and physical examination with standard laboratory tests will usually suffice to make the diagnosis. However, careful follow-up is necessary.

References

1. Nascher, I.L. *Geriatrics: The Diseases of Old Age and Their Treatment*. New York: Arno Press, 1979. (Reprint of the 1914 edition originally published by P. Blackiston's, Philadelphia.)
2. Ahkee, S., Srinath, L., and Ramirez, J. (1997). Community-acquired pneumonia in the elderly: association of mortality with lack of fever and leukocytosis. *Southern Medical Journal* **90**, 863–4.
3. Isaacs, B. *The Challenge of Geriatric Medicine*. Oxford: Oxford University Press, 1992.
4. Castle, S.C. et al. (1991). Fever response in elderly nursing home residents: are the older truly colder? *Journal of the American Geriatrics Society* **39**, 853–7.
5. Hazzard, W.R. et al., ed. *Principles of Geriatric Medicine and Gerontology* 4th edn. New York: McGraw-Hill, 1999.
6. Wasserman, M. et al. (1989). Utility of fever, white blood cells, and differential count in predicting bacterial infections in the elderly. *Journal of the American Geriatrics Society* **37**, 537–43.
7. Bentley, D.W. et al. (2001). Practice guideline for evaluation of fever and infection in long-term care facilities. *Journal of the American Geriatrics Society* **49**, 210–22.
8. King, D. (1996). Diagnosis and management of heart failure in the elderly. *Postgraduate Medicine* **72**, 577–80.
9. Dwolatzky, T., Sonnenblick, M., and Nesher, G. (1997). Giant cell arteritis and polymyalgia rheumatica: clues to early diagnosis. *Geriatrics* **52**, 38–44.

16.5 Dementia

Howard Bergman, David B. Hogan,
Christopher Patterson, Howard Chertkow,
and A. Mark Clarfield

Dementia is a clinical syndrome which can be diagnosed when multiple cognitive deficits are observed. They must include impairment in memory as well as in one or more of the following domains: language, praxis, perception, and executive function. These deficits must cause significant impairment in the usual social and occupational function of the person and represent significant decline from a previous level of function in the absence of depression or delirium.[1] It is a complex clinical problem with multiple potential causes leading to significant social and economic repercussions for affected individuals, families, and the community.

Providing comprehensive, coordinated, and timely care over the duration of the illness from the early phases of initial diagnosis and treatment through the late phases of caring in the home and institution is particularly challenging. In collaboration with a variety of providers and agencies, primary care physicians need to work in an interdisciplinary manner with medical consultants, nurses, social workers, psychologists, and other professional and support staff.

Epidemiology, risk factors, and prevention

Dementia is one of the most important disorders affecting older individuals. Although rare in people less than 65 years old, it affects 8–10 per cent of those over 65 and 35–40 per cent of those over 85 years and over. Prevalence increases with age and varies across cultures.[2] Alzheimer's disease (AD) accounts for at least 60 per cent of dementia cases in Europe and North America, while in China and Japan, vascular dementia (VaD) is predominant. Across cultures, differences exist in the approach to dementing illnesses. In some cultures, the concept of dementia does not exist and cognitive changes are attributed to 'senility' or natural ageing.[3]

The incidence of dementia is declining in the developed world, possibly due, at least in part, to more effective prevention of cerebrovascular disease. However, the incidence appears lower in some developing countries than in the United States. For example, the age-standardized incidence is 1.35 per cent in Nigeria versus 3.24 per cent in African-Americans. In both developing and developed countries, the growth in the total number of older persons will result in an increase in the absolute number of cases of dementia.

The societal and economic burden of dementia is enormous. In developed countries, the majority of affected individuals residing in the community will have mild to moderate disease. They require increased supervision and care at home resulting in increased burden for caregivers in whom psychiatric symptoms, especially depression are common. Caregivers may have to leave their employment or rely on paid caregivers or formal support provided by the health care system. A diagnosis of dementia in a community-dwelling person increases the probability of acute hospitalization and may result in prolonged hospital stay. Individuals with dementia are at greater risk of motor vehicle collision and household injuries (e.g. falls, burns). Rates of institutional admission vary widely between countries but the risk of admission is much higher in people with dementia than in those without. In most long-term care facilities, the prevalence of dementia exceeds 50 per cent.

Genetic factors influence AD, frontotemporal (FTD), and Huntington's dementias. The rare genetic (autosomal dominant) forms of AD usually present early, in the fifth and sixth decades. In AD, the presence of one and particularly two apoE4 allele on chromosome 19 significantly increases the risk of AD even in later years. Other risk factors for AD, in common with VaD, include age, family history, significant head injury, vascular risk factors (atrial fibrillation, hypertension, hyperlipidaemia, diabetes mellitus), and depression. Interestingly, education may be a protective factor.

With this expanding knowledge of the risk factors for dementia (in particular AD), primary prevention is becoming a possibility. When clinical conditions that can lead to dementia (e.g. alcohol abuse) are detected, they should be treated. Management of vascular risk factors (e.g. hypertension) would be reasonably expected to decrease the likelihood of vascular dementias, mixed dementias, and possibly AD. The evidence does not support the use of antioxidants, anti-inflammatories, and oestrogen replacement therapy in the prevention of AD. Higher educational attainment, avoidance of head injuries, regular physical activity, and extensive social networks are associated with a lower likelihood of dementia. If the onset of AD could be delayed by as little as 1 year, this would result in 800 000 fewer cases after 50 years in the United States.

Aetiology and natural history

Elderly individuals vary widely in their degree of cognitive ability. About 5 per cent of elderly individuals demonstrate a memory capacity that exceeds that of younger subjects. More commonly, elderly individuals note a decline when compared with their performance at a younger age. The most commonly noted changes include memory problems, specifically difficulty recalling proper names of occasional acquaintances. While not infrequently of concern to patients, these subjective alterations are unaccompanied by objective impairment on formal mental status testing, and are of no particular prognostic significance. These subjective changes are often termed 'normal cognitive ageing'. When a patient complains of memory problems with normal performance on delayed memory tests (e.g. recall of three words), a likely cause is depression or anxiety.

Other elderly individuals manifest mild memory loss both subjectively and on objective formal testing. These are the patients or their families who usually complain that their memory has deteriorated over recent years but without significant decline in daily function. In many cases this degree of impairment, often termed mild cognitive impairment (MCI), is insufficient to make a clear diagnosis of dementia. Some within this heterogeneous group have a benign course and do not progress to dementia. Over the course of a year, about 15 per cent per year of MCI subjects do progress to dementia, usually AD. Persons with MCI should not be labelled as demented neither should they be dismissed as having 'normal ageing'. They are at increased risk of developing dementia and should be reviewed regularly.[4]

Rarely, dementia may have reversible causes. The main aetiologies have been found to be medications such as sedatives, depression, and metabolic abnormalities. Other rarer causes include subdural haematomas (SDH) and normal pressure hydrocephalus (NPH). Truly reversible dementia is rare with fully reversible dementia encountered in less than 3 per cent of cases.

The most common cause of dementia is AD, accounting in most series for 55–65 per cent of all dementias. Typically, such patients are brought to the physician by family members concerned about their short-term memory loss. Long-term memory is initially preserved, but recall of recent events or ability to learn new lists of items may be severely impaired. Attention (e.g. serial seven subtractions) remains intact initially. It typically presents insidiously with subsequent progressive, gradual decline affecting other domains of cognition.

In the middle stages, executive function declines (sequencing and planning of complex tasks) leading to difficulties with instrumental and later basic activities of daily living. In the later stages of AD as in the other forms of dementia, behavioural abnormalities (e.g. aggression, agitation, apathy, disinhibition) commonly arise. Death is usually preceded by motor changes including rigidity and flexion contractures, but often results from an intercurrent illness such as pneumonia. The time from first symptoms to death has been estimated at 7–10 years, although recent evidence suggests that the median duration of AD may be as short as 3.1 years.[5]

While memory is usually the predominant problem, there are atypical cases where language, behaviour, or recognition of objects are the major domains affected. FTD is the currently accepted broad term encompassing what was previously termed Pick's disease. This condition, accounting for approximately 10 per cent of the dementias, can present with prominent early behavioural or language changes with relative sparing of memory. Core diagnostic features include loss of personal hygiene, disinhibition and loss of social awareness, impulsivity, and loss of behavioural control.

Some dementia patients have abnormal motor signs such as focal weakness or rigidity and bradykinesia. VaD from multiple cerebrovascular accidents accounts for 10–20 per cent of cases. At times, AD and VaD coexist (termed mixed dementia) which represents the third most reported category. Lewy body dementia (LBD) is accompanied by psychiatric complaints such as visual hallucinations, and there are early and prominent parkinsonian features such as rigidity and bradykinesia. Such patients often show large day-to-day fluctuations in the severity of their deficit. Thus, the presence of motor features early in the disease, should prompt a search for a diagnosis other than AD.

Diagnosis and investigation

Although community or office screening of all elderly patients may not be justified, a high index of suspicion should be maintained concerning any behaviour reported or observed suggesting cognitive decline (decreased medication or appointment compliance, personal neglect, social withdrawal, etc.).

The diagnosis of dementia is essentially a clinical one that for the most part can be determined in primary care. Through history, physical examination, and investigation the clinician will be able to determine whether or not dementia is present and what is the likely underlying aetiology. There are presently no reliable biological, genetic, or imaging diagnostic markers recommended for routine clinical use.

The most important element of the diagnosis is the history, which should always be corroborated by someone who knows the patient well. The history should include a family history, past evidence of cardiovascular disease, head injury, depression and/or other psychiatric problems, substance or alcohol abuse, and the use of prescribed and over-the-counter medications (in particular any medication with anticholinergic or sedative properties).

The onset, evolution, and characteristics of the cognitive changes and accompanying functional decline will usually point to the presence and cause of the dementia. In all cases, it is essential to elicit a history of significant decline from previous levels of functional abilities. Clinicians may use a scale such as the Functional Assessment Questionnaire (FAQ). Early in the disease, it is important to elicit evidence of decline in the ability to manage finances, grocery shopping, meal preparation, and medications, or carry out hobbies and social activities. As well, it is useful to query the family or caregiver as to whether they believe the patient could live on his/her own for several weeks or months. Finally, the clinician should assess how the caregiver is coping.

The physical examination should aim to detect evidence of any systemic disease, which could affect cognition as well as other co-morbid conditions. The neurological examination should seek the presence of extrapyramidal or motor abnormalities suggestive of a non-Alzheimer aetiology such as NPH, VaD, or LBD.

The mental status examination is the next essential step. Many instruments are available but the Folstein Mini-Mental State Examination (MMSE)[6] is the most commonly used. It examines orientation, memory, calculation, language, praxis, and visuo-spatial ability. Although a score of 24/30 has been suggested as a cut-off for the diagnosis of dementia, it is more useful to interpret the MMSE in the clinical context. In general, a score below 20 is very highly suggestive of the presence of dementia and a score above 27 is strongly indicative of its absence (although the MMSE may be normal early in the course of FTD). Limited education, language skills, cultural factors, and poor hearing may all produce an artificially low score. While the MMSE represents the best available tool, physicians should also assess long-term memory (e.g. dates of weddings, birthdays), insight, judgement, and executive function (usually from history). Finally, the physician should assess for behavioural abnormalities and psychiatric features such as depression or aggression.

Once the diagnosis is determined, the objectives of the investigations (laboratory tests and neuroimaging) are to detect co-morbid conditions,

which may affect cognition, to detect the rare cases of potentially reversible dementia, and to confirm the type of dementia.

Most recent evidence-based consensus guidelines agree that only a limited number of laboratory tests (complete blood count, thyroid simulating hormone, serum electrolytes, serum calcium, serum glucose) should be carried out in cases typical of AD with additional tests being ordered if indicated by the history, physical examination, and initial investigations.

There is more controversy on the use of neuroimaging, which has a role in the diagnosis of certain causes of dementia (e.g. vascular) or in detecting rare reversible causes (e.g. meningioma, NPH, SDH). The 1998 Canadian Consensus Conference on Dementia[7] recommended limiting the use of computer tomography (CT) scanning to people who meet specific clinical criteria such as early onset, atypical presentation and progression, recent head trauma, localizing or unexplained neurological signs, history of cancer, use of anticoagulants, urinary incontinence, or gait disturbance suggestive of NPH. Other guidelines that may not necessarily be appropriate for primary care, such as those proposed by the American Academy of Neurology, do recommend neuroimaging for all cases of dementia.[8]

In most cases, using accepted diagnostic criteria and on the basis of the history, physical examination, and investigation, the primary care physician will be able to determine the diagnosis of dementia and establish a plan for treatment. This is, however, not a simple process (see Fig. 1) and rarely

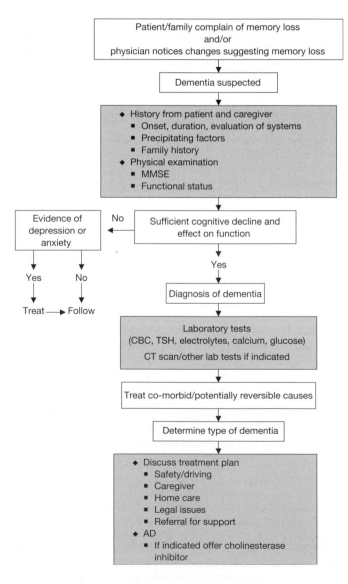

Fig. 1 Diagnosis, investigation, and treatment of dementia.

possible to complete in a single visit. A multiple visit strategy is usually necessary and in fact desirable in that it permits the clinician to carry out a careful assessment, detect variation in performance and establish a relationship with the patient and caregiver.

Referral may be indicated in certain situations such as continued uncertainty as to the diagnosis or appropriate treatment, the presence of significant depression or behaviour problems, a request for a second opinion, the need for genetic counselling, or the need for multidisciplinary intervention. The patient can be referred to a geriatrician, neurologist, or geriatric psychiatrist or to a multidisciplinary dementia clinic when available.

Management

The initial approach includes discussion of the diagnosis as well as management options. At least in North America, disclosure to families and caregivers has long been accepted as essential. There is increasing consensus on the desirability of disclosure to the patient as well. These decisions will be influenced by the stage of the disease, as well as by family dynamics and the cultural setting. Initial discussion should include home help, safety issues, and legal questions such as power of attorney and the use of advance directives. The patient's ability to drive should be discussed and, when indicated, measures to withdraw the driver's permit should be undertaken.

Caregivers are often the 'hidden patients'.[9] Helping them to cope effectively will often allow a longer residence in the community. Caregivers should be routinely asked about burden and should be advised on coping strategies and how to deal with problem behaviours. Community resources such as home care, day programmes, and respite can be used to relieve the caregiver. Referral to voluntary agencies such as the local Alzheimer's Society for information and support is often beneficial.

While true reversibility is rare, treatment of co-morbid conditions may enhance function and quality of life of the person with dementia. When appropriate, medications which adversely affect cognition should be discontinued.

Cholinesterase inhibitors (e.g. donepezil, galantamine, rivastigmine) are now available for the treatment of AD. These medications can have a symptomatic effect but there is little evidence of disease modification. Modest cognitive, functional, and behavioural benefits can be seen in a significant proportion of treated patients but not all respond.[10] These agents are indicated for those patients, preferably with caregivers, in the mild to moderate stages of the illness in the absence of contraindications. At the present time, they are not indicated for MCI or severe dementia. There is growing evidence that these drugs may also be helpful in LBD. According to some authors,[11] addition of vitamin E for patients with AD may help slow progression.

It is important to manage patient and caregiver expectations by explaining the potential effectiveness and side-effects. These medications need to be titrated up to the maximum tolerated maintenance dose. During titration, side-effects, such as nausea, vomiting, anorexia, and muscle cramps may occur and require monitoring. Once the maintenance dose is reached, regular 6-month review is necessary to evaluate medication effect and the progress of the disease. The evolution of the MMSE score, functional status changes, and the overall impression of the caregiver compared to pretreatment levels comprise useful 'yardsticks'. Although it is uncertain how long the medication should be maintained, in the absence of side-effects, treatment should continue if there is improvement, stabilization, or even a decreased rate of decline compared to the pre-treatment status.

As the disease progresses, the behavioural and psychological symptoms of dementia become increasingly common and comprise a major cause of morbidity and caregiver burden. Depression, agitation, psychotic features, and other behavioural challenges often respond to a combined nonpharmacological and pharmacological approach (low-dose antidepressants or neuroleptics). Underlying causes of the problem behaviour such as delirium or uncontrolled pain should be sought and treated with before prescribing any psychoactive drugs. Issues such as incontinence, falls, complications of immobility, and end-of-life issues need to be addressed.

Dementia increases the complexity of any acute illness, as it lowers the threshold for delirium, diminishes decision-making capacity, complicates both diagnosis (inaccurate or misleading history) and treatment (impaired adherence to prescribed medications, poor tolerance of hospital environment) and can delay recovery.[12]

Primary care physicians need to be familiar with and work in collaboration with available specialized geriatric and geriatric psychiatry services as well as with the available community resources (home care, day programmes, respite, etc.). This would include, when appropriate, facilitating institutional admission by planning ahead with caregivers and community resources.

Conclusions

Dementia is a common syndrome, especially in the very elderly. The absolute number of cases will grow over the next half century, especially in the less developed regions of the world. Despite the complexity of the syndrome, diagnosis and treatment are certainly within the purview of the primary care physician working in an interdisciplinary manner with other professionals. In most cases, diagnosis can be made on the basis of history, physical and simple laboratory tests. In a small minority of cases, more extensive testing and referral may be required. Management must address all aspects of the problem. Drug therapy is now available and is modestly effective in a significant proportion of AD patients. Taking into account both potential benefits and costs, it is essential that drug therapy be initiated in patients for whom a confident diagnosis has been made and for whom regular assessment of benefits and side-effects will be provided. In addition, it is critical that the caregiver be supported in all phases of the disease. Much professional satisfaction can be had in helping patients and their families to cope at each stage of the illness.

Keypoints

- ◆ Dementia affects 8–10% of people over 61 years old and up to 35–40% of people 85 years and over.

- ◆ Risk factors for Alzheimer's disease include age, family history, significant head injury, vascular risk factors, and depression. Education may be a protective factor. Genetic factors influence Alzheimer's disease, frontotemporal dementia (FTD), and Huntington's dementias.

- ◆ Alzheimer's disease is the most common form of dementia. Mixed dementia, vascular dementia, FTD, and Lewy Body dementia (LBD) need to be recognized.

- ◆ Older persons with subjective and objective findings of memory impairment who do not meet criteria for dementia may have mild cognitive impairment (MCI) and have increased risk to progress to dementia.

- ◆ The diagnosis of dementia is essentially clinical (history, physical, and mental status examinations) and for the most part can be determined in primary care.

- ◆ Once the diagnosis is determined, the objectives of the investigation (laboratory tests and neuroimaging) are to detect co-morbid conditions which may affect cognition, to detect rare causes of reversible dementia, and to confirm the cause of the dementia.

- ◆ The approach to management is interdisciplinary and includes caring for the caregiver.

- ◆ Cholinesterase inhibitors (donepezil, reminyl, rivastigmine) are indicated for persons with mild to moderate Alzheimer's disease. Effects are systematic with modest cognitive, behavioural, and functional effects in a significant proportion of treated persons. Regular assessment of cognitive and functional status must be carried out.

References

1. **American Psychiatric Association.** *Diagnostic and Statistical Manual of Mental Disorders (DSM IV)* 4th edn. (abbreviated from). Washington DC: *American Psychiatric Association,* 1994.

2. **Fratiglioni, L., De Ronchi, D., and Aguero-Torres, H.** (1999). Worldwide prevalence and incidence of dementia. *Drugs & Aging* **15** (5), 365–75.

3. **Herbert, C.P.** (2001). Cultural aspects of dementia. *The Canadian Journal of Neurological Sciences* **28** (Suppl. 1), S77–82.

4. **Chertkow, H.** et al. (2001). Assessment of suspected dementia. *The Canadian Journal of Neurological Sciences* **28** (Suppl. 1), S28–41.

5. **Wolfson, C.** et al. (2001). A reevaluation of the duration of survival after the onset of dementia. *New England Journal of Medicine* **344** (15), 1111–16.

6. **Folstein, M.F., Folstein, S.E., and McHugh, P.R.** (1975). Mini-mental state: a practical method for grading the cognitive state of patient for the clinician. *Journal of Psychiatric Research* **12**, 196–8.

7. **Patterson, C.** et al. (1999). The recognition, assessment and management of dementing disorders: conclusions from the Consensus Conference on Dementia. *Canadian Medical Association Journal* **160** (Suppl. 12), S1–15.

8. **Knopman, D.S.** et al. (2001). Practice parameter: diagnosis of dementia (an evidence-based review). *Neurology* **56**, 1143–53.

9. **Parks, S.M. and Novielli, K.D.** (2000). A practical guide to caring for caregivers. *American Family Physician* **62**, 2613–20.

10. **O'Brien, J.T. and Ballard, C.G.** (2001). Drugs for Alzheimer's Disease. *British Medical Journal* **323**, 123–4.

11. **Doody, R.S.** et al. (2001). Practice parameter: management of dementia (an evidence-based review). *Neurology* **56**, 1154–66.

12. **Brauner, D.J., Muir, J.C., and Sachs, G.A.** (2000). Treating nondementia illnesses in patients with dementia. *Journal of the American Medical Association* **283**, 3230–5.

Further reading

Canadian Consensus Conference on Dementia (2001). *The Canadian Journal of Neurological Sciences* **28** (Suppl. 1), S1–123. (An in-depth evidence-based series of articles on all aspects of dementia.)

Patterson, C. et al. (1999). Canadian Consensus Conference on Dementia: a physician's guide to using the recommendations. *Canadian Medical Association Journal* **160**, 1738–42. (A practical case based approach to the diagnosis and treatment of various forms of dementia.)

16.6 Urinary incontinence

Toine Lagro-Janssen

Epidemiology

Urinary incontinence, defined as the involuntary loss of urine, is a major problem that affects many elderly people. In addition, urinary incontinence, together with confusion, falling, and immobility, is one of the most prevalent non-specific expressions of an underlying disorder in elderly patients.[1] It is estimated that, depending on the definition, 15–30 per cent of elderly people living independently suffer from incontinence;[2] this rate increases to 50 per cent in the elderly in retirement homes, to 90 per cent in the elderly in nursing homes.[3] Almost twice as many elderly women suffer from urinary incontinence as elderly men; 14 per cent of women aged 65 years and older are troubled daily by incontinence.[4] Urinary incontinence is considered to be one of the most important reasons to admit patients to retirement homes or nursing homes. In elderly people with incontinence, there is a high prevalence of co-morbidity and functional limitations. These concern disorders that can play a contributory role in incontinence, such as decreased mobility, arthrosis, cerebrovascular accidents, chronic coughing, and visual impairment. The onset or deterioration of incontinence can be caused by such disorders localized outside the urinary tract. Incontinence is transient in 30–50 per cent of the elderly. Generally, elderly people suffer from urge incontinence or mixed incontinence. In many cases, the origin of urine loss is multifactorial and there are also mobility, cognitive, and communication disorders.

Presentation

About half of elderly people with incontinence consult their GP.[5] Many elderly people are poorly informed about what incontinence is and what can be done about it.[6] They view the disorder as a normal part of growing old, or as an untreatable consequence of being a woman and giving birth to children. Treatment is not expected to be effective, or absorbent products have already been purchased.

Data from the Nijmegen Continuous Morbidity Registration show a prevalence of 3.6 per cent of women and 1.9 per cent of men who consult their GP about incontinence and an incidence of 0.8 in women and 0.3 in men.[7] The largest quantitative group of patients with urinary incontinence in general practice comprises women of 65 years and older. Owing to the fact that few people seek professional help themselves, it is important for the GP or district nurse to ask their elderly patients about urinary incontinence and bladder problems in general. Sometimes, the smell of urine might be noticed during physical examination or a home visit. The greater the severity of the incontinence, the greater the likelihood that the patient will seek help from the GP.[5]

Possible causes

During ageing, various changes occur in the lower urinary tract.[2] Bladder capacity, the ability to postpone micturition, and bladder contractility all decrease. Uninhibited detrusor contractions increase and there is a slight rise in the residual volume. In women, the maximum urethral closure pressure and the length of the urethra decrease; in the majority of elderly men, the prostate becomes enlarged and the urine outflow decreases. Another important change occurs in the pattern of fluid excretion: young people excrete the greatest volume of their daily fluid intake during the day, whereas many elderly people excrete the greatest volume of their daily fluid intake during the night. None of these age-dependant changes cause incontinence, but each of them predisposes to incontinence.

In most cases, involuntary urine loss is related to disturbances in the continence mechanism of the bladder itself. This applies to urge incontinence, stress incontinence, mixed incontinence, and overflow incontinence.[8] In contrast, functional incontinence is characterized by insufficient control over micturition as a result of disturbances and disorders outside the bladder.

Urge incontinence

Urge incontinence is the involuntary loss of urine concomitant with a sudden intense urge to urinate (severe urgency). Other common symptoms are frequency and nocturia. Urge incontinence is usually accompanied by urodynamic findings of *detrusor hyperactivity*. If a neurological disorder is involved (upper motor neurone lesion, CVA, Alzheimer's disease, Parkinson's disease), there will be *detrusor hyper-reflexia*. If there are no associated neurological disorders, then we speak in terms of *detrusor instability*. The latter can be caused by local irritation of the bladder, for example, by a stone, infection, or tumour.

Another urodynamic finding in elderly patients that can accompany the symptom of urge incontinence is detrusor hyperactivity with decreased bladder contractility (DHIC: detrusor hyperactivity with impaired bladder contractility). Patients with DHIC have involuntary detrusor contractions, but they have to bear down in order to empty their bladder completely or partially. Clinically, these patients have symptoms of urge incontinence, with an increased residual volume. However, they can also present with symptoms of obstruction, stress incontinence, or overflow incontinence.

Stress incontinence

Stress incontinence is the involuntary loss of urine during coughing, sneezing, laughing, or other physical activities that cause an increase in intra-abdominal pressure. This symptom can be made urodynamically objective by the observation of urine loss simultaneously with an increase in intra-abdominal pressure, in the absence of detrusor contractions or an overfull bladder. The most common cause of stress incontinence is *hypermobility of the urethra and bladder neck*. This is the result of a weak pelvic floor, probably caused by childbirth and decreased post-menopausal oestrogen levels.

Mixed incontinence

Many elderly people have a combination of stress and urge incontinence, referred to as mixed incontinence. Mixed incontinence has the same causes as those mentioned under the separate headings of stress and urge incontinence.

Overflow incontinence

Overflow incontinence is involuntary urine loss accompanied by overfilling of the bladder. These patients generally suffer from very frequent to continuous loss of small volumes of urine (continuous leakage). Other symptoms can include 'bearing-down' while urinating, incomplete voiding and weak stream.

Overflow incontinence can be caused by two factors: (i) a hyperactive or non-active detrusor; or (ii) bladder neck or urethral obstruction. A hyperactive or non-active detrusor can be caused by for example, medication, faecal impaction, neurological disorders such as diabetic neuropathy and spinal lesions, or surgical intervention in the lower pelvis. In men, obstruction is mostly caused by prostate hypertrophy, but less commonly by prostate cancer, urethral stricture, or faecal impaction. In women, obstruction is rare, but it can occur after incontinence surgery or in the case of a giant cystocoele or uterus prolapse.

Functional incontinence

When involuntary urine loss is caused by factors outside the lower urinary tract, such as limitations in physical or cognitive functioning, this is referred to as functional incontinence. Hip arthrosis, muscle weakness, hand problems, and tremors can hinder the elderly person's self-care: climbing out of bed unaided, going to the toilet, undoing clothes, and sitting down to urinate. This also applies to communication and cognitive disturbances. An elderly person must be able to adequately feel the urge to urinate or if necessary, make it clearly apparent to others.

Making a diagnosis

History

The clinical history serves to establish the nature and cause of the incontinence and gives an indication of the severity and consequences. Obtaining a good outline of the incontinence pattern is essential for constructing the most suitable treatment plan. In a prospective study by Resnick, the urodynamic cause of urinary incontinence could be predicted on the basis of thorough history and physical examination in 90 per cent of the cases.[9]

The characteristic clinical symptom of stress incontinence is the loss of small volumes of urine during activities that increase the intra-abdominal pressure, such as sneezing, coughing, jumping, laughing, lifting, and sport. The patient does not feel the urge to urinate before leakage occurs. As soon as the increased pressure ceases, the urine loss also ceases. The remaining micturition pattern is normal.

In urge incontinence, the patients feel such an urgent need to urinate that they can no longer reach the toilet in time. Once micturition has started, it is very difficult to stop the flow. Urge incontinence is often accompanied by

Table 1 Reversible and other contributing factors in incontinence[8]

Possible reversible factors:

Conditions: delirium, faecal impaction, depression, symptomatic UTI, oedema

Environment: impaired locomotion, lack of access to toilet, restraints, restrictive clothing

Excessive intake of caffeinated beverages or other bladder irritants

Diagnoses: diabetes, CHF, CVA, Parkinson's disease, and other neurological diseases affecting motor skills

Medication: diuretics, antiparkinsonian medication, disopyramide, antispasmodics, antihistamines, and other anticholinergics

Drugs that stimulate or block sympathetic nervous system: calcium-channel blockers, narcotics

Psychoactive medication: antipsychotics, antianxiety agents, antidepressants, hypnotics

Other contributing factors:

Conditions: pain, excessive or inadequate urine output, atrophic vaginitis, cancer of the bladder or prostate, urethral obstruction, disorders of the brain or spinal cord

Abnormal laboratory values: elevated blood glucose or calcium

other complaints, such as frequency and nocturia. Pain does not form part of incontinence, but when present, forms more of an indication of infection. The nature of the symptoms must be established carefully, because each particular symptom can have various causes. In the case of frequency, a patient might be going to the toilet so often to prevent involuntary urine loss, but this symptom does not say anything about the cause of the incontinence. Frequency due to a sharp urge to urinate indicates detrusor hyperactivity.

In the case of nocturia, it is important to know how long a person sleeps. Someone can wake up and go to the toilet out of habit. Moreover, elderly people can urinate several times a night without having any pathology. The latter is associated with greater fluid excretion at night. Besides detrusor hyperactivity, nocturia can also have metabolic and cardiac causes. These can usually be distinguished with the aid of the history and a micturition diary.

The clinical history in elderly people with incontinence not only targets micturition patterns, but also their independent functioning, determined by cognition, mobility, and communication. For the purpose of judging the consequences of incontinence for the patients and their environment, collateral history can be indispensable. In addition, a thorough search should be made for disorders that can cause (transient) incontinence and for side-effects from any medication being taken by the patient (Table 1).[8]

It is also important for the GP to ask each individual patient about the meaning of incontinence and its psycho-social consequences.

Examination

Physical examination aims to detect any relevant disorders within and outside the urinary tract.

- Abdomen: attention should be paid to scars from surgical interventions, abnormal resistance, suprapubic pressure pain, and a palpable bladder.

- In women, vaginal palpation and speculum examination should be performed. Attention should be paid to signs of atrophic vaginitis. The patient is asked to contract her pelvic floor muscles ('as if you were trying to hold back your urine'). Further, the GP should be on the look out for uterine prolapse or cystocoele/rectocoele, the presence of tumours, abnormal swellings, fistulae, vaginal discharge, and signs of infection.

- Rectal palpation: attention should be paid to the tone of the sphincter. The voluntary control of the sphincter should be established by asking the patient to contract the sphincter ('as if you were trying to hold back your faeces'). Some elderly people will not be able to do this although there is no pathology. If the patient is able to contract the sphincter, then this is strong evidence against disrupted innervation of the bladder neck and bladder. N.B: the same sacral roots innervate the external urethra and the anal sphincter. Attention should be paid to faecal impaction in the rectum.

In men, the surface and consistency of the prostate should be examined. The size of the prostate is of less importance, because of the poor correlation with the extent of outflow obstruction. Attention should be paid to the presence of abnormal resistance in the rectum.

Additional tests

Patients with incontinence should be tested for urinary tract infection by means of urine sedimentation and if necessary, culture. Keeping a micturition diary is one of the most valuable tools in diagnosing urinary incontinence. In this way, the symptoms are made objective, the information can give indications about the cause of the incontinence and about the capacity of the bladder (normal value: 300–600 ml). Moreover, the diary can provide starting points for designing individual treatment.

In a micturition diary, records are kept of the time of urination, the time and volume (drops, small volume, total void) of involuntary urine loss, and any accompanying symptoms or circumstances.

It is recommended to exclude urine retention. In care facilities, ultrasound scanning of the bladder is a better alternative to exclude urine retention than once-off catheterization.[8,9] Laboratory tests are seldom indicated. If obstruction or retention is suspected, kidney function tests should be performed and in the case of polyuria and/or nocturia, glucose and electrolytes should be monitored. However, the value of the latter has not been established in randomized trials. Urodynamic examination is only worthwhile if the results might influence treatment, such as in patients being considered for surgical procedures; the examination is stressful for the patient, relatively expensive, and difficult to interpret in the elderly.[10] Furthermore, the extent to which additional examinations are performed depends on the amount of trouble the incontinence causes to the patient and care providers, the motivation and cooperation of the patient, the prognosis, and life-expectancy of the patient.[10]

Management

In the majority of cases, a distinction can be made between reversible forms of incontinence and chronic incontinence with the aid of clinical history, incontinence-oriented physical examination, a micturition diary and possible residual volume determination. Treatment is designed according to these findings.

In elderly people, quality of life improves after treatment for incontinence.[11,12] Firstly, the provoking factors are addressed.[13] Medication is reviewed and constipation, a urinary tract infection or atrophic vaginitis are treated. In the case of limited mobility, physiotherapy can be considered or a walking aid, or the layout of the bathroom can be modified or a commode provided. Clothing should be simple and quick to undo and do up again. It is of great importance that the toilet is easily accessible (no obstacles en route), practical, (high and spacious), and easy to use (simple clothing). Mood disorders or delirium are dealt with adequately. If the incontinence persists after the provoking factors have been treated and the condition is chronic, then treatment should focus on the bladder disturbance. The motivation of the elderly patient, co-morbidity, and life-expectancy to a large extent determine further management. It is better to consider functional limitations as contributing factors to the incontinence than as the sole cause, because several small improvements in the separate risk areas can lead to major general improvement.

Urge incontinence

Controlled trials have shown that non-medicinal treatments, such as a micturition time-table and bladder training, are also effective in the elderly and take preference as primary care treatment. The reason for the bladder training and its aim are explained to the patient and the patient is given an assignment to carry out over a period of 6 weeks: during the day, urination must be postponed for 15 min. It is very important to motivate the patient to persevere, because in the early stages, bladder training is difficult and effects cannot be expected until after 6 weeks.

If non-medicinal treatment does not have sufficient effect, trial medication can be tried with urospasmolytics. However, anticholinergic side-effects can lead to problems in the elderly, not only a dry mouth, constipation, and

urine retention, but also confusion and falls if the patient already has a cognitive disorder. Progress is reviewed after 2 weeks. Flavoxate did not prove to be effective in placebo controlled trials, but oxybutinin was effective.[8] In many cases, the advantages do not outweigh the disadvantages.

Stress incontinence

Stress incontinence is very rare in men and in fact only occurs after the sphincter has been damaged during surgery. Therefore, stress incontinence chiefly affects women. Elderly women generally suffer from mixed incontinence.

The basic principle behind treatment for stress incontinence is returning the bladder–urethra region to abdominal control. During vaginal palpation, the patient is asked to contract her pelvic floor as if she is trying to hold back her urine. She is instructed how to contract her pelvic floor muscles in the correct manner, without contracting her abdominal muscles, gluteal muscles, or adductors. Contracting the pelvic floor muscles must be repeated at least five times in succession, up to a total of 50 times per day. The greater the compliance of the patient to the exercise schedule, the better the results. If the patient is unable to contract the correct muscles, a physiotherapist can be asked to provide assistance.

Medicinal treatment for stress incontinence is not worthwhile. Furthermore, at present, there is too little evidence that oestrogen therapy is effective in post-menopausal women.[14]

In the case of uterus prolapse or a troublesome cystocoele, a pessary or reversed Hodge technique may be effective. The disadvantage of a pessary in an atrophic vagina is an increase in vaginal discharge, sometimes with decubitus ulceration in the posterior fornix. The application of a vaginal cream containing oestrogen is then indicated.

As a final resort, patients can undergo surgery. A great many operations have been described for the treatment of stress incontinence in women. The most common procedure is colpo-suspension (Burch), with a long-term success rate (more than 5 years) of between 55 and 90 per cent.[14] In elderly patients, surgery is usually a major intervention. Fairly recently, a new less invasive treatment has become available: tension-free vaginal tape. Results in the short-term are very encouraging, but not yet sufficiently clear in the longer term.

Mixed incontinence

As the urge component of mixed incontinence is usually the most troublesome feature, treatment generally starts with bladder training, after which, depending on the amount of progress, pelvic floor muscle exercises can be added.

Absorbent products

Absorbent products can considerably decrease the handicap and ensuing problems, such as soiled clothes, bedding and furniture. The pharmacy, practice assistant or district nurse can give advice about the best choice of absorbent pads. In men, condom catheters can form a solution in some situations, for example, at night.

The use of indwelling catheters should be avoided as much as possible, unless after being informed of the risks, the patient chooses this approach. Indwelling catheters not only increase the risk of urinary tract infection, but also the risk of injury and stricture of the urinary tract.

Long-term prevention

Nothing is known about primary prevention of urinary incontinence in the elderly, who generally have a complex form of incontinence. However, information is available about secondary prevention, especially about improving co-morbid conditions and identifying specific risk factors that contribute to the incontinence (Table 1). Limiting these non-urological disorders, for example, by increasing mobility, can decrease the severity of the incontinence or even put an end to it.[3]

In practice, however, goal-oriented prevention of incontinence is not very common. Moreover, incontinence in the elderly far too often leads to providing absorbent products, instead of making an adequate diagnosis and prescribing treatment.

Conclusions

In conclusion, a great deal is still unknown, both about preventive measures and the most effective treatments. Research into the degree to which separate factors contribute to incontinence in the elderly, with a study on the effectiveness of one intervention per factor, is urgently required. Data are also missing on the effectiveness of instruction for pelvic floor muscle exercises and bladder training by the general practitioner. In addition, and most importantly, we know very little about what elderly patients themselves wish to do or have done about the incontinence.

Key points

1. Urinary incontinence is a common problem in the elderly.

2. The clinical history provides a good guide to the likely cause of incontinence.

3. It is important to search for reversible factors contributing to incontinence.

4. Non-medical approaches to management are often successful, and should precede drug therapy.

References

1. Brocklehurst, J.C. (1990). Urinary incontinence in old age: helping the general practitioner to make a diagnosis. *Gerontology* **36** (Suppl. 2), 3–7.

2. Resnick, N.M. (1992). Urinary incontinence in older adults. *Hospital Practice* **15**, 490–504.

3. Valk, M. Urinary incontinence in psychogeriatric nursing home patients. Prevalence and determinants. Thesis, University of Utrecht, Utrecht, 1999.

4. Rekers, H., Drogendijk, A.C., Valkenburg, H., and Riphagen, F. (1992). Urinary incontinence in women from 35 to 79 years of age: prevalence and consequences. *European Journal of Gynaecology and Reproductive Biology* **43**, 229–34.

5. Branch, L.G. et al. (1994). Urinary incontinence knowledge among community-dwelling people 65 years of age and older. *Journal of the American Geriatrics Society* **42**, 1257–63.

6. Lagro-Janssen, A.L.M., Smits, A.J.A., and Weel, C. (1990). Women with urinary incontinence: self-perceived worries and general practitioners' knowledge of the problem. *British Journal of General Practice* **40**, 331–4.

7. Van de Lisdonk, E.H., van den Bosch, W.J.H.M., Huygen, F.J.A., and Lagro-Janssen, A.L.M. *Ziekten in de huisartspraktijk (Illness in general practice)*. Maarssen: Elzevier/Bunge, 1999.

8. Fantl, J.A. et al. *Urinary Incontinence in Adults: Acute and Chronic Management*. Clinical Practice Guideline No. 2. Rockville MD: US Department of Health and Human Services. Public Health Service, Agency for Health Care Policy and Research; (AHCPR Publication No. 96-0682), 1996.

9. Resnick, N.M. (1990). Noninvasive diagnosis of the patient with complex incontinence. *Gerontology* **36** (Suppl. 2), 8–18.

10. Abram, P. (2000). Assessment and treatment of urinary incontinence. *Lancet* **355**, 2153–8.

11. Fonda, D. et al. (1995). Sustained improvement of subjective quality of life in older community-dwelling people after treatment of urinary incontinence. *Age and Ageing* **24**, 283–6.

12. Wyman, J.J. et al. (1997). Quality of life following bladder training in older women with urinary incontinence. *International Urogynaecology Journal of Pelvic Floor Dysfunction* **8**, 223–9.

13. Lagro-Janssen, A.L.M. et al. (1995). NHG-standaard Incontinentie voor urine. *Huisarts en Wetenschap* **38** (2), 71–80.

14. Cooper, J. (2002). Stress incontinence in clinical evidence. In *The International Source of the Best Available Evidence for Effective Health Care* (ed. S. Barton), pp. 1772–83. London: BMJ Publishing Group.

16.7 Functional assessment of the elderly

Kathleen A. Bell-Irving

Definition, epidemiology, gender, and cultural differences

In primary care medicine, functional assessment in old age refers to the assessment of the individual's personal capacity and actual performance in the activities necessary to sustain life, maintain health, and minimize the impact of ageing and disease. The goal is to maintain involvement in the various activities that are deemed to make the individual's life worthwhile. Functional assessment is a core element of comprehensive geriatric assessment.[1,2]

Health-related 'functioning' includes a number of domains of function: physical, cognitive, mental, social, economic, and spiritual.[2] The purpose of functional assessment is to assess and monitor the integrated output of these domains as represented within the context of the patient's living environment.

Each individual has several roles: personal, family, cultural, and community.[3,4] Each role activity is achieved through contributions from functional domains. With ageing, each area of functional domain is susceptible to malfunction due to the onset of disease, disuse, or injury. 'Malfunction' leads to the development of disability and dependency. Disability is the second strongest predictor of adverse health outcome, after age.[5]

Activities of daily living (ADLs)

Core activities have been identified that represent the skills and abilities required for basic human survival and the successful achievement of personal life roles. These core activities have been called 'Activities of Daily Living' or 'ADLs'. The concept was initially developed in the 1960s in the acute care setting, motivated by a need to evaluate treatment and rehabilitation protocols in very ill and disabled elderly patients.[6]

ADLs break down into the basic, physical, self-maintaining ADLs, called 'BADLs', and the more physically, cognitively, and organizationally complex, 'Instrumental' ADLs, or 'IADLs'. BADLs include: toileting, feeding, dressing, grooming and hygiene, physical ambulation, and bathing. IADLs traditionally include such activities as: the ability to use the telephone, shopping, food preparation, housekeeping and home-maintenance, laundry, mode of transportation, responsibility for own medications, and the ability to handle finances.[7,8] Leisure and occupation-related activities in old age are an extension of the identified core IADLs, and should be included in the overall assessment of daily functioning.[9,10]

Each ADL/IADL activity can be viewed as a battery of interactive physical and cognitive tasks.[6,11] Basic ADLs were first incorporated into an assessment tool by Katz et al.[8] IADLs were subsequently formulated within an ADL assessment tool proposed by Lawton and Brody.[7] Many functional assessment tools have since been developed.[11,12] All have, as a basis, the tasks included in these two original tools.

Historical

ADL assessment tools were intended to represent reliable and valid tools to measure rehabilitation potential and response to rehabilitation protocols as part of acute care and academic medicine. They were quickly adopted by hospital, and community-based, home care assessors to predict need, and establish eligibility, for subsidized home-supports and institutionalization.

ADL assessment is now being incorporated into mandated clinical assessment protocols in community care settings, with ongoing funding hinging on completion of these tools. The 'Minimal Data Set' is the first such initiative.[13,14] Originating in the United States, and now translated into 11 languages, it is being utilized in various clinical assessment settings around the world.[15] The primary care physician (PCP) contributes to these mandated clinical assessments.

ADLs: hierarchical or multidimensional?[16]

BADLs and IADLs were originally felt to represent a hierarchy of neuropsychological and primary physical development. IADL items were felt to be at a higher developmental level than BADLs. Items were believed to have equal weighing within each level, following the properties of a Guttman scale. Recent studies question this initial belief.[5,17–19]

Each BADL/IADL activity item has physical and cognitive requirements for successful completion. Inequity among items is clear when consideration is given to comparative grading of difficulty in the independent performances of the various items.[16,17] Inequity makes sense, clinically, recognizing that individuals may become disabled through different mechanisms.[16]

IADLs have been found to be the most strongly correlated with cognitive functioning.[16,17] Four of these, use of the telephone, transportation, medication management, and financial management, appear to be of higher neuropsychological complexity than the other IADLs. Transportation is recognized to involve both memory and orientation skills.[17] The handling of finances is the most heavily cognitively mediated of the IADLs.[17] This finding has clinical implications for detecting dementia at a 'pre-clinical' stage when deficits are first noticed in these more complex activities.[17]

The physical requirements within BADL and IADL tasks are also not equal. Stair climbing, included in the Barthel ADL Index, has been found to be the most physically demanding of the BADLs,[20] while bathing and walking are the next most physically demanding.[16]

Cultural differences

Life circumstance, personal and cultural values and practices, personal experience, education, knowledge, skills, and attitudes, will all affect BADL/IADL task components; influencing what is considered standard for any individual.

The original BADL/IADL tools were developed with a 'Western' culture in mind. Studies across cultures indicate that ADLs are not valued equally. Differences arise related to variability in the nature of the basic tasks. For example, studies based in the United Kingdom, Japan, and Canada ranked bathing as the most difficult activity; while in the United States bathing ranked fifth among the BADLs.[21] This likely reflects differences in the physical requirements of getting into a bath as compared with a shower.

The United Kingdom ranked feeding as the most difficult, while in the United States and Japan it was regarded as the easiest activity; indicative of comparative differences in the manner of eating: cutting with knife and fork together, as compared with picking up pre-cut pieces with a fork, chop-sticks or fingers.[16,21] Differences in diet require variable manual skills to ingest food. A diet of mostly rice, lentils, and breads will not require the use of knife and fork.[21]

'Bathing', describing the Western-style of washing in a bath or shower, is not universal. A Turkish study changed the term to 'wash-all-over' to make it relevant to their study population.[22] This change proved equally valid. 'Toileting' on an 'Eastern-style' toilet requires squatting. This is clearly more physically demanding than using a raised 'Western-style' toilet.[23]

Gender differences

Males have greater muscle mass and overall fitness than females, which will lead to differences in the relative rate of onset of disability in physically dependent tasks.[24–26]

Females of the current cohort of elderly have tended to be responsible for household activities and so may score better than males in these tasks.[27] In some cultures, the females will be responsible, throughout adulthood, for performing many of the IADL items for their spouse.[28]

These cultural and gender-based differences impact the interpretation of what constitutes baseline performance. Ultimately, BADL/IADL tasks need to be completed by self, or other, to sustain life, preserve safety, and maintain an acceptable quality of life (QOL).

Natural history of ADLs with ageing

While ageing, individuals progressively develop 'functional limitation' in ADL performance; that is, adapted performance that preserves independence.[20,29,30] There is a continuum from functional limitation to 'disability', whereby successful or safe performance requires assistance.[1,26] There is, however, nothing pre-destined in the onset, course, or nature of functional limitation with ageing.[31,32] Functional limitation represents abnormality and puts the individual at increased risk of disability.

The role for ADL assessment in primary care medicine

1. Represents the integrated performance of all body systems.

2. Baseline performance, prior to old age, suggests the norm for each individual, and will help to guide end-of-life care-planning and decision-making.

3. Case-finding: identifying a change from baseline allows for early detection of disease, injury, and/or age-related consequences of disuse.[1,31] Provides opportunity to identify changes in health at a 'pre-clinical' state.[17]

4. Focus of tertiary prevention: minimize premature morbidity and mortality, and minimize discomfort, disability, and dependency.[31,33]

5. Provides a context, meaningful to the patient, in which to:

    (i) explain the pathology/physiology of the consequences of ageing and disease;

    (ii) help the patient understand the value and role of proposed investigations or referrals.

6. Provides a patient-centred context in which to explain potential interventions:

    (i) recommendations for treatment of identified disease; whether curative, preventive, or palliative;

    (ii) recommendations for physical or cognitive rehabilitation;

    (iii) recommendations for strategies to augment home supports.

7. Basis for assessment of personal and financial capacity,[34] and overall safety, 'everyday' capacity.[29,35]

8. Basis for assessment of caregiver strain, and risk for neglect or abuse.[36]

Making a diagnosis of functional impairment or disability in ADLs

History-taking

Guide to the elements to be considered and monitored

1. Define baseline behaviour and performance: normal performance throughout adulthood. Identify positive/negative health habits/attitudes.

    Changes from baseline need explanation. The 'negative' are opportunities for education; the 'positive' might assist care planning strategies.

2. Clarify social and cultural factors influencing baseline performance, choices made, and expressed desired outcome.

    PCPs cannot assume they share the patient's/carer's same values regarding desired outcome performance in each area of BADL/IADL.[37]

3. Identify areas of functional limitation or frank disability.

    Clarify level at which task process becomes impaired.

4. Confirm or clarify contributing aetiology:

    (i) Does known disease profile account for limitation/disability detected?

(ii) Identify areas for further assessment and/or treatment adjustment.

(iii) Is referral to specialty physician, allied health care professional (AHCP), or tertiary care geriatric assessment team, required to complete assessment?

5. Clarify patient's/carer's insight regarding deterioration in function, and long-term functional goals.

6. Identify areas where additional support may make living situation more tenable.

7. Is family conflict or caregiver strain negatively influencing functional status? Is their any indication of neglect or abuse of patient by carer, or vice versa.

The role of the functional assessment screening tool in history-taking

The diagnosis of functional limitation and disability is made by interview and/or direct assessment of performance in BADL/IADLs, and in leisure/occupational activities. The overall functional picture is developed progressively with each doctor–patient/carer encounter contributing.

A BADL/IADL functional assessment screening tool will provide the basis of assessment. Use of a standardized tool will increase the reliability and validity of the initial, and repeat, assessments.[2,7,11,12] The comparative patient-specific data collected can be reassessed by the PCP annually, and is useful to detect decline, and when providing an opinion regarding financial/personal capacity, rate of decline, prognosis, and treatment options.

The tool can be adapted for use in direct patient interview, or provided to the patient/carer to complete prior to the interview. A self-reporting tool should include space for the patient/carer to indicate baseline performance, including any variability from the options provided in the tool.

Gathering collateral perspectives from primary carers, friends, community support personnel, and/or AHCPs is critical to obtain a reliable and valid picture of baseline functioning and any change therein, especially when cognitive impairment is suspected. Collateral information should be gathered employing ethical process that allows for collection of detail, yet maintaining patient privacy. The proxy providing collateral, must actually see the patient's performance at a given task, and must have the cognitive capacity to interpret performance, and report accurately, to the interviewer.[11]

History-taking strategies; role in diagnosis

Understanding the potential task breakdown for each BADL and IADL item will facilitate history taking. 'Task breakdown' refers to the various physical and organizational steps that make up each activity.[7,12] This approach is critical, as without prompting, the patient/carer may not recognize they are not performing a task as well as previously. For example, if asked only if they make their meals, the patient/carer may report to the affirmative; even though more in-depth consideration would reveal that the meals made were often burned, or were unreliable in content. Additional questioning may reveal that the patient becomes so short of breath that while they can make healthy meals, they have no energy left to eat them. Detailing elements of task performance will help to detect dysfunction, narrow down the differential diagnosis, and direct treatment planning and priority.

The PCP should select, and adapt, a tool for office use that contains task elements for each BADL/IADL item.[7,10,12,25]

Principles of management

Teamwork, including patient, physicians, carers, and AHCPs, is key to the process of functional assessment, and to its application to treatment planning and the establishment of 'functional goals'.[38] These should be individualized and reflect the patient's values and life goals. It is important to include representative family and community carers in the planning process.

Functional assessment in long-term and continuing care

ADL assessment is an integral part of tools used to establish home support needs and eligibility for institutionalization.[39]

The PCP has a key role to assure that appropriate medical interpretation accompanies the clinical assessments of eligibility.[13,40] All tools are not equal, and interpretation can differ significantly depending upon the clinical experience and area of interest of the AHCP selecting or administering the tool.[40,41]

Valid and reliable serial functional assessments promote early intervention and proactive care-planning, in addition, can indicate an individual's rate of decline and prognosis.

Future implications

Current research into the role of functional assessment in old age medicine has rested in the domains of geriatricians and geriatric psychiatrists. It has yet to be determined what functional and economic gain, and tertiary prevention, can be achieved if functional assessment is a regular part of primary care medicine. This is a new area for primary care medical research.

Key points

Functional assessment in the elderly:

1. Assessment of 'activities of daily living' plus leisure and remaining occupational activities.

2. Purpose: detect functional limitation and disability. Baseline functioning establishes individual's norm. Directs tertiary prevention.

3. Role: provides framework to detect disease, injury, or de-conditioning. Identify rehabilitation potential: physical, cognitive, and environmental. Quantifies need: home support/institutionalization.

4. Framework for capacity assessment, end-of-life care-planning and decision-making.

5. Detect caregiver strain; risk for neglect/abuse.

References

1. Palmer, R. (1999). Geriatric assessment. *Medical Clinics of North America* **83** (6), 1503–23.

2. Fillenbaum, G.G. *The Wellbeing of the Elderly. Approaches to Multidimensional Assessment.* Geneva: A Publication of the World Health Organization, 1984, pp. 1–99.

3. Mechanic, D. (1995). Sociological dimensions of illness behaviour. *Social Science and Medicine* **41** (9), 1207–16.

4. Ostbye, T. et al. (1997). Reported activities of daily living: agreement between elderly subjects with and without dementia and their caregivers. *Age and Ageing* **26**, 99–106.

5. Guralnik, J.M., Fried, L.P., and Salive, M.E. (1996). Disability as a public health outcome in the aging population. *Annual Review of Public Health* **17**, 25–46.

6. Lazaridis, E.N. et al. (1994). Do activities of daily living have a hierarchical structure? An analysis using the longitudinal study of aging. *Journal of Gerontology: Medical Sciences* **49** (2), M47–51.

7. Lawton, M.P. and Brody, E.M. (1969). Assessment of older people: self-maintaining and instrumental activities of daily living. *The Gerontologist* **9**, 179–86.

8. Katz, S. et al. (1963). Studies of illness in the aged: the index of ADL. A standardized measure of biological and psychosocial function. *Journal of the American Medical Association* **185** (12), 94–9.

9. Berg, K. and Norman, K.E. (1996). Functional assessment of balance and gait. *Clinics in Geriatric Medicine* **12** (4), 705–23.

10. Bucks, R.S. et al. (1996). Assessment of activities of daily living in dementia: development of the Bristol Activities of Daily Living Scale. *Age and Ageing* **25**, 113–20.

11. Guralnik, J.M. et al. (1989). Physical performance measures in aging research. *Journal of Gerontology: Medical Sciences* **44** (5), M141–6.

12. Burns, A., Lawlor, B., and Craig, S. *Assessment Scales in Old Age Psychiatry.* London: Martin Dunitz Ltd., 1999.

13. Kane, R.L. and Kane, R.A. (2000). Assessment in long-term care. *Annual Review of Public Health* **21**, 659–86.

14. Landi, F. et al. (2000). Minimum data set for home care. A valid instrument to assess frail older people living in the community. *Medical Care* **38** (12), 1184–90.

15. Fries, B. et al. (1997). Approaching cross-national comparisons of nursing home residents. *Age and Ageing* **26-S2**, 13–18.

16. Salazar Thomas, V., Rockwood, K., and McDowell, I. (1998). Multi-dimensionality in instrumental and basic activities of daily living. *Journal of Clinical Epidemiology* **51** (4), 315–21.

17. Barberger-Gateau, P. et al. (1999). Neuropsychological correlates of self-reported performance in instrumental activities of daily living and prediction of dementia. *Journal of Gerontology: Psychological Sciences* **54B** (5), 293–303.

18. Spector, W.D. et al. (1987). The hierarchical relationship between activities of daily living and instrumental activities of daily living. *Journal of Chronic Diseases* **40** (6), 481–9.

19. Kempen, G.I.J.M., Myers, A.M., and Powell, L.E. (1995). Hierarchical structure in ADL and IADL: analytical assumptions and applications for clinicians and researchers. *Journal of Clinical Epidemiology* **48** (11), 1299–305.

20. Startzell, J.K. et al. (2000). Stair negotiation in older people: a review. *Journal of the American Geriatrics Society* **48**, 567–80.

21. Chino, N. (1990). Efficacy of Barthel Index in evaluating activities of daily living in Japan, the United States, and United Kingdom. *Stroke* **21** (Suppl. II), II64–5.

22. Kucukdeveci, A.A. et al. (2000). Adaptation of the Modified Barthel Index for use in physical medicine and rehabilitation in Turkey. *Scandinavian Journal of Rehabilitation Medicine* **32**, 87–92.

23. Yukawa, M. (2000). Culture specific implications for decline in ADL and IADL. *Journal of the American Geriatrics Society* **48**, 1527–8.

24. Manandhar, M.C. (1995). Functional ability and nutritional status of free-living elderly people. *Proceedings of the Nutrition Society* **54**, 677–91.

25. Pfeffer, R.I. et al. (1982). Measurement of functional activities in older adults in the community. *Journal of Gerontology* **37**, 323–9.

26. Chandler, J.M. and Hadley, E.C. (1996). Exercise to improve physiologic and functional performance in old age. *Clinics in Geriatric Medicine* **12** (4), 761–84.

27. Hachisuka, K. et al. (1999). Gender-related differences in scores of the Barthel Index and Frenchay Activities Index in randomly sampled elderly persons living at home in Japan. *Journal of Clinical Epidemiology* **52** (11), 1089–94.

28. Hsieh, R.L. et al. (1995). Disability among the elderly of Taiwan. *American Journal of Physical Medicine & Rehabilitation* **74** (5), 370–4.

29. Wahl, H.W., Oswald, F., and Zimprich, D. (1999). Everyday competence in visually impaired older adults: a case for person–environment perspectives. *The Gerontologist* **39** (2), 140–9.

30. Clark, D.O., Stump, T.E., and Wolinsky, F.D. (1997). A race- and gender-specific replication of five dimensions of functional limitation and disability. *Journal of Aging and Health* **9** (1), 28–42.

31. Goldberg, T. and Chavin, S.I. (1997). Preventive medicine and screening in older adults. *Journal of the American Geriatrics Society* **45**, 344–54.

32. Stuck, A.E. et al. (1993). Comprehensive geriatric assessment: a meta-analysis of controlled trials. *The Lancet* **342**, 1032–6.

33. Evans, W.J. (1995). Effects of exercise on body composition and functional capacity of the elderly. *The Journals of Gerontology Series A* **50A** (special issue), 147–50.

34. MacKay, M.J. (1989). Financial and personal competence in the elderly. The position of the Canadian Psychiatric Association. *Canadian Journal of Psychiatry* **34**, 829–32.

35. Oliver, R. et al. (1993). Development of the Safety Assessment of Function and the Environment for Rehabilitation (SAFER) tool. *Canadian Journal of Occupational Therapy* **60** (2), 78–82.

36. Markson, E.W. (1997). Functional, social, and psychological disability as causes of loss of weight and independence in older community-living people. *Clinics in Geriatric Medicine* **13** (4), 639–52.

37. Kane, R.L. et al. (1998). Differences in valuation of functional status components among consumers and professionals in Europe and the United States. *Journal of Clinical Epidemiology* **51** (8), 657–66.

38. Stolee, P. et al. (1999). An individualized approach to outcome measurement in geriatric rehabilitation. *Journal of Gerontology: Medical Sciences* **54A** (12), M641–7.

39. Miller, E.A. and Weissert, W.G. (2000). Predicting elderly people's risk for nursing home placement, hospitalization, functional impairment, and mortality: a synthesis. *Medical Care Research and Review* **57** (3), 259–97.

40. Stewart, K. et al. (1999). Assessment approaches for older people receiving social care: content and coverage. *International Journal of Geriatric Psychiatry* **14**, 147–56.

41. Neuhaus, B.E. and Miller, P. (1995). Status of functional assessment in occupational therapy with the elderly. *Journal of Allied Health* **Winter**, 29–40.

Further reading

Burns, A., Lawlor, B., and Craig, S. *Assessment Scales in Old Age Psychiatry.* London: Martin Dunitz Ltd., 1999. (A comprehensive resource summarizing clinical assessment scales/tools covering a broad range of areas in old age psychiatry, including ADL assessment, depression, neuropsychological tests, quality-of-life, mental health, caregiver assessments, delirium, and memory function. Provides the PCP with an appreciation of the scales available, a visual example of each scale, indication for use and level of tested validity and reliability. Original references are provided. This is useful for clinical practice as well as research or programme development.)

Fillenbaum, G.G. *The Wellbeing of the Elderly. Approaches to Multidimensional Assessment.* Geneva: A Publication of the World Health Organization, 1984, pp. 1–99. (The recommendations laid out in this document have yet to be achieved world-wide, and remain the overall guide. As such it is an important read for family physicians involved in primary care and primary care program development. Functional assessment is presented as a key element of comprehensive medical care for the elderly.)

Kane, R.L. and Kane, R.A. (2000). Assessment in long-term care. *Annual Review of Public Health* **21**, 659–86. (Outlines principles enabling the PCP to be prepared to evaluate tool utility, using the minimum data set, and be an advocate for their institutionalized patient.)

Mechanic, D. (1995). Sociological dimensions of illness behaviour. *Social Science and Medicine* **41** (9), 1207–16. (Presented as a departure from the traditional diagnostic disease model, uses the disability process to review considerations relevant to promoting function and maintaining quality of life. Practical implications for primary care medicine in the elderly.)

Startzell, J.K. et al. (2000). Stair negotiation in older people: a review. *Journal of the American Geriatrics Society* **48**, 567–80. (This article, and the ones by Evans,[33] and Chandler and Hadley,[26] utilize principles of exercise physiology, tested in the elderly, to indicate impact on function by disease processes and reduced physical performance measures. Evidence for benefit from training, well into old age, is presented, and related to ADLs.)

16.8 Drugs in the elderly

Munir Pirmohamed

Introduction

In the Western World, the proportion of the population above the age of 65 years is increasing steadily.[1] For example, in the United Kingdom,

6.7 million individuals are currently above 70 years of age, an increase of 2 million since 1985. While the proportion of the population above 70 years of age is currently steady, those above 80 years is still increasing and reached 1.1 million (1.9 per cent of the population) in 2001. In the United States, by 2030, people over the age of 65 years will constitute 21 per cent of the population, compared with 11 per cent currently.[2]

The elderly are the major users of the health service, and consumption of drugs is a major component of this. Figures in the United Kingdom for 2000 show that 54 per cent of all prescriptions dispensed by community pharmacists were for the elderly (men aged 65 years and above, and women aged 60 years and above). The number of prescription items dispensed by community pharmacists per head of population for the elderly has increased from 17.3 in 1990 to 26.5 in 2000; this is four to six times higher than in the other age groups.[3] These figures relate largely to prescribing in primary care; it is therefore incumbent on the general practitioner (GP) to be aware of the problems associated with the use of drugs in the elderly. The elderly are more susceptible to adverse effects, to drug–drug interactions as a result of polypharmacy, and overall are subject to more overuse and inappropriate use of drugs than any other age group in the population.

The purpose of the chapter is to highlight some of these issues, and to provide possible solutions that can be used to improve drug prescribing in the elderly.

Age-related changes in pharmacokinetics and pharmacodynamics

A drug given to an elderly patient often produces a response that is different and unexpected when compared with the response observed in a younger patient of the same body weight given the same drug at the same dose. This can often be explained by age-related changes in pharmacokinetic (what the body does to the drug) and pharmacodynamic (how the drug interacts with targets in the body) parameters.[4] For each drug, either pharmacokinetic and/or pharmacodynamic parameters may be responsible for producing an altered drug response in the elderly.

Pharmacokinetic changes

There is a reduction in the clearance of many drugs in the elderly. This may have two possible consequences:

- no effect, particularly if the drug has a wide therapeutic index;
- prolonged duration of action, which may be manifested as an adverse effect.

Pharmacokinetic changes in the elderly can affect the processes of absorption, distribution, metabolism, and excretion (Fig. 1). In general, changes in absorption and distribution have little effect on drug disposition, and hence on drug action in the elderly.

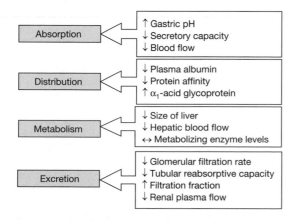

Fig. 1 Age-related changes in pharmacokinetic parameters.

In relation to metabolism, the changes observed are dependent on both the individual and drug being considered. Although the changes are minor in most cases, the overall effect at a population level is greater interindividual variability in metabolic pathways in the elderly population when compared with younger patients. Any changes that are observed usually affect the phase I pathways that are catalyzed by the cytochrome P450 enzymes, rather than the phase II conjugative pathways. In this respect, concomitant disease may be an important determinant of enzyme activity.[5] Frailty, which can be defined as the dependence on others for activities of daily living in persons over 65 years old, is known to be associated with reduced metabolism of drugs such as aspirin, theophylline, paracetamol, and metoclorpramide. The reason for this is unclear, but seems to be related to down-regulation of enzyme expression by cytokines.

Old age is associated with a reduction in glomerular filtration rate, a decrease in renal plasma flow and decreased tubular reabsorptive capacity. The net effect of this is a decrease in renal clearance of drugs that are hydrophilic in nature, for example digoxin. Such drugs should either be avoided or given at lower dosages. It is important to note that a normal serum creatinine does not exclude renal impairment in the elderly. The Cockcroft–Gault formula[6] (shown below) can be used to estimate the creatinine clearance:

Calculated creatinine clearance
$$= \frac{(140 - \text{patient's age}) \times \text{patient's weight (in kg)}}{72 \times \text{patient's serum creatinine concentration (in mmol/l)}}$$

Pharmacodynamic changes

Much less is known about pharmacodynamic changes that occur with age when compared with pharmacokinetic changes.[4] The same drug concentration at a receptor site can have a completely different action in an elderly person when compared with a younger individual. This may be due to a change in the

- affinity of the drug with the target protein;
- number of target proteins;
- signal transduction processes;
- cellular response; and
- homeostatic mechanisms.

The net effect may be either an increase or a decrease in sensitivity to the drug. For example, chronotropic and inotropic responses to β-adrenergic agents decrease with age, which is probably related to changes in signal transduction mechanisms. By contrast, sensitivity to benzodiazepines increases with age; these effects can be seen even after single doses. The molecular mechanisms underlying this increase in sensitivity are unclear; animal studies suggest that it may be due to an increase in benzodiazepine binding sites in the CNS.

Epidemiology of drug use in the elderly

Approximately 50 per cent of the NHS drug bill in the United Kingdom is spent on drugs for the elderly. At least 80 per cent of patients above the age of 75 years are on at least one prescribed medicine, while 36 per cent take four or more medicines.[1] Women are generally prescribed more medicines than men. There has been an increase in prescribing in the elderly over the last two decades; reasons for this are listed in Table 1.

A survey of 805 people was particularly informative regarding the use of drugs in the elderly in the United Kingdom:[7]

- most of the drugs being taken by the elderly are prescribed on a long-term basis, with 59 per cent having been prescribed for more than 2 years;
- eighty-eight per cent of all drugs prescribed were by repeat prescription; and
- forty per cent had not discussed their treatment with their doctor in the last 6 months.

Table 1 Possible reasons for increased prescribing in the elderly

Evidence showing benefits of drug use in the elderly, e.g. the use of warfarin in patients with atrial fibrillation

Increase in the numbers of elderly and very elderly patients, with a consequent increase in morbidity

Increase in screening and detection of asymptomatic conditions, e.g. hypertension

Increased patient expectations

The practice of defensive medicine

Reproduced with permission from the BMJ Publishing Group. Walley, T. and Scott, A.K. (1995). Prescribing in the elderly. *Postgraduate Medicine Journal* **71**, 466–71.

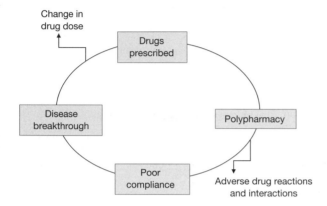

Fig. 2 The inter-relationship between polypharmacy and poor compliance, resulting in a vicious cycle that leads to a prescribing cascade.

Worryingly, 28 per cent of drugs prescribed by GPs were not known to the patients, while 36 per cent of drugs reported by patients were not known to the GP. This largely reflects poor communication between different health care settings. It is known that full medication histories are often not provided to hospitals. Medication is often changed while in hospital; unfortunately this is often poorly communicated to the patient's GP. This leads to continuation of a medicine in primary care that may have been deemed to be ineffective, or occasionally duplication of treatment (e.g. the use of medicine prescribed by both generic and trade names). Such difficulties in communication are likely to get worse as different health care personnel such as pharmacists and nurses are allowed to prescribe drugs. Another reason for the discrepancies between the intake of medicines and GP records may be due to hoarding of medicines by the elderly and use on an 'as required basis'. A factor blamed for hoarding of medicines in the United Kingdom is the repeat prescription system, which may suffer from lack of regular review.

Clearly, the elderly suffer from multiple pathologies, each of which necessarily requires the prescription of drugs of different therapeutic classes. The net effect of both the appropriate and inappropriate use of medicines in the elderly is polypharmacy. This, in turn, predisposes the elderly to adverse drug reactions and drug–drug interactions. Furthermore, the prescription of several drugs will also adversely affect compliance with the medications, which if not identified and corrected, will lead to inadequate control of the disease process, and further addition to the pill burden, thereby leading to a vicious cycle (Fig. 2).

Inappropriate prescribing in the elderly

Inappropriate prescribing in the elderly is a problem not only in the United Kingdom, but also in most other European countries and in the United

Table 2 Reasons for inappropriate prescribing in the elderly

Incremental prescribing, with side-effects being treated with other drugs, rather than discontinuation of the original drug

Therapeutic enthusiasm, with use of drugs as first line treatment without considering the use of non-drug therapies

Failure to adequately assess patients' needs and individualize treatment

Unrealistic expectations on the part of both patient and doctor

Giving in to pressure from relatives, patients and other health care professionals to prescribe

Inadequate review of medicines, leading to continuation of drugs that are no longer necessary

Governmental pressure to meet targets

Reproduced with permission from the BMJ Publishing Group. Walley, T. and Scott, A.K. (1995). Prescribing in the elderly. *Postgraduate Medicine Journal* **71**, 466–71.

Box 1 A theoretical case illustrating the problem of incremental prescribing

A 75-year-old woman was diagnosed as having hypertension. She was started on bendrofluazide by her doctor. Two weeks later, a routine blood test showed her to have a potassium level of 2.9 mmol/l. She was prescribed potassium replacement therapy in form of slow release potassium tablets to be taken together with bendrofluazide. At the next visit 2 weeks later, her potassium level had come up to 3.4 mmol/l, and she was continued on slow potassium. She presented 2 months later with a history of severe heartburn; a gastroscopy showed her to have an oesophageal ulcer. This was blamed on slow potassium, which was stopped. The patient was started on omeprazole. Unfortunately, after a few days treatment she developed diarrhoea. The doctor continued the omeprazole in order to relieve the oesophageal ulcer, and prescribed codeine phosphate for the diarrhoea. After two doses of codeine phosphate, the patient developed dizziness, had a fall, and was admitted to a hospital with a fractured left hip.

States. There are several possible reasons for this (Table 2). An example of inappropriate prescribing includes the use of drugs at doses higher or lower than recommended by the manufacturers. For instance, hypnotic use has been shown to be consistently inappropriate in the elderly, with higher than recommended doses being used in at least one-third of patients. Conversely, in the treatment of depression, tricyclic antidepressants are not only more commonly used in the elderly than the relatively safer selective serotonin re-uptake inhibitors, but the doses used are often lower than required to achieve a mood-elevating effect (this may obviously reflect the apprehension of the prescribers as to the possibility of inducing dose-dependent adverse effects; see below). Other examples of inappropriate prescribing include the use of drugs where there is no evidence for their effectiveness, duplicate prescribing, concomitant prescribing of two or more drugs with potentially dangerous interactions, and failure to use safer alternatives with equivalent or superior efficacy. Incremental prescribing, where drugs are added sequentially to treat the side-effects of a drug that may have been used appropriately, also seems to be a particular problem in the elderly (Box 1). It is important to note that such inappropriate prescribing occurs in all age groups, but given the higher prevalence of illnesses in the elderly and the greater use of drugs, the problem is proportionately much greater in the elderly. Particular care should be taken when prescribing hypnotics, diuretics, non-steroidal anti-inflammatory drugs, antiparkinsonian medicines, antihypertensives, psychotropics, and digoxin in the elderly. Regular review of all medications being taken by the elderly may be all that is needed to reduce the problem of inappropriate prescribing. Clearly, GPs are under increasing time pressure, and such reviews are time-consuming particularly when there is a high proportion of elderly patients in the practice. However, there are ways to overcome this, for example, by employing or working closely with a pharmacist, who by undertaking a regular review of medicines being taken by the elderly, and improving repeat prescribing systems within a practice, have been shown to be cost-effective.

Overuse of drugs in the elderly

Overuse of drugs in the elderly has been shown to be of major concern in nursing homes in the United Kingdom, other European countries and the United States.[2] In the United Kingdom, approximately, 0.7 per cent of the population live in nursing homes. Almost 90 per cent of patients in long-term homes are on long-term medication, receiving a median of three drugs per day. A review of drug usage in these patients will usually show that the patients have been on the drugs long-term, and the original indication for prescribing the drug may no longer be valid. Medication review performed by either GPs or pharmacists have been shown to be highly effective in reducing drug consumption. For example, a single visit by the GP in one study resulted in a drug being stopped in half of the patients, a change in medication to a cheaper alternative in 25 per cent of patients, and a decrease in the median number of prescriptions;[8] this was found to be cost-effective. Similarly, pharmacist review has been shown to result in discontinuation of medicines in 50 per cent of patients. There is always a worry that stopping of medicines may lead to recurrence or inadequate control of the disease for which the drug was originally prescribed. However, in most cases, the evidence points to the contrary, in that reduction in numbers of drugs taken by the elderly has no adverse impact on morbidity and mortality, and reduces the frequency of drug toxicity.[9] In the United States, all care homes are required by law to employ a pharmacist who reviews the medicines prescribed and provides advice on appropriate drug choices and dosages. Such prescribing advice is accepted and welcomed by doctors and staff looking after the care homes. Training of staff in itself may lead to a reduction in drug use in the elderly in nursing homes. This is particularly important, and has been shown to work, in relation to the use of psychotropics. These drugs are perhaps the most commonly used drugs in nursing homes: studies have shown that up to 25 per cent of patients are given these drugs, and in 90 per cent of cases their use can be considered to be inappropriate.[2] Such widespread use of these drugs can lead to many adverse effects ranging from being a factor in falls to a hastening of cognitive decline in patients with dementia.

Underuse of drugs in the elderly

Given the enormous usage of drugs in the elderly, it is perhaps surprising to note that for some conditions, there is evidence of underuse of drugs. Two specific examples that merit further discussion are the treatment of systolic hypertension and the use of anticoagulants in atrial fibrillation, both of which are important in preventing strokes in the elderly.

Treatment of systolic hypertension

Isolated systolic hypertension is predominantly a disease of the elderly with a prevalence of 8 per cent in those aged 70 years and older, and 25 per cent in those aged above 80 years. Treatment of 1000 patients for 5 years with either calcium channel blockers, thiazide diuretics or ACE inhibitors may prevent 29 strokes or 53 major cardiovascular disorders. Furthermore, a meta-analysis of outcome trials has shown that absolute benefit was greater in men, and in patients over the age of 70 years.[10] Treatment of isolated systolic hypertension also decreases the incidence of dementia: 1000 patients treated for 5 years would prevent 19 cases of dementia. Such

benefits of treatment may not be widely appreciated in the elderly, in many of whom hypertension is either inadequately treated or worse still, not treated at all.

Anticoagulation in atrial fibrillation

The prevalence of atrial fibrillation rises from less than 1 per cent in individuals between 50 and 59 years to 9 per cent in those between 80 and 89 years. The use of warfarin reduces the risk of stroke in patients with atrial fibrillation by 68 per cent, compared with a reduction of 21 per cent with the use of aspirin.[11] Despite such evidence, there is underuse of warfarin in patients where there are no obvious contraindications. This may reflect anxiety regarding the potential of warfarin to cause bleeding, particularly in the frail elderly, those with a history of falls and forgetfulness, and those on medicines known to interact with warfarin. The risk of warfarin-related haemorrhage is greater in the elderly, and careful assessment of individual risks and benefits are required. Certainly, in those patients with a previous history of stroke, thromboembolism, hypertension, heart failure, diabetes mellitus, or structural heart disease, warfarin should be used unless there are known contraindications.

Compliance with medications

Adherence to medications is poor in the elderly. Up to 75 per cent of elderly may be non-compliant with medication, leading to disease breakthrough in 25 per cent. Reasons for non-compliance include poor instructions, difficulty in reading labels, excessively complicated drug regimens, adverse drug reactions, poor perception of the importance of treating the disease, lack of confidence in the doctor, and inconvenience.[12] Non-compliance may also be due to the inability to use devices such as inhalers. Inadequate control of symptoms or signs should always raise the suspicion of non-compliance. Compliance with medicines can be improved by simplifying drug regimens, avoiding polypharmacy, providing clear written instructions of how to take medicines and the importance of taking them, and in some cases, by using once-a-day formulations. Pharmacists may be able to assist by dispensing medicines in devices such as reminder boxes.

Adverse drug reactions

An adverse drug reaction (ADR) can be defined as 'an appreciably harmful or unpleasant reaction, resulting from an intervention related to the use of a medicinal product, which predicts hazard from future administration and warrants prevention or specific treatment, or alteration of the dosage regimen, or withdrawal of the product'.[13] ADRs in general are more common in the elderly. The incidence of ADRs while in hospital ranges from 6 to 19 per cent, while ADRs account for the 5–17 per cent of admissions in the elderly.[14] There are many reasons for this including age-related changes in pharmacokinetics and pharmacodynamics, multiple pathology, and polypharmacy.

ADRs can be divided in to two basic types, A and B. Type A reactions are predictable from the known pharmacology of the drug and often represent an exaggeration of the known primary and/or secondary pharmacology of the drug. In contrast, type B ADRs are bizarre reactions that are unpredictable from the known pharmacology of the drug, and show no apparent dose–response relationship.[15] Type A reactions are more common accounting for 80 per cent of all ADRs. Type A ADRs represent a particular problem in the elderly; however there are some type B ADRs, for example, hyponatraemia with selective serotonin re-uptake inhibitors, and agranulocytosis with mianserin, that are also known to occur more commonly in the elderly.

Lack of appreciation that the elderly have impaired homeostatic mechanisms is responsible for many type A ADRs (Table 3). A group of drugs to use with caution in the elderly are those with anticholinergic effects, which can have a wide range of effects (Table 4).

Table 3 Altered homeostatic mechanisms as a cause of adverse effects in the elderly

Drug	Adverse effect
Anticholinergics	Urinary retention
Anticoagulants	Haemorrhage
Antihypertensives	Postural hypotension Falls
Antipsychotics	Extrapyramidal effects
β-Blocker	Cardiac failure Bradycardia
Benzodiazepines	Confusion Falls
Diuretics	Postural hypotension Renal impairment Falls
Non-steroidal anti-inflammatory drugs	Renal impairment
Vasodilators	Vascular steal

Table 4 Anticholinergic agents in the elderly

Drug class	Drug example
Drugs with anticholinergic actions	
Antivertigo	Prochlorperazine
Antiparkinsonian	Benztropine
Antispasmodic	Oxybutinin
Bronchodilator	Ipratropium
Mydriatic	Tropicamide
Drugs with anticholinergic adverse effects	
Antiarrhythmics	Disopyramide
Antidiarrhoeals	Diphenoxylate
Antihistamines	Diphenhydramine
Antidepressants	Amitriptyline
Antipsychotics	Clozapine
Anticholinergic adverse effects	
Dry mouth	
Urinary retention	
Blurred vision	
Constipation	
Tachycardia	

Table 5 Classification and examples of drug–drug interactions

Mechanism	Drug affected	Interacting drug	Consequence
Pharmacokinetic interactions			
Absorption	Digoxin	Cholestyramine	Reduced digoxin absorption
Distribution	Warfarin	Non-steroidal anti-inflammatory drugs	Haemorrhage[a]
Metabolism	Terfenadine	Erythromycin	QT prolongation and torsades de pointes
Excretion	Digoxin	Verapamil	Digoxin toxicity
Pharmacodynamic interactions			
Synergistic	Diazepam	Alcohol	Increased sedation
Antagonistic	Bendrofluazide	Non-steroidal anti-inflammatory drugs	Reduced hypotensive effect

[a] Protein binding displacement does not usually lead to interactions, unless compensatory mechanisms are also affected. In the specific example cited, although non-steroidal anti-inflammatory drugs displace warfarin from protein binding sites, there may also be inhibition of warfarin metabolism and reduction in platelet adhesiveness.

Summary: A strategy to improve prescribing in the elderly

- Careful clinical assessment of the patient and an evaluation of the risk–benefit ratio of starting drug therapy.

- Start at low doses, and increase dose gradually. Remember that the elderly often require lower doses.

- Use one drug if possible, and avoid polypharmacy.

- Keep the drug prescribing regime simple.

- Give clear, and if possible, written instructions on how to take the medicines.

- Use sources of information such as formularies in order to appropriately prescribe in patients with renal and liver impairment, and to avoid the use of interacting drugs. Remember that in the elderly, a normal serum creatinine does not indicate normal renal function.

- Undertake a regular review of medications, and stop medicines when necessary.

- Review and improve repeat prescribing system, if necessary. Let patients know what to do when their medicines run out, and how to dispose of medicines that are no longer necessary.

- Consider drug(s) as the cause of new symptoms and signs arising in the patient.

- Ensure communication between hospital and primary care is up-to-date. In the future, this may be facilitated by the use of individual smart cards or electronic patient records.

- Multidisciplinary team working with pharmacists and nurses will help in many of the objectives outlined above.

Between 6 and 30 per cent of all ADRs are due to drug–drug interactions. Interactions increase in prevalence with the number of drugs prescribed, and this, together with age-related changes in pharmacokinetic and pharmacodynamic changes, puts the elderly at high risk of developing interactions. A classification of drug–drug interactions is provided in Table 5. Drugs particularly liable to be involved in interactions in the elderly include digoxin, warfarin, theophylline, lithium and psychotropic agents.

Most ADRs in the elderly are dose-dependent and predictable, and therefore potentially preventable. Careful choice of drug and dose, slower dose titration, avoidance of interacting medicines, better communication between all health care professionals involved in the care of the patient, regular review of medications, and in general, a more critical attitude to prescribing, are all needed to reduce the problem of ADRs in the elderly. It is important to remember that ADRs may present in a non-specific way in the elderly, for example, constipation or postural hypotension. Evaluation of the occurrence of new symptoms in the elderly should always include ADRs in the differential diagnosis. This is important to avoid the problem of incremental prescribing (Box 1).

Conclusions

In summary, the proportion of the population that is elderly is increasing. The elderly suffer from multiple pathologies and consequently often require the use of more than one drug. It is widely acknowledged that the quality of prescribing is poor in the elderly. This is compounded by the age-related changes in pharmacokinetic and pharmacodynamic parameters. Taken together, this greatly increases the risk of drug-related morbidity and mortality. Prescribing in the elderly needs to be improved; the box provides some simple rules and possible avenues by which we may be able to attain this goal.

References

1. **Walley, T. and Scott, A.K.** (1995). Prescribing in the elderly. *Postgraduate Medicine Journal* **71**, 466–71.

2. **Dhall, J., Larrat, E.P., and Lapane, K.L.** (2002). Use of potentially inappropriate drugs in nursing homes. *Pharmacotherapy* **22** (1), 88–96.

3. **Department of Health.** *Prescriptions Dispensed in the Community Statistics 1990 to 2000.* London: Department of Health, 2000.

4. **Hammerlein, A., Derendorf, H., and Lowenthal, D.T.** (1988). Pharmacokinetic and pharmacodynamic changes in the elderly. Clinical implications. *Clinical Pharmacokinetics* **35** (1), 49–64.

5. **Kinirons, M.T. and Crome, P.** (1997). Clinical pharmacokinetic considerations in the elderly. An update. *Clinical Pharmacokinetics* **33** (4), 302–12.

6. **Cockcroft, D.W. and Gault, M.H.** (1976). Prediction of creatinine clearance from serum creatinine. *Nephron* **16** (1), 31–41.

7. **Cartwright, A. and Smith, C.** *Elderly People: Their Medicines and Their Doctors.* London: Routledge, 1988.

8. **Khunti, K. and Kinsella, B.** (2000). Effect of systematic review of medication by general practitioner on drug consumption among nursing-home residents. *Age and Ageing* **29** (5), 451–3.

9. **Department of Health.** Medicines and older people. In *Implementing Medicines-Related Aspects on the National Service Framework for Older People.* London: Department of Health, 2001.

10. **Staessen, J.A.** et al. (2000). Risks of untreated and treated isolated systolic hypertension in the elderly: meta-analysis of outcome trials. *Lancet* **355** (9207), 865–72.

11. **Atrial Fibrillation Investigators** (1994). Risk factors for stroke and efficacy of antithrombotic therapy in atrial fibrillation. Analysis of pooled data from five randomized controlled trials. *Archives of Internal Medicine* **154** (13), 1449–57.

12. **McElnay, J.C., McCallion, C.R., al-Deagi, F., and Scott, M.** (1997). Self-reported medication non-compliance in the elderly. *European Journal of Clinical Pharmacology* **53** (3–4), 171–8.

13. **Edwards, I.R. and Aronson, J.K.** (2000). Adverse drug reactions: definitions, diagnosis, and management. *Lancet* **356** (9237), 1255–9.

14. **McMurdo, M.E.** (2000). Adverse drug reactions. *Age and Ageing* **29** (1), 5–6.

15. **Pirmohamed, M., Breckenridge, A.M., Kitteringham, N.R., and Park, B.K.** (1998). Adverse drug reactions. *British Medical Journal* **316** (7140), 1295–8.

Further reading

Department of Health. Medicines and older people. In *Implementing Medicines-Related Aspects of the National Service Framework for Older People.* London: Department of Health, 2001. (A very well-produced document that highlights the problems of prescribing in the elderly, and comes up with practical suggestions for improving the situation.)

16.9 Influenza

Th.M.E. Govaert and G.A. van Essen

Introduction

Although influenza often seems to be a harmless illness, its in industrialized countries is enormous, both socially and economically.

We all know of the three pandemics in the twentieth century which saw millions of deaths, worldwide: the Spanish flu, in 1918 with some 40 million deaths,[1] the Asian flu in 1957, and the Hong Kong flu in 1968. And in 1997 there was the threat of a new pandemic: in Hong Kong we had a chicken flu with an unknown antigen structure H5N1 for humans, in which six of 18 infected persons died.

Economically, influenza has a significant impact, resulting in considerable health care cost and costs lost production. In 1997, estimated costs due to influenza were in Germany approximately 2 billion Deutschmarks, in 1989 in France 14 billion Francs and in the United States costs were approximately 11 up to 18 billion dollars each year.[2]

Every year, 5–10 per cent of the population suffers from influenza. The incidence of influenza is relatively high among children and young adults, but serious complications occur more among the elderly, 65 years of age or more.[3]

Epidemiology

From reports of former chroniclers we can see that even in the Middle Ages large flu epidemics had occurred, and may be even further back.[4]

Epidemics arise from changes in the antigen structure of the virus, the haemagglutinin and neurominidase spikes of glucoproteins. A small change of the antigen structure of the virus is called an antigenic drift. That occurs once in 2–3 years. Large antigenic changes are called an antigenic shift. They are responsible for epidemics and occur every 8–12 years. In that case it is mostly a change of the haemagglutinin component, sometimes of the neurominidase component, that has occurred. When the virus develops a totally different antigenic structure, which means both the haemagglutinin and the neurominidase component have changed, a pandemic can occur. This complete change of the antigen structure of the virus occurs once in every 30–40 years and can cause a pandemic because a high proportion of the population lacks immunity to the new virus.

Surveillance

In 1847, William Farr, director of the Department of Statistics of the General Register Office in England, published the first incidence figures of influenza in the *International Journal of Epidemiology*. At that time, it was already clear to Farr that many deaths, attributed to bronchitis or pneumonia, in fact should be attributed to influenza and that deaths diagnosed as bronchitis or pneumonia were in fact a complication of influenza.

The word 'surveillance' was introduced, comprising a number of measures to control a disease.[5] In 1947, the World Health Organization (WHO) established an international network for the surveillance of influenza. Now the network consists of about 110 national centres all over the world and four main centres for registration and research in Atlanta, London, Melbourne, and Tokyo.[6]

In many of these countries, a network of general practitioners and hospitals registers and reports influenza-like illnesses. They also collect virus material (nose-swab, throat-wash) for the national centres. The national influenza centres report the findings to one of the four WHO centres.

The virus

The influenza virus belongs to the family orthomyxoviridae and consists of an RNH-nucleus, enveloped by an inner protein layer and an outer lipoid layer (Fig. 1). The RNH nucleus and the inner protein layer determine the types of the virus: influenza A, B, or C. On the surface of the outer lipoid layer are glucoprotein spikes, consisting of haemagglutinin (HA) and neuraminidase (NA) components. They are responsible for the antigen structure of the virus, for example, H1N2 or H3N2. There are 15 sub-types of HA (H1–H15) and nine sub-types of NA (N1–N9). Influenza A viruses circulate among humans as well as among animals (pigs, horses, fowl, ducks, turkeys, terns, whales) and show the most antigenic variation. Type B is only pathogenic in humans. Type C is restricted to humans and pigs.

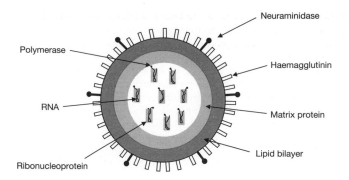

Fig. 1 Diagram of influenza A or B virus.

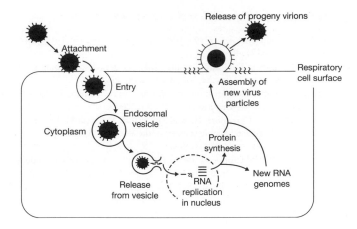

Fig. 2 Replicative cycle of the influenza virus showing the key role of neuraminidase.

Type C shows the less antigenic variation and causes harmless respiratory track infections in children. The nomenclature of the influenza viruses contains the type and data about the place of isolation, the registration number, the year of isolation and, for the A-viruses, the antigenic description of the haemagglutinin and neuraminidase, for example, A/New Caledonia/20/99 (H1N1), A/Panama/ 2007/99 (H3N2), B/Sichuan/379/99.

Replication of the virus

Influenza viruses penetrate the epithelial cells of the airways by binding the haemagglutinin of the virus to sialic acid, which coats the cell surface (Fig. 2). This binding induces the cell to take up the virus. Inside the epithelial cell the virus falls into pieces. Newly made proteins and RNH strands assemble into new virus copies or particles, coated with sialic acid. The haemagglutinin molecules on one particle attach to the sialic acid on other particles and on the cell, causing the new viruses to clump together. However, the neuraminidase of the virus can cleave this sialic acid barrier, leaving the new viruses free to travel and invade other cells.

Vaccine

After the discovery of the influenza virus in 1933,[7] many studies were performed to develop a vaccine. In 1937 after several attempts, Smith and his colleagues succeeded in preparing a useful formalin-treated inactivated vaccine. However, that vaccine was not potent enough. After the discovery in 1942 of manufacturing concentrated vaccines by high-speed centrifugation and producing vaccines by growing the virus on the chorioallantoic membrane of chicken eggs,[8] full production of potent vaccines became possible.

This inactivated 'whole' virus vaccine contained a lot of contaminating egg protein causing significant local and systemic reactions. More purified vaccines were prepared by using better isolation techniques to separate the vaccine from contaminating egg proteins.[9] Since 1970, split virus vaccines and later on surface antigen (sub-unit) vaccines are used. Split vaccines consist of disrupted virus particles which still contain the most important antigenic materials. Therefore, the efficacy of the split vaccines are nearly the same as the whole virus vaccines, with less side-effects. The sub-unit vaccines consist of purified surface proteins, haemagglutinin, and neuraminidase, which are the most immunogenic proteins of the influenza virus. Since these two vaccines are not as immunogenic as whole virus vaccines in unprimed populations, such as young children, a second booster dose is required.

Live attenuated vaccines have been used for many years in Russia. The live viruses are attenuated by cooling (cold adapted) and administered intranasally. These cold-adapted vaccines give a good immune response but the risk exists that the attenuated virus will return to the original, non-attenuated form. Another problem is that the reaction to infection with an attenuated virus is not the same for each individual, thus causing different

immunity. Adjuvants are compounds to enhance the immune response to vaccination, for example, aluminium hydroxide in tetanus vaccine. In the case of influenza vaccines mostly oil components are used. They form cages or envelopes from which the vaccine can be released (controlled release).

The production of vaccine, which requires hatched chicken eggs, is time-consuming. That can be a major problem, especially in the case of a pandemic. An important development in this field is the possibility of propagating the virus in cell cultures. Cell cultures such as Madins Darby Canine Kidney (MDCK)-cells, yield high titres of virus in a short time. The latest developments are the 'high-tech' vaccines manufactured by recombinant techniques. This method is still under development.

Clinical picture and diagnosis

As long as there is no reliable, fast, and simple laboratory test for the diagnosis of influenza the physician has to rely on the clinical symptomatology. Sometimes there are no physical signs except red eyes and a running nose. The characteristic symptoms are acute onset, fever, coughing, malaise, rigor or chills, headache, myalgia, lost appetite, chest pain, sore throat, nasal and eye problems. According to the criteria of the International Classification of Health Problems in Primary Care (ICHPPC-2),[10] the diagnosis of influenza can be made if six of the nine symptoms occur (Table 1); in case of an influenza epidemic four symptoms are enough. The clinical diagnosis can be confirmed by viral culture or serological evidence.

Many influenza-like illnesses, caused, for example, by the parainfluenza virus, the respiratory syncytial virus, the adenovirus, the rhinovirus, the corona-virus, the herpes simplex virus, or *Mycoplasma pneumoniae*, are clinically indistinguishable from influenza. Furthermore, a wide range of unrelated pyrexial illnesses can mimic influenza, for example, malaria, pyelitis, tonsillitis, psittacosis, and acute bacterial endocarditis. However, when influenza is suspected and an influenza outbreak exists, and when clinical findings do not explicitly relate to another disease, the triad of fever, acute onset, and coughing will be helpful in confirming the diagnosis of influenza.

Usually, influenza is a harmless illness and lasts 3–5 days but complete recovery can take 2–3 weeks. Because the influenza viruses damage the epithelial cells of the airways a secondary bacterial infection, bronchitis or (broncho) pneumonia can arise. Sometimes such an infection occurs within the first days of the illness. *Streptococcus pneumoniae* (pneumococcus), sometimes *Staphylococcus aureus* and, far less frequently, *Streptococcus pyogenes* and *Haemophilus influenzae* are bacterial causes of a pneumonia. They can also cause sepsis and meningitis. Staphylococcal pneumonia is a very dangerous complication. An influenza virus pneumonia is an

Table 1 Criteria for diagnosis of influenza and influenza-like illness, according to the ICHPPC-2

Inclusion requires *one* of the following:
(a) Viral culture or serological evidence of influenza virus infection
(b) Influenza epidemic, plus *four* of the criteria in (c)
(c) *Six* of the following:
   Sudden onset (within 12 h)
   Cough
   Rigors or chills
   Fever
   Prostration and weakness
   Headache
   Myalgia, widespread aches and pains
   No significant physical signs other than redness of nasal mucous membrane and throat
   Influenza in close contacts

Table 2 Recommendation for vaccination according to the WHO guidelines

1. Persons aged 65 years or older
2. Residents of nursing homes who have chronic medical conditions
3. Children and adults who have chronic disorders of the pulmonary or cardiovascular systems, including asthma
4. Children and adults who have required regular medical follow-up or hospitalization during the preceding year because of chronic metabolic diseases (including diabetes mellitus), renal dysfunction, haemoglobinopathies, or immunosupression
5. Children and adolescents aged 6 months to 18 years, who are long-term users of salicylates
6. Women who will be in the second or third trimester of pregnancy during the influenza season

uncommon, but very serious, complication which can develop within 48 h after the onset of the illness.

Influenza-related complications can occur at any age. However, elderly and people with a risk factor such as cardiovascular and pulmonary diseases or diabetes mellitus are more likely to develop serious complications than younger, healthy people.

To confirm the clinical diagnosis of influenza we need a positive culture or a four-fold increase of the antibody titre in paired sera.

Sputum, naso-pharyngeal washes, or a combined nose and throat swab are transported in a suitable medium and inoculated in embryonated chicken eggs or in mammalian or avian tissue cultures. This process takes about 4–5 days. There are more rapid tests (1–3 days), which detect viruses in cultured cells by immunological methods, as immunofluorescence, enzyme immunosorbent assays, and polymerase chain reaction (PCR). Rapid 'near patient' testing is commercially available, but the predictive value is not very high.

The best known serological tests are the haemagglutinin inhibition (HI) test, the complement fixation (CF) test, and the more modern enzyme-linked immunosorbent assay (ELISA). In most laboratories, HI is the test of choice. Because the need for paired sera (acute and after 2 weeks) serological tests are not appropriate for immediate clinical management. They are used to confirm the diagnosis afterwards when, for example, virus culture has failed, for the surveillance and epidemiology of influenza and in research studies.

Vaccination

Based on studies among military recruits and healthy adult civilians, influenza vaccination has a protective effect of 40–90 per cent, depending on a poor or good match between vaccine and circulating virus strains.[11] Ninety-five per cent of deaths due to influenza occur among people aged 60 years and older[3] but it is widely believed that elderly persons have a diminished response to vaccination. A meta-analysis of studies regarding the efficacy of vaccination in elderly persons demonstrated a vaccine efficacy in the observational studies of 56 per cent for preventing respiratory illness, 53 per cent for preventing pneumonia, 50 per cent for preventing hospitalization, and 68 per cent for preventing death. Vaccine efficacy in the case-controlled studies ranged from 32 to 45 per cent for preventing hospitalization for pneumonia and 31–65 per cent for preventing hospital deaths from pneumonia and influenza.[12] A randomized double-blind placebo-controlled trial in 1992 among 1838 elderly individuals (>69 years), of which 27 per cent belonged to the patients at risk, demonstrated 58 per cent reduction in laboratory confirmed influenza. Considering these studies we have to conclude that in the elderly influenza vaccination has a good protective effect. Several recent studies have confirmed the effectiveness of repeated influenza vaccinations.[13] Influenza vaccine must be administered each year because of the frequent antigenic changes in circulating

strains of influenza viruses. Unvaccinated children up to 6 years, as well as patients with immunodeficiencies, are recommended to receive two complete doses with an interval of 4 weeks.

Immunization is recommended for people of all ages with chronic diseases that place them at increased risk of complications of influenza, and all those aged 65 years and older (Table 2). It is also important to vaccinate all health care workers involved in the direct care of patients, because they can infect their patients and become infected themselves.

Although immunization against influenza is strongly recommended for high-risk patients, the vaccination rate remains low in many countries. Patients are often concerned about the side-effects of vaccination and there is disagreement about how frequently they occur. Since the introduction of modern vaccines, side-effects of vaccination have been reduced. Most studies have found a low incidence of local (up to 20 per cent) and systemic (up to 5 per cent) adverse reactions to influenza. All side-effects were mild in nature and transitory. Local reactions were mostly tenderness at the site of injection, erythema, and induration. The most important systemic reactions were myalgia, headache, and fever. Women reported more side-effects than men and patients who had never received vaccine before showed more systemic reactions.

Vaccination of persons allergic to chicken eggs should be avoided, and should in patients who have reacted adversely to previous vaccination. It is also advisable to delay vaccination when persons are febrile or have an acute infection.

During the influenza season 1976–1997, there was an increased incidence of Guillain–Barré syndrome (GBS) in vaccinated persons which could not be explained. Therefore, vaccination should also be avoided in persons with a history of GBS.

Treatment

Vaccination has its limitations. Because of the relatively low efficacy of influenza vaccination, one out of every two vaccinated persons can still develop influenza. Moreover, there is always a possibility of a mismatch between the vaccine and the circulating strain of the virus.

To reduce the burden of influenza we have, apart from vaccination, the option of treatment of influenza by antiviral drugs. Amantadine and rimantadine have been on the market for many years. Recently neuraminidase inhibitors like zanamivir and oseltamivir have been developed.

Amantadine and rimantadine are only effective against influenza A. They block the action of the virus protein M2, an enzyme necessary for the replication of the influenza virus, existing only in the influenza A virus. After using it a short time, resistance can develop. Side-effects of amantadine and rimantadine concern the cardiovascular system, the nervous system, and the digestive system. Moreover, they can interfere with other medications.

The neuraminidase inhibitors are a new class of antivirals. By blocking neuraminidase they inhibit viral spreading and thereby break the cycle of infection. They are effective against influenza A and B. There have been several randomized, double-blind, placebo-controlled studies, which show a shortening of the illness by 1–2 days.[14] The problem is that these drugs have to be administered within 48 h from the onset of symptoms (zanamivir by inhalation, oseltamivir orally). The efficacy is not proven sufficiently in high-risk patients. There has not been any recorded resistance of the virus to neuraminidase inhibitors. They are well tolerated and can be used together with other medicaments. Patients with a history of asthma or COPD can develop acute bronchospasm or decline of respiratory function after use of zanamivir. These patients should be told to have a quick-acting bronchodilator at hand.

Patients at risk could benefit from treatment with these neuraminidase inhibitors if they develop influenza in spite of vaccination and when vaccination has been omitted. Other options for the use of antiviral medicaments are mismatching of the vaccine and the circulating virus, and the shortage of vaccine in the case of a pandemic. Non-vaccinated patients outside the risk groups could be treated on request.

Finally, neuraminidase inhibitors are effective in preventing influenza among healthy adults. They are approximately 70 per cent effective in preventing influenza, the same figure as vaccination. However, neuraminidase inhibitors cannot substitute for vaccination. For prevention, they can be useful in specific situations, for example, for a short period of exposure when travelling or when there is a local outbreak of influenza in a nursing house, a community, or even in a family.

Organization of vaccination programme

Depending on the demographic distribution, 20–25 per cent of the population has an indication for vaccination, either on account of their age or other risk factors. The vaccination rate varies widely between countries. In the 1999–2000 season in Sweden, 7 per cent of the population was immunized, compared to 17 per cent in the Netherlands. Nevertheless, most countries acknowledge the WHO indications for vaccination.

In countries where general practice is based on a list system, the GP can send an invitation to the patients at risk. The practice can make up a list of these patients or use computer software to select them from the electronical medical records on the basis of coded diagnoses, flags, or prescribed medication, pointing to certain risk groups. The invitation can offer a vaccination administered by the practice nurse at a special vaccination session. A small leaflet with a description of the procedure and the few side-effects can be enclosed. It is efficient to have the vaccine at the surgery. In that case the patient does not have to visit the pharmacy before coming to the practice.

In countries where the vaccination is given free to patients at risk, the vaccination rate is higher than in countries where the patient has to pay for the vaccination himself/herself. Adequate reimbursement for the GP seems to have a stimulating effect on the vaccination rate.

Key points

- Fever, acute onset and coughing during an influenza outbreak is indicative of influenza.

- Vaccination is recommended for all people at risk, including those of 65 years and older.

- The efficacy of influenza vaccination in elderly persons amounts to 50–70% if there is a good match between the vaccine and the circulating virus strains.

- Flu management consists of prevention by vaccination and treatment by antiviral drugs and antibiotics in the case of secondary bacterial infection.

Combining the influenza vaccination with pneumococcal vaccination (once every 5 years) does not lower the vaccination rate for influenza and could be a very cost-efficient measure. These two vaccines are indicated for the same risk groups.

References

1. Patterson, K.D. and Pyle, G.F. (1991). The geography and mortality of the 1918 influenza pandemic. *Bulletin of the History of Medicine* **65**, 4–21.
2. Szucs, T.D. (1999). Influenza, the role of burden-of-illness research. *Pharmacoeconomics* **16** (Suppl. 1), 28–9.
3. Sprenger, M.J.W., Mulder, P.G.H., Beyer, W.E.P., van Strik, R., and Masurel, N. (1993). Impact of influenza on mortality regarding age and entity of underlying disease, during the period 1967 to 1989. *International Journal of Epidemiology* **22**, 333–9.
4. Vanghan, W.T. (1921). Influenza—an epidemiology study. *American Journal of Hygiene* Monograph **1**, 1.
5. Langmuir, A.D. (1971). Evolution of the concept of surveillance in the United States. *Proceedings of the Royal Society of Medicine* **64**, 681–4.
6. Hampson, A.W. and Cox, N.J. (1996). Global surveillance for pandemic influenza: are we prepared? In *Options for the Control of Influenza* Vol. 3 (ed. L.E. Brown, A.W. Hampson, and R.G. Webster), pp. 37–8. Amsterdam: Elsevier.
7. Smith, W., Andrewes, C.H., and Laidlaw, C.H. (1933). A virus obtained from influenza patients. *Lancet* **ii**, 66–8.
8. Hirst, G.K., Rikard, E.R., Whitman, L., and Horsfall, F.L. (1942). Antibody response of human beings following vaccination with influenza viruses. *Journal of Experimental Medicine* **75**, 495–511.
9. Reimer, C.B. (1996). Comparison of techniques for influenza virus purification. *Journal of Bacteriology* **92**, 1271–2.
10. Classification Committee of Wonca. *ICHPPC-2-defined. Inclusion Criteria for the Use of the Rubrics of the International Classification of Health Problems in Primary Care.* Oxford: Oxford University Press, 1983.
11. Meiklejohn, C. (1983). Viral respiratory disease at Lowry Air Force Base in Denver, 1952–1982. *The Journal of Infectious Diseases* **147**, 775–84.
12. Gross, P.A., Hermogenes, A.W., Sacks, H.S., Lau, J., and Levandowski, R.A. (1995). The efficacy of influenza vaccine in elderly persons. A meta-analysis and review of the literature. *Annals of Internal Medicine* **123**, 518–27.
13. Keitel, W.A., Cate, T.R., and Couch, R.B. (1986). Efficacy of sequential annual vaccination with inactivated influenza virus vaccine. *American Journal of Epidemiology* **127**, 353–64.
14. Monto, A.S., Webster, A., and Keene, O. (1999). Randomised, placebo-controlled studies of inhaled zanamivir in the treatment of influenza A and B: pooled efficacy analysis. *Journal of Antimicrobial Chemotherapy* **44**, 23–9.

Further reading

Nicholson, K.G., Webster, R.G., and Hay, A.J. *Textbook of Influenza.* Oxford: Blackwell Science, 1998. (This textbook gives a complete survey about influenza.)

Nicholson, K.G. *Managing Influenza in Primary Care.* Oxford: Blackwell Science, 1999.

Websites

Centres for Disease Control and Prevention: http://www.cdc.gov/ncidod/diseases/flu/fluvirus.htm.

NIMR Influenza Bibliography: http://www.nimr.mrc.ac.uk/Library/flu.

FluNet: http://oms.b3e.jussieu.fr/flunet/.

17

Palliative care

17 Palliative care

17.1 The dying patient and their family

Irene J. Higginson, Massimo Costantini, Polly Edmonds, and Paola Viterbori

Epidemiology and future trends

The epidemiologically based needs assessment for palliative and terminal care estimates the numbers of patients who will die and their symptoms and problems (see Further reading, ref. 4). It has been used in the United Kingdom, the United States, Australia, and many European countries. Data also are available from government statistics, such as the Office of National Statistics or local health authorities, and primary care clinicians may have their own records. Table 1 estimates the number of deaths during 1 year in

Table 1 Number of deaths in the population during 1 year for the most common causes

Cause of death	Men	Women	Total
Neoplasms	1 464	1 341	2 805
Lip, oral pharynx, larynx	41	34	75
Digestive and peritoneum	449	339	788
Trachea, bronchus, lung	394	291	685
Female breast	0	255	255
Genitourinary	243	178	421
Lymphatic and haematopoietic	154	54	208
Other, unspecified	7	7	14
Circulatory system	2 429	2 624	5 053
Respiratory system	595	626	1 221
Chronic liver and cirrhosis	34	26	60
Nervous system and sense organs	88	88	176
Parkinson's disease	37	28	65
Multiple sclerosis	1	1	2
Meningitis	4	4	8
Senile and pre-senile organic conditions	22	22	44
Endocrine, nutritional, metabolic, immunity	187	123	310
Total of these diseases	4 819	4 850	9 669
Total deaths from all causes	5 356	5 644	11 000

Total population = 1 million, because of small numbers for some categories in 10 000. Deaths in those aged under 28 days excluded.

Note: Countries will vary.

a population of 1 million and similar to England and Wales. There would be roughly equal numbers of men and women who died, the numbers would be roughly constant over the years. A typical age distribution for England and Wales would be: less than 15 years, less than 1 per cent; 16–35 years, 3 per cent; 36–64 years, 19 per cent; 65–74 years, 21 per cent; 75+ years, 56 per cent. The numbers of older people will increase in the next decades.

How commonly do primary care clinicians encounter dying and what are the causes?

Within an average population, such as that of England and Wales, of 1 million people, there would be 11 000 deaths, and most of these deaths would be from cancers (2800), circulatory disorders (5000), and respiratory conditions (1200) (Table 1). Thus, in a smaller population, such as a group practice serving 10 000 people, there would be 110 deaths per year, and most, about 95, would be from conditions where the death occurred following a period where it became more and more apparent that the illness was progressing. Of these, almost 30 would be from cancer, about 50 from circulatory disorders, particularly stroke and heart disease, and 10 or so from respiratory conditions. Death rates can vary considerably, and will be higher in elderly communities or in those groups where disease is prevalent. Thus, it is advisable to obtain local data.

Applying the prevalence of symptoms from epidemiological assessments (see Further reading, ref. 4) to these data gives estimates of numbers of people with different problems that the primary team is likely to encounter. Thus, of the 28 patients who would die from cancer, 23 would have pain, 13 breathlessness, 14 vomiting or feeling sick, 20 loss of appetite, and nine where the patient and seven where the family had severe anxiety or worries which was seriously affecting their daily life and concentration. As for cancer patients, estimates of the prevalence of symptoms and other problems can be applied to determine the numbers of people with these problems at the end of life. The number of people affected is more that double those for cancer.

In the next 20 years, more and more people will die from chronic rather than acute diseases. The main causes of mortality now and for the next 20 years will be heart disease, cerebrovascular disorders, chronic respiratory disease, and the cancers. Thus, increasingly, the primary care physician will have to deal with the management of progressive illness, and care of the dying following a progressive illness.

Assessment and diagnosis

When is a patient dying?

It can be extremely difficult to identify when a patient is dying, but an awareness that a patient might die and when that might be can be very important for patients, families, and health care professionals. Many

(a) Common pattern of deterioration in cancer: gradual deterioration over weeks to months

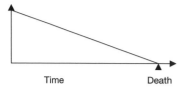

(b) Common pattern of deterioration in many non-malignant conditions: stepwise deterioration over months to years

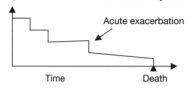

(c) Alternative pattern, a swinging trajectory

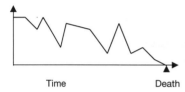

(d) Stable disease followed by sudden deterioration and subsequent death

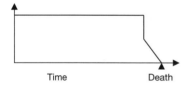

Fig. 1 Possible trajectories experienced by patients.

patients will ask about prognosis ('How long have I got?'), but it is usually better not to be too specific—all health care professionals are notoriously inaccurate at predicting how long an individual has to live, even close to death. Even among hospice patients in the United States, although the median survival was 36 days, almost 15 per cent lived longer than 6 months and 5 per cent lived more than 2 years.

Common signs of impending death include profound weakness, being confined to bed, drowsiness for extended periods, lack of interest in food and fluids, disorientation with respect to time, limited attention span, and difficulty in swallowing medication. However, some patients do make a partial recovery following deterioration and a wide range of different trajectories can occur (Fig. 1). It is sometimes helpful to discuss likely scenarios with the patient and the family, and as Teno argues to plan for both the best and the worst possible outcomes.[1]

What is an 'appropriate' or 'good' death?

Experts in different countries have defined the principles of a 'good' death, but rarely were patients consulted. The domains identified by patients and experts differ; there are also differences between and within countries and cultures (Table 2). Pain and symptom control and ensuring dignity are common domains. There is no 'right' way to die and all studies identify the importance of an individual dying 'in character'. Thus, it is probably better to think of an 'appropriate', rather than a 'good', death. This needs to be reflected in individualized approaches to meeting need and care, taking account of culture, background, circumstances, and preferences.

Assessment and diagnosis of individual symptoms, problems, or syndromes

Assessment and diagnosis are just as important in the dying as in acute care, intensive care, and any other time in care. This assessment should be of those things that are important to the patient and family (see Chapter 7.8, Vol. 1).

Accurate assessment of the aetiology of new symptoms can be more difficult in the dying, when patients are weak or find it difficult or uncomfortable to move. Unnecessary or excessive tests, if uncomfortable, can increase rather than reduce suffering. Clinicians should always carefully assess patients to identify potentially reversible symptoms. Investigations should only be undertaken, however, where they are likely to inform management decisions and if further tests are in line with the patients' wishes.

Attention to detail, reassessment, and ensuring treatments and interventions are individualized are the cornerstones of successful management. Assessment can be aided by using standardized audit or assessment schedules (see Chapter 7.8, Vol. 1), especially if these are incorporated in a care pathway or protocol. Choose assessment schedules that are intended for the end of life and do not burden the patient.

In the dying patient, especially if she/he is unconscious, particular attention needs to be paid to mouth and pressure areas, comfort, and dignity. The family or nearest carer needs and their coping also need to be assessed; often, their perception of the symptoms and comfort is important.

The principles of management

The patient and family as the unit of care

Care for both the patient and family is an essential element in the care of people who are dying. The term family is meant in its broad sense and encompasses close relatives (often a spouse, children, or siblings), a partner, and close friend(s) who are significant for the patient. They should have every available option to meet their choices, with expert recognition of their cultural and individual needs. This includes acknowledging the concerns of the family or friends, and finding mechanisms for these to be heard and discussed.

Changing gear

Evidence-based guidelines have reviewed the need to 'change gear' when managing the care of patients who are dying. During the terminal phase, the goals of care are re-defined towards the alleviation of symptoms and distress and support for the patient and family at the time of death. Existing symptoms may change or new symptoms may arise, which require management. Patients often need more time to express what is important to them, and clinicians have to 'slow down' when dealing with the patient and family, and listening to their concerns.

A review of medication is needed. Some medications, such as those for pre-existing heart or respiratory disorders, or any other non-essential mediation, may become inappropriate, particularly if these are difficult for the patient to take.

Planning of end-of-life care

Anticipatory planning of care, once it has been identified that a patient is likely to die, is crucial in order to facilitate patient and family choices. Factors that need to be considered are:

◆ *Symptom control*—anticipation of symptoms that might occur, particularly outside of normal working hours and the development of effective management plans to address these (including the prescribing of appropriate medication).

◆ *Information and communication*—it is vital that patients and families are given frequent opportunities to have questions answered and outstanding issues addressed.

Table 2 Common features of a 'good death' from recent studies and reports

Payne et al. (1996)	UK	Patients (n = 18)	Dying in one's sleep
			Dying quietly
			Dignity
			Pain free
		Health professionals (n = 20)	Symptom control
			Family involvement
			Peacefulness
			Lack of distress
Kelleher (1990)	Australia	Cancer patients (n not known)	Social life
			Open awareness
			Social adjustment
			Personal and public preparation
			Farewells
Steinhauser et al. (2000)	US	Nurses (n = 27), patients (n = 14), social workers (n = 10), hospice volunteers (n = 8), others (n = 14)	Pain and symptom management
			Clear decision-making
			Preparation for death
			Completion
			Contributing to others
			Affirmation of the whole person
Singer et al. (1999)	Canada	Dialysis patients (n = 48), HIV patients (n = 40), residents of a long-term care facility (n = 38)	Receiving adequate pain and symptom management
			Avoiding inappropriate prolongation of dying
			Achieving a sense of control
			Relieving burden
			Strengthening relationships
Debate of the Age Health and Care Study Group	UK	Workgroup of experts	To know when death is coming, and to understand what can be expected
			To be able to retain control of what happens
			To be afforded dignity and privacy
			To have control over pain relief and other symptom control
			To have choice and control over where death occurs (at home or elsewhere)
			To have access to information and expertise of whatever kind is necessary
			To have access to any spiritual or emotional support required
			To have access to hospice care in any location, not only in hospital
			To have control over who is present and who shares the end
			To be able to issue advance directives which ensure wishes are respected
			To have time to say goodbye, and control over other aspects of timing
			To be able to leave when it is time to go, and not to have life prolonged pointlessly

- *End-of-life decisions*—these can include treatment options or choices in place of care and of death. Advance discussion and documentation of patients' wishes can reduce distress and facilitate appropriate care.

- *Equipment*—as appropriate to facilitate safe care in all settings.

Pain and symptom management in the dying

Pain and symptom management are essential. Detailed guidance on symptom management is given in Chapters 17.2 and 17.6, and much of this applies to the dying patient. The subsections below provide some additional guidance on the management of symptoms in the last days or hours of life.

Oral and subcutaneous medication

A common difficulty is that patients become too weak to swallow oral medication. Ambulatory infusion devices, syringe drivers, and other continuous delivery systems are useful in this situation. They allow either a continuous or regular infusion of opioid and other suitable medications, thus avoiding repeated injection. Patient controlled and spring operated delivery systems are also available and are particularly useful in countries where batteries to operate the delivery system cannot be obtained. The 24-h dose for subcutaneous delivery should be calculated based on prior treatment. The most useful sites to insert the butterfly needle for subcutaneous infusions are the upper chest, outer aspect of the outer arm,

abdomen, and thighs. Patients should undergo frequent assessment of pain, cognition, and other symptoms. Common symptoms in dying patients and their subcutaneous drug treatments are shown in Table 3.

Pain control

While patients are dying, and even when they become unconscious, pain control using regular analgesics is still required if it was needed at an earlier stage of illness. For patients receiving strong opioids, the 24-h morphine dose can then be recalculated to provide the equivalent dose subcutaneously. The dose of opioids and other adjuvants should be frequently titrated in order to prevent metabolite accumulation or drug interactions contributing to agitated delirium.

Feeding and hydration

In general, as death approaches appetite reduces and many patients find it more comfortable to eat less, or little at all. This can cause great anxiety to families and, less commonly, patients. Explanation of the normality of reduced oral intake at the end of life, alongside a general 'shutting down' of the systems, is often required to support families.

There is no evidence that artificial feeding in patients with a progressive illness prolongs life, and insertion of intravenous, percutaneous, and nasogastric feeding devices can cause iatrogenic disease.

The evidence regarding hydration is less clear. The sensation of thirst is probably not related to hydration or to sodium levels, and can be relieved

Table 3 Common drugs for use in syringe drivers

Indication	Drug	Dose in syringe driver (over 24 h)	PRN dose	Comments
Pain	Diamorphine (UK) [or Hydromorphone (US, Canada)]	5–20 mg diamorphine or 1–5 mg hydromorphone if no previous strong opioid (e.g. morphine), and pain is severe. Patients on morphine: divide total daily dose of oral morphine by 3 for 24 h diamorphine dose; patients on hydromorphone: divide total daily dose of oral hydromorphone by 5 for 24 h hydromorphone dose	Diamorphine—2.5–5 mg as required. One-sixth total daily dose of opioid as required	Diamorphine and hydromorphone are better absorbed s.c. than morphine. No 'maximum' dose
Sedation	Midazolam	10–30 mg/24 h	2.5–5 mg as required	Max dose 200 mg/24 h
	Levomepromazine	25–200 mg/24 h	6.25–25 mg as required	Not in patients with cerebral metastases or history of fits
Antiemetic	Haloperidol	3–5 mg/24 h	1.5–3 mg as required	Can be sedating
	Cyclizine	150 mg/24 h	—	Can precipitate
	Levomepromazine	6.25–25 mg/24 h	6.25 mg as required	Sedating in increased doses
Retained oro-pharyngeal secretions	Glycopyrronium	0.6 mg/24 h	0.2 mg as required	More potent than hyoscine hydrobromide and does not cross blood brain barrier (BBB)
	Buscopan	60–180 mg/24 h	20 mg as required	Antispasmodic; does not cross BBB

Patients' individual opioid requirements can vary greatly and opioid dose should be titrated against the pain, for more details see http://www.vh.org/adult/provider/radiology/lungtumors/treatment/symptom/paincontrol.html or see specialist advice.

by good mouth care, and sips of water or wetting the lips and mouth. Equally, intravenous hydration can be uncomfortable and restrictive in a dying patient, and can easily tip a patient into fluid overload. However, research has also shown that dehydration has been associated with increased confusion at the end of life, and giving relatively small amounts of fluid (e.g. 1 l/day) subcutaneously can reduce this. Thus, subcutaneous hydration may have a role for some patients.

Nursing care

Good nursing care of the dying patient is particularly important, especially in maintaining dignity. This includes care of pressure areas, mouth and skin care, bathing, as well as assessment and management of symptoms and support of the patient and family. Alongside these, care needs to be orientated towards enabling the patient to 'live' with dignity until death. This can involve a wide and very individual range of aspects, in the last weeks or even days of life there may be new achievable activities, the creative activities of day care, attention to appearance (e.g. hair, teeth), the environment and surroundings, family gatherings or attending important functions, a reconciliation of existential and spiritual meanings.

Delirium

Delirium is a very distressing symptom for patients and family. Patients experiencing delirium are often aware and they and their family are very anxious. Sometimes referred to as acute confusional state, terminal restlessness, or acute brain syndrome, it is characterized by acute onset cognitive impairment. Thresholds of detecting delirium vary, but some cognitive impairment, changing sleep–wake cycle, and fluctuating consciousness are common in the terminal stages. Delirium is frequently undiagnosed and it is important to check the more distressing manifestations of delirium, such as misinterpretations, psycho-motor agitation, hallucinations, delusions, and other abnormalities of perception. Frequent causes include: urinary retention, infection, dehydration, constipation, metabolic abnormalities, toxicity of opioids, benzodiazepines and other drugs, and cytokine production. Where appropriate, underlying causes should be sought and actively treated.

Haloperidol is indicated in the symptomatic management of patients presenting with hyperactive forms of delirium, including psycho-motor agitation, delusions, or hallucinations. It can be given orally or by subcutaneous infusion. Haloperidol should be considered a temporary measure while other strategies such as change in the type of opioid, hydration, or the management of metabolic or infectious complications are introduced. If haloperidol fails to control symptoms, midazolam, which also can be included in a subcutaneous infusion, can be used.

Communication and information

Towards the end of life, patients, their families, and those close to them may have specific concerns that they wish to discuss, or at least express. These may relate to the diagnosis, prognosis, or to particular things that she/he wishes to achieve or resolve before death. The skills needed for effective communication in palliative care include: listening, assessment, facilitation, techniques for handling difficult questions, and self-awareness (see Chapter 7.8, Vol. 1). When they are dying, patients may need more time to express their concerns. Concerns can range widely, but some of the difficult issues may relate to fears about the process of death, how dying will happen, what will happen afterwards. Some people may wish to plan their funerals in advance, but others may not wish to discuss death at all.

Psychological and emotional concerns

All of the emotional reactions found in palliative and terminal care (see Chapter 7.8, Vol. 1) can be found in the patient who is dying. Fear of loss of control can be increased at this time. Fear of dying is a common and normal reaction. Nevertheless, a patient may be particularly upset or concerned by specific aspects of dying, the recognition of which allows the professional to intervene properly. Their fears may be about physical illness and suffering, treatments and their consequences, family, finances, and social status, existential and religious concerns.

In order to understand the emotional process in response to dying, Buckman proposes a three-stage model:

1. The patient faces the threat of death and exhibits a combination of reactions, which depend on his/her previous personality and way of coping.

2. The second phase is characterized by resolution of the initial emotional response. The intensity of emotions may diminish, but depression and withdrawal can be common.

3. The final stage is defined by acceptance of death. Nevertheless, acceptance and full awareness of dying are not essential, especially if the patient is not distressed, has adequate relationships with family and friends, and can make decisions as she/he wishes.

Care of the family

The emotional concerns of family members or carers escalate as death approaches, and they are often more anxious than the patient. Those families most at risk of escalating anxiety are those who have been very anxious before. Other factors include: being a spouse of the patient, a patient diagnosis of breast cancer, young patient age, shorter time from diagnosis, and low patient mobility.[2]

The needs of the family are all too often overlooked; indeed, family members and carers often feel ambiguous about asking for support. A recent study among the family members of patients who were close to death found that many report that they have put their own needs and life 'on hold', but at the same time they recognize that they long for support or a break (Harding and Higginson, personal communication). As for the patient, communication and information about particular concerns or worries is important. It is likely that the family will need some time alone. In some instances, support groups or services have been found to help carers, and practical support and respite are important when patients are at home. Support after the death is considered further in Chapter 17.3.

Euthanasia, living wills, and advance directives

Euthanasia, living wills, and advance directives are being debated in different ways in different countries. Physician-assisted suicide (PAS) has been legalized in Oregon State in the United States and Euthanasia in the Netherlands. PAS was legalized and then the law reversed in the Northern Territories of Australia. Contrary to some fears, data from the United States and the Netherlands suggest that it is younger patients who opt for euthanasia or PAS because of a wish for control and the desire not to be a burden to others. Longitudinal and other studies suggest that the feeling of being a burden on the family, the presence of pain, shortness of breath, and depression are associated with an increased desire for death and in some instances suicide in patients with progressive illness.[3] Concerns must be discussed and if possible problems alleviated. Data on whether advance directives and living wills improve care is controversial, although these are being adopted particularly in the United States.

End-of-life decision-making

Discussions regarding end-of-life decisions are commonly encountered when dealing with dying patients and their families. These can include decisions regarding the withdrawal or withholding of treatment (e.g. chemotherapy, other potentially life-prolonging treatment such as antibiotics or fluids, or cardiopulmonary resuscitation), or choices in place of care and death. It is good practice for health care professionals involved in caring for dying patients to encourage and support discussions regarding patient and family wishes for care at the end of life. This may minimize anxieties and conflicts as death approaches.

Where patients are competent they should always be given the opportunity to be involved in these decisions. A patient may be regarded as competent if they are able to understand the information given to them and retain that information over time, and if there is no evidence of coercion affecting decision-making. In discussions with patients, it is important to be seen to act in the patient's best interests, that is, to provide treatments only if they allow an overall net benefit to the patient.

If a patient becomes unconscious, it is important to establish the family's role and status in decision-making. In England and Wales, and many other countries, proxies have no legal status and the responsibility for decision-making rests with the clinician in charge of the patients care (e.g. the GP or hospital consultant). Where this is the case, it is good practice to involve families in the decision-making process, enabling them to express their views and those of the patient (where known), but the lead clinician must always act in what she/he perceives is the patient's best interest. If possible it is best to try to elicit patient choices whilst she/he is still competent, though subsequently family views can influence decision-making.

Care and death at home

Trends and preferences

Much of the care in the last year of life occurs at home, although there has been an increasing trend towards the hospitalization of death in many countries. In England, during the second half of the twentieth century, deaths in hospital increased and deaths at home decreased. However, during the last decade deaths at home have stabilized and deaths in nursing homes and other settings (including hospices for cancer patients) have begun to replace some of the hospital deaths (see Chapter 17.5 for more details).

A systematic literature review including 15 studies of preferences, in different developed countries, found that between 50 and 70 per cent of patients preferred to be cared for at home for as long as possible and to die at home.[4] Family members often have slightly lower preferences for home care than do patients, and in a few recent studies there has been an increasing preference for hospice care among both patients and families. Health professionals also usually favour home care, although views vary. However, studies have often not included patients from a broad range of ethnic groups or cultural backgrounds, those living in deprived areas, or very elderly patients.

It is important to discuss with patients who wish to die at home, and their families, what equipment and support is available in the community to help facilitate this. Advance discussion of the patient's wishes and end-of-life decisions is needed. It is important to plan for expected, and unexpected, eventualities. This may include the provision of appropriate medication for use by subcutaneous injection or a syringe driver once the patient becomes unable to swallow, appropriate equipment, and occasionally an emergency box if it is anticipated that the patient is at a risk of an acute event, such as haemorrhage. Table 4 provides a planning checklist for a home death.

Factors associated with an increased likelihood of a home death include:[5] younger patient, strong informal carer system, preference for home death, higher socio-economic status, longer disease trajectory, good symptom control, and good advance planning.

Advising families about patient's death at home

The family or carers need to know what to do once the patient dies. This includes calling the physician (usually the primary care doctor) to certify death and complete the death certificate, laying out of the body—relatives may wish to do this in conjunction with the district nurse (or palliative care nurse), but bodies may also be laid out at the funeral directors—calling the funeral director, and registering the death.

If families are unsure of what to do in the event of a patient's death, they will be more likely to panic and call an ambulance in the event of deterioration or death (see Chapter 17.5). Ambulance staff may commence resuscitation, which they must continue until a doctor tells them to stop; this may involve transfer of a body to the nearest Accident and Emergency Department, causing increased distress for all involved.

Long-term planning and opportunities for prevention

The primary care physician needs to have services in place that can respond quickly to the changing needs of those patients within their practice who die each year from progressive illnesses. This will include the professionals, services, and equipment in Table 4. The number of dying patients needing care can be predicted quite accurately, as the sections on epidemiology

Table 4 Checklist of things to consider when planning to facilitate dying at home

Advance care planning and decision-making
Are the patient's wishes for end-of-life treatments and place of care and death known?
If yes, have these been discussed with the patient, family, and health care professionals and recorded in relevant documentation?
If no, is it possible to begin a discussion, at least to ascertain if and to what extent the patient wishes to make decisions, and what role they wish their family and professionals to play?
Have any other end-of-life issues or matters the patient wishes to achieve been considered

Symptom control
Are a patient's symptoms adequately controlled?
If yes, how often do they require review and by whom?
If no, is it possible to optimize symptom control further and where would this best be achieved (home, hospital, hospice)?
What is the most appropriate route of drug administration, e.g. oral, subcutaneous (syringe driver)?
Who will administer medication at home?

Emotional needs
Have you adequately explored all of the patient's concerns regarding home death?
Have you adequately explored all of the family's concerns regarding home death?
What is the patient/family's support network in the community?
Who will support the family?
Is any further psychological support required?

Social needs
What is the patient's accommodation like, e.g. flat, house, stairs, lift access?
Is there space at home for appropriate equipment?
What can the patient do, e.g. self-caring, needing help with personal care?
Who will shop, cook, clean?
Will the patient require any aids/equipment?

Other health care professionals to consider involving in planning home deaths
Specialist palliative care team (hospital ± community/hospice team)
District nurse
Occupational therapist, physiotherapist
Social worker
Home care nursing service, e.g. Marie Curie Nursing Service
Other, e.g. Crossroads, respite nursing team, religious organizations

Equipment to consider
Commode, bath seat, toilet seat
Walking aids, stair rails, stair lift
Hospital bed, pressure-relieving mattresses, hoist

show. Therefore, there is a great opportunity for the primary care team to ensure appropriate plans are in place for their population. As described in Chapter 7.8 (Vol. 1), a specialist palliative care team can often help in caring for patients who are dying, working alongside the primary care physician. These can provide the needed multiprofessional approach, including doctors, nurses, social workers, chaplains, therapists, and psychologists or psychiatrists.

Several levels of prevention are important. Good anticipatory care can prevent problems for patients and families in the short-term. Bereavement outcomes can be improved by good prior care (see Chapter 17.3). In the longer term, a well managed death reduces future fears about death among families and their children. A bad experience of a death results in increased fear and bad memories when another family member suffers from a progressive illness. In addition, this major life event often leads family members to re-appraise their lives. A good experience with health professionals can offer an opportunity for future health promotion contacts, and lifestyle or other changes.

Implications

During the last century, new treatments and social changes have lengthened life and provided treatments for many diseases. While this is a positive development, as a consequence medicine became less and less concerned with care of the dying. At younger ages death may be seen as a rarity, unfair, a tragedy, a problem, something society should strive to prevent; even at older ages it can be seen as something unexpected and unwelcome and much effort and resources are devoted to trying to postpone it. Death is taboo in many societies and in medicine it is commonly seen as failure. These attitudes affect patients, their families, carers, friends and children, and staff in health, social, and other services. The consequences can be that doctors and nurses withdraw from a patient who is dying, fail to make appropriate detailed clinical assessments, or make heroic attempts at curative treatment that increases suffering.

Although death is an inevitable part of life, much of the suffering that is so often endured by patients and families before death is not (see Further reading, ref. 3). Developments in the management of symptoms, and emotional and social problems during the last 30 years has meant that many problems can be alleviated. There is a great need now to make best practice more universally available. Research into the management of many other symptoms and problems has been largely neglected and needs urgent support particularly in community settings. Similarly, continuing education is needed. Patients who have diseases other than cancer, but are dying, often do not receive care from specialist palliative care services; this must be a special priority in general practice.

Social changes mean that our ageing population will increasingly live separately from their children. But the fall in birth rate, leading to fewer people able to provide care, for example, in nursing, in the health professions presents a major challenge. Medical treatments and technologies are changing, and now are more and more geared to increasing survival or improving quality of life, and few treatments are developed that cure, rather than ameliorate disease. Attitudes in society are increasing in favour of greater autonomy and provision of information, and patients obtain information from a wide range of sources. Care of the dying will be part of this debate, although patients at the end of life often have most difficulty in expressing their autonomy and choice.

Key points

- The number of patients who are likely to die in general practice populations and the symptoms and problems they will experience can be predicted.

- Assessment, accurate diagnosis, skilled management, and anticipatory care are the cornerstones to successful management.

- In the dying, there is a need to change gear, review medications, stopping those that are not essential, sometimes changing to subcutaneous routes, and providing excellent nursing care and communication.

- The family and those close to the patient also have practical and psychological needs.

- Home death is a common preference, but requires careful planning and anticipatory care.

References

1. **Teno, J.M.** (1999). Lessons learned and not learned from the SUPPORT project (editorial). *Palliative Medicine* **13** (2), 91–3.
2. **Higginson, I.J. and Priest, P.** (1996). Predictors of family anxiety in the weeks before bereavement. *Social Science and Medicine* **43** (11), 1621–5.

3. Chochinov, H.M., Tataryn, D., Clinch, J.J., and Dudgeon, D. (1999). Will to live in the terminally ill. *Lancet* **354**, 816–19.
4. Higginson, I.J. and Sen-Gupta, G.J.A. (2000). Place of care in advanced cancer: a qualitative systematic review of patient preferences. *Journal of Palliative Medicine* **3**, 287–300.
5. Karlsen, S. and Addington-Hall, J. (1995). How do cancer patients who die at home differ from those who die elsewhere? *Palliative Medicine* **12**, 279–86.

Further reading

Addington-Hall, J.A. and Higginson, I.J., ed. *Palliative Care in Non-Malignant Disease*. Oxford: Oxford University Press, 2001. (First main text book on palliative care for a whole range of non-malignant diseases.)

Cartwright, A. (1996). Dying. In *Epidemiology in Old Age* Vol. 44 (ed. S. Ebrahim and A. Kalache), pp. 408–14. London: BMJ Publications. (Major epidemiological text on dying.)

Foley, K. and Gelband, H. *Improving Palliative Care for Cancer. Summary and Recommendations*. National Academy Press, 2001. (Authoritative summary of main issues and recommendations from the United States.)

Higginson, I.J. (1997). Palliative and terminal care. In *DHA Project: Research Programme. Epidemiologically-Based Needs Assessment* Series 2 (ed. A. Stevens and J. Raffery), Oxford: Radcliffe Medical Press. (The basis for forming epidemiologically based needs assessment, and local palliative and terminal care plans.)

Working Party on Clinical Guidelines in Palliative Care. *Changing Gear. Guidelines for Managing Patients at the End of Life*. London: National Council for Hospice and Specialist Palliative Care Services, 1997. (Evidence-based guidelines for care at the end of life.)

17.2 Pain concepts and pain control in palliative care

Rodger Charlton and Gary Smith

Introduction

This chapter provides basic knowledge in assessing pain, which analgesic to use, the theories concerning adjuvant analgesia, the use of opiates, and non-pharmacological methods of pain control. Most patients respond to pharmacological measures, but on occasions specialist help and other therapies are also required and these are discussed. Most GPs consider palliative care to be a core element of general practice involving patients in their care. On average, a GP will care for about five patients dying of cancer at home each year and also a similar number of patients dying with disease other than cancer. The aim of care for people with life-threatening illnesses is to cure sometimes, to relieve often, to comfort always.

> But pain is perfect miserie, the worst
> Of evils, and excessive, overturnes
> All patience.
>
> (Milton, Paradise Lost)

Pain, and the fear that accompanies it, are common features, in particular of people with incurable cancer. The causes of pain are complex and not purely physical, as it may be modified by coexistent psychological and emotional processes. To control pain, the first priority is adequate communication including explanation, neglect of which will lead to anxiety and fear, which lower the pain threshold.

Dame Cicely Saunders (the founder of the modern hospice movement) stated that pain control in cancer patients should be of a level such that the fear of pain is removed, hence enabling a patient to 'live until they die'. Alleviation and prevention of pain improves quality of life, but also alleviation of associated fear, enhanced mobility, increased appetite, improved sleep, and an increased sense of well-being.

What is pain?

Pain is an extraordinarily complex experience that profoundly affects both the psychology and physiology of the person who experiences it. It involves a combination of sensory, affective, and cognitive dimensions which are unique to each person.

Pain is an unpleasant sensory and emotional experience associated with actual or potential tissue damage, or described in terms of such damage.

Perception of pain

The description of an unpleasant distressing sensation or sensations in one or several parts of the body vary according to the sufferer's reaction to them.

Some centres use body charts, where individual pains may be identified and the effect of analgesia monitored. Unfortunately, there tends to be a discrepancy between the pain subjectively perceived by the patient and attempts at objective charting by the doctor, particularly when the pain is severe. It is the significance of pain to the patient that should be of dominating importance and the analgesia prescribed should be sufficient to allow them to function effectively.

Why treat pain?

Pain is one of the most frightening aspects of dying for many patients and their families. Unrelieved pain causes both physical and psychological suffering and can lead patients to reject active treatment programmes or even to request euthanasia. A sound basis in pain management is the cornerstone of good palliative care; by minimizing pain, we give patients more control over their quality of life and reduce their fears.

Emotional pain

There may often be a psychological component to pain. However, some physicians, patients, and policy makers conceive of illness purely in biological terms. According to this view, social, psychological, spiritual, economic, and legal forces are irrelevant to symptoms and behaviour. And yet, factors such as depressed mood exacerbates pain, not to mention loss of capacity for enjoyment, loss of long-held interests, hopelessness, the loneliness, and isolation of severe illness that must impact on the perception of pain and thus its severity.

All these factors can affect the pain experience and so the 'pain threshold' through tremendous emotional anxiety and anguish. Depression is a predominant aspect of cancer pain occurring in at least 20 per cent of cancer patients.

Teachers of medical students and neuroscience graduate students can unintentionally impart the erroneous assumption that pain is a simple, unpleasant sensation originating in injured tissues. Perhaps, Aristotle's belief that pain is above all else a powerful and demanding feeling state is a more appropriate approach.

Pain management

> Let a sufferer try to describe a pain in his head to a doctor and at once language runs dry.
>
> (Virginia Woolf)

Pain is entirely subjective and, because of this, successful pain management in palliative care requires carefully tailored pain control for each individual patient, as what is bearable to one patient may be insufferable to another. To do this one must

- accurately determine the cause and nature of a patient's pain;
- decide upon appropriate analgesic and adjuvant agents;
- consider other non-medication pain-relief measures;
- frequently reassess pain control and make necessary adjustments.

Pain tends to increase with progression of malignant disease and is often disproportionate in its intensity to the size of a tumour. It also varies according to the location and type of cancer or disease condition. Some diseases are frequently associated with pain, for example, bone cancer, and some are not, for example, leukaemia. Cancer is not synonymous with pain. In general terms, two-thirds of patients with cancer will have pain at some time, but the percentage increases with advanced disease. Also significant numbers of cancer patients (80 per cent with advanced cancer) will have two or more pains. So, assessment should be applied to each pain in order to provide relief.

Assessment

Due to the individual subjectivity of pain, the patient should be the prime assessor of the pain. Patient self-report is the gold standard in pain assessment.

Assessment should include a detailed history of temporal features (onset, pattern, and course); location (primary sites and patterns of radiation); severity using a simple formal assessment tool in the ongoing assessment of pain (e.g. usually measured with a verbal rating scale such as mild moderate, severe, or a 0–10 numeric scale); quality (e.g. sharp, burning, etc.); and factors that exacerbate or relieve pain. Aetiology of the pain should be determined to help in problem-based planning of analgesic therapy.

Pain scoring can be useful in monitoring pain control, with for example, the McGill Pain Questionnaire, although a shortened version should be used for simplicity. Due to the complexity of pain assessment, one should also determine the psychological and social state of the patient, looking particularly for anxiety and depression as these are known factors to affect pain perception.

Several self-report measures assess patients' ability to engage in functional activities where efficacy can be monitored by three basic goals of pain relief:

- ability to sleep through the night undisturbed by pain;
- pain-free at rest during the day;
- pain-free on moving.

Understanding and appropriately treating a patient with pain, whether acute or chronic, requires an accurate assessment of the tissue damage and the many factors discussed that can influence a patient's subjective experience.

Pain control options

This is an essential part of pain management. Patients and their families should be counselled carefully about the range of pain relief options. Actively involving patients with regular and open communication in their own care reduces fear and thereby enhances effectiveness in pain control. This should include explanation of the various methods of pain control therapies available to them, including pharmacological and non-pharmacological techniques. Details of efficacy and side-effects should be emphasized, exploring their understanding and anxieties so that they do not feel helpless or out of control. This will promote trust, allowing for more effective care in the future.

Making decisions

Knowledge of the benefits and burdens associated with each therapy through open communication will enable informed consent about these issues.

Box 1 Types of pain

- Somatic pain—tissue injury
- Visceral pain—from the viscera
- Neuropathic pain—nerve damage

Types of pain

Three physiological processes are identifiable and often co-exist (Box 1).

Somatic pain

Somatic pain occurs due to the activation of nociceptors by what is presumed to be continual tissue injury. This includes bone, joint, and muscle. Bone pain is generally caused by metastases, and is usually well localized and severe in nature. By far the most common tumour in the production of bone pain is breast cancer. Management of bone pain may require a number of different therapies as it is only partially responsive to morphine and other opioids. Commonly, treatment involves NSAIDs, radiotherapy, bisphosphonates, and occasionally orthopaedic intervention.

Visceral pain

Visceral pain arises from the nociceptors of internal sympathetically innervated organs within the body cavities. It is often poorly localized, dull, aching pain and difficult to describe, often referred to dermatomes of the same nerve root. It may be associated with unpleasant sensations such as bloating and nausea. Usually, it will respond to conventional opioid analgesics although in some cases invasive nerve block techniques may be indicated.

Neuropathic pain

Neuropathic pain originates from malignant or chemical nerve damage. It can cause dull aching pain as well as sharp excruciating or burning pains. Neuropathic pain responds poorly to opioid drugs, unless they are given in high doses, which may bring about unnecessary sedation. This indicates a need for other therapies such as adjuvant drugs, tricyclic antidepressants in low doses, anticonvulsants in low doses, and corticosteroids.

The coexistence of these three processes can be a source of confusion in the objective assessment of the pain.

Breakthrough pain and incident pain

Breakthrough pain describes transient pain that is not relieved by the normal daily dose of medication. Thus, it 'breaks through' regular analgesia. Breakthrough pain indicates that the current level of daily analgesia is inadequate and needs increase.

Incident pain is the transient pain associated with voluntary actions such as walking or sitting up. A rescue dose may be prescribed for incident pain analgesia, which should be administered before the pain provoking activity is undertaken. However, this may be the most difficult pain to control pharmacologically without unacceptable side-effects, and may require other approaches where possible.

Which analgesic?

Analgesics may be divided into three categories: non-opioid, weak opioid, and strong opioid, where opioid means any naturally occurring or synthetic drug, whose effects are counteracted by the morphine antagonist, naloxone. The pain suffered by palliative care patients is continuous and for this reason analgesia should be prescribed prophylactically using a regular regime in accordance with duration, drug action, and formulation. This should be explained carefully to the patient, who may otherwise wait for pain to come back and so make control more difficult.

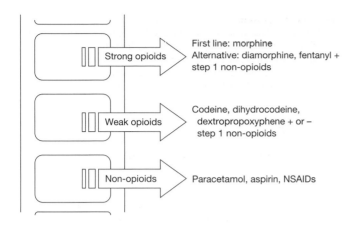

Fig. 1 World Health Organization analgesic ladder.

A useful principle to apply when prescribing to palliative care patients is that the total number of drugs given should be as few as possible and regularly reviewed and rationalized. The patient at home should be supplied with a sheet or card clearly stating which tablet is to be taken and when. In addition, for older patients, those who are forgetful or have impaired vision, dosset boxes or medidose containers, of which many types are available, should be used to separate tablets for each day of the week and time intervals during the day, for example, morning, lunch, tea, and night-time.

The World Health Organization 'analgesic ladder' is widely accepted as sound basis for pharmacological intervention to pain control (see Fig. 1). It describes how analgesic treatment should progress through the three steps from non-opioids, to weak opioids, and on to strong opioids according to the type and severity of pain.

The analgesia prescribed should not necessarily move up the ladder in a stepwise progression, starting with non-opioids and moving up until pain is controlled. Instead, the step of the ladder chosen should be decided according to pain assessment and one's own judgement. There is now general encouragement to begin treatment with opioids at an earlier stage. This is preferred to trying a number of different non-opioid analgesics to control pain. In a climate forever altered by the convicted ex-GP, Harold Shipman, who murdered patients through morphine overdose, acceptance of opiate use by patients and carers is only going to be achieved if those advocating it have a good evidence base.

Non-opioid

The first step is administration of a non-opioid, for example, paracetamol. Its singular advantage is a relative absence of side-effects and it may be given 6 hourly. Furthermore, it is available in tablets or a soluble form and 125 mg suppositories for children. Paracetamol is also useful as an antipyretic and for headache, which often responds poorly to opiates. Side-effects are unusual at recommended doses. All other analgesics have potential or actual side-effects.

The other important non-opioid analgesics are the non-steroidal anti-inflammatory drugs (NSAIDs). These are particularly useful for mild to moderate pain or for bone pain uncontrolled with paracetamol. These work by blocking the cyclo-oxygenase pathway, stopping prostaglandin production. Prostaglandins are released in tissue damage and they sensitize and activate nociceptors. Side-effects associated with NSAIDs include gastrointestinal bleeding and ulceration, and very rarely kidney damage. A good example of an NSAID is ibuprofen, which should be taken with food to minimize gastric side-effects. Concomitant medication may be required to prevent gastrointestinal haemorrhage on NSAIDs. A similar approach should be considered with the elderly and therapies including steroids and warfarin.

Box 2 Adjuvant medication

- Psychotropic medication—where fear is prominent
- Tricyclic antidepressants—if neuropathic pain is present
- Corticosteroids—for nerve compression, and for its adjuvant effect on appetite, mood, and analgesia

Weak opioid

For pain uncontrolled by non-opioids, the second step in the ladder is weak opioids, for example, dextropropoxyphene, codeine phosphate, and dihydrocodeine tartrate. If any of these are given in combination with paracetamol or NSAIDs, this will give additive analgesia, but less dose-related side-effects due to reduced dose of the opioid. These combinations produce co-proxamol, co-codamol, and co-dydramol, respectively. However, all three can cause drowsiness, nausea, and constipation and the patient should be warned of these (see section on Side-effects).

Adjuvants

At any step of the analgesic ladder, an adjuvant to the analgesic may be added, although these drugs tend to be administered after opioid therapy has been optimized. This is any drug whose primary indication is other than for pain. However, in combination with an analgesic, an adjuvant may enhance its effect or become analgesic itself in certain conditions (Box 2).

Anticonvulsants

Anticonvulsants, such as carbamazepine and gabapentin, reduce the spontaneous activity in dysfunctional neural afferent pathways. They are effective in non-malignant neuropathic pain, usually reducing the sharp excruciating pains.

Tricyclic antidepressants

Tricyclic antidepressants, such as amitriptyline, inhibit the uptake of endogenous noradrenaline and serotonin. These are effective in treating persistent neuropathic pain. The effective doses required for analgesic effects are much smaller than those used in the treatment of depression; their analgesic effects have been shown to be independent of any effects on mood and begin to take effect within 48–72 h, rather than the 10–14-day timescale of antidepressant action. Side-effects of tricyclic antidepressants include constipation, urinary retention, sedation, and postural hypotension, but most reduce with time.

Corticosteroids

Many studies have been performed using corticosteroids as adjuvant analgesics. However, the way they work in this situation is largely unknown, but their effects can be dramatic. They are not beneficial to all patients, but are worth considering in patients with persistent pain as a result of advanced cancer or nerve compression. Their additional advantages are in creating a feeling of well-being, reducing anorexia, and malaise and so improving quality of life. However, their disadvantages can be severe including skin breakdown (bed sores), candidiasis, infection, peptic ulceration, and hyperglycaemia. Dexamethasone is the drug of choice as it is seven times as potent as prednisolone and thus fewer tablets are needed to be taken. A suggested starting dosage of 8 mg daily may be tried and this may be reduced or increased according to response. Most palliative care centres use a once daily morning dose except in high-dose regimes for brain tumour oedema where divided doses may be required. In either case the last dose should not be given in the evening as it can cause insomnia. In addition, benefit is unlikely to be long-term, so dose reduction is important in patients with prognosis of a few months in order to reduce side-effects. Also if no therapeutic effects occur after a week at 8 mg, it is probably not worth continuing.

Psychotropic drugs

To control pain it is sometimes necessary to control the associated anxiety and psychotropic drugs may be used. Useful drugs for this purpose are methotrimeprazine and diazepam. Methotrimeprazine may be especially beneficial through its antiemetic effect if nausea or vomiting are present. Diazepam is also useful for associated muscle spasm. Both, however, may cause drowsiness. In the long-term, spending time with the patient, listening to their concerns, and if available, recommending a patient support group may be just as beneficial and sometimes more.

Strong opioid

When stronger opioids are needed to control pain, morphine and its derivatives should be considered as the next step. Roughly 80–90 per cent of pain due to cancer can be relieved relatively simply with oral analgesics and adjuvant drugs. Initiation of morphine should be given with careful explanation and that it is not the 'end', as this is what it is often associated with, but rather a very effective analgesic.

Oral morphine

Oral administration of drugs is the preferred route, with morphine still the gold standard. When prescribing these drugs in step three of the analgesic ladder, it is important to overcome the notion that there is a dose limit. There is little risk of addiction or tolerance. This is borne out in clinical practice with palliative care patients who do not take morphine for its euphoric effect and can be maintained on the same dose for many weeks. They seldom experience withdrawal when it is stopped, if it is no longer required. If a higher dose is required, it is likely to be due to the natural progression of cancer and so increased pain. This information must be fully shared with the patient.

The prescriber must also be reassured that oral morphine has been repeatedly shown in clinical practice not to depress respiration, even in patients with chest disease, despite a theoretical risk. (Pain is the physiological antagonist of opioids' depressant effect.) This also applies to parenteral morphine, provided the patient has already been on oral morphine. It is often beneficial where dyspnoea is encountered. The dose should be increased gradually and the patient not given a large initial dose, unless it is required to treat overwhelming pain. However, an exception exists if pain is suddenly relieved, for example, through a surgical procedure.

Dose titration

The *starting dose* is chosen according to the pain severity, age, and previous analgesia used. For example, 5–10 mg of morphine may be given if weak analgesics such as co-proxamol were being used or 10–20 mg if stronger analgesics such as co-dydramol were being used. Particular care should be taken in those with decreased renal function.

Ideally, the first dose should be given by mouth if the patient's condition allows. Each day the pain control should be reassessed and the total dose of morphine used in the last 24 h including 'rescue doses' used should be calculated. This dose should then be divided by six and this provides the 4-hourly dosage required for the next day. The *rescue dose* should then be adjusted accordingly. If the patient has refused to use rescue doses then titration requires the dosage to be increased by 30–50 per cent. The increase should be made if breakthrough pain is experienced regularly and

the patient reassessed frequently. This enables the practitioner to titrate the lowest possible dose required to alleviate the pain fully with minimum side-effects. Titration is usually performed with normal release morphine elixir, which has an effect within 20 min and reaches peak effect in about 60 min. Modified release morphine does not achieve its peak effect for at least 4 h and can be as long as 8.5 h when using once daily treatments. These are inadequate for titration purposes.

Once the dose is established, the patient should be converted to one of the modified release morphine preparation such as MST Continus (twice daily) or MXL capsules (once daily). The same total daily dose is required, but should be given as one when using MXL capsules and divided by two, for each dose if using MST Continus (Table 1).

Once a 12 or 24-hourly regime is established, breakthrough pain must be alleviated with a short-acting morphine preparation of tablets or elixir. The dose for *incident pain* and *breakthrough pain* is one-sixth of the total 24-h dosage. The patient should then be regularly reassessed and the 12 or 24-hourly dosage increased, as opposed to increasing the frequency of administration. The increase in dose will vary from 30 to 100 per cent of the original dose and will depend upon the severity of pain and how much additional morphine has been required for breakthrough pain where the background dose is insufficient and so not lasting for the 12- or 24-h period. This may not apply, however, to incident pain that may be momentary, for example, walking to the shops. In this way the lowest necessary dose may be calculated.

Subcutaneous diamorphine

The preferred alternative route of oral administration is usually subcutaneous infusion. A change in route of administration may be necessary for a number of reasons:

- persistent nausea,
- vomiting,
- difficulty swallowing,
- drowsiness,
- unable to cooperate,
- excessive quantities of tablet or liquid required for a dose.

It is important to avoid painful intramuscular 4-hourly injections and a continuous subcutaneous infusion should be considered.

This may be delivered through a *syringe driver*—a small battery operated infusion pump, which is used to deliver the medication to subcutaneous tissues. The injection site should be changed every 2–3 days to avoid skin irritation. Diamorphine is most commonly used because it is about 10 times more soluble than morphine and so there is little restriction on the dose than can be delivered through the syringe driver. When converting from an oral to a parenteral preparation the relative potency is 3 : 1 whereas subcutaneous diamorphine is one-third of the 24-h dose of oral morphine.

A conversion table is helpful to relate the different preparations (Table 2). The formulations listed in Table 2 are approximate equivalents. Note, however, that these are approximate only, and that patients should be carefully monitored and doses may need to be adjusted according to response, particularly when patients have been taking longer-acting opioids that may be still active.

Table 1 Morphine preparations for cancer pain management[1]

Normal release	12-h release	24-h release
Oramorph liquid[a]	MST Continus tablets	Morcap SR capsules[b]
Sevredol liquid	Oramorph SR tablets	MXL capsules[b]
Sevredol tablets	Zomorph capsules[b]	

[a] Contains alcohol.

[b] Contains gelatin.

Table 2 Conversion table

Formulation	Strength (mg)	Total dose in 24 h (mg)
Modified release morphine once daily	180	180
Modified release morphine twice daily	90	180
Oral morphine solution 4 hourly	30	180
Subcutaneous diamorphine over 24 h	60	60

If required, a bolus loading dose of diamorphine prior to commencing subcutaneous diamorphine (of 60 mg over 24 h) in a syringe driver is 10 mg. This level of dose (one-sixth of the 24-h dose) may also be given for breakthrough pain. It is kinder to give this subcutaneously, rather than IV or IM.

Very often patients will require other drugs to be administered concomitantly through the syringe driver (see Chapter 17.1 for more information). Special caution should be taken to ensure drug compatibility. It is important to review this situation regularly if further adjustment of dose is required.

Transdermal fentanyl

Fentanyl is a synthetic opioid that is up to 100 times more potent than morphine. It is a powerful μ-receptor agonist. Due to its lipid and water solubility, it is able to permeate the skin allowing it to be used as a transdermal patch. The patch requires replacement every 72 h. Fentanyl can take about 6–12 h to take effect and is suitable for the control of stable pain.

Fentanyl may lead to reduced constipation in many patients previously on oral morphine. The patch size of fentanyl is related to the number of micrograms it delivers per hour. Further analgesia may be needed for rescue doses in the case of incident pain.

A 25-μg fentanyl patch over 72 h is roughly equivalent to 90 mg of oral morphine over 24 h. However, this can have a range of approximate equivalence from 30 to 135 mg of oral morphine over 24 h. For a person who has not had fentanyl previously, caution in relation to potential side-effects should, therefore, be considered. If converting a patient from morphine to fentanyl, no gap in therapy is required and for a short time a short-acting morphine may be continued until fentanyl takes its effect. However, if converting from fentanyl to morphine, the morphine should not be commenced until the patch has been taken off for 8–12 h. If there is uncontrolled pain in the situation, specialist help should be sought.

Side-effects

Palliative care patients will seek to strike a balance between good pain relief and the desire to avoid troublesome side-effects (Box 3). In many cases, they are willing to tolerate pain to avoid these, particularly those affecting the central nervous system. Individualization of the dose is the key principle in opioid therapy. The goal is to achieve a favourable balance between analgesia and side-effects through gradual adjustment of the dose.

Nausea and vomiting

Nausea and even vomiting may be a problem initially and can be treated with a suitable antiemetic such as metoclopramide. Some patients experience drowsiness initially, but this will wear off after a few days.

Sedation

Drowsiness and confusion may occur in the first few days of opioid use, and effects are increased with concomitant use of other drugs. The symptoms may also occur in patients who have been stabilized on a dose of morphine and have had palliative radiotherapy or chemotherapy. The resultant reduction of tumour size and these symptoms indicate that the dose of morphine needs to be reduced.

The patient may also suffer from a dry mouth and should be informed educated about the need for good dental hygiene.

Constipation

The usage of opiates always induces side-effects such as constipation and this must be anticipated by prophylactic prescription of stool softening and bulking agents such as lactulose, as well as stimulant laxatives. Bowel habit must be discussed when reviewing a patient's analgesia. Unlike nausea and drowsiness, this is likely to be an ongoing issue and requires regular review.

Caution should be exercised in patients with renal or hepatic failure, where a smaller dose is required and it can often be reduced by 50 per cent. Caution is also required in the elderly. Opioid dose should be titrated against the patient's pain. If patients are failing to achieve pain control from the opioid despite increasing doses and yet are experiencing side-effects, then the reasons for this must be explored. It may be that the pain is poorly responsive to opioids and co-analgesics or other therapies will play a more important role.

Problems with opioids

Addiction is not an issue in palliative care. Tolerance may occur but more often reflects increased pain as previously mentioned. Respiratory depression is a theoretical but not a practical problem (Box 4). The most common side-effects are related to gastrointestinal function (constipation, nausea, and vomiting) and neuropsychological function (somnolence and impairment of cognition).

Opioid toxicity may present as subtle agitation, seeing shadows at the periphery of the visual field, vivid dreams, visual and auditory hallucinations, confusion, and myoclonic jerks. It should be pointed out that patients may experience hallucinations with one opioid but not another, and occasionally with different formulations of the same opioid—so consider changing opioid if problems occur, or formulation if the analgesia is effective.

Negative attitudes to using morphine still exist and many patients express fears, for example, fear of addiction in about one-third of patients. Ethnic minority patients might not be receiving acceptable doses of opioid analgesia because of the social stigma attached to their use. Physicians need to communicate more effectively regarding opioids.

Non-cancer pain

The use of opioids in the treatment of non-cancer pain is controversial. Many GPs have anxieties about initiating modified release morphine in suitable patients. This is an effect of the strict regulations surrounding the prescription of these drugs in the past and fears over their addictive nature, which is in reality minimal, with a risk of addiction estimated at less than 4 per cent.

Evidence now suggests that opioid therapy should be initiated in non-cancer pain sufferers when all other attempts at reasonable analgesia have failed. However, if it becomes clear that a patient receives no subjective improvement in pain control, or suffers further deterioration in daily function, then they should not continue with the therapy. This is an area where training, gaining experience, and seeking specialist support is important.

Specialist therapy

A wide variety of specialist treatments must be considered when pain is difficult to control and it is resistant to the analgesics and adjuvants described in the three steps of the analgesic ladder.

Box 3 Side-effects of opioids

- Initially in some patients—nausea and drowsiness
- Always constipation—administer with a laxative
- Morphine elixir has a bitter taste

Box 4 Fears and myths about morphine

- Risk of addiction and tolerance
- An upper dose limit
- Depression of respiration
- A last resort used only in the last 24 h of life
- It can never be stopped

Anaesthetics

Most pain can be controlled by the means outlined. However, on occasions, the pain attributed to nerve compression or damage may be better treated with an anaesthetic block. It may be that the first-line treatment with opioids causes persistent drowsiness and clouding of consciousness but not a complete alleviation of the pain.

Local anaesthetic or neurolysis may be used to block a peripheral nerve or sympathetic nerve block, for example, a coeliac plexus block in the case of pancreatic carcinoma and other upper abdominal malignancies.

Cordotomy is useful in treating unilateral pain which is well localized. It can provide effective analgesia to areas of opioid resistant pain in two out of three patients if carefully selected. Pain relief using this method seldom lasts longer than 1 year.

Epidural and intrathecal opioid administration decrease central nervous system reception and transmission of pain signals and achieve excellent analgesia. The dose of opioid required to produce effective analgesia using these methods is very low and so reduces side-effects. The use of these methods requires skilled practitioners, usually pain clinic anaesthetists.

Radiotherapy

Radiotherapy is considered the most effective oncological treatment in relieving pain. In particular, it may be used to treat the severe and often sudden onset and specific pain of bony metastases, and when used in this context produce few side-effects. It can be useful before pain becomes severe, especially in patients with a poor prognosis, for example, lung cancer, where repeat treatments are unlikely to be required. Bisphosphonates can also be considered to provide pain relief and reduce fracture rate for bony secondaries.

Radiotherapy may also be used as an emergency in:

◆ the case of cord compression, to preserve vital neurological function;

◆ in superior vena cava obstruction.

Chemotherapy

While used less frequently than radiotherapy, chemotherapy also has a role in pain relief. It can be used to reduce tumour mass in chemosensitive tumours and reduce pressure on surrounding tissues, which is causing pain, for example, in locally recurrent head and neck cancer or liver secondaries in breast cancer.

Endocrine therapy

Endocrine therapy is used in the treatment of breast and prostate cancer. It is well tolerated but slow response rates mean that it may be ineffective for pain control in the short-term. However, it is very useful for palliating the disease in the long-term.

Surgery

Surgery may also be considered, such as a bypass procedure for intestinal obstruction or fixation of a pathological fracture.

Non-pharmacological and complementary therapy

Such therapies include hypnotherapy, hydrotherapy, homeopathy, special diets, and faith healing. Aromatherapy and massage have been shown to reduce anxiety and pain scores in a randomized trial. Two therapies commonly available from pain clinics or specialists are transcutaneous electrical nerve stimulation (TENS) and acupuncture. These are usually used in treating short lived or fluctuating pain.

TENS

TENS may be used at pulsed low frequency (1–2 Hz) for neuropathic pain or continuous high frequency (40–150 Hz) for somatic pain due to tissue damage. Initially, as many as 80 per cent of patients may respond and there are few side-effects. It is applied using surface electrodes connected to a small portable battery to stimulate large diameter nerves in the skin. However, after a year of treatment, only 35 per cent of patients still derive benefit from TENS.

Acupuncture

Here, a mildly painful stimulus is administered through a fine needle at carefully defined acupuncture points to relieve pain. Acupuncture has been shown to be a useful approach to pain relief in western medical practice and is, of course, widely used in other cultures. Its effectiveness is reliant on the availability of a local skilled practitioner.

Team approach to pain

Many members of the health care team should be involved in treating pain, as well as doctors and nurses, to provide care that encompasses the physical, psychological, social, and spiritual aspects of suffering. An occupational therapist may be able to improve quality of life and regain function through the use of aids and physiotherapy may increase mobility and reduce the pain caused by stiffness. A psychologist may help a patient to develop coping skills, reduce fear and anxiety, which can decrease the pain threshold. A member of the clergy may be useful in helping to deal with an individual who appears to be expressing spiritual pain or need.

Conclusion

Failure to achieve pain control may be due to many reasons, which are not necessarily physical. There may be failures of communication or assessment. Review may be too infrequent to treat the recurrence of pain and the patient may have unresolved emotional, psychological, or spiritual conflicts. Pain control should not be seen as an insurmountable challenge, but a rewarding aspect of medical practice in improving the quality of life of those patients with pain as a result of progressive incurable disease.

Acknowledgements

Thanks to Dr Mandy Barnett, Consultant in Palliative Medicine, Coventry, and Senior Lecturer, Centre for Primary Health Care Studies, University of Warwick, for her specialist advice and comments regarding this chapter.

Key points

◆ Pain involves a combination of sensory, affective, and cognitive dimensions, making it unique to each individual.

◆ Determine the cause and nature of a patient's pain and then decide upon appropriate analgesic and adjuvant agents.

◆ Opioid dose should be titrated against a patient's pain.

◆ Consider non-medication pain relief measures, for example, acupuncture, TENS.

◆ Treatment of a patient's pain should involve many members of the health care team, for example, physiotherapist, occupational therapist, psychologist.

◆ Pain control can be a rewarding part of medical practice.

Reference

1. Faull, C. (2000–2001). Palliative care: pain control and other aspects. In *Members' Reference Book*, pp. 227–8. London UK: Campden Publishing Ltd.

Further reading

Forbes, K. and Faull, C. (1998). The principles of pain management. In *Handbook of Palliative Care* (ed. C. Faull, Y. Carter, and R. Woof), pp. 99–133. Oxford: Blackwell Science Ltd.

O'Neill, B. and Fallon, M. (1997). ABC of palliative care: principles of palliative care and pain control. *British Medical Journal* 315, 801–4.

Sykes, J., Johnson, R., and Hanks, G.W. (1997). ABC of palliative care: difficult pain problems. *British Medical Journal* 315, 867–9.

Portenroy, R.K. and Lesage, P. (1999). Management of cancer pain. *The Lancet* 353, 1695–700.

Virik, K. and Glare, P. (2000). Pain management in palliative care. *Australian Family Physician* 29, 1027–33.

Scottish Intercollegiate Guidelines Network and Scottish Cancer Therapy Network. *Control of Pain in Patients with Cancer*. Edinburgh: SIGN, 2000. (http://www.sign.ac.uk).

Shannon, C.N. and Baranowski, A.P. (1997). Use of opioids in non-cancer pain. *British Journal of Hospital Medicine* 58, 459–63.

McQuay, H. (2001). Opioids in chronic non-malignant pain. *British Medical Journal* 322, 1134–5.

17.3 Bereavement and grief

Victoria H. Raveis

Bereavement, experiencing the death of a loved one, is a universal occurrence. It is also a particularly potent and stressful life event. Death represents a multifaceted challenge for the survivors, who must deal with their grief over the loss of their loved ones, adapt to the social and economic readjustments emerging from the death, and come to terms with changes in self-identity resulting from their loss. Bereavement and loss in palliative care are pervasive occurrences. An understanding of what constitutes normal grief and an appreciation of the special circumstances of bereavement in palliative care may aid clinicians in attending families facing the impending loss of a loved one.

Overview of the grief process

Grieving has been conceptualized as a process comprising a series of stages or phases consisting of: numbness, searching and pining, depression, and recovery.[1] In the immediate period following the death, even if the death has been anticipated, the bereaved is usually in a state of shock, feeling numb, and experiencing disbelief over the event. Cognitions may be impacted and the bereaved may experience a sense of confusion and have difficulty concentrating.[2,3] During the acute grieving period, these initial responses give way to intense feelings of loss and longing for the deceased. It is not uncommon for the bereaved to experience a sense of the deceased's presence or auditory or visual hallucinations about the deceased.[3] The bereaved may also exhibit restless behaviour, revisit places that relate to the deceased, and treasure or revere objects belonging to the deceased.[3,4] As the realization of the loss becomes more evident, the bereaved may experience frequent crying spells, have difficulty sleeping, withdraw from other people, show little interest in outside activities, and experience a loss of appetite.[1–3]

For recovery or resolution to be achieved, it is necessary that the bereaved: (a) accept the reality of the loss (i.e. face the reality that the person is dead, will not return, and that reunion is impossible);[1,3,4] (b) acknowledge and work through the emotional and behavioural pain associated with the loss;[3] (c) adjust to an environment in which the deceased is missing[2,3] (for the widowed this involves coming to terms with living alone, facing an empty house, and managing finances alone); and (d) withdraw emotional energy from the deceased and reinvest it in other relationships.[2–4] While there is debate as to whether these stages are experienced in sequence and without overlap, it is widely acknowledged that even in situations of uncomplicated grief, the process of grieving occurs gradually over time. Individuals vary at the rate at which they progress through these stages or phases of grief. Most bereaved return to a normal level of functioning 1–2 years after their loss.[5]

Symptoms of grief

Individuals who are grieving can exhibit a constellation of psychological and physiological reactions of varying intensity and duration.[1,3,5] The emotions most commonly expressed include shock, numbness, sadness, anxiety, loneliness, fatigue, anger, relief, and guilt. It is also commonplace for bereaved individuals to experience somatic complaints such as weakness, lethargy, loss of appetite, tightness in throat or chest, shortness of breath, and sleeplessness.

Grief-related distress is generally highest the first year following the loss, although elevated rates of distress can persist for more than 2 years following the loss.[5] Increased distress is often associated with the anniversary of the death or with significant events previously shared with the deceased, such as birthdays or wedding anniversaries.[4] While there can be much individual variation in how grief is expressed, normal or uncomplicated grief is distinguished from pathological or complicated grief by the duration and intensity of these psychological and physiological reactions. Pathological grief may be chronic (indefinite prolongation of grief), inhibited (partial or distorted expression of grief), or delayed.[1]

Bereavement in palliative care

In palliative care, grief and bereavement are inexorably tied up with the losses experienced during the illness and the dying process. The terminal period of an illness is an extremely stressful and particularly vulnerable time for families of dying patients. While bereavement is usually the specific event that precipitates the grieving process, for deaths that occur in the context of palliative care, a variety of circumstance occurring prior to the death are likely to impact the grief experienced. Foremost is the fact that often in palliative care, death can be anticipated. Advance knowledge of the death provides an opportunity for the survivors to prepare for the impending death and for the palliative care team to intervene preventively to reduce adverse bereavement outcomes.

Anticipatory grief

Anticipatory grief is the process whereby survivors begin grieving prior to the death. This process permits rehearsal of the bereaved role and the initiation of working through the emotional changes associated with a death.[6] It is believed that anticipatory grief mitigates the intensity of the grief reaction following the actual death and leaves the survivor less vulnerable to maladaptive reactions. However, the evidence on the adaptive value of being forewarned that a death will occur is inconsistent.[7] While some studies have found that bereaved who have had opportunity for anticipatory grief adjusted better to their loss, others have found no differences. The beneficial value of being able to anticipate and prepare for a death may be lessened by circumstances leading up to the death (e.g. extensive caregiving), which may impede the bereaved's ability to initiate preparations for the death or deplete their resources for coping with this impending loss.

When death is preceded by a chronic illness, survivors will have experienced a variety of losses that will also need to be mourned. These losses include altered relationships, changes in lifestyle, the forfeit of future dreams that will never be realized, as well as losses related to illness-induced changes (i.e. progressive debilitation, increasing dependence, and excessive pain).[6] At the same time, the multiple stresses and demands the illness and its treatment have imposed on the survivors increase their risk for morbid bereavement outcomes.

Caregiving

A factor in palliative care situations that may adversely impact on the grieving process is the family's involvement in the patient's care.[8] The family often becomes a care-partner with the health care team and performs a vital role in providing informal support and assistance to the ill relative. While the benefits to the patient of familial caregiving are readily apparent, this care provision is not without cost to the care providers. The gains of forewarning of the impending death may be counteracted by the stresses emerging from the caregiving situation. Financial stress, neglect of their own health, physical and psychological exhaustion from providing care, and the social isolation resulting from restricting outside activities to carry out caregiving responsibilities are some of the routine consequences endured by families providing illness-related support and care. In addition, during the final illness period, families often direct all their energy and attention towards tending to the patient, thus delaying or inhibiting any advance psychological preparation for the death. As one spousal caregiver related: 'I have to take care of him. I'm the one that's going to do it. I've resigned myself to keeping and doing as much as I can for him. Keep the level and quality of his life at a certain peak, and live with it. And I'll deal with it, and my loss and my despair, ultimately. Right now, I'm not going to wallow in what's coming. I have a job to do'.

Protracted illness

The duration of the terminal illness may also mitigate any benefits derived from advance forewarning of the death. Researchers have found that bereaved relatives whose loved one suffered a long, lingering illness actually adjusted more poorly to bereavement than those whose loved one died after a short illness.[8] These differences may be due to the impact of providing informal support and care during an extended illness and the stresses of living with a protracted illness. These consequences are illustrated in the comments made by the wife of a patient who survived a series of cerebral haemorrhages over a 2-year period: 'This pattern of alive, not-alive, is very difficult to cope with. It's gone on for too long and it tires one out. It's like a slow leak. I'm completely exhausted'.

Cause of death

The illness and its disease trajectory are additional factors that can impact bereavement reactions. Conditions that impact on the patients' functioning and quality of life, such as severe, chronic pain, are particularly difficult for family members. It is distressing to observe a loved one suffering, but this strain is exacerbated when families also feel helplessness in alleviating or managing the conditions. In such situations, the bereaved can experience more severe grief reactions post-death.[1] The anguish families experience is reflected in the words of one woman anxiously contemplating her husband's impending death: 'As long as he lingers without his knowing it, or having the pain, I'm not afraid. I'm only afraid if he's going to be conscious, experiencing whatever . . . It's his being in pain, and seeing him, and, I have to do something for him to put him out of that pain'.

When death is from an illness that is stigmatized or associated with unhealthy or socially unacceptable lifestyles, such as alcoholism or drug abuse, the bereaved may experience conflicting emotions or encounter difficulty resolving their feelings about the deceased. The family may be less open about the cause of death or the circumstances leading up to the event. Support to the bereaved may be less forthcoming. In communicable illnesses such as HIV/AIDS, the bereaved may be infected as well and are, therefore, confronting issues related to their own mortality. They may also be dealing with multiple deaths or the serious illness of several members of their social network. In these contexts, the bereavement process can become more complicated.

Vulnerability factors for adverse grief reactions

The clinical and research literature on bereavement suggests a constellation of individual and situational factors that are likely to affect the course and outcome of the grieving process.[1,5,9,10] The bereaved's pre-existing physical health condition, history of substance abuse, and/or premorbid mental illness can contribute to adverse bereavement outcomes. Personality characteristics, such as low self-esteem or a low internal sense of control, are also associated with increased distress post-death. Men are at higher risk for bereavement-related mortality; women experience more affective distress. Limited financial resources pre-death or declining income as a consequence of the death can precipitate problems in grieving. Deficits in social support or restricted social resources can also contribute to adverse grief outcomes.

The nature of the loss is another important factor. The death of a spouse is considered to be one of the most stressful life events, although the loss of a child is regarded as particularly problematic for the survivor to resolve. A high level of dependency or an ambivalent relationship (feelings of love/hate, need/resentment) between the deceased and the bereaved often culminates in a severe grief reaction and difficulty in accepting and resolving the loss. Vulnerability to poor adjustment is also increased by the occurrence of additional severe stresses concurrent to the bereavement, such as multiple losses or concurrent life changes. Prior losses, if they have not been successfully resolved, may need to be worked through before resolution can be achieved regarding the current bereavement. Sudden death or death following a long-term illness are also associated with problematic outcomes for the survivor, as are stigmatized, violent, or untimely deaths.

The distribution of these vulnerability factors frequently clusters, creating subgroups at increased risk for morbid outcomes. Older bereaved spouses are an example of a vulnerable group. Although death is more anticipated in the elderly, the survivor envisions less of a future, and has less motivation to suffer the pain of mourning and relinquishing the spouse. In addition, old age is a time when stressful life events converge and physical illness and disability are more likely. Spousal death may follow closely upon other deaths or losses (e.g. retirement, change in housing) still being mourned. Social networks and support systems are constricted as well. As a consequence, widowhood can have especially adverse economic, social, and psychological ramifications for older adults and bereavement reactions may be severe.[8]

Health-related consequences of bereavement

Bereavement can predispose people to physical and mental illness, precipitate suicide and death, and aggravate existing health conditions.[5] The recently bereaved have been shown to display an increased incidence of depressive symptoms and somatic complaints, as well as manifest changes in their endocrine, immune, and cardiovascular systems. They have higher rates of utilization of medical and mental health care services (i.e. increased hospitalizations, prescribed drug use, and physician and mental health clinician visits). For some individuals, bereavement is not a transient life crisis but can have enduring negative consequences. For example, it is associated with an increase in behaviours that can be injurious to health, such as alcohol or substance abuse. An excellent review of the epidemiological evidence of bereavement-related health consequences can be found in Osterweis et al.[5]

Presentation of the bereavement-related problems in primary care

The impact of bereavement-induced depression and/or somatization on the health care system can be considerable. Based on findings from the National Hospice Study, researchers have estimated that among the approximately 216 000 bereaved spouses in the United States annually who are depressed, the health care utilization that accompanies bereavement-related depression may represent an excess of 648 000 physician visits during the first year of bereavement.[11] Bereavement-related somatization can also result in inappropriate hospitalizations, tests, and surgeries, particularly among the elderly.

Patient and family as the unit of care in palliative settings

It is important to acknowledge that family members are not just a part of the patient care team, but are also impacted by the illness and the impending death. The delivery of palliative care offers the health care practitioner opportunity to attend to the well-being of affected family members prior to the patient's death. Clinicians can make an effort to address the informational, emotional, and practical support needs of the family without diverting primary attention from the care and management of the dying patient. Such efforts may make the dying experience less stressful for the family, facilitate their grieving, and reduce their risk of adverse bereavement outcomes. Supporting the family members during this period will also enable them to remain actively involved in assisting the care team in meeting the patient's needs.

Enable open discussion of illness and death-related concerns

The palliative care team should be available and willing to address family concerns about the patient's condition and care. Reassurance that therapeutic and ameliorative measures are being utilized appropriately to care for the patient will comfort families and reduce the potential for future guilt. Encouraging open communication and facilitating opportunity to discuss emerging concerns will prevent survivors from later engaging in self-recrimination or regrets about how these events should have been handled, facilitating their grieving process.

Provide emotional support

Supporting survivors' grief work in the terminal phase of the illness is a means of facilitating adjustment after the death. In palliative care situations, most families are aware of the nature of their relative's condition and its prognosis. Families experience a diverse range of feelings (e.g. anger, sadness, regret, resentment, or guilt) regarding the illness and loss of function in their relative, the consequent burdens they are required to assume, and the impending death. They may also feel isolated and alone. Families need to be given permission to express their feelings and be reassured that these feelings are normal. Some individuals may benefit from individual or group counselling or peer support groups during this period to normalize their experiences and support their grief. Many palliative care programmes provide access to some type of supportive counselling or include a mental

health or pastoral counsellor as part of the care team. Referral to existing lay or professional support services in the community may also be beneficial. Once a death occurs, the family's contact with the health care team often ceases abruptly. The impact of the loss of this source of emotional support can be eased by a condolence card or brief sympathy call from a member of the care team.

Facilitate practical assistance

The family may benefit from assistance by the palliative care team in ensuring that any issues related to the dying patient's finances and legal matters are attended to and that procedures for adhering to the patient's preferences for care at end of life are established (e.g. advance directives, health care proxy). Families often become very involved in the dying patient's care, neglecting their own health and setting unreasonable expectations of what they expect to be able to accomplish. It is common for families to isolate themselves, curtailing outside activities, afraid to leave the patient for any length of time. The palliative care team may need to advocate for families setting limits on their personal efforts, and encourage them to respect and attend to their own needs. Arranging for respite services, where they are available, or suggesting ways to mobilize other network members, with the goal of reducing the care burden on the family, are means of facilitating needed practical assistance. The families' perception of the adequacy of practical services available during the period of terminal illness is another factor that can contribute to their bereavement adjustment.

Respect cultural, ethnic, and religious practices

Religion and culture can exert a significant influence on the way loss is perceived and experienced. Mourning rituals provide for the sanctioned public articulation of private distress and reaffirm the bereaved's solidarity with the group.[5] Clinicians need to become aware of any special needs or requirements associated with the mourning rituals practiced by the bereaved, so as to ensure that the circumstances at the time of death will permit adherence to these customs and practices. The inability to properly perform these rites may complicate the grieving experience for the bereaved family.

Management of bereavement-related problems

Health care professionals need to be aware of the lay and professional resources available in the community for those bereaved who are in need of and desire support. Implementing screens for vulnerability factors during case review or family conferences may be a means of assisting the bereaved in the context of routine health care. Most bereaved individuals will not require mental health treatment. However, persistent depressive or somatic symptoms that do not lessen in intensity over time, prolonged social withdrawal, expressed difficulty adjusting to the loss, and/or engaging in health-endangering behaviour, such as drug or alcohol abuse, should trigger referral to a mental health professional for evaluation.[5]

Pharmacologic treatment of bereavement reactions

Antidepressants, tranquillizers, and sedatives are often prescribed to lessen the intensity of a variety of persistent and severe bereavement-related reactions (e.g. depression, anxiety, sleeplessness) that impair functioning and exacerbate the bereaved's distress. While it may be clinically indicated to intervene pharmacologically to remediate intense bereavement-related reactions, such treatments warrant discretion. Medically suppressing the grief experience may lead to adverse consequences later. There is an absence of clinical evidence on the short- and long-term benefits and consequences of medication use on the grief process.[5] In prescribing medications, clinicians need to consider also the heightened potential for alcohol abuse in bereaved populations.

Supportive services and bereavement programmes

Bereavement services can reduce grief-related physical and mental symptoms and improve the quality of life of the bereaved.[5] A variety of treatment modalities have been developed to help the bereaved adjust to their loss. These include services provided by trained clinicians; services in which volunteers are selected, trained and supported by professionals, such as the 'Widow-to-Widow' programme in the United States; and self-help or mutual support groups in which the bereaved help each other, with or without professional supervision. Cruse Bereavement Care, a national charity in Great Britain, offers counselling, information, and social support groups to bereaved individuals throughout the United Kingdom. Most professionally administered bereavement programmes focus on facilitating grieving, as well as providing support and practical assistance. Informally organized mutual support or self-help groups provide friendship and the special empathy of shared status. Hospice programmes routinely offer families pre- and post-death support services, although there is great variability in the type and extent of bereavement services provided.

Many grief specialists recommend intervening pre-death with the family to prevent pathological responses to the death.[1,3,4,6] Research on bereaved widows and hospice programmes indicate the value of supportive services during final illness stages.[1,5] The advantage of preventive interventions initiated pre-bereavement is that they can prevent problems in mourning from developing, while programmes implemented after a death occurs can only attempt to remedy the difficulties after the event.[6] Oftentimes, bereavement support programmes initiated during the terminal illness period, such as those provided through hospice programmes, continue into the post-death period. A post-death programme component is useful because a number of issues regarding reactions and adjustment to the loss cannot be effectively raised before the death or dealt with during the terminal phase of the illness.

Preventive bereavement-focused services provided on the basis of a predetermined set of risk criteria have been shown to be beneficial in reducing adverse bereavement-related outcomes in vulnerable populations.[1] Given the scarcity of supportive services and the cost of this type of care, targeting those who are in need and can benefit from the support is cost-effective as well. In this regard, screening tools have been helpful in identifying individuals in need of services. Parkes' bereavement work with St Christopher's Hospice in London, England, is an early example of implementing such an approach. Hospice nurses at St Christopher's completed the Index of Bereavement Risk, developed by Parkes and his colleagues,[1] on the family member most affected by the patient's impending death. Those who scored 'high risk' were then offered a bereavement support programme that Parkes introduced at the hospice.

Summary

Clinicians involved in primary care are often in contact with families who are approaching or have experienced bereavement. These families are at a point of heightened vulnerability. In time, most bereaved do make a successful psychosocial adjustment to their loss. The provision of emotional support and compassionate care by the health care team during this stressful period may facilitate families' grieving process and reduce adverse bereavement consequences. An understanding and appreciation of the individual and situational factors that inform the bereavement process will also aid clinicians in determining when professional intervention is indicated.

Key points

- Grieving is a process comprised of numbness, searching and pining, depression and recovery.

- Grief is expressed with a constellation of psychological and physiological reactions.

- Bereavement predisposes people to physical and mental illness, and precipitates death.

- Individual and situational factors increase vulnerability to adverse bereavement outcomes.

- Services and support can reduce adverse symptoms and prevent pathological responses.

- Benefits of anticipatory grief mitigated by care provision, illness duration, and cause of death.

- Patients and families are the unit of care in palliative setting.

- Palliative care team should provide support, facilitate assistance, and respect mourning practices.

References

1. **Parkes, C.M. and Weiss, R.S.** *Recovery from Bereavement.* New York: Basic Books, 1983.
2. **Shuchter, S.R.** *Dimensions of Grief: Adjusting to the Death of a Spouse.* San Francisco CA: Jossey-Bass Publishers, 1986.
3. **Worden, J.W.** *Grief Counseling and Grief Therapy: A Handbook for the Mental Health Practitioner* 2nd edn. New York: Springer, 1991.
4. **Raphael, B.** *The Anatomy of Bereavement.* New York: Basic Books, Inc, 1983.
5. **Osterweis, M., Solomon, F., and Green, M.,** ed. *Bereavement: Reactions, Consequences, and Care. A Report of the Institute of Medicine, National Academy of Sciences.* Washington DC: National Academy Press, 1984.
6. **Rando, T.A.** (1986). Understanding and facilitating anticipatory grief in the loved ones of the dying. In *Loss & Anticipatory Grief* (ed. T.A. Rando), pp. 97–130. Lexington MA: Lexington Books.
7. **Siegel, K. and Weinstein, L.** (1984–1985). Anticipatory grief reconsidered. *Journal of Psychosocial Oncology* **1**, 61–73.
8. **Raveis, V.H.** (1999). Facilitating older spouses adjustment to widowhood: a preventive intervention program. *Social Work in Health Care* **29** (4), 12–32.
9. **Sanders, C.** *Grief: The Mourning After Dealing with Adult Bereavement.* New York: John Wiley and Sons, Inc, 1989.
10. **Vachon, M.L.S., Rogers, J., Lyall, W.A., Lancee, W.J., Sheldon, A.R., and Freeman, S.J.J.** (1982). Predictors and correlates of adaptation to conjugal bereavement. *American Journal of Psychiatry* **139** (8), 998–1002.
11. **McHorney, C.A. and Mor, V.** (1988). Predictors of bereavement depression and its health services consequences. *Medical Care* **26**, 882–93.

Further reading

Kelly, B., Edwards, P., Synott, R., Neil, C., Baillie, R., and Battistutta, D. (1999). 'Predictors of bereavement outcome for family carers of cancer patients.' *Psycho-Oncology* **8**, 237–49. (Prospective study identified clinical risk factors in familial caregivers for adverse bereavement outcomes that could be assessed in palliative care programmes. Findings describe a potential basis for palliative care programmes to intervene preventively to enhance familial caregivers' outcomes.)

Zisook, S. (2000). 'Understanding and managing bereavement in palliative care.' In *Handbook of Psychiatry in Palliative Medicine* (ed. H.M. Chochinov and W. Breitbart), pp. 321–34. New York: Oxford University Press. (Comprehensive discussion of the multidimensional approach to bereavement and review of the clinical literature on grief. Provides an overview of current approaches to the treatment of grief. Contains an extensive reference list.)

17.4 Death of a child

Kimberley A. Widger,
Vincent E. MacDonald, and Gerri Frager

The challenge

A primary care physician may be faced with:

◆ a distraught couple who have been enthusiastically awaiting their newborn and deliver a stillborn infant;

◆ a call from a school about a 10-year-old child acting out following the death of his younger sister from an unusual inborn error of metabolism;

◆ a father with a previous history of depression exacerbated by his 6-year-old son's accidental death;

◆ a 14-year-old who presents with somatic complaints mirroring the nausea and vomiting that she witnessed throughout her best friend's treatment for ultimately fatal osteogenic sarcoma.

What is expected? What is unusual? How can the parents, siblings, and others impacted by the death of a child best be supported by their physician?

The birth of a child adds new meaning and purpose to the lives of parents, and when a child dies, the parents experience a life storm like no other. Siblings are affected by the death compounded by how the parents cope with and grieve the death. Grandparents grieve both for their grandchild and for their own children whom they could not protect from the pain of losing a child. Other family members as well as peers of the deceased child and of the siblings also grieve the loss. The impact of the death of a child is great and affects many different people in many different ways. The focus of this chapter is on the role of the family physician in supporting parents and grieving children following the death of a child. Chapter 17.3 deals with more general aspects of bereavement. Statistics on childhood deaths in developing and developed countries are presented to promote an understanding of the scope of the issue. Suggestions for the assessment, management, and continuing care of grieving parents and children are presented along with the long-term implications of the experience of the death of a child. Requiring a realistic scope, the focus for this chapter is on the developed countries and a general, practical approach to lessen the distress of those impacted by a child's death.

Demographics and epidemiology

The typical practising physician may consider the likelihood of encountering a situation involving the death of a child to be very low. Relative to deaths in the adult population, particularly in developed countries, deaths in the paediatric population are far less numerous.

Throughout the world, greater than 11 million children younger than 5 years of age die each year. Malnutrition contributes to more than half of the deaths in developing countries where infections assume a prominent role, with pneumonia, diarrhoea, malaria, and measles accounting for close to 4.9 million deaths. In the past 20 years, nearly 4 million children have died worldwide from HIV and AIDS. In typical developed societies, perinatal factors head the causes with approximately 3 million foetuses and infants born each year with major congenital malformations. US statistics for childhood deaths mirror the pattern for the developed world whereby congenital abnormalities, prematurity, and infection initially predominate (from 0 to 1 year of age), changing to cancer, accidents, and homicides (from 1 to 14 years of age) followed by accidents, homicides, and cancer (14–19 years of age). The number of deaths that occur before a live birth, as in stillbirths, second trimester terminations, and spontaneous abortions, are not included in childhood death statistics. They do, nevertheless, represent a considerable degree of parental suffering, often largely unrecognized and poorly supported by their family, friends, and community, including health care professionals.

The illnesses causing childhood deaths in developed countries are notably diverse with regards to the type of the illness and compounded by the variability imposed by age and developmental stage. For example, muscular dystrophy may seem like three different entities when considering the physical aspects and needs of the child and family at the time of diagnosis initially as a toddler, as an 11-year-old child with progressive motor impairment, and then as a wheelchair ambulant young man requiring assistance for his personal care. Disease progression in the growing child is a pattern largely reserved for developed countries where children are afforded the opportunity to grow older through such interventions as artificial nutrition via a feeding tube or frequent antibiotic administration.

Canadian statistics have estimated that for every death, approximately five more individuals are significantly affected. When the death is that of a child's, the impact is vast. For the parent, grief following the death of a child is known to be profound, far-reaching, and long lasting. This depth of parental grief holds true whether the parent is 90 and the child is 70 or the parent is 30 and the child is 4.

Grieving parents

Assessment

The grief experience after the death of a child is never static. The parent wonders how they will be perceived, how they will be understood, and how they will fit back into the larger community. Initially, the parent lives through a filter of confusion and uncertainty, a world inconceivable to others not directly impacted. It is important for health care professionals to have some understanding of a bereaved parent's pain.

A conversation may begin with open-ended questions or statements such as 'Tell me about your day/week'. 'What has it been like for you since the death or funeral?' 'Can you tell me about what you have been through lately.' If the physician did not know the child, the parent could be asked to talk about who their child was, and what that child meant to them ('Tell me what Scott was like.'). Effective listening skills can be used to help a bereaved parent feel safe enough to tell his/her story. Listening skills include minimizing interruptions, being aware of non-verbal behaviour (eye contact, posture, facial expressions, tone of voice), paraphrasing ('I hear you saying . . . '), asking clarifying questions ('Can you tell me more about . . . '), and interpreting feelings ('It sounds as though you feel . . . '). Avoid saying 'I know how you feel' as this statement minimizes the parent's experience.

Manifestations of grief

Initially, bereaved parents may experience shock and denial, even if the death was anticipated. This reaction can protect parents from confronting the death of their child without being overwhelmed. These grief reactions, although a part of a normal process, can lead non-grieving people to believe that the parents are either holding up well or are incapable of expressing feelings. The initial grief reactions of disbelief, confusion, restlessness, numbness, shock, and feeling helpless may last for days, weeks, or even months. While some parents express their feelings, others may suppress theirs because the pain may feel too difficult to manage. This difference is not an indication of the degree of the parent's pain, or the amount of love they had for the child, but rather is a different coping style. A mother and father will often have completely different styles of coping with grief and may find it difficult to understand and support each other. Thus, parents should be told that they each might grieve differently. As Chapter 17.3 shows, bereaved individuals may swing from one state to the other, varying the process both within individuals and in time. This has been referred to as the dual process of coping with bereavement, where one approach is aligned with confronting the loss and the other seeks relief through concepts and activities focused in areas other than the loss. The grieving individual copes by moving between the two approaches.[1]

Components of assessment include: the parent's relationship with the child, the circumstances of the death, previous experiences with death, availability of support systems, the parents' personality and emotional health, religious or cultural backgrounds, and the gender of the survivor (women may be seen as more expressive in their grief relative to men). The typical grief reactions of parents will be varied and influenced by many of these factors.

When grief may be complicated

Difficulty with grief, previously labelled pathologic grief, is often referred to as complicated grief. It is important to identify those individuals who may be at risk for complicated grief in order to provide more regular assessments of how the parent is doing and make referrals as needed. A parent may be at risk for complicated grief when there is:

◆ a history of family abuse, violence, or addictions, which could result in poor coping or problem-solving skills;

◆ inadequate support systems (i.e. friends, family, spouse/partner, or faith communities);

◆ previous mental health or psychiatric problems (i.e. depression, anxiety, or psychosis);

◆ history of multiple losses or unresolved losses;

◆ ambiguous losses, where there is uncertainty about a child's return or the absence of a body as evidence of death (i.e. a missing child who is presumed dead);

◆ any loss in which the relationship with the child was persistently problematic, ambivalent, conflicted, or dependent (i.e. a single mother caring for her chronically ill and only child);

◆ inadequate parental understanding of their own ability to solve problems or resolve issues, or having little or no hope that their life will ever be better;

◆ benefit for not resolving their grief, perpetuating a pattern of seeking attention and sympathy;

◆ an inability to share grief publicly (i.e. a teenage mother who miscarries but had not told others of her pregnancy);

◆ an unresolved litigious situation involving an accident or murder, preserving details of the death in the parents' minds.

Specific signals may indicate that a bereaved parent is having difficulty with the death of their child.[2] Each signal should not be taken in isolation as indicative of complicated grief. Rather, the presence of persistent signals in the setting of poor functioning in all aspects of life warrants concern. The signals include:

◆ years after the death of their child, a parent still experiences fresh and intense grief when the child's name is mentioned;

◆ minor events or news events trigger apparently intense and exaggerated grief reactions;

◆ long after a child has died, conversations consistently focus on death, pain, or loss;

◆ long-term depression, guilt, anger, insomnia, or anxiety;

◆ avoidance of funerals, memorial services, visitations, or the attendance or participation in any death-related rituals;

◆ alcohol or substance abuse;

◆ parents who meticulously maintain their child's bedroom in the exact same condition for years or those who quickly and completely redecorate the child's room and remove all traces of the child from their lives warrant extra vigilance in follow-up.

It is often difficult to make a clear distinction between normal grief responses and clinical depression, and to know when healthy functioning has returned. Table 1 presents examples of common emotions, thoughts, behaviours, and physical symptoms for each situation.

Management

Bereaved parents need to have validation of their myriad emotions and the life and death of their child. There may be a tendency to minimize the impact of the death of a profoundly cognitively impaired child, by referring to the death as 'a blessing' or 'a relief' for the parent. Parents may see these references as devaluing the life of their child (i.e. this child was not worth as much as a normal child was) and minimizing the profound grief that the parent will likely experience.

The pain of a grieving parent may be very painful for another person to listen to and to be present for. It is natural to want to try and find fast relief for the distress, such as prescribing medications. But the use of medication to treat grief may obstruct the working through of the grief. Grief creates a state of physical and emotional exhaustion and while sedatives, tranquillizers, or antidepressants may be calming, there must be care not to delay, mask, or short-circuit the grief process. It is alright for parents not to be alright. The parents need to be reassured that they are not going crazy when

Table 1 Parental grief responses

	Normal grief	Depression	Signs of healing
Affective	Feelings of anger, guilt, and sadness Feelings are openly expressed	Feelings of helplessness or hopelessness Feelings of anger, guilt, or sadness are generally reflected back to themselves and may be masked	Able to enjoy humour without feeling guilty Can talk about child without being overwhelmed Minimal anxiety, irritability, or crying spells
Cognitive	Thoughts focused on the child's death Decision-making skills may be limited Forgetful	Poor self-worth Little or no hope for the future Unable to make decisions Absence of coping skills	Looks forward to future events Able to think of things other than the child's death Able to problem-solve and make decisions Able to concentrate, less forgetful
Behavioural	Able to both share and withdraw from emotional pain Minimal socialization Less participation in previously enjoyed activities	Do not initiate contacts or interactions No enthusiasm for life or life's pleasures	Able to be with and enjoy friends Can effectively parent surviving children Can complete the tasks of daily living Involved in meaningful activities
Physiologic	Intermittent somatic symptoms Temporary or periodic disruption in sleeping or eating habits	Persistent somatic symptoms Chronic disruption of sleeping and eating patterns	Able to pay attention to personal appearance Feeling rested with more energy Sleeping and eating without difficulty Absence of drug or alcohol use as a way of coping

they think they see their child in the mall or hear his/her voice on occasion, for example. In order to get *through* the pain of the loss a parent must be allowed to experience it. The use of medication may be appropriate when used to reduce anxiety or to regulate sleep that has become disturbed and irregular but they do not take away the pain of grief.

Grief has been described as the inner feelings of pain and loss, while mourning is the outward expression of that grief.[3] A bereaved parent can be assisted through their grief by creating a safe environment in which mourning can occur. Wolfelt has identified six needs of mourning central to the process of healing and these are discussed in the context of the death of a child.

1. *Acknowledging the reality of the death.* Slow and gentle confrontation that their child has died and will never physically come back to life is one way the parent comes to acknowledge the full reality of their loss. This process may occur over weeks to months. The parents may want to tell the story of their child's life and death over and over again in order to make the events seem more real, and to acknowledge the fact that the child is gone. The physician should allow time to meet with the parent on a regular basis and actively listen to the story without judgement. This requires time and a longer than usual office visit should be allocated whether for a specific bereavement follow-up visit or for a medically focused visit. Optimal scheduling of the appointment should take into account that these visits may be emotionally draining for the physician. It may be helpful to start the visit by advising the parent of the length of time available to meet. As the allotted time ends, one might say: 'In the few minutes we have left, is there anything else you would like to raise that we haven't talked about? We can talk for a few moments now and then address that issue further at the start of our next meeting'.

   In addition to these follow-up visits, it is advisable to offer a scheduled visit approximately 3 or more months following the child's death with the intent of 'debriefing' with the parents and older siblings. This meeting serves the purpose of probing for unresolved concerns and answering remaining questions. As well as reviewing and clarifying circumstances related to the death, this time presents an opportunity for the physician to air emotional burdens relating to questions of delayed diagnosis, the decisions made about various treatment options, and other management. There may be some aspect of culpability best addressed through sensitive and honest exploration. Such an approach may require the physician to *first* conduct a somewhat painful but necessary and mutually beneficial reflective self-examination.

2. *Feeling the pain of the loss.* It is natural for parents to not want to experience this pain. It is easier to avoid, delay, or deny the pain. Physicians can learn to listen to the parent's thoughts, emotions, and experiences without judging or trying to eliminate the pain. People often rely on old clichés to explain a death or comfort a parent. Clichés may make the person who said them feel better, but tend to minimize the importance of the parent's unique grief and his or her need to mourn. Simply saying a heartfelt 'I'm sorry' or 'I care' can be very supportive and may help to create a healing relationship.

3. *Remembering the person who died.* Parents continue a relationship with their child through their memories. Precious memories are remembered in dreams and through objects such as photos and other symbols that embrace the physical aspect of the relationship with the dead child. With time, many parents rely less on these external representations of their child and more on an internal image of their child. Families appreciate when the physician speaks about the deceased child using his or her name and shares his/her own memories of the child.

4. *Developing a new self-identity.* Parents change with a child's death, as it is impossible to stay the same. The parent of an only child who has died may struggle with whether they are still considered a parent. Parents can be encouraged in their exploration of this new identity but be cautioned to take their time (i.e. not pursue a pregnancy, career change, or relocation immediately after the death).

5. *Searching for meaning.* Bereaved parents may question the meaning and purpose of life. Parents ponder what life will be like without their child. Feeling empty, they may be faced with finding meaning in going on with their lives. The death of a child may be pivotal to how bereaved parents live their lives (e.g. after her child's death one mother went on to found MADD—Mother's Against Drunk Driving). They need to feel that they and the world are richer because their child lived. Discovering a new life's purpose can be a very difficult task and may take many years. Some will lose their faith or spirituality and others will strengthen or find new faith as they search for an answer to the seemingly unanswerable question— 'why my child?' Unfortunately, these questions are unanswerable, so none need be attempted. Clichés such as 'It was God's will' are not helpful.

6. *Receiving ongoing support from others.* The healing of parental grief takes place best in a supportive community comprised of family, friends, colleagues, faith community, and health professionals. Healing is not done alone. Because mourning is a process that takes place over time, support and encouragement for bereaved parents to mourn continues for months and years after a child's death.

Most parents can cope with the death of their child with the support of people around them, including their family physician, who are able to listen to and respect their pain, say the child's name, honour stories and memories about the child, and comfort the bereaved parent with gestures of kindness and presence. Parents have related that alternative activities such as journalling, painting, poetry, or other creative expressions provided relief, as one parent stated, 'I could no longer find words'. Familiar places that provide comfort and happy memories that include their child are also of benefit.

A grief counsellor may be able to assist with a parent who is having difficulty in coping with the 'typical' grief experience. Grief counselling often involves providing some education about the grief process, problem-solving, and decision-making. Parents may also receive some advice about their own unique concerns and feelings. A support group can be helpful for some parents to receive grief counselling and support from other parents who have been through similar experiences. Grief therapy with a trained professional, on the other hand, is indicated when a parent is experiencing complicated grief as outlined in the section on Assessment.[4] Local palliative care or hospice services, health centres, community agencies, or spiritual centres may be the best resources for knowing the availability of local community supports.

Continuing care

Bereaved parents will always hurt. They never get over or recover from the death of a child. The parent will always be a bereaved parent. In continuing to support grieving parents, sending a card at the anniversaries of the birth and death of the child or on the date that the child would have been born in the case of a miscarriage, is very much valued by the parent. In a busy office, 'thinking of you' cards may be sent out by support staff on behalf of the office. Periodic phone calls at these same times or others are also greatly appreciated, quite disproportionate to the small expenditure of effort.

A common misperception is that divorce is more common in couples who experience the death of a child. A recent survey on behalf of Compassionate Friends (a bereaved parent support group) found that 72 per cent of parents were still married to the person that they were married to at the time of their child's death. While parents need to understand that they will likely grieve differently from their spouse and they may need to make extra effort to keep communication lines open, losing a child does not mean that their marriage is destined to fail. The divorce rate in bereaved parents may in fact be lower than that of the general population.[5]

Grieving children

Assessment

The grief of children can often be overlooked or forgotten. However, the death of a child impacts on a number of other children directly or indirectly connected with that child. The children impacted may include siblings, cousins, friends, classmates, schoolmates, and particularly in small communities, every child in the community may be affected by the death of a child. The family physician should be aware of the impact on a number of other children in the practice. A proactive approach should be taken to touch base with these children and their families and to give parents some guidance on how to identify problems and support their children in grief. It may be practical for some offices to provide this guidance as written material mailed out to the families with an invitation for follow-up.

Manifestations of grief

The emotions that children experience in their grief are similar to those of an adult—sadness, anger, guilt, fear, relief, etc. A child is different in that he/she is often unable to verbally express those emotions. Instead, the emotions are evident through art or play activities or changes in behaviour. Typical expressions of grief in a child include: dwelling on things he/she used to do with the person who died, being disruptive in school, inability to concentrate, appearing unaffected at times by the death, declining or improving grades at school, physical complaints, eating or sleeping disturbances, regressive behaviour, and increasing risk-taking behaviour. Children are very good at taking time out from their grief, which may lead others to believe that either they are coping well or are not grieving at all.

Some factors may alert a physician to be particularly watchful of a child affected by the death. Such factors would include death through murder or suicide, a death that the child played some role in (i.e. a child playing with a gun who accidentally shot his sibling), multiple deaths, or other factors similar to the parent risks for complicated grief.

Identifying signs indicative of complicated grief

Most children will handle their grief with the love and support of their peers and adults around them. It is important to be aware of signs that a child is having more difficulty with their grief and to seek professional counselling for the child. The red flags include:

♦ destructive or negative behaviour that is persistent or recurrent;

♦ disturbing changes in behaviour;

♦ suicidal thoughts or actions;

♦ persistent denial in a developmentally appropriate child that the death occurred;

♦ persistent somatic complaints after any other cause has been ruled out;

♦ depression.

Management

A child's understanding of death

A child's depth of understanding of death will depend on his/her previous experiences with death, verbal ability, ethnic and cultural background, religious beliefs and practices, and exposure to the popular culture and the media. Table 2 lists the understanding that a typical child of various developmental ages would have about death.[6] This is only a guide and children should be assessed individually. Just as with talking to adults, it is important to start by asking children what they know, or think about all that has been going on around them (i.e. 'Can you tell me what you know about what made your sister so sick?'). Pacing is important with children. If they have questions, it is important to find out exactly what they are wondering about before launching into a long answer (i.e. a child who asks 'What happens to the body?' may simply want to know how it gets from the hospital to the funeral home or how cremation is done, rather than the spiritual aspects related to death). It is important to use accurate language. For example, referring to death as 'being like sleep' will make it difficult for a young child to understand that unlike sleep, death is permanent, and may cause the child to have difficulties going to sleep for fear of never waking up. It may be helpful to provide an opportunity to talk with the child on their own as a parent may be too overwhelmed with their own grief to realize that their surviving children are suffering. Also, a child may not volunteer his/her distress for fear of upsetting the parent.

Supporting children through their grief

While it is important for a physician to be involved in supporting a grieving child, it is also important that a child be supported in their home environment by the people who are with them on a regular basis. The family physician may best be involved by helping parents to support their children and to interpret a child's behaviour as part of normal grief. The physician may be asked for advice on such things as whether or not to take children to funerals. Every child over the age of 2 or 3 years can be given the option of attending the funeral. It is important that the funeral be explained in terms of who will be there, what will happen, what they will see, and what they will hear. The child should be told about the options for not attending the

Table 2 Children's understanding and support

Developmental age	Understanding of death	How to support
0–2 years old	Aware of loss through separation Experiences the world through the senses Affected by emotions of caregivers	Provide an article of clothing or toy from sibling as linking object Maintain usual routines and consistent caregiver
2–6 years old	Views death as a reversible event Associates death with external causes such as a car accident or 'the bogey man' Tends to have 'magical thinking' May feel guilty/responsible	Provide honest answers to questions, but do not give more information than they are really asking for Allow for repeated questions Written resource: Prestine, J.S. (1993). *Someone Special Died*. Fearon Teacher Aids, Torrance, California
6–12 years old	Understands that death is permanent but may believe it only happens to others Younger child: associates death with external causes of death Older child: aware of internal (i.e. illness) and external causes of death Often wants the 'gory' details of the death	Provide honest information Encourage normal activities Involve in family rituals related to death Model appropriate ways of expressing grief Written resource: Brown, L.K. and Brown, M. (1996). *When Dinosaurs Die*. Little, Brown and Company, Boston
Adolescent	May consider themselves invincible But . . . aware of universality of death Fairly adult-like understanding	Provide honest information Allow 'space', but also include in family rituals Encourage expression of emotions without judgement Ensure availability of peer support Written resource: Dower, L. (2001). *I Will Remember You*. Scholastic Inc., New York

funeral (i.e. staying with a neighbour). Wherever the child is, they need a support person with them who is not actively grieving, to be available to take them out of the funeral if they need a break, or to bring them to the funeral if they change their mind. Children can be encouraged to participate by making a card or necklace or writing a letter that can be placed into the coffin or given a special place in the home.

Table 2 also lists interventions that may be useful for supporting children of different developmental ages. Generally, children need to be allowed to ask questions repeatedly and have them answered honestly. They benefit from being encouraged to create and be involved in rituals, to act out their feelings through play or art, and to have fun, even when mourning. Wolfelt[3] suggests that children of any age have the same mourning needs as adults and can be supported in similar ways to meet these needs. A physician's office can be stocked with a few stuffed toys, puppets, crayons, and paper as useful media for communication. Children are more likely to enter into a conversation about how they are feeling indirectly through a puppet than directly with an adult. Children can be encouraged to draw pictures while the physician talks to the parent. The pictures provide a great opportunity to ask the child questions about what is happening in the picture.

Children may experience physical symptoms in response to their grief including headaches, abdominal pains, fatigue, lack of appetite, shortness of breath, or general nervousness. All physical complaints should be taken seriously and a history and physical examination completed to rule out any specific cause. A child may have misperceptions about the cause of another child's death or may believe that he/she may be dying if they have similar symptoms. Hearing from a doctor after a complete examination that they are in fact healthy may help to alleviate fears. Young children often have magical thinking whereby they believe that wishing someone dead or not being a 'good boy' can cause someone's death. Offering experiences that other children have had may help a child open up about such 'unspeakable' thoughts (i.e. 'I know some children who have a sister die worry that something they said or thought or did, made that person die. Then pause for their response, prompt with 'I wonder if you ever had any worries like that?' After waiting for their response, follow with 'We know that your sister died because of her cancer and the doctors just could not make her better. I really want you to know it had nothing to do with anything you did or thought or said.').

The way a family grieves and copes with a death impacts greatly on the way a child will grieve and cope with a death. Children look to others for cues on how one is supposed to grieve. Encourage the family to be open and honest about the death (children's imaginations can create scenarios far worse than the most difficult situations), to freely bring up the name of the person who died, to talk about family stories that include the deceased child, to have happy times together, and to demonstrate and discuss the emotions that family members are feeling. Let parents know that it is alright to cry in their children's presence provided the child is not burdened with that grief or forced to assume the role of comforter on a consistent basis.

Continuing care

Children will often 'revisit' a death as they reach new levels of maturity and ability to understand past events. It is normal for intense sadness to recur for the child during special events, which would have been shared with a sibling, such as graduation or marriage. On the other hand, when a child seems to cope very well with a death and then years later demonstrates typical grief behaviours, it may be that the child did not feel safe enough to grieve until his/her parents had moved on enough in their own grief. By this time, family members and teachers may not attribute the behaviour to the death. In this situation, it is important that the child receive additional support from a counsellor to deal with delayed grief.

Implications

The potential sequelae of grief run large and deep. It is known that grief will impact on the parent and surviving child's capacity to work, play, and

interact. Physicians may need to advocate for the parents in their workplace or for siblings at their school.

The gaps in the understanding about bereavement following a child's death are significant as much of what is known about complicated bereavement relates to adults impacted by the death of adults. Bereaved parents have highlighted the helpfulness of having access to their physicians, being provided with medical information, general support, assistance with confronting denial, and counselling related to their grief.[7] Bereaved children are known to consult the primary health team more frequently than their age-matched controls.[8] Somatic complaints, a frequent manifestation of grief in bereaved children, were noted to be significantly impacted upon by a bereavement support group.[9] However, there is an overall paucity of studies looking at outcomes from interventions to prevent or treat the sequelae of complicated grief following a child's death.

The personal impact of a child's death

Physicians need to be aware that supporting a grieving person may increase memories of their own losses and raise apprehensions regarding any potential losses. For example, a physician with an infant of his/her own may become hyper-vigilant about checking that child when faced with a parent who recently lost a child to Sudden Infant Death Syndrome. As a physician giving care to a bereaved parent or child, it is also important to give care to oneself through caring and supportive relationships both at home and at work. A receptive work environment may enable a physician to discuss the circumstances and personal impact of a death with a colleague. The importance of setting and maintaining realistic limits on the support provided to an individual bereaved parent or child needs to be recognized. It is an unattainable goal to try and extinguish another person's grief, but by listening and nurturing self and the bereaved parent or child, a physician can make a difference.

The potential to 'do good' in the face of tragedy

The primary care physician, who provides support and follow-up to all those in their practice, is alert to those at risk for complicated grief, and knows when to refer for additional help is a truly valuable resource. The approach can be modified and enhanced by incorporating the results of future research documenting the beneficial outcomes of specific interventions. Although not without personal impact, the caring physician will welcome these opportunities of being able to do good in the time of life's great tragedies. One of life's great mysteries is that even in the face of profound pain, there is growth. As stated by a bereaved parent speaking of her adult daughter's death 8 years ago, 'Although a part of me had died, another came to life in ways that I never would have dreamed possible'.

Key points

1. A bereaved parent is forever a bereaved parent regardless of their age or their child's age.

2. There are many patterns of grief. The difference between normal and complicated grief relates to the degree and duration of distress and level of function in all spheres of life.

3. Children can be helped by guiding the family to be honest, talk about the deceased child, and model and share their emotions.

4. Children tend to express their emotions through activities in art or play, facilitated by providing a few stuffed toys, puppets, crayons, and paper in one's office.

5. It is an unattainable goal to try and eliminate a person's grief. Yet, simple measures of follow-up phone calls, cards, and listening provide substantial and integral support.

6. Working with bereaved parents and children can be painful. All health care staff should be aware of the personal impact.

References

1. Stroebe, M. and Shut, H. (1999). The dual process model of coping with bereavement: rationale and description. *Death Studies* 23 (3), 197–224.

2. Rando, T.A. *Treatment of Complicated Mourning.* Champaign IL: Research Press, 1993. (An extensive source for any practitioner who wishes to understand, assess, and treat complicated mourning.)

3. Wolfelt, A.D. *Healing a Parent's Grieving Heart; Healing your Grieving Heart for Kids; Healing your Grieving Heart for Teens; Healing a Friend's Grieving Heart; Healing a Child's Grieving Heart; Healing a Teen's Grieving Heart.* Fort Collins CO: Companion Press, 2001. (Six small books in 'The 100 Ideas' Series. Three of the books are written for the grieving child, teen, or parent to provide practical ideas for coping with grief. The other three books are written for families, friends, or caregivers offering ideas on how to support a grieving child, teen, or adult.)

4. Worden, J.W. G*rief Counseling and Grief Therapy: A Handbook for the Mental Health Practitioner.* New York: Springer, 1991. (An excellent resource for any practitioner who seeks an understanding of the practical issues of normal and complicated grief. This volume will assist and inform the professional when to make referrals for further counselling.)

5. The Compassionate Friends Inc. (1999). When a child dies: a survey of bereaved parents. *The Forum Newsletter* 25 (6), 1, 10–11.

6. Stevens, M.M. (1998). Psychological adaptation of the dying child. In *Oxford Textbook of Palliative Medicine* (ed. D. Doyle, G.W.C. Hanks, and N. MacDonald), pp. 1046–55. Oxford: Oxford University Press.

7. Harper, M.B. and Wisian, N.B. (1994). Care of bereaved parents. A study of patient satisfaction. *Journal of Reproductive Medicine* 39 (2), 80–6.

8. Lloyd-Williams, M., Wilkinson, C., and Lloyd-Williams, F.F. (1998). Do bereaved children consult the primary health care team more frequently? *European Journal of Cancer Care* 7 (2), 12–24.

9. Opie, N.D., Goodwin, T., Finke, L.M., Beaty, J.M., Lee, B., and van Epps, J. (1992). The effect of bereavement group experience on bereaved children's and adolescents affective and somatic distress. *Child and Adolescent Psychiatric Mental Health Nursing* 5 (1), 20–6.

Further reading

Adams, D. and Deveau, E., ed. *Beyond the Innocence of Childhood.* Amityville, New York: Baywood Publishing Company, Inc, 1995. (A three-volume collection to assist educators and other professionals to help children and adolescents cope with dying, death, and bereavement including information on funerals, different cultures, AIDS, traumatic deaths, use of play, art, stories, humour, and pets in supporting children. Describes palliative care, spirituality and the long-term effects of grief.)

Growth House (http://www.growthhouse.org). (A comprehensive website that provides professionals and the public with a wealth of information with links to other websites and books related to end-of-life care, grief, and bereavement.)

Klass, D., Silverman, P.R., and Nickman, S.L. *Continuing Bonds: New Understandings of Grief.* Washington DC: Taylor & Francis, 1996. (Over 20 scholars and practitioners show through experience and research that a continuing bond with the deceased is necessary for healthy functioning and development.)

Larson, D.G. *The Helper's Journey.* Champaign IL: Research Press, 1993. (Helpful guidelines and suggestions are given to improve the quality of caregiving, while attending to the caregivers' own need for self-care and nurturance.)

McCracken, A. and Semel, M. *A Broken Heart Still Beats.* Center City, Minnesota: Hazeldon Information and Educational Services, 1998. (An inspiring collection of poetry, fiction and essays on what it means to lose a child. Both authors are bereaved parents who offer wisdom, comfort, insight, and hope to other bereaved parents.)

Smith, S.C. and Pennells, M., ed. *Interventions with Bereaved Children.* London: Jessica Kingsley Publishers Limited, 1995. (The authors suggest effective strategies for working in schools, hospitals, and residential settings using treatment methods that encompass individual, group, or family work.)

17.5 Hospice and home care

Frederick I. Burge

There is a desire by the majority of patients with advanced progressive disease to spend much of their time at home. The doctor should assess the patient's and family's capacity to remain at home. Engaging other community-based primary care providers and palliative care specialists to provide team-based care at home should enhance care and support the family doctor. It is important to anticipate the needs of patients and families in these settings and to outline mechanisms to access care 'out of hours'. Hospice or palliative care units may be an appropriate alternative care setting for some patients.

In the early twentieth century, most deaths occurred at home. By the 1980s, 70–90 per cent of deaths were occurring in hospital, and by the end of the twentieth century the pendulum had begun to swing back again towards deaths occurring at home.[1,2] Depending on the country, options for location of terminal care include the patient's home, a long-term care setting, a 'free-standing' hospice, a hospice or palliative care inpatient unit in an acute care hospital, and acute in-hospital care.[3] Research regarding cancer patients' 'preferred' location of care overwhelmingly favours home.[1] The preferred location of death also favours the home setting, with approximately 50–80 per cent of patients choosing that location.[4–6] Such preferences are less clear for those dying of other diseases. Many factors intervene to prevent patients from achieving their goal of dying at home. For the average family physician, the thought of providing 24 h per day, 7 days per week continuous medical care to a patient with a progressive illness can be daunting. Countering that concern are two studies of death in family practice which found that there were only two to three anticipated deaths at home per year per physician practice.[7,8]

Currently, the most common causes of anticipated deaths in hospices and home include cancer, cardiovascular disease (particularly congestive heart failure), neurologic disease (such as multiple sclerosis, amyotrophic lateral sclerosis, and dementias), chronic obstructive pulmonary disease, and acquired immunodeficiency syndrome (AIDS).[9] All represent chronic diseases and most will be found in family practices today.

Assessing the desire and capacity for the patient to remain at home

Dying at home is not for everyone as the previously reported numbers tell us. However, many patients want to remain at home for some time, even if they do not want to die at home. The first step in assessment is to ask the patient which location is preferred. This must be reassessed over time.[10] The strong desire of the patient to remain at home is one of the single greatest predictors of success.[11] Once this has been declared, the next step is to estimate the emotional and physical capacity of the family to help the patient achieve this wish. Care for the dying at home places substantial responsibility on the family. Indeed, without a supportive family member, success is unlikely.[11,12] Not only must the family be in agreement, but also they must be prepared to bring resources to the task. This will often entail financial resources to pay for equipment, drugs, or professional home services. In some home settings, these costs are sometimes provided for by the state or through the patient's privately held insurance plan. They may also be provided by charities. The family physician should make referral to community social services to assess the financial resources of families and to see what can be provided to the family and what they will need to bare the cost themselves. These costs can be a significant deterrent for many families and may necessitate admission to hospital or other care setting.

In addition to the physical/financial requirements, families will need substantial emotional or psychological capacity to care for someone and in particular have someone die at home. Women, the elderly, and those of lower socio-economic status are all less likely to be cared for and to die at home, perhaps because these groups in society are less likely to have someone able to care for them.[13] The family doctor has a substantial role to support the home caregiver emotionally, with positive encouragement, by providing information, with practical support by putting in place other professionals who can help in the home, and by ensuring that patient suffering is kept to a minimum. It is vital that the family physician cares for both the patient and their family or lay caregivers. Marked anxiety, stress, and even depression are commonly found in the caregivers. Respite care, provided by professionals, other family members, or volunteers, may be a critical step to keep the primary caregiver well. The health of the caregiver, if a patient of the family physician, should be assessed regularly along with that of the patient. It will be important to care for the family whether patients are at home or admitted to a hospice, as this is an emotionally demanding time for the family. More information of providing care for the dying patient is given in Chapter 17.1.

Knowing and working with community resources

The family physician should not work in isolation in caring for patients with progressive illness. Most communities have other professionals who are part of the primary home care team. These may include, at a minimum, home care nurses and home health care workers. In some jurisdictions, this team may be much larger and include physiotherapists, occupational therapists, nutritionists, pharmacists, and others. Sharing the primary care of the patient at home with these members of the team make the work easier for the doctor, and provide much needed information and care for patients that the family is unable to provide on their own. The home care nurse is able to assess symptom control, emotional well-being, and the status of the family. This nurse will often be in a position to make suggestions to the family doctor about needed changes, to triage the need for home visits, or to adjust medications with the doctor's support and advice. A knowledgeable pharmacist is also an important resource with respect to achieving optimal symptom control.

In some communities, there may be specialized teams that care for those with progressive illness and those at the end of life. These teams may include palliative care teams, hospice-in-the-home teams, specialized palliative care nursing organizations, and others. The family physician may make a referral to these teams to provide special assessment and interventions in the home. This may be needed when the primary care team is unable to meet all of the needs, when the family requests, or in order for the primary care team to simply share the work of supporting families at home. Each team functions somewhat differently. Some provide only an advisory service whereas, at the other end of the continuum, some will provide total care.

Working with hospices and palliative care units

There are now hospices or palliative care units in 90 countries of the world. These may be inpatient units, home care services (often linked to an inpatient unit), day care units, or inpatient units within an acute hospital (see Chapter 7.8, Vol. 1). The staff of hospices usually have specialist training in palliative care; palliative medicine is a recognized specialty in the United Kingdom. The environment of a hospice seeks to be more home like and staff have expertise in symptom control, nursing care, and emotional and spiritual support. Staff-to-patient ratios are often higher than in hospitals, so patients and their families have more time with staff. Patients usually stay for fairly short periods of time in the inpatient units (on average around 13 days), and may be discharged home again or die in the hospice. Those who are discharged home may go on to die at home or may be re-admitted several times. They may also receive support from the palliative care home care team or attend the day centre. Thus, hospices and

palliative care services can be an important community resource for the family doctor, as patients who cannot remain at home all the time, but want an environment different to hospital and who need expertise in palliative care, may be cared for in a hospice (see Chapter 7.8, Vol. 1). Hospice and palliative care services should not be reserved until patients are in the last days of life. In many countries, palliative care teams are becoming involved at earlier stages of care, especially in the last 3–6 months of life.

Providing good symptom control

An uncontrolled symptom is one of the most frequent reasons patients return to hospital or are admitted to a hospice. The other common reason is caregiver stress. Control of symptoms is discussed in detail in Chapters 17.2 and 17.6. However, common problems leading to urgent hospitalization include confusion or delirium, severe pain, unrelieved cough, faecal incontinence, and malodourous lesions.[3] In addition, emergencies near the end of life may include haemorrhage, superior vena cava obstruction, spinal cord compression, hypercalcaemia, haemorrhage, and seizures. Anticipating these situations in patients who have conditions that might lead to them may prevent hospitalization and family distress. Some of the symptoms may not be ameliorated, such as haemorrhage. However, with gentle advance discussion, explanations, and emergency contact information, family caregivers can often manage an otherwise very difficult situation. Another common situation to precipitate hospitalization may occur when the patient is no longer able to take anything by mouth, including symptom control medications such as morphine. Anticipating this time by having a syringe driver or subcutaneous butterfly ready, injectable forms of the medication readily available and the caregiver taught how to manage these will save an urgent visit by ambulance to the emergency department (see Chapter 17.1).

Equipment at home

In order to succeed at home, as the patient grows weaker common pieces of equipment may be helpful. These include walkers, commode chairs, bath or shower chairs, and hand rails, a hospital bed, fans to help alleviate breathlessness, emesis basins, and more. Such equipment may be paid for through local home health services in some countries, by insurance in some, or through local 'equipment lending cupboards' in still others. In addition, many procedures can be performed in the home today that might not have been available several years ago. These include home intravenous infusions, hypodermoclysis, percutaneous gastrostomy feeding, and abdominal paracentesis.

Providing continuity of care

Some believe that family physicians should be available 24 h a day for patient's with progessive illness and those who are dying. If you are a physician who practices in this pattern, the ability to provide continuity of medical care becomes relatively straightforward (although, potentially, exhausting). For others, however, family life, other responsibilities, or simply a belief in how the practice should run, necessitates 'handing over' care at times to a 'covering' physician. It is imperative to anticipate these times and to inform the patient and family as well as the 'covering' physician of the situation. Ensuring the patient and family know how to reach the 'covering' physician is important. An update on the current symptom control, the caregiver situation, and the anticipation of any likely needs will help the 'covering' physician provide care. It is important to be clear what might be expected should the patient become sicker and need a home visit or assessment. Such negotiation should take place between the professionals before the patient or family find themselves in these situations trying to negotiate care from the 'covering' physician. Ideally, the family physician has an active 'on-call' group that knows each other and practices in a similar style. In addition, the community-based team (nurses, palliative care team, etc.) should know of the 'covering' arrangements should the need arise. Out-of-hours crises and the inability to get help are, as mentioned before, one of the most common reasons dying patients end up in an emergency room for assessment.

Communication

At no other time in a patient's life is there greater need for open, accurate, and clear communication than as death approaches. It is important to establish early on with the patient just 'who' is to be part of the information-sharing process. Likely this will include spouses and immediate family members but this should not be assumed. Determining what kind of information and to what extent the patient wishes to know the information is also important. This may change as time goes on. Using the 'patient-centred clinical method'[14] as the basis for the doctor–patient encounters will allow better health outcomes including patient satisfaction. This model is based on six components: understanding the disease and the illness experienced by the patient, the context of the patient (including life story and family context), finding common ground on goals and who will play what roles, enhancing the doctor–patient relationship, and being realistic in what can be accomplished and by whom.

The need for excellence in communication is not unique to the home setting but particular circumstances apply specifically at home. First, it is unlikely that members of the health care team are in the home 24 h per day as in hospital. Therefore, patients and families must hold on to their questions until the next visit or contact the health professional by phone. Leaving contact phone numbers and perhaps even instructions on the best time of day to place such calls to the practice may be helpful. Helping patients and families know which questions to direct to different members of the health care team may be challenging at first, but usually, with practice they come to learn who is the most appropriate person for each issue.

Secondly, because a professional is not always present, providing anticipatory information can be helpful, such as what symptoms may be expected, the possible causes of them, how they may be ameliorated including the specifics of medications (when and how to take and what adverse effects are likely), and possible psychological reactions patients or caregivers may have. As death nears, a careful explanation of what to expect in physical changes and how to contact the doctor/home care nurse is vital to relieve concern and prevent urgent transfers to the emergency department of the hospital.

At times it may be difficult to be certain about some issues without the usually available information in the hospital setting. For example, one may not be sure if worsening dyspnoea is due to heart failure or progressing lung cancer. Without access to a chest X-ray, the doctor may be left speculating and treating empirically. Honesty about such situations is usually appreciated if the goal of care to stay at home is the paramount one for the patient and family. It is often important to decide to treat symptoms, and to undertake tests only if the diagnosis will make a difference to the symptomatic treatment.

Finally, there is the issue of communication among the health care team. In a busy practice setting it can be difficult to take phone calls from other members of the health care team but doing so may make the flow of information and decision-making better and more consistent for the patient and family. At the same time, the family physician should not hesitate to contact other members of the team to facilitate care. This may include clarifying events that took place in hospital on previous occasions.

Managing transitions in location of care

Despite the best efforts of the professional and family caregivers there may be a need to transfer the patient to hospital or hospice for a day procedure, clinic visit, or short hospital stay. Usually, this comes about by revisiting the goals of care, although sometimes respite admissions may be planned. Although the goal of staying at home may be important, it can be superceded by the need for effective symptom assessment and control or the inability of the family to cope with the situation at home. These should not be seen as failures but rather meeting the patient's needs in the best possible way.

Ensuring smooth transitions between locations of care requires timely and accurate information transfer between the care team at home and that at the hospital/hospice/clinic. In addition, the goal of the stay should be clear among all. Once in a specialized setting, it can be tempting to start down a path of multiple investigations or interventions and lose sight of the goals of care.

Spiritual care

The family physician may not feel comfortable or knowledgeable to approach spiritual issues with patients at home. Nevertheless, the patient should be given the opportunity to discuss these concerns and a referral made should it be desired. Ministers, priests, or other spiritual advisors known to the family may be more than willing to visit in the home. In addition, some communities will have specialized individuals attached to home palliative care or hospice teams who could be consulted.

Caring for yourself

Providing home-based terminal care can, on occasion, be very wearing for the family physician. Trying to meet the symptom control needs of patients, the psychological needs of families, making home visits, helping to coordinate professionals and services coming to the home, while trying to manage a busy primary care practice exacts a toll as the physician may feel torn between the competing demands. At the same time, the physician is, in all likelihood, losing a patient who may have been in the practice for some time. This long relationship with its complex layers of knowledge of both the patient and family can make terminal care both rewarding and draining. The physician is also grieving and the physician, the physician's colleagues, or family does not often recognize this. I believe it is important to share the work with other members of the team and, in my view, take time out with adequate coverage for the patient and family. How the physician balances the needs of the dying patient with his/her own personal and family needs is a matter of personal decision but must be done so knowing the long-term consequences.

References

1. Higginson, I.J. and Sen-Gupta, G.J.A. (2000). Place of care in advanced cancer: a qualitative systematic literature review of patient preferences. *Journal of Palliative Medicine* **3** (3), 287.

2. Wilson, D.M. et al. *Social and Health Care Trends Influencing Palliative Care and the Location of Death in Twentieth-Century Canada.* Final NHRDP Report. Edmonton: University of Alberta, 1998.

3. Doyle, D., Hanks, W.C., and MacDonald, N., ed. *Oxford Textbook of Palliative Medicine.* Oxford: Oxford University Press, 1998.

4. Dunlop, R.J., Davies, R.J., and Hockley, J.M. (1989). Preferred versus actual place of death: a hospital palliative care support team experience. *Palliative Medicine* **3**, 197–201.

5. Rural Palliative Home Care Staff and Consultants. A rural palliative home care model: the development and evaluation of an integrated palliative care program in Nova Scotia and Prince Edward Island. A Federal Health Transition Fund Project Report. Nova Scotia: Communications Nova Scotia, 2001.

6. Dudgeon, D.J. and Kristjanson, L. (1995). Home versus hospital death: assessment of preferences and clinical challenges. *Canadian Medical Association Journal* **152** (3), 337–40.

7. Barritt, P.W. (1984). Care of the dying in one practice. *Journal of the Royal College of General Practitioners* **34**, 446–8.

8. Blyth, A.C. (1990). Audit of terminal care in a general practice. *British Medical Journal* **300**, 983–6.

9. Haupt, B.J. and Jones, A. *National Home and Hospice Care Survey: Annual Summary, 1996.* Vital Health Stat 13(141). Hyattsville MD, Washington DC: US Department of Health and Human Services, Centers for Disease Control and Prevention, National Center for Health Statistics, 1999.

10. Billings, J.A. and Stoeckle, J.D. *The Clinical Encounter: A Guide to the Medical Interview and Case Presentation.* Chicago: Year Book Medical Publishers, Inc., 1989.

11. Cantwell, P. et al. (2000). Predictors of home death in palliative care cancer patients. *Journal of Palliative Care* **16** (1), 23–8.

12. Burge, F.I. et al. (2001). Palliative care by Canadian physicians in the 1990s: resiliency amid reform. *Canadian Family Physician* **47** (Oct), 1989–95.

13. Grande, G.E., Addington-Hall, J.M., and Todd, C.J. (1998). Place of death and access to home care services: are certain patient groups at a disadvantage? *Social Science and Medicine* **47** (5), 565–79.

14. Stewart, M. et al. *Patient-Centered Medicine: Transforming the Clinical Method.* Thousand Oaks: Sage Publications, 1995.

Table 1 Prevalence of symptoms in advanced cancer patients

Symptom	Total palliative care population (%)[2]	Mean % at referral to palliative care service[3–9]	Mean % in last week of life[6–8,10,11]
Pain	57	63 (41–100)	49 (15–99)
Anorexia	30	62 (8–79)	43 (6–80)
Weakness	51	43 (13–77)	50 (20–82)
Breathlessness	19	32 (15–53)	33 (21–47)
Confusion	8	18 (8–30)	36 (9–68)
Nausea	21	25 (12–44)	28 (13–71)
Vomiting		14 (8–25)	6 (2–10)
Constipation	23	33 (3–54)	21 (1–55)
Dry mouth/xerostomia		54 (27–73)	70
Anxiety		28 (11–51)	31 (18–45)
Depression		37 (8–53)	21 (4–39)

Table 2 Symptom prevalence for patients dying of chronic heart and lung diseases

Symptom	Chronic heart failure[11],a (%)	Chronic lung diseases[12,13],a (%)
Pain	78	68–77
Anorexia	43	36–67
Breathlessness	61	94–95
Nausea and vomiting	32	47
Constipation	37	27–44
Dry mouth/xerostomia		59–67
Insomnia	45	55–65
Low mood	59	71

a Data refer to the last year of life.

17.6 Symptoms and palliation

Polly Edmonds and Sarah Cox

Introduction

Symptom control is a central issue to patients, carers, and health care professionals facing life-threatening illnesses. There is some evidence to suggest that good symptom control may enhance quality of life and facilitate achievement of a home death, if that is a patient's choice. This chapter explores the prevalence of symptoms in patients with advanced disease and discusses a framework for effective symptom management. The management of pain is discussed in detail in Chapter 17.2.

Epidemiology

As many as 70 per cent of patients say that they would like to die at home, but fewer achieve this. However, in 1995 approximately 38 per cent of cancer and 40 per cent of non-cancer deaths occurred under the care of the primary health care team.[1] Approximately 50 per cent of cancer patients are under the care of a community palliative care team at some stage in their final illness, but the number is negligible for patients dying from diseases other than cancer. As most patients with advanced disease will spend a large proportion of the last year of life in the community, under the care of the primary health care team, it is important for all members of the team to have a basic understanding of symptom control.

Prevalence of symptoms

At present little is known of the frequency of symptoms experienced by patients with life-threatening illnesses other than cancer. Table 1 summarizes data from 10 studies addressing symptom prevalence for patients with advanced cancer.[2–11] This demonstrates that there are marked differences in reported symptom prevalence, although the commonest symptoms at referral to specialist palliative care services appear to be pain and the anorexia/cachexia syndrome, with weakness the commonest symptom in the last week of life. These studies demonstrate that patients with advanced cancer have multiple symptoms, many of which are closely inter-related.

Table 2 outlines symptom prevalence for patients with chronic heart and lung diseases in the last year of life.[12–14] As can be seen, there are remarkably few differences in the frequency of symptoms from those reported for cancer patients and these patients are also reported to have multiple symptoms. Much less is known about the prevalence of symptoms for patients with other non-cancer diagnoses; indeed, the symptoms experienced may to an extent be specific for different disease processes. For example, patients with neurodegenerative diseases are frequently reported to experience pain, dysphagia, pooling or dribbling of saliva, breathlessness, dysarthria, bladder and bowel dysfunction, and depression/anxiety.[15] Patients with end-stage renal or liver disease may develop alterations in consciousness, confusion, nausea and vomiting, ascites, and peripheral oedema. Despite the occurrence of symptoms specific to certain disease processes, there appear to be more similarities than differences in the symptom burden experienced by patients with advanced disease at the end of life.

Some of the variations in symptom frequencies reported in these patient populations arise from differences in study methodology, such as whether the information was obtained directly from patients or by using proxies. Staff, family members, or friends can act as a proxy for the patient. However, staff ratings have been shown to be more similar to patients' than ratings provided by a member of the patients' family.[16] The similarity between patient- and proxy-generated scores are strongest when measuring physical symptoms, whereas psycho-social aspects of quality of life seem to be more difficult for proxies to assess and show poor correlation with patients' own scores.[17] Nevertheless, research suggests that proxy assessments can provide valuable and valid data when evaluating services, when assessing observable symptoms, and when measuring levels of satisfaction.[18]

Aetiology of symptoms in advanced disease

Symptoms in a patient with advanced disease may be caused by

- the underlying disease,
- by treatment(s),
- general debility,
- by concurrent illnesses.

An example of all the factors contributing to the development of symptoms in a patient with advanced disease is given in Table 3, using nausea and vomiting as an example.

Patients with advanced disease typically experience multiple symptoms, many of which are inter-related. A patient with advanced cancer and pain may also experience nausea, constipation, and drowsiness from opioid analgesics. The nausea may result in early satiety from gastric stasis with resulting anorexia; weakness, poor oral intake, and immobility due to pain may contribute to constipation.

Symptom assessment

Effective symptom control for patients with advanced diseases requires the accurate assessment of all contributing factors in an individual patient at

Table 3 Aetiology of symptoms—nausea and vomiting

Underlying disease
Cancer—hypercalcaemia, liver metastases, brain metastases, malignant bowel obstruction, gastric stasis
Chronic heart failure—liver congestion, gastric stasis
Chronic lung disease—liver congestion from right heart failure, gastric stasis
Neurodegenerative disease—gastric stasis

Treatment
Cancer—drugs (e.g. opioid analgesics), constipation, chemotherapy
Non-cancer—drugs (e.g. digoxin, antibiotics), immobility, enteral feeding

Concurrent illness/co-morbidity
Gastroenteritis
Motion sickness
Constipation

any given time. The general principles for the systematic assessment of symptoms can be summarized as follows, and are demonstrated in Fig. 1:

- detailed history and examination;
- appropriate investigations to guide clinical decision-making;
- treat potentially reversible causes;
- explanation;
- pro-active and skilful treatment;
- regular monitoring.

It is important to take a detailed history and to examine patients in order to identify a pattern of symptoms that will inform subsequent investigations and management. This could include the differentiation of a specific pain syndrome in a cancer patient, or of the aetiology of nausea and vomiting that will guide antiemetic use. As stated above, symptoms in patients with advanced disease may be inter-related, and an understanding of the development of symptoms(s) in relation to other symptoms can be an important factor in successful management.

Useful factors to identify when taking a symptom history include:

- time course;
- symptom pattern;
- relation to new drugs or other symptoms;
- effect of medication or other management strategies;
- exacerbating factors;
- psychological factors, for example, fear and/or anxiety or the meaning of a symptom for a patient and/or family; cancer patients who develop pain or breathlessness often equate this to starting to die, which may not necessarily be true;
- social history, for example, stairs, equipment, family support, ability to perform activities of daily living.

Investigations should be targeted to identifying the underlying cause of a symptom wherever possible. Decisions to investigate or not should be individualized and taken in the context of a patient's overall clinical condition. Tests should generally only be undertaken where they will inform treatment decisions or end-of-life decision-making. If a patient is too unwell for the results of tests to be acted upon, then they are rarely indicated.

Principles of symptom management
General

The majority of patients and their carers benefit from a full explanation of the reason(s) for a symptom occurring. Patients and carers may become

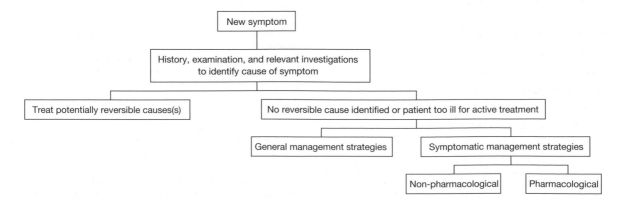

Fig. 1 Assessment and management of symptoms in advanced disease.

Table 4 Risk and benefits from palliative and symptomatic treatments

Potential risks from treatment	Potential benefits
Direct injury from treatment, e.g. NSAID induced gastritis	Symptomatic benefit
Burden of medication	Increased longevity
Discomfort from intervention, e.g. intravenous cannulation	
Treatment uses time for which patient has other priorities, e.g. hospital visits	

more anxious when the aetiology of a symptom is unclear and may also attach great importance to the development or progression of symptoms such as pain or breathlessness. Taking time to explain your thoughts to a patient and their family and to outline a plan of action may alleviate anxiety.

Wherever possible, the health care professional should discuss treatment options with the patient and their carer. Enlisting the cooperation of carers in treatment management strategies may improve compliance considerably.

Palliative treatment and symptom control should be

- active—aiming for maximum comfort;
- individualized to the patient's priorities;
- reviewed as frequently as possible.

Symptomatic or palliative management embraces an enormous range of interventions from teaching breathing techniques to disease-modifying management like surgery. The common intention with such treatment is not to make the patient well but to make them better, if only for a while. This principle can be applied to every management decision and used to weigh risks against the potential benefit (see Table 4). Treatment decisions need to be individualized. Some patients may be too unwell to tolerate or benefit from specific treatments and in these situations treatment should be geared towards comfort measures. Patients will often have multiple problems and can be involved in prioritizing them.

Disease-modifying palliative treatment

In the treatment of cancer, surgery, radiotherapy, chemotherapy, and hormone therapy are amongst the most commonly used forms of disease-modifying treatment. They may be offered even when cure is not possible to improve quality of life or because they offer the chance of prolonged life. In a patient with lung cancer causing bronchial obstruction, radiotherapy may offer the best relief of breathlessness even where metastases are present and treatment cannot cure.

In the palliation of non-malignant disease, this principle also applies. A patient with advanced left ventricular failure will obtain symptomatic benefit from 'disease-modifying' diuretics that may need to be continued when other, no longer appropriate medications, are being stopped.

Principles of symptom management

- Assess each symptom to diagnose and treat the cause.
- Tailor symptomatic management to the cause.
- Consider pharmacological and non-pharmacological therapy.
- Review treatment frequently.
- Increase dose of symptomatic drug to maximum.
- Change treatment if not effective.

Symptomatic treatments may be either non-pharmacological or pharmacological. Examples of non-pharmacological treatment approaches include:

- breathing control techniques for breathlessness;
- relaxation techniques for anxiety;
- dietary modifications for anorexia;
- provision of a pressure-relieving mattress for debilitated patients;
- acupuncture or TENS for the relief of pain;
- provision of a quiet and supportive environment for agitated or distressed patients.

Principles of prescribing in advanced disease

There are several basic principles that should guide all prescribing for symptoms for patients with advanced disease:

- prescribe drugs proactively for persistent symptoms;
- each new drug should be perceived to have benefits that outweigh potential side-effects (burdens) in the context of the patient's condition;
- consider drug interactions;
- appropriate route of administration;
- avoid polypharmacy—stop medications that are no longer appropriate or have not worked;
- regular review.

Improving compliance in advanced disease

Both patients and carers need clear concise guidelines to ensure maximum cooperation. Drug regimens should ideally be written out in full for patients and families and patient's self-medication charts are a useful adjunct to this. Where patients and families are easily confused by treatment regimens, this should be reviewed to reduce the number of drugs/tablets. Compliance may be further aided by the use of a dossette box, which can be filled by a relative, district nurse, or pharmacist.

Patients and carers also benefit from a clear plan of action should a current management plan not be working and know who to contact and how to contact them.

Regular review is essential for effective symptom control.

Management of specific symptoms

Anorexia and cachexia

Cancer cachexia or anorexia–cachexia is a syndrome that occurs commonly in patients with advanced malignant disease and non-suppressed HIV infection. It presents as loss of appetite and weight, and is often associated with lethargy and weakness. Changes in carbohydrate, fat, protein, and energy metabolism can be demonstrated, causing sometimes dramatic wasting with loss of skeletal muscle and fat. Anorexia–cachexia makes patients feel unwell with fatigue, weakness, and consequences of weight loss, including a change in body image. It also affects the ability to tolerate anticancer therapy. It has been reported as a major contributing factor to death in up to 50 per cent cancer deaths. The syndrome is especially marked in certain solid tumours such as pancreatic cancer and some lung cancers.

Efforts to reverse the cachexia by nutritional support have proved largely ineffective. The body of evidence shows that the use of TPN or enteral feeding support does not prolong survival, improve tumour response to treatment, or reduce its toxicity.[19] Some evidence supporting pre-operative nutritional support has been contrasted by other studies, which do not show any benefit either in post-operative complications or mortality. Most importantly, there is no evidence that artificial nutritional support improves the quality of patient's lives.

Eating is a social interaction. Not eating can be a cause of distress to patients and their families who may feel that their relative is being allowed to starve to death. Sensitive explanation of the syndrome and what might and might not be helpful can reduce conflict. Patients should be encouraged to try small meals or snacks when desired rather than attempting three

Table 5 Management of nausea and vomiting

Cause	Assessment	Treatment
Poor gastric emptying, e.g. pyloric obstruction, hepatomegaly, pancreatic cancer, gastritis	Little nausea Effortless vomiting Large vomitus	Metoclopromide 10–20 mg tds orally or subcutaneously
Drug induced or metabolic, e.g. hypercalcaemia, digoxin, renal failure	Prominent nausea ± metabolic flap Onset with drug therapy	Antidopaminergic drug, e.g. haloperidol 1.5–3 mg nocte or 2.5–5 mg sc
Raised intracranial pressure	Morning headache Drowsiness Confusion Papilloedema	Cyclizine 50 mg tds or subcutaneously
Malignant bowel obstruction	Constipation Distension ± vomiting Colicky ± constant abdominal pain	Stop stimulant laxatives Consider surgery Parenteral control with strong opioid, cyclizine ± haloperidol ± hyoscine butylbromide

large meals a day. Taste changes and a dry mouth can make some foods unpalatable.

Symptomatic treatment of anorexia–cachexia syndrome with drug therapy is directed towards helping appetite.

Corticosteroids improve anorexia and can also give a feeling of well-being. Their prescription should be considered carefully in view of the side-effects associated with them. Positive effects are not persistent after discontinuing treatment. Corticosteroids may be appropriate if prognosis is short and side-effects less likely to cause problems or to improve symptoms temporarily, around a family celebration, for instance.

Progestogens such as megestrol acetate and medroxyprogesterone acetate produce improved appetite and weight gain, and are generally well tolerated. Side-effects including fluid retention, thrombosis, and impotence in men can restrict their use. Maximal effect may take some weeks and the response appears to be dose-related.

Cyproheptadine, hydrazine sulfate, and cannabinoids have also been demonstrated to improve appetite, and sometimes reduce weight loss, in patients with advanced cancer. Other drug treatments that may be effective include omega-3 fatty acids and thalidomide.[20]

Breathlessness

It is important to remember that breathlessness in patients with advanced disease may arise from reversible causes, such as infection, pulmonary emboli, anaemia, left ventricular failure, and pleural effusion.

Difficulty breathing is often associated with a high level of anxiety that exacerbates the problem. There may be particular concerns, such as not choking to death, about which specific reassurance can be offered. Upright positioning in the bed or chair and a stream of air from an open window or a fan can both be helpful. Teaching breathing exercises can give some feeling of control and have been demonstrated with a variety of other interventions to improve breathlessness.

Patients may need to reduce their expectations and adapt their home environment to make daily activities more manageable.

Oxygen can be helpful, especially where there is hypoxia, but similar effects can be achieved by a stream of air that produces less practical difficulties. If there is some reversible airways obstruction bronchodilators may be useful.

Opioids can improve exercise tolerance in advanced airways limitation and reduce the sensation of breathlessness. *Benzodiazepines* are central sedatives and also relieve the unpleasant feeling of dyspnoea.

Nausea and vomiting

If a patient is experiencing moderate to severe nausea and vomiting, the oral route may be ineffective. Consider using parenteral routes early (e.g. intermittent or continuous subcutaneous injection). Management strategies for the common causes of nausea and vomiting are shown in Table 5.

Constipation

Constipation is a common cause of discomfort in palliative care. Management should be preventative, but treatment of acute constipation is often required. Patients who are able to should be encouraged to drink plenty of fluids, eat appropriately, and move about. These measures are usually inadequate by themselves.

Management of constipation usually requires a combination of a softening and a stimulant laxative (except in bowel obstruction). Remember that with faecal impaction rectal intervention will be required as well to initiate bowel movement. Microlette enemas are only slightly less effective than phosphate enemas but better tolerated by patients.

Key points

1. The commonest symptoms in patients with advanced disease are: anorexia and cachexia, pain, and weakness.

2. Patients with advanced disease frequently have multiple symptoms, many of which may be inter-related.

3. Symptom assessment should identify the underlying cause(s) of a new symptom.

4. Symptom management is focused on treating any potentially reversible underlying cause(s).

5. Regular review of both pharmacological and non-pharmacological measures for symptom palliation is required.

References

1. **Office for National Statistics Mortality Data** www.statistics.gov.uk/CCI/nscl.asp?ID=6444/ (England and Wales, 1997).

2. **Vainio, A. and Auvinen, A.** (1996). Prevalence of symptoms among patients with advanced cancer: an international collaborative study. *Journal of Pain and Symptom Management* **12**, 3–10.

3. **Reuben, D.B., Mor, V., and Hiris, J.** (1988). Clinical symptoms and length of survival in patients with terminal cancer. *Archives of Internal Medicine* **148**, 1586–91.

4. **Donnelly, S., Walsh, D., and Rybicki, L.** (1995). The symptoms of advanced cancer: identification of clinical and research priorities by assessment of prevalence and severity. *Journal of Palliative Care* **11**, 27–32.

5. Curtis, E.B., Krech, R., and Walsh, T.D. (1991). Common symptoms in patients with advanced cancer. *Journal of Palliative Care* 7, 25–9.

6. Connill, C., Verger, E., Henriquez, I., Saiz, N., Espier, M., Lugo, F., and Garrigos, A. (1997). Symptom prevalence in the last week of life. *Journal of Pain and Symptom Management* 14, 328–31.

7. Coyle, N., Adelhardt, J., Foley, K.M., and Portenoy, R.K. (1990). Character of terminal illness in advanced cancer patient: pain and other symptoms during the last four weeks of life. *Journal of Pain and Symptom Management* 5, 83–93.

8. Higginson, I. and McCarthy, M. (1989). Measuring symptoms in terminal cancer: are pain and dyspnoea controlled? *Journal of the Royal Society of Medicine* 82, 264–7.

9. Edmonds, P.M., Stuttaford, J.M., Penny, J., Lynch, A.M., and Chamberlain, J. (1998). Do hospital palliative care teams improve symptom control? Use of a modified STAS as an evaluation tool. *Palliative Medicine* 12, 345–51.

10. Licter, I. and Hunt, E. (1990). The last 48 hours of life. *Journal of Palliative Care* 6, 7–15.

11. Fainsinger, R., Miller, M.J., Bruera, E., Hanson, J., and Maceachern, T. (1991). Symptom control during the last week of life on a palliative care unit. *Journal of Palliative Care* 7, 5–11.

12. McCarthy, M., Lay, M., and Addington-Hall, J. (1996). Dying from heart disease. *Journal of the Royal College of Physicians* 30, 325–8.

13. Skilbeck, J., Mott, L., Page, H., Smith, D., Hjelmeland-Ahmedzai, S., and Clark, D. (1998). Palliative care in chronic obstructive airways disease: a needs assessment. *Palliative Medicine* 12, 245–54.

14. Edmonds, P., Karlsen, S., Khan, S., and Addington-Hall, J. (2001). A comparison of the palliative care needs of patients dying from chronic respiratory diseases and lung cancer. *Palliative Medicine* 15, 287–95.

15. O'Brien, T. (2001). Neurodegenerative disease. In *Palliative Care for Non-Cancer Patients* (ed. J.M. Addington-Hall and I.J. Higginson), pp. 44–55. Oxford: Oxford University Press.

16. Higginson, I.J. and McCarthy, M. (1994). A comparison of two measures of quality of life; their sensitivity and validity for patients with advanced cancer. *Palliative Medicine* 29, 282–90.

17. Rothman, M.L., Hedrick, S.C., Bulcroft, K.A., Hickam, D.H., and Rubenstein, L.Z. (1991). The validity of proxy-generated scores as a measure of patient health status. *Medical Care* 29, 115–24.

18. Hinton, J. (1996). How reliable are relatives' reports of terminal illness? Patients and relatives compared. *Social Science and Medicine* 43, 1229–36.

19. Koretz, R. (1984). Parenteral nutrition: is it oncologically logical? *Journal of Clinical Oncology* 2, 534–8.

20. Lopinzi, C.L. (1998). The pharmacological manipulation of appetite. In *Topics in Palliative Care* Vol. 2 (ed. R.R. Portenoy and E. Breura), pp. 131–40. New York: Oxford University Press.

Index

Main index entries are given in **bold**.
Page numbers in *italics* refer to tables.